OPTUM 360°®

PROFESSIONAL

HCPCS Level II

A resourceful compilation of HCPCS codes Supports HIPAA compliance

D0774954

2020

THE NEW WEBSITE HAS
LAUNCHED!
VISIT OPTUM360CODING.COM

Publisher's Notice

The Optum360 2020 *HCPCS Level II* is designed to be an accurate and authoritative source of information about this government coding system. Every effort has been made to verify the accuracy of the listings, and all information is believed reliable at the time of publication. Absolute accuracy cannot be guaranteed, however. This publication is made available with the understanding that the publisher is not engaged in rendering legal or other services that require a professional license.

Our Commitment to Accuracy

Optum360 is committed to producing accurate and reliable materials. To report corrections, please email accuracy@optum.com. You can also reach customer service by calling 1.800.464.3649, option 1.

To view Optum360 updates/correction notices, please visit http://www.optum360coding.com/ProductUpdates/

Acknowledgments

Gregory A. Kemp, MA, *Product Manager*

Karen Schmidt, BSN, *Technical Director*

Stacy Perry, *Manager, Desktop Publishing*

Lisa Singley, *Project Manager*

Elizabeth Leibold, RHIT, *Clinical/Technical Editor*

Regina Magnani, RHIT, *Clinical/Technical Editor*

Jacqueline Petersen, RHIA, CHDA, CPC, *Clinical/Technical Editor*

Tracy Betzler, *Senior Desktop Publishing Specialist*

Hope M. Dunn, *Senior Desktop Publishing Specialist*

Katie Russell, *Desktop Publishing Specialist*

Jean Parkinson, *Editor*

Copyright

Property of Optum360, LLC. Optum360 and the Optum360 logo are trademarks of Optum360, LLC. All other brand or product names are trademarks or registered trademarks of their respective owner.

© 2019 Optum360, LLC. All rights reserved.

Made in the USA

HB 978-1-62254-554-4

Technical Editors

Elizabeth Leibold, RHIT

Ms. Leibold has more than 25 years of experience in the health care profession. She has served in a variety of roles, ranging from patient registration to billing and collections, and has an extensive background in both physician and hospital outpatient coding and compliance. She has worked for large health care systems and health information management services companies, and has wide-ranging experience in facility and professional component coding, along with CPT expertise in interventional procedures, infusion services, emergency department, observation, and ambulatory surgery coding. Her areas of expertise include chart-to-claim coding audits and providing staff education to both tenured and new coding staff. She is an active member of the American Health Information Management Association (AHIMA).

Regina Magnani, RHIT

Ms. Magnani has more than 30 years of experience in the healthcare industry in both health information management and patient financial services. Her areas of expertise include facility revenue cycle management, patient financial services, CPT/HCPCS and ICD-10-CM coding, the outpatient prospective payment system (OPPS), and chargemaster development and maintenance. She is an active member of the Healthcare Financial Management Association (HFMA) and the American Health Information Management Association (AHIMA).

Jacqueline Petersen, RHIA, CHDA, CPC

Ms. Petersen is a Clinical/Technical editor with Optum360. She has served as Senior Clinical Product Research Analyst with Optum360 developing business requirements for edits to support correct coding and reimbursement for claims processing applications. Her experience includes development of data-driven and system rules for both professional and facility claims and in-depth analysis of claims data inclusive of ICD-10-CM, CPT, HCPCS, and modifiers. Her background also includes consulting work for Optum, serving as a SME, providing coding and reimbursement education to internal and external clients. Ms. Petersen is a member of the American Academy of Professional Coders (AAPC), and the American Health Information Management Association (AHIMA).

OPTUM360®

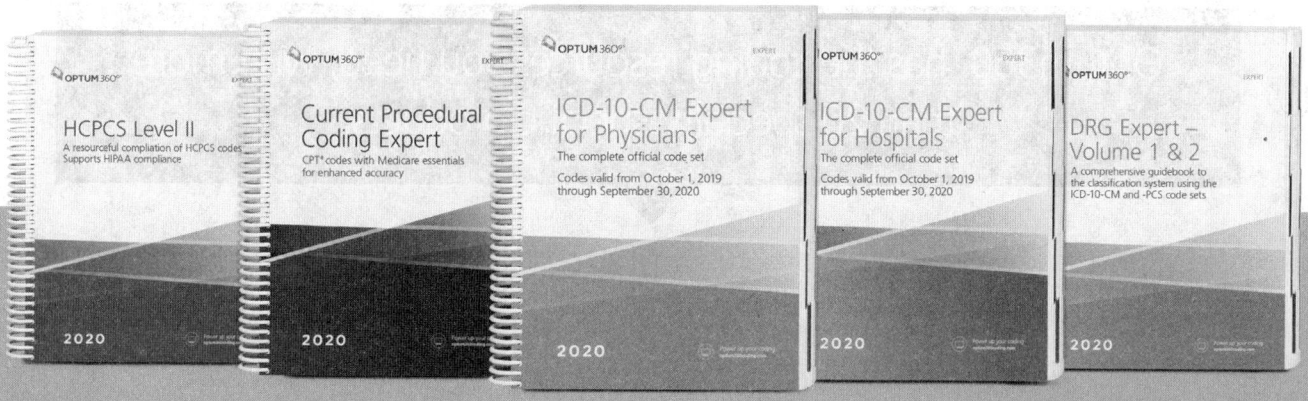

Keep your go-to coding resources up to date

Stay current and compliant with our 2020 edition code books. With more than 30 years in the coding industry, Optum360® is proud to be your trusted resource for coding, billing and reimbursement resources. Our 2020 editions include tools for ICD-10-CM/PCS, CPT®, HCPCS, DRG, specialty-specific coding and much more.

SAVE UP TO 25% ON ADDITIONAL CODING RESOURCES

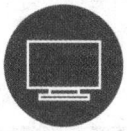

Visit us at optum360coding.com and enter promo code **FOBA20ED** to save 25%.

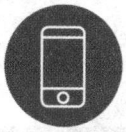

Call 1-800-464-3649, option 1, and be sure to mention promo code **FOBA20ED** to save 20%.

CPT is a registered trademark of the American Medical Association.

Excludes custom fee and bookstore items, data files, online coding tools and educational courses. Cannot be combined with any other offer.
Offer not valid for Partner or Medallion accounts.
© 2019 Optum360, LLC. All rights reserved. WF1175922 SPRJ5816

OPTUM360®

Optum360® has the coding resources you need, with more than 20 specialty-specific products.

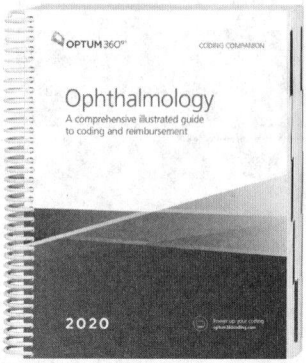

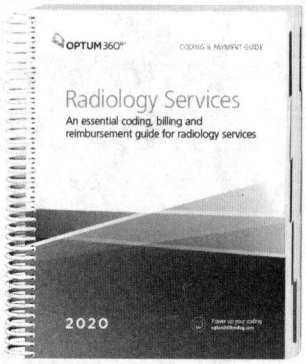

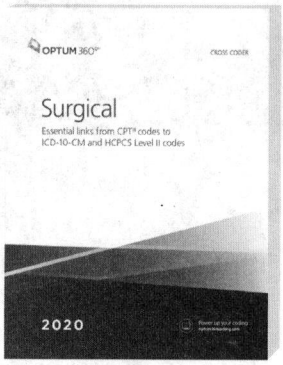

Coding Companions/Coding and Payment Guides

Comprehensive and easy to use, these guides include 2020 CPT®, HCPCS and ICD-10-CM code sets specific to your specialty. Each procedure code includes both official and lay descriptions, coding tips, cross-coding to common ICD-10-CM codes, with relative value units, *CPT® Assistant* references, CCI and other Medicare edits.

Cross Coders

These resources provide the specialty-specific crosswalks that billing and coding staff need, so you code it right the first time.

Coding Companion® specialties:

Cardiology/Cardiothoracic/Vascular Surgery
ENT/Allergy/Pulmonology
General Surgery/Gastroenterology
Neurosurgery/Neurology
OB/GYN
Ophthalmology
Orthopaedics: Hips & Below
Orthopaedics: Spine & Above
Plastics/Dermatology
Podiatry
Primary Care/Pediatrics/Emergency Medicine
Urology/Nephrology

Coding and Payment Guide specialties:

Anesthesiology/ Pain Management
Behavioral Health
Dental
Medical Oncology/Hematology
OMS (Coding Guide)
For the Physical Therapist
Radiology

Cross Coder specialties:

Anesthesia (CPT® to ICD-10-CM/ HCPCS Level II codes)
Procedural (ICD-10-PCS to CPT®/ HCPCS Level II codes)
Surgical (CPT® to ICD-10-CM/ HCPCS Level II codes)

SAVE UP TO 30% ON 2020 SPECIALTY RESOURCES*

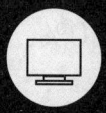

Visit us at optum360coding.com and enter promo code **SPEC2020** at checkout **to save 30%**.

Call 1-800-464-3649, option 1, and be sure to mention promo code **SPEC2020** to **save 20%**.

*Discount excludes the 2020 Coding Guide for OMS.
CPT is a registered trademark of the American Medical Association.

© 2019 Optum360, LLC. All rights reserved. WF1150897 04/19

Contents

Introduction i

Index ..... Index — 1

A Codes 1

Transportation Services Including Ambulance 1

Medical and Surgical Supplies 2

B Codes 18

Enternal and Parenteral Therapy 18

C Codes 21

Outpatient PPS 21

E Codes 29

Durable Medical Equipment 29

G Codes 45

Procedures/Professional Services (Temporary) 45

H Codes 87

Alcohol and Drug Abuse Treatment Services 87

J Codes 89

J Codes Drugs 89

J Codes Chemotherapy Drugs 103

K Codes 107

Temporary Codes 107

L Codes 111

Orthotic Devices and Procedures 111

Prosthetic Procedures 123

M Codes 135

Medical Services 135

Quality Measures 135

P Codes 138

Pathology and Laboratory Services 138

Q Codes 140

Q Codes (Temporary) 140

R Codes 149

Diagnostic Radiology Services 149

S Codes 151

Temporary National Codes (Non-Medicare) 151

T Codes 163

National T Codes Established for State Medicaid Agencies 163

V Codes 165

Vision Services 165

Hearing Services 167

Appendixes

Appendix 1 — Table of Drugs ..... Appendixes — 1

Appendix 2 — Modifiers ..... Appendixes — 29

Appendix 3 — Abbreviations and Acronyms ..... Appendixes — 35

Appendix 4 — Internet-only Manuals (IOMs) ..... Appendixes — 37

Appendix 5 — HCPCS Changes for 2020 ..... Appendixes — 207

Appendix 6 — Place of Service and Type of Service ..... Appendixes — 215

© 2019 Optum360, LLC

Introduction

Organization of HCPCS

The Optum360 2020 *HCPCS Level II* contains mandated changes and new codes for use as of January 1, 2020. Deleted codes have also been indicated and cross-referenced to active codes when possible. New codes have been added to the appropriate sections, eliminating the time-consuming step of looking in two places for a code. However, keep in mind that the information in this book is a reproduction of the 2020 HCPCS; additional information on coverage issues may have been provided to Medicare contractors after publication. All contractors periodically update their systems and records throughout the year. If this book does not agree with your contractor, it is either because of a mid-year update or correction, or a specific local or regional coverage policy.

Index

Because HCPCS is organized by code number rather than by service or supply name, the index enables the coder to locate any code without looking through individual ranges of codes. Just look up the medical or surgical supply, service, orthotic, or prosthetic in question to find the appropriate codes. This index also refers to many of the brand names by which these items are known.

Table of Drugs and Biologicals

The brand names of drugs and biologicals listed are examples only and may not include all products available for that type. The table lists HCPCS codes from any available section including A codes, C codes, J codes, S codes, and Q codes under brand and generic names with amount, route of administration, and code numbers. While every effort is made to make the table comprehensive, it is not all-inclusive.

Color-coded Coverage Instructions

The Optum360 *HCPCS Level II* book provides colored symbols for each coverage and reimbursement instruction. A legend to these symbols is provided on the bottom of each two-page spread.

HOW TO USE OPTUM360 HCPCS LEVEL II BOOKS

Green Color Bar—Special Coverage Instructions

A green bar for "special coverage instructions" over a code means that special coverage instructions apply to that code. These special instructions are also typically given in the form of Medicare Internet Only Manuals (IOM) reference numbers. The appendixes provide the full text of the cited Medicare IOM.

A4336 **Incontinence supply, urethral insert, any type, each**

Yellow Color Bar—Carrier Discretion

Issues that are left to "carrier discretion" are covered with a yellow bar. Contact the carrier for specific coverage information on those codes.

A9581 **Injection, gadoxetate disodium, 1 ml**

Pink Color Bar—Not Covered by or Invalid for Medicare

Codes that are not covered by or are invalid for Medicare are covered by a pink bar. The pertinent Medicare Internet-only Manuals (IOMs) reference numbers are also given explaining why a particular code is not covered. These numbers refer to the appendixes, where the Medicare references are listed.

A4264 **Permanent implantable contraceptive intratubal occlusion device(s) and delivery system**

Codes in the Optum360 *HCPCS Level II* follow the AMA CPT book conventions to indicate new, revised, and deleted codes.

- A black circle (●) precedes a new code.
- A black triangle (▲) precedes a code with revised terminology or rules.
- A circle (○) precedes a recycled/reinstated code.
- Codes deleted from the current active codes appear with a strike-out.

●	**K1003**	**Whirlpool tub, walk in, portable**
▲	**B4185**	**Parenteral nutrition solution, not otherwise specified, 10 g lipids**
○	**J3245**	**Injection, tildrakizumab, 1 mg**
	~~**M1000**~~	~~**Pain screened as moderate to severe**~~

☑ Quantity Alert

Many codes in HCPCS report quantities that may not coincide with quantities available in the marketplace. For instance, a HCPCS code for an ostomy pouch with skin barrier reports each pouch, but the product is generally sold in a package of 10; "10" must be indicated in the quantity box on the CMS claim form to ensure proper reimbursement. This symbol indicates that care should be taken to verify quantities in this code. These quantity alerts do not represent Medicare Unlikely Edits (MUEs) and should not be used for MUEs.

☑ **J0120** **Injection, tetracycline, up to 250 mg**

© 2019 Optum360, LLC

♀ Female Only
This icon identifies procedures that some payers may consider female only.

A4261 **Cervical cap for contraceptive use** ♀

♂ Male Only
This icon identifies procedures that some payers may consider male only.

A4326 **Male external catheter with integral collection chamber, anytype, each** ♂

Q2037 **Influenza virus vaccine, split virus, when administered to individuals 3 years of age and older, for intramuscular use (FLUVIRIN)** A

A Age Edit
This icon denotes codes intended for use with a specific age group, such as neonate, newborn, pediatric, and adult. Carefully review the code description to ensure that the code reported most appropriately reflects the patient's age.

H1001 **Prenatal care, at-risk enhanced service; antepartum management** M

M Maternity
This icon identifies procedures that by definition should only be used for maternity patients generally between 12 and 55 years of age.

G0105 **Colorectal cancer screening; colonoscopy on individual at high risk** A2

A2–Z3 ASC Payment Indicators
Codes designated as being paid by ASC groupings that were effective at the time of printing are denoted by the group number.

E0988 **Manual wheelchair accessory, lever-activated, wheel drive, pair** ♿

♿ DMEPOS
Use this icon to identify when to consult the CMS durable medical equipment, prosthetics, orthotics, and supplies (DMEPOS) for payment of this durable medical item. For modifiers NU, RR, and UE: These modifiers are for use when DME equipment is either new, used, or rented. The RR modifiers must also be used in conjunction with rental modifiers KH, KI, or KJ.

A4653 **Peritoneal dialysis catheter anchoring device, belt, each** ⊘

⊘ Skilled Nursing Facility (SNF)
Use this icon to identify certain items and services excluded from SNF consolidated billing. These items may be billed directly to the Medicare contractor by the provider or supplier of the service or item.

C9254 **Injection, lacosamide, 1 mg**
Use this code for VIMPAT.

Drugs commonly reported with a code are listed underneath by brand or generic name.

CMS does not use consistent terminology when a code for a specific procedure is not listed. The code description may include any of the following terms: unlisted, not otherwise classified (NOC), unspecified, unclassified, other, and miscellaneous. If unsure there is no code for the service or supply provided or used, provide adequate documentation to the payer. Check with the payer for more information.

A0999 **Unlisted ambulance service**

For a new, revised, or deleted code, the specific effective quarter is shown to the right of the code.

● **J9199[Jan]** **Injection, gemcitabine HCl (Infugem), 200 mg**

© 2019 Optum360, LLC

OPPS Status Indicators

A-Y Status indicators identify how individual HCPCS Level II codes are paid or not paid under the OPPS. The same status indicator is assigned to all the codes within an ambulatory payment classification (APC). Consult the payer or resource to learn which CPT codes fall within various APCs. Status indicators for HCPCS and their definitions follow:

A Services furnished to a hospital outpatient that are paid under a fee schedule or payment system other than OPPS, for example:
- Ambulance Services
- Clinical Diagnostic Laboratory Services
- Non-Implantable Prosthetic and Orthotic Devices
- Physical, Occupational, and Speech Therapy
- Diagnostic Mammography
- Screening Mammography

B Codes that are not recognized by OPPS when submitted on an outpatient hospital Part B bill type (12x and 13x)

C Inpatient Procedures

E1 Items, Codes, and Services:
- Not covered by any Medicare outpatient benefit category
- Statutorily excluded by Medicare
- Not reasonable and necessary

F Corneal Tissue Acquisition; Certain CRNA Services and Hepatitis B Vaccines

G Pass-Through Drugs and Biologicals

H Pass-Through Device Categories

J1 Hospital Part B services paid through a comprehensive APC

K Nonpass-Through Drugs and Nonimplantable Biologicals, Including Therapeutic Radiopharmaceuticals

L Influenza Vaccine; Pneumococcal Pneumonia Vaccine

M Items and Services Not Billable to the MAC

N Items and Services Packaged into APC Rates

P Partial Hospitalization

Q1 STVX-Packaged Codes

Q2 T-Packaged Codes

Q3 Codes That May Be Paid Through a Composite APC

Q4 Conditionally packaged laboratory tests

R Blood and Blood Products

S Significant Procedure, Not Discounted when Multiple

T Significant Procedure, Multiple Procedure Reduction Applies

U Brachytherapy Sources

V Clinic or Emergency Department Visit

Y Nonimplantable Durable Medical Equipment

A	**L8440**	**Prosthetic shrinker, below knee, each**
B	**Q4005**	**Cast supplies, long arm cast, adult (11 years +), plaster**
C	**G0341**	**Percutaneous islet cell transplant, includes portal vein catheterization and infusion**
E1	**A0021**	**Ambulance service, outside state per mile, transport (Medicaid only)**
F	**V2785**	**Processing, preserving and transporting corneal tissue**
G	**C9460**	**Injection, cangrelor, 1 mg**
H	**C2613**	**Lung biopsy plug with delivery system**
K	**J1750**	**Injection, iron dextran, 50 mg**
L	**Q2036**	**Influenza virus vaccine, split virus, when administered to individuals 3 years of age and older, for intramuscular use (FLULAVAL)**
M	**G0333**	**Pharmacy dispensing fee for inhalation drug(s); initial 30-day supply as a beneficiary**
N	**A4220**	**Refill kit for implantable infusion pump**
P	**G0129**	**Occupational therapy services requiring the skills of a qualified occupational therapist, furnished as a component of a partial hospitalization treatment program, per session (45 minutes or more)**
Q3	**C8935**	**Magnetic resonance angiography without contrast, upper extremity**
R	**P9010**	**Blood (whole), for transfusion, per unit**
S	**G0117**	**Glaucoma screening for high risk patients furnished by an optometrist or ophthalmologist**
T	**C9727**	**Insertion of implants into the soft palate; minimum of 3 implants**
U	**A9527**	**Iodine I-125, sodium iodide solution, therapeutic, per millicurie**
V	**G0101**	**Cervical or vaginal cancer screening; pelvic and clinical breast examination**
Y	**A5500**	**For diabetics only, fitting (including follow-up), custom preparation and supply of off-the-shelf depth-inlay shoe manufactured to accommodate multidensity insert(s), per shoe**

© 2019 Optum360, LLC

ASC Payment Indicators

A2–Z3 This icon identifies the ASC status payment indicators. They indicate how the ASC payment rate was derived and/or how the procedure, item, or service is treated under the ASC payment system. For more information about these indicators and how they affect billing, consult Optum360's *Outpatient Billing Editor*.

- A2 Surgical procedure on ASC list in CY 2007 or later; payment based on OPPS relative payment weight
- C5 Inpatient procedure
- F4 Corneal tissue acquisition, hepatitis B vaccine; paid at reasonable cost
- G2 Non-office-based surgical procedure added in CY 2008 or later; payment based on OPPS relative payment weight
- H2 Brachytherapy source paid separately when provided integral to a surgical procedure on ASC list; payment based on OPPS rate
- J7 OPPS pass-through device paid separately when provided integral to a surgical procedure on ASC list; payment based on OPPS rate
- J8 Device-intensive procedure paid at adjusted rate
- K2 Drugs and biologicals paid separately when provided integral to a surgical procedure on ASC list; payment based on OPPS rate
- K7 Unclassified drugs and biologicals; payment contractor-priced
- L1 Influenza vaccine; pneumococcal vaccine; packaged item/service; no separate payment made
- L6 New Technology Intraocular Lens (NTIOL); special payment
- N1 Packaged service/item; no separate payment made
- P2 Office-based surgical procedure added to ASC list in CY 2008 or later with MPFS nonfacility PE RVUs; payment based on OPPS relative payment weight
- P3 Office-based surgical procedure added to ASC list in CY 2008 or later with MPFS nonfacility PE RVUs; payment based on MPFS nonfacility PE RVUs
- R2 Office-based surgical procedure added to ASC list in CY 2008 or later without MPFS nonfacility PE RVUs; payment based on OPPS relative payment weight
- Z2 Radiology service paid separately when provided integral to a surgical procedure on ASC list; payment based on OPPS relative payment weight
- Z3 Radiology service paid separately when provided integral to a surgical procedure on ASC list; payment based on MPFS nonfacility PE RVUs

F4 **V2785** **Processing, preserving and transporting corneal tissue**

H2 **A9527** **Iodine I-125, sodium iodide solution, therapeutic per millicurie**

J7 **C1841** **Retinal prosthesis, includes all internal and external components**

K2 **C9132** **Prothrombin complex concentrate (human), Kcentra, per IU of Factor IX activity**

K7 **C9399** **Unclassified drugs or biologicals**

L1 **Q2037** **Influenza virus vaccine, split virus, when administered to individuals 3 years of age and older, for intramuscular use (FLUVIRIN)**

N1 **C9353** **Microporous collagen implantable slit tube (NeuraWrap Nerve Protector), per cm length**

Z3 **G0130** **Single energy x-ray absorptiometry (SEXA) bone density study, one or more sites; appendicular skeleton (peripheral) (e.g., radius, wrist, heel)**

Z2 **C8911** **Magnetic resonance angiography without contrast followed by with contrast, chest (excluding myocardium)**

CMS: This notation precedes an instruction pertaining to this code in the CMS Internet-only Manuals (IOMs) electronic manual or in a National Coverage Determination (NCD). These CMS sources, formerly called the Medicare Carriers Manual (MCM) and Coverage Issues Manual (CIM), present the rules for submitting these services to the federal government or its contractors and are included in the appendix of this book.

A4618 **Breathing circuits**

CMS: 100-04, 20, 100.2

AHA: American Hospital Association Coding Clinic® for HCPCS citations help in finding expanded information about specific codes and their usage.

A4290 **Sacral nerve stimulation test lead, each**

AHA: 1Q, '02, 9

© 2019 Optum360, LLC

About HCPCS Codes

HCPCS Level II codes are developed and maintained by the Centers for Medicare and Medicaid Services (CMS). Optum360 does not change the code descriptions other than correcting typographical errors. For 2020, there are some codes that appear to be duplicates. CMS has indicated that each of the codes is used to report a specific condition or service. At press time, CMS had not provided further clarification regarding these codes. Additional information may be found on the CMS website, https://www.cms.gov/Medicare/Coding/HCPCSReleaseCodeSets/index.html.

Any supplier or manufacturer can submit a request for coding modification to the HCPCS Level II national codes. A document explaining the HCPCS modification process, as well as a detailed format for submitting a recommendation for a modification to HCPCS Level II codes, is available on the HCPCS website at https://www.cms.gov/MedHCPCSGenInfo/01a_Application_Form_and_Instructions.asp#TopOfPage. Besides the information requested in this format, a requestor should also submit any additional descriptive material, including the manufacturer's product literature and information that is believed would be helpful in furthering CMS's understanding of the medical features of the item for which a coding modification is being recommended. The HCPCS coding review process is an ongoing, continuous process.

Requests for coding modifications should be sent to the following address:

Felicia Eggleston, CMS HCPCS Workgroup Coordinator
Centers for Medicare and Medicaid Services
C5-08-27
7500 Security Blvd
Baltimore, Maryland 21244-1850

The dental (D) codes are not included in the official 2020 HCPCS Level II code set. The American Dental Association (ADA) holds the copyright on those codes and instructed CMS to remove them. As a result, Optum360 has removed them from this product; however, Optum360 has additional resources available for customers requiring the dental codes. Please visit www.optum360coding.com or call 1.800.464.3649.

How to Use HCPCS Level II

Coders should keep in mind, that the insurance companies and government do not base payment solely on what was done for the patient. They need to know why the services were performed. In addition to using the HCPCS coding system for procedures and supplies, coders must also use the ICD-10-CM coding system to denote the diagnosis. This book will not discuss ICD-10-CM codes, which can be found in a current ICD-10-CM code book for diagnosis codes. To locate a HCPCS Level II code, follow these steps:

1. Identify the services or procedures that the patient received.

   Example:

   Patient administered PSA exam.

2. Look up the appropriate term in the index.

   Example:

   Screening
   prostate specific antigen test (PSA)

   Coding Tip: Coders who are unable to find the procedure or service in the index can look in the table of contents for the type of procedure or device to narrow the code choices. Also, coders should remember to check the unlisted procedure guidelines for additional choices.

3. Assign a tentative code.

   Example:

   Code G0103

   Coding Tip: To the right of the terminology, there may be a single code or multiple codes, a cross-reference, or an indication that the code has been deleted. Tentatively assign all codes listed.

4. Locate the code or codes in the appropriate section. When multiple codes are listed in the index, be sure to read the narrative of all codes listed to find the appropriate code based on the service performed.

   Example:

   G0103 Prostate cancer screening; prostate specific antigen test (PSA)

5. Check for color bars, symbols, notes, and references.

   Example:

   G0103 Prostate cancer screening; prostate specific antigen test (PSA) ♂ A

6. Review the appendixes for the reference definitions and other guidelines for coverage issues that apply.

7. Determine whether any modifiers should be used.

8. Assign the code.

   Example:

   The code assigned is G0103.

Coding Standards

Levels of Use

Coders may find that the same procedure is coded at two or even three levels. Which code is correct? There are certain rules to follow if this should occur.

When both a CPT and a HCPCS Level II code have virtually identical narratives for a procedure or service, the CPT code should be used. If, however, the narratives are not identical (e.g., the CPT code narrative is generic, whereas the HCPCS Level II code is specific), the Level II code should be used.

Be sure to check for a national code when a CPT code description contains an instruction to include additional information, such as describing a specific medication. For example, when billing Medicare or Medicaid for supplies, avoid using CPT code 99070 Supplies and materials (except spectacles), provided by the physician over and above those usually included with the office visit or other services rendered (list drugs, trays, supplies, or materials provided). There are many HCPCS Level II codes that specify supplies in more detail.

Special Reports

Submit a special report with the claim when a new, unusual, or variable procedure is provided or a modifier is used. Include the following information:

- A copy of the appropriate report (e.g., operative, x-ray), explaining the nature, extent, and need for the procedure
- Documentation of the medical necessity of the procedure
- Documentation of the time and effort necessary to perform the procedure

© 2019 Optum360, LLC

A

Abdomen/abdominal
dressing holder/binder, A4461, A4463
pad, low profile, L1270
Abduction
control, each, L2624
pillow, E1399
rotation bar, foot, L3140-L3170
Ablation
prostate, transrectal
high intensity focused ultrasound, C9747
robotic, waterjet, C2596
transbronchial, C9751
ultrasound, C9734
Abortion, S0199, S2260-S2267
Absorption dressing, A6251-A6256
Access system, A4301
Accessories
ambulation devices, E0153-E0159
artificial kidney and machine (*see also* ESRD), E1510-E1699
beds, E0271-E0280
Medicare IVIG demonstration, Q2052
oxygen, E1352, E1354-E1358
retinal prosthesis, L8608
total artificial heart, L8698
ventricular assist device, Q0477, Q0501-Q0509
wheelchairs, E0950-E1012, E1050-E1298, E2201-E2231, E2295, E2300-E2367, K0001-K0108
AccuChek
blood glucose meter, E0607
test strips, box of 50, A4253
Accurate
prosthetic sock, L8420-L8435
stump sock, L8470-L8485
Acetate concentrate for hemodialysis, A4708
Acid concentrate for hemodialysis, A4709
ACO Model, G9868-G9870
Action Patriot manual wheelchair, K0004
Action Xtra, Action MVP, Action Pro-T, manual wheelchair, K0005
Active Life
convex one-piece urostomy pouch, A4421
flush away, A5051
one-piece
drainable custom pouch, A5061
pre-cut closed-end pouch, A5051
stoma cap, A5055
Activity therapy, G0176
Adaptor
electric/pneumatic ventricular assist device, Q0478
neurostimulator, C1883
pacing lead, C1883
Addition
cushion AK, L5648
cushion BK, L5646
harness upper extremity, L6675-L6676
to halo procedure, L0861
to lower extremity orthotic, K0672, L2750-L2760, L2780-L2861
to lower extremity prosthesis, L5970-L5990
to upper extremity orthotic, L3891
wrist, flexion, extension, L6620
Adhesive
barrier, C1765
catheter, A4364
disc or foam pad, A5126
medical, A4364
Nu-Hope
1 oz bottle with applicator, A4364
3 oz bottle with applicator, A4364
ostomy, A4364
pads, A6203-A6205, A6212-A6214, A6219-A6221, A6237-A6239, A6245-A6247, A6254-A6256
remover, A4455, A4456
support, breast prosthesis, A4280
tape, A4450, A4452
tissue, G0168
Adjunctive blue light cystoscopy, C9738
Adjustabrace 3, L2999
Adjustment
bariatric band, S2083
Administration
aerosolized drug therapy, home, S9061
chemotherapy infusion
continued in community, G0498
hepatitis B vaccine, G0010
influenza virus vaccine, G0008
medication, T1502-T1503
direct observation, H0033
pneumococcal vaccine, G0009
Adoptive immunotherapy, S2107
Adrenal transplant, S2103
AdvantaJet, A4210
Affinity, Q4159
AFO, E1815, E1830, L1900-L1990, L4392, L4396
Aimsco Ultra Thin syringe, 1 cc or 1/2 cc, each, A4206
Air bubble detector, dialysis, E1530
Air fluidized bed, E0194
Air pressure pad/mattress, E0186, E0197
Air travel and nonemergency transportation, A0140
Aircast air stirrup ankle brace, L1906
Airlife Brand Misty-Neb nebulizer, E0580
AirSep, E0601
Airway device, E0485-E0486
Alarm
device, A9280
enuresis, S8270
pressure, dialysis, E1540
Albumarc, P9041
Albumin, human, P9041, P9045-P9047
Alcohol
abuse service, H0047
assessment, G0396-G0397, G2011, H0001
pint, A4244
testing, H0048
wipes, A4245
Alert device, A9280
Algiderm, alginate dressing, A6196-A6199
Alginate dressing, A6196-A6199
Algosteril, alginate dressing, A6196-A6199
Alkaline battery for blood glucose monitor, A4233-A4236
AlloDerm, Q4116
AlloGen, Q4212
Allogenic cord blood harvest, S2140
Allograft
small intestine and liver, S2053
AlloPatch HD, Q4128
AlloSkin, Q4115
AlloSkin AC, Q4141
AlloSkin RT, Q4123
AlloWrap DS, Q4150
Alternating pressure mattress/pad, E0181, E0277
pump, E0182
Alternative communication device, i.e., communication board, E1902
Ambulance, A0021-A0999
air, A0436
disposable supplies, A0382-A0398
non-emergency, S9960-S9961
oxygen, A0422
response, treatment, no transport, A0998
Ambulation device, E0100-E0159
Ambulation stimulator
spinal cord injured, E0762
Aminaid, enteral nutrition, B4154
Amirosyn-RF, parenteral nutrition, B5000
Ammonia test paper, A4774
Amnio Bio, Q4211
AmnioArmor, Q4168
AmnioBand, Q4151, Q4168
AmnioExcel, AmnioExcel Plus, Q4137
AmnioMatrix, Q4139
AmnioPro, Q4163
AmnioPro Flow, Q4162
AmnioWound, Q4181
AmnioWrap2, Q4221
Amputee
adapter, wheelchair, E0959
prosthesis, L5000-L7510, L7520, L8400-L8465
stump sock, L8470
Amputee — *continued*
wheelchair, E1170-E1190, E1200
Analysis
dose optimization, S3722
gene sequence
hypertrophic cardiomyopathy, S3865, S3866
semen, G0027
Anchor, screw, C1713
Anesthesia
dialysis, A4736-A4737
monitored (MAC), G9654
Angiography
fluorescent
nonocular, C9733
iliac artery, G0278
magnetic resonance, C8901-C8914, C8918-C8920
reconstruction, G0288
Ankle foot system, L5973
Ankle orthosis, L1902, L1904, L1907
Ankle–foot orthotic (AFO), L1900, L1906, L1910-L1940, L2106-L2116
Dorsiwedge Night Splint, A4570, L2999, L4398
Specialist
Ankle Foot Orthotic, L1930
Tibial Pre-formed Fracture Brace, L2116
Surround Ankle Stirrup Braces with Foam, L1906
Annual wellness visit, G0438-G0439
Antenna
replacement
diaphragmatic/phrenic nerve stimulator, L8696
Anterior-posterior orthotic
lateral orthotic, L0700, L0710
Antibiotic home infusion therapy, S9494-S9504
Antibiotic regimen, G9286-G9287
Antibody testing, HIV-1, S3645
Anticoagulation clinic, S9401
Antifungal home infusion therapy, S9494-S9504
Antimicrobial prophylaxis, G9196-G9198
Antiseptic
chlorhexidine, A4248
Antisperm antibodies, S3655
Antiviral home infusion therapy, S9494-S9504
Apheresis
low density lipid, S2120
Apligraf, Q4101
Apnea monitor, E0618-E0619
electrodes, A4556
lead wires, A4557
with recording feature, E0619
Appliance
cleaner, A5131
pneumatic, E0655-E0673
Application
skin substitute, C5271-C5278
tantalum rings, S8030
Appropriate Use Criteria
Clinic Decision Support Mechanism, G1000-G1011
AquaPedic sectional gel flotation, E0196
Aqueous
shunt, L8612
Arch support, L3040-L3100
Architect, Architect PX, or Architect FX, Q4147
Arm
sling
deluxe, A4565
mesh cradle, A4565
universal
arm, A4565
elevator, A4565
wheelchair, E0973
Arrow, power wheelchair, K0014
Artacent AC (fluid), Q4189
Artacent AC, Q4190
Artacent Cord, Q4216
Artacent Wound, Q4169
Arteriovenous fistula creation, C9754-C9755
Arthroereisis
subtalar, S2117
ArthroFlex, Q4125
Arthroscopy
knee
harvest of cartilage, S2112
removal loose body, FB, G0289
shoulder
with capsulorrhaphy, S2300
Artificial
kidney machines and accessories (*see also* Dialysis), E1510-E1699
larynx, L8500
saliva, A9155
Ascent, Q4213
Assertive community treatment, H0039-H0040
Assessment
alcohol and/or substance, G0396-G0397, G2011, H0001
audiologic, V5008-V5020
chronic care management services
comprehensive, G0506
family, H1011
functional outcome, G9227
geriatric, S0250
mental health, H0031
online
qualified nonphysician professional, G2061-G2063
pain, G8442
speech, V5362-V5364
wellness, S5190
Assisted living, T2030-T2031
Assistive listening device, V5268-V5274
alerting device, V5269
cochlear implant assistive device, V5273
FM/DM, V5281
accessories, V5283-V5290
system, V5281-V5282
supplies and accessories, V5267
TDD, V5272
telephone amplifier, V5268
television caption decoder, V5271
Asthma
education, S9441
kit, S8097
Attendant care, S5125-S5126
Attends, adult diapers, A4335
Audiologic assessment, V5008-V5020
Audiometry, S0618
Auditory osseointegrated device, L8690, L8691, L8692-L8693
Autoclix lancet device, A4258
Auto-Glide folding walker, E0143
Autolance lancet device, A4258
Autolet lancet device, A4258
Autolet Lite lancet device, A4258
Autolet Mark II lancet device, A4258
AxoBioMembrane, Q4211
Axolotl Ambient, Axolotl Cryo, Q4215
Axolotl Graft, Axolotl DualGraft, Q4210

B

Babysitter, child of parents in treatment, T1009
Back school, S9117
Back supports, L0450-L0710
Bacterial sensitivity study, P7001
Bag
drainage, A4357
irrigation supply, A4398
resuscitation bag, S8999
spacer, for metered dose inhaler, A4627
urinary, A4358, A5112
Balken, fracture frame, E0946
Ballistocardiogram, S3902
Bandage
adhesive, A6413
compression
high, A6452
light, A6448-A6450
medium, A6451
padding, S8430
roll, S8431
conforming, A6442-A6447
Orthoflex elastic plastic bandages, A4580
padding, A6441
self-adherent, A6413, A6453-A6455

© 2019 Optum360, LLC

Bandage — *continued*
specialist plaster bandages, A4580
zinc paste impregnated, A6456
Bariatric
bed, E0302-E0304
brief/diaper, T4543
surgery, S2083
Barium enema, G0106
cancer screening, G0120
Barrier
4 x 4, A4372
adhesion, C1765
with flange, A4373
Baseball finger splint, A4570
Bath chair, E0240
Bathtub
chair, E0240
heat unit, E0249
stool or bench, E0245
transfer bench, E0247, E0248
transfer rail, E0246
wall rail, E0241, E0242
Battery, L7360, L7364
blood glucose monitor, A4233-A4236
charger, L7362, L7366, L7368, L8695, L8699, Q0495
cochlear implant device
alkaline, L8622
lithium, L8623-L8624
zinc, L8621
hearing device, V5266
infusion pump, external, A4602, K0601-K0605
lithium, A4601-A4602, L7367, Q0506
charger, L7368
replacement
charger, L7368
ear pulse generator, A4638
external defibrillator, K0607
external infusion pump, A4602, K0601-K0605
six volt battery, L7360
TENS, A4630
twelve volt battery, L7364
ventilator, A4611-A4613
ventricular assist device, Q0496, Q0503
wheelchair, E2358-E2359, E2397, K0733
Bayer chemical reagent strips, box of 100 glucose/ketone urine test strips, A4250
BCPI home visit, G9187
BCW 600, manual wheelchair, K0007
BCW Power, power wheelchair, K0014
BCW recliner, manual wheelchair, K0007
B-D alcohol swabs, box, A4245
B-D disposable insulin syringes, up to 1 cc, per syringe, A4206
B-D lancets, per box of 100, A4258
Bebax, foot orthotic, L3160
Bed
accessory, E0315
air fluidized, E0194
cradle, any type, E0280
drainage bag, bottle, A4357, A5102
extra size for bariatric patients, E0302-E0304
hospital, E0250-E0270
full electric, home care, without mattress, E0297
manual, without mattress, E0293
pediatric, E0328-E0329
safety enclosure frame/canopy, E0316
semi-electric, without mattress, E0295
pan, E0275, E0276
Moore, E0275
rail, E0305, E0310
safety enclosure frame/canopy, hospital bed, E0316
Behavioral health, H0002-H0030
day treatment, H2013
Medicaid certified health clinic services, T1040-T1041
per hour, H2012
residential treatment program, T2048
BellaCell HD, Q4220
Bell-Horn
prosthetic shrinker, L8440-L8465
Belt
adapter, A4421
extremity, E0945
Little Ones Sur-Fit pediatric, A4367
ostomy, A4367
pelvic, E0944
ventricular assist device, Q0499
wheelchair, E0978, K0098
Bench, bathtub — *see also* Bathtub, E0245
Benesch boot, L3212-L3214
Berkeley shell, foot orthotic, L3000
Beta-blocker therapy, G9188-G9192
Betadine, A4246
swabs/wipes, A4247
Bicarbonate concentration for hemodialysis, A4706-A4707
Bifocal, glass or plastic, V2200-V2299
Bilirubin (phototherapy) light, E0202
Binder
extremity, nonelastic, A4465
Bio Flote alternating air pressure pump, pad system, E0181, E0182
bio-ConneKt Wound Matrix, Q4161
BioDExcel, Q4137
BioDFence, Q4140
BioDFence DryFlex, Q4138
BioDMatrix, Q4139
Biofeedback device, E0746
Biopsy
bone marrow
biopsy needle, C1830
lung
non small cell, G9282-G9285, G9288-G9290
plug, C2613
non-lung, G9285, G9291
other, G9292-G9295
BioSkin, Q4163
BioSkin Flow, Q4162
BIOVANCE, Q4154
BioWound, BioWound Plus, BioWound Xplus, Q4217
Birth control pills, S4993
Birthing classes, S9436-S9439, S9442
Bite disposable jaw locks, E0700
Blinded procedure
interatrial shunt/placebo control, C9758
Blood
Congo red, P2029
cryoprecipitate, P9012
glucose monitor, A4258, E0607
disposable, A9275
receiver, K0554
supply allowance, 1 month, K0553
with integrated lancing system, E2101
with voice synthesizer, E2100
glucose test strips, A4253
granulocytes, pheresis, P9050
ketone test strips, A4252
leak detector, dialysis, E1560
leukocyte reduced, P9016, P9040, P9050, P9054, P9056-P9058
mucoprotein, P2038
not otherwise specified, P9099
pressure equipment, A4660, A4663, A4670
pump, dialysis, E1620
red blood cells, P9016, P9021-P9022, P9038, P9040, P9057-P9058
split unit, P9011
strips
blood glucose test or reagent strips, A4253
blood ketone test or reagent strip, A4252
testing supplies, A4770
transfusion, home, S9538
tubing, A4750, A4755
whole, P9010, P9051, P9056
Bock Dynamic, foot prosthesis, L5972
Body jacket
scoliosis, L1300, L1310
Body sock, L0984
Body wrap
foam positioners, E0191
therapeutic overlay, E0199
Bond or cement, ostomy, skin, A4364
Boot
pelvic, E0944
surgical, ambulatory, L3260
walking
nonpneumatic, L4386-L4387
pneumatic, L4360-L4361
Boston type spinal orthotic, L1200
Brachytherapy
cesium 131, C2642-C2643
cesium-131 chloride solution, C2644
gold 198, C1716
iodine 125, A9527
iridium 192
high dose, C1717
nonhigh dose, C1719
low dose rate (LDR), prostate, G0458
needle, C1715
nonhigh dose rate iridium 192, C1719
nonstranded
cesium-131, C2643
gold-198, C1716
iodine-125, C2634, C2639
iridium-192, C1717, C1719
NOS, C2699
palladium-103, C2635-C2636, C2641
ytterbium-169, C2637
yttrium-90, C2616
palladium-103, C2645
placement of endorectal intracavitary applicator, C9725
radioelements, Q3001
stranded
cesium-131, C2642
iodine-125, C2638
NOS, C2698
palladium-103, C2640
Brake attachment, wheeled walker, E0159
Breast
exam (with pelvic exam), G0101
exam (without pelvic exam), S0613
milk collection, K1005
milk processing, T2101
placement/removal applicator, C9726
prosthesis, L8000-L8035, L8031, L8600
adhesive skin support, A4280
nipple, L2006
pump, E0602-E0604
supplies, A4281-A4286
reconstruction, S2066-S2068
Breathing circuit, A4618
Brief
adult, T4521-T4524
bariatric, T4543
pediatric, T4529-T4530
Broncho-Cath endobronchial tubes, with CPAP system, E0601
Bronchoscopy, C9751
Buck's, traction
frame, E0870
stand, E0880
Bulb for therapeutic light box, A4634
Bulking agent
anal, L8605
vocal cord, L8607
Burn
garment, A6501, A6512-A6513
matrix, Q4103
Bus, nonemergency, A0110

C

Calibrator solution, A4256
Camisole, post mastectomy, S8460
Camping therapy, T2036-T2037
Cancer screening
barium enema, G0106, G0120, G0122
breast exam, G0101
cervical
exam, G0101
HPV infectious agent detection by DNA/RNA, G0476
colorectal, G0104-G0106, G0120-G0122, G0328
Cancer screening — *continued*
prostate, G0102-G0103
Cane, E0100, E0105
accessory, A4636, A4637
Easy-Care quad, E0105
quad canes, E0105
Quadri-Poise, E0105
wooden, E0100
Canister
disposable, used with suction pump, A7000
non-disposable, used with suction pump, A7001
Cannula
fistula, set (for dialysis), A4730
nasal, A4615
tracheostomy, A4623
Carbon filter, A4680
Cardiac contractility modulation generator, C1824
Cardiac event, recorder implantable, C1764, E0616
Cardiac monitoring, transesophageal doppler, G9157
Cardiac rehabilitation, G0422-G0423
program, S9472
Cardiointegram, S9025
Cardiokymography, Q0035
Cardiovascular services, M0300-M0301
Cardioverter-defibrillator, C1721, C1722, C1882
Care
attendant, S5125-S5126
companion, S5135-S5136
coordination
cancer treatment, S0353-S0354
day care, S5100-S5105
foster, S5140-S5141, S5145-S5146
home infusion catheter, S5497-S5502
personal care item, S5199
planning
chronic care management services, G0506
respite, S5150-S5151
Care management, CMMI Model, G0076-G0087
Carelet safety lancet, A4258
Carex
adjustable bath/shower stool, E0245
aluminum crutches, E0114
cane, E0100
folding walker, E0135
shower bench, E0245
Cartridge
digestive enzyme(s), B4105
Case management, G9012, T1016-T1017
per month, T2022
targeted, T2023
Casec, enteral nutrition, B4155
Cast
body cast, Q4001-Q4002
gauntlet, Q4013-Q4016
hand restoration, L6900-L6915
hip spica, Q4025-Q4028
long arm, Q4005-Q4008
long leg, Q4029-Q4036
materials, special, A4590
plaster, A4580
short arm, Q4009-Q4012
short leg, Q4037-Q4040
shoulder, Q4003-Q4004
supplies, A4580, A4590, Q4050
body cast, Q4001-Q4002
Delta-Cast Elite Casting Material, A4590
Delta-Lite Conformable Casting Tape, A4590
Delta-Lite C-Splint Fibreglass Immobilizer, A4590
Delta-Lite "S" Fibreglass Casting Tape, A4590
Flashcast Elite Casting Material, A4590
Orthoflex Elastic Plaster Bandages, A4580
Orthoplast Splints (and Orthoplast II Splints), A4590
Specialist Plaster Bandages, A4580

© 2019 Optum360, LLC

Cast — *continued*
supplies — *continued*
Specialist Plaster Roll Immobilizer, A4580
Specialist Plaster Splints, A4580
thermoplastic, L2106, L2126
Caster, wheelchair, E2214, E2219, E2395-E2396
Catheter, A4300-A4364
anchoring device, A4333, A4334
percutaneous, A5200
balloon, C1727
brachytherapy, C1728
cap, disposable (dialysis), A4860
diagnostic, C1730, C1731
ablation, C1732, C1733
drainage, C1729
electrophysiology, C2630
external collection device, A4326-A4330
extravascular tissue ablation, C1886
guiding, C1887
hemodialysis, C1750, C1752
implantable access, A4301
implantable intraspinal, E0785
indwelling, A4338-A4346
infusion, C1752
insertion
centrally inserted infusion, C1751
midline, infusion, C1751
midline venous, home health, S5523
peripherally inserted infusion, C1751
tray, A4354
intermittent, with insertion supplies, A4353
intracardiac echocardiography, C1759
intradiscal, C1754
intraspinal, C1755
intravascular ultrasound, C1753
irrigation supplies, A4355
lubricant, A4332
male, A4326, A4349
noncardiac ablation, C1888
nonvascular balloon dilatation, C1726
occlusion, C2628
intermittent, C1982
oropharyngeal suction, A4628
pacing, transesophageal, C1756
pressure generating, C1982
specimen collection, P9612, P9615
suprapubic, cystoscopic, C2627
thrombectomy, emobolectomy, C1757
tracheal suction, A4605, A4624
transluminal
angioplasty
laser, C1885
nonlaser, C1725, C2623
atherectomy
directional, C1714
rotational, C1724
ureteral, C1758
CBC, G0306-G0307
Cellesta, Cellesta Duo, Q4184
Cellesta Cord, Q4214
Cellesta Flowable Amnion, Q4185
Cellular therapy, M0075
Cement, ostomy, A4364
Centrifuge, for dialysis, E1500
Cephalin flocculation, blood, P2028
Certified nurse assistant, S9122
Cerumen removal, G0268
Cervical
collar, L0120, L0130, L0140, L0150, L0170
halo, L0810-L0830
head harness/halter, E0942
helmet, A8000-A8004
orthotic, L0180-L0200
traction equipment, not requiring frame, E0855
Cervical cap contraceptive, A4261
Cervical-thoracic-lumbar-sacral orthotic (CTLSO), L0700, L0710, L1000, L1001
Cesium-131, C2642-C2643
Chair
adjustable, dialysis, E1570
bathtub, E0240
commode, E0163-E0165
lift, E0627, E0629
rollabout, E1031
Chair — *continued*
shower or bath, E0240
sitz bath, E0160-E0162
Challenger manual wheelchair, K0009
Champion 1000 manual wheelchair, K0004
Champion 30000, manual wheelchair, K0005
CheckMate Plus blood glucose monitor, E0607
Chelation therapy, M0300
home infusion, administration, S9355
Chemical endarterectomy, M0300
Chemistry and toxicology tests, P2028-P3001
Chemodenervation
vocal cord, S2340-S2341
Chemotherapy
administration
both infusion and other technique, Q0085
home infusion, continuous, S9325-S9379, S9494-S9497
infusion, Q0084
continued in community, G0498
other than infusion, Q0083
Chemstrip bG, box of 50 blood glucose test strips, A4253
Chemstrip K, box of 100 ketone urine test strips, A4250
Chemstrip UGK, box of 100 glucose/ ketone urine test strips, A4250
Chest shell (cuirass), E0457
Chest wrap, E0459
Childbirth, S9442
cesarean birth, S9438
class, S9442
early induction, G9355-G9356
elective delivery, G9355-G9356
Lamaze, S9436
postpartum education, G9357-G9358
postpartum evaluation, G9357-G9358
postpartum screening, G9357-G9358
preparation, S9436
refresher, S9437
VBAC (vaginal birth after cesarean), S9439
Childcare, T2026-T2027
parents in treatment, T1009
Chin
cup, cervical, L0150
strap (for CPAP device), A7036
Chlorhexidine, A4248
Chondrocyte cell harvest, arthroscopic, S2112
Chopart prosthetic
ankle, L5050, L5060
below knee, L5100
Chore services, S5130-S5131
Christian Science provider services, S9900
Chromic phosphate, A9564
Chronic care management, G2058
Chux, A4554
Clamp
external urethral, A4356
Clarix 100, Q4156
Clarix Cord, Q4148
Clarix Flo,, Q4155
Classes, S9441-S9446
asthma, S9441
birthing, S9442
exercise, S9451
infant safety, S9447
lactation, S9443
nutrition, S9452
parenting, S9444
smoking cessation, S9453
stress management, S9454
weight management, S9449
Clavicle
splint, L3650
Cleaning solvent, Nu-Hope
16 oz bottle, A4455
4 oz bottle, A4455
Cleanser, wound, A6260
Cleft palate, feeder, S8265
Clevis, hip orthotic, L2570, L2600, L2610
Clinic visit/encounter, T1015
hospital outpatient, G0463
multidisciplinary, child services, T1025
Clinical Decision Support Mechanism, G1000-G1011
Clinical trials
lodging costs, S9994
meals, S9996
phase II, S9990
phase III, S9991
service, S9988
transportation costs, S9992
Closure device, vascular, C1760
Clotting time tube, A4771
Clubfoot wedge, L3380
CMMI Model, G0076-G0087, G2001-G2009, G2013-G2015
CMS Innovation Center Model
assessment, G9490
care managment, G0076-G0087
in-home visit, G2001-G2009, G2013-G2015
remote in-home visit, G9481-G9489, G9978-G9987
Cochlear implant, L8614
battery
alkaline, L8622
lithium, L8623-L8624
zinc, L8621
external recharging system, L8625
external sound processor, L8691
headset, L8615
microphone, L8616
replacement, L8619
transducer/actuator, replacement, L8625
transmitter cable, L8618
transmitting coil, L8617
zinc, L8621
Coil, imaging, C1770
Cold fluid bottle/wrap, A9273
Collagen
implant, urinary tract, L8603
microporous nonhuman origin, C9352-C9353
skin test, Q3031
wound dressing, A6021-A6024, Q4164
Collar
cervical
contour (low, standard), L0120
multiple post, L0180-L0200
nonadjustable foam, L0120
Philadelphia tracheotomy, L0172
Philly one-piece extraction, L0150
tracheotomy, L0172
traction, E0856
turtle neck safety, E0942
Coll-e-Derm, Q4193
Colonoscopy, G9659-G9661
cancer screening
patient at high risk, G0105
patient not at high risk, G0121
consultation, prescreening, S0285
Coloplast
closed pouch, A5051
drainable pouch, A5061
closed, A5054
small, A5063
skin barrier
4 x 4, A4362
6 x 6, A5121
8 x 8, A5122
stoma cap, A5055
Coma stimulation, S9056
Combo-Seat universal raised toilet seat, E0244
Commode, E0160-E0171
chair, E0163-E0165, E0170-E0171
lift, E0172, E0625
pail, E0167
seat, wheelchair, E0968
Communication board, E1902
Companion care, S5135-S5136
Composite
dressing, A6203-A6205
Comprehensive care management, G2064-G2065
Compressed gas system, E0424-E0480
Compression
bandage
high, A6452
light, A6448
Compression — *continued*
bandage — *continued*
medium, A6451
burn garment, A6501-A6512
burn mask, A6513
stockings, A6530-A6549
wrap, A6545
Compressogrip prosthetic shrinker, L8440-L8465
Compressor, E0565, E0570, E0650-E0652, E0670, K0738
Computer aided detection
breast MRI image, C8937
Concentrator
oxygen, E1390-E1392
rental, E1392
Condom
female, A4268
male, A4267
Conductive
garment (for TENS), E0731
paste or gel, A4558
Conductivity meter (for dialysis), E1550
Conference
interdisciplinary team, G0175
Conforming bandage, A6442-A6447
Congenital torticollis orthotic, L0112
Congo red, blood, P2029
Consultation
telehealth, G0406-G0408, G0425-G0427, G0508-G0509
Contact layer, A6206-A6208
Contact lens, S0500, S0512-S0514, V2500-V2599
Continent device, A5081, A5082
Continuous intraoperative neurophysiology monitoring, G0453
Continuous, monitor
blood glucose, S1030-S1031
receiver, K0554
supply allowance, 1 month, K0553
Continuous passive motion exercise device, E0936
Continuous positive airway pressure (CPAP) device, E0601
chin strap, A7036
face mask, A7030-A7031
filter, A7038-A7039
headgear, A7035
nasal application accessories, A7032-A7034
oral interface, A7044
tubing, A7037
Contraceptive
cervical cap, A4261
condom
female, A4268
male, A4267
diaphragm, A4266
etonogestrel, implant, J7307
foam, A4269
gel, A4269
hormone patch, J7304
implant, A4264, J7306-J7307
intratubal occlusion device, A4264
intrauterine
copper contraceptive, J7300
etonogestrel, J7307
levonorgestrel-releasing, J7296-J7298, S4981
other, S4989
Progestacert, S4989
Levonorgestrel, implants and supplies, J7296-J7298, J7301, J7306
pills, S4993
spermicide, A4269
vaginal ring, J7303
Contracts, maintenance, ESRD, A4890
Contrast material
high osmolar, Q9958-Q9964
injection during MRI, A9575-A9579, Q9953
low osmolar, Q9951, Q9965-Q9967
nonradioactive NOC, A9698
oral MRI, Q9954
Controlyte, enteral nutrition, B4155
Convulsive therapy, G2000
Coordinated care fee
home monitoring, G9006

Coordinated care fee — *continued*
initial rate, G9001
maintenance rate, G9002
physician oversight, G9008
risk adjusted, G9003-G9005
scheduled team conference, G9007
Copying fee, medical records, S9981-S9982
Corn, trim or remove, S0390
Corneal tissue processing, V2785
Coronary artery bypass surgery, direct
with coronary arterial and venous grafts
single, each, S2208
two arterial and single venous, S2209
with coronary arterial grafts, only
single, S2205
two grafts, S2206
with coronary venous grafts, only
single, S2207
Corset, spinal orthotic, L0970-L0976
Cough stimulation device, E0482
Counseling
alcohol, G0443
cardiovascular disease risk, G0446
end of life, S0257
genetic, S0265
lung cancer screening, G0296
obesity, G0447
group (2-10), G0473
prevention
sexually transmitted infection, G0445
Coupling gel/paste, A4559
Cover, shower
ventricular assist device, Q0501
Cover, wound
alginate dressing, A6196-A6198
foam dressing, A6209-A6214
hydrocolloid dressing, A6234-A6239
hydrogel dressing, A6242-A6248
specialty absorptive dressing, A6251-A6256
CPAP (continuous positive airway pressure) device, E0601
chin strap, A7036
exhalation port, A7045
face mask, A7030-A7031
headgear, A7035
humidifier, E0561-E0562
nasal application accessories, A7032-A7034
oral interface, A7044
supplies, E0470-E0472, E0561-E0562
tubing, A7037
Cradle, bed, E0280
Creation
arteriovenous fistula, C9754-C9755
Crisis intervention, H2011, S9484-S9485, T2034
Criticare HN, enteral nutrition, B4153
Crutch
substitute
lower leg platform, E0118
Crutches, E0110-E0116
accessories, A4635-A4637, E2207
aluminum, E0114
articulating, spring assisted, E0117
forearm, E0111
Ortho-Ease, E0111
underarm, other than wood, pair, E0114
Quikfit Custom Pack, E0114
Red Dot, E0114
underarm, wood, single, E0113
Ready-for-use, E0113
wooden, E0112
Cryoprecipitate, each unit, P9012
CTLSO, L0700, L0710, L1000-L1120
Cuirass, E0457
Culture sensitivity study, P7001
Culture, urine, bacterial, P7001
Curasorb, alginate dressing, A6196-A6199
Cushion
decubitus care, E0190
Oral/Nasal, A7029
positioning, E0190
wheelchair
AK addition, L5648
BK addition, L5646
Custom
DME, K0900
Custom — *continued*
wheelchair/base, K0008, K0013
Custom Masterhinge Hip Hinge 3, L2999
Customized item (in addition to code for basic item), S1002
Cyanocobalamin cobalt, A9546, A9559
Cycler
disposable set, A4671
Cycler dialysis machine, E1594
Cygnus, Q4170
Cylinder tank carrier, E2208
Cymetra, Q4112
Cystoscopy, blue light, C9738
Cystourethroscopy
for ureteral calculi, S2070
with insertion of transprostatic implant; 1 to 3 implants, C9739
with insertion of transprostatic implant; 4 or more implants, C9740
Cytal, Q4166
Cytopathology, screening, G0123, G0124, G0141, G0143-G0148

D

Day care services, S5100-S5102, S5105
Decompression
disc, S2348
hip core, S2325
lumbar
percutaneous image guided (pild), G0276
vertebral axial, S9090
Decubitus care equipment, E0181
cushion or pillow, E0190
mattress
AquaPedic Sectional Gel Flotation, E0196
Iris Pressure Reduction/Relief, dry, E0184
PressureGuard II, air, E0186
TenderFlo II, E0187
TenderGel II, E0196
pressure pads, overlays, E0197-E0199
Body Wrap, E0199
Geo-Matt, E0199
Iris, E0199
PressureKair, E0197
Richfoam Convoluted and Flat, E0199
pressure pads, with pumps, E0181
Bio Flote, E0181
KoalaKair, E0181
protectors
heel or elbow, E0191
Body Wrap Foam Positioners, E0191
Pre-Vent, E0191
pump, E0182
Bio Flote, E0182
Pillo, E0182
TenderCloud, E0182
Deionizer, water purification system, E1615
Delivery system
kidney, E1510
oxygen, topical, E0446
Delivery to high risk area requiring escort, S9381
Delivery/set-up/dispensing, A9901
Delta-Cast Elite Casting Material, A4590
Delta-Lite Conformable Casting Tape, A4590
Delta-Lite C-Splint Fiberglass Immobilizer, A4590
Delta-Lite "S" Fiberglass Casting Tape, A4590
Deluxe item, S1001
Demonstration project
clinic, extended stay, G9140
CMS Innovation Center Model, G0076-G0087, G2001-G2009, G2013-G2015, G9481-G9490, G9978-G9987
ESRD, G9013-G9014
Medicare Care Choice Model (MCCM), G9480
oncology, G9050-G9139, G9678
smoking, G9016
Dennis Browne, foot orthotic, L3140, L3150
Depression, G9212-G9213, G9232
Derata injection device, A4210
DermACELL, DermACELL AWM, DermACELL AWM Porous, Q4122
Derma-Gide, Q4203
Dermagraft, Q4106
DermaPure, Q4152
DermaSpan, Q4126
Dermavest, Q4153
Destruction
intraosseous basivertebral nerve, C9752-C9753
lesion, G0186
tumor, S2095
Detector, blood leak, dialysis, E1560
Device
auditory osseointegrated, L8691, L8695
continuous passive motion, E0936
drug matrix, C1734
electrical stimulation device for cancer treatment, E0766
endoscope colonoscope implantable, C1749
eversion/inversion, A9285
hygienic, any type, A9286
implantable/insertable, C1889-C1890
intermittent limb compression, E0676
joint, C1776
medication management, T1505
occlusive device placement, G0269
ocular, C1784
orthopedic, C1734
range of motion, E1841, L8701-L8702
reaching/grabbing, A9281
retrieval, C1773
speech generating, E2500
tissue localization and excision, C1819
urinary incontinence repair, C1771, C2631
ventricular assist device
supply, Q0477, Q0507-Q0509
Dextrostick, A4772
Diabetes
alcohol swabs, per box, A4245
battery for blood glucose monitor, A4233-A4236
bent needle set for insulin pump infusion, A4231
blood glucose monitor, E0607, S1030-S1031
receiver, K0554
supply allowance, 1 month, K0553
with integrated lancer, E2101
with voice synthesizer, E2100
blood glucose test strips, box of 50, A4253
drugs
Humalin, J1815, J1817
Humalog, J1817, S5551
insulin, J1815, J1817, S5551
Novolin, J1815, J1817
evaluation and management LOPS, G0245
injection device, needle-free, A4210
insulin pump, external, E0784, E0787
infusion set, A4231
supplies, maintenance, A4226
syringe with needle, A4232
lancet device, A4258
lancets, box of 100, A4259
MDPP, G9873-G9891
non-needle cannula for insulin infusion, A4232
retinal exam, S3000
self management training
group, G0109
individual, G0108
shoe
fitting, A5500
inlay, A5508
insert, A5512-A5514
modification, A5503-A5507
syringe, disposable
box of 100, S8490
each, A4206
urine glucose/ketone test strips, box of 100, A4250
Diabetic management program
dietitian visit, S9465
E/M of sensory neuropathy, G0246-G0247
Diabetic management program — *continued*
follow-up visit to MD provider, S9141
follow-up visit to non-MD provider, S9140
foot care, G0247
group session, S9455
insulin pump initiation, S9145
MDPP, G9873-G9891
nurse visit, S9460
Dialet lancet device, A4258
Dialysate
concentrate additives, A4765
peritoneal dialysis solution, A4720-A4726, A4766
solution, A4728
testing solution, A4760
Dialysis
access system, C1881
air bubble detector, E1530
anesthetic, A4736-A4737
bath conductivity, meter, E1550
blood leak detector, E1560
centrifuge, E1500
cleaning solution, A4674
concentrate
acetate, A4708
acid, A4709
bicarbonate, A4706-A4707
documentation, G9231
drain bag/bottle, A4911
emergency treatment, G0257
equipment, E1510-E1699
ESRD facility
acute kidney injury without ESRD, G0491-G0492
extension line, A4672-A4673
filter, A4680
fluid barrier, E1575
heating pad, E0210
hemostats, E1637
home equipment repair, A4890
infusion pump, E1520
mask, surgical, A4928
peritoneal
clamps, E1634
pressure alarm, E1540
scale, E1639
shunt accessory, A4740
supplies, A4671-A4918
surgical mask, A4928
syringe, A4657
tourniquet, A4929
unipuncture control system, E1580
Dialyzer, artificial kidney, A4690
Diaper service, T4538
Diaphragm, contraceptive, A4266
Diathermy, home use, K1004
Dietary education, S9449, S9452
Disarticulation
lower extremities, prosthesis, L5000-L5999
upper extremities, prosthesis, L6000-L6692
Discharge, patient, G9254-G9255
Disease management program, S0315, S0317, S0320
Disetronic
glass cartridge syringe for insulin pump, each, A4232
H-Tron insulin pump, E0784
insulin infusion set with bent needle, with or without wings, each, A4231
Disk decompression, lumbar, S2348
Diskard head halter, E0940
Diskectomy, lumbar, S2350, S2351
single interspace, S2350
Dispensing fee
BICROS, V5240
binaural, V5160
CROS, V5200
monaural hearing aid, V5241
new spectacle lenses, S0595
pharmacy
inhalation drugs, G0333, Q0513-Q0514
Disposable
diapers, A4335
glucose monitor, A9275

© 2019 Optum360, LLC

Disposable — *continued*
supplies, ambulance, A0382-A0398
underpads, A4554
DNA analysis, S3840
Dome
and mouthpiece (for nebulizer), A7016
Don-Joy
cervical support collar, L0150
deluxe knee immobilizer, L1830
wrist forearm splint, L3984
Donor cadaver
harvesting multivisceral organs, with allografts, S2055
Doppler, transesophageal, G9157
Dornix Plus, E0601
Dorsiwedge Night Splint, A4570, L2999, L4398
Dose optimization, for infusion, S3722
Dosimeter, implantable radiation, ea, A4650
Double bar
AK, knee-ankle-foot orthotic, L2020, L2030
BK, ankle-foot orthotic, L1990
Drainage
bag, A4357, A4358, A4911
board, postural, E0606
bottle, A4911, A5102
vacuum, A7048
Dressing — *see also* Bandage, A6021-A6404
absorptive, for use with suction pump, K0744-K0746
alginate, A6196-A6199
composite, A6203-A6205
contact layer, A6206-A6208
film, A6257-A6259
foam, A6209-A6215
gauze, A6216-A6230, A6402-A6404
holder/binder, A4461, A4463
hydrocolloid, A6234-A6241
hydrogel, A6242-A6248
resorbable, A6460-A6461
specialty absorptive, A6251-A6256
tape, A4450, A4452
transparent film, A6257-A6259
tubular, A6457
Dropper, A4649
Drug confirmation, G0480-G0483
Drug delivery implant
non-biodegradable
insertion, G0516
removal, G0517-G0518
Drug delivery system
controlled dose delivery system, K0730
disposable, A4306
Drug testing, G0480-G0483, G0659
Drugs — *see* Table of Drugs
administered through a metered dose inhaler, J3535
disposable delivery system, 5 ml or less per hour, A4306
disposable delivery system, 50 ml or greater per hour, A4305
infusion supplies, A4221, A4222, A4230-A4232
not otherwise classified, J3490, J7599, J7699, J7799, J8499, J8999, J9999
Part B drug CAP NOC, Q4082
Dry pressure pad/mattress, E0184, E0199
DSM IV criteria major depressive disorder, G9212-G9213
Dunlap
heating pad, E0210
Duolock curved tail closures, A4421
Durable medical equipment (DME), E0100-E8002
Durr-Fillauer
cervical collar, L0140
Pavlik harness, L1620

E

Ear wax removal, G0268
Easy Care
folding walker, E0143
quad cane, E0105
ECG
initial Medicare ECG, G0403-G0405
Echocardiogram
transesophageal, C8925-C8928
Echocardiogram — *continued*
transthoracic, C8921-C8924, C8929-C8930
Echosclerotherapy, S2202
Economy knee splint, L1830
Edetate
calcium disodium, J0600
edetate disodium, J3520
Education
asthma, S9441
birthing, S9436-S9439, S9442
chronic kidney disease, G0420-G0421
diabetes, S9145
exercise, S9451
family planning
individualized programs, school based, T1018
nonmedical, H1010
infant safety, S9447
lactation, S9443
Lamaze, S9436
mental health problems, G0177
parenting, S9444
smoking cessation, S9453
stress management, S9454
weight management, S9449
Eggcrate dry pressure pad/mattress, E0184, E0199
Elastic support, A6530-A6549
Elbow
brace, universal rehabilitation, L3720
disarticulation, endoskeletal, L6450
Masterhinge Elbow Brace 3, L3999
orthotic
EO, E1800, L3702-L3740, L3760-L3762
EWHO, L3764-L3766
protector, E0191
Electric hand
adult, L7007
independently articulating digits, L6880
pediatric, L7008
Electric heat pad for peritoneal dialysis, E0210
Electric hook, L7009
Electric stimulator supplies, A4595
Electrical stimulation, S8930
Electrical stimulation device for cancer treatment, E0766
Electrical work, dialysis equipment, A4870
Electrode
Electrodes, per pair, A4556
Electrode/transducer, A4555
Electrodes, per pair, A4556
Electromagnetic therapy, G0295, G0329
Electron beam computed tomography, S8092
Electrotherapy stimulation, cranial, K1002
Elevating leg rest, K0195
Elevator, air pressure, heel, E0370
Embolization, protection system, C1884
for tumor destruction, S2095
Embryo
cryopreserved transferred, S4037
monitor/store cryopreserved, S4040
storage, S4027
Emergency response system, S5160-S5162
EMG
biofeedback device, E0746
surface, S3900
Encounter, clinic, T1015
End of life care planning, S0257
Endarterectomy, chemical, M0300
Endoscope
colonoscope device (implantable), C1749
sheath, A4270
Endoscopy
nasal, C9745, S2342
Endoskeletal system, addition, L5925, L5984
Enema
bag, reusable, A4458
barium, G0106
cancer screening, G0120
manual pump system, A4459
Enrich, enteral nutrition, B4150
Ensure, enteral nutrition, B4150
HN, B4150
Plus, B4152
Plus HN, B4152
Ensure, enteral nutrition — *continued*
powder, B4150
Enteral
administration services, feeding, S9340-S9343
digestive enzyme(s), B4105
feeding supply kit (syringe) (pump) (gravity), B4034-B4036
fiber or additive, B4104
formulae, B4150-B4162
electrolytes, B4102, B4103
for metabolic disease, B4157
intact nutrients, B4149, B4150, B4152
pediatric, B4158-B4162
gastronomy tube, B4087-B4088
nutrition infusion pump, any type, B9002
supplies, not otherwise classified, B9998
Enterostomal therapy, S9474
Enzyme(s)
enteral feeding, B4105
Eosinophil count, S3630
EpiCord, Q4187
EpiFix (injectable), Q4145
EpiFix, Q4186
Equestrian/hippotherapy, S8940
ESRD End Stage Renal Disease — *see also* Dialysis
bundle demo/basic, G9013
expanded, G9014
documentation, G9231
ESRD facility
acute kidney injury without ESRD, G0491-G0492
machines and accessories, E1510-E1699
plumbing, A4870
supplies, A4651-A4913
Evaluation
comprehensive, multi-discipline, H2000
for power mobility device, G0372
ocularist, S9150
remote, images/video, G2010
risk factors, G9298-G9299
self assessment, depression, S3005
team for handicapped, T1024
Evaluation device, remote
cardiovascular, G2066
Eversion device, A9285
Exactech lancet device, A4258
Examination
breast, S0613
breast and pelvic, G0101
diabetic for LOPS, G0245-G0246
for college, S0622
initial Medicare, G0402
related to surgical procedure, S0260
Excellagen, Q4149
Excision, tissue localization, C1819
Exercise
class, S9451
continuous passive motion device, E0936
equipment, A9300
Exo-Static overdoor traction unit, E0860
External
ambulatory infusion pump, E0781, E0784
counterpulsation, G0166
power, battery components, L7360-L7499
power, elbow, L7191
External defibrillator
battery replacement, K0607
electrode replacement, K0609
garment replacement, K0608
Extracorporeal shock wave lithotripsy, S0400
Extremity belt/harness, E0945
Eye
lens (contact) (spectacle), S0500-S0514, V2100-V2615
pad, A6410-A6411
patch, A6410-A6412
prosthetic, C1839, V2623-V2629
service (miscellaneous), V2700-V2799
E-Z Lite wheelchair, E1250
EZ-Derm, Q4136
E-ZJect disposable insulin syringes, up to 1 cc, per syringe, A4206
E-ZJect Lite Angle lancets, box of 100, A4259
E-Z-lets lancet device, A4258

F

Face tent, oxygen, A4619
Family stabilization, S9482
FDG, A9552
Fecal microbiota, preparation/instillation, G0455
Fee, coordinated care
coordinated care, G9001
Fern test, Q0114
Fertility services
donor service (sperm or embryo), S4025
in vitro fertilization, S4013-S4022
ovulation induction, S4042
sperm procurement, S4026, S4030-S4031
Fertilization
in vitro, S4011
Fetal surgery, repair teratoma, S2405
Fetoscopic laser therapy, S2411
Filler
bone, C9359
wound
alginate, A6199
foam, A6215
hydrocolloid, A6240-A6241
hydrogel, A6248
not elsewhere classified, A6261-A6262
Film
dressing, A6257-A6259
Filter
aerosol compressor, A7013
carbon, A4680
CPAP device, A7038-A7039
dialysis carbon, A4680
ostomy, A4368
tracheostoma, A4481
ultrasonic generator, A7013
vena cava, C1880
ventricular assist device, Q0500
Finasteride, S0138
Finger
orthotic (FO), L3933-L3935
splint
baseball, A4570
fold-over, A4570
four-pronged, A4570
static, Q4049
Fisher&Paykel HC220, E0601
Fistula
arteriovenous, C9754-C9755
cannulation set, A4730
Fitness club membership, S9970
Flashcast Elite casting material, A4590
Flex HD, Q4128
Flow rate meter, peak, A4614
FlowerAmnioFlo, Q4177
FlowerAmnioPatch, Q4148
FlowerDerm, Q4179
Flowmeter, E0440, E0555, E0580
Fluid barrier, dialysis, E1575
Fluid Flow, Fluid GF, Q4206
Fluorescent imaging
blue light cystoscopy, C9738
Fluorine-18 fluorodeoxyglucose
contrast material, A9552
imaging using dual-head coincidence detection system, S8085
Flutamide, S0175
Flutter device, S8185
Foam
dressing, A6209-A6215
pad adhesive, A5126
Folding walker, E0135, E0143
Fold-over finger splint, A4570
Foley catheter, A4312-A4316, A4338-A4346
Follitropin
beta, S0128
Food supplement, S9434
Food thickener, B4100
Foot care, routine, G0247, S0390
Foot, cast boot
Specialist Closed-Back Cast Boot, L3260
Specialist Gaitkeeper Boot, L3260
Specialist Open-Back Cast Boot, L3260

© 2019 Optum360, LLC

Foot, cast boot — *continued*
Specialist Toe Insert for Specialist Closed-Back Cast Boot and Specialist Health/Post Operative Shoe, A9270
Foot exam, G9225-G9226
Foot impression casting, S0395
Foot insert, L2180, L3000-L3003, L3031, L5000
Foot, insoles/heel cups
Specialist Heel Cups, L3485
Specialist Insoles, L3510
Foot, soles
Masterfoot Walking Cast Sole, L3649
Solo Cast Sole, L3540
Footdrop splint, L4398
Footplate, E0175, E0970
Footwear, orthopedic, L3201-L3265
Forearm crutches, E0110, E0111
Fortex, alginate dressing, A6196-A6199
Foster care, H0041-H0042, S5140-S5146
Four Poster, fracture frame, E0946
Four-pronged finger splint, A4570
Fracture
bedpan, E0276
frame, E0920, E0930, E0946-E0948
orthotic, L2106-L2136
orthotic additions, L3995
pelvic bone, G0412-G0415
specialist pre-formed humeral fracture brace, L3980-L3981
Frame
meaning spectacles, V2020, V2025
sales tax, S9999
safety, for hospital bed, E0316
sit-to-stand, E0637
standing system, E0638, E0641-E0642
FreAmine HBC, parenteral nutrition, B5200
Frejka, hip orthotic, L1600
replacement cover, L1610
Functional outcome assessment, G9227

G

Gait trainer
pediatric
anterior, E8002
posterior, E8000
upright, E8001
GammaGraft, Q4111
Ganirelix acetate, S0132
Garment breast prosthesis, L8015
Garment covering, A4467
Gas system
compressed, E0424, E0425
gaseous, E0430, E0431, E0441, E0443
liquid, E0434-E0440, E0442, E0444
Gasket, prosthetic socket insert, L7700
Gastric
band adjustment, S2083
Gastric suction pump, E2000
Gastrostomy tube, B4087-B4088
Gauze, A6216-A6230, A6266
impregnated, A6222-A6230, A6266
nonimpregnated, A6216, A6221, A6402
pads, A6216-A6230, A6402-A6404
Johnson&Johnson, A6402
Kendall, A6402
Moore, A6402
Gel
conductive, A4558
coupling for ultrasound, A4559
pressure pad, E0185, E0196
sheet, dermal or epidermal, A6025
Generator
cardiac, C1824
neurostimulator
nonrechargeable, C1767, C1823
with rechargeable battery/charging sys
high frequency, C1822
nonhigh frequency, C1820
Genesis Amniotic Membrane, Q4198
Genetic
counseling, S0265
testing, S3800, S3840-S3842, S3844-S3846, S3849-S3850, S3852-S3854, S3861-S3870
Genetic — *continued*
testing — *continued*
hypertrophic cardiomyopathy, S3865, S3866
Genmould Creamy Plaster, A4580
Geo-Matt
therapeutic overlay, E0199
Geronimo PR, power wheelchair, K0011
Gerval Protein, enteral nutrition, B4155
Gestational home visit
for diabetes, S9214
for hypertension, S9211
for preeclampsia, S9213
GIFT, S4013
Glasses
air conduction, V5070
binaural, V5120-V5150
bone conduction, V5080
frames, V2020, V2025
hearing aid, V5150, V5190, V5230
lens, V2100-V2499, V2610, V2718, V2730, V2755, V2770, V2780
Glaucoma screening, G0117-G0118
Global fee, urgent care center, S9083
Gloves
dialysis, A4927
non-sterile, A4927
sterile, A4930
Glucometer
3 blood glucose meter, E0607
3 blood glucose test strips, box of 50, A4253
II blood glucose meter, E0607
II blood glucose test strips, box of 50, A4253
Glucose
monitor device, continuous, noninvasive, S1030-S1031
receiver, K0554
supply allowance, 1 month, K0553
receiver, A9278, K0554
sensor, A9276
test strips, A4253, A4772
transmitter, A9277
Gluteal pad, L2650
Gold
sodium thiomalate, J1600
Gomco
aspirators, E0600
Grab bar, trapeze, E0910, E0940
Grade-aid, wheelchair, E0974
Gradient pressure aids, S8420-S8429
Grafix Core, GrafixPL Core, Q4132
Grafix Prime, GrafixPL Prime, Q4133
Graft
vascular, C1768
GRAFTJACKET, Q4107
GRAFTJACKET XPRESS, Q4113
Gravity traction device, E0941
Gravlee jet washer, A4470
Greissing, foot prosthesis, L5978
Guardian, Q4151
Guidance
Stereoscopic, radiation therapy delivery, G6002
Ultrasonic, radiation therapy fields, G6001
Guide wire, C1769
Guilford multiple-post collar, cervical orthotic, L0190

H

Haberman Feeder, S8265
Habilitation, T2012-T2021
Hair analysis (excluding arsenic), P2031
Hallus-valgus dynamic splint, L3100
Hallux prosthetic implant, L8642
Halo procedures, L0810-L0859, L0861
Halter, cervical head, E0942
Hand
electric, L6880, L7007-L7008
mechanical, L6708-L6709
orthotic (WHFO), E1805, E1825, L3808, L3900-L3923
partial prosthesis, L6000-L6020
restoration, L6900-L6915
rims, wheelchair, E0967
Handgrip (cane, crutch, walker), A4636
Harness, E0942, E0944, E0945
Harvest
multivisceral organs, cadaver donor, S2055
peripheral stem cell, S2150
Harvey arm abduction orthotic, L3960
Health club membership, S9970
Hearing devices, L8614, V5030-V5299
accessories/supplies, V5267
analog, V5242-V5251
assistive listening device, V5268-V5274, V5281-V5290
battery, V5266
BICROS, V5211-V5215, V5221, V5230
binaural, V5120-V5150, V5211-V5215, V5221, V5248-V5249
body worn, V5030, V5040, V5100
CROS, V5171-V5172, V5181, V5190
digital, V5250-V5261
dispensing fee, V5241
BICROS, V5240
bilateral, V5110
binaural, V5160
CROS, V5200
monaural, V5241
unspecified, V5090
disposable, V5262-V5263
ear impression, V5275
ear mold/insert, V5264-V5265
glasses, V5070-V5080, V5190-V5230
middle ear prosthesis, V5095
monaural, V5030-V5060, V5171-V5172
programmable
binaural, V5250-V5253
monaural, V5244-V5247
Heat
application, E0200-E0239
lamp, E0200, E0205
pad, E0210, E0215, E0217, E0249
units, E0239
Hydrocollator, mobile, E0239
Thermalator T-12-M, E0239
Heater (nebulizer), E1372
Heating pad, Dunlap, E0210
for peritoneal dialysis, E0210
Heel
elevator, air, E0370
loop/holder, E0951
pad, L3480, L3485
protector, E0191
shoe, L3430-L3485
stabilizer, L3170
Helicoll, Q4164
Helicopter, ambulance — *see also* Ambulance, A0431
Helmet
cervical, A8000-A8004
custom, A8002-A8003
hard, A8001, A8003
interface replacement, A8004
prefabricated, A8000-A8001
soft, A8000, A8002
Hemalet lancet device, A4258
Hematopoietic hormone administration, S9537
Hemilaminectomy, C9757
Hemipelvectomy prosthesis, L5280
Hemi-wheelchair, E1083-E1086
Hemodialysis
acetate concentrate, A4708
acid solution, A4709
bicarbonate concentrate, A4706-A4707
catheter, C1750, C1752
drain bag/bottle, A4911
machine, E1590
maintenance, G9264-G9266
mask, surgical, A4928
protamine sulfate, A4802
surgical mask, A4928
tourniquet, A4929
vascular access not catheter, G9241
vascular access per catheter, G9239-G9240
Hemodialyzer, portable, E1635
Hemostats, for dialysis, E1637
Hemostix, A4773
Heparin
infusion pump (for dialysis), E1520
HepatAmine, parenteral nutrition, B5100
Hepatic-aid, enteral nutrition, B4154
Hepatitis B screening
non-pregnant, high-risk individual, G0499
Hexalite, A4590
Hexior power wheelchair, K0014
High frequency
chest wall oscillation equipment, A7025-A7026, E0483
neurostimulator generator with battery and charging system, C1822
High osmolar contrast
150-199 mg iodine, Q9959
200-249 mg iodine, Q9960
250-299 mg iodine, Q9961
300-349 mg iodine, Q9962
350-399 mg iodine, Q9963
400 or greater mg iodine, Q9964
up to 149 mg iodine, Q9958
Hip
Custom Masterhinge Hip Hinge 3, L2999
disarticulation prosthesis, L5250, L5270
Masterhinge Hip Hinge 3, L2999
orthotic (HO), L1600-L1686
Hip-knee-ankle-foot orthotic (HKAFO), L2040-L2090
History and physical
related to surgical procedure, S0260
HIV-1 antibody testing, S3645
HIV-1 or HIV-2 screening, G0432-G0435
HKAFO, L2040-L2090
hMatrix, Q4134
Holder
heel, E0951
surgical dressing, A4461, A4463
toe, E0952
Hole cutter tool, A4421
Hollister
belt adapter, A4421
closed pouch, A5051, A5052
colostomy/ileostomy kit, A5061
drainable pouches, A5061
with flange, A5063
medical adhesive, A4364
pediatric ostomy belt, A4367
remover, adhesive, A4455
skin barrier, A4362, A5122
skin cleanser, A4335
skin conditioning cream, A4335
skin gel protective dressing wipes, A5120
stoma cap, A5055
two-piece pediatric ostomy system, A5054, A5063, A5073
urostomy pouch, A5071, A5072
Home
delivered meals, S5170
modifications, S5165
ventilator, any type
invasive interface, E0465
multifunction, E0467
non-invasive interface, E0466
Home health
aerosolized drug therapy, S9061
aide, S9122, T1030-T1031
home health setting, G0156
bundled payment, G9187
care
attendant care, S5125-S5126
certified nurse assistant, S9122, T1021
home health aide, S9122, T1021
home health care, Q5001-Q5002, Q5009
management
episodic, S0272
hospice, S0271
standard, S0270
nursing care, G0299-G0300, S9122-S9124, T1030-T1031
outside capitation arrangement, S0273-S0274
re-certification, G0179-G0180
training, S5108-S5116

© 2019 Optum360, LLC

Home health — *continued*
contracted services, T1022
gestational
assessment, T1028
delivery supplies, S8415
diabetes, S9214
hypertension, S9211
pre-eclampsia, S9213
preterm labor, S9208-S9209
hydration therapy, S9373-S9379
infusion therapy, S5035-S5036, S9325-S9379, S9494-S9497, S9537-S9810
catheter care, S5497-S5498, S5517-S5518
corticosteroid infusion, S9490
insertion midline venous catheter, S5523
insertion PICC line, S5520, S5522
supplies, S5517-S5521
nursing services, G0162, G0490, G0493-G0496, S0274, S9212-S9213
physician services, S0270-S0273
postpartum hypertension, S9212
respiratory therapy, S5180-S5181
services of
clinical social worker, G0155
occupational therapist, G0152
physical therapist, G0151
skilled nurse, G0299-G0300
speech/language pathologist, G0153
speech/language pathologist, G0153, G0161
therapy, G0151-G0152, G0157-G0160
transfusion, blood products, S9538
venipuncture, S9529
wound care, S9097
Home uterine monitor, S9001
Hook
electric, L7009
mechanical, L6706-L6707
Hospice
care, Q5001-Q5010, S9126, T2042-T2046
care coordinator, G9477
chaplain, G9473
dietary counselor, G9474
evaluation and counseling services, G0337
nursing services, G0162, G0299-G0300, G0493-G0496
other counselor, G9475
other qualified pharmacist, G9479
other qualified therapist, G9478
referral visit, S0255
speech/language pathologist, G0153
therapy, G0151-G0152, G0157-G0158
volunteer, G9476
Hospital
observation
direct admit, G0379
per hour, G0378
outpatient clinic visit, G0463
readmission, G9309-G9310
Hospitalist services, S0310
Hot fluid bottle/wrap, A9273
Houdini security suit, E0700
Housing, supported, H0043-H0044
Hoyer patient lifts, E0621, E0625, E0630
H-Tron insulin pump, E0784
H-Tron Plus insulin pump, E0784
Hudson
adult multi-vent venturi style mask, A4620
nasal cannula, A4615
oxygen supply tubing, A4616
UC-BL type shoe insert, L3000
Human amniotic tissue allograft, Q4163
Human placental tissue matrix, Q4162
Humidifier, E0550-E0560
water chamber, A7046
Hyalomatrix, Q4117
Hydration therapy, S9373-S9379
Hydraulic patient lift, E0630
Hydrocollator, E0225, E0239
Hydrocolloid dressing, A6234-A6241
Hydrocortisone
acetate, J1700
sodium phosphate, J1710
sodium succinate, J1720
Hydrocortone
acetate, J1700
phosphate, J1710
Hydrogel dressing, A6242-A6248
Hydroxyurea, S0176
Hygienic device/item, A9286
Hyperbaric oxygen chamber
full body, G0277
topical, A4575
Hypo-Let lancet device, A4258
Hypothermia
intragastric, M0100

I

Ice cap/collar, A9273
Ilfeld, hip orthotic, L1650
Imaging, C1770
coil, MRI, C1770
Implant
access system, A4301
aqueous shunt, L8612
auditory device
brainstem, S2235
middle ear, S2230
breast, L8600
cochlear, L8614, L8627-L8628
collagen
meniscus, knee, G0428
urinary, L8603
contraceptive, A4264, J7306
device, C1734
dextranomer/hyaluronic acid copolymer, urinary tract, L8604, L8605
drug delivery, G0516-G0518
drug matrix, C1734
endoscope colonoscope device, C1749
ganciclovir, J7310
goserelin acetate, J9202
hallux, L8642
infusion pump, E0782-E0783
injectable bulking agent
anal, L8605
urinary tract, L8606
vocal cord, L8607
interatrial shunt/placebo control, C9758
interspinous process distraction device, C1821
joint, L8630
lacrimal duct, A4262-A4263
levonorgestrel, J7306
metacarpophalangeal joint, L8630
metatarsal joint, L8641
Mometasone sinus, J7401
nasal
vestibular lateral wall, C9749
neurostimulator
nonrechargeable, C1767, C1823
with rechargeable battery/charging sys
high frequency, C1822
nonhigh frequency, C1820
Norplant, J7306
not otherwise specified, L8699
ocular, L8610
drainage assist device, C1783
orthopedic, C1734
ossicular, L8613
osteogenesis stimulator, E0749
percutaneous access system, A4301
porcine, C9364
prosthetic device, C9899, G9303-G9304
sinus, J7401
urinary tract, L8603-L8604
vascular access portal, A4300
vascular graft, L8670
yttrium 90, S2095
Zoladex, J9202
Implantable radiation dosimeter, ea, A4650
Impregnated gauze dressing, A6222-A6230
In vitro fertilization, S4011
Incontinence
appliances and supplies, A4310, A4336, A5051-A5093, A5102-A5114, A5120-A5200
brief or diaper, T4521-T4528, T4543-T4544
disposable/liner, T4535
Incontinence — *continued*
garment, A4520
pediatric
brief or diaper, T4529-T4530
pull-on protection, T4531-T4532
penile wrap, T4545
rectal insert, A4337
reusable
diaper or brief, T4539
pull-on protection, T4536
underpad, A4553
underpad
disposable, T4541, T4542
reusable, A4553, T4537, T4540
youth
brief or diaper, T4533
pull-on protection, T4534
Indium 111
capromab pendetide, A9507
ibritumomab tiuxetan, A9542
labeled
platelets, A9571
white blood cells, A9570
oxyguinoline, A9547
pentetate, A9548, A9572
pentetreotide, A9572
satumomab pendetide, A4642
Infant safety, CPR, training, S9447
Infection, G9311-G9312
Infusion
catheter, C1751
dose optimization, for infusion, S3722
IV, OPPS, C8957
pump, C1772, C2626
ambulatory, with administrative equipment, E0781
epoprostenol, K0455
heparin, dialysis, E1520
implantable, E0782, E0783
implantable, refill kit, A4220
insulin, E0784
mechanical, reusable, E0779, E0780
nonprogrammable, C1891
supplies, A4221, A4222, A4226, A4230-A4232
Versa-Pole IV, E0776
Sipuleucel-T autologous CD54+, Q2043
supplies, A4222, A4223
syringe cartridge, non-insulin pump, K0552
therapy, home, S9347, S9351, S9497-S9504
Inhalation drugs
acetylcysteine, J7608
albuterol, J7609, J7610, J7611
Alupent, J7668-J7669
atropine, J7635-J7636
Atrovent, J7644
Azmacort, J7684
beclomethasone, J7622
betamethasone, J7624
bitolterol mesylate, J7628-J7629
Brcanyl, J7680-J7681
Brethine, J7680-J7681
budesonide, J7626-J7627, J7633-J7634
colistimethate sodium, S0142
cromolyn sodium, J7631
dexamethasone, J7637-J7638
dornase alpha, J7639
flunisolide, J7641
formoterol, J7606, J7640
Gastrocrom, J7631
glycopyrrolate, J7642-J7643
iloprost, Q4074
Intal, J7631
ipratropium bromide, J7644-J7645
isoetharine HCl, J7647-J7650
isoproterenol HCl, J7657-J7660
levalbuterol, J7607, J7614, J7615
metaproterenol sulfate, J7667-J7670
methacholine chloride, J7674
Mucomyst, J7608
Mucosil, J7608
Nasalcrom, J7631
NOC, J7699
pentamidine isethionate, J7676
Pulmicort Respules, J7627
Inhalation drugs — *continued*
terbutaline sulfate, J7680-J7681
Tobi, J7682
tobramycin, J7682, J7685
Tornalate, J7628-J7629
triamcinolone, J7683-J7684
Initial
ECG, Medicare, G0403-G0405
physical exam, Medicare, G0402
Injectable
bulking agent
urinary tract, L8603-L8606
vocal cord, L8607
Injection — *see also* Table of Drugs
adjustment, bariatric band, S2083
bulking agent
urinary tract, L8603-L8606
vocal cord, L8607
contrast material, during MRI, A9576-A9579, Q9953
dermal filler for LDS, G0429
sacroiliac joint, G0259-G0260
supplies for self-administered, A4211, A4224-A4225
Inpatient telehealth pharmacologic management, G0459
Insert
convex, for ostomy, A5093
diabetic, for shoe, A5512-A5514
foot insert/plate, L3031
implant
prosthetic socket, gasket or seal, L7700
soft palate, C9727
Insertion
cardioverter-defibrillator system, G0448
intrauterine system, S4981
tray, A4310-A4316
Instillation fecal microbiota, G0455
Integra
Bilayer Matrix Wound Dressing, Q4104
Dermal Regeneration Template, Q4105
Flowable, Q4114
Matrix, Q4108
Meshed Bilayer Wound Matrix, C9363
MOZAIK Osteoconductive Scaffold Putty, C9359
MOZAIK Osteoconductive Scaffold Strip, C9362
IntegoPLY, Q4126
Interface
cough stimulating device, A7020
oral with suction pump, A7047
Interfyl, Q4171
Intermittent
limb compression device, E0676
peritoneal dialysis system, E1592
positive pressure breathing (IPPB) machine, E0500
Interphalangeal joint, prosthetic implant, L8658
Interrogation, remote evaluation
cardiovascular, G2066
Interscapular thoracic prosthesis
endoskeletal, L6570
upper limb, L6350-L6370
Interspinous process distraction device, C1821
Intervention
alcohol and/or drug, H0050
leak of endoluminal contents, G9305-G9306
Intrafallopian transfer
complete cycle, gamete, S4013
complete cycle, zygote, S4014
donor egg cycle, S4023
incomplete cycle, S4017
Intraocular lenses, C1780, C1840, Q1004-Q1005, S0596, V2630-V2632
new technology
category 4, Q1004
category 5, Q1005
presbyopia correcting function, V2788
refractive correcting, S0596
telescopic, C1840

© 2019 Optum360, LLC

Intraoperative
near-infrared fluorescence lymphatic mapping, C9756
Intraosseous basivertebral nerve destruction, C9752-C9753
Intratubal occlusion device, A4264
Intrauterine device
copper contraceptive, J7300
etonogestrel, J7307
levonorgestrel-releasing, J7296-J7298, S4981
other, S4989
Progestacert, S4989
Introducer sheath
guiding, C1766, C1892, C1893
other than guiding, C1894, C2629
Inversion device, A9285
Iodine 125, A9527, A9532, C2638-C2639
Iodine I-131
albumin, A9524
iobenguane sulfate, A9508
sodium iodide, A9517
Iodine swabs/wipes, A4247
IPD
system, E1592
IPPB machine, E0500
delivery device, A9274, E0784, S5560-S5561, S5565-S5571
home infusion administration, S9353
intermediate acting, S5552
long acting, S5553
NPH, J1815, S5552
outpatient IV treatment, G9147
rapid onset, S5550-S5551
Ipratropium bromide
administered through DME, J7644-J7645
Iris Preventix pressure relief/reduction mattress, E0184
Iris prosthesis, C1839
Iris therapeutic overlays, E0199
IRM ankle-foot orthotic, L1950
Iron
sucrose, J1756
Irrigation supplies, A4320, A4322, A4355, A4397-A4400
Surfit
irrigation sleeve, A4397
night drainage container set, A5102
Visi-flow irrigator, A4398, A4399
Irrigation/evacuation system, bowel
control unit, E0350
disposable supplies for, E0352
Islet cell transplant
laparoscopy, G0342
laparotomy, G0343
percutaneous, G0341
Isocal, enteral nutrition, B4150
HCN, B4152
Isoetharine
inhalation solution
concentrated, J7647
unit dose, J7649-J7650
Isolates, B4150, B4152
Isoproterenol HCl
administered through DME, J7657-J7660
Isosulfan blue, Q9968
Isotein, enteral nutrition, B4153
IV, G0459
administration set, non-PVC, S1016
infusion, OPPS, C8957
pole, E0776, K0105
solution
10% LMD, J7100
5% dextrose/normal saline, J7042
D-5-W, J7070
dextran, J7100, J7110
Gentran, J7100, J7110
normal saline, A4217, J7030-J7040, J7050
Rheomacrodex, J7100
Ringer's lactate, J7120
tubing extension set, S1015

J

Jace tribrace, L1832
Jacket
scoliosis, L1300, L1310
J-cell battery, replacement for blood glucose monitor, A4234
Jejunostomy tube, B4087-B4088
Joint device, C1776
transcutaneous electrical stimulation, E0762

K

Kaltostat, alginate dressing, A6196-A6199
Kartop Patient Lift, toilet or bathroom (*see also* Lift), E0625
Keramatrix, Kerasorb, Q4165
Keratectomy photorefractive, S0810
Keratoprosthesis, C1818
Kerecis Omega3, Q4158
Keroxx, Q4202
Keto-Diastix, box of 100 glucose/ketone urine test strips, A4250
Key-Pred
-25,-50, J2650
Kidney
ESRD supply, A4651-A4913
system, E1510
wearable artificial, E1632
Kingsley gloves, above hands, L6890
Kits
asthma, S8097
enteral feeding supply (syringe) (pump) (gravity), B4034-B4036
fistula cannulation (set), A4730
parenteral nutrition, B4220-B4224
surgical dressing (tray), A4550
tracheostomy, A4625
Knee
Adjustabrace 3, L2999
disarticulation, prosthesis, L5150-L5160, L5312
extension/flexion device, E1812
immobilizer, L1830
joint, miniature, L5826
Knee-O-Prene Hinged Wraparound Knee Support, L1810
locks, L2405-L2425
Masterbrace 3, L2999
Masterhinge Adjustabrace 3, L2999
orthotic (KO), E1810, L1810, L1820, L1830-L1860, L1851-L1852
Knee Support, L2000-L2038, L2126-L2136
Knee-O-Prene Hinged Knee Sleeve, L1810
Knee-O-Prene Hinged Wraparound Knee Support, L1810
KnitRite
prosthetic
sheath, L8400-L8415
sock, L8420-L8435
stump sock, L8470-L8485
K-Y Lubricating Jelly, A4332, A4402
Kyphosis pad, L1020, L1025

L

Labor care (not resulting in delivery), S4005
Laboratory tests
chemistry, P2028-P2038
miscellaneous, Q0111-Q0115
Lacrimal duct implant
permanent, A4263
temporary, A4262
Laminotomy, C9757
Lancet, A4258, A4259
Laparoscopy, surgical
esophagomyotomy, S2079
Laryngectomy
tube, A7520-A7522
Larynx, artificial, L8500
Laser
application, S8948
assisted uvulopalatoplasty (LAUP), S2080
in situ keratomileusis, S0800
myringotomy, S2225
Laser skin piercing device, for blood collection, E0620
replacement lens, A4257
LAUP, S2080
Lead
adaptor
neurostimulator, C1883
pacing, C1883
cardioverter, defibrillator, C1777, C1895, C1896
environmental, home evaluation, T1029
neurostimulator, C1778
neurostimulator/test kit, C1897
pacemaker, C1779, C1898, C1899
ventricular, C1900
Leg
bag, A4358, A5112
extensions for walker, E0158
Nextep Contour Lower Leg Walker, L2999
Nextep Low Silhouette Lower Leg Walkers, L2999
rest, elevating, K0195
rest, wheelchair, E0990
strap, A5113, A5114, K0038, K0039
Legg Perthes orthotic, A4565, L1700-L1755
Lens
aniseikonic, V2118, V2318
contact, V2500-V2599
deluxe feature, V2702
eye, S0504-S0508, S0580-S0590, S0596, V2100-V2615, V2700-V2799
intraocular, C1780, C1840, V2630-V2632
low vision, V2600-V2615
mirror coating, V2761
occupational multifocal, V2786
polarization, V2762
polycarbonate, V2784
progressive, V2781
skin piercing device, replacement, A4257
telescopic, C1840
tint, V2744
addition, V2745
Lenticular lens
bifocal, V2221
single vision, V2121
trifocal, V2321
Lerman Minerva spinal orthotic, L0174
Lesion
destruction, G0186
Leukocyte
poor blood, each unit, P9016
Levine, stomach tube, B4087-B4088
Levonorgestrel, contraceptive implants and supplies, J7296-J7298, J7301, J7306
Lice infestation treatment, A9180
Lifescan lancets, box of 100, A4259
Lifestand manual wheelchair, K0009
Lifestyle modification program, coronary heart disease, S0340-S0342
Lift
combination, E0637
patient, and seat, E0621-E0635
Hoyer
Home Care, E0621
Partner All-Purpose, hydraulic, E0630
Partner Power Multifunction, E0625
separate seat mechanism, any type, E0627, E0629
shoe, L3300-L3334
standing frame system, E0638
Lift-Aid patient lifts, E0621
Light box, E0203
Lispro insulin, S5551
Lithium battery for blood glucose monitor, A4233-A4236
Lithotripsy, gallstones, S9034
Little Ones
drainable pouch, A5063
mini-pouch, A5054
one-piece custom drainable pouch, A5061
one-piece custom urostomy pouch, A5071
pediatric belt, A4367
pediatric urine collector, A4335
urostomy pouch, transparent, A5073
Lively, knee-ankle-foot orthotic, L2038
Lobectomy, lung, donor, S2061
Lodging
NOS, S9976
Lodging — *continued*
recipient, escort nonemergency transport, A0180, A0200
transplant-related, S9975
Lomustine, S0178
Lonalac powder, enteral nutrition, B4150
Low cost, application of skin substitute, C5271-C5278
Low osmolar contrast
100-199 mgs iodine, Q9965
200-299 mgs iodine, Q9966
300-399 mgs iodine, Q9967
400 or greater mgs iodine, Q9951
Lower limb, prosthesis, addition, L5968
LPN services, T1003
Lubricant, A4332, A4402
Lumbar
orthotic, L0625-L0627
pad, L1030, L1040
sacral orthotic (LSO), L0628-L0640
Lung biopsy plug, C2613
Lung volume reduction surgery services, G0302-G0305
LVRS services, G0302-G0305
Lymphatic
mapping, intraoperative, near-infrared fluorescence, C9756
Lymphedema therapy, S8950

M

Madamist II medication compressor/nebulizer, E0570
Magnacal, enteral nutrition, B4152
Magnetic
resonance angiography, C8900, C8901-C8914, C8918-C8920, C8931-C8936
resonance cholangiopancreatography, S8037
resonance imaging, low field, S8042
source imaging, S8035
Maintenance contract, ESRD, A4890
Male erection system, L7900
Malibu cervical turtleneck safety collar, L0150
Management
advanced illness, S0311
disease, S0316-S0317
Mapping
topographic brain, S8040
Marker
tissue, A4648
Mask
burn compression, A6513
CPAP, A7027
oxygen, A4620
surgical, for dialysis, A4928
Mastectomy
bra, L8002
camisole, S8460
form, L8020
prosthesis, L8000-L8039, L8600
sleeve, L8010
Masterbrace 3, L2999
Masterfoot Walking Cast Sole, L3649
Masterhinge Adjustabrace 3, L2999
Masterhinge Elbow Brace 3, L3999
Masterhinge Hip Hinge 3, L2999
Masterhinge Shoulder Brace 3, L3999
Masters 2 step, S3904
Matrion, Q4201
MatriStem, Q4118
Matrix HD, Q4128
Mattress
air pressure, E0186, E0197
alternating pressure, E0277
pad, Bio Flote, E0181
pad, KoalaKair, E0181
AquaPedic Sectional, E0196
decubitus care, E0196
dry pressure, E0184
flotation, E0184
gel pressure, E0196
hospital bed, E0271, E0272
non-powered, pressure reducing, E0373
Iris Preventix pressure relief/reduction, E0184

© 2019 Optum360, LLC

Mattress — *continued*
Overlay, E0371-E0372
pressure reducing, E0181
TenderFlor II, E0187
TenderGel II, E0196
water pressure, E0187, E0198
powered, pressure reducing, E0277
MCCM, G9480
MCP, multi-axial rotation unit, L5986
MCT Oil, enteral nutrition, B4155
MDPP, G9873-G9891
Meals
adults in treatment, T1010
per diem NOS, S9977
Mechanical
hand, L6708-L6709
hook, L6706-L6707
wound suction, A9272
Medialization material for vocal cord, C1878
Medical and surgical supplies, A4206-A6404
Medical conference, S0220-S0221
Medical food, S9435
Medical home program, S0280-S0281
Medical records copying fee, S9981-S9982
Medical visit, G0463, G9246-G9247
Medicare Care Choice Model (MCCM), G9480
Medicare Diabetes Prevention Program (MDPP), G9873-G9891
Medicare "welcome"
ECG, G0403-G0405
physical, G0402
Medication management device, T1505
Medication services
comprehensive, H2010
reminder, S5185
Medi-Jector injection device, A4210
MediSense 2 Pen blood glucose monitor, E0607
Mediskin, Q4135
Medralone
40, J1030
80, J1040
Membrane Graft, Membrane Wrap, Q4205
MemoDerm, Q4126
Menotropins, S0122
Mental health
assessment, H0031
education, G0177
hospitalization, H0035
peer services, H0038
self-help, H0038
service plan, H0032
services, NOS, H0046
supportive treatment, H0026-H0037
training, G0177
Meritene, enteral nutrition, B4150
powder, B4150
MESA, S4028
Mesh, C1781
Metabolism error, food supplement, S9434
Metacarpophalangeal joint prosthesis, L8630
Metatarsal joint, prosthetic implant, L8641
Meter, bath conductivity, dialysis, E1550
Methylene blue injection, Q9968
Methylprednisolone
acetate, J1020-J1040
oral, J7509
sodium succinate, J2920, J2930
Meunster Suspension, socket prosthesis, L6110
Microbiology test, P7001
Microcapillary tube, A4651
sealant, A4652
Micro-Fine
disposable insulin syringes, up to 1 cc, per syringe, A4206
lancets, box of 100, A4259
Microlipids, enteral nutrition, B4155
Mileage, ambulance, A0380, A0390
Milk, breast
processing, T2101
Milwaukee spinal orthotic, L1000
Minerva, spinal orthotic, L0700, L0710
Mini-bus, nonemergency transportation, A0120
Minimed
3 cc syringe, A4232
506 insulin pump, E0784
insulin infusion set with bent needle wings, each, A4231
Sof-Set 24" insulin infusion set, each, A4230
Miroderm Biologic Wound Matrix, Q4175
Mitotic rate, G9292-G9294
Mobilite hospital beds, E0293, E0295, E0297
Moderate sedation, G0500
Moducal, enteral nutrition, B4155
Moisture exchanger for use with invasive mechanical ventilation, A4483
Moisturizer, skin, A6250
Monitor
apnea, E0618
blood glucose, E0607
Accu-Check, E0607
device, continuous, S1030-S1031
receiver, K0554
supply allowance, 1 month, K0553
Tracer II, E0607
blood pressure, A4670
device, A9279
pacemaker, E0610, E0615
ultrafiltration, S9007
Monoject disposable insulin syringes, up to 1 cc, per syringe, A4206
Monojector lancet device, A4258
Morcellator, C1782
Mouthpiece (for respiratory equipment), A4617
MRCP, S8037
MRI
contrast material, A9576-A9579, Q9954
low field, S8042
Mucoprotein, blood, P2038
Mucus trap, S8210
Multidisciplinary services, children, T1026
Multifetal pregnancy reduction, ultrasound guidance, S8055
Multiple post collar, cervical, L0180-L0200
Multipositional patient support system, E0636
Muscular dystrophy, genetic test, S3853
Myotonic muscular dystrophy, genetic test, S3853
MyOwn Skin, Q4226
Myringotomy, S2225

N

Nail trim, G0127, S0390
Narrowing device, wheelchair, E0969
Nasal
application device (for CPAP device), A7032-A7034
endoscopy, C9745, S2342
repair
vestibular lateral wall, C9749
vaccine inhalation, J3530
Nasogastric tubing, B4081, B4082
Nebulizer, E0570-E0585
aerosol mask, A7015
aerosols, E0580
Airlife Brand Misty-Neb, E0580
Power-Mist, E0580
Up-Draft Neb-U-Mist, E0580
Up-Mist hand-held nebulizer, E0580
compressor, with, E0570
Madamist II medication compressor/nebulizer, E0570
Pulmo-Aide compressor/nebulizer, E0570
Schuco Mist nebulizer system, E0570
corrugated tubing
disposable, A7010, A7018
distilled water, A7018
filter
disposable, A7013
non-disposable, A7014
heater, E1372
large volume
disposable, prefilled, A7008
disposable, unfilled, A7007
not used with oxygen
durable glass, A7017
Nebulizer — *continued*
pneumatic, administration set, A7003, A7005, A7006
pneumatic, nonfiltered, A7004
portable, E0570
small volume, E0574
spacer or nebulizer, S8100
with mask, S8101
ultrasonic, dome and mouthpiece, A7016
ultrasonic, reservoir bottle
nondisposable, A7009
water, A7018
water collection device large volume nebulizer, A7012
distilled water, A7018
Needle, A4215
biopsy
bone marrow, C1830
brachytherapy, C1715
non-coring, A4212
with syringe, A4206-A4209
Negative pressure wound therapy
dressing set, A6550
pump, E2402
NeoPatch, Q4176
Neox 100, Q4156
Neox 1K, Neox Cord 1K, Neox Cord RT, Q4148
Neox Flo, Q4155
NephrAmine, parenteral nutrition, B5000
Neuromuscular stimulator, E0745
ambulation of spinal cord injured, E0762
Neurophysiology monitoring, G0453
Neuro-Pulse, E0720
Neurostimulator
functional transcutaneous, E0764
generator
nonrechargeable, C1767, C1823
with rechargeable battery/charging system
high frequency, C1822
nonhigh frequency, C1820
implantable
electrode, L8680
pulse generator, L8679, L8685-L8688
receiver, L8682
lead, C1778
patient programmer, C1787, L8681
receiver and/or transmitter, C1816
transmitter
external, L8683-L8684
Newington
Legg Perthes orthotic, L1710
Newport Lite hip orthotic, L1685
Next Generation ACO Model, G9868-G9870
Nextep Contour Lower Leg Walker, L2999
Nextep Low Silhouette Lower Leg Walkers, L2999
Nicotine
gum, S4995
patches, S4990-S4991
Niemann-Pick disease, genetic test, S3849
Nipple prosthesis, L2006, L8032
Noncovered services, A9270, G0293-G0294
Nonemergency transportation, A0080-A0210
Nonimpregnated gauze dressing, A6216, A6221, A6402, A6404
Nonprescription drug, A9150
Nonthermal pulsed high frequency radiowaves treatment device, E0761
Northwestern Suspension, socket prosthesis, L6110
Not medically necessary service, S9986
Not otherwise specified supply, T5999
NovaFix, Q4208
NuHope
adhesive, 1 oz bottle with applicator, A4364
adhesive, 3 oz bottle with applicator, A4364
cleaning solvent, 16 oz bottle, A4455
cleaning solvent, 4 oz bottle, A4455
hole cutter tool, A4421
Nursing care, in home
licensed practical nurse, G0494, G0496, S9124
nursing visit (FQHC, RHC), G0490
registered nurse, G0493, G0495, S9123
Nursing services, G0493-G0496, S9211-S9212, T1000-T1004
nursing facility resident
evaluation and management, G9685
treatment, G9679-G9684
NuShield, Q4160
Nutri-Source, enteral nutrition, B4155
Nutrition
counseling
dietary, S9452
enteral formulae, B4150-B4162
enteral infusion pump, B9002
medical food, S9433
parenteral infusion pump, B9004, B9006
parenteral solution, B4164-B5200
Nutritional counseling, dietitian visit, S9470

O

O&P Express
above knee, L5210
ankle-foot orthotic with bilateral uprights, L1990
anterior floor reaction orthotic, L1945
below knee, L5105
elbow disarticulation, L6200
hip disarticulation, L5250
hip-knee-ankle-foot orthotic, L2080
interscapular thoracic, L6370
knee disarticulation, L5150, L5160
knee-ankle-foot orthotic, L2000, L2010, L2020, L2036
Legg Perthes orthotic, Patten bottom type, L1755
Legg Perthes orthotic, Scottish Rite, L1730
partial foot, L5000, L5020
plastic foot drop brace, L1960
supply/accessory/service, L9900
OASIS
Burn Matrix, Q4103
Ultra Tri-Layer Matrix, Q4124
Wound Matrix, Q4102
Observation service
direct admission, G0379
per hour, G0378
Occipital/mandibular support, cervical, L0160
Occlusive device placement, G0269
Occupational multifocal lens, V2786
Occupational therapist
home health setting, G0152
Occupational therapy, G0129, S9129
OCM, G9678
Octafluoropropae microspheres, Q9956
Ocular device, C1783, C1784
Ocular prosthetic implant, L8610
Offobock cosmetic gloves, L6895
Ofloxacin, S0034
Ohio Willow
prosthetic sheath
above knee, L8410
below knee, L8400
upper limb, L8415
prosthetic sock, L8420-L8435
stump sock, L8470-L8485
OIVIT, G9147
Olanzapine, S0166
Omegaven, B4187
Omnicardiogram, S9025
Oncology
breast cancer, G9071-G9075, G9131
gene profiling, S3854
chronic myelogenous leukemia, G9139
colon cancer, G9083-G9089
coordination of care, G9054
demonstration project, G9050-G9139, G9678
esophageal cancer, G9096-G9099
evaluation, G9050
expectant management, G9053
gastric cancer, G9100-G9104
head and neck, G9109-G9112
management
adheres to guidelines, G9056
differs from guidelines, G9057-G9060, G9062
not addressed by guidelines, G9061
management of care, G9054

© 2019 Optum360, LLC

Oncology — *continued*
multiple myeloma, G9128-G9130
no directed therapy, G9053
non-Hodgkin's lymphoma, G9123-G9125, G9134-G9138
nonsmall cell lung cancer, G9063-G9070
ovarian cancer, G9113-G9117, G9126
pancreatic cancer, G9105-G9108
prostate cancer, G9077-G9083, G9132-G9133
rectal cancer, G9090-G9095
staging, G9050
supervising care, G9054
surveillance for recurrence, G9052
treatment decision making, G9051
unspecified service, G9055
work up, G9050
Oncology Care Model (OCM) Monthly Enhanced Oncology Svc (MEOS), G9678
Oncoscint, A4642
One Touch
Basic blood glucose meter, E0607
Basic test strips, box of 50, A4253
Profile blood glucose meter, E0607
One-Button foldaway walker, E0143
Online assessment
qualified nonphysician professional, G2061-G2063
Oral
cushion replacement, A7028
interface for respiratory suction pump, A7047
interpreter or sign language services, T1013
Organ donor procurement, S2152
Oropharyngeal suction catheter, A4628
Ortho-Ease forearm crutches, E0111
Orthoflex Elastic Plaster Bandages, A4580
Orthoguard hip orthotic, L1685
Orthomedics
ankle-foot orthotic, L1900
pediatric hip abduction splint, L1640
plastic foot drop brace, L1960
single axis shoe insert, L2180
ultralight airplane arm abduction splint, L3960
upper extremity fracture orthotic
combination, L3763
humeral, L3980-L3981
radius/ulnar, L3982
Orthomerica
below knee test socket, L5620
pediatric hip abduction splint, L1640
plastic foot drop brace, L1960
single axis shoe insert, L2180
upper extremity fracture orthotic
humeral, L3980-L3981
radius/ulnar, L3982
Orthopedic devices, E0910-E0948
cervical
Diskard head halters, E0942
Turtle Neck safety collars, E0942
Orthopedic shoes
arch support, L3040-L3100
footwear, L3201-L3265
insert, L3000-L3030
lift, L3300-L3334
miscellaneous additions, L3500-L3595
positioning device, L3140-L3170
transfer, L3600-L3649
wedge, L3340-L3420
Orthoplast Splints (and Orthoplast II Splints), A4590
Orthotic additions
ankle/foot, L5969
carbon graphite lamination, L2755
cervical congenital torticollis, L0112
electric lock, L6638
electronic elbow with microprocessor, L7181
endoskeletal knee-shin system, L5848
with microprocessor, L5856, L5857
fracture, L2180-L2192, L3995
halo, L0859
lock mechanism for elbow, L6698
lower extremity, K0672, L2200-L2999, L5646-L5648, L5781-L5782, L5984
Orthotic additions — *continued*
ratchet lock, L2430
removable soft interface, K0672
replacement strap, L4002
rocker bottom for ankle, L2232
scoliosis, L1010-L1120, L1210-L1290
shoe, L3300-L3595, L3649
shoulder lock, L6646-L6648
socket insert for elbow, L6694-L6697
spinal, L0970-L0999
suspension sleeve for knee, L5685
upper extremity joint, L3956
upper limb, E2631-E2633, L3956, L3995
vacuum pump, L5781-L5782
Orthotic devices
additions, L1005-L1120, L1210-L1290, L5961, L5988-L5990, L6611, L6624
ankle-foot (*see also* Orthopedic shoes), E1815, E1830, L1900-L1990, L2108-L2116, L3160, L4396-L4397, L4631
anterior-posterior-lateral, L0700, L0710
cervical, L0112, L0180-L0200
cervical-thoracic-lumbar-sacral, L0700, L0710, L1000-L1001
congenital torticollis, L0112
cranial remolding, S1040
cranial-cervical, L0113
elbow, E1800, L3702-L3740, L3761
finger, L3925, L3927
fracture, L3980-L3984
halo, L0810-L0830
hand, E1805, E1825, L3900-L3930
hip, L1600-L1686
hip-knee-ankle-foot, L2040-L2090
interface material, E1820
knee, E1810, L1810-L1820, L1830-L1860, L1851-L1852
knee-ankle-foot, L2000-L2038, L2126-L2136
Legg Perthes, A4565, L1700-L1755
lumbar, L0625-L0627
lumbar-sacral, L0628-L0651
lumbar-sacral, hip, femur, L1690
multiple post collar, L0180-L0200
not otherwise specified, L0999, L1499, L2999, L3999, L5999, L7499, L8039
pneumatic splint, L4350-L4370
preparatory below knee, L5535
repair or replacement, L4000-L4210
replace soft interface material, L4392-L4394
sacroiliac, L0621-L0624
scoliosis, L1000, L1200, L1300-L1499
shoulder, L3650-L3671, L3674-L3678
shoulder-elbow-wrist-hand, L3960-L3962
spinal, cervical, L0112, L0180-L0200
thoracic belt, L0220
thoracic-lumbar-sacral, L0450-L0492, L1200
toe, E1830
transfer (shoe orthotic), L3600-L3640
walking splint, nonpneumatic, L4386
wrist hand, L3150, L3905-L3908, L3916
wrist hand finger, L3806-L3809, L3900-L3904, L3931
Osmolite, enteral nutrition, B4150
HN, B4150
Ossicula prosthetic implant, L8613
Osteogenic stimulator, E0747-E0749, E0760
Osteotomy, periacetabular, S2115
Ostomy
absorbent material, A4422
accessories, A5093
adhesive remover wipes, A4456
appliance belt, A4367
clamp, A4363
cone/catheter, A4399
filter, A4368
irrigation supply, A4398, A4399
pediatric one-piece system, A5061, A5062
pediatric two-piece drainable pouch, A5063
pouch, A4416-A4420, A4423-A4434
drainable, A4412-A4413, A5056-A5057
pediatric, A5061-A5062
skin barrier, A4411, A4414-A4415
Ostomy — *continued*
skin barrier — *continued*
extended wear, A4407-A4410
paste, A4405-A4406
wipes or swabs, A5120
vent, A4366
Otto Bock prosthesis
battery charger, six volt, L7362
battery, six volt, L7360
hook adapter, L6628
lamination collar, L6629
pincher tool, L6810
wrist, L6629
Outpatient hospital clinic visit, G0463
Overlay, mattress, E0371-E0373
Ovulation induction, S4042
Owens & Minor
cervical collar, L0140
cervical helmet, L0120
Oximeter, E0445
probe, A4606
Oxi-Uni-Pak, E0430
Oxygen
accessory, E1352
ambulance, A0422
battery
charger, E1357
pack, E1356
chamber, hyperbaric, topical, A4575
concentrator, E1390, E1391
portable, rental, E1392
gaseous, K0738, S8120
liquid, S8121
mask, A4620
medication supplies, A4611-A4627
portable, E0433, E0443-E0444, E0447, K0738
power adapter, E1358
rack/stand, E1355
regulator, E1353
respiratory equipment/supplies, A4611-A4627, E0424-E0480
Oxi-Uni-Pak, E0430
supplies and equipment, E0425-E0444, E0433, E0455, E1353-E1406
tent, E0455
tubing, A4616
water vapor enriching system, E1405, E1406
wheeled cart, E1354

P

Pacemaker
dual chamber
non-rate responsive, C2619
rate responsive, C1785
lead, C1779, C1898, C1899
monitor, E0610, E0615
other than single or dual chamber, C2621
single chamber
non-rate responsive, C2620
rate responsive, C1786
Pacer manual wheelchair, K0003
Packing strips, A6407
Pad
abdominal, L1270
adhesive, A6203-A6205, A6212-A6214, A6219-A6221, A6237-A6239, A6245-A6247, A6254-A6256
alginate, A6196-A6199
alternating pressure, E0181
arm, K0019
Asis, L1250
condylar, L2810
crutch, A4635
fluid circulating, cold, with pump, E0218
gel pressure, E0185, E0196
gluteal, L2650
gradient pressure pads, S8421-S8429
heating, E0210, E0215, E0217, E0249
heel, L3480, L3485
kyphosis, L1020, L1025
lumbar, L1030, L1040, L1240
Pad — *continued*
nonadhesive (dressing), A6209-A6211, A6216-A6218, A6222-A6224, A6228-A6230, A6234-A6236, A6242-A6244
orthotic device interface, E1820
pressure, E0181-E0182
replacement, infrared heat system, A4639
rib gusset, L1280
sheepskin, E0188, E0189
shoe, L3430-L3485
stabilizer, L3170
sternal, L1050
thoracic, L1060, L1260
triceps, L6100
trochanteric, L1290
truss, L8320, L8330
water circulating, heat, unit, E0249
water circulating, heat, with pump, E0217
water pressure, E0198
Pail, for use with commode chair, E0167
Pain, G9250-G9251
PalinGen Flow or ProMatrX (fluid), Q4174
PalinGen or PalinGen XPlus Membrane, Q4173
Palladium, C2640-C2641
Pan, for use with commode chair, E0167
Pancreas, S1034-S1037
artificial device system, S1034
replacement external receiver, S1037
replacement external transmitter, S1036
replacement invasive disposable subcutaneous sensor, S1035
Pantoprazole sodium, C9113, S0164
Papanicolaou (Pap) screening smear, P3000, P3001, Q0091
Paraffin, A4265
bath unit, E0235
Paramedic intercept, S0207-S0208
Paranasal sinus ultrasound, S9024
Parenteral nutrition
administration kit, B4224
home infusion therapy, S9364-S9368
pump, B9004, B9006
solution, B4164-B5200
supplies, not otherwise classified, B9999
supply kit, B4220, B4222
Parenting class, S9444
infant safety, S9447
Parking fee, nonemergency transport, A0170
Partial hospitalization, S0201
PASRR, T2010-T2011
Passive motion
continuous exercise device, E0936
Paste, conductive, A4558
conductive, A4558
coupling for ultrasound, A4559
Pathogen(s)
reduced, platelets, P9073
test for platelets, P9100
Pathology and laboratory tests
molecular pathology, G0452
surgical
prostate, G0416
Pathology screening tests, P3000-P3001, Q0091
Patient
complications, G9267-G9270
daily aspirin regimen, G9277-G9278
death, G9256, G9260, G9262
decision making, G9296-G9297
discharged to home, G9254-G9255
stroke, G9257-G9259
survival, G9259, G9261, G9263
tobacco non-user, G9276
tobacco user, G9275
Patient lift, E0625, E0637, E0639, E0640
Patten Bottom, Legg Perthes orthotic, L1755
Pavlik harness, hip orthotic, L1650
Payment, home health bundled care improvement initiative, G9187
Peak flow meter, S8110
portable, S8096
Pediatric hip abduction splint
Orthomedics, L1640
Orthomerica, L1640
Pediculosis treatment, A9180

© 2019 Optum360, LLC

PEFR, peak expiratory flow rate meter, A4614
Pelvic and breast exam, G0101
Pelvic belt/harness/boot, E0944
Penicillin G
potassium, J2540
procaine, aqueous, J2510
Penlet II lancet device, A4258
Penlet lancet device, A4258
Percussor, E0480
Percutaneous
access system, A4301
image-guided lumbar decompression (PILD), G0276
transluminal coronary atherectomy, C9602-C9603
transluminal revascularization, C9604-C9608
Perflexane lipid microspheres, Q9955
Perflutren lipid microsphere, Q9957
Peripheral
catheter infusion, C1751
Perlstein, ankle-foot orthotic, L1920
Permacol, C9364
Peroneal strap, L0980
Peroxide, A4244
Personal care item, S5199
Personal care services, T1019-T1020
Pessary, A4561-A4562
PET imaging
any site, NOS, G0235
breast, G0252
whole body, G0219
Pharmacy
compounding and dispensing, S9430
dispensing fee
inhalation drugs
per 30 days, Q0513
per 90 days, Q0514
supply fee
initial immunosuppressive drugs, Q0510
oral anticancer antiemetic or immunosuppressive drug, Q0511-Q0512
Pharmaplast disposable insulin syringes, per syringe, A4206
Phelps, ankle-foot orthotic, L1920
Pheresis, platelets, P9034-P9037, P9053
pathogen reduced, P9073
Philadelphia tracheotomy cervical collar, L0172
Philly One-piece Extrication collar, L0150
pHisoHex solution, A4246
Photocoagulation, G0186
Phototherapy
home visit service (Bili-Lite), S9098
keratectomy (PKT), S0812
light (bilirubin), E0202
Physical exam
for college, S0622
related to surgical procedure, S0260
Physical therapy, S8990
shoulder stretch device, E1841
Physical therapy/therapist
home health setting, G0151, S9131
Physician management
home care
episodic, S0272
hospice monthly, S0271
standard monthly, S0270
Physician quality reporting system (PQRS)
See Quality payment program (QPP)
Physician review
home INR testing, G0250
Physician supervision, G0181-G0182
Pillow
abduction, E1399
decubitus care, E0190
nasal, A7029
positioning, E0190
Pinworm examination, Q0113
Placement
applicator, breast, C9726
interstitial device radiotherapy, other than prostate, C9728
occlusive, G0269
Plan of care, T2024
Planning
cancer treatment, S0353-S0354
Plasma
autologous platelet rich plasma, G0460
cryoprecipitate reduced, P9044
frozen, P9058-P9060
multiple donor, pooled, frozen, P9023, P9070-P9071
protein fraction, P9043, P9048
single donor, fresh frozen, P9017
Plastazote, L3002, L3252, L3253, L3265, L5654-L5658
Plaster
bandages
Orthoflex Elastic Plaster Bandages, A4580
Specialist Plaster Bandages, A4580
Genmould Creamy Plaster, A4580
Specialist J-Splint Plaster Roll Immobilizer, A4580
Specialist Plaster Roll Immobilizer, A4580
Specialist Plaster Splints, A4580
Platelets, P9019-P9020, P9031-P9037, P9052-P9053, P9055
apheresis/pheresis, P9052, P9055
concentrate, each unit, P9019
pathogen(s)
reduced, platelets, P9073
test, P9100
pheresis, P9034-P9037, P9053
pathogen reduced, P9073
rich plasma, each unit, P9020
Platform attachment
forearm crutch, E0153
walker, E0154
Platform, for home blood glucose monitor, A4255
Plumbing, for home ESRD equipment, A4870
Plurivest, Q4153
Pneumatic nebulizer
administration set
small volume
disposable, A7004
filtered, A7006
non-disposable, A7005
non-filtered, A7003
Polaris, E0601
Polaris Lt, E0601
Polycose, enteral nutrition
liquid, B4155
powder, B4155
Poor blood, each unit, P9016
Port
indwelling, C1788
Portable
equipment transfer, R0070-R0076
hemodialyzer system, E1635
home suction pump, K0743
nebulizer, E0570
oxygen contents
gaseous, E0443
liquid, E0444, E0447
oxygen system
gaseous, E0430-E0431
liquid, E0433-E0435
x-ray equipment, Q0092
Portagen Powder, enteral nutrition, B4150
Posey restraints, E0700
Positive airway pressure device supply, A7046
Postcoital examination, Q0115
Postdischarge services
LVRS surgery, G0305
Postural drainage board, E0606
Potassium
hydroxide (KOH) preparation, Q0112
Pouch
Active Life convex one-piece urostomy, A4421
closed, A4387, A5052
drainable, A4388-A4389, A5056-A5057, A5061
fecal collection, A4330
Little Ones Sur-fit mini, A5054
Pouch — *continued*
ostomy, A4375-A4378, A4387-A4391, A4416-A4420, A4423-A4434, A4435, A5051-A5054, A5061-A5063
pediatric, drainable, A5061
Pouchkins pediatric ostomy system, A5061, A5062, A5073
Sur-Fit, drainable, A5063
urinary, A4379-A4383, A4391, A5071-A5073
urostomy, A5073
Power
mist nebulizer, E0580
mobility device, K0800-K0812, K0899
wheelchair, K0813-K0898
pediatric, E1239
Power mobility device
does not meet criteria, K0899
group 1, K0800-K0802, K0813-K0816
group 2, K0806-K0808, K0820-K0843
group 3, K0849-K0864
group 4, K0868-K0886
group 5, K0890-K0891
not coded by DME PDAC, K0899
not otherwise classified (NOC), K0812, K0898
Power operated vehicle
group 1, K0800-K0802
group 2, K0806-K0808
not otherwise classified (NOC), K0812
Precision, enteral nutrition
HN, B4153
Isotonic, B4153
Prednisolone
acetate, J2650
oral, J7510
Pregnancy care, H1000-H1005
Pregnancy documentation, G9231
Premium knee sleeve, L1830
Prenatal care, H1000-H1005
Preoperative Services
LVRS surgery, G0302-G0304
Preparatory prosthesis, L5510-L5595
Prescription drug
brand, S5001
generic, S5000
Pressure
alarm, dialysis, E1540
pad, E0181-E0182
PressureGuard II, E0186
PressureKair mattress overlay, E0197
Prestige blood glucose monitor, E0607
Pre-Vent heel & elbow protector, E0191
Prevention, developmental delay, H2037
Preventive
foot care, S0390
health Medicare
ECG, G0403-G0405
exam, G0402
prolonged services, G0513-G0514
PriMatrix, Q4110
Probe
cryoablation, C2618
oximeter, A4606
percutaneous lumbar discectomy, C2614
Processing
breast milk, T2101
Procurement, organ donor, S2152
Procuren, S9055
Professional services, G0068-G0070
ProgenaMatrix, Q4222
Prolonged services
preventive, G0513-G0514
Prolotherapy, M0076
ProMatrX wound matrix, Q4174
Promix, enteral nutrition, B4155
Pronation/supination device, forearm, E1802
Propac, enteral nutrition, B4155
Prophylaxis
antibiotic, G9300-G9302
antimicrobial prophylaxis, G9196-G9198
Prostate
high intensity focused ultrasound transrectal, C9747
low dose rate (LDR) brachytherapy, G0458
specific antigen test (PSA), G0103
Prostate — *continued*
surgical pathology, G0416
Prosthesis
addition
lower extremity prosthesis, L5858, L5859
breast, C1789, L2006, L8000-L8031, L8035-L8039, L8600
eye, C1839, L8610, V2623-V2629
finger joint, L8659
fitting, L5400-L5460, L6380-L6388
grasper, L6881
hand, L6000-L6020, L6708-L6709, L7007-L7008
hemifacial, L8044
hook, L6703-L6707, L7009
implants, L8600-L8699
iris, C1839
larynx, L8500, L8505
lower extremity, L5700-L5999, L8642
maxillofacial, provided by a nonphysician, L8040-L8048
metacarpal, L8631
midfacial, L8041
miscellaneous service, L8499
nasal
septal, L8047
nipple, L2006, L8032
partial facial, L8046
penile
inflatable, C1813
non-inflatable, C2622
repair, L7520
repair or modification, maxillofacial, L8048-L8049
retinal, C1841-C1842
accessory/component/supply, L8608
socks (shrinker, sheath, stump sock), L8400-L8480
tracheoesophageal, L8511-L8514
tracheo-esophageal, L8507-L8509
tracheoesophageal gelatin capsule, L8515
tracheostomy speaking, L8501
unspecified maxillofacial, L8048
upper extremity, L6000-L6915
urinary sphincter, C1815
vacuum erection system, L7900
Prosthetic
additions
lower extremity, L5610
device, implanted, C9899
donning sleeve, L7600
hand, L6708-L6709, L6713-L6714, L6722
hook, L6706-L6707, L6711-L6712, L6721, L6722, L7009
shrinker, L8440-L8465
Prosthetic shrinker, L8440-L8465
Protectant, skin, A6250
Protector, heel or elbow, E0191
PSA, G0103
Psychiatric care, H0036-H0037, H2013-H2014, S9480
Psychological services
CORF, G0409
Psychotherapy
group, G0410-G0411
PTK, S0812
Pulmo-Aide compressor
nebulizer, E0570
Pulmonary rehabilitation, G0424
program, S9473
Pulse generator
ear, E2120
battery, A4638
Pump
alternating pressure pad, E0182
ambulatory infusion, E0781
ambulatory insulin, E0784
Bio Flote alternating pressure pad, E0182
blood, dialysis, E1620
breast, E0602-E0604
supplies, A4281-A4286
Broncho-Cath endobronchial tubes, with CPAP, E0601
enteral infusion, B9002
supply, K0552

© 2019 Optum360, LLC

Pump — *continued*
fluid/water circulating pad, E0217, E0218, E0236
gastric suction, E2000
Gomco lightweight mobile aspirator, E0600
Gomco portable aspirator, E0600
heparin infusion, E1520
implantable infusion, E0782, E0783
implantable infusion, refill kit, A4220
infusion
nonprogrammable, C1891, C2626
supplies, A4230-A4232
insulin, external, E0784, E0787
instruction, S9145
supplies, A4226
negative pressure wound therapy, E2402
parenteral infusion, B9004, B9006, K0455
Pillo alternating pressure pad, E0182
portable home suction, K0743
suction
CPAP, E0601
gastric, E2000
portable, E0600, K0743
TenderCloud alternating pressure pad, E0182
PuraPly, PuraPly AM, PuraPly XT, Q4195-Q4197
Purification system, E1610, E1615
Pyeloscopy
for ureteral calculi, S2070

Q

Quad cane, E0105
Quadri-Poise canes, E0105
Quality assurance, G9148-G9153
Quality Payment Program (QPP)
abdominal imaging, G9547-G9548, G9550-G9551
ACE or ARB therapy, G8473-G8475, G8506, G8935-G8937
adenoma, G9933-G9935
admission
Medicare care choice model program (MCCM), G9480
alcohol use, G9621-G9624
AMI, G9798
amoxicillin with/without clavulanate as first line antibiotic, G9313-G9315
androgen deprivation therapy, G9894-G9897
anesthesia, post procedure body temperature, G9771-G9773
anesthetic, inhalation
for induction, G9955
antibiotic regimen, G8708-G8712, G8916-G8918, G9286-G9287, G9301-G9302, G9498, G9505, G9558-G9560, G9701, G9703, G9712
anticoagulation, G8967-G8969, G9724, G9927-G9928
antiemetic agents, G9775-G9777, G9956-G9958
antimicrobial
prophylaxis, G9196-G9198
systemic, G9959-G9961
antiplatelet/antithrombotic/aspirin therapy, G2128, G8598-G8599, G9277-G9278, G9609-G9611, G9794, M1055-M1057
anti-TNF therapy, G8869, G9504, G9912-G9914
aortic aneurysm, G9598-G9600
Appropriate Use Criteria
Clinic Decision Support Mechanism, G1000-G1011
assessment, patient
bone loss, G8863
functional outcomes, G8942
pain, G8732, G8939
asthma, G9432, G9434, G9799, G9808, G9810-G9811
atherosclerotic cardiovascular disease (ASCVD), G9662, G9674
atrial fibrillation (AF), G9746
back pain, G2136-G2139, G9943, G9946
beta-blocker, G8450-G8452, G9188-G9192, G9800, G9803-G9804

Quality Payment Program (QPP) — *continued*
beta-lactam antibiotic, G9558-G9560
biologic immune response modifier, G9506
biologic treatment, G9765
biopsy, G8872-G8874, G8878, G8880, G8882-G8885, G8946, G9282-G9285, G9288-G9291, G9939
bipolar disorder, G9717
birth year
1945-1965, G9448
bladder injury, G9625-G9627
blood pressure, G2129, G8476-G8478, G8752-G8756, G8783-G8785, G8950-G8952, G9273-G9274, G9788-G9790
blunt head trauma, G9529-G9537, G9593-G9597
BMI, G8417-G8422, G8938, G9716
bone loss, G8863
bowel injury, G9628-G9630
brain imaging, G9529-G9530, G9532-G9533, G9537
breast cancer, G8875-G8877, G8881, G8946, G9911
AJCC stage, G9704-G9705, G9831-G9832
breastfeeding, G9779
bronchodilator, inhaled, G9695-G9699
cancer diagnosis (other than basal cell or melanoma), M1018
cardiac implantable device
not readmitted, G9411, G9413
readmission within 180 days, G9410, G9412
cardiac stress test imaging, G8961-G8966
cardiac tamponade, G9408-G9409
care improvement initiative home visit, G9187
care management, CMMI Model, G0076-G0087
case management service NEC, G9012
cataract, G0916-G0918
postoperative refraction, G9519-G9520
cataract surgery, G0915-G0916, G0918, G8627-G8628
postoperative refraction, G9519-G9520
cause
transient or reversible AF, G9929
CEA, G8838, G9258, G9260-G9261
cervical cytology, G9806-G9807
chemotherapy, G9829, G9847-G9848
chlamydia screening, G9820-G9821
CMMI Model
assessment, G9490
care managment, G0076-G0087
in-home visit, G2001-G2009, G2013-G2015
remote in-home visit, G9481-G9489, G9978-G9987
colectomy, total, G9711
colonoscopy, G9612-G9614, G9659-G9661, G9933, G9935-G9937
colorectal cancer, G9711
comfort care only, G9930
complications, G9267-G9270
coordinated care fee
home monitoring, G9006
initial rate, G9001
maintenance rate, G9002
physician oversight, G9008
risk adjusted, G9003-G9005, G9009-G9011
scheduled team conference, G9007
corticosteroids, G9468-G9470
CT studies
reported to a radiation dose index registry, G9326-G9327
sinuses, G9348
current medications, G8427-G8428
death, nursing home resident, G9394

Quality Payment Program (QPP) — *continued*
demonstration project, G0076-G0087, G2001-G2009, G2013-G2015, G9013-G9014, G9016, G9050-G9139, G9140, G9480-G9490, G9678, G9978-G9987
depression, G8431-G8433, G8510-G8511, G8959-G8960, G9212-G9213, G9232, G9717, M1019-M1020, M1023-M1024
DEXA, DXA, G8399-G8400, G9471
diabetes, G9676
dialysis documentation, G9231
dialysis, palliative, G9747, G9749
Dicom format image data, G9329, G9340
discharge, patient, G8818, G8825-G8826, G8833-G8834, G8838, G9254-G9255, G9263
follow up, G9402-G9407
door to puncture time, G9580-G9582
dose reduction techniques, G9637-G9638
durable medical equipment (DME), G0454
dysthymia, M1019-M1020, M1023-M1024
ear drainage, G8560, G8562
early induction, G9355-G9356
ED admitted patients, G9426-G9427
elder maltreatment, G8535-G8536, G8733-G8735, G8941
elective delivery, G9355-G9356
elective surgery, G9643
embolization, G9962-G9963
emergency department visits, G9521-G9522, G9850-G9851
emergency surgery, G9752
emergent cases, M1142
end of life, G9380-G9382
endometrial
ablation/sampling, G9822-G9824
episode of care, M1106, M1111, M1116, M1121, M1126, M1135-M1136
ESRD documentation, G9231
exam
dilated macula, G9892-G9893, G9974-G9977
dilated retina, G2102
fall risk, M1069-M1070
female unable to bear children, M1016
filter placement/removal, G9539-G9544
final treatment and evaluation, M1009-M1015
follow up
colon polyp, 10-year interval, G9862
follow up imaging, G9548-G9550, G9554-G9556, G9755
foot exam, G9225-G9226, G9502
footwear evaluation, G8410, G8415-G8416
fraility, G2090-G2091, G2098-G2101, G2106-G2107, G2109-G2110, G2114-G2118, G2123-G2127, G2131-G2135
FS PROM, G2166, G9726-G9739
functional outcome, G8539-G8543, G9227
functional status, G2142-G2145, G9916-G9918, M1141
ankle, foot, lower leg, G8655-G8658
elbow, wrist or hand, G8667-G8670
hip, G8651-G8654
knee, G8647-G8650
low back, G8569-G8662
neck, cranium or mandible, G8671-G8674
Oswestry Disability Index (ODI) measurement, G2142-G2145
other general orthopedic impairment, G8671-G8674
Oxford Knee Score (OKS), M1141
shoulder, G8663-G8666
thoracic spine or ribs, G8671-G8674
gene mutation
RAS (KRAS, NRAS), G9840-G9843
HCV infection screening, G9383-G9386, G9451-G9454
hearing loss, G8565, G8567
hemodialysis, G8956, G9239-G9241, G9264-G9266, G9523

Quality Payment Program (QPP) — *continued*
hemoglobin, G8973-G8976
hepatitis B (HBV), G8869, G9504, G9912-G9913, G9915
hepatocellular cancer screening (HCC), G9455-G9457
HER2, G9825, G9827-G9828, G9830
herpes zoster, G2160-G2162
high risk medication, G9365-G9368, G9637-G9638
history
blood transfusion before 1992, G9449
injection drug use, G9450
HIV screening
antigen/antibody combination assay, G0475
HIV-1 or HIV-2, G0432-G0433, G0435
home health agency (HHA) specimen collection, G0471
home health nursing visit, G0490
hospice, G2153, G9524-G9526, G9687-G9694, G9700, G9702, G9707, G9709-G9710, G9713-G9715, G9718, G9720, G9723, G9725, G9740-G9741, G9758, G9760-G9761, G9768, G9802, G9805, G9809, G9819, G9856-G9861, G9868-G9870, G9930, M1022, M1025-M1026, M1059, M1067
hospital readmission, G9309-G9310
HPV
test, G9806-G9807
vaccine, G9762-G9763
hybrid procedure, G9640
hypercholesterolemia, G9782
hypertension, G8950-G8952, G9744-G9745
hysterectomy, G9774
hysteroscopy, G9823-G9824
imaging documentation, G9457, G9753, M1027-M1031
immunosuppressive therapy, M1063
incidental findings, G9547, G9552, G9754
induction, G9361
influenza vaccination, G2163-G2165, G8482-G8484
injection drug use, G9518
intensive care unit, G9853-G9854
interval and modality follow up, G9755
intervention, leak of endoluminal contents, G9305-G9306
intraoperative cystoscopy, G9606-G9608
kidney transplant, G9748, G9750
KRAS testing, G9840-G9841, G9843
left ventricular ejection fraction (LVEF), G8395-G8396, G8450-G8452, G8694, G8923, G8934
leg pain, G2140-G2141, G2146-G2147, M1052
lumbar spine
procedure same date as discectomy/laminotomy, G9942, G9948
related to
cancer, fracture, infection, G9945
idiopathic, congenital scoliosis, G9945
lung cancer screening, G0296-G0297
lymph node, G8878, G8880, G8882
major amputation, G9639, G9641
mastectomy, G9708
medical visit, G0463, G9246-G9247
medication assisted treatment, G2067-G2080, G2112-G2113, G2119-G2120, M1034-M1035
medication list/review, G8427-G8430
melanoma, G8749, G8944
meningococcal vaccine, G9414-G9415
metastatic disease, G9834, G9838, G9842
mitotic rate, G9292-G9294
mitral stenosis, G9746
modified Rankin scale (MRS), G9646-G9648
monitored anesthesia (MAC), G9654

© 2019 Optum360, LLC

Quality Payment Program (QPP) — *continued*
monoclonal antibody therapy, G9839, G9844-G9845
neck impairment, M1143
neurological condition, G2151, M1107, M1112, M1117, M1122, M1127, M1131, M1137
neurological exam, G8404-G8405, G9529-G9537, G9594, G9646-G9648
nonambulatory patient, G9719, G9721, M1008
nonsmall cell lung cancer, G9418-G9425
nursing home resident, M1058
nursing services
Christian science, journal-listed, per hour, S9901
home health nursing visit, G0490
ongoing care, M1108-M1110, M1113-M1115, M1118-M1120, M1123-M1125, M1128-M1130, M1132-M1134, M1138-M1140, M1144
open surgical bypass, G9639, G9641
opioid therapy, G2067-G2088, G9561-G9563, G9577-G9579, G9583-G9585, M1032-M1036
oral systemic/biologic therapy, G9765
osteoporosis, G8635, G8863, G9769
otology referrals, G8559, G8561, G8563-G8564, G8566, G8568, G8856-G8858
P2Y12 antagonists, G9609-G9611
pain, G8442, G8509, G8730-G8732, G9250-G9251, G9949
multimodal, G2148-G2150
palliative care, M1017, M1059
paranasal sinus CT
at time of or within 28 days of diagnosis, G9348-G9350
more than once within 90 days of diagnosis, G9351-G9354
pathology, G9428-G9429, G9431, G9784-G9786
performed by same biopsy clinician, G9939
report, G9428-G9429, G9431, G9784-G9786
second opinion, G9784
patient alive, G9787
patient care survey, G0914, G0917
patient category, G9428-G9429, G9431
patient death, G9256, G9260, G9262, G9751, G9812-G9817, G9846, G9849, G9852, M1060
patient decision making, G9296-G9297
patient has at time of procedure
lumbar spine cancer, M1037, M1041, M1051
lumbar spine fracture, M1038, M1041, M1051
lumbar spine infection, M1039, M1041, M1051
scoliosis, M1040-M1041, M1051
patient health questionnaire (PHQ), G9393, G9395-G9396, G9509-G9511, G9573-G9574
patient immunocompromised, M1062
patient referred to another provider, G9968-G9970
patient stroke, G9257-G9259
patient survey score, G9603-G9605
patient survival, G9259, G9261
patient-specific risk assessment, G9316-G9317
PECARN prediction, G9593, G9597
pediatric head trauma, G9593, G9596-G9597
performance, G2150, G2152, G2167
peripheral nerve block (PNB), G9770
pharmacological therapy, G8633-G8635, M1032-M1036
PHQ-9/PHQ-9M score, G9393, G9395-G9396, G9509-G9511, G9573-G9574, M1019-M1020, M1023-M1024
pneumococcal vaccine, G2157-G2159, G8864-G8867, G9279-G9280

Quality Payment Program (QPP) — *continued*
positive airway pressure, G8845, G8849-G8855
posterior capsule rupture, G9389-G9390, G9759
postoperative assessment, G9540
postoperative discharge, G9601-G9602
postpartum education, G9357-G9358
postpartum evaluation, G9357-G9358
postpartum screening, G9357-G9358
pregnancy documentation, G9231, G9778, M1061
pregnancy location, G8806
preoperative assessment, G9497, G9615-G9617
preoperative order, IV antibiotic, G8916-G8918
prolonged intubation, G8569-G8570
proportion of days covered (PDC), G9512-G9513
prostate cancer, G8465, G9706
prosthetic heart valve, G9746
prosthetic implant, G9303-G9305
psoriasis
assessment, G9649, G9651
treatment, G9764-G9765
psychiatric symptoms, G2121-G2122
quality of life assessment, G9634-G9636
RA, M1007-M1008
radiation exposure indices, G9500-G9501
recommended guidelines for incidental pulmonary nodule, G9345-G9347
reexploration, G8577-G8578
refraction, G9519-G9520
remission (PHQ-9 score), G9509-G9511, G9573-G9574
renal failure, G8575-G8576, G9722
renal transplant documentation, G9231
rendering treatment in place, G2021-G2022
respiratory, G8842-G8846, G8849-G8855
retinopathy, G8397-G8398
return to the operating room, G9307-G9308, G9514-G9515
Rh immune globulin (RhoGam), G8809-G8811
rhabdomyolysis, G9780
risk adjusted functional status, G8648-G8674
risk factor
evaluation, G8648-G8674
postoperative vomiting, G9954
risk score
CHA2DS2-VASc, G9931
safety concerns, G9922-G9926
screening, G9919-G9921
alcohol use, G9624
delays, children, G9966-G9968
mammography, G9899-G9900
tobacco use, G9902-G9905
search for patient prior imaging studies, G9341-G9344
sexual activity, G9818
sexually transmitted disease, G9228-G9230
Shingrix vaccine, M1064-M1066
silicone oil use, surgical procedures, G9756-G9757
sinusitis
caused by bacterial infection, G9364
skilled nursing facility (SNF) specimen collection, G0471
sleep apnea, G8839-G8855
special needs plans (SNP)
institutional, G2081, G2105, G2108, G2130, G9898, G9901, G9910, G9938
specimen site, G8797-G8798, G9295, G9430
spine or other procedure same date as discectomy/laminotomy, G9942, G9948, M1071
spirometry, G8924-G8926
staged procedure, G9640
standard nomenclature for imaging study, G9318-G9319

Quality Payment Program (QPP) — *continued*
statin therapy, G8815-G8817, G9507-G9508, G9663-G9666, G9675-G9676, G9781, G9783, G9796-G9797, G9940
stereoscopic photos, G2103-G2104
stroke/CVA/TIA, G8573-G8574, G9257-G9259, G9261, G9580-G9582, G9766-G9767
surgical site infection, G9311-G9312
tamsulosin hydrochloride, G9503
TB screening, M1003-M1006
Td/Tdap vaccination, G2154-G2156
test, gene mutation, G9840-G9841
tetanus, diphtheria, pertussis vaccine (Tdap), G9416-G9417
thromboembolism risk factor, G8970
thyroid, G9552-G9553, G9557
tobacco use, G9275-G9276, G9458-G9460, G9642, G9644-G9645, G9791-G9792, G9902-G9909
TPA, G8602
transfer
anesthetizing location to PACU/non-ICU, G9656
hospital to non-acute care facility, G9801
to practice after initiation of chemotherapy, G9826, G9833
transfer of care protocol, G9655-G9658
trastuzumab administration, G9835-G9837
treatment choices, G9399-G9401
tuberculosis screening, G9359-G9360, G9932
tumor, G8721-G8724
ultrasound, G8806-G8808
ureter injury, G9631-G9633
urgent care, M1021, M1054
uterine malignancy screening, G9618-G9620
vaccination, G2154-G2165, G9279-G9281, G9762-G9763
viral load, G9242-G9243
visual acuity, G9516-G9517
visual analog scale (VAS), G2136-G2141, G2146-G2147, G9949, M1052
visual function, G0913, G0915
volume management, G8955, G8958
well-child visit, G9964-G9965
wheelchair evaluation, G9156
wound infection, G8571-G8572
Quality reporting measures
See Quality payment program (QPP)
Quick Check blood glucose test strips, box of 50, A4253
Quick release restraints, E0700
Quikfit crutch, E0114
Quik-Fold Walkers, E0141, E0143

R

Rack/stand, oxygen, E1355
Radiation
compensator based, G6016
intensity modulated, G6015
intra-fraction, G6017
treatment delivery
single area
11-19mev, G6005
20mev or greater, G6006
6-10mev, G6004
up to 5mev, G6003
three or more areas
11-19mev, G6013
20mev or greater, G6014
6-10mev, G6012
up to 5mev, G6011
two separate areas
11-19mev, G6009
20mev or greater, G6010
6-10mev, G6008
up to 5mev, G6007
Radiation dosimeter, implantable, ea, A4650
Radioelements for brachytherapy, Q3001
Radiofrequency
radiofrequency transmitter, sacral root neurostimulator, replacement, L8684
Radioimmunoscintigraphy, S8080
Radiolabeled product provided during inpatient stay, C9898
Radiology service, R0070-R0076
Radiopharmaceutical
ammonia N-13, A9526
chromic phosphate P32, A9564
cyanocobalamin cobalt Co 57, A9559
diagnostic imaging agent, A4641, A4642, A9597-A9598, A9604
gallium Ga 67, A9556
indium I-111
ibitumomab tiuxetan, A9542
pentreotide, A9572
satumomab pendetide, A4642
inpatient, C9898
non-tumor identification, A9598
not otherwise classified, A9597-A9598, A9699
PET, diagnostic, A9597-A9598
radium ra-223 dischloride, A9606
rubidium RB-82, A9555
sodium
fluoride F-18, diagnostic, A9580
iodide I-131, A9528-A9531
phosphate, A9563
technetium Tc 99m
arcitumomab, A9568
bicisate, A9557
depreotide, A9536
disofenin, A9510
exametazime, A9521, A9569
fanolesomab, A9566
glucepatate, A9550
labeled red blood cells, A9560
macroaggregated albumin, A9540
mebrofenin, A9537
medronate, A9503
mertiatide, A9562
oxidronate, A9561
pentetate, A9539, A9567
pertechnetate, A9512
sestamibi, A9500
sulfur colloid, A9541
teboroxime, A9501
tetrofosmin, A9502
tilmanocept, A9520
therapeutic, A9517, A9543, A9600, A9604
tumor identification, PET, A9597
xenon Xe 133, A9558
yttrium 90 ibritumomab tiuxetan, A9543
Rail
bathtub, E0241, E0242, E0246
bed, E0305, E0310
toilet, E0243
Rancho hip action, hip orthotic, L1680
Range of motion device
elbow, hand, wrist, L8702
shoulder, E1841
Rascal, power wheelchair, K0010
Ready-For-Use wooden crutches, E0113
Reassessment, nutrition therapy, G0270-G0271
Receiver
interstitial glucose monitor, A9278
Recombinant
ankle splints, L4392-L4398
DNA insulin, J1815, J1817
Reconstruction
breast, S2066-S2067
Rectal control system, A4563
Red blood cells, P9038-P9040
Red blood cells, each unit, P9021, P9022
Red Dot
crutches, E0114
folding walkers, E0135, E0143
Regulator, oxygen, E1353
Rehabilitation
intensive cardiac, G0422-G0423
program, H2001
pulmonary, G0424
service
juveniles, H2033

© 2019 Optum360, LLC

Rehabilitation — *continued*
service — *continued*
mental health clubhouse, H2030-H2031
psychosocial, H2017-H2018
social work and psychological, G0409
substance abuse, H2034-H2036
supported employment, H2023-H2024
vestibular, S9476
Removal
applicator, breast, C9726
corns/calluses, S0390
impacted cerumen, G0268
soft interspace, K0672
sutures, S0630
RemRes, E0601
REMStar, E0601
Renacidin, Q2004
RenAmin, parenteral nutrition, B5000
Renu, enteral nutrition, B4150
Repair
contract, ERSD, A4890
DME, K0739
oxygen, K0740
fetal
congenital malformation NOC, S2409
cystic adenomatoid malformation, S2402
extralobar pulmonary sequestration, S2403
myelomeningocele, S2404
sacrococcygeal teratoma, S2405
urinary tract, S2401
hearing aid, V5014, V5336
hernia
diaphragmatic
fetus, S2400
home dialysis equipment, A4890
nasal
vestibular lateral wall, C9749
orthotic, L4000-L4130
prosthetic, L7510, L7520
Replacement
battery, A4233-A4236, A4630
ear pulse generator, A4638
external infusion pump, K0601-K0605
cardioverter-defibrillator system, G0448
handgrip for cane, crutch, walker, A4636
oral cushion, A7028
ostomy filters, A4421
sleeve, intermittent limb compression device, A4600
tip for cane, crutch, walker, A4637
underarm pad for crutch, A4635
Rep-Pred
40, J1030
80, J1040
Repriza, Q4143
ResCap headgear, A7035
Reservoir
metered dose inhaler, A4627
Residential care, T2032-T2033
ResMed Sb Elite, E0601
Resource-intensive services
mobility-assistive technology, G0501
Respiratory therapy, G0237-G0238
home, S5180-S5181
Respite care, T1005
in home, S9125
not in home, H0045
Restorative
injection
face, G0429
Restorigin (fluid), Q4192
Restorigin, Q4191
Restraint
any type, E0710
belts
Posey, E0700
Secure-All, E0700
Bite disposable jaw locks, E0700
body holders
Houdini security suit, E0700
Quick Release, one piece, E0700
Restraint — *continued*
body holders — *continued*
Secure-All, one piece, E0700
System2 zippered, E0700
UltraCare vest-style
with sleeves, E0700
hand
Secure-All finger control mitt, E0700
limb holders
Posey, E0700
Quick Release, E0700
Secure-All, E0700
pelvic
Secure-All, E0700
Resurfacing
total hip, S2118
Retail therapy item, miscellaneous, T1999
Retinal
device, intraoperative, C1784
exam for diabetes, S3000
prosthesis, C1841-C1842
accessory/component/supply, L8608
tamponade, C1814
Retinoblastoma, genetic test, S3841
Retrieval device, insertable, C1773
Revascularization, percutaneous transluminal, C9604-C9608
Revita, Q4180
Revitalon, Q4157
Rib belt
thoracic, L0220
Rice ankle splint, L1904
Richfoam convoluted & flat overlays, E0199
Ride Lite 200, Ride Lite 9000, manual wheelchair, K0004
Ring, ostomy, A4404
Riveton, foot orthotic, L3140, L3150
RN services, T1002
Road Savage power wheelchair, K0011
Road Warrior power wheelchair, K0011
Robotic surgical system, S2900
Rocking bed, E0462
Rollabout chair, E1031
Rubidium RB-82, A9555
Rural health clinic (RHC)
behavioral health integration services, G0511
chronic care management services, G0511
psychiatric COCM services, G0512
technology based services, G0071

S

Sabre power wheelchair, K0011
Sacral nerve stimulation test
lead, each, A4290
Sacroiliac
injection, G0259-G0260
orthotic, L0621-L0624
Safe, hand prosthesis, L5972
Safety
enclosure frame/canopy, for hospital bed, E0316
equipment, E0700
eyeglass frames, S0516
vest, wheelchair, E0980
Saline, A4216-A4217
hypertonic, J7131
solution, J7030-J7050
Saliva
artificial, A9155
Saliva test, hormone level
during menopause, S3650
preterm labor risk, S3652
Sam Brown, Legg Perthes orthotic, A4565
Sansibar Plus, E0601
Saquinavir, S0140
Satumomab pendetide, A4642
Scale, for dialysis, E1639
Schuco
mist nebulizer system, E0570
vac aspirator, E0600
Scintimammography, S8080
Scleral application tantalum rings, S8030
Scleral lens bandage, S0515
Scoliosis, L1000, L1200, L1300-L1499
additions, L1010-L1120, L1210-L1290
Scott ankle splint, canvas, L1904
Scott-Craig, stirrup orthotic, L2260
Scottish-Rite, Legg Perthes orthotic, L1730
Screening
alcohol and/or drug, G0442, H0049
cervical or vaginal, G0101, G0476
Chlamydia, gonorrhea, syphilis, G9228-G9230
colorectal cancer, G0104-G0106, G0120-G0122
cytopathology, G0123-G0124, G0141, G0143-G0148
depression, G0444
early periodic screening diagnosis and treatment (EPSDT), S0302
glaucoma, G0117-G0118
gynecological
established patient, S0612
new patient, S0610
hepatitis B
non-pregnant, high-risk individual, G0499
hepatitis C antibody, high risk, G0472
HIV
antigen/antibody combination assay, G0475
HIV-1 or HIV-2, G0432-G0433, G0435
lung cancer
counseling visit to discuss CT screening, G0296
low dose CT scan (LDCT), G0297
newborn metabolic, S3620
ophthalmological, including refraction
established patient, S0621
new patient, S0620
pneumococcal, G9279
preadmission, T2010-T2011
proctoscopy, S0601
program participation, T1023
prostate
digital, rectal, G0102
prostate specific antigen test (PSA), G0103
vaccination not given, G9281
Seal, prosthetic socket insert, L7700
Sealant
pulmonary, liquid, C2615
skin, A6250
Seat
attachment, walker, E0156
insert, wheelchair, E0992
lift (patient), E0621, E0627-E0629
positioning, T5001
power system, wheelchair, E1002-E1012
Seattle Carbon Copy II, foot prosthesis, L5976
Secure-All
restraints, E0700
universal pelvic traction belt, E0890
Sedation, moderate, G0500
Sensitivity study, P7001
Sensor
invasive blood glucose monitor, A9276
pulmonary artery, wireless, C2624
Sensory nerve conduction test, G0255
Septal defect implant system, C1817
Sermorelin acetate, Q0515
Serum clotting time tube, A4771
Service assessment, T2024
Services
attendant, S5125-S5126
behavioral, H2019-H2020
by Christian Science practitioner, S9900-S9901
chore services, S5120-S5121
community support, H2015-H2016
community-based wrap-around, H2021-H2022
homemaker services, S5130-S5131
laundry, S5175
Medicare IVIG demonstration, Q2052
medication reminder, S5185
provided outside USA, S9989
psychoeducational, H2027
sexual offender treatment, H2028-H2029
SEWHO, L3960-L3962
Sexa, G0130
Sheath
introducer
guiding, C1766, C1892, C1893
other than guiding, C1894, C2629
Sheepskin pad, E0188, E0189
Shoes
arch support, L3040-L3100
for diabetics, A5500-A5508, A5510, A5512-A5513
insert, L3000-L3030
for diabetics, A5512-A5513
lift, L3300-L3334
miscellaneous additions, L3500-L3595
orthopedic (*see* Orthopedic shoes), L3201-L3265
positioning device, L3140-L3170
post-operative
Specialist Health/Post Operative Shoe, A9270
transfer, L3600-L3649
wedge, L3340-L3485
Shoulder
abduction positioner, L3999
braces, L3999
Masterhinge Shoulder Brace 3, L3999
disarticulation, prosthetic, L6300-L6320, L6550
orthotic (SO), L3650-L3677
spinal, cervical, L0112
Shoulder-elbow-wrist-hand orthotic (SEWHO), L3960-L3978
Shower chair, E0240
Shunt accessory for dialysis, A4740
aqueous, L8612
Sickle cell anemia, genetic test, S3850
Sierra wrist flexion unit, L6805
Sigmoidoscopy, cancer screening, G0104, G0106
Sign language or oral interpreter services, T1013
Sildenafil citrate, S0090
Silenzio Elite, E0601
Single bar "AK," ankle-foot orthotic, L2000, L2010
Single bar "BK," ankle-foot orthotic, L1980
Sinus
sinus implant (Mometasone), J7401
Sitz bath, E0160-E0162
Skilled nurse, G0128, G0493-G0496
Skin
barrier, ostomy, A4362, A4369, A4385
bond or cement, ostomy, A4364
gel protective dressing wipes, A5120
sealant, protectant, moisturizer, A6250
Skin substitute
Affinity, Q4159
AlloDerm, Q4116
AlloGen, Q4212
AlloPatch HD, Q4128
AlloSkin, Q4115
AlloSkin AC, Q4141
AlloSkin RT, Q4123
AlloWrap DS, Q4150
Amnio Bio, Q4211
AmnioArmor, Q4188
AmnioBand, Q4151, Q4168
AmnioExcel, AmnioExcel Plus, Q4137
AmnioMatrix, Q4139
AmnioPro, Q4163
AmnioPro Flow, Q4162
AmnioWound, Q4181
AmnioWrap2, Q4221
Apligraf, Q4101
Architect, Architect PX, or Architect FX, Q4147
Artacent AC (fluid), Q4189
Artacent AC, Q4190
Artacent Cord, Q4216
Artacent Wound, Q4169
ArthroFlex, Q4125
Ascent, Q4213
AxoBioMembrane, Q4211
Axolotl Ambient, Axolotl Cryo, Q4215
Axolotl Graft, Axolotl DualGraft, Q4210
BellaCell HD, Q4220
bio-ConneKt Wound Matrix, Q4161

© 2019 Optum360, LLC

Skin substitute — *continued*
BioDExcel, Q4137
BioDFence, Q4140
BioDFence DryFlex, Q4138
BioDMatrix, Q4139
BioSkin, Q4163
BioSkin Flow, Q4162
Biovance, Q4154
BioWound, BioWound Plus, BioWound Xplus, Q4217
Cellesta, Cellesta Duo, Q4184
Cellesta Cord, Q4214
Cellesta Flowable Amnion, Q4185
Clarix 100, Q4156
Clarix Cord, Q4148
Clarix Flo, Q4155
Coll-e-Derm, Q4193
Cygnus, Q4170
Cymetra, Q4112
Cytal, Q4166
DermACELL, DermACELL AWM, DermACELL AWM Porous, Q4122
Derma-Gide, Q4203
Dermagraft, Q4106
DermaPure, Q4152
DermaSpan, Q4126
Dermavest, Q4153
EpiCord, Q4187
EpiFix (injectable), Q4145
EpiFix, Q4186
Excellagen, Q4149
EZ-Derm, Q4136
Flex HD, Q4128
FlowerAmnioFlo, Q4177
FlowerAmnioPatch, Q4178
FlowerDerm, Q4179
Fluid Flow, Fluid GF, Q4206
GammaGraft, Q4111
Genesis Amniotic Membrane, Q4198
Grafix Core, GrafixPL Core, Q4132
Grafix Prime, GrafixPL Prime, Q4133
GRAFTJACKET, Q4107
GRAFTJACKET XPRESS, Q4113
Guardian, Q4151
Helicoll, Q4164
hMatrix, Q4134
Hyalomatrix, Q4117
Integra
Bilayer Matrix Wound Dressing, Q4104
Dermal Regeneration Template, Q4105
Flowable, Q4114
Matrix, Q4108
Meshed Bilayer Wound Matrix, C9363
MOZAIK Osteoconductive Scaffold Putty, C9359
MOZAIK Osteoconductive Scaffold Strip, C9362
IntegoPLY, Q4126
Interfyl, Q4171
Keramatrix, Kerasorb, Q4165
Kerecis Omega3, Q4158
Keroxx, Q4202
low cost, application of, C5271-C5278
Matrion, Q4201
MatriStem, Q4118
Matrix HD, Q4128
Mediskin, Q4135
Membrane Graft, Membrane Wrap, Q4205
MemoDerm, Q4126
Miroderm, Q4175
MyOwn Skin, Q4226
NeoPatch, Q4176
Neox 100, Q4156
Neox 1K, Neox Cord 1K, Neox Cord RT, Q4148
Neox Flo, Q4155
NovaFix, Q4208
NuShield, Q4160
Oasis
Burn Matrix, Q4103
Ultra Tri-Layer Matrix, Q4124
Wound Matrix, Q4102
PalinGen or PalinGen XPlus, Q4173

Skin substitute — *continued*
PalinGen or ProMatrX (fluid), Q4174
Plurivest, Q4153
PriMatrix, Q4110
ProgenaMatrix, Q4222
PuraPly, PuraPly AM, PuraPly XT, Q4195-Q4197
Repriza, Q4143
Restorigin (fluid), Q4192
Restorigin, Q4191
Revita, Q4180
Revitalon, Q4157
SkinTE, Q4200
Strattice, Q4130
Stravix, StravixPL, Q4133
SureDerm, Q4220
SurgiCORD, Q4218
SurgiGRAFT, Q4183
SurgiGRAFT-Dual, Q4219
SurgiMend, C9358
SurGraft, Q4209
Talymed, Q4127
Tensix, Q4146
TheraSkin, Q4121
TranCyte, Q4182
TranZgraft, Q4126
TruSkin, Q4167
WoundEx, Q4163
WoundEx Flow, Q4162
WoundFix, WoundFix Plus, WoundFix Xplus, Q4217
XCM Biologic Tissue Matrix, Q4142
XWRAP, Q4204
SkinTE, Q4200
Sleep apnea treatment, K1001
Sleep study
home, G0398-G0400
Sleeve
intermittent limb compression device, A4600
mastectomy, L8010
Sling, A4565
axilla, L1010
Legg Perthes, A4565
lumbar, L1090
patient lift, E0621, E0630, E0635
pelvic, L2580
Sam Brown, A4565
trapezius, L1070
Smoking cessation
classes, S9453
counseling, G9016
SNCT, G0255
Social worker
CORF, G0409
home health setting, G0155
nonemergency transport, A0160
visit in home, S9127
Sock
body sock, L0984
prosthetic sock, L8420-L8435, L8480, L8485
stump sock, L8470-L8485
Sodium
chromate Cr-51, A9553
ferric gluconate in sucrose, J2916
iothalamate I-125, A9554
sodium iodide I-131
diagnostic imaging agent, A9528, A9531
therapeutic agent, A9530
succinate, J1720
Soft Touch II lancet device, A4258
Soft Touch lancets, box of 100, A4259
Softclix lancet device, A4258
Solo Cast Sole, L3540
Solo LX, E0601
Solution
calibrator, A4256
dialysate, A4728, A4760
enteral formulae, B4150-B4155
parenteral nutrition, B4164-B5200
S.O.M.I. brace, L0190, L0200
S.O.M.I. multiple-post collar, cervical orthotic, L0190
Sorbent cartridge, ESRD, E1636
Sorbsan, alginate dressing, A6196-A6198

Source
brachytherapy
gold 198, C1716
iodine 125, C2638-C2639
non-high dose rate iridium 192, C1719
palladium-103, C2640-C2641, C2645
yttrium 90, C2616
Spacer
interphalangeal joint, L8658
Specialist Ankle Foot Orthotic, L1930
Specialist Closed-Back Cast Boot, L3260
Specialist Gaitkeeper Boot, L3260
Specialist Health/Post Operative Shoe, A9270
Specialist Heel Cups, L3485
Specialist Insoles, L3510
Specialist J-Splint Plaster Roll Immobilizer, A4580
Specialist Open-Back Cast Boot, L3260
Specialist Plaster Bandages, A4580
Specialist Plaster Roll Immobilizer, A4580
Specialist Plaster Splints, A4580
Specialist Pre-Formed Humeral Fracture Brace, L3980-L3981
Specialist Pre-Formed Ulnar Fracture Brace, L3982
Specialist Tibial Pre-formed Fracture Brace, L2116
Specialist Toe Insert for Specialist Closed-Back Cast Boot and Specialist Health/Post Operative Shoe, A9270
Specialized mobility technology
resource-intensive services, G0501
Specialty absorptive dressing, A6251-A6256
Specimen, G9291, G9295
Spectacles, S0504-S0510, S0516-S0518
dispensing, S0595
Speech and language pathologist
home health setting, G0153
Speech assessment, V5362-V5364
speech generating device
software, E2511
supplies, E2500-E2599
Speech generating device, E2500
Speech therapy, S9128, S9152
Spenco shoe insert, foot orthotic, L3001
Sperm
aspiration, S4028
donor service, S4025
sperm procurement, S4026, S4030-S4031
Sphygmomanometer/blood pressure, A4660
Spinal orthotic
Boston type, L1200
cervical, L0112, L0180-L0200
cervical-thoracic-lumbar-sacral orthotic (CTLSO), L0700, L0710, L1000
halo, L0810-L0830
Milwaukee, L1000
multiple post collar, L0180-L0200
scoliosis, L1000, L1200, L1300-L1499
torso supports, L0970-L0999
Spirometer
electronic, E0487
nonelectronic, A9284
Splint
ankle, L4392-L4398, S8451
digit, prefabricated, S8450
dynamic, E1800, E1805, E1810, E1815
elbow, S8452
finger, static, Q4049
footdrop, L4398
hallus valgus, L3100
long arm, Q4017-Q4020
long leg, L4370, Q4041-Q4044
pneumatic, L4350, L4360, L4370
short arm, Q4021-Q4024
short leg, Q4045-Q4048
Specialist Plaster Splints, A4580
supplies, Q4051
Thumb-O-Prene Splint, L3999
toad finger, A4570
wrist, S8451
Spoke protectors, each, K0065
Sports supports hinged knee support, L1832
Standing frame system, E0638, E0641-E0642
Star Lumen tubing, A4616

Stat
laboratory request, S3600-S3601
Sten, foot prosthesis, L5972
Stent
coated
with delivery system, C1874
without delivery system, C1875
with delivery system, C1876
without delivery system, C1877
noncoronary
temporary, C2617, C2625
Stent placement
intracoronary, C9600-C9601
with percutaneous transluminal coronary atherectomy, C9602-C9603
Stereotactic radiosurgery
therapy, G0339, G0340
Sterile water, A4216-A4218
Stimulated intrauterine insemination, S4035
Stimulation
electrical, E0740, G0281-G0283
acupuncture, S8930
electromagnetic, G0295
Stimulators
cough, device, E0482
electric, supplies, A4595
interferential current, S8130-S8131
joint, E0762
neuromuscular, E0744, E0745, E0764
osteogenesis, electrical, E0747-E0749
pelvic floor, E0740
salivary reflex, E0755
transcutaneous, E0770
ultrasound, E0760
Stocking
gradient compression, A6530-A6549
Stoma
cap, A5055
catheter, A5082
cone, A4399
plug, A5081
Stomach tube, B4083
Stomahesive
skin barrier, A4362, A5122
sterile wafer, A4362
strips, A4362
Storm Arrow power wheelchair, K0014
Storm Torque power wheelchair, K0011
Strattice, Q4130
Stravix, StravixPL, Q4133
Stress management class, S9454
Stretch device, E1801, E1811, E1816, E1818, E1831, E1841
Strip(s)
blood, A4253
glucose test, A4253, A4772
Nu-Hope
adhesive, 1 oz bottle with applicator, A4364
adhesive, 3 oz bottle with applicator, A4364
urine reagent, A4250
Stroke, G9257-G9258
Study
gastrointestinal fat absorption, S3708
sleep, G0398-G0400
Stump sock, L8470-L8485
Stylet, A4212
Substance abuse
ambulatory settings, S9475
assessment, G2011
other than tobacco, G0396-G0397
treatment, T1006-T1012
Suction
wound, A9272, K0743
Sulfamethoxazole and trimethoprim, S0039
Sullivan
CPAP, E0601
Sumacal, enteral nutrition, B4155
Sunbeam moist/dry heat pad, E0215
Sunglass frames, S0518
Supplies
infection control NOS, S8301
insulin pump, external, A4226

Supplies — *continued*
Medicare IVIG demonstration, Q2052
miscellaneous DME, A9999
ventricular assist device, Q0477, Q0507-Q0509
Supply allowance
continuous glucose monitor, K0553
Supply fee
pharmacy
anticancer oral antiemetic or immunosuppressive drug, Q0511-Q0512
immunosuppressive drugs, Q0510
Supply/accessory/service, A9900
Support
arch, L3040-L3090
cervical, L0120
elastic, A6530-A6549
ongoing to maintain employment, H2025-H2026
spinal, L0970-L0999
vaginal, A4561-A4562
Supported housing, H0043-H0044
Supportive device
foot pressure off loading, A9283
Supreme bG Meter, E0607
SureDerm, Q4220
Sure-Gait folding walker, E0141, E0143
Sure-Safe raised toilet seat, E0244
SureStep blood glucose monitor, E0607
Sur-Fit
closed-end pouch, A5054
disposable convex inserts, A5093
drainable pouch, A5063
flange cap, A5055
irrigation sleeve, A4397
urostomy pouch, A5073
Sur-Fit/Active Life tail closures, A4421
Surgical
arthroscopy
knee, G0289, S2112
shoulder, S2300
boot, L3208-L3211
mask, for dialysis, A4928
procedure, return/no return to OR, G9307-G9308
site infection, G9311-G9312
stocking, A4490-A4510
supplies, miscellaneous, A4649
tray, A4550
SurgiCORD, Q4218
SurgiGRAFT, Q4183
SurgiGRAFT-Dual, Q4219
SurgiMend, fetal bovine, C9358
SurgiMend, neonatal bovine, C9360
SurGraft, Q4209
Survival, G9259, G9261, G9263
Sustacal, enteral nutrition, B4150
HC, B4152
Sustagen Powder, enteral nutrition, B4150
Swabs, betadine or iodine, A4247
Swede, ACT, Cross, or Elite manual wheelchair, K0005
Swede Basic F# manual wheelchair, K0004
Swedish knee orthotic, L1850
Swivel adaptor, S8186
Syringe, A4213
dialysis, A4657
insulin, box of 100, S8490
with needle, A4206-A4209
System2 zippered body holder, E0700

T

Table
bed, E0274, E0315
sit-to-stand, E0637
standing, E0637-E0638, E0641-E0642
Tachdijan, Legg Perthes orthotic, L1720
Talymed, Q4127
Tamoxifen citrate, S0187
Tamponade
retinal, C1814
Tantalum rings scleral application, S8030
Tape
nonwaterproof, A4450
waterproof, A4452
Taxi, nonemergency transportation, A0100
Tc-99 from non-highly enriched uranium, Q9969
Team conference, G0175, G9007, S0220-S0221
TechneScan, A9512
Technetium Tc 99
arcitumomab, A9568
biscate, A9557
depreotide, A9536
disofenin, A9510
exametazime, A9521, A9569
fanolesomab, A9566
glucepatate, A9550
labeled red blood cells, A9560
macroaggregated albumin, A9540
mebrofenin, A9537
medronate, A9503
mertiatide, A9562
oxidronate, A9561
pentetate, A9539, A9567
pertechretate, A9512
pyrophosphate, A9538
sestamibi, A9500
succimer, A9551
sulfur colloid, A9541
teboroxime, A9501
tetrofosmin, A9502
tilmanocept, A9520
Technol
Colles splint, L3763
wrist and forearm splint, L3906
Technology based services
FQHC or RHC, G0071
Telehealth
consultation
emergency department, G0425-G0427
inpatient, G0406-G0408, G0425-G0427
critical care, G0508-G0509
facility fee, Q3014
inpatient pharmacologic management, G0459
transmission, T1014
Telemonitoring
patient in home, includes equipment, S9110
Television
amplifier, V5270
caption decoder, V5271
TenderCloud electric air pump, E0182
TenderFlo II, E0187
TenderGel II, E0196
Tenderlet lancet device, A4258
TenoGlide Tendon Protector Sheet, C9356
TENS, A4595, E0720-E0749
Neuro-Pulse, E0720
Tensix, Q4146
Tent, oxygen, E0455
Terminal devices, L6703-L6715, L6721-L6722
Terumo disposable insulin syringes, up to 1 cc, per syringe, A4206
Test materials, home monitoring, G0249
Testing
comparative genomic hybridization, S3870
developmental, G0451
drug, G0480-G0483, G0659
genetic, S3800, S3840-S3842, S3844-S3846, S3849-S3850, S3852-S3853, S3861
Warfarin responsiveness, genetic technique, G9143
Thalassemia, genetic test
alpha, S3845
hemoglobin E beta, S3846
Thallous chloride Tl 201, A9505
Therapeutic
agent, A4321
procedures, respiratory, G0239
Therapeutic radiopharmaceutical
sodium iodide I-131, A9530
Therapy
activity, G0176, H2032
beta-blocker, G9188-G9192
convulsive, G2000
infusion, Q0081
lymphedema, S8950
Therapy — *continued*
nutrition, reassessment, G0270-G0271
respiratory, G0237-G0239
TheraSkin, Q4121
Thermalator T-12-M, E0239
Thermometer
oral, A4931
rectal, A4932
Thickener, food, B4100
Thinning solvent, NuHope, 2 oz bottle, A4455
Thomas
heel wedge, foot orthotic, L3465, L3470
Thoracic-lumbar-sacral orthotic (TLSO)
flexible with trunk support, L0450-L0457
sagittal control, L0466-L0467
sagittal-coronal control, L0468-L0469, L0490-L0492
scoliosis, L1200-L1290
triplanar control, L0458-L0464, L0470-L0488
Threshold
current perception, G0255
Thumb-O-Prene Splint, L3999
Thymol turbidity, blood, P2033
Thyrotropin
alpha, J3240
Tibia
Specialist Tibial Pre-formed Fracture Brace, L2116
Toad finger splint, A4570
Ticarcillin disodium and clavulanate potassium, S0040
Tip (cane, crutch, walker) replacement, A4637
Tire, wheelchair, E2214, E2220
Tissue
connective
human, C1762
non-human, C1763
localization and excision device, C1819
marker, A4648
Tissue marker, A4648
TLSO, L0450-L0492, L1200-L1290
Tobramycin
inhalation solution, J7682, J7685
sulfate, J3260
unit dose, J7682
Toe
holder, E0952
Specialist Toe Insert for Specialist Closed-Back Cast Boot and Specialist Health/Post Operative Shoe, A9270
Toilet accessories, E0167-E0175, E0243, E0244, E0625
raised toilet seat, E0244
Combo-Seat Universal, E0244
Moore, E0244
Sure-Safe, E0244
seat lift, E0172
transfer bench, E0247, E0248
Toll, non-emergency transport, A0170
Tomosynthesis, diagnostic, G0279
Topical hyperbaric oxygen chamber, A4575
Topographic brain mapping, S8040
Toronto, Legg Perthes orthotic, L1700
Total hip resurfacing, S2118
Total Universal Buck's Boot, E0870
Tourniquet, for dialysis, A4929
TPN, home infusion therapy, S9364-S9368
Tracer blood glucose
meter, E0607
strips, box of 50, A4253
Tracer II Diabetes Care System, E0607
Tracer Wheelchairs, E1240, E1250, E1260, E1270, E1280, E1285, E1290, E1295
Tracheal suction catheter, A4624
Tracheoesophageal prosthesis supplies, L8511-L8514
Tracheostoma
adhesive disc, A7506
filter, A7504
filter holder, A7503, A7507, A7509
housing, A7505, A7508
replacement diaphragm, faceplate, A7502
valve, A7501
Tracheostomy
care kit, A4629
Tracheostomy — *continued*
filter, A4481
mask, A7525
speaking valve, L8501
supplies, A4623-A4626, A4628, A4629, A7523-A7526, S8189
tube, A7520-A7522
Traction equipment, E0840-E0948
cervical equipment
not requiring frame, E0855
stand or frame, E0849
device
cervical, E0856
extremity, E0870, E0880
Total Universal Buck's Boot, E0870
head harness/halter, cervical, E0942
occipital-pull head halter, E0942
overdoor, cervical, E0860
Exo-Static, E0860
pelvic, E0890, E0900
Secure-All universal, belt, E0890
Training
child development, T1027
diabetes, G0108, G0109
home care, S5108-S5116
INR monitoring device, G0248
medication, H0034
skills, H2014
Tramacal, enteral nutrition, B4154
TranCyte, Q4182
Transbronchial ablation, C9751
Transcutaneous electrical nerve stimulator (TENS), E0720-E0749
Transducer protector, dialysis, E1575
Transesophageal doppler, G9157
Transfer (shoe orthoses), L3600-L3640
Transfer board or device, E0705
Transfer system, E1036
Transfusion, blood products, at home, S9538
Transmitter
interstitial glucose monitor, A9277
Transmitting coil/cable, L8629
Transparent film (for dressing), A6257-A6259
Transplant
autologous chondrocyte, J7330
bone marrow, allogeneic, S2150
islet cell, G0341-G0343
islet cell tissue, allogeneic, S2102
lobar lung, S2060
multivisceral organs, S2054
pancreas/kidney, S2065
renal, documentation, G9231
small intestine and liver allografts, S2053
stem cell, S2142
Transport chair, E1037-E1038
heavy weight, E1039
Transportation
ambulance, A0021-A0999
corneal tissue, V2785
EKG (portable), R0076
extra attendant, A0424
handicapped, A0130
nonemergency, A0080-A0210, T2001-T2005, T2049
mileage, S0215
parking fees, A0170
service, including ambulance, A0021-A0999
taxi, nonemergency, A0100
toll, nonemergency, A0170
volunteer, nonemergency, A0080, A0090
waiting time, T2007
x-ray (portable), R0070, R0075
TranZgraft, Q4126
Trapeze bar, E0910-E0912, E0940
Trauma response team, G0390
Traum-aid, enteral nutrition, B4154
Travasorb, enteral nutrition, B4150
Hepatic, B4154
HN, B4153
MCT, B4154
Renal, B4154
Travel allowance, P9603-P9604
Traveler manual wheelchair, K0001
Tray
insertion, A4310-A4316, A4354
irrigation, A4320

© 2019 Optum360, LLC

Tray — *continued*
surgical (*see also* kits), A4550
wheelchair, E0950
Treatment
fracture
pelvic bone, G0412-G0415
nursing facility acute care, G9679-G9684
outpatient IV insulin, G9147
Treatment planning and care coordination
cancer, S0353-S0354
comprehensive, advanced illness, S0311
Trifocal, glass or plastic, V2300-V2399
Trim nails, G0127
Truform prosthetic shrinker, L8440-L8465
TruSkin, Q4167
Truss, L8300-L8330
Tub
transfer bench, E0247-E0248
Tube/Tubing
anchoring device, A5200
blood, A4750, A4755
chest
drain valve, A7040
drainage container, A7041
CPAP device, A7037
gastrostomy/jejunostomy, B4087-B4088
irrigation, A4355
microcapillary, calibrated, A4651
sealant, A4652
nasogastric, B4081, B4082
oxygen, A4616
serum clotting time, A4771
stomach, B4083
suction pump, each, A7002
tire, E2212-E2213, E2215
tracheostomy or laryngotomy plug, A7527
urinary drainage, A4331
with integrated heating element, A4604
Tumor
destruction
embolization, S2095
infiltrating lymphocyte therapy, S2107
Turtle Neck safety collars, E0942

U

Ulcers
electromagnetic therapy, G0329
Ultra Blood Glucose
monitor, E0607
test strips, box of 50, A4253
UltraCare vest-style body holder, E0700
Ultrafast computed tomography, S8092
Ultrafine disposable insulin syringes, per syringe, A4206
Ultralightweight wheelchair, K0005
Ultrasound
ablation, C9734
prostate, C9747
uterine, C9734
aerosol generator, E0574
guidance
multifetal pregnancy reduction, S8055
radiation therapy field placement, G6001
paranasal sinus, S9024
therapeutic intervention, C9734
Ultraviolet light-therapy
bulb, A4633
cabinet, E0691-E0694
system panel, E0691-E0693
Underpads, disposable, A4554
Unilet lancet device, A4258
Unipuncture control system, dialysis, E1580
Unistik lancet device, A4258
Universal
remover for adhesives, A4455
socket insert
above knee, L5694
below knee, L5690
telescoping versarail bed rail, E0310
Up-Draft Neb-U-Mist, E0580
Upper extremity addition, locking elbow, L6693
Upper extremity fracture orthotic, L3980-L3999
Upper limb prosthesis, L6000-L7499
Ureteroscopy
for ureteral calculi, S2070
Urethral clamp/compression device, A4360
Urethral insert, A4336
Urgent care, S9088
global fee, S9083
Urinal, E0325, E0326
Urinary
catheter, A4338-A4346, A4351-A4353
catheter irrigation, A4321
collection and retention (supplies), A4310-A4358
incontinence repair device, C1771, C2631
incontinence supplies, A4310-A4421, A4423-A4434, A5051-A5093, A5102-A5114, A5120-A5200
leg bag, A5105, A5112
tract implant, collagen, L8603
Urine
collector, A4335
sensitivity study, P7001
tests, A4250
Urostomy pouch, A5073
USMC
hinged Swedish knee cage, L1850
universal knee immobilizer, L1830
U-V lens, V2755
Uvulopalatoplasty, laser assisted, S2080

V

V Elite, E0601
Vabra aspirator, A4480
Vaccination, administration
hepatitis B, G0010
influenza virus, G0008
pneumococcal, G0009, G9279
Not Given
Before Discharge, G9280
Not Indicated, G9281
Refused, G9281
Vacuum erection system, L7900
tension ring replacement, L7902
Vaginal
contraceptive ring, J7303
Vaporizer, E0605
Vascular
catheter (appliances and supplies), A4300-A4306
closure device, C1760
synthetic, L8670
Venous thromboembolism prophylaxis, G9298-G9299
Vent
ostomy, A4366
Ventilator
battery, A4611-A4613
home
any type with invasive interface, E0465
any type with non-invasive interface, E0466
multifunction, E0467
moisture exchanger, disposable, A4483
Ventilator tray
wheelchair, E1029-E1030
Ventricular assist device
accessory, Q0507-Q0509
battery, Q0496, Q0503
charger, Q0495
clips, Q0497
belt, Q0499
driver, Q0480
emergency
hand pump, Q0494
power cable, Q0492-Q0493
power source, Q0490-Q0491
filter, Q0500
holster, Q0498
leads, Q0487-Q0488
microprocessor control unit, Q0481-Q0482
miscellaneous supply, Q0503, Q0507-Q0509
mobility cart, Q0502
monitor
control cable, Q0485-Q0486
Ventricular assist device — *continued*
monitor — *continued*
display module, Q0483-Q0484
power
back base, Q0489
adapter, Q0504
emergency
power source, Q0490-Q0491
power supply cable, Q0492-Q0493
module, cable, Q0477
power adapter/module, Q0478-Q0479
shower cover, Q0501
supply, Q0507-Q0509, Q0507-Q0509
vest, Q0499
Versa-Pole IV pole, E0776
Vertebral axial decompression, S9090
Vest, E0980
safety, wheelchair, E0980
ventricular assist device, Q0499
Vestibular rehabilitation, S9476
Viral load , G9242-G9243
Visi wheelchair tray, E0950
Visi-flow
irrigation, A4367, A4397, A4398, A4399, A4402, A4421
stoma cone, A4399
Vision service, S0500-S0592, V2020-V2799
Visit
emergency department
established patient, G0467
type B, G0380-G0384
FQHC
behavioral health integration services, G0511
chronic care management services, G0511
established patient, G0467
IPPE or AWV, G0468
mental health, established patient, G0470
mental health, new patient, G0469
new patient, G0466
psychiatric COCM services, G0512
technology based services, G0071
home by nurse practitioner, S0274
home by physician, S0273
hospital outpatient clinic, G0463
medical, G9246-G9247
FQHC established patient, G0467
FQHC IPPE or AWV, G0468
FQHC mental health, established patient, G0470
FQHC mental health, new patient, G0469
FQHC new patient, G0466
nurse home, T1031
RHC
behavioral health integration services, G0511
chronic care management services, G0511
psychiatric COCM services, G0512
technology based services, G0071
Vitajet, A4210
Vital HN, enteral nutrition, B4153
Vitamin
multiple, A9153
prenatal 30-day supply, S0197
single, A9152
supplement in ESRD, S0194
Vivonex, enteral nutrition
HN, B4153
T.E.N., B4153
Vocal cord
chemodenervation, S2341
injectable bulking agent, L8607
medialization material, implantable, C1878
Voice amplifier, L8510
Von Hippel-Lindau disease, genetic test, S3842
Von Rosen, hip orthotic, L1630
Vortex power wheelchair, K0014
VPlus, E0601

W

Waiver services, T2024-T2041
Walker, E0130-E0144
accessories, A4636, A4637
attachments, E0153-E0159
enclosed with wheels, E0144
folding
Auto-Glide, E0143
Easy Care, E0143
framed with wheels, E0144
heavy duty
with wheels, E0148
without wheels, E0149
heavy duty, multiple braking system, E0141
One-Button, E0143
Quik-Fold, E0141, E0143
Red Dot, E0135, E0143
Sure-Gait, E0141, E0143
Water
ambulance, A0429
distilled (for nebulizer), A7018
for nebulizer, A7018
pressure pad/mattress, E0187, E0198
purification system (ESRD), E1610, E1615
softening system (ESRD), E1625
treated, A4714
Water chamber
humidifier, A7046
Wedge, positioning, E0190
Wedges, shoe, L3340-L3420
Weight management class, S9449
Wellness
annual visit, G0438-G0439
assessment, S5190
Wet mount, Q0111
Wheel attachment, rigid pickup walker, E0155
Wheelchair, E0950-E1298, K0001-K0108
accessories, E0950-E1031, E1036-E1295, E2358-E2359, E2398, E2627-E2633
elevating legrest, E0990, K0046-K0047, K0195
wheel lock, E2206
tray, E0950
Visi, E0950
amputee, E1170-E1200
base, E2358-E2359, E2627-E2633, K0008, K0013
battery, E2358-E2359, E2397, K0733
bearings, any type, E2210
braking system and lock, E2228
component or accessory, NOS, K0108
control hand or chin, E2373-E2374
controller, E2375-E2377
crutch and cane holder, E2207
cushion
back, E2291, E2293, E2605, E2606, E2608-E2617, E2620, E2621
custom, E2609
seat, E2610, E2622-E2625
general, E2601, E2602
positioning, E2605, E2606, E2607
replacement cover, E2619
skin protection, E2603, E2604, E2607, E2622-E2625
cylinder tank carrier, E2208
elevating proximal arm, E2631
foot box, E0954
hand rim, E0967, E2205
heavy-duty
shock absorber, E1015-E1016
Tracer, E1280, E1285, E1290, E1295
lightweight, E1240-E1270
EZ Lite, E1250
Tracer, E1240, E1250, E1260, E1270
manual, adult, E1161
accessories, E2201-E2295, E2300-E2392, E2394-E2397
motorized, E1239, K0010-K0898
narrowing device, E0969
pediatric, E1229, E1231-E1238
back
contoured, E2293
planar, E2291
modification, E1011
power, E1239
power, NOS, E1239

© 2019 Optum360, LLC

Wheelchair — *continued*
pediatric — *continued*
seat
contoured, E2294
planar, E2292
power, accessories, E2300-E2397, E2378, E2394-E2397, K0098
battery, E2358-E2359
gear box, E2369
motor, E2368
motor and gear box, E2370
power seating system
addition to power seating system
leg elevation system
center mount, complete, any type, each, E1012
mechanically linked, including pushrod and legrest, each, E1009
power, including legrest, pair, E1010
recline only
with mechanical shear reduction, E1004
with power shear reduction, E1005
without shear reduction, E1003
tilt and recline
with mechanical shear reduction, E1007
with power shear reduction, E1008

Wheelchair — *continued*
power seating system — *continued*
tilt and recline — *continued*
without shear reduction, E1006
tilt only, E1002
reclining back, E1014
residual limb support, E1020
rocker arm, E2632
seat or back cushion, K0669
specially sized, E1220-E1230
supinator, E2633
support, E0953-E0954, E1020, E2626-E2633
tire, E2211, E2214, E2220-E2222, E2381-E2392
transfer board or device, E0705
transport chair, E1037-E1038
van, nonemergency, A0130, S0209
wheel, E2227, E2394-E2395
wheel drive, E0988
WHFO, with inflatable air chamber, L3807
Whirlpool equipment, E1300-E1310, K1003
Wig, A9282
Wipes, A4245, A4247
Adhesive remover, A4456
Allkare protective barrier, A5120
Wire, guide, C1769
WIZZ-ard manual wheelchair, K0006
Wooden canes, E0100
Wound
cleanser, A6260
cover
alginate dressing, A6196-A6198
collagen dressing, A6021-A6024
foam dressing, A6209-A6214
hydrocolloid dressing, A6234-A6239

Wound — *continued*
cover — *continued*
hydrogel dressing, A6242-A6248
packing strips, A6407
specialty absorptive dressing, A6251-A6256
warming card, E0232
warming device, E0231
non-contact warming cover, A6000
electrical stimulation, E0769
filler
alginate, A6199
foam, A6215
gel/paste, A6011
hydrocolloid, A6240-A6241
hydrogel, A6242-A6248
not elsewhere classified, A6261-A6262
healing
other growth factor preparation, S9055
matrix, Q4100-Q4204
packing strips, A6407
pouch, A6154
warming device, E0231
cover, A6000
warming card, E0232
suction, A9272
suction pump, K0743
therapy
negative pressure supplies, A6550
Wound matrix, Q4100-Q4226
WoundEx, Q4163
WoundEx Flow, Q4162

WoundFix, WoundFix Plus, WoundFix Xplus, Q4217
Wrap
abdominal aneurysm, M0301
cold/heat, A9273
compression, A6545
Wrist
brace, cock-up, L3908
disarticulation prosthesis, L6050, L6055
hand/finger orthotic (WHFO), E1805, E1825, L3806-L3808
Specialist Pre-Formed Ulnar Fracture Brace, L3982

X

Xcaliber power wheelchair, K0014
XCM Biologic Tissue Matrix, Q4142
Xenon Xe-133, A9558
X-ray
equipment
portable, Q0092, R0070, R0075
XWRAP, Q4204

Y

Y set tubing for peritoneal dialysis, A4719
Yttrium 90
ibritumomab tiuxeton, A9543
microsphere
brachytherapy, C2616
procedure, S2095

Z

ZIFT, S4014

© 2019 Optum360, LLC

Transportation Services Including Ambulance A0021-A0999

This code range includes ground and air ambulance, nonemergency transportation (taxi, bus, automobile, wheelchair van), and ancillary transportation-related fees.

HCPCS Level II codes for ambulance services must be reported with modifiers that indicate pick-up origins and destinations. The modifier describing the arrangement (QM, QN) is listed first. The modifiers describing the origin and destination are listed second. Origin and destination modifiers are created by combining two alpha characters from the following list. Each alpha character, with the exception of X, represents either an origin or a destination. Each pair of alpha characters creates one modifier. The first position represents the origin and the second the destination. The modifiers most commonly used are:

D	Diagnostic or therapeutic site other than "P" or "H" when these are used as origin codes
E	Residential, domiciliary, custodial facility (other than 1819 facility)
G	Hospital-based ESRD facility
H	Hospital
I	Site of transfer (e.g., airport or helicopter pad) between modes of ambulance transport
J	Free standing ESRD facility
N	Skilled nursing facility (SNF)
P	Physician's office
R	Residence
S	Scene of accident or acute event
X	Intermediate stop at physician's office on way to hospital (destination code only)

Note: Modifier X can only be used as a destination code in the second position of a modifier. See S0215. For Medicaid, see T codes and T modifiers.

Ambulance Transport and Supplies

A0021 **Ambulance service, outside state per mile, transport (Medicaid only)** E
CMS: 100-04,15,20.4

A0080 **Nonemergency transportation, per mile - vehicle provided by volunteer (individual or organization), with no vested interest** E
CMS: 100-04,15,20.4

A0090 **Nonemergency transportation, per mile - vehicle provided by individual (family member, self, neighbor) with vested interest** E
CMS: 100-04,15,20.4

A0100 **Nonemergency transportation; taxi** E
CMS: 100-04,15,20.4

A0110 **Nonemergency transportation and bus, intra- or interstate carrier** E
CMS: 100-04,15,20.4

A0120 **Nonemergency transportation: mini-bus, mountain area transports, or other transportation systems** E
CMS: 100-04,15,20.4

A0130 **Nonemergency transportation: wheelchair van** E
CMS: 100-04,15,20.4

A0140 **Nonemergency transportation and air travel (private or commercial) intra- or interstate** E
CMS: 100-04,15,20.4

A0160 **Nonemergency transportation: per mile - caseworker or social worker** E
CMS: 100-04,15,20.4

A0170 **Transportation ancillary: parking fees, tolls, other** E
CMS: 100-04,15,20.4

A0180 **Nonemergency transportation: ancillary: lodging-recipient** E
CMS: 100-04,15,20.4

A0190 **Nonemergency transportation: ancillary: meals, recipient** E
CMS: 100-04,15,20.4

A0200 **Nonemergency transportation: ancillary: lodging, escort** E
CMS: 100-04,15,20.4

A0210 **Nonemergency transportation: ancillary: meals, escort** E
CMS: 100-04,15,20.4

A0225 **Ambulance service, neonatal transport, base rate, emergency transport, one way** E
CMS: 100-02,10,10.1.2; 100-02,10,10.2.1; 100-02,10,30.1; 100-02,10,30.1.1; 100-04,15,20.4

A0380 **BLS mileage (per mile)** E ☑
See code(s): A0425
CMS: 100-02,10,10.1.2; 100-02,10,10.2.1; 100-02,10,10.3.3; 100-02,10,30.1; 100-02,10,30.1.1; 100-04,15,20.4; 100-04,15,30.2

A0382 **BLS routine disposable supplies** E
CMS: 100-02,10,10.1.2; 100-02,10,10.2.1; 100-02,10,30.1; 100-02,10,30.1.1; 100-04,15,20.4

A0384 **BLS specialized service disposable supplies; defibrillation (used by ALS ambulances and BLS ambulances in jurisdictions where defibrillation is permitted in BLS ambulances)** E
CMS: 100-02,10,10.1.2; 100-02,10,10.2.1; 100-02,10,30.1; 100-02,10,30.1.1; 100-04,15,20.4

A0390 **ALS mileage (per mile)** E ☑
See code(s): A0425
CMS: 100-02,10,10.1.2; 100-02,10,10.2.1; 100-02,10,10.3.3; 100-02,10,30.1; 100-02,10,30.1.1; 100-04,15,20.4; 100-04,15,30.2

A0392 **ALS specialized service disposable supplies; defibrillation (to be used only in jurisdictions where defibrillation cannot be performed in BLS ambulances)** E
CMS: 100-02,10,10.1.2; 100-02,10,10.2.1; 100-02,10,30.1; 100-02,10,30.1.1; 100-04,15,20.4

A0394 **ALS specialized service disposable supplies; IV drug therapy** E
CMS: 100-02,10,10.1.2; 100-02,10,10.2.1; 100-02,10,30.1; 100-02,10,30.1.1; 100-04,15,20.4

A0396 **ALS specialized service disposable supplies; esophageal intubation** E
CMS: 100-02,10,10.1.2; 100-02,10,10.2.1; 100-02,10,30.1; 100-02,10,30.1.1; 100-04,15,20.4

A0398 **ALS routine disposable supplies** E
CMS: 100-02,10,10.1.2; 100-02,10,10.2.1; 100-02,10,30.1; 100-02,10,30.1.1; 100-04,15,20.4

Waiting Time

Units	Time
1	1/2 to 1 hr.
2	1 to 1-1/2 hrs.
3	1-1/2 to 2 hrs.
4	2 to 2-1/2 hrs.
5	2-1/2 to 3 hrs.
6	3 to 3-1/2 hrs.
7	3-1/2 to 4 hrs.
8	4 to 4-1/2 hrs.
9	4-1/2 to 5 hrs.
10	5 to 5-1/2 hrs.

A0420 **Ambulance waiting time (ALS or BLS), one-half (1/2) hour increments** E
CMS: 100-02,10,10.1.2; 100-02,10,10.2.1; 100-02,10,30.1; 100-02,10,30.1.1; 100-04,15,20.4

© 2019 Optum360, LLC

Other Ambulance Services

A0422 **Ambulance (ALS or BLS) oxygen and oxygen supplies, life sustaining situation** E
CMS: 100-02,10,10.1.2; 100-02,10,10.2.1; 100-02,10,30.1; 100-02,10,30.1.1; 100-04,15,20.4

A0424 **Extra ambulance attendant, ground (ALS or BLS) or air (fixed or rotary winged); (requires medical review)** E
Pertinent documentation to evaluate medical appropriateness should be included when this code is reported.
CMS: 100-02,10,10.1.2; 100-02,10,10.2.1; 100-02,10,30.1; 100-02,10,30.1.1; 100-04,15,20.4; 100-04,15,30.2.1

A0425 **Ground mileage, per statute mile** A ☑
CMS: 100-02,10,10.1.2; 100-02,10,10.2.1; 100-02,10,10.2.2; 100-02,10,10.3.3; 100-02,10,20; 100-02,10,30.1; 100-02,10,30.1.1; 100-02,10.20; 100-04,15,10.3; 100-04,15,20.1.4; 100-04,15,20.4; 100-04,15,20.6; 100-04,15,30; 100-04,15,30.1.2; 100-04,15,30.2.1; 100-04,15,40
AHA: 4Q, '12, 1

A0426 **Ambulance service, advanced life support, nonemergency transport, level 1 (ALS 1)** A
CMS: 100-02,10,10.1.2; 100-02,10,10.2.1; 100-02,10,10.2.2; 100-02,10,10.3.3; 100-02,10,20; 100-02,10,30.1; 100-02,10,30.1.1; 100-02,10.20; 100-04,15,10.3; 100-04,15,20.1.4; 100-04,15,20.4; 100-04,15,30; 100-04,15,30.1.2; 100-04,15,30.2; 100-04,15,30.2.1; 100-04,15,40
AHA: 4Q, '12, 1

A0427 **Ambulance service, advanced life support, emergency transport, level 1 (ALS 1 - emergency)** A
CMS: 100-02,10,10.1.2; 100-02,10,10.2.1; 100-02,10,10.2.2; 100-02,10,10.3.3; 100-02,10,20; 100-02,10,30.1; 100-02,10,30.1.1; 100-02,10.20; 100-04,15,10.3; 100-04,15,20.1.4; 100-04,15,20.4; 100-04,15,30; 100-04,15,30.1.2; 100-04,15,30.2; 100-04,15,30.2.1; 100-04,15,40
AHA: 4Q, '12, 1

A0428 **Ambulance service, basic life support, nonemergency transport, (BLS)** A
CMS: 100-02,10,10.1.2; 100-02,10,10.2.1; 100-02,10,10.2.2; 100-02,10,10.3.3; 100-02,10,20; 100-02,10,30.1; 100-02,10,30.1.1; 100-02,10.20; 100-04,15,10.3; 100-04,15,20.1.4; 100-04,15,20.4; 100-04,15,20.6; 100-04,15,30; 100-04,15,30.1.2; 100-04,15,30.2; 100-04,15,30.2.1; 100-04,15,40
AHA: 4Q, '12, 1

A0429 **Ambulance service, basic life support, emergency transport (BLS, emergency)** A
CMS: 100-02,10,10.1.2; 100-02,10,10.2.1; 100-02,10,10.2.2; 100-02,10,10.3.3; 100-02,10,20; 100-02,10,30.1; 100-02,10,30.1.1; 100-02,10.20; 100-04,15,10.3; 100-04,15,20.1.4; 100-04,15,20.4; 100-04,15,30; 100-04,15,30.1.2; 100-04,15,30.2; 100-04,15,30.2.1; 100-04,15,40
AHA: 4Q, '12, 1

A0430 **Ambulance service, conventional air services, transport, one way (fixed wing)** A
CMS: 100-02,10,10.1.2; 100-02,10,10.2.1; 100-02,10,10.2.2; 100-02,10,10.3.3; 100-02,10,20; 100-02,10,30.1; 100-02,10,30.1.1; 100-02,10.20; 100-04,15,10.3; 100-04,15,20.1.4; 100-04,15,20.3; 100-04,15,20.4; 100-04,15,30; 100-04,15,30.1.2; 100-04,15,30.2; 100-04,15,30.2.1; 100-04,15,40
AHA: 4Q, '12, 1

A0431 **Ambulance service, conventional air services, transport, one way (rotary wing)** A
CMS: 100-02,10,10.1.2; 100-02,10,10.2.1; 100-02,10,10.2.2; 100-02,10,10.3.3; 100-02,10,20; 100-02,10,30.1; 100-02,10,30.1.1; 100-02,10.20; 100-04,15,10.3; 100-04,15,20.1.4; 100-04,15,20.3; 100-04,15,20.4; 100-04,15,30; 100-04,15,30.1.2; 100-04,15,30.2; 100-04,15,30.2.1; 100-04,15,40
AHA: 4Q, '12, 1

A0432 **Paramedic intercept (PI), rural area, transport furnished by a volunteer ambulance company which is prohibited by state law from billing third-party payers** A
CMS: 100-02,10,10.1.2; 100-02,10,10.2.1; 100-02,10,10.2.2; 100-02,10,10.3.3; 100-02,10,20; 100-02,10,30.1; 100-02,10,30.1.1; 100-02,10.20; 100-04,15,10.3; 100-04,15,20.1.4; 100-04,15,20.4; 100-04,15,30; 100-04,15,30.1.2; 100-04,15,30.2; 100-04,15,30.2.1; 100-04,15,40
AHA: 4Q, '12, 1

A0433 **Advanced life support, level 2 (ALS 2)** A
CMS: 100-02,10,10.1.2; 100-02,10,10.2.1; 100-02,10,10.2.2; 100-02,10,10.3.3; 100-02,10,20; 100-02,10,30.1; 100-02,10,30.1.1; 100-02,10.20; 100-04,15,10.3; 100-04,15,20.1.4; 100-04,15,20.4; 100-04,15,30; 100-04,15,30.1.2; 100-04,15,30.2; 100-04,15,30.2.1; 100-04,15,40
AHA: 4Q, '12, 1

A0434 **Specialty care transport (SCT)** A
CMS: 100-02,10,10.1.2; 100-02,10,10.2.1; 100-02,10,10.2.2; 100-02,10,10.3.3; 100-02,10,20; 100-02,10,30.1; 100-02,10,30.1.1; 100-02,10.20; 100-04,15,10.3; 100-04,15,20.1.4; 100-04,15,20.4; 100-04,15,30; 100-04,15,30.1.2; 100-04,15,30.2; 100-04,15,30.2.1; 100-04,15,40
AHA: 4Q, '12, 1

A0435 **Fixed wing air mileage, per statute mile** A
CMS: 100-02,10,10.1.2; 100-02,10,10.2.1; 100-02,10,10.2.2; 100-02,10,10.3.3; 100-02,10,20; 100-02,10,30.1; 100-02,10,30.1.1; 100-02,10.20; 100-04,15,10.3; 100-04,15,20.1.4; 100-04,15,20.3; 100-04,15,20.4; 100-04,15,30; 100-04,15,30.1.2; 100-04,15,30.2; 100-04,15,30.2.1; 100-04,15,40
AHA: 4Q, '12, 1

A0436 **Rotary wing air mileage, per statute mile** A
CMS: 100-02,10,10.1.2; 100-02,10,10.2.1; 100-02,10,10.2.2; 100-02,10,10.3.3; 100-02,10,20; 100-02,10,30.1; 100-02,10,30.1.1; 100-02,10.20; 100-04,15,10.3; 100-04,15,20.1.4; 100-04,15,20.3; 100-04,15,20.4; 100-04,15,30; 100-04,15,30.1.2; 100-04,15,30.2; 100-04,15,30.2.1; 100-04,15,40
AHA: 4Q, '12, 1

A0888 **Noncovered ambulance mileage, per mile (e.g., for miles traveled beyond closest appropriate facility)** E
CMS: 100-02,10,10.1.2; 100-02,10,10.2.1; 100-02,10,20; 100-02,10,30.1; 100-02,10,30.1.1; 100-04,15,20.4; 100-04,15,30.1.2; 100-04,15,30.2.4

A0998 **Ambulance response and treatment, no transport** E
CMS: 100-02,10,10.1.2; 100-02,10,10.2.1; 100-02,10,30.1; 100-02,10,30.1.1; 100-04,15,20.4

A0999 **Unlisted ambulance service** A
CMS: 100-02,10,10.1; 100-02,10,10.1.2; 100-02,10,10.2.1; 100-02,10,20; 100-02,10,30.1; 100-02,10,30.1.1; 100-04,15,20.4

Medical and Surgical Supplies A4206-A9999

This section covers a wide variety of medical, surgical, and some durable medical equipment (DME) related supplies and accessories. DME-related supplies, accessories, maintenance, and repair required to ensure the proper functioning of this equipment is generally covered by Medicare under the prosthetic devices provision.

Injection Supplies

A4206 **Syringe with needle, sterile, 1 cc or less, each** N ☑

A4207 **Syringe with needle, sterile 2 cc, each** N ☑

A4208 **Syringe with needle, sterile 3 cc, each** N ☑

A4209 **Syringe with needle, sterile 5 cc or greater, each** N ☑

A4210 **Needle-free injection device, each** E ☑
Sometimes covered by commercial payers with preauthorization and physician letter stating need (e.g., for insulin injection in young children).

© 2019 Optum360, LLC

A4211 **Supplies for self-administered injections** N
When a drug that is usually injected by the patient (e.g., insulin or calcitonin) is injected by the physician, it is excluded from Medicare coverage unless administered in an emergency situation (e.g., diabetic coma).

A4212 **Noncoring needle or stylet with or without catheter** N

A4213 **Syringe, sterile, 20 cc or greater, each** N ☑

A4215 **Needle, sterile, any size, each** N

A4216 **Sterile water, saline and/or dextrose, diluent/flush, 10 ml** N ☑ ♿

A4217 **Sterile water/saline, 500 ml** N ☑ ♿ (AU)
CMS: 100-04,20,30.9

A4218 **Sterile saline or water, metered dose dispenser, 10 ml** N ☑

A4220 **Refill kit for implantable infusion pump** N

A4221 **Supplies for maintenance of noninsulin drug infusion catheter, per week (list drugs separately)** N ♿

A4222 **Infusion supplies for external drug infusion pump, per cassette or bag (list drugs separately)** N ♿

A4223 **Infusion supplies not used with external infusion pump, per cassette or bag (list drugs separately)** N ☑

A4224 **Supplies for maintenance of insulin infusion catheter, per week** N ♿

A4225 **Supplies for external insulin infusion pump, syringe type cartridge, sterile, each** N ♿

● **A4226**[Jan] **Supplies for maintenance of insulin infusion pump with dosage rate adjustment using therapeutic continuous glucose sensing, per week**

A4230 **Infusion set for external insulin pump, nonneedle cannula type** N ☑
Covered by some commercial payers as ongoing supply to preauthorized pump.

A4231 **Infusion set for external insulin pump, needle type** N ☑
Covered by some commercial payers as ongoing supply to preauthorized pump.

A4232 **Syringe with needle for external insulin pump, sterile, 3 cc** E ☑
Covered by some commercial payers as ongoing supply to preauthorized pump.

Batteries

A4233 **Replacement battery, alkaline (other than J cell), for use with medically necessary home blood glucose monitor owned by patient, each** E ☑ ♿ (NU)
CMS: 100-04,23,60.3

A4234 **Replacement battery, alkaline, J cell, for use with medically necessary home blood glucose monitor owned by patient, each** E ☑ ♿ (NU)
CMS: 100-04,23,60.3

A4235 **Replacement battery, lithium, for use with medically necessary home blood glucose monitor owned by patient, each** E ☑ ♿ (NU)
CMS: 100-04,23,60.3

A4236 **Replacement battery, silver oxide, for use with medically necessary home blood glucose monitor owned by patient, each** E ☑ ♿ (NU)
CMS: 100-04,23,60.3

Other Supplies

A4244 **Alcohol or peroxide, per pint** N ☑

A4245 **Alcohol wipes, per box** N ☑

A4246 **Betadine or pHisoHex solution, per pint** N ☑

A4247 **Betadine or iodine swabs/wipes, per box** N ☑

A4248 **Chlorhexidine containing antiseptic, 1 ml** N ☑

A4250 **Urine test or reagent strips or tablets (100 tablets or strips)** E ☑
CMS: 100-02,15,110

Reference chart

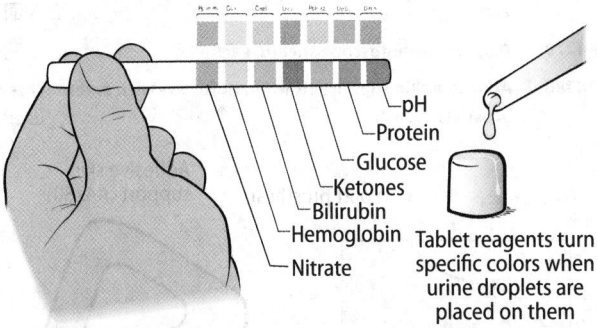

Dipstick urinalysis: The strip is dipped and color-coded squares are read at timed intervals (e.g., pH immediately; ketones at 15 seconds, etc.). Results are compared against a reference chart

A4252 **Blood ketone test or reagent strip, each** E ☑

A4253 **Blood glucose test or reagent strips for home blood glucose monitor, per 50 strips** N ☑ ♿ (NU)
Medicare covers glucose strips for diabetic patients using home glucose monitoring devices prescribed by their physicians.
CMS: 100-04,23,60.3

A4255 **Platforms for home blood glucose monitor, 50 per box** N ☑ ♿
Some Medicare contractors cover monitor platforms for diabetic patients using home glucose monitoring devices prescribed by their physicians. Some commercial payers also provide this coverage to noninsulin dependent diabetics.

A4256 **Normal, low, and high calibrator solution/chips** N ♿
Some Medicare contractors cover calibration solutions or chips for diabetic patients using home glucose monitoring devices prescribed by their physicians. Some commercial payers also provide this coverage to noninsulin dependent diabetics.
CMS: 100-04,23,60.3

A4257 **Replacement lens shield cartridge for use with laser skin piercing device, each** E ☑ ♿
AHA: 1Q, '02, 5

A4258 **Spring-powered device for lancet, each** N ☑ ♿
Some Medicare contractors cover lancing devices for diabetic patients using home glucose monitoring devices prescribed by their physicians. Medicare jurisdiction: DME regional contractor. Some commercial payers also provide this coverage to noninsulin dependent diabetics.
CMS: 100-04,23,60.3

A4259 **Lancets, per box of 100** N ☑ ♿
Medicare covers lancets for diabetic patients using home glucose monitoring devices prescribed by their physicians. Medicare jurisdiction: DME regional contractor. Some commercial payers also provide this coverage to noninsulin dependent diabetics.
CMS: 100-04,23,60.3

A4261 **Cervical cap for contraceptive use** M ♀ E

A4262 **Temporary, absorbable lacrimal duct implant, each** N ☑
Always report concurrent to the implant procedure.

A4263 **Permanent, long-term, nondissolvable lacrimal duct implant, each** N ☑
Always report concurrent to the implant procedure.

© 2019 Optum360, LLC

A4264 **Permanent implantable contraceptive intratubal occlusion device(s) and delivery system** M ♀ E ☑

A4265 **Paraffin, per pound** N ☑ ♿

A4266 **Diaphragm for contraceptive use** M ♀ E

A4267 **Contraceptive supply, condom, male, each** ♂ E ☑

A4268 **Contraceptive supply, condom, female, each** M ♀ E ☑

A4269 **Contraceptive supply, spermicide (e.g., foam, gel), each** M ♀ E ☑

A4270 **Disposable endoscope sheath, each** N ☑

A4280 **Adhesive skin support attachment for use with external breast prosthesis, each** N ☑ ♿

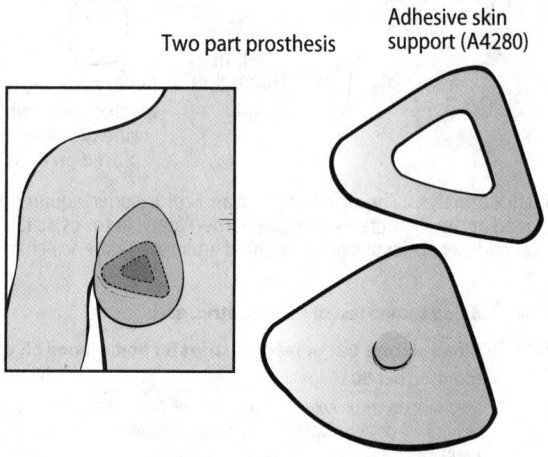

Any of several breast prostheses fits over skin support

A4281 **Tubing for breast pump, replacement** M ♀ E

A4282 **Adapter for breast pump, replacement** M ♀ E

A4283 **Cap for breast pump bottle, replacement** M ♀ E

A4284 **Breast shield and splash protector for use with breast pump, replacement** M ♀ E

A4285 **Polycarbonate bottle for use with breast pump, replacement** M ♀ E

A4286 **Locking ring for breast pump, replacement** M ♀ E

A4290 **Sacral nerve stimulation test lead, each** N ☑

CMS: 100-04,32,40.1
AHA: 1Q, '02, 9

Vascular Catheters and Drug Delivery Systems

A4300 **Implantable access catheter, (e.g., venous, arterial, epidural subarachnoid, or peritoneal, etc.) external access** N

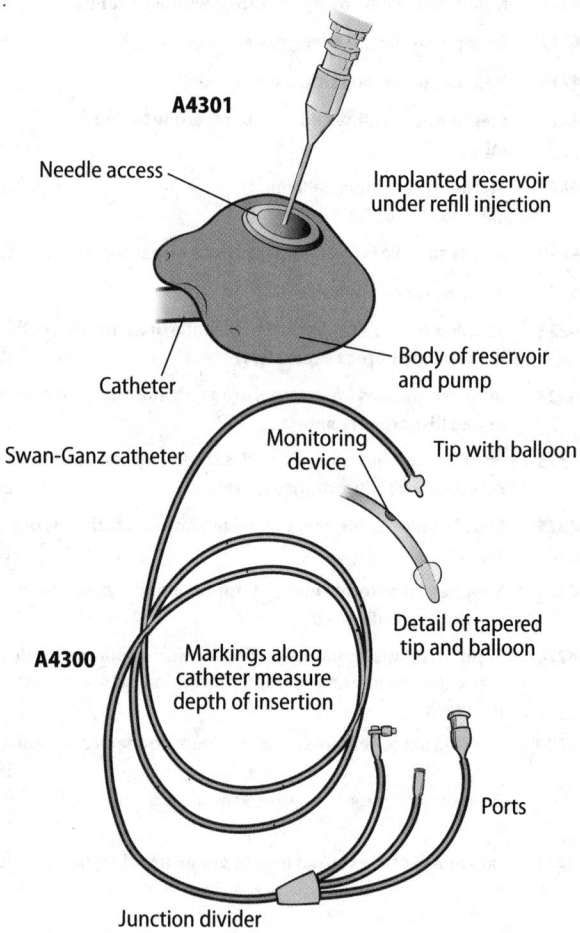

A4301 **Implantable access total catheter, port/reservoir (e.g., venous, arterial, epidural, subarachnoid, peritoneal, etc.)** N

A4305 **Disposable drug delivery system, flow rate of 50 ml or greater per hour** N ☑

A4306 **Disposable drug delivery system, flow rate of less than 50 ml per hour** N ☑

Incontinennce Appliances and Care Supplies

Covered by Medicare when the medical record indicates incontinence is permanent, or of long and indefinite duration.

A4310 **Insertion tray without drainage bag and without catheter (accessories only)** N ♿

A4311 **Insertion tray without drainage bag with indwelling catheter, Foley type, two-way latex with coating (Teflon, silicone, silicone elastomer or hydrophilic, etc.)** N ♿

A4312 **Insertion tray without drainage bag with indwelling catheter, Foley type, two-way, all silicone** N ♿

A4313 **Insertion tray without drainage bag with indwelling catheter, Foley type, three-way, for continuous irrigation** N ♿

A4314 **Insertion tray with drainage bag with indwelling catheter, Foley type, two-way latex with coating (Teflon, silicone, silicone elastomer or hydrophilic, etc.)** N ♿

© 2019 Optum360, LLC

A4315 Insertion tray with drainage bag with indwelling catheter, Foley type, two-way, all silicone N ♿

A4316 Insertion tray with drainage bag with indwelling catheter, Foley type, three-way, for continuous irrigation N ♿

A4320 Irrigation tray with bulb or piston syringe, any purpose N ♿

A4321 Therapeutic agent for urinary catheter irrigation N ♿

A4322 Irrigation syringe, bulb or piston, each N ☑ ♿

A4326 Male external catheter with integral collection chamber, any type, each ♂ N ☑ ♿

A4327 Female external urinary collection device; meatal cup, each ♀ N ☑ ♿

A4328 Female external urinary collection device; pouch, each A ♀ N ☑ ♿

A4330 Perianal fecal collection pouch with adhesive, each N ☑ ♿

A4331 Extension drainage tubing, any type, any length, with connector/adaptor, for use with urinary leg bag or urostomy pouch, each N ☑ ♿

A4332 Lubricant, individual sterile packet, each N ☑ ♿

A4333 Urinary catheter anchoring device, adhesive skin attachment, each N ☑ ♿

A4334 Urinary catheter anchoring device, leg strap, each N ☑ ♿

A4335 Incontinence supply; miscellaneous N

A4336 Incontinence supply, urethral insert, any type, each N ☑ ♿

A4337 Incontinence supply, rectal insert, any type, each N

A4338 Indwelling catheter; Foley type, two-way latex with coating (Teflon, silicone, silicone elastomer, or hydrophilic, etc.), each N ☑ ♿

A4340 Indwelling catheter; specialty type, (e.g., Coude, mushroom, wing, etc.), each N ☑ ♿

A4344 Indwelling catheter, Foley type, two-way, all silicone, each N ☑ ♿

A4346 Indwelling catheter; Foley type, three-way for continuous irrigation, each N ☑ ♿

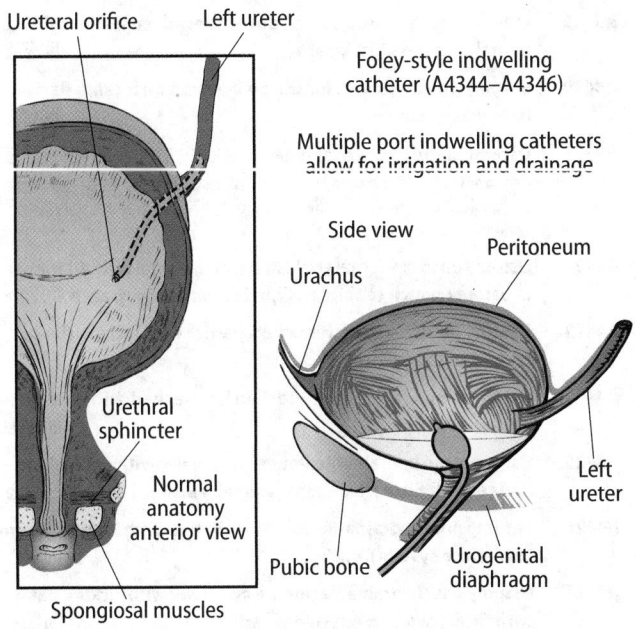

A4349 Male external catheter, with or without adhesive, disposable, each ♂ N ☑ ♿

A4351 Intermittent urinary catheter; straight tip, with or without coating (Teflon, silicone, silicone elastomer, or hydrophilic, etc.), each N ☑ ♿

A4352 Intermittent urinary catheter; Coude (curved) tip, with or without coating (Teflon, silicone, silicone elastomeric, or hydrophilic, etc.), each N ☑ ♿

A4353 Intermittent urinary catheter, with insertion supplies N ♿

A4354 Insertion tray with drainage bag but without catheter N ♿

A4355 Irrigation tubing set for continuous bladder irrigation through a three-way indwelling Foley catheter, each N ☑ ♿

A4356 External urethral clamp or compression device (not to be used for catheter clamp), each N ☑ ♿

A4357 Bedside drainage bag, day or night, with or without antireflux device, with or without tube, each N ☑ ♿

A4358 Urinary drainage bag, leg or abdomen, vinyl, with or without tube, with straps, each N ☑ ♿

A4360 Disposable external urethral clamp or compression device, with pad and/or pouch, each N ☑ ♿

Ostomy Supplies

A4361 Ostomy faceplate, each N ☑ ♿

A4362 Skin barrier; solid, 4 x 4 or equivalent; each N ☑ ♿

A4363 Ostomy clamp, any type, replacement only, each E ♿

A4364 Adhesive, liquid or equal, any type, per oz N ☑ ♿

A4366 Ostomy vent, any type, each N ☑ ♿

A4367 Ostomy belt, each N ☑ ♿

A4368 Ostomy filter, any type, each N ☑ ♿

A4369 Ostomy skin barrier, liquid (spray, brush, etc.), per oz N ☑ ♿

A4371 Ostomy skin barrier, powder, per oz N ☑ ♿

A4372 Ostomy skin barrier, solid 4 x 4 or equivalent, standard wear, with built-in convexity, each N ☑ ♿

A4373 Ostomy skin barrier, with flange (solid, flexible or accordion), with built-in convexity, any size, each N ☑ ♿

Faceplate flange and skin barrier combination (A4373)

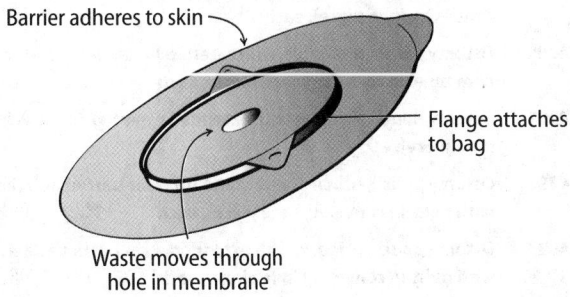

A4375 Ostomy pouch, drainable, with faceplate attached, plastic, each N ☑ ♿

© 2019 Optum360, LLC

A4376 **Ostomy pouch, drainable, with faceplate attached, rubber, each** N ☑ ♿

Colostomy pouch with faceplate and drain (A4376)

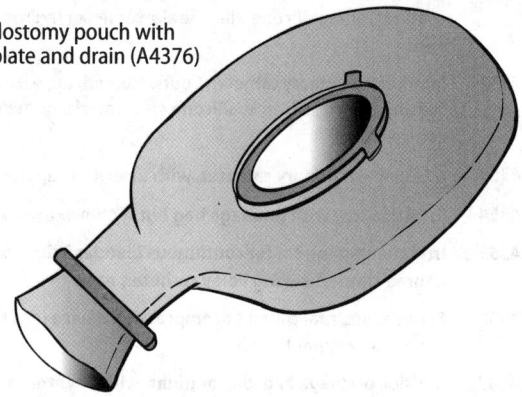

A4377 **Ostomy pouch, drainable, for use on faceplate, plastic, each** N ☑ ♿

A4378 **Ostomy pouch, drainable, for use on faceplate, rubber, each** N ☑ ♿

A4379 **Ostomy pouch, urinary, with faceplate attached, plastic, each** N ☑ ♿

A4380 **Ostomy pouch, urinary, with faceplate attached, rubber, each** N ☑ ♿

A4381 **Ostomy pouch, urinary, for use on faceplate, plastic, each** N ☑ ♿

A4382 **Ostomy pouch, urinary, for use on faceplate, heavy plastic, each** N ☑ ♿

A4383 **Ostomy pouch, urinary, for use on faceplate, rubber, each** N ☑ ♿

A4384 **Ostomy faceplate equivalent, silicone ring, each** N ☑ ♿

A4385 **Ostomy skin barrier, solid 4 x 4 or equivalent, extended wear, without built-in convexity, each** N ☑ ♿

A4387 **Ostomy pouch, closed, with barrier attached, with built-in convexity (one piece), each** N ☑ ♿

A4388 **Ostomy pouch, drainable, with extended wear barrier attached, (one piece), each** N ☑ ♿

A4389 **Ostomy pouch, drainable, with barrier attached, with built-in convexity (one piece), each** N ☑ ♿

A4390 **Ostomy pouch, drainable, with extended wear barrier attached, with built-in convexity (one piece), each** N ☑ ♿

A4391 **Ostomy pouch, urinary, with extended wear barrier attached (one piece), each** N ☑ ♿

A4392 **Ostomy pouch, urinary, with standard wear barrier attached, with built-in convexity (one piece), each** N ☑ ♿

A4393 **Ostomy pouch, urinary, with extended wear barrier attached, with built-in convexity (one piece), each** N ☑ ♿

A4394 **Ostomy deodorant, with or without lubricant, for use in ostomy pouch, per fl oz** N ☑ ♿

A4395 **Ostomy deodorant for use in ostomy pouch, solid, per tablet** N ☑ ♿

A4396 **Ostomy belt with peristomal hernia support** N ♿

A4397 **Irrigation supply; sleeve, each** N ☑ ♿

A4398 **Ostomy irrigation supply; bag, each** N ☑ ♿

A4399 **Ostomy irrigation supply; cone/catheter, with or without brush** N ♿

A4400 **Ostomy irrigation set** N ♿

A4402 **Lubricant, per oz** N ☑ ♿

A4404 **Ostomy ring, each** N ☑ ♿

A4405 **Ostomy skin barrier, nonpectin-based, paste, per oz** N ☑ ♿

A4406 **Ostomy skin barrier, pectin-based, paste, per oz** N ☑ ♿

A4407 **Ostomy skin barrier, with flange (solid, flexible, or accordion), extended wear, with built-in convexity, 4 x 4 in or smaller, each** N ☑ ♿

A4408 **Ostomy skin barrier, with flange (solid, flexible or accordion), extended wear, with built-in convexity, larger than 4 x 4 in, each** N ☑ ♿

A4409 **Ostomy skin barrier, with flange (solid, flexible or accordion), extended wear, without built-in convexity, 4 x 4 in or smaller, each** N ☑ ♿

A4410 **Ostomy skin barrier, with flange (solid, flexible or accordion), extended wear, without built-in convexity, larger than 4 x 4 in, each** N ☑ ♿

A4411 **Ostomy skin barrier, solid 4 x 4 or equivalent, extended wear, with built-in convexity, each** N ☑ ♿

A4412 **Ostomy pouch, drainable, high output, for use on a barrier with flange (two-piece system), without filter, each** N ☑ ♿

A4413 **Ostomy pouch, drainable, high output, for use on a barrier with flange (two-piece system), with filter, each** N ☑ ♿

A4414 **Ostomy skin barrier, with flange (solid, flexible or accordion), without built-in convexity, 4 x 4 in or smaller, each** N ☑ ♿

A4415 **Ostomy skin barrier, with flange (solid, flexible or accordion), without built-in convexity, larger than 4 x 4 in, each** N ☑ ♿

A4416 **Ostomy pouch, closed, with barrier attached, with filter (one piece), each** N ☑ ♿

A4417 **Ostomy pouch, closed, with barrier attached, with built-in convexity, with filter (one piece), each** N ☑ ♿

A4418 **Ostomy pouch, closed; without barrier attached, with filter (one piece), each** N ☑ ♿

A4419 **Ostomy pouch, closed; for use on barrier with nonlocking flange, with filter (two piece), each** N ☑ ♿

A4420 **Ostomy pouch, closed; for use on barrier with locking flange (two piece), each** N ☑ ♿

A4421 **Ostomy supply; miscellaneous** N

Determine if an alternative HCPCS Level II or a CPT code better describes the service being reported. This code should be used only if a more specific code is unavailable.

A4422 **Ostomy absorbent material (sheet/pad/crystal packet) for use in ostomy pouch to thicken liquid stomal output, each** N ☑ ♿

A4423 **Ostomy pouch, closed; for use on barrier with locking flange, with filter (two piece), each** N ☑ ♿

A4424 **Ostomy pouch, drainable, with barrier attached, with filter (one piece), each** N ☑ ♿

A4425 **Ostomy pouch, drainable; for use on barrier with nonlocking flange, with filter (two-piece system), each** N ☑ ♿

A4426 **Ostomy pouch, drainable; for use on barrier with locking flange (two-piece system), each** N ☑ ♿

A4427 **Ostomy pouch, drainable; for use on barrier with locking flange, with filter (two-piece system), each** N ☑ ♿

© 2019 Optum360, LLC

A4428 **Ostomy pouch, urinary, with extended wear barrier attached, with faucet-type tap with valve (one piece), each** N ☑ ♿

A4429 **Ostomy pouch, urinary, with barrier attached, with built-in convexity, with faucet-type tap with valve (one piece), each** N ☑ ♿

A4430 **Ostomy pouch, urinary, with extended wear barrier attached, with built-in convexity, with faucet-type tap with valve (one piece), each** N ☑ ♿

A4431 **Ostomy pouch, urinary; with barrier attached, with faucet-type tap with valve (one piece), each** N ☑ ♿

A4432 **Ostomy pouch, urinary; for use on barrier with nonlocking flange, with faucet-type tap with valve (two piece), each** N ☑ ♿

A4433 **Ostomy pouch, urinary; for use on barrier with locking flange (two piece), each** N ☑ ♿

A4434 **Ostomy pouch, urinary; for use on barrier with locking flange, with faucet-type tap with valve (two piece), each** N ☑ ♿

A4435 **Ostomy pouch, drainable, high output, with extended wear barrier (one-piece system), with or without filter, each** N ♿

Miscellaneous Supplies

A4450 **Tape, nonwaterproof, per 18 sq in** N ☑ ♿ (AU, AV, AW)
See also code A4452.
CMS: 100-04,20,30.9

A4452 **Tape, waterproof, per 18 sq in** N ☑ ♿ (AU, AV, AW)
See also code A4450.
CMS: 100-04,20,30.9

A4455 **Adhesive remover or solvent (for tape, cement or other adhesive), per oz** N ☑ ♿

A4456 **Adhesive remover, wipes, any type, each** N ☑ ♿

A4458 **Enema bag with tubing, reusable** N

A4459 **Manual pump-operated enema system, includes balloon, catheter and all accessories, reusable, any type** N

A4461 **Surgical dressing holder, nonreusable, each** N ☑ ♿

A4463 **Surgical dressing holder, reusable, each** N ☑ ♿

A4465 **Nonelastic binder for extremity** N

A4467 **Belt, strap, sleeve, garment, or covering, any type** E

A4470 **Gravlee jet washer** N

A4480 **VABRA aspirator** ♀ N
CMS: 100-03,230.6; 100-03,240.4

A4481 ~~**Tracheostoma filter, any type, any size, each**~~ N ☑ ♿

A4483 **Moisture exchanger, disposable, for use with invasive mechanical ventilation** N ♿

A4490 **Surgical stockings above knee length, each** E ☑
CMS: 100-02,15,110

A4495 **Surgical stockings thigh length, each** E ☑
CMS: 100-02,15,110

A4500 **Surgical stockings below knee length, each** E ☑
CMS: 100-02,15,110

A4510 **Surgical stockings full-length, each** E ☑
CMS: 100-02,15,110

A4520 **Incontinence garment, any type, (e.g., brief, diaper), each** E ☑

A4550 **Surgical trays** B

A4553 **Nondisposable underpads, all sizes** E

A4554 **Disposable underpads, all sizes** E ☑

A4555 **Electrode/transducer for use with electrical stimulation device used for cancer treatment, replacement only** E

A4556 **Electrodes (e.g., apnea monitor), per pair** N ☑ ♿
If service is not separately payable, or incident to a physician's service, bill through the local carrier. If other, bill the DME MAC.
Some payers only cover apnea monitors for newborn or pediatric use. Review specific carrier policy for apnea monitors and supplies.

A4557 **Lead wires (e.g., apnea monitor), per pair** N ☑ ♿
If service is not separately payable, or incident to a physician's service, bill through the local carrier. If other, bill the DME MAC.
Some payers only cover apnea monitors for newborn or pediatric use. Review specific carrier policy for apnea monitors and supplies.

A4558 **Conductive gel or paste, for use with electrical device (e.g., TENS, NMES), per oz** N ☑ ♿

A4559 **Coupling gel or paste, for use with ultrasound device, per oz** N ☑ ♿

A4561 **Pessary, rubber, any type** ♀ N ♿

A4562 **Pessary, nonrubber, any type** ♀ N ♿
Medicare jurisdiction: DME regional contractor.

A4563 **Rectal control system for vaginal insertion, for long term use, includes pump and all supplies and accessories, any type each**

A4565 **Slings** N ♿

A4566 **Shoulder sling or vest design, abduction restrainer, with or without swathe control, prefabricated, includes fitting and adjustment** E

A4570 **Splint** E
Dressings applied by a physician are included as part of the professional service.

A4575 **Topical hyperbaric oxygen chamber, disposable** A

A4580 **Cast supplies (e.g., plaster)** E
See Q4001-Q4048.

A4590 **Special casting material (e.g., fiberglass)** E
See Q4001-Q4048.

A4595 **Electrical stimulator supplies, 2 lead, per month, (e.g., TENS, NMES)** N ♿
CMS: 100-03,10.2

A4600 **Sleeve for intermittent limb compression device, replacement only, each** E ☑

A4601 **Lithium-ion battery, rechargeable, for nonprosthetic use, replacement** E

A4602 ~~**Replacement battery for external infusion pump owned by patient, lithium, 1.5 volt, each**~~ N ♿ (NU)

A4604 **Tubing with integrated heating element for use with positive airway pressure device** N ♿ (NU)
CMS: 100-04,23,60.3; 100-04,36,50.14

A4605 **Tracheal suction catheter, closed system, each** N ☑ ♿ (NU)

A4606 **Oxygen probe for use with oximeter device, replacement** N

A4608 **Transtracheal oxygen catheter, each** N ☑ ♿
CMS: 100-04,23,60.3

Supplies for Oxygen and Related Respiratory Equipment

A4611 **Battery, heavy-duty; replacement for patient-owned ventilator** E

A4612 **Battery cables; replacement for patient-owned ventilator** E

A4613 **Battery charger; replacement for patient-owned ventilator** E ☑

© 2019 Optum360, LLC

A4614 **Peak expiratory flow rate meter, hand held** N ♿

A4615 **Cannula, nasal** N ♿
CMS: 100-04,20,100.2; 100-04,23,60.3

A4616 **Tubing (oxygen), per foot** N ☑ ♿
CMS: 100-04,20,100.2; 100-04,23,60.3

A4617 **Mouthpiece** N ♿
CMS: 100-04,20,100.2; 100-04,23,60.3

A4618 **Breathing circuits** N ♿ (NU, RR, UE)
CMS: 100-04,20,100.2

A4619 **Face tent** N ♿ (NU)
CMS: 100-04,20,100.2

A4620 **Variable concentration mask** N ♿
CMS: 100-04,20,100.2; 100-04,23,60.3

A4623 **Tracheostomy, inner cannula** N ♿

A4624 **Tracheal suction catheter, any type other than closed system, each** N ☑ ♿ (NU)

A4625 **Tracheostomy care kit for new tracheostomy** N ♿

A4626 **Tracheostomy cleaning brush, each** N ☑ ♿

A4627 **Spacer, bag or reservoir, with or without mask, for use with metered dose inhaler** E
CMS: 100-02,15,110

A4628 **Oropharyngeal suction catheter, each** N ☑ ♿ (NU)

A4629 **Tracheostomy care kit for established tracheostomy** N ♿

Replacement Supplies for DME

A4630 **Replacement batteries, medically necessary, transcutaneous electrical stimulator, owned by patient** E ☑ ♿ (NU)

A4633 **Replacement bulb/lamp for ultraviolet light therapy system, each** E ☑ ♿ (NU)

A4634 **Replacement bulb for therapeutic light box, tabletop model** N

A4635 **Underarm pad, crutch, replacement, each** E ☑ ♿ (NU, RR, UE)

A4636 **Replacement, handgrip, cane, crutch, or walker, each** E ☑ ♿ (NU, RR, UE)
CMS: 100-04,23,60.3; 100-04,36,50.15

A4637 **Replacement, tip, cane, crutch, walker, each** E ☑ ♿ (NU, RR, UE)
CMS: 100-04,23,60.3; 100-04,36,50.15

A4638 **Replacement battery for patient-owned ear pulse generator, each** E ☑ ♿ (NU, RR, UE)

A4639 **Replacement pad for infrared heating pad system, each** E ☑ ♿ (RR)

A4640 **Replacement pad for use with medically necessary alternating pressure pad owned by patient** E ♿ (NU, RR, UE)

Radiopharmaceuticals

A4641 **Radiopharmaceutical, diagnostic, not otherwise classified** N ☑
CMS: 100-04,13,60.3; 100-04,13,60.3.1; 100-04,13,60.3.2
AHA: 4Q, '05, 1-6; 3Q, '04, 1-10

A4642 **Indium In-111 satumomab pendetide, diagnostic, per study dose, up to 6 mCi** N ☑
Use this code for Oncoscint.
AHA: 4Q, '05, 1-6; 3Q, '04, 1-10; 2Q, '02, 8-9

Miscellaneous Supplies

A4648 **Tissue marker, implantable, any type, each** N ☑ ⊘
AHA: 3Q, '13, 9

A4649 **Surgical supply; miscellaneous** N
Determine if an alternative HCPCS Level II or a CPT code better describes the service being reported. This code should be used only if a more specific code is unavailable.

A4650 **Implantable radiation dosimeter, each** N ☑ ⊘

A4651 **Calibrated microcapillary tube, each** N ☑ ⊘
AHA: 1Q, '02, 5

A4652 **Microcapillary tube sealant** N ⊘
AHA: 1Q, '02, 5

Dialysis Supplies

A4653 **Peritoneal dialysis catheter anchoring device, belt, each** N ☑ ⊘

A4657 **Syringe, with or without needle, each** N ☑ ⊘
CMS: 100-04,8,60.4.4; 100-04,8,60.4.6.3
AHA: 1Q, '02, 5

A4660 **Sphygmomanometer/blood pressure apparatus with cuff and stethoscope** N ⊘

A4663 **Blood pressure cuff only** N ⊘

A4670 **Automatic blood pressure monitor** E

A4671 **Disposable cycler set used with cycler dialysis machine, each** B ☑ ⊘

A4672 **Drainage extension line, sterile, for dialysis, each** B ☑ ⊘

A4673 **Extension line with easy lock connectors, used with dialysis** B ⊘

A4674 **Chemicals/antiseptics solution used to clean/sterilize dialysis equipment, per 8 oz** B ☑ ⊘

A4680 **Activated carbon filter for hemodialysis, each** N ☑ ⊘

A4690 **Dialyzer (artificial kidneys), all types, all sizes, for hemodialysis, each** N ☑ ⊘

A4706 **Bicarbonate concentrate, solution, for hemodialysis, per gallon** N ☑ ⊘
AHA: 1Q, '02, 5

A4707 **Bicarbonate concentrate, powder, for hemodialysis, per packet** N ☑ ⊘
AHA: 1Q, '02, 5

A4708 **Acetate concentrate solution, for hemodialysis, per gallon** N ☑ ⊘
AHA: 1Q, '02, 5

A4709 **Acid concentrate, solution, for hemodialysis, per gallon** N ☑ ⊘
AHA: 1Q, '02, 5

A4714 **Treated water (deionized, distilled, or reverse osmosis) for peritoneal dialysis, per gallon** N ☑ ⊘

A4719 **"Y set" tubing for peritoneal dialysis** N ⊘
AHA: 1Q, '02, 5

A4720 **Dialysate solution, any concentration of dextrose, fluid volume greater than 249 cc, but less than or equal to 999 cc, for peritoneal dialysis** N ☑ ⊘
AHA: 1Q, '02, 5

A4721 **Dialysate solution, any concentration of dextrose, fluid volume greater than 999 cc but less than or equal to 1999 cc, for peritoneal dialysis** N ☑ ⊘
AHA: 1Q, '02, 5

A4722 **Dialysate solution, any concentration of dextrose, fluid volume greater than 1999 cc but less than or equal to 2999 cc, for peritoneal dialysis** N ☑ ⊘
AHA: 1Q, '02, 5

© 2019 Optum360, LLC

A4723 Dialysate solution, any concentration of dextrose, fluid volume greater than 2999 cc but less than or equal to 3999 cc, for peritoneal dialysis N ☑ ⊘
AHA: 1Q, '02, 5

A4724 Dialysate solution, any concentration of dextrose, fluid volume greater than 3999 cc but less than or equal to 4999 cc, for peritoneal dialysis N ☑ ⊘
AHA: 1Q, '02, 5

A4725 Dialysate solution, any concentration of dextrose, fluid volume greater than 4999 cc but less than or equal to 5999 cc, for peritoneal dialysis N ☑ ⊘
AHA: 1Q, '02, 5

A4726 Dialysate solution, any concentration of dextrose, fluid volume greater than 5999 cc, for peritoneal dialysis N ☑ ⊘
AHA: 1Q, '02, 5

A4728 Dialysate solution, nondextrose containing, 500 ml B ☑ ⊘

A4730 Fistula cannulation set for hemodialysis, each N ☑ ⊘

A4736 Topical anesthetic, for dialysis, per g N ☑ ⊘
AHA: 1Q, '02, 5

A4737 Injectable anesthetic, for dialysis, per 10 ml N ☑ ⊘
AHA: 1Q, '02, 5

A4740 Shunt accessory, for hemodialysis, any type, each N ⊘

A4750 Blood tubing, arterial or venous, for hemodialysis, each N ☑ ⊘

A4755 Blood tubing, arterial and venous combined, for hemodialysis, each N ☑ ⊘

A4760 Dialysate solution test kit, for peritoneal dialysis, any type, each N ☑ ⊘

A4765 Dialysate concentrate, powder, additive for peritoneal dialysis, per packet N ☑ ⊘

A4766 Dialysate concentrate, solution, additive for peritoneal dialysis, per 10 ml N ☑ ⊘
AHA: 1Q, '02, 5

A4770 Blood collection tube, vacuum, for dialysis, per 50 N ☑ ⊘

A4771 Serum clotting time tube, for dialysis, per 50 N ☑ ⊘

A4772 Blood glucose test strips, for dialysis, per 50 N ☑ ⊘

A4773 Occult blood test strips, for dialysis, per 50 N ☑ ⊘

A4774 Ammonia test strips, for dialysis, per 50 N ☑ ⊘

A4802 Protamine sulfate, for hemodialysis, per 50 mg N ☑ ⊘
AHA: 1Q, '02, 5

A4860 Disposable catheter tips for peritoneal dialysis, per 10 N ☑ ⊘

A4870 Plumbing and/or electrical work for home hemodialysis equipment N ⊘

A4890 Contracts, repair and maintenance, for hemodialysis equipment N ⊘

A4911 Drain bag/bottle, for dialysis, each N ☑ ⊘
AHA: 1Q, '02, 5

A4913 Miscellaneous dialysis supplies, not otherwise specified N ⊘
Pertinent documentation to evaluate medical appropriateness should be included when this code is reported. Determine if an alternative HCPCS Level II or a CPT code better describes the service being reported. This code should be used only if a more specific code is unavailable.

A4918 Venous pressure clamp, for hemodialysis, each N ☑ ⊘

A4927 Gloves, nonsterile, per 100 N ☑ ⊘

A4928 Surgical mask, per 20 N ☑ ⊘
AHA: 1Q, '02, 5

A4929 Tourniquet for dialysis, each N ☑ ⊘
AHA: 1Q, '02, 5

A4930 Gloves, sterile, per pair N ☑ ⊘

A4931 Oral thermometer, reusable, any type, each N ☑ ⊘

A4932 Rectal thermometer, reusable, any type, each N ☑

Ostomy Pouches and Supplies

A5051 Ostomy pouch, closed; with barrier attached (one piece), each N ☑ ♿

A5052 Ostomy pouch, closed; without barrier attached (one piece), each N ☑ ♿

A5053 Ostomy pouch, closed; for use on faceplate, each N ☑ ♿

A5054 Ostomy pouch, closed; for use on barrier with flange (two piece), each N ☑ ♿

A5055 Stoma cap N ♿

A5056 Ostomy pouch, drainable, with extended wear barrier attached, with filter, (one piece), each N ☑ ♿

A5057 Ostomy pouch, drainable, with extended wear barrier attached, with built in convexity, with filter, (one piece), each N ☑ ♿

A5061 Ostomy pouch, drainable; with barrier attached, (one piece), each N ☑ ♿

A5062 Ostomy pouch, drainable; without barrier attached (one piece), each N ☑ ♿

A5063 Ostomy pouch, drainable; for use on barrier with flange (two-piece system), each N ☑ ♿

A5071 Ostomy pouch, urinary; with barrier attached (one piece), each N ☑ ♿

A5072 Ostomy pouch, urinary; without barrier attached (one piece), each N ☑ ♿

A5073 Ostomy pouch, urinary; for use on barrier with flange (two piece), each N ☑ ♿

A5081 Stoma plug or seal, any type N ♿

A5082 Continent device; catheter for continent stoma N ♿

A5083 Continent device, stoma absorptive cover for continent stoma N ♿

A5093 Ostomy accessory; convex insert N ♿

Incontinence Supplies

A5102 Bedside drainage bottle with or without tubing, rigid or expandable, each N ☑ ♿

A5105 Urinary suspensory with leg bag, with or without tube, each N ☑ ♿

A5112 Urinary drainage bag, leg or abdomen, latex, with or without tube, with straps, each N ☑ ♿

A5113 Leg strap; latex, replacement only, per set E ☑ ♿

A5114 Leg strap; foam or fabric, replacement only, per set E ☑ ♿

A5120 Skin barrier, wipes or swabs, each N ☑ ♿ (AU, AV)

A5121 Skin barrier; solid, 6 x 6 or equivalent, each N ☑ ♿

A5122 Skin barrier; solid, 8 x 8 or equivalent, each N ☑ ♿

A5126 Adhesive or nonadhesive; disk or foam pad N ♿

A5131 Appliance cleaner, incontinence and ostomy appliances, per 16 oz N ☑ ♿

A5200 Percutaneous catheter/tube anchoring device, adhesive skin attachment N ♿

© 2019 Optum360, LLC

Diabetic Shoes, Fitting, and Modifications

According to Medicare, documentation from the prescribing physician must certify the diabetic patient has one of the following conditions: peripheral neuropathy with evidence of callus formation; history of preulcerative calluses; history of ulceration; foot deformity; previous amputation; or poor circulation. The footwear must be fitted and furnished by a podiatrist, pedorthist, orthotist, or prosthetist.

A5500 **For diabetics only, fitting (including follow-up), custom preparation and supply of off-the-shelf depth-inlay shoe manufactured to accommodate multidensity insert(s), per shoe** Y ☑ ♿
CMS: 100-02,15,140

A5501 **For diabetics only, fitting (including follow-up), custom preparation and supply of shoe molded from cast(s) of patient's foot (custom molded shoe), per shoe** Y ☑ ♿
CMS: 100-02,15,140

A5503 **For diabetics only, modification (including fitting) of off-the-shelf depth-inlay shoe or custom molded shoe with roller or rigid rocker bottom, per shoe** Y ☑ ♿
CMS: 100-02,15,140

A5504 **For diabetics only, modification (including fitting) of off-the-shelf depth-inlay shoe or custom molded shoe with wedge(s), per shoe** Y ☑ ♿
CMS: 100-02,15,140

A5505 **For diabetics only, modification (including fitting) of off-the-shelf depth-inlay shoe or custom molded shoe with metatarsal bar, per shoe** Y ☑ ♿
CMS: 100-02,15,140

A5506 **For diabetics only, modification (including fitting) of off-the-shelf depth-inlay shoe or custom molded shoe with off-set heel(s), per shoe** Y ☑ ♿
CMS: 100-02,15,140

A5507 **For diabetics only, not otherwise specified modification (including fitting) of off-the-shelf depth-inlay shoe or custom molded shoe, per shoe** Y ☑ ♿
CMS: 100-02,15,140

A5508 **For diabetics only, deluxe feature of off-the-shelf depth-inlay shoe or custom molded shoe, per shoe** Y ☑
CMS: 100-02,15,140

A5510 **For diabetics only, direct formed, compression molded to patient's foot without external heat source, multiple-density insert(s) prefabricated, per shoe** N ☑
CMS: 100-02,15,140
AHA: 1Q, '02, 5

A5512 **For diabetics only, multiple density insert, direct formed, molded to foot after external heat source of 230 degrees Fahrenheit or higher, total contact with patient's foot, including arch, base layer minimum of 1/4 inch material of Shore A 35 durometer or 3/16 inch material of Shore A 40 durometer (or higher), prefabricated, each** Y ☑ ♿

A5513 **For diabetics only, multiple density insert, custom molded from model of patient's foot, total contact with patient's foot, including arch, base layer minimum of 3/16 inch material of Shore A 35 durometer (or higher), includes arch filler and other shaping material, custom fabricated, each** Y ☑ ♿

A5514 **For diabetics only, multiple density insert, made by direct carving with CAM technology from a rectified CAD model created from a digitized scan of the patient, total contact with patient's foot, including arch, base layer minimum of 3/16 inch material of Shore A 35 durometer (or higher), includes arch filler and other shaping material, custom fabricated, each**

Dressings

A6000 **Noncontact wound-warming wound cover for use with the noncontact wound-warming device and warming card** E
AHA: 1Q, '02, 5

A6010 **Collagen based wound filler, dry form, sterile, per g of collagen** N ☑ ♿
AHA: 1Q, '02, 5

A6011 **Collagen based wound filler, gel/paste, per g of collagen** N ☑ ♿

A6021 **Collagen dressing, sterile, size 16 sq in or less, each** N ☑ ♿

A6022 **Collagen dressing, sterile, size more than 16 sq in but less than or equal to 48 sq in, each** N ☑ ♿

A6023 **Collagen dressing, sterile, size more than 48 sq in, each** N ☑ ♿

A6024 **Collagen dressing wound filler, sterile, per 6 in** N ☑ ♿

A6025 **Gel sheet for dermal or epidermal application, (e.g., silicone, hydrogel, other), each** N ☑

A6154 **Wound pouch, each** N ☑ ♿

A6196 **Alginate or other fiber gelling dressing, wound cover, sterile, pad size 16 sq in or less, each dressing** N ☑ ♿

A6197 **Alginate or other fiber gelling dressing, wound cover, sterile, pad size more than 16 sq in but less than or equal to 48 sq in, each dressing** N ☑ ♿

A6198 **Alginate or other fiber gelling dressing, wound cover, sterile, pad size more than 48 sq in, each dressing** N ☑

A6199 **Alginate or other fiber gelling dressing, wound filler, sterile, per 6 in** N ☑ ♿

A6203 **Composite dressing, sterile, pad size 16 sq in or less, with any size adhesive border, each dressing** N ☑ ♿

A6204 **Composite dressing, sterile, pad size more than 16 sq in, but less than or equal to 48 sq in, with any size adhesive border, each dressing** N ☑ ♿

A6205 **Composite dressing, sterile, pad size more than 48 sq in, with any size adhesive border, each dressing** N ☑

A6206 **Contact layer, sterile, 16 sq in or less, each dressing** N ☑

A6207 **Contact layer, sterile, more than 16 sq in but less than or equal to 48 sq in, each dressing** N ☑ ♿

A6208 **Contact layer, sterile, more than 48 sq in, each dressing** N ☑

A6209 **Foam dressing, wound cover, sterile, pad size 16 sq in or less, without adhesive border, each dressing** N ☑ ♿

A6210 **Foam dressing, wound cover, sterile, pad size more than 16 sq in but less than or equal to 48 sq in, without adhesive border, each dressing** N ☑ ♿

A6211 **Foam dressing, wound cover, sterile, pad size more than 48 sq in, without adhesive border, each dressing** N ☑ ♿

A6212 **Foam dressing, wound cover, sterile, pad size 16 sq in or less, with any size adhesive border, each dressing** N ☑ ♿

A6213 **Foam dressing, wound cover, sterile, pad size more than 16 sq in but less than or equal to 48 sq in, with any size adhesive border, each dressing** N ☑

A6214 **Foam dressing, wound cover, sterile, pad size more than 48 sq in, with any size adhesive border, each dressing** N ☑ ♿

A6215 **Foam dressing, wound filler, sterile, per g** N ☑

A6216 **Gauze, nonimpregnated, nonsterile, pad size 16 sq in or less, without adhesive border, each dressing** N ☑ ♿

© 2019 Optum360, LLC

A6217 Gauze, nonimpregnated, nonsterile, pad size more than 16 sq in but less than or equal to 48 sq in, without adhesive border, each dressing N ☑ ♿

A6218 Gauze, nonimpregnated, nonsterile, pad size more than 48 sq in, without adhesive border, each dressing N ☑

A6219 Gauze, nonimpregnated, sterile, pad size 16 sq in or less, with any size adhesive border, each dressing N ☑ ♿

A6220 Gauze, nonimpregnated, sterile, pad size more than 16 sq in but less than or equal to 48 sq in, with any size adhesive border, each dressing N ☑ ♿

A6221 Gauze, nonimpregnated, sterile, pad size more than 48 sq in, with any size adhesive border, each dressing N ☑

A6222 Gauze, impregnated with other than water, normal saline, or hydrogel, sterile, pad size 16 sq in or less, without adhesive border, each dressing N ☑ ♿

A6223 Gauze, impregnated with other than water, normal saline, or hydrogel, sterile, pad size more than 16 sq in but less than or equal to 48 sq in, without adhesive border, each dressing N ☑ ♿

A6224 Gauze, impregnated with other than water, normal saline, or hydrogel, sterile, pad size more than 48 sq in, without adhesive border, each dressing N ☑ ♿

A6228 Gauze, impregnated, water or normal saline, sterile, pad size 16 sq in or less, without adhesive border, each dressing N ☑

A6229 Gauze, impregnated, water or normal saline, sterile, pad size more than 16 sq in but less than or equal to 48 sq in, without adhesive border, each dressing N ☑ ♿

A6230 Gauze, impregnated, water or normal saline, sterile, pad size more than 48 sq in, without adhesive border, each dressing N ☑

A6231 Gauze, impregnated, hydrogel, for direct wound contact, sterile, pad size 16 sq in or less, each dressing N ☑ ♿

A6232 Gauze, impregnated, hydrogel, for direct wound contact, sterile, pad size greater than 16 sq in but less than or equal to 48 sq in, each dressing N ☑ ♿

A6233 Gauze, impregnated, hydrogel, for direct wound contact, sterile, pad size more than 48 sq in, each dressing N ☑ ♿

A6234 Hydrocolloid dressing, wound cover, sterile, pad size 16 sq in or less, without adhesive border, each dressing N ☑ ♿

A6235 Hydrocolloid dressing, wound cover, sterile, pad size more than 16 sq in but less than or equal to 48 sq in, without adhesive border, each dressing N ☑ ♿

A6236 Hydrocolloid dressing, wound cover, sterile, pad size more than 48 sq in, without adhesive border, each dressing N ☑ ♿

A6237 Hydrocolloid dressing, wound cover, sterile, pad size 16 sq in or less, with any size adhesive border, each dressing N ☑ ♿

A6238 Hydrocolloid dressing, wound cover, sterile, pad size more than 16 sq in but less than or equal to 48 sq in, with any size adhesive border, each dressing N ☑ ♿

A6239 Hydrocolloid dressing, wound cover, sterile, pad size more than 48 sq in, with any size adhesive border, each dressing N ☑

A6240 Hydrocolloid dressing, wound filler, paste, sterile, per oz N ☑ ♿

A6241 Hydrocolloid dressing, wound filler, dry form, sterile, per g N ☑ ♿

A6242 Hydrogel dressing, wound cover, sterile, pad size 16 sq in or less, without adhesive border, each dressing N ☑ ♿

A6243 Hydrogel dressing, wound cover, sterile, pad size more than 16 sq in but less than or equal to 48 sq in, without adhesive border, each dressing N ☑ ♿

A6244 Hydrogel dressing, wound cover, sterile, pad size more than 48 sq in, without adhesive border, each dressing N ☑ ♿

A6245 Hydrogel dressing, wound cover, sterile, pad size 16 sq in or less, with any size adhesive border, each dressing N ☑ ♿

A6246 Hydrogel dressing, wound cover, sterile, pad size more than 16 sq in but less than or equal to 48 sq in, with any size adhesive border, each dressing N ☑ ♿

A6247 Hydrogel dressing, wound cover, sterile, pad size more than 48 sq in, with any size adhesive border, each dressing N ☑ ♿

A6248 Hydrogel dressing, wound filler, gel, per fl oz N ☑ ♿

A6250 Skin sealants, protectants, moisturizers, ointments, any type, any size N

Surgical dressings applied by a physician are included as part of the professional service. Surgical dressings obtained by the patient to perform homecare as prescribed by the physician are covered.

A6251 Specialty absorptive dressing, wound cover, sterile, pad size 16 sq in or less, without adhesive border, each dressing N ☑ ♿

A6252 Specialty absorptive dressing, wound cover, sterile, pad size more than 16 sq in but less than or equal to 48 sq in, without adhesive border, each dressing N ☑ ♿

A6253 Specialty absorptive dressing, wound cover, sterile, pad size more than 48 sq in, without adhesive border, each dressing N ☑ ♿

A6254 Specialty absorptive dressing, wound cover, sterile, pad size 16 sq in or less, with any size adhesive border, each dressing N ☑ ♿

A6255 Specialty absorptive dressing, wound cover, sterile, pad size more than 16 sq in but less than or equal to 48 sq in, with any size adhesive border, each dressing N ☑ ♿

A6256 Specialty absorptive dressing, wound cover, sterile, pad size more than 48 sq in, with any size adhesive border, each dressing N ☑

A6257 Transparent film, sterile, 16 sq in or less, each dressing N ☑ ♿

Surgical dressings applied by a physician are included as part of the professional service. Surgical dressings obtained by the patient to perform homecare as prescribed by the physician are covered. Use this code for Polyskin, Tegaderm, and Tegaderm HP.

A6258 Transparent film, sterile, more than 16 sq in but less than or equal to 48 sq in, each dressing N ☑ ♿

Surgical dressings applied by a physician are included as part of the professional service. Surgical dressings obtained by the patient to perform homecare as prescribed by the physician are covered.

A6259 Transparent film, sterile, more than 48 sq in, each dressing N ☑ ♿

Surgical dressings applied by a physician are included as part of the professional service. Surgical dressings obtained by the patient to perform homecare as prescribed by the physician are covered.

A6260 Wound cleansers, any type, any size N

Surgical dressings applied by a physician are included as part of the professional service. Surgical dressings obtained by the patient to perform homecare as prescribed by the physician are covered.

A6261 Wound filler, gel/paste, per fl oz, not otherwise specified N ☑

Surgical dressings applied by a physician are included as part of the professional service. Surgical dressings obtained by the patient to perform homecare as prescribed by the physician are covered.

A6262 Wound filler, dry form, per g, not otherwise specified N ☑

© 2019 Optum360, LLC

A6266 **Gauze, impregnated, other than water, normal saline, or zinc paste, sterile, any width, per linear yd** N ☑ ♿

Surgical dressings applied by a physician are included as part of the professional service. Surgical dressings obtained by the patient to perform homecare as prescribed by the physician are covered.

A6402 **Gauze, nonimpregnated, sterile, pad size 16 sq in or less, without adhesive border, each dressing** N ☑ ♿

Surgical dressings applied by a physician are included as part of the professional service. Surgical dressings obtained by the patient to perform homecare as prescribed by the physician are covered.

A6403 **Gauze, nonimpregnated, sterile, pad size more than 16 sq in but less than or equal to 48 sq in, without adhesive border, each dressing** N ☑ ♿

Surgical dressings applied by a physician are included as part of the professional service. Surgical dressings obtained by the patient to perform homecare as prescribed by the physician are covered.

A6404 **Gauze, nonimpregnated, sterile, pad size more than 48 sq in, without adhesive border, each dressing** N ☑

A6407 **Packing strips, nonimpregnated, sterile, up to 2 in in width, per linear yd** N ☑ ♿

A6410 **Eye pad, sterile, each** N ☑ ♿

A6411 **Eye pad, nonsterile, each** N ☑ ♿

A6412 **Eye patch, occlusive, each** N ☑

A6413 **Adhesive bandage, first aid type, any size, each** E ☑

A6441 **Padding bandage, nonelastic, nonwoven/nonknitted, width greater than or equal to 3 in and less than 5 in, per yd** N ☑ ♿

A6442 **Conforming bandage, nonelastic, knitted/woven, nonsterile, width less than 3 in, per yd** N ☑ ♿

A6443 **Conforming bandage, nonelastic, knitted/woven, nonsterile, width greater than or equal to 3 in and less than 5 in, per yd** N ☑ ♿

A6444 **Conforming bandage, nonelastic, knitted/woven, nonsterile, width greater than or equal to 5 in, per yd** N ☑ ♿

A6445 **Conforming bandage, nonelastic, knitted/woven, sterile, width less than 3 in, per yd** N ☑ ♿

A6446 **Conforming bandage, nonelastic, knitted/woven, sterile, width greater than or equal to 3 in and less than 5 in, per yd** N ☑ ♿

A6447 **Conforming bandage, nonelastic, knitted/woven, sterile, width greater than or equal to 5 in, per yd** N ☑ ♿

A6448 **Light compression bandage, elastic, knitted/woven, width less than 3 in, per yd** N ☑ ♿

A6449 **Light compression bandage, elastic, knitted/woven, width greater than or equal to 3 in and less than 5 in, per yd** N ☑ ♿

A6450 **Light compression bandage, elastic, knitted/woven, width greater than or equal to 5 in, per yd** N ☑ ♿

A6451 **Moderate compression bandage, elastic, knitted/woven, load resistance of 1.25 to 1.34 ft lbs at 50% maximum stretch, width greater than or equal to 3 in and less than 5 in, per yd** N ☑ ♿

A6452 **High compression bandage, elastic, knitted/woven, load resistance greater than or equal to 1.35 ft lbs at 50% maximum stretch, width greater than or equal to 3 in and less than 5 in, per yd** N ☑ ♿

A6453 **Self-adherent bandage, elastic, nonknitted/nonwoven, width less than 3 in, per yd** N ☑ ♿

A6454 **Self-adherent bandage, elastic, nonknitted/nonwoven, width greater than or equal to 3 in and less than 5 in, per yd** N ☑ ♿

A6455 **Self-adherent bandage, elastic, nonknitted/nonwoven, width greater than or equal to 5 in, per yd** N ☑ ♿

A6456 **Zinc paste impregnated bandage, nonelastic, knitted/woven, width greater than or equal to 3 in and less than 5 in, per yd** N ☑ ♿

A6457 **Tubular dressing with or without elastic, any width, per linear yd** N ♿

A6460 **Synthetic resorbable wound dressing, sterile, pad size 16 sq in or less, without adhesive border, each dressing**

A6461 **Synthetic resorbable wound dressing, sterile, pad size more than 16 sq in but less than or equal to 48 sq in, without adhesive border, each dressing**

Compression Garments

A6501 **Compression burn garment, bodysuit (head to foot), custom fabricated** N ♿

A6502 **Compression burn garment, chin strap, custom fabricated** N ♿

A6503 **Compression burn garment, facial hood, custom fabricated** N ♿

A6504 **Compression burn garment, glove to wrist, custom fabricated** N ♿

A6505 **Compression burn garment, glove to elbow, custom fabricated** N ♿

A6506 **Compression burn garment, glove to axilla, custom fabricated** N ♿

A6507 **Compression burn garment, foot to knee length, custom fabricated** N ♿

A6508 **Compression burn garment, foot to thigh length, custom fabricated** N ♿

A6509 **Compression burn garment, upper trunk to waist including arm openings (vest), custom fabricated** N ♿

A6510 **Compression burn garment, trunk, including arms down to leg openings (leotard), custom fabricated** N ♿

A6511 **Compression burn garment, lower trunk including leg openings (panty), custom fabricated** N ♿

A6512 **Compression burn garment, not otherwise classified** N

A6513 **Compression burn mask, face and/or neck, plastic or equal, custom fabricated** B ♿

A6530 **Gradient compression stocking, below knee, 18-30 mm Hg, each** E ☑

A6531 **Gradient compression stocking, below knee, 30-40 mm Hg, each** N ☑ ♿ (AW)

A6532 **Gradient compression stocking, below knee, 40-50 mm Hg, each** N ☑ ♿ (AW)

A6533 **Gradient compression stocking, thigh length, 18-30 mm Hg, each** E ☑

A6534 **Gradient compression stocking, thigh length, 30-40 mm Hg, each** E ☑

A6535 **Gradient compression stocking, thigh length, 40-50 mm Hg, each** E ☑

A6536 **Gradient compression stocking, full-length/chap style, 18-30 mm Hg, each** E ☑

A6537 **Gradient compression stocking, full-length/chap style, 30-40 mm Hg, each** E ☑

A6538 **Gradient compression stocking, full-length/chap style, 40-50 mm Hg, each** E ☑

A6539 **Gradient compression stocking, waist length, 18-30 mm Hg, each** E ☑

© 2019 Optum360, LLC

A6540 Gradient compression stocking, waist length, 30-40 mm Hg, each [E] ☑

A6541 Gradient compression stocking, waist length, 40-50 mm Hg, each [E] ☑

A6544 Gradient compression stocking, garter belt [E]

A6545 Gradient compression wrap, nonelastic, below knee, 30-50 mm Hg, each [N] ☑ ♿ (AW)

A6549 Gradient compression stocking/sleeve, not otherwise specified [E]

A6550 Wound care set, for negative pressure wound therapy electrical pump, includes all supplies and accessories [N] ☑ ♿
CMS: 100-02,7,40.1.2.8; 100-02,7,50.4.4; 100-04,23,60.3

Respiratory Supplies

A7000 Canister, disposable, used with suction pump, each [Y] ☑ ♿ (NU)
CMS: 100-04,23,60.3

A7001 Canister, nondisposable, used with suction pump, each [Y] ☑ ♿ (NU)

A7002 Tubing, used with suction pump, each [Y] ☑ ♿ (NU)

A7003 Administration set, with small volume nonfiltered pneumatic nebulizer, disposable [Y] ♿ (NU)

A7004 Small volume nonfiltered pneumatic nebulizer, disposable [Y] ♿ (NU)

A7005 Administration set, with small volume nonfiltered pneumatic nebulizer, nondisposable [Y] ♿ (NU)

A7006 Administration set, with small volume filtered pneumatic nebulizer [Y] ♿ (NU)

A7007 Large volume nebulizer, disposable, unfilled, used with aerosol compressor [Y] ♿ (NU)

A7008 Large volume nebulizer, disposable, prefilled, used with aerosol compressor [Y] ♿ (NU)

A7009 Reservoir bottle, nondisposable, used with large volume ultrasonic nebulizer [Y] ♿ (NU)

A7010 Corrugated tubing, disposable, used with large volume nebulizer, 100 ft [Y] ☑ ♿ (NU)

A7012 Water collection device, used with large volume nebulizer [Y] ♿ (NU)

A7013 Filter, disposable, used with aerosol compressor or ultrasonic generator [Y] ♿ (NU)

A7014 Filter, nondisposable, used with aerosol compressor or ultrasonic generator [Y] ♿ (NU)

A7015 Aerosol mask, used with DME nebulizer [Y] ♿ (NU)

A7016 Dome and mouthpiece, used with small volume ultrasonic nebulizer [Y] ♿ (NU)

A7017 Nebulizer, durable, glass or autoclavable plastic, bottle type, not used with oxygen [Y] ♿ (NU, RR, UE)

A7018 Water, distilled, used with large volume nebulizer, 1000 ml [Y] ☑ ♿

A7020 Interface for cough stimulating device, includes all components, replacement only [Y] ♿ (NU)

A7025 High frequency chest wall oscillation system vest, replacement for use with patient-owned equipment, each [N] ☑ ♿ (RR)

A7026 High frequency chest wall oscillation system hose, replacement for use with patient-owned equipment, each [Y] ☑ ♿ (NU)

A7027 Combination oral/nasal mask, used with continuous positive airway pressure device, each [Y] ☑ ♿ (NU)

A7028 Oral cushion for combination oral/nasal mask, replacement only, each [Y] ☑ ♿ (NU)

A7029 Nasal pillows for combination oral/nasal mask, replacement only, pair [Y] ☑ ♿ (NU)

A7030 Full face mask used with positive airway pressure device, each [Y] ☑ ♿ (NU)
CMS: 100-04,23,60.3; 100-04,36,50.14

A7031 Face mask interface, replacement for full face mask, each [Y] ☑ ♿ (NU)
CMS: 100-04,23,60.3; 100-04,36,50.14

A7032 Cushion for use on nasal mask interface, replacement only, each [Y] ☑ ♿ (NU)
CMS: 100-03,240.4; 100-04,23,60.3; 100-04,36,50.14

A7033 Pillow for use on nasal cannula type interface, replacement only, pair [Y] ☑ ♿ (NU)
CMS: 100-03,240.4; 100-04,23,60.3; 100-04,36,50.14

A7034 Nasal interface (mask or cannula type) used with positive airway pressure device, with or without head strap [Y] ♿ (NU)
CMS: 100-03,240.4; 100-04,23,60.3; 100-04,36,50.14

A7035 Headgear used with positive airway pressure device [Y] ♿ (NU)
CMS: 100-03,240.4; 100-04,23,60.3; 100-04,36,50.14

A7036 Chinstrap used with positive airway pressure device [Y] ♿ (NU)
CMS: 100-03,240.4; 100-04,23,60.3; 100-04,36,50.14

A7037 Tubing used with positive airway pressure device [Y] ♿ (NU)
CMS: 100-03,240.4; 100-04,23,60.3; 100-04,36,50.14

A7038 Filter, disposable, used with positive airway pressure device [Y] ♿ (NU)
CMS: 100-04,23,60.3; 100-04,36,50.14

A7039 Filter, nondisposable, used with positive airway pressure device [Y] ♿ (NU)
CMS: 100-04,23,60.3; 100-04,36,50.14

A7040 One way chest drain valve [N] ♿

A7041 Water seal drainage container and tubing for use with implanted chest tube [N] ♿

A7044 Oral interface used with positive airway pressure device, each [Y] ☑ ♿ (NU)
CMS: 100-03,240.4; 100-04,23,60.3; 100-04,36,50.14

A7045 Exhalation port with or without swivel used with accessories for positive airway devices, replacement only [Y] ♿ (NU, RR, UE)
CMS: 100-03,240.4; 100-04,23,60.3; 100-04,36,50.14

A7046 Water chamber for humidifier, used with positive airway pressure device, replacement, each [Y] ☑ ♿ (NU)
CMS: 100-04,23,60.3; 100-04,36,50.14

A7047 Oral interface used with respiratory suction pump, each [N] ☑ ♿ (NU)

A7048 Vacuum drainage collection unit and tubing kit, including all supplies needed for collection unit change, for use with implanted catheter, each [N] ♿

Tracheostomy Supplies

A7501 Tracheostoma valve, including diaphragm, each [N] ☑ ♿

A7502 Replacement diaphragm/faceplate for tracheostoma valve, each [N] ☑ ♿

A7503 Filter holder or filter cap, reusable, for use in a tracheostoma heat and moisture exchange system, each [N] ☑ ♿

© 2019 Optum360, LLC

A7504 Filter for use in a tracheostoma heat and moisture exchange system, each N ☑ ♿

A7505 Housing, reusable without adhesive, for use in a heat and moisture exchange system and/or with a tracheostoma valve, each N ☑ ♿

A7506 Adhesive disc for use in a heat and moisture exchange system and/or with tracheostoma valve, any type each N ☑ ♿

A7507 Filter holder and integrated filter without adhesive, for use in a tracheostoma heat and moisture exchange system, each N ☑ ♿

A7508 Housing and integrated adhesive, for use in a tracheostoma heat and moisture exchange system and/or with a tracheostoma valve, each N ☑ ♿

A7509 Filter holder and integrated filter housing, and adhesive, for use as a tracheostoma heat and moisture exchange system, each N ☑ ♿

A7520 Tracheostomy/laryngectomy tube, noncuffed, polyvinyl chloride (PVC), silicone or equal, each N ☑ ♿

A7521 Tracheostomy/laryngectomy tube, cuffed, polyvinyl chloride (PVC), silicone or equal, each N ☑ ♿

A7522 Tracheostomy/laryngectomy tube, stainless steel or equal (sterilizable and reusable), each N ☑ ♿

A7523 Tracheostomy shower protector, each N ☑

A7524 Tracheostoma stent/stud/button, each N ☑ ♿

A7525 Tracheostomy mask, each N ☑ ♿

A7526 Tracheostomy tube collar/holder, each N ☑ ♿

A7527 Tracheostomy/laryngectomy tube plug/stop, each N ☑ ♿

Protective Helmet

A8000 Helmet, protective, soft, prefabricated, includes all components and accessories Y ♿ (NU, RR, UE)

A8001 Helmet, protective, hard, prefabricated, includes all components and accessories Y ♿ (NU, RR, UE)

A8002 Helmet, protective, soft, custom fabricated, includes all components and accessories Y ♿ (NU, RR, UE)

A8003 Helmet, protective, hard, custom fabricated, includes all components and accessories Y ♿ (NU, RR, UE)

A8004 Soft interface for helmet, replacement only Y ♿ (NU, RR, UE)

Other Supplies and Devices

A9150 Nonprescription drugs B

A9152 Single vitamin/mineral/trace element, oral, per dose, not otherwise specified E ☑

A9153 Multiple vitamins, with or without minerals and trace elements, oral, per dose, not otherwise specified E ☑

A9155 Artificial saliva, 30 ml B ☑

A9180 Pediculosis (lice infestation) treatment, topical, for administration by patient/caretaker E

A9270 Noncovered item or service E
CMS: 100-04,11,100.1; 100-04,20,30.9
AHA: 1Q, '14, 7; 3Q, '04, 1-10

A9272 Wound suction, disposable, includes dressing, all accessories and components, any type, each E ☑

A9273 Cold or hot fluid bottle, ice cap or collar, heat and/or cold wrap, any type E

A9274 External ambulatory insulin delivery system, disposable, each, includes all supplies and accessories E ☑

A9275 Home glucose disposable monitor, includes test strips E

A9276 Sensor; invasive (e.g., subcutaneous), disposable, for use with interstitial continuous glucose monitoring system, 1 unit = 1 day supply E ☑

A9277 Transmitter; external, for use with interstitial continuous glucose monitoring system E

A9278 Receiver (monitor); external, for use with interstitial continuous glucose monitoring system E

A9279 Monitoring feature/device, stand-alone or integrated, any type, includes all accessories, components and electronics, not otherwise classified E

A9280 Alert or alarm device, not otherwise classified E

A9281 Reaching/grabbing device, any type, any length, each E ☑

A9282 Wig, any type, each E ☑

A9283 Foot pressure off loading/supportive device, any type, each E ☑

A9284 Spirometer, nonelectronic, includes all accessories N

A9285 Inversion/eversion correction device A

A9286 Hygienic item or device, disposable or nondisposable, any type, each E

A9300 Exercise equipment E

Radiopharmaceuticals

A9500 Technetium Tc-99m sestamibi, diagnostic, per study dose N NI ☑ ⊘
Use this code for Cardiolite.
AHA: 2Q, '06, 5; 4Q, '05, 1-6; 3Q, '04, 1-10

A9501 Technetium Tc-99m teboroxime, diagnostic, per study dose N NI ☑ ⊘

A9502 Technetium Tc-99m tetrofosmin, diagnostic, per study dose N NI ☑ ⊘
Use this code for Myoview.
AHA: 2Q, '06, 5; 4Q, '05, 1-6; 3Q, '04, 1-10

A9503 Technetium Tc-99m medronate, diagnostic, per study dose, up to 30 mCi N NI ☑ ⊘
Use this code for CIS-MDP, Draximage MDP-10, Draximage MDP-25, MDP-Bracco, Technetium Tc-99m MPI-MDP.
AHA: 4Q, '05, 1-6; 3Q, '04, 1-10; 2Q, '02, 8-9

A9504 Technetium Tc-99m apcitide, diagnostic, per study dose, up to 20 mCi N NI ☑ ⊘
Use this code for Acutect.
AHA: 4Q, '05, 1-6; 3Q, '04, 1-10; 2Q, '02, 8-9; 4Q, '01, 5

A9505 Thallium Tl-201 thallous chloride, diagnostic, per mCi N NI ☑ ⊘
Use this code for MIBG, Thallous Chloride USP.
AHA: 4Q, '05, 1-6; 3Q, '04, 1-10; 2Q, '02, 8-9

A9507 Indium In-111 capromab pendetide, diagnostic, per study dose, up to 10 millicuries N NI ☑ ⊘
Use this code for Prostascint.
AHA: 4Q, '05, 1-6; 3Q, '04, 1-10

A9508 Iodine I-131 iobenguane sulfate, diagnostic, per 0.5 mCi N NI ☑ ⊘
Use this code for MIBG.
AHA: 4Q, '05, 1-6; 3Q, '04, 1-10; 2Q, '02, 8-9

A9509 Iodine I-123 sodium iodide, diagnostic, per mCi N NI ☑ ⊘

A9510 Technetium Tc-99m disofenin, diagnostic, per study dose, up to 15 mCi N NI ☑ ⊘
Use this code for Hepatolite.
AHA: 4Q, '05, 1-6; 3Q, '04, 1-10

© 2019 Optum360, LLC

A9512 **Technetium Tc-99m pertechnetate, diagnostic, per mCi** N N1 ☑ ⊘
Use this code for Technelite, Ultra-Technelow.
AHA: 4Q, '05, 1-6; 3Q, '04, 1-10

A9513 **Lutetium Lu 177, dotatate, therapeutic, 1 mCi**
Use this code for Lutathera.

A9515 **Choline C-11, diagnostic, per study dose up to 20 mCi** G N1 ☑

A9516 **Iodine I-123 sodium iodide, diagnostic, per 100 mcCi, up to 999 mcCi** N N1 ☑ ⊘
AHA: 4Q, '05, 1-6; 3Q, '04, 1-10

A9517 **Iodine I-131 sodium iodide capsule(s), therapeutic, per mCi** K ☑ ⊘
AHA: 3Q, '08, 6; 4Q, '05, 1-6; 3Q, '04, 1-10

A9520 **Technetium Tc-99m, tilmanocept, diagnostic, up to 0.5 mCi** N N1 ☑

A9521 **Technetium Tc-99m exametazime, diagnostic, per study dose, up to 25 mCi** N N1 ☑ ⊘
Use this code for Ceretec.
AHA: 4Q, '05, 1-6; 3Q, '04, 1-10

G9537 **Documentation of system reason(s) for obtaining imaging of the head (CT or MRI) (i.e., needed as part of a clinical trial; other clinician ordered the study)** M

A9524 **Iodine I-131 iodinated serum albumin, diagnostic, per 5 mcCi** N N1 ☑ ⊘
AHA: 4Q, '05, 1-6; 3Q, '04, 1-10

A9526 **Nitrogen N-13 ammonia, diagnostic, per study dose, up to 40 mCi** N N1 ☑ ⊘
CMS: 100-04,13,60.3; 100-04,13,60.3.1; 100-04,13,60.3.2
AHA: 4Q, '05, 1-6; 3Q, '04, 1-10

A9527 **Iodine I-125, sodium iodide solution, therapeutic, per mCi** U H2 ☑ ⊘
AHA: 3Q, '16, 11

A9528 **Iodine I-131 sodium iodide capsule(s), diagnostic, per mCi** N N1 ☑ ⊘
AHA: 4Q, '05, 1-6; 3Q, '04, 1-10

A9529 **Iodine I-131 sodium iodide solution, diagnostic, per mCi** N N1 ☑ ⊘
AHA: 4Q, '05, 1-6; 3Q, '04, 1-10

A9530 **Iodine I-131 sodium iodide solution, therapeutic, per mCi** K ☑ ⊘
AHA: 4Q, '05, 1-6; 3Q, '04, 1-10

A9531 **Iodine I-131 sodium iodide, diagnostic, per mcCi (up to 100 mcCi)** N N1 ☑ ⊘
AHA: 4Q, '05, 1-6; 3Q, '04, 1-10

A9532 **Iodine I-125 serum albumin, diagnostic, per 5 mcCi** N N1 ☑ ⊘
AHA: 4Q, '05, 1-6; 3Q, '04, 1-10

A9536 **Technetium Tc-99m depreotide, diagnostic, per study dose, up to 35 mCi** N N1 ☑ ⊘
AHA: 4Q, '05, 1-6

A9537 **Technetium Tc-99m mebrofenin, diagnostic, per study dose, up to 15 mCi** N N1 ☑ ⊘
AHA: 4Q, '05, 1-6

A9538 **Technetium Tc-99m pyrophosphate, diagnostic, per study dose, up to 25 mCi** N N1 ☑ ⊘
Use this code for CIS-PYRO, Phosphostec, Technescan Pyp Kit.
AHA: 4Q, '05, 1-6

A9539 **Technetium Tc-99m pentetate, diagnostic, per study dose, up to 25 mCi** N N1 ☑ ⊘
Use this code for AN-DTPA, DTPA, MPI-DTPA Kit-Chelate, MPI Indium DTPA IN-111, Pentate Calcium Trisodium, Pentate Zinc Trisodium.
AHA: 4Q, '05, 1-6

A9540 **Technetium Tc-99m macroaggregated albumin, diagnostic, per study dose, up to 10 mCi** N N1 ☑ ⊘
AHA: 4Q, '05, 1-6

A9541 **Technetium Tc-99m sulfur colloid, diagnostic, per study dose, up to 20 mCi** N N1 ☑ ⊘
AHA: 4Q, '05, 1-6

A9542 **Indium In-111 ibritumomab tiuxetan, diagnostic, per study dose, up to 5 mCi** N N1 ☑ ⊘
Use this code for Zevalin.
AHA: 4Q, '05, 1-6

A9543 **Yttrium Y-90 ibritumomab tiuxetan, therapeutic, per treatment dose, up to 40 mCi** K ☑ ⊘
AHA: 4Q, '05, 1-6

A9546 **Cobalt Co-57/58, cyanocobalamin, diagnostic, per study dose, up to 1 mcCi** N N1 ☑ ⊘
AHA: 4Q, '05, 1-6

A9547 **Indium In-111 oxyquinoline, diagnostic, per 0.5 mCi** N N1 ☑ ⊘
AHA: 4Q, '05, 1-6

A9548 **Indium In-111 pentetate, diagnostic, per 0.5 mCi** N N1 ☑ ⊘
AHA: 4Q, '05, 1-6

A9550 **Technetium Tc-99m sodium gluceptate, diagnostic, per study dose, up to 25 mCi** N N1 ☑ ⊘
AHA: 4Q, '05, 1-6

A9551 **Technetium Tc-99m succimer, diagnostic, per study dose, up to 10 mCi** N N1 ☑ ⊘
Use this code for MPI-DMSA Kidney Reagent.
AHA: 4Q, '05, 1-6

A9552 **Fluorodeoxyglucose F-18 FDG, diagnostic, per study dose, up to 45 mCi** N N1 ☑ ⊘
CMS: 100-03,220.6.13; 100-03,220.6.17; 100-04,13,60.15; 100-04,13,60.16; 100-04,13,60.3.2
AHA: 3Q, '08, 7, 8; 4Q, '05, 1-6

A9553 **Chromium Cr-51 sodium chromate, diagnostic, per study dose, up to 250 mcCi** N N1 ☑ ⊘
Use this code for Chromitope Sodium.
AHA: 4Q, '05, 1-6

A9554 **Iodine I-125 sodium iothalamate, diagnostic, per study dose, up to 10 mcCi** N N1 ☑ ⊘
Use this code for Glofil-125.
AHA: 4Q, '05, 1-6

A9555 **Rubidium Rb-82, diagnostic, per study dose, up to 60 mCi** N N1 ☑ ⊘
Use this code for Cardiogen 82.
CMS: 100-03,220.6.1; 100-04,13,60.3.2
AHA: 4Q, '05, 1-6

A9556 **Gallium Ga-67 citrate, diagnostic, per mCi** N N1 ☑ ⊘
AHA: 4Q, '05, 1-6

A9557 **Technetium Tc-99m bicisate, diagnostic, per study dose, up to 25 mCi** N N1 ☑ ⊘
Use this code for Neurolite.
AHA: 4Q, '05, 1-6

A9558 **Xenon Xe-133 gas, diagnostic, per 10 mCi** N N1 ☑ ⊘
AHA: 4Q, '05, 1-6

© 2019 Optum360, LLC

A9559 **Cobalt Co-57 cyanocobalamin, oral, diagnostic, per study dose, up to 1 mcCi** N N1 ☑ ⊘
AHA: 4Q, '05, 1-6

A9560 **Technetium Tc-99m labeled red blood cells, diagnostic, per study dose, up to 30 mCi** N N1 ☑ ⊘
AHA: 3Q, '08, 7, 8; 4Q, '05, 1-6

A9561 **Technetium Tc-99m oxidronate, diagnostic, per study dose, up to 30 mCi** N N1 ☑ ⊘
Use this code for TechneScan.
AHA: 4Q, '05, 1-6

A9562 **Technetium Tc-99m mertiatide, diagnostic, per study dose, up to 15 mCi** N N1 ☑ ⊘
Use this code for TechneScan MAG-3.
AHA: 4Q, '05, 1-6

A9563 **Sodium phosphate P-32, therapeutic, per mCi** K ☑ ⊘
AHA: 4Q, '05, 1-6

A9564 **Chromic phosphate P-32 suspension, therapeutic, per mCi** E ☑ ⊘
Use this code for Phosphocol (P32).
AHA: 4Q, '05, 1-6

A9566 **Technetium Tc-99m fanolesomab, diagnostic, per study dose, up to 25 mCi** N N1 ☑ ⊘
AHA: 4Q, '05, 1-6

A9567 **Technetium Tc-99m pentetate, diagnostic, aerosol, per study dose, up to 75 mCi** N N1 ☑ ⊘
Use this code for AN-DTPA, DTPA, MPI-DTPA Kit-Chelate, MPI Indium DTPA IN-111, Pentate Calcium Trisodium, Pentate Zinc Trisodium.
AHA: 4Q, '05, 1-6

A9568 **Technetium Tc-99m arcitumomab, diagnostic, per study dose, up to 45 mCi** N N1 ☑ ⊘
Use this code for CEA Scan.

A9569 **Technetium Tc-99m exametazime labeled autologous white blood cells, diagnostic, per study dose** N N1 ☑ ⊘
AHA: 1Q, '08, 6

A9570 **Indium In-111 labeled autologous white blood cells, diagnostic, per study dose** N N1 ☑ ⊘

A9571 **Indium In-111 labeled autologous platelets, diagnostic, per study dose** N N1 ☑ ⊘

A9572 **Indium In-111 pentetreotide, diagnostic, per study dose, up to 6 mCi** N N1 ☑ ⊘
Use this code for Ostreoscan.

A9575 **Injection, gadoterate meglumine, 0.1 ml** N N1 ☑
Use this code for Dotarem.
AHA: 1Q, '14, 6

A9576 **Injection, gadoteridol, (ProHance multipack), per ml** N N1 ☑

A9577 **Injection, gadobenate dimeglumine (MultiHance), per ml** N N1 ☑
AHA: 1Q, '08, 6

A9578 **Injection, gadobenate dimeglumine (MultiHance multipack), per ml** N N1 ☑

A9579 **Injection, gadolinium-based magnetic resonance contrast agent, not otherwise specified (NOS), per ml** N N1 ☑
Use this code for Omniscan, Magnevist.
CMS: 100-03,1,220.2
AHA: 1Q, '08, 6

A9580 **Sodium fluoride F-18, diagnostic, per study dose, up to 30 mCi** N N1 ☑ ⊘
CMS: 100-03,220.6.19; 100-04,13,60.18; 100-04,13,60.3.2

A9581 **Injection, gadoxetate disodium, 1 ml** N N1 ☑
Use this code for Eovist.

A9582 **Iodine I-123 iobenguane, diagnostic, per study dose, up to 15 mCi** N N1 ☑

A9583 **Injection, gadofosveset trisodium, 1 ml** N N1 ☑
Use this code for Ablavar, Vasovist.

A9584 **Iodine I-123 ioflupane, diagnostic, per study dose, up to 5 mCi** N N1 ☑
Use this code for DaTscan.

A9585 **Injection, gadobutrol, 0.1 ml** N N1 ☑
Use this code for Gadavist.

A9586 **Florbetapir F18, diagnostic, per study dose, up to 10 mCi** N K2 ☑
Use this code for Amyvid.
CMS: 100-04,17, 80.12
AHA: 3Q, '14, 7; 1Q, '14, 6

A9587 **Gallium Ga-68, dotatate, diagnostic, 0.1 mCi** G K2 ☑
Use this code for Netspot.
CMS: 100-04,13,60.3.2
AHA: 1Q, '17, 9-10

A9588 **Fluciclovine F-18, diagnostic, 1 mCi** G K2 ☑
Use this code for Axumin.
CMS: 100-04,13,60.3.2
AHA: 1Q, '17, 9-10

A9589 **Instillation, hexaminolevulinate HCl, 100 mg**
Use this code for Cysview.
CMS: 100-04,13,60.3.2

● **A9590** Jan **Iodine I-131, iobenguane, 1 mCi**
Use this code for Azedra.
CMS: 100-04,13,60.3.2

A9597 **Positron emission tomography radiopharmaceutical, diagnostic, for tumor identification, not otherwise classified** N N1 ☑
CMS: 100-04,13,60.3.2
AHA: 1Q, '17, 9-10; 1Q, '17, 8

A9598 **Positron emission tomography radiopharmaceutical, diagnostic, for nontumor identification, not otherwise classified** N N1 ☑
CMS: 100-04,13,60.3.2
AHA: 1Q, '17, 9-10; 1Q, '17, 8

A9600 **Strontium Sr-89 chloride, therapeutic, per mCi** K ☑ ⊘
Use this code for Metastron.
AHA: 4Q, '05, 1-6; 3Q, '04, 1-10; 2Q, '02, 8-9

A9604 **Samarium Sm-153 lexidronam, therapeutic, per treatment dose, up to 150 mCi** K ☑
Use this code for Quadramet.

A9606 **Radium RA-223 dichloride, therapeutic, per mcCi** K ☑
Use this code for Xofigo.

A9698 **Nonradioactive contrast imaging material, not otherwise classified, per study** N N1 ☑ ⊘
AHA: 1Q, '17, 8; 4Q, '05, 1-6

A9699 **Radiopharmaceutical, therapeutic, not otherwise classified** N ☑ ⊘
AHA: 4Q, '05, 1-6; 3Q, '04, 1-10

A9700 **Supply of injectable contrast material for use in echocardiography, per study** N N1
AHA: 1Q, '17, 8; 2Q, '03, 7; 4Q, '01, 5

Miscellaneous

A9900 **Miscellaneous DME supply, accessory, and/or service component of another HCPCS code** Y

© 2019 Optum360, LLC

A9901 **DME delivery, set up, and/or dispensing service component of another HCPCS code** [A]

A9999 **Miscellaneous DME supply or accessory, not otherwise specified** [Y]

© 2019 Optum360, LLC

Enteral and Parenteral Therapy B4034-B9999

This section includes codes for supplies, formulae, nutritional solutions, and infusion pumps.

Enteral Formulae and Enteral Medical Supplies

B4034 **Enteral feeding supply kit; syringe fed, per day, includes but not limited to feeding/flushing syringe, administration set tubing, dressings, tape** Y ☑
CMS: 100-03,180.2; 100-04,20,160.2; 100-04,23,60.3

B4035 **Enteral feeding supply kit; pump fed, per day, includes but not limited to feeding/flushing syringe, administration set tubing, dressings, tape** Y ☑
CMS: 100-03,180.2; 100-04,20,160.2; 100-04,23,60.3

B4036 **Enteral feeding supply kit; gravity fed, per day, includes but not limited to feeding/flushing syringe, administration set tubing, dressings, tape** Y ☑
CMS: 100-03,180.2; 100-04,20,160.2; 100-04,23,60.3

B4081 **Nasogastric tubing with stylet** Y
CMS: 100-03,180.2; 100-04,20,160.2; 100-04,23,60.3

Many types of stylets are used. Some may be fitted with lights or optics. Others are used as guides

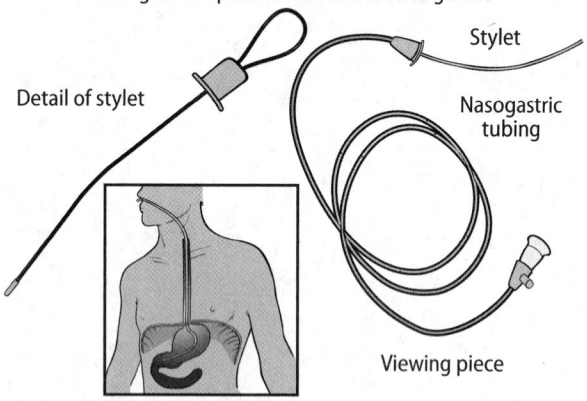

B4082 **Nasogastric tubing without stylet** Y
CMS: 100-03,180.2; 100-04,20,160.2; 100-04,23,60.3

B4083 **Stomach tube - Levine type** Y
CMS: 100-03,180.2; 100-04,20,160.2; 100-04,23,60.3

B4087 **Gastrostomy/jejunostomy tube, standard, any material, any type, each** A ☑
CMS: 100-03,180.2; 100-04,23,60.3

B4088 **Gastrostomy/jejunostomy tube, low-profile, any material, any type, each** A ☑
CMS: 100-03,180.2; 100-04,23,60.3

B4100 **Food thickener, administered orally, per oz** E ☑
CMS: 100-03,180.2

B4102 **Enteral formula, for adults, used to replace fluids and electrolytes (e.g., clear liquids), 500 ml = 1 unit** Y ☑
CMS: 100-03,180.2

B4103 **Enteral formula, for pediatrics, used to replace fluids and electrolytes (e.g., clear liquids), 500 ml = 1 unit** Y ☑
CMS: 100-03,180.2

B4104 **Additive for enteral formula (e.g., fiber)** E
CMS: 100-03,180.2

B4105 **In-line cartridge containing digestive enzyme(s) for enteral feeding, each**
CMS: 100-03,180.2

B4149 **Enteral formula, manufactured blenderized natural foods with intact nutrients, includes proteins, fats, carbohydrates, vitamins and minerals, may include fiber, administered through an enteral feeding tube, 100 calories = 1 unit** Y ☑
CMS: 100-03,180.2; 100-04,23,60.3

B4150 **Enteral formula, nutritionally complete with intact nutrients, includes proteins, fats, carbohydrates, vitamins and minerals, may include fiber, administered through an enteral feeding tube, 100 calories = 1 unit** Y ☑
Use this code for Enrich, Ensure, Ensure HN, Ensure Powder, Isocal, Lonalac Powder, Meritene, Meritene Powder, Osmolite, Osmolite HN, Portagen Powder, Sustacal, Renu, Sustagen Powder, Travasorb.
CMS: 100-03,180.2; 100-04,20,160.2; 100-04,23,60.3

B4152 **Enteral formula, nutritionally complete, calorically dense (equal to or greater than 1.5 kcal/ml) with intact nutrients, includes proteins, fats, carbohydrates, vitamins and minerals, may include fiber, administered through an enteral feeding tube, 100 calories = 1 unit** Y ☑
Use this code for Magnacal, Isocal HCN, Sustacal HC, Ensure Plus, Ensure Plus HN.
CMS: 100-03,180.2; 100-04,20,160.2; 100-04,23,60.3

B4153 **Enteral formula, nutritionally complete, hydrolyzed proteins (amino acids and peptide chain), includes fats, carbohydrates, vitamins and minerals, may include fiber, administered through an enteral feeding tube, 100 calories = 1 unit** Y ☑
Use this code for Criticare HN, Vivonex t.e.n. (Total Enteral Nutrition), Vivonex HN, Vital (Vital HN), Travasorb HN, Isotein HN, Precision HN, Precision Isotonic.
CMS: 100-03,180.2; 100-04,20,160.2; 100-04,23,60.3

B4154 **Enteral formula, nutritionally complete, for special metabolic needs, excludes inherited disease of metabolism, includes altered composition of proteins, fats, carbohydrates, vitamins and/or minerals, may include fiber, administered through an enteral feeding tube, 100 calories = 1 unit** Y ☑
Use this code for Hepatic-aid, Travasorb Hepatic, Travasorb MCT, Travasorb Renal, Traum-aid, Tramacal, Aminaid.
CMS: 100-03,180.2; 100-04,20,160.2; 100-04,23,60.3

B4155 **Enteral formula, nutritionally incomplete/modular nutrients, includes specific nutrients, carbohydrates (e.g., glucose polymers), proteins/amino acids (e.g., glutamine, arginine), fat (e.g., medium chain triglycerides) or combination, administered through an enteral feeding tube, 100 calories = 1 unit** Y ☑
Use this code for Propac, Gerval Protein, Promix, Casec, Moducal, Controlyte, Polycose Liquid or Powder, Sumacal, Microlipids, MCT Oil, Nutri-source.
CMS: 100-03,180.2; 100-04,20,160.2; 100-04,23,60.3

B4157 **Enteral formula, nutritionally complete, for special metabolic needs for inherited disease of metabolism, includes proteins, fats, carbohydrates, vitamins and minerals, may include fiber, administered through an enteral feeding tube, 100 calories = 1 unit** Y ☑
CMS: 100-03,180.2

B4158 **Enteral formula, for pediatrics, nutritionally complete with intact nutrients, includes proteins, fats, carbohydrates, vitamins and minerals, may include fiber and/or iron, administered through an enteral feeding tube, 100 calories = 1 unit** Y ☑
CMS: 100-03,180.2

B4159 **Enteral formula, for pediatrics, nutritionally complete soy based with intact nutrients, includes proteins, fats, carbohydrates, vitamins and minerals, may include fiber and/or iron, administered through an enteral feeding tube, 100 calories = 1 unit** Y ☑
CMS: 100-03,180.2

© 2019 Optum360, LLC

B4160 **Enteral formula, for pediatrics, nutritionally complete calorically dense (equal to or greater than 0.7 kcal/ml) with intact nutrients, includes proteins, fats, carbohydrates, vitamins and minerals, may include fiber, administered through an enteral feeding tube, 100 calories = 1 unit** Y ☑
CMS: 100-03,180.2

B4161 **Enteral formula, for pediatrics, hydrolyzed/amino acids and peptide chain proteins, includes fats, carbohydrates, vitamins and minerals, may include fiber, administered through an enteral feeding tube, 100 calories = 1 unit** Y ☑
CMS: 100-03,180.2

B4162 **Enteral formula, for pediatrics, special metabolic needs for inherited disease of metabolism, includes proteins, fats, carbohydrates, vitamins and minerals, may include fiber, administered through an enteral feeding tube, 100 calories = 1 unit** Y ☑
CMS: 100-03,180.2

Parenteral Nutrition Solutions and Supplies

B4164 **Parenteral nutrition solution: carbohydrates (dextrose), 50% or less (500 ml = 1 unit), home mix** Y ☑
CMS: 100-03,180.2; 100-04,20,160.2

B4168 **Parenteral nutrition solution; amino acid, 3.5%, (500 ml = 1 unit) - home mix** Y ☑
CMS: 100-03,180.2; 100-04,20,160.2

B4172 **Parenteral nutrition solution; amino acid, 5.5% through 7%, (500 ml = 1 unit) - home mix** Y ☑
CMS: 100-03,180.2; 100-04,20,160.2

B4176 **Parenteral nutrition solution; amino acid, 7% through 8.5%, (500 ml = 1 unit) - home mix** Y ☑
CMS: 100-03,180.2; 100-04,20,160.2

B4178 **Parenteral nutrition solution: amino acid, greater than 8.5% (500 ml = 1 unit) - home mix** Y ☑
CMS: 100-03,180.2; 100-04,20,160.2

B4180 **Parenteral nutrition solution: carbohydrates (dextrose), greater than 50% (500 ml = 1 unit), home mix** Y ☑
CMS: 100-03,180.2; 100-04,20,160.2

▲ **B4185**[Jan] **Parenteral nutrition solution, not otherwise specified, 10 g lipids** B ☑
CMS: 100-03,180.2

● **B4187**[Jan] **Omegaven, 10 g lipids**
CMS: 100-03,180.2

B4189 **Parenteral nutrition solution: compounded amino acid and carbohydrates with electrolytes, trace elements, and vitamins, including preparation, any strength, 10 to 51 g of protein, premix** Y ☑
CMS: 100-03,180.2; 100-04,20,160.2

B4193 **Parenteral nutrition solution: compounded amino acid and carbohydrates with electrolytes, trace elements, and vitamins, including preparation, any strength, 52 to 73 g of protein, premix** Y ☑
CMS: 100-03,180.2; 100-04,20,160.2

B4197 **Parenteral nutrition solution; compounded amino acid and carbohydrates with electrolytes, trace elements and vitamins, including preparation, any strength, 74 to 100 g of protein - premix** Y ☑
CMS: 100-03,180.2; 100-04,20,160.2

B4199 **Parenteral nutrition solution; compounded amino acid and carbohydrates with electrolytes, trace elements and vitamins, including preparation, any strength, over 100 g of protein - premix** Y ☑
CMS: 100-03,180.2; 100-04,20,160.2

B4216 **Parenteral nutrition; additives (vitamins, trace elements, Heparin, electrolytes), home mix, per day** Y
CMS: 100-03,180.2; 100-04,20,160.2

B4220 **Parenteral nutrition supply kit; premix, per day** Y
CMS: 100-03,180.2; 100-04,20,160.2

B4222 **Parenteral nutrition supply kit; home mix, per day** Y
CMS: 100-03,180.2; 100-04,20,160.2

B4224 **Parenteral nutrition administration kit, per day** Y
CMS: 100-03,180.2; 100-04,20,160.2

B5000 **Parenteral nutrition solution: compounded amino acid and carbohydrates with electrolytes, trace elements, and vitamins, including preparation, any strength, renal - Amirosyn RF, NephrAmine, RenAmine - premix** Y
Use this code for Amirosyn-RF, NephrAmine, RenAmin.
CMS: 100-03,180.2; 100-04,20,160.2

B5100 **Parenteral nutrition solution compounded amino acid and carbohydrates with electrolytes, trace elements, and vitamins, including preparation, any strength, hepatic-HepatAmine-premix** Y
Use this code for FreAmine HBC, HepatAmine.
CMS: 100-03,180.2; 100-04,20,160.2

B5200 **Parenteral nutrition solution compounded amino acid and carbohydrates with electrolytes, trace elements, and vitamins, including preparation, any strength, stress-branch chain amino acids-FreAmine-HBC-premix** Y
CMS: 100-03,180.2; 100-04,20,160.2

Enteral and Parenteral Pumps

B9002 **Enteral nutrition infusion pump, any type** Y
CMS: 100-03,180.2; 100-04,20,160.2; 100-04,23,60.3

B9004 **Parenteral nutrition infusion pump, portable** Y
CMS: 100-03,180.2; 100-04,20,160.2

B9006 **Parenteral nutrition infusion pump, stationary** Y
CMS: 100-03,180.2; 100-04,20,160.2

B9998 **NOC for enteral supplies** Y
CMS: 100-03,180.2

B9999 **NOC for parenteral supplies** Y
Determine if an alternative HCPCS Level II or a CPT code better describes the service being reported. This code should be used only if a more specific code is unavailable.
CMS: 100-03,180.2

© 2019 Optum360, LLC

Outpatient PPS C1713-C9899

This section reports drug, biological, and device codes that must be used by OPPS hospitals. Non-OPPS hospitals, Critical Access Hospitals (CAHs), Indian Health Service Hospitals (HIS), hospitals located in American Samoa, Guam, Saipan, or the Virgin Islands, and Maryland waiver hospitals may report these codes at their discretion. The codes can only be reported for facility (technical) services.

The C series of HCPCS may include device categories, new technology procedures, and drugs, biologicals and radiopharmaceuticals that do not have other HCPCS codes assigned. Some of these items and services are eligible for transitional pass-through payments for OPPS hospitals, have separate APC payments, or are items that are packaged. Hospitals are encouraged to report all appropriate C codes regardless of payment status.

C1713 **Anchor/screw for opposing bone-to-bone or soft tissue-to-bone (implantable)** N N1
AHA: 3Q, '16, 15-19; 3Q, '16, 10-15; 3Q, '15, 2; 2Q, '10, 3; 3Q, '02, 4-5; 1Q, '01, 6

C1714 **Catheter, transluminal atherectomy, directional** N N1
AHA: 3Q, '16, 10-15; 4Q, '04, 4-5; 4Q, '03, 8; 3Q, '02, 4-5; 1Q, '01, 6

C1715 **Brachytherapy needle** N N1 ⊘
AHA: 3Q, '16, 10-15; 3Q, '02, 4-5; 1Q, '01, 6

C1716 **Brachytherapy source, nonstranded, gold-198, per source** U H2 ☑ ⊘
AHA: 3Q, '16, 11; 3Q, '16, 10-15; 2Q, '07, 11; 4Q, '04, 8; 2Q, '04, 10; 3Q, '02, 4-5; 1Q, '01, 6

C1717 **Brachytherapy source, nonstranded, high dose rate iridium-192, per source** U H2 ☑ ⊘
AHA: 3Q, '16, 11; 3Q, '16, 10-15; 2Q, '07, 11; 4Q, '04, 8; 2Q, '04, 10; 3Q, '02, 4-5; 1Q, '01, 6

C1719 **Brachytherapy source, nonstranded, nonhigh dose rate iridium-192, per source** U H2 ☑ ⊘
AHA: 3Q, '16, 11; 3Q, '16, 10-15; 2Q, '07, 11; 4Q, '04, 8; 2Q, '04, 10; 3Q, '02, 4-5; 1Q, '01, 6

C1721 **Cardioverter-defibrillator, dual chamber (implantable)** N N1
CMS: 100-04,14,40.8
AHA: 3Q, '16, 10-15; 4Q, '04, 4-5; 3Q, '02, 4-5; 1Q, '01, 6

C1722 **Cardioverter-defibrillator, single chamber (implantable)** N N1
CMS: 100-04,14,40.8
AHA: 3Q, '16, 10-15; 2Q, '06, 11; 4Q, '04, 4-5; 3Q, '02, 4-5; 1Q, '01, 6

C1724 **Catheter, transluminal atherectomy, rotational** N N1
AHA: 3Q, '16, 9; 3Q, '16, 10-15; 4Q, '04, 4-5; 4Q, '03, 8; 3Q, '02, 4-5; 1Q, '01, 6

C1725 **Catheter, transluminal angioplasty, nonlaser (may include guidance, infusion/perfusion capability)** N N1
To appropriately report drug-coated transluminal angioplasty catheters, use HCPCS code C2623.
AHA: 3Q, '16, 15-19; 3Q, '16, 10-15; 4Q, '04, 4-5; 4Q, '03, 8; 3Q, '02, 4-5; 1Q, '01, 6

C1726 **Catheter, balloon dilatation, nonvascular** N N1
AHA: 3Q, '16, 15-19; 3Q, '16, 10-15; 3Q, '02, 4-5; 1Q, '01, 6

C1727 **Catheter, balloon tissue dissector, nonvascular (insertable)** N N1
AHA: 3Q, '16, 15-19; 3Q, '16, 10-15; 3Q, '02, 4-5; 1Q, '01, 6

C1728 **Catheter, brachytherapy seed administration** N N1 ⊘
AHA: 3Q, '16, 10-15; 3Q, '02, 4-5; 1Q, '01, 6

C1729 **Catheter, drainage** N N1
AHA: 3Q, '16, 15-19; 3Q, '16, 10-15; 3Q, '02, 4-5; 1Q, '01, 6

C1730 **Catheter, electrophysiology, diagnostic, other than 3D mapping (19 or fewer electrodes)** N N1
AHA: 3Q, '16, 15-19; 3Q, '16, 10-15; 4Q, '04, 4-5; 3Q, '02, 4-5; 3Q, '01, 4-5; 1Q, '01, 6

C1731 **Catheter, electrophysiology, diagnostic, other than 3D mapping (20 or more electrodes)** N N1
AHA: 3Q, '16, 15-19; 3Q, '16, 10-15; 4Q, '04, 4-5; 3Q, '02, 4-5; 1Q, '01, 6

C1732 **Catheter, electrophysiology, diagnostic/ablation, 3D or vector mapping** N N1
AHA: 3Q, '16, 15-19; 3Q, '16, 10-15; 4Q, '04, 4-5; 3Q, '02, 4-5; 3Q, '01, 4-5; 1Q, '01, 6

C1733 **Catheter, electrophysiology, diagnostic/ablation, other than 3D or vector mapping, other than cool-tip** N N1
AHA: 3Q, '16, 15-19; 3Q, '16, 10-15; 4Q, '04, 4-5; 3Q, '02, 4-5; 3Q, '01, 4-5; 1Q, '01, 6

● **C1734** Jan **Orthopedic/device/drug matrix for opposing bone-to-bone or soft tissue-to bone (implantable)**

C1749 **Endoscope, retrograde imaging/illumination colonoscope device (implantable)** N N1
AHA: 3Q, '16, 10-15

C1750 **Catheter, hemodialysis/peritoneal, long-term** N N1
AHA: 3Q, '16, 10-15; 4Q, '15, 6; 4Q, '12, 9; 4Q, '03, 8; 3Q, '02, 4-5; 1Q, '01, 6

C1751 **Catheter, infusion, inserted peripherally, centrally or midline (other than hemodialysis)** N N1
AHA: 3Q, '16, 10-15; 3Q, '14, 5; 4Q, '04, 4-5; 4Q, '03, 8; 3Q, '02, 4-5; 3Q, '01, 4-5; 1Q, '01, 6

C1752 **Catheter, hemodialysis/peritoneal, short-term** N N1
AHA: 3Q, '16, 10-15; 4Q, '03, 8; 3Q, '02, 4-5; 1Q, '01, 6

C1753 **Catheter, intravascular ultrasound** N N1
AHA: 3Q, '16, 10-15; 4Q, '03, 8; 3Q, '02, 4-5; 1Q, '01, 6

C1754 **Catheter, intradiscal** N N1
AHA: 3Q, '16, 10-15; 4Q, '03, 8; 3Q, '02, 4-5; 1Q, '01, 6

C1755 **Catheter, intraspinal** N N1
AHA: 3Q, '16, 10-15; 4Q, '03, 8; 3Q, '02, 4-5; 1Q, '01, 6

C1756 **Catheter, pacing, transesophageal** N N1
AHA: 4Q, '03, 8; 3Q, '02, 4-5; 1Q, '01, 6

C1757 **Catheter, thrombectomy/embolectomy** N N1
AHA: 3Q, '16, 10-15; 4Q, '03, 8; 3Q, '02, 4-5; 1Q, '01, 6

C1758 **Catheter, ureteral** N N1
AHA: 3Q, '16, 10-15; 4Q, '03, 8; 3Q, '02, 4-5; 1Q, '01, 6

C1759 **Catheter, intracardiac echocardiography** N N1
AHA: 3Q, '16, 10-15; 4Q, '03, 8; 3Q, '02, 4-5; 3Q, '01, 4-5; 1Q, '01, 6

C1760 **Closure device, vascular (implantable/insertable)** N N1
AHA: 3Q, '16, 15-19; 3Q, '16, 10-15; 4Q, '03, 8; 3Q, '02, 4-5; 1Q, '01, 6

C1762 **Connective tissue, human (includes fascia lata)** N N1
AHA: 3Q, '16, 9; 3Q, '16, 15-19; 3Q, '16, 10-15; 3Q, '15, 2; 4Q, '03, 8; 3Q, '03, 11; 3Q, '02, 4-5; 1Q, '01, 6

C1763 **Connective tissue, nonhuman (includes synthetic)** N N1
AHA: 3Q, '16, 9; 3Q, '16, 15-19; 3Q, '16, 10-15; 4Q, '10, 1; 2Q, '10, 3; 4Q, '03, 8; 3Q, '03, 11; 3Q, '02, 4-5; 1Q, '01, 6

C1764 **Event recorder, cardiac (implantable)** N N1
CMS: 100-04,14,40.8
AHA: 3Q, '16, 10-15; 2Q, '15, 8; 4Q, '03, 8; 3Q, '02, 4-5; 1Q, '01, 6

C1765 **Adhesion barrier** N N1
AHA: 3Q, '16, 15-19; 3Q, '16, 10-15

C1766 **Introducer/sheath, guiding, intracardiac electrophysiological, steerable, other than peel-away** N N1
AHA: 3Q, '16, 10-15; 4Q, '04, 4-5; 3Q, '02, 4-5; 3Q, '01, 4-5

© 2019 Optum360, LLC

C1767 **Generator, neurostimulator (implantable), nonrechargeable** N N1
CMS: 100-04,14,40.8; 100-04,32,40.1
AHA: 3Q, '16, 10-15; 4Q, '06, 4; 4Q, '04, 4-5; 4Q, '03, 8; 3Q, '02, 4-5; 1Q, '02, 9; 1Q, '01, 6

C1768 **Graft, vascular** N N1
AHA: 3Q, '16, 10-15; 4Q, '03, 8; 3Q, '02, 4-5; 1Q, '01, 6

C1769 **Guide wire** N N1
AHA: 3Q, '16, 10-15; 3Q, '16; 3Q, '14, 5; 2Q, '07, 6; 4Q, '03, 8; 3Q, '02, 4-5; 3Q, '01, 4-5; 1Q, '01, 6

C1770 **Imaging coil, magnetic resonance (insertable)** N N1
AHA: 3Q, '16, 10-15; 4Q, '03, 8; 3Q, '02, 4-5; 1Q, '01, 6

C1771 **Repair device, urinary, incontinence, with sling graft** N N1
CMS: 100-04,14,40.8
AHA: 3Q, '16, 15-19; 3Q, '16, 10-15; 4Q, '03, 8; 3Q, '02, 4-5; 3Q, '01, 4-5; 1Q, '01, 6

C1772 **Infusion pump, programmable (implantable)** N N1
CMS: 100-04,14,40.8
AHA: 3Q, '16, 10-15; 4Q, '04, 4-5; 3Q, '02, 4-5; 1Q, '01, 6

C1773 **Retrieval device, insertable (used to retrieve fractured medical devices)** N N1
AHA: 3Q, '16, 15-19; 3Q, '16, 10-15; 4Q, '03, 8; 3Q, '02, 4-5; 1Q, '01, 6

C1776 **Joint device (implantable)** N N1
CMS: 100-04,14,40.8
AHA: 3Q, '16, 3; 3Q, '16, 15-19; 3Q, '16, 10-15; 3Q, '10, 6; 4Q, '08, 6, 8; 3Q, '02, 4-5; 3Q, '01, 4-5; 1Q, '01, 6

C1777 **Lead, cardioverter-defibrillator, endocardial single coil (implantable)** N N1
AHA: 3Q, '16, 10-15; 2Q, '06, 11; 4Q, '04, 4-5; 3Q, '02, 4-5; 1Q, '01, 6

C1778 **Lead, neurostimulator (implantable)** N N1
CMS: 100-04,14,40.8; 100-04,32,40.1
AHA: 3Q, '16, 10-15; 4Q, '11, 10; 3Q, '02, 4-5; 1Q, '02, 9; 1Q, '01, 6

C1779 **Lead, pacemaker, transvenous VDD single pass** N N1
CMS: 100-04,14,40.8
AHA: 3Q, '16, 15-19; 3Q, '16, 10-15; 4Q, '04, 4-5; 3Q, '02, 4-5; 1Q, '01, 6

C1780 **Lens, intraocular (new technology)** N N1
AHA: 3Q, '16, 15-19; 3Q, '16, 10-15; 3Q, '02, 4-5; 1Q, '01, 6

C1781 **Mesh (implantable)** N N1
Use this code for OrthADAPT Bioimplant.
AHA: 3Q, '16, 15-19; 3Q, '16, 10-15; 2Q, '12, 3; 2Q, '10, 3; 2Q, '10, 2, 3; 3Q, '02, 4-5; 1Q, '01, 6

C1782 **Morcellator** N N1
AHA: 3Q, '16, 15-19; 3Q, '16, 10-15; 3Q, '02, 4-5; 1Q, '01, 6

C1783 **Ocular implant, aqueous drainage assist device** N N1
AHA: 1Q, '17, 5; 3Q, '16, 10-15

C1784 **Ocular device, intraoperative, detached retina** N N1
AHA: 3Q, '16, 15-19; 3Q, '16, 10-15; 3Q, '02, 4-5; 1Q, '01, 6

C1785 **Pacemaker, dual chamber, rate-responsive (implantable)** N N1
CMS: 100-04,14,40.8; 100-04,21,320.4.7; 100-04,32,320.4.1; 100-04,32,320.4.2; 100-04,32,320.4.4; 100-04,32,320.4.6; 100-04,32,320.4.7
AHA: 3Q, '16, 10-15; 4Q, '03, 8; 3Q, '02, 4-5; 1Q, '01, 6

C1786 **Pacemaker, single chamber, rate-responsive (implantable)** N N1
CMS: 100-04,14,40.8; 100-04,21,320.4.7; 100-04,32,320.4.1; 100-04,32,320.4.2; 100-04,32,320.4.4; 100-04,32,320.4.6; 100-04,32,320.4.7
AHA: 3Q, '16, 10-15; 4Q, '04, 4-5; 4Q, '03, 8; 3Q, '02, 4-5; 1Q, '01, 6

C1787 **Patient programmer, neurostimulator** N N1
AHA: 3Q, '16, 15-19; 3Q, '16, 10-15; 4Q, '03, 8; 3Q, '02, 4-5; 1Q, '01, 6

C1788 **Port, indwelling (implantable)** N N1
AHA: 3Q, '16, 10-15; 3Q, '14, 5; 4Q, '04, 4-5; 4Q, '03, 8; 3Q, '02, 4-5; 3Q, '01, 4-5; 1Q, '01, 6

C1789 **Prosthesis, breast (implantable)** N N1
AHA: 3Q, '16, 10-15; 4Q, '03, 8; 3Q, '02, 4-5; 1Q, '01, 6

C1813 **Prosthesis, penile, inflatable** N N1
CMS: 100-04,14,40.8
AHA: 3Q, '16, 10-15; 4Q, '03, 8; 3Q, '02, 4-5; 1Q, '01, 6

C1814 **Retinal tamponade device, silicone oil** N N1
AHA: 3Q, '16, 15-19; 3Q, '16, 10-15; 2Q, '06, 12

C1815 **Prosthesis, urinary sphincter (implantable)** N N1
CMS: 100-04,14,40.8
AHA: 3Q, '16, 10-15; 4Q, '03, 8; 3Q, '02, 4-5; 1Q, '01, 6

C1816 **Receiver and/or transmitter, neurostimulator (implantable)** N N1
AHA: 3Q, '16, 10-15; 4Q, '03, 8; 3Q, '02, 4-5; 1Q, '01, 6

C1817 **Septal defect implant system, intracardiac** N N1
AHA: 3Q, '16, 15-19; 3Q, '16, 10-15; 4Q, '03, 8; 3Q, '02, 4-5; 1Q, '01, 6

C1818 **Integrated keratoprosthesis** N N1
AHA: 3Q, '16, 15-19; 3Q, '16, 10-15; 4Q, '03, 4-5

C1819 **Surgical tissue localization and excision device (implantable)** N N1
AHA: 3Q, '16, 10-15; 1Q, '04, 10

C1820 **Generator, neurostimulator (implantable), with rechargeable battery and charging system** N N1
Use to report neurostimulator generators that are not high frequency.
CMS: 100-04,14,40.8; 100-04,4,10.12
AHA: 3Q, '16, 10-15; 2Q, '16, 7; 1Q, '16, 9

C1821 **Interspinous process distraction device (implantable)** N N1
AHA: 3Q, '16, 10-15; 2Q, '09, 1

C1822 **Generator, neurostimulator (implantable), high frequency, with rechargeable battery and charging system** N N1
Use to report neurostimulator generators that are high frequency.
AHA: 3Q, '16, 10-15; 2Q, '16, 7; 1Q, '16, 9

C1823 **Generator, neurostimulator (implantable), nonrechargeable, with transvenous sensing and stimulation leads** J7
CMS: 100-04,4,260.1; 100-04,4,260.1.1

● **C1824** Jan **Generator, cardiac contractility modulation (implantable)**

C1830 **Powered bone marrow biopsy needle** N N1
AHA: 3Q, '16, 10-15; 4Q, '11, 10

● **C1839** Jan **Iris prosthesis**

C1840 **Lens, intraocular (telescopic)** N N1
AHA: 3Q, '16, 10-15; 3Q, '12, 10; 4Q, '11, 10

C1841 **Retinal prosthesis, includes all internal and external components** N J7
AHA: 1Q, '17, 6; 3Q, '16, 10-15

C1842 **Retinal prosthesis, includes all internal and external components; add-on to C1841** E J7
In the ASC setting, C1842 must be reported with C1841 and CPT code 0100T.
AHA: 1Q, '17, 6

C1874 **Stent, coated/covered, with delivery system** N N1
AHA: 3Q, '16, 15-19; 3Q, '16, 10-15; 4Q, '04, 4-5; 3Q, '04, 11-13; 4Q, '03, 8; 3Q, '02, 7; 3Q, '02, 4-5; 3Q, '01, 4-5; 1Q, '01, 6

C1875 **Stent, coated/covered, without delivery system** N N1
AHA: 3Q, '16, 15-19; 3Q, '16, 10-15; 4Q, '04, 4-5; 4Q, '03, 8; 3Q, '02, 7; 3Q, '02, 4-5; 1Q, '01, 6

© 2019 Optum360, LLC

C1876 **Stent, noncoated/noncovered, with delivery system** N N1
AHA: 3Q, '16, 15-19; 3Q, '16, 10-15; 4Q, '04, 4-5; 4Q, '03, 8; 3Q, '02, 7; 3Q, '02, 4-5; 3Q, '01, 4-5; 1Q, '01, 6

C1877 **Stent, noncoated/noncovered, without delivery system** N N1
AHA: 3Q, '16, 10-15; 4Q, '04, 4-5; 4Q, '03, 8; 3Q, '02, 7; 3Q, '02, 4-5; 3Q, '01, 4-5; 1Q, '01, 6

C1878 **Material for vocal cord medialization, synthetic (implantable)** N N1
AHA: 3Q, '16, 15-19; 3Q, '16, 10-15; 3Q, '02, 4-5; 1Q, '01, 6

C1880 **Vena cava filter** N N1
AHA: 3Q, '16, 10-15; 4Q, '03, 8; 3Q, '02, 4-5; 1Q, '01, 6

C1881 **Dialysis access system (implantable)** N N1
CMS: 100-04,14,40.8
AHA: 3Q, '16, 10-15; 4Q, '03, 8; 3Q, '02, 4-5; 1Q, '01, 6

C1882 **Cardioverter-defibrillator, other than single or dual chamber (implantable)** N N1
CMS: 100-04,14,40.8
AHA: 3Q, '16, 15-19; 3Q, '16, 10-15; 2Q, '12, 9; 2Q, '06, 11; 4Q, '04, 4-5; 3Q, '02, 4-5; 1Q, '01, 6

C1883 **Adaptor/extension, pacing lead or neurostimulator lead (implantable)** N N1
CMS: 100-04,32,40.1
AHA: 3Q, '16, 15-19; 3Q, '16, 10-15; 3Q, '02, 4-5; 1Q, '02, 9; 1Q, '01, 6

C1884 **Embolization protective system** N N1
AHA: 3Q, '16, 15-19; 3Q, '16, 10-15; 3Q, '14, 5

C1885 **Catheter, transluminal angioplasty, laser** N N1
AHA: 3Q, '16, 15-19; 3Q, '16, 10-15; 1Q, '16, 5; 4Q, '04, 4-5; 4Q, '03, 8; 3Q, '02, 4-5; 1Q, '01, 6

C1886 **Catheter, extravascular tissue ablation, any modality (insertable)** N N1
AHA: 3Q, '16, 10-15

C1887 **Catheter, guiding (may include infusion/perfusion capability)** N N1
AHA: 3Q, '16, 15-19; 3Q, '16, 10-15; 4Q, '04, 4-5; 3Q, '02, 4-5; 3Q, '01, 4-5; 1Q, '01, 6

C1888 **Catheter, ablation, noncardiac, endovascular (implantable)** N N1
AHA: 3Q, '16, 15-19; 3Q, '16, 10-15

C1889 **Implantable/insertable device, not otherwise classified** N N1

C1890 **No implantable/insertable device used with device-intensive procedures** J7
CMS: 100-04,4,260.1; 100-04,4,260.1.1

C1891 **Infusion pump, nonprogrammable, permanent (implantable)** N N1
CMS: 100-04,14,40.8
AHA: 3Q, '16, 10-15; 4Q, '04, 4-5; 4Q, '03, 8; 3Q, '02, 4-5; 1Q, '01, 6

C1892 **Introducer/sheath, guiding, intracardiac electrophysiological, fixed-curve, peel-away** N N1
AHA: 3Q, '16, 15-19; 3Q, '16, 10-15; 4Q, '04, 4-5; 3Q, '02, 4-5; 1Q, '01, 6

C1893 **Introducer/sheath, guiding, intracardiac electrophysiological, fixed-curve, other than peel-away** N N1
AHA: 3Q, '16, 10-15; 4Q, '04, 4-5; 3Q, '02, 4-5; 3Q, '01, 4-5; 1Q, '01, 6

C1894 **Introducer/sheath, other than guiding, other than intracardiac electrophysiological, nonlaser** N N1
AHA: 3Q, '16, 9; 3Q, '16, 10-15; 3Q, '02, 4-5; 1Q, '01, 6

C1895 **Lead, cardioverter-defibrillator, endocardial dual coil (implantable)** N N1
AHA: 3Q, '16, 10-15; 2Q, '06, 11; 4Q, '04, 4-5; 3Q, '02, 4-5; 1Q, '01, 6

C1896 **Lead, cardioverter-defibrillator, other than endocardial single or dual coil (implantable)** N N1
AHA: 3Q, '16, 10-15; 2Q, '06, 11; 4Q, '04, 4-5; 3Q, '02, 4-5; 1Q, '01, 6

C1897 **Lead, neurostimulator test kit (implantable)** N N1
CMS: 100-04,14,40.8; 100-04,32,40.1
AHA: 3Q, '16, 10-15; 3Q, '02, 4-5; 1Q, '02, 9; 1Q, '01, 6

C1898 **Lead, pacemaker, other than transvenous VDD single pass** N N1
CMS: 100-04,14,40.8
AHA: 3Q, '16, 10-15; 3Q, '02, 8; 3Q, '02, 4-5; 3Q, '01, 4-5; 1Q, '01, 6

C1899 **Lead, pacemaker/cardioverter-defibrillator combination (implantable)** N N1
AHA: 3Q, '16, 10-15; 4Q, '04, 4-5; 3Q, '02, 4-5; 1Q, '01, 6

C1900 **Lead, left ventricular coronary venous system** N N1
CMS: 100-04,14,40.8
AHA: 3Q, '16, 15-19; 3Q, '16, 10-15; 4Q, '04, 4-5

● **C1982**[Jan] **Catheter, pressure generating, one-way valve, intermittently occlusive**

● **C2596**[Jan] **Probe, image guided, robotic, waterjet ablation**

C2613 **Lung biopsy plug with delivery system** N N1
AHA: 3Q, '16, 10-15; 3Q, '15, 7

C2614 **Probe, percutaneous lumbar discectomy** N N1
AHA: 3Q, '16, 10-15

C2615 **Sealant, pulmonary, liquid** N N1
AHA: 3Q, '16, 15-19; 3Q, '16, 10-15; 4Q, '03, 8; 3Q, '02, 4-5; 1Q, '01, 6

C2616 **Brachytherapy source, nonstranded, yttrium-90, per source** U P2 ☑ ⊘
AHA: 3Q, '16, 11; 3Q, '16, 10-15; 2Q, '07, 11; 4Q, '04, 8; 2Q, '04, 10; 3Q, '03, 11; 3Q, '02, 4-5

C2617 **Stent, noncoronary, temporary, without delivery system** N N1
AHA: 3Q, '16, 15-19; 3Q, '16, 10-15; 3Q, '16; 4Q, '04, 4-5; 4Q, '03, 8; 3Q, '02, 4-5; 1Q, '01, 6

C2618 **Probe/needle, cryoablation** N N1
AHA: 3Q, '16, 10-15; 4Q, '04, 4-5; 4Q, '03, 8; 3Q, '02, 4-5; 1Q, '01, 6

C2619 **Pacemaker, dual chamber, nonrate-responsive (implantable)** N N1
CMS: 100-04,14,40.8; 100-04,21,320.4.7; 100-04,32,320.4.1; 100-04,32,320.4.2; 100-04;32,320.4.4; 100-04,32,320.4.6; 100-04,32,320.4.7
AHA: 3Q, '16, 10-15; 3Q, '02, 4-5; 3Q, '01, 4-5; 1Q, '01, 6

C2620 **Pacemaker, single chamber, nonrate-responsive (implantable)** N N1
CMS: 100-04,14,40.8; 100-04,21,320.4.7; 100-04,32,320.4.1; 100-04,32,320.4.2; 100-04,32,320.4.4; 100-04,32,320.4.6; 100-04,32,320.4.7
AHA: 3Q, '16, 10-15; 4Q, '04, 4-5; 4Q, '03, 8; 3Q, '02, 4-5; 1Q, '01, 6

C2621 **Pacemaker, other than single or dual chamber (implantable)** N N1
CMS: 100-04,14,40.8
AHA: 3Q, '16, 15-19; 3Q, '16, 10-15; 4Q, '03, 8; 3Q, '02, 8; 3Q, '02, 4-5; 1Q, '01, 6

C2622 **Prosthesis, penile, noninflatable** N N1
CMS: 100-04,14,40.8
AHA: 3Q, '16, 10-15; 4Q, '03, 8; 3Q, '02, 4-5; 1Q, '01, 6

C2623 **Catheter, transluminal angioplasty, drug-coated, nonlaser** N N1
AHA: 3Q, '16, 10-15

C2624 **Implantable wireless pulmonary artery pressure sensor with delivery catheter, including all system components** N N1
AHA: 3Q, '16, 10-15; 3Q, '15, 1-2

© 2019 Optum360, LLC

C2625 **Stent, noncoronary, temporary, with delivery system** N N1
AHA: 3Q, '16, 15-19; 3Q, '16, 10-15; 2Q, '15, 9; 4Q, '04, 4-5; 4Q, '03, 8; 3Q, '02, 4-5; 1Q, '01, 6

C2626 **Infusion pump, nonprogrammable, temporary (implantable)** N N1
CMS: 100-04,14,40.8
AHA: 3Q, '16, 15-19; 3Q, '16, 10-15; 4Q, '04, 4-5; 3Q, '02, 4-5; 1Q, '01, 6

C2627 **Catheter, suprapubic/cystoscopic** N N1
AHA: 3Q, '16, 15-19; 3Q, '16, 10-15; 4Q, '03, 8; 3Q, '02, 4-5; 1Q, '01, 6

C2628 **Catheter, occlusion** N N1
AHA: 3Q, '16, 10-15; 4Q, '04, 4-5; 4Q, '03, 8; 3Q, '02, 4-5; 1Q, '01, 6

C2629 **Introducer/sheath, other than guiding, other than intracardiac electrophysiological, laser** N N1
AHA: 3Q, '16, 10-15; 3Q, '02, 4-5; 1Q, '01, 6

C2630 **Catheter, electrophysiology, diagnostic/ablation, other than 3D or vector mapping, cool-tip** N N1
AHA: 3Q, '16, 15-19; 3Q, '16, 10-15; 3Q, '02, 4-5; 1Q, '01, 6

C2631 **Repair device, urinary, incontinence, without sling graft** N N1
CMS: 100-04,14,40.8
AHA: 3Q, '16, 15-19; 3Q, '16, 10-15; 4Q, '03, 8; 3Q, '02, 4-5; 1Q, '01, 6

C2634 **Brachytherapy source, nonstranded, high activity, iodine-125, greater than 1.01 mCi (NIST), per source** U H2 ☑ ⊘
AHA: 3Q, '16, 11; 2Q, '07, 11; 2Q, '05, 8; 4Q, '04, 8

C2635 **Brachytherapy source, nonstranded, high activity, palladium-103, greater than 2.2 mCi (NIST), per source** U H2 ☑ ⊘
AHA: 3Q, '16, 11; 2Q, '07, 11; 2Q, '05, 8; 4Q, '04, 8

C2636 **Brachytherapy linear source, nonstranded, palladium-103, per 1 mm** U H2 ☑ ⊘
AHA: 3Q, '16, 11; 2Q, '07, 11; 4Q, '04, 8

C2637 **Brachytherapy source, nonstranded, ytterbium-169, per source** B ☑ ⊘
AHA: 3Q, '16, 11; 2Q, '07, 11; 3Q, '05, 7

C2638 **Brachytherapy source, stranded, iodine-125, per source** U H2 ☑
AHA: 3Q, '16, 11

C2639 **Brachytherapy source, nonstranded, iodine-125, per source** U H2 ☑ ⊘
AHA: 3Q, '16, 11

C2640 **Brachytherapy source, stranded, palladium-103, per source** U H2 ☑
AHA: 3Q, '16, 11

C2641 **Brachytherapy source, nonstranded, palladium-103, per source** U H2 ☑ ⊘
AHA: 3Q, '16, 11

C2642 **Brachytherapy source, stranded, cesium-131, per source** U H2 ☑
AHA: 3Q, '16, 11

C2643 **Brachytherapy source, nonstranded, cesium-131, per source** U H2 ☑ ⊘
AHA: 3Q, '16, 11

C2644 **Brachytherapy source, cesium-131 chloride solution, per mCi** U ☑
AHA: 3Q, '16, 11

C2645 **Brachytherapy planar source, palladium-103, per sq mL** U H2 ☑
AHA: 3Q, '16, 11

C2698 **Brachytherapy source, stranded, not otherwise specified, per source** U H2 ☑
AHA: 3Q, '16, 11

C2699 **Brachytherapy source, nonstranded, not otherwise specified, per source** U H2 ☑
AHA: 3Q, '16, 11

C5271 **Application of low cost skin substitute graft to trunk, arms, legs, total wound surface area up to 100 sq cm; first 25 sq cm or less wound surface area** T G2 ☑

C5272 **Application of low cost skin substitute graft to trunk, arms, legs, total wound surface area up to 100 sq cm; each additional 25 sq cm wound surface area, or part thereof (list separately in addition to code for primary procedure)** N N1 ☑

C5273 **Application of low cost skin substitute graft to trunk, arms, legs, total wound surface area greater than or equal to 100 sq cm; first 100 sq cm wound surface area, or 1% of body area of infants and children** T G2 ☑

C5274 **Application of low cost skin substitute graft to trunk, arms, legs, total wound surface area greater than or equal to 100 sq cm; each additional 100 sq cm wound surface area, or part thereof, or each additional 1% of body area of infants and children, or part thereof (list separately in addition to code for primary procedure)** N N1 ☑

C5275 **Application of low cost skin substitute graft to face, scalp, eyelids, mouth, neck, ears, orbits, genitalia, hands, feet, and/or multiple digits, total wound surface area up to 100 sq cm; first 25 sq cm or less wound surface area** T G2 ☑

C5276 **Application of low cost skin substitute graft to face, scalp, eyelids, mouth, neck, ears, orbits, genitalia, hands, feet, and/or multiple digits, total wound surface area up to 100 sq cm; each additional 25 sq cm wound surface area, or part thereof (list separately in addition to code for primary procedure)** N N1 ☑

C5277 **Application of low cost skin substitute graft to face, scalp, eyelids, mouth, neck, ears, orbits, genitalia, hands, feet, and/or multiple digits, total wound surface area greater than or equal to 100 sq cm; first 100 sq cm wound surface area, or 1% of body area of infants and children** T G2 ☑

C5278 **Application of low cost skin substitute graft to face, scalp, eyelids, mouth, neck, ears, orbits, genitalia, hands, feet, and/or multiple digits, total wound surface area greater than or equal to 100 sq cm; each additional 100 sq cm wound surface area, or part thereof, or each additional 1% of body area of infants and children, or part thereof (list separately in addition to code for primary procedure)** N N1 ☑

C8900 **Magnetic resonance angiography with contrast, abdomen** Q3 Z2 ⊘
CMS: 100-04,13,40.1.1; 100-04,13,40.1.2

C8901 **Magnetic resonance angiography without contrast, abdomen** Q3 Z2 ⊘
CMS: 100-04,13,40.1.1; 100-04,13,40.1.2

C8902 **Magnetic resonance angiography without contrast followed by with contrast, abdomen** Q3 Z2 ⊘
CMS: 100-04,13,40.1.1; 100-04,13,40.1.2

C8903 **Magnetic resonance imaging with contrast, breast; unilateral** Q3 Z2 ⊘

C8905 **Magnetic resonance imaging without contrast followed by with contrast, breast; unilateral** Q3 Z2 ⊘

C8906 **Magnetic resonance imaging with contrast, breast; bilateral** Q3 Z2 ⊘

C8908 **Magnetic resonance imaging without contrast followed by with contrast, breast; bilateral** Q3 Z2 ⊘

© 2019 Optum360, LLC

C8909 **Magnetic resonance angiography with contrast, chest (excluding myocardium)** Q3 Z2 ⊘
CMS: 100-04,13,40.1.1; 100-04,13,40.1.2

C8910 **Magnetic resonance angiography without contrast, chest (excluding myocardium)** Q3 Z2 ⊘
CMS: 100-04,13,40.1.1; 100-04,13,40.1.2

C8911 **Magnetic resonance angiography without contrast followed by with contrast, chest (excluding myocardium)** Q3 Z2 ⊘
CMS: 100-04,13,40.1.1; 100-04,13,40.1.2

C8912 **Magnetic resonance angiography with contrast, lower extremity** Q3 Z2 ⊘
CMS: 100-04,13,40.1.1; 100-04,13,40.1.2

C8913 **Magnetic resonance angiography without contrast, lower extremity** Q3 Z2 ⊘
CMS: 100-04,13,40.1.1; 100-04,13,40.1.2

C8914 **Magnetic resonance angiography without contrast followed by with contrast, lower extremity** Q3 Z2 ⊘
CMS: 100-04,13,40.1.1; 100-04,13,40.1.2

C8918 **Magnetic resonance angiography with contrast, pelvis** Q3 Z2 ⊘
CMS: 100-04,13,40.1.1; 100-04,13,40.1.2
AHA: 4Q, '03, 4-5

C8919 **Magnetic resonance angiography without contrast, pelvis** Q3 Z2 ⊘
CMS: 100-04,13,40.1.1; 100-04,13,40.1.2
AHA: 4Q, '03, 4-5

C8920 **Magnetic resonance angiography without contrast followed by with contrast, pelvis** Q3 Z2 ⊘
CMS: 100-04,13,40.1.1; 100-04,13,40.1.2
AHA: 4Q, '03, 4-5

C8921 **Transthoracic echocardiography with contrast, or without contrast followed by with contrast, for congenital cardiac anomalies; complete** S
CMS: 100-04,4,200.7.2
AHA: 3Q, '12, 8; 2Q, '08, 9

C8922 **Transthoracic echocardiography (TEE) with contrast, or without contrast followed by with contrast, for congenital cardiac anomalies; follow-up or limited study** S
AHA: 2Q, '08, 9

C8923 **Transthoracic echocardiography (TEE) with contrast, or without contrast followed by with contrast, real-time with image documentation (2D), includes M-mode recording, when performed, complete, without spectral or color doppler echocardiography** S
AHA: 2Q, '08, 9

C8924 **Transthoracic echocardiography (TEE) with contrast, or without contrast followed by with contrast, real-time with image documentation (2D), includes M-mode recording when performed, follow-up or limited study** S
AHA: 2Q, '08, 9

C8925 **Transesophageal echocardiography (TEE) with contrast, or without contrast followed by with contrast, real time with image documentation (2D) (with or without M-mode recording); including probe placement, image acquisition, interpretation and report** S
AHA: 2Q, '08, 9

C8926 **Transesophageal echocardiography (TEE) with contrast, or without contrast followed by with contrast, for congenital cardiac anomalies; including probe placement, image acquisition, interpretation and report** S
AHA: 2Q, '08, 9

C8927 **Transesophageal echocardiography (TEE) with contrast, or without contrast followed by with contrast, for monitoring purposes, including probe placement, real time (2D) image acquisition and interpretation leading to ongoing (continuous) assessment of (dynamically changing) cardiac pumping function and to therapeutic measures on an immediate time basis** S
AHA: 2Q, '08, 9

C8928 **Transthoracic echocardiography (TEE) with contrast, or without contrast followed by with contrast, real-time with image documentation (2D), includes M-mode recording, when performed, during rest and cardiovascular stress test using treadmill, bicycle exercise and/or pharmacologically induced stress, with interpretation and report** S
AHA: 2Q, '08, 9

C8929 **Transthoracic echocardiography (TEE) with contrast, or without contrast followed by with contrast, real-time with image documentation (2D), includes M-mode recording, when performed, complete, with spectral doppler echocardiography, and with color flow doppler echocardiography** S

C8930 **Transthoracic echocardiography (TEE) with contrast, or without contrast followed by with contrast, real-time with image documentation (2D), includes M-mode recording, when performed, during rest and cardiovascular stress test using treadmill, bicycle exercise and/or pharmacologically induced stress, with interpretation and report; including performance of continuous electrocardiographic monitoring, with physician supervision** S
AHA: 3Q, '12, 8

C8931 **Magnetic resonance angiography with contrast, spinal canal and contents** Q3 Z2

C8932 **Magnetic resonance angiography without contrast, spinal canal and contents** Q3 Z2

C8933 **Magnetic resonance angiography without contrast followed by with contrast, spinal canal and contents** Q3 Z2

C8934 **Magnetic resonance angiography with contrast, upper extremity** Q3 Z2

C8935 **Magnetic resonance angiography without contrast, upper extremity** Q3 Z2

C8936 **Magnetic resonance angiography without contrast followed by with contrast, upper extremity** Q3 Z2

C8937 **Computer-aided detection, including computer algorithm analysis of breast MRI image data for lesion detection/characterization, pharmacokinetic analysis, with further physician review for interpretation (list separately in addition to code for primary procedure)**

C8957 **Intravenous infusion for therapy/diagnosis; initiation of prolonged infusion (more than 8 hours), requiring use of portable or implantable pump** S
CMS: 100-04,4,230.2
AHA: 3Q, '08, 7, 8; 4Q, '05, 15

~~**C9035**~~ Jan ~~**Injection, aripiprazole lauroxil (Aristada Initio), 1 mg**~~
To report, see ~J1943

~~**C9036**~~ Jan ~~**Injection, patisiran, 0.1 mg**~~
To report, see ~J0222

~~**C9037**~~ Jan ~~**Injection, risperidone (Perseris), 0.5 mg**~~
To report, see ~J2798

~~**C9038**~~ Jan ~~**Injection, mogamulizumab-kpkc, 1 mg**~~
To report, see ~J9204

~~**C9039**~~ Jan ~~**Injection, plazomicin, 5 mg**~~
To report, see ~J0291

~~**C9040**~~ Jan ~~**Injection, fremanezumab-vfrm, 1 mg**~~
To report, see ~J3031

© 2019 Optum360, LLC

● **C9041**[Jan] **Injection, coagulation Factor Xa (recombinant), inactivated (Andexxa), 10 mg** K2

~~**C9042**[Jan] **Injection, bendamustine HCl (Belrapzo), 1 mg**~~
To report, see ~J9036

~~**C9043**[Jan] **Injection, levoleucovorin, 1 mg**~~
To report, see ~J0641

~~**C9044**[Jan] **Injection, cemiplimab-rwlc, 1 mg**~~
To report, see ~J9119

~~**C9045**[Jan] **Injection, moxetumomab pasudotox-tdfk, 0.01 mg**~~
To report, see ~J9313

● **C9046**[Jan] **Cocaine HCl nasal solution for topical administration, 1 mg** K2
Use this code for Goprelto.

● **C9047**[Jan] **Injection, caplacizumab-yhdp, 1 mg** K2
Use this code for Cablivi.

~~**C9048**[Jan] **Dexamethasone, lacrimal ophthalmic insert, 0.1 mg**~~
To report, see ~J1096

~~**C9049**[Jan] **Injection, tagraxofusp-erzs, 10 mcg**~~
To report, see ~J9269

~~**C9050**[Jan] **Injection, emapalumab-lzsg, 1 mg**~~
To report, see ~J9210

~~**C9051**[Jan] **Injection, omadacycline, 1 mg**~~
To report, see ~J0121

~~**C9052**[Jan] **Injection, ravulizumab-cwvz, 10 mg**~~
To report, see ~J1303

● **C9054**[Jan] **Injection, lefamulin (Xenleta), 1 mg**

● **C9055**[Jan] **Injection, brexanolone, 1 mg**
Use this code for Zulresso.

C9113 **Injection, pantoprazole sodium, per vial** N N1 ☑
Use this code for Protonix.
AHA: 1Q, '02, 5

C9132 **Prothrombin complex concentrate (human), Kcentra, per IU of Factor IX activity** K K2 ☑

~~**C9141**[Jan] **Injection, Factor VIII, (antihemophilic factor, recombinant), pegylated-aucl (Jivi), 1 IU**~~
To report, see ~J7208

C9248 **Injection, clevidipine butyrate, 1 mg** N K2 ☑
Use this code for Cleviprex.

C9250 **Human plasma fibrin sealant, vapor-heated, solvent-detergent (Artiss), 2 ml** K K2 ☑

C9254 **Injection, lacosamide, 1 mg** N N1 ☑
Use this code for VIMPAT.

C9257 **Injection, bevacizumab, 0.25 mg** K K2 ☑
Use this code for Avastin.
CMS: 100-03,110.17
AHA: 3Q, '13, 9

C9285 **Lidocaine 70 mg/tetracaine 70 mg, per patch** N N1 ☑
Use this code for SYNERA.
AHA: 3Q, '11, 9

C9290 **Injection, bupivacaine liposome, 1 mg** N K2 ☑
Use this code for EXPAREL.
AHA: 2Q, '12, 7

C9293 **Injection, glucarpidase, 10 units** K K2 ☑
Use this code for Voraxaze.

C9352 **Microporous collagen implantable tube (NeuraGen Nerve Guide), per cm length** N N1 ☑
AHA: 1Q, '08, 6

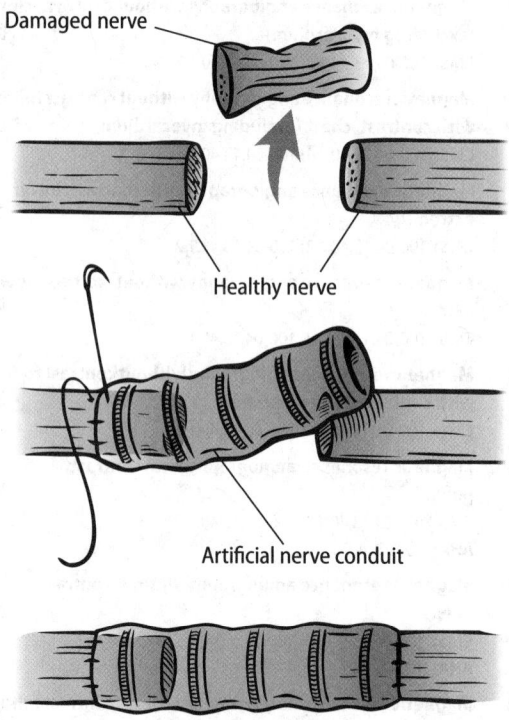

A synthetic "bridge" is affixed to each end of a severed nerve with sutures. This procedure is performed using an operating microscope

C9353 **Microporous collagen implantable slit tube (NeuraWrap Nerve Protector), per cm length** N N1 ☑
AHA: 1Q, '08, 6

C9354 **Acellular pericardial tissue matrix of nonhuman origin (Veritas), per sq cm** N N1 ☑
AHA: 1Q, '08, 6

C9355 **Collagen nerve cuff (NeuroMatrix), per 0.5 cm length** N N1 ☑
AHA: 1Q, '08, 6

C9356 **Tendon, porous matrix of cross-linked collagen and glycosaminoglycan matrix (TenoGlide Tendon Protector Sheet), per sq cm** N N1 ☑
AHA: 3Q, '08, 6

C9358 **Dermal substitute, native, nondenatured collagen, fetal bovine origin (SurgiMend Collagen Matrix), per 0.5 sq cm** N N1 ☑
AHA: 2Q, '12, 7; 3Q, '08, 6

C9359 **Porous purified collagen matrix bone void filler (Integra Mozaik Osteoconductive Scaffold Putty, Integra OS Osteoconductive Scaffold Putty), per 0.5 cc** N N1 ☑
AHA: 3Q, '15, 2

C9360 **Dermal substitute, native, nondenatured collagen, neonatal bovine origin (SurgiMend Collagen Matrix), per 0.5 sq cm** N N1 ☑
AHA: 2Q, '12, 7

C9361 **Collagen matrix nerve wrap (NeuroMend Collagen Nerve Wrap), per 0.5 cm length** N N1 ☑

C9362 **Porous purified collagen matrix bone void filler (Integra Mozaik Osteoconductive Scaffold Strip), per 0.5 cc** N N1 ☑
AHA: 2Q, '10, 8

© 2019 Optum360, LLC

C9363 **Skin substitute (Integra Meshed Bilayer Wound Matrix), per sq cm** N N1 ☑
CMS: 100-04,4,260.1; 100-04,4,260.1.1
AHA: 2Q, '12, 7; 2Q, '10, 8

C9364 **Porcine implant, Permacol, per sq cm** N N1 ☑

C9399 **Unclassified drugs or biologicals** A K7
CMS: 100-02,15,50.5; 100-04,17,90.3; 100-04,4,260.1; 100-04,4,260.1.1
AHA: 1Q, '17, 8; 1Q, '17, 1-3; 4Q, '16, 10; 4Q, '14, 5; 2Q, '14, 8; 2Q, '13, 5; 1Q, '13, 9; 1Q, '08, 6; 4Q, '05, 7, 9; 4Q, '04, 3

~~**C9407**~~ Jan ~~**Iodine I-131 iobenguane, diagnostic, 1 mCi**~~
To report, see ~A9590

~~**C9408**~~ Jan ~~**Iodine I-131 iobenguane, therapeutic, 1 mCi**~~
To report, see ~A9590

~~**C9447**~~ Jan ~~**Injection, phenylephrine and ketorolac, 4 ml vial**~~

C9460 **Injection, cangrelor, 1 mg** G K2 ☑
Use this code for Kengreal.
AHA: 1Q, '16, 6-8

C9462 **Injection, delafloxacin, 1 mg** G K2
Use this code for Baxdela.

C9482 **Injection, sotalol HCl, 1 mg** G K2 ☑
AHA: 4Q, '16, 9

C9488 **Injection, conivaptan HCl, 1 mg** G K2 ☑
Use this code for Vaprisol.

C9600 **Percutaneous transcatheter placement of drug eluting intracoronary stent(s), with coronary angioplasty when performed; single major coronary artery or branch** J

C9601 **Percutaneous transcatheter placement of drug-eluting intracoronary stent(s), with coronary angioplasty when performed; each additional branch of a major coronary artery (list separately in addition to code for primary procedure)** N

C9602 **Percutaneous transluminal coronary atherectomy, with drug eluting intracoronary stent, with coronary angioplasty when performed; single major coronary artery or branch** J

C9603 **Percutaneous transluminal coronary atherectomy, with drug-eluting intracoronary stent, with coronary angioplasty when performed; each additional branch of a major coronary artery (list separately in addition to code for primary procedure)** N

C9604 **Percutaneous transluminal revascularization of or through coronary artery bypass graft (internal mammary, free arterial, venous), any combination of drug-eluting intracoronary stent, atherectomy and angioplasty, including distal protection when performed; single vessel** J

C9605 **Percutaneous transluminal revascularization of or through coronary artery bypass graft (internal mammary, free arterial, venous), any combination of drug-eluting intracoronary stent, atherectomy and angioplasty, including distal protection when performed; each additional branch subtended by the bypass graft (list separately in addition to code for primary procedure)** N

C9606 **Percutaneous transluminal revascularization of acute total/subtotal occlusion during acute myocardial infarction, coronary artery or coronary artery bypass graft, any combination of drug-eluting intracoronary stent, atherectomy and angioplasty, including aspiration thrombectomy when performed, single vessel** J
CMS: 100-04,4,260.1; 100-04,4,260.1.1

C9607 **Percutaneous transluminal revascularization of chronic total occlusion, coronary artery, coronary artery branch, or coronary artery bypass graft, any combination of drug-eluting intracoronary stent, atherectomy and angioplasty; single vessel** J

C9608 **Percutaneous transluminal revascularization of chronic total occlusion, coronary artery, coronary artery branch, or coronary artery bypass graft, any combination of drug-eluting intracoronary stent, atherectomy and angioplasty; each additional coronary artery, coronary artery branch, or bypass graft (list separately in addition to code for primary procedure)** N

C9725 **Placement of endorectal intracavitary applicator for high intensity brachytherapy** T G2 ⊘
AHA: 3Q, '05, 7

C9726 **Placement and removal (if performed) of applicator into breast for intraoperative radiation therapy, add-on to primary breast procedure** N N1
AHA: 2Q, '07, 10

C9727 **Insertion of implants into the soft palate; minimum of three implants** T G2 ☑

C9728 **Placement of interstitial device(s) for radiation therapy/surgery guidance (e.g., fiducial markers, dosimeter), for other than the following sites (any approach): abdomen, pelvis, prostate, retroperitoneum, thorax, single or multiple** S J8

C9733 **Nonophthalmic fluorescent vascular angiography** Q2

C9734 **Focused ultrasound ablation/therapeutic intervention, other than uterine leiomyomata, with magnetic resonance (MR) guidance** J
AHA: 3Q, '13, 9; 2Q, '13, 9

C9738 **Adjunctive blue light cystoscopy with fluorescent imaging agent (list separately in addition to code for primary procedure)** N N1

C9739 **Cystourethroscopy, with insertion of transprostatic implant; one to three implants** ♂ J J8
AHA: 2Q, '14, 8

C9740 **Cystourethroscopy, with insertion of transprostatic implant; four or more implants** ♂ J J8
AHA: 2Q, '14, 8

C9745 **Nasal endoscopy, surgical; balloon dilation of eustachian tube** J J8

~~**C9746**~~ Jan ~~**Transperineal implantation of permanent adjustable balloon continence device, with cystourethroscopy, when performed and/or fluoroscopy, when performed**~~
To report, see ~0548T

C9747 **Ablation of prostate, transrectal, high intensity focused ultrasound (HIFU), including imaging guidance** J G2

C9749 **Repair of nasal vestibular lateral wall stenosis with implant(s)** J J8

C9751 **Bronchoscopy, rigid or flexible, transbronchial ablation of lesion(s) by microwave energy, including fluoroscopic guidance, when performed, with computed tomography acquisition(s) and 3D rendering, computer-assisted, image-guided navigation, and endobronchial ultrasound (EBUS) guided transtracheal and/or transbronchial sampling (e.g., aspiration[s]/biopsy[ies]) and all mediastinal and/or hilar lymph node stations or structures and therapeutic intervention(s)**
CMS: 100-04,4,260.1; 100-04,4,260.1.1

C9752 **Destruction of intraosseous basivertebral nerve, first two vertebral bodies, including imaging guidance (e.g., fluoroscopy), lumbar/sacrum** J8
CMS: 100-04,4,260.1; 100-04,4,260.1.1

© 2019 Optum360, LLC

C9753 **Destruction of intraosseous basivertebral nerve, each additional vertebral body, including imaging guidance (e.g., fluoroscopy), lumbar/sacrum (list separately in addition to code for primary procedure)** N1

CMS: 100-04,4,260.1; 100-04,4,260.1.1

C9754 **Creation of arteriovenous fistula, percutaneous; direct, any site, including all imaging and radiologic supervision and interpretation, when performed and secondary procedures to redirect blood flow (e.g., transluminal balloon angioplasty, coil embolization, when performed)** J8

CMS: 100-04,4,260.1; 100-04,4,260.1.1

C9755 **Creation of arteriovenous fistula, percutaneous using magnetic-guided arterial and venous catheters and radiofrequency energy, including flow-directing procedures (e.g., vascular coil embolization with radiologic supervision and interpretation, when performed) and fistulogram(s), angiography, venography, and/or ultrasound, with radiologic supervision and interpretation, when performed** J8

CMS: 100-04,4,260.1; 100-04,4,260.1.1

● **C9756**[Jan] **Intraoperative near-infrared fluorescence lymphatic mapping of lymph node(s) (sentinel or tumor draining) with administration of indocyanine green (ICG) (List separately in addition to code for primary procedure)**

● **C9757**[Jan] **Laminotomy (hemilaminectomy), with decompression of nerve root(s), including partial facetectomy, foraminotomy and excision of herniated intervertebral disc, and repair of annular defect with implantation of bone anchored annular closure device, including annular defect measurement, alignment and sizing assessment, and image guidance; 1 interspace, lumbar**

● **C9758**[Jan] **Blinded procedure for NYHA Class III/IV heart failure; transcatheter implantation of interatrial shunt or placebo control, including right heart catheterization, transesophageal echocardiography (TEE)/intracardiac echocardiography (ICE), and all imaging with or without guidance (e.g., ultrasound, fluoroscopy), performed in an approved investigational device exemption (IDE) study**

C9898 **Radiolabeled product provided during a hospital inpatient stay** N

CMS: 100-04,4,260.1; 100-04,4,260.1.1

C9899 **Implanted prosthetic device, payable only for inpatients who do not have inpatient coverage** A

© 2019 Optum360, LLC

Durable Medical Equipment E0100-E8002

E codes include durable medical equipment such as canes, crutches, walkers, commodes, decubitus care, bath and toilet aids, hospital beds, oxygen and related respiratory equipment, monitoring equipment, pacemakers, patient lifts, safety equipment, restraints, traction equipment, fracture frames, wheelchairs, and artificial kidney machines.

Canes

E0100 **Cane, includes canes of all materials, adjustable or fixed, with tip** Y ♿ (NU, RR, UE)
White canes for the blind are not covered under Medicare.

E0105 **Cane, quad or three-prong, includes canes of all materials, adjustable or fixed, with tips** Y ♿ (NU, RR, UE)

Crutches

E0110 **Crutches, forearm, includes crutches of various materials, adjustable or fixed, pair, complete with tips and handgrips** Y ☑ ♿ (NU, RR, UE)

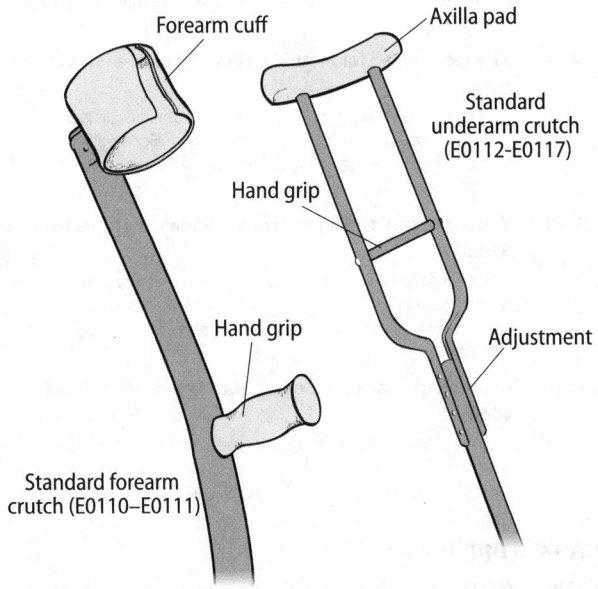

E0111 **Crutch, forearm, includes crutches of various materials, adjustable or fixed, each, with tip and handgrips** Y ☑ ♿ (NU, RR, UE)

E0112 **Crutches, underarm, wood, adjustable or fixed, pair, with pads, tips, and handgrips** Y ☑ ♿ (NU, RR, UE)

E0113 **Crutch, underarm, wood, adjustable or fixed, each, with pad, tip, and handgrip** Y ☑ ♿ (NU, RR, UE)

E0114 **Crutches, underarm, other than wood, adjustable or fixed, pair, with pads, tips, and handgrips** Y ☑ ♿ (NU, RR, UE)
AHA: 2Q, '02, 1-3

E0116 **Crutch, underarm, other than wood, adjustable or fixed, with pad, tip, handgrip, with or without shock absorber, each** Y ☑ ♿ (NU, RR, UE)

E0117 **Crutch, underarm, articulating, spring assisted, each** Y ☑ ♿ (RR)

E0118 **Crutch substitute, lower leg platform, with or without wheels, each** E ☑
Medicare covers walkers if patient's ambulation is impaired.

Walkers

E0130 **Walker, rigid (pickup), adjustable or fixed height** Y ♿ (NU, RR, UE)
CMS: 100-04,23,60.3; 100-04,36,50.15

E0135 **Walker, folding (pickup), adjustable or fixed height** Y ♿ (NU, RR, UE)
Medicare covers walkers if patient's ambulation is impaired.
CMS: 100-04,23,60.3; 100-04,36,50.15

E0140 **Walker, with trunk support, adjustable or fixed height, any type** Y ♿ (RR)
CMS: 100-04,23,60.3; 100-04,36,50.15

E0141 **Walker, rigid, wheeled, adjustable or fixed height** Y ♿ (NU, RR, UE)
Medicare covers walkers if patient's ambulation is impaired.
CMS: 100-04,23,60.3; 100-04,36,50.15

E0143 **Walker, folding, wheeled, adjustable or fixed height** Y ♿ (NU, RR, UE)
Medicare covers walkers if patient's ambulation is impaired.
CMS: 100-04,23,60.3; 100-04,36,50.15

E0144 **Walker, enclosed, four-sided framed, rigid or folding, wheeled with posterior seat** Y ♿ (RR)
CMS: 100-04,23,60.3; 100-04,36,50.15

E0147 **Walker, heavy-duty, multiple braking system, variable wheel resistance** Y ♿ (NU, RR, UE)
Medicare covers safety roller walkers only in patients with severe neurological disorders or restricted use of one hand. In some cases, coverage will be extended to patients with a weight exceeding the limits of a standard wheeled walker.
CMS: 100-04,23,60.3; 100-04,36,50.15

E0148 **Walker, heavy-duty, without wheels, rigid or folding, any type, each** Y ☑ ♿ (NU, RR, UE)
CMS: 100-04,23,60.3; 100-04,36,50.15

E0149 **Walker, heavy-duty, wheeled, rigid or folding, any type** Y ♿ (RR)
CMS: 100-04,23,60.3; 100-04,36,50.15

Attachments

E0153 **Platform attachment, forearm crutch, each** Y ☑ ♿ (NU, RR, UE)

E0154 **Platform attachment, walker, each** Y ☑ ♿ (NU, RR, UE)
CMS: 100-04,23,60.3; 100-04,36,50.14; 100-04,36,50.15

E0155 **Wheel attachment, rigid pick-up walker, per pair** Y ☑ ♿ (NU, RR, UE)
CMS: 100-04,23,60.3; 100-04,36,50.15

E0156 **Seat attachment, walker** Y ♿ (NU, RR, UE)
CMS: 100-04,23,60.3; 100-04,36,50.14; 100-04,36,50.15

E0157 **Crutch attachment, walker, each** Y ☑ ♿ (NU, RR, UE)
CMS: 100-04,23,60.3; 100-04,36,50.14; 100-04,36,50.15

E0158 **Leg extensions for walker, per set of four** Y ☑ ♿ (NU, RR, UE)
CMS: 100-04,23,60.3; 100-04,36,50.14; 100-04,36,50.15

E0159 **Brake attachment for wheeled walker, replacement, each** Y ☑ ♿ (NU, RR, UE)
CMS: 100-04,23,60.3; 100-04,36,50.15

Commodes

E0160 **Sitz type bath or equipment, portable, used with or without commode** Y ♿ (NU, RR, UE)
Medicare covers sitz baths if medical record indicates that the patient has an infection or injury of the perineal area and the sitz bath is prescribed by the physician.

© 2019 Optum360, LLC

E0161 **Sitz type bath or equipment, portable, used with or without commode, with faucet attachment(s)** Y ♿ (NU, RR, UE)
Medicare covers sitz baths if medical record indicates that the patient has an infection or injury of the perineal area and the sitz bath is prescribed by the physician.

E0162 **Sitz bath chair** Y ♿ (NU, RR, UE)
Medicare covers sitz baths if medical record indicates that the patient has an infection or injury of the perineal area and the sitz bath is prescribed by the physician.

E0163 **Commode chair, mobile or stationary, with fixed arms** Y ♿ (NU, RR, UE)
Medicare covers commodes for patients confined to their beds or rooms, for patients without indoor bathroom facilities, and to patients who cannot climb or descend the stairs necessary to reach the bathrooms in their homes.

E0165 **Commode chair, mobile or stationary, with detachable arms** Y ♿ (RR)
Medicare covers commodes for patients confined to their beds or rooms, for patients without indoor bathroom facilities, and to patients who cannot climb or descend the stairs necessary to reach the bathrooms in their homes.

E0167 **Pail or pan for use with commode chair, replacement only** Y ♿ (NU, RR, UE)
Medicare covers commodes for patients confined to their beds or rooms, for patients without indoor bathroom facilities, and to patients who cannot climb or descend the stairs necessary to reach the bathrooms in their homes.

E0168 **Commode chair, extra wide and/or heavy-duty, stationary or mobile, with or without arms, any type, each** Y ☑ ♿ (NU, RR, UE)

E0170 **Commode chair with integrated seat lift mechanism, electric, any type** Y ♿ (RR)

E0171 **Commode chair with integrated seat lift mechanism, nonelectric, any type** Y ♿ (RR)

E0172 **Seat lift mechanism placed over or on top of toilet, any type** E

E0175 **Footrest, for use with commode chair, each** Y ☑ ♿ (NU, RR, UE)

Decubitus Care Equipment

E0181 **Powered pressure reducing mattress overlay/pad, alternating, with pump, includes heavy-duty** Y ♿ (RR)
For Medicare coverage, a detailed written order must be received by the supplier before a claim is submitted.

E0182 **Pump for alternating pressure pad, for replacement only** Y ♿ (RR)
For Medicare coverage, a detailed written order must be received by the supplier before a claim is submitted.

E0184 **Dry pressure mattress** Y ♿ (NU, RR, UE)
For Medicare coverage, a detailed written order must be received by the supplier before a claim is submitted.

E0185 **Gel or gel-like pressure pad for mattress, standard mattress length and width** Y ♿ (NU, RR, UE)
For Medicare coverage, a detailed written order must be received by the supplier before a claim is submitted.

E0186 **Air pressure mattress** Y ♿ (RR)
For Medicare coverage, a detailed written order must be received by the supplier before a claim is submitted.

E0187 **Water pressure mattress** Y ♿ (RR)
For Medicare coverage, a detailed written order must be received by the supplier before a claim is submitted.

E0188 **Synthetic sheepskin pad** Y ♿ (NU, RR, UE)
For Medicare coverage, a detailed written order must be received by the supplier before a claim is submitted.

E0189 **Lambswool sheepskin pad, any size** Y ♿ (NU, RR, UE)
For Medicare coverage, a detailed written order must be received by the supplier before a claim is submitted.

E0190 **Positioning cushion/pillow/wedge, any shape or size, includes all components and accessories** E

E0191 **Heel or elbow protector, each** Y ☑ ♿ (NU, RR, UE)

E0193 **Powered air flotation bed (low air loss therapy)** Y ♿ (RR)
CMS: 100-04,23,60.3

E0194 **Air fluidized bed** Y ♿ (RR)
An air fluidized bed is covered by Medicare if the patient has a stage 3 or stage 4 pressure sore and, without the bed, would require institutionalization. For Medicare coverage, a detailed written order must be received by the supplier before a claim is submitted.

E0196 **Gel pressure mattress** Y ♿ (RR)
Medicare covers pads if physicians supervise their use in patients who have decubitus ulcers or susceptibility to them. For Medicare coverage, a detailed written order must be received by the supplier before a claim is submitted.

E0197 **Air pressure pad for mattress, standard mattress length and width** Y ♿ (RR)
Medicare covers pads if physicians supervise their use in patients who have decubitus ulcers or susceptibility to them. For Medicare coverage, a detailed written order must be received by the supplier before a claim is submitted.

E0198 **Water pressure pad for mattress, standard mattress length and width** Y ♿ (RR)
Medicare covers pads if physicians supervise their use in patients who have decubitus ulcers or susceptibility to them.For Medicare coverage, a detailed written order must be received by the supplier before a claim is submitted.

E0199 **Dry pressure pad for mattress, standard mattress length and width** Y ♿ (NU, RR, UE)
Medicare covers pads if physicians supervise their use in patients who have decubitus ulcers or susceptibility to them. For Medicare coverage, a detailed written order must be received by the supplier before a claim is submitted.

Heat/Cold Application

E0200 **Heat lamp, without stand (table model), includes bulb, or infrared element** Y ♿ (NU, RR, UE)

E0202 **Phototherapy (bilirubin) light with photometer** Y ♿ (RR)

E0203 **Therapeutic lightbox, minimum 10,000 lux, table top model** E

E0205 **Heat lamp, with stand, includes bulb, or infrared element** Y ♿ (NU, RR, UE)

E0210 **Electric heat pad, standard** Y ♿ (NU, RR, UE)

E0215 **Electric heat pad, moist** Y ♿ (NU, RR, UE)

E0217 **Water circulating heat pad with pump** Y ♿ (NU, RR, UE)

E0218 **Fluid circulating cold pad with pump, any type** Y

E0221 **Infrared heating pad system** Y
AHA: 1Q, '02, 5

E0225 **Hydrocollator unit, includes pads** Y ♿ (NU, RR, UE)

E0231 **Noncontact wound-warming device (temperature control unit, AC adapter and power cord) for use with warming card and wound cover** E
AHA: 1Q, '02, 5

E0232 **Warming card for use with the noncontact wound-warming device and noncontact wound-warming wound cover** E
AHA: 1Q, '02, 5

© 2019 Optum360, LLC

E0235 **Paraffin bath unit, portable (see medical supply code A4265 for paraffin)** Y ♿ (RR)

E0236 **Pump for water circulating pad** Y ♿ (RR)

E0239 **Hydrocollator unit, portable** Y ♿ (NU, RR, UE)

Bath and Toilet Aids

E0240 **Bath/shower chair, with or without wheels, any size** E

E0241 **Bathtub wall rail, each** E ☑

E0242 **Bathtub rail, floor base** E

E0243 **Toilet rail, each** E ☑

E0244 **Raised toilet seat** E

E0245 **Tub stool or bench** E

E0246 **Transfer tub rail attachment** E

E0247 **Transfer bench for tub or toilet with or without commode opening** E

E0248 **Transfer bench, heavy-duty, for tub or toilet with or without commode opening** E

E0249 **Pad for water circulating heat unit, for replacement only** Y ♿ (NU, RR, UE)

Hospital Beds and Accessories

E0250 **Hospital bed, fixed height, with any type side rails, with mattress** Y ♿ (RR)
CMS: 100-04,23,60.3

E0251 **Hospital bed, fixed height, with any type side rails, without mattress** Y ♿ (RR)
CMS: 100-04,23,60.3

E0255 **Hospital bed, variable height, hi-lo, with any type side rails, with mattress** Y ♿ (RR)
CMS: 100-04,23,60.3

E0256 **Hospital bed, variable height, hi-lo, with any type side rails, without mattress** Y ♿ (RR)
CMS: 100-04,23,60.3

E0260 **Hospital bed, semi-electric (head and foot adjustment), with any type side rails, with mattress** Y ♿ (RR)
CMS: 100-04,23,60.3

E0261 **Hospital bed, semi-electric (head and foot adjustment), with any type side rails, without mattress** Y ♿ (RR)
CMS: 100-04,23,60.3

E0265 **Hospital bed, total electric (head, foot, and height adjustments), with any type side rails, with mattress** Y ♿ (RR)
CMS: 100-04,23,60.3

E0266 **Hospital bed, total electric (head, foot, and height adjustments), with any type side rails, without mattress** Y ♿ (RR)
CMS: 100-04,23,60.3

E0270 **Hospital bed, institutional type includes: oscillating, circulating and Stryker frame, with mattress** E

E0271 **Mattress, innerspring** Y ♿ (NU, RR, UE)
CMS: 100-04,23,60.3; 100-04,36,50.14

E0272 **Mattress, foam rubber** Y ♿ (NU, RR, UE)
CMS: 100-04,23,60.3; 100-04,36,50.14

E0273 **Bed board** E

E0274 **Over-bed table** E

E0275 **Bed pan, standard, metal or plastic** Y ♿ (NU, RR, UE)
Reusable, autoclavable bedpans are covered by Medicare for bed-confined patients.

E0276 **Bed pan, fracture, metal or plastic** Y ♿ (NU, RR, UE)
Reusable, autoclavable bedpans are covered by Medicare for bed-confined patients.

E0277 **Powered pressure-reducing air mattress** Y ♿ (RR)
CMS: 100-04,23,60.3

E0280 **Bed cradle, any type** Y ♿ (NU, RR, UE)
CMS: 100-04,23,60.3; 100-04,36,50.14

E0290 **Hospital bed, fixed height, without side rails, with mattress** Y ♿ (RR)
CMS: 100-04,23,60.3

E0291 **Hospital bed, fixed height, without side rails, without mattress** Y ♿ (RR)
CMS: 100-04,23,60.3

E0292 **Hospital bed, variable height, hi-lo, without side rails, with mattress** Y ♿ (RR)
CMS: 100-04,23,60.3

E0293 **Hospital bed, variable height, hi-lo, without side rails, without mattress** Y ♿ (RR)
CMS: 100-04,23,60.3

E0294 **Hospital bed, semi-electric (head and foot adjustment), without side rails, with mattress** Y ♿ (RR)
CMS: 100-04,23,60.3

E0295 **Hospital bed, semi-electric (head and foot adjustment), without side rails, without mattress** Y ♿ (RR)
CMS: 100-04,23,60.3

E0296 **Hospital bed, total electric (head, foot, and height adjustments), without side rails, with mattress** Y ♿ (RR)
CMS: 100-04,23,60.3

E0297 **Hospital bed, total electric (head, foot, and height adjustments), without side rails, without mattress** Y ♿ (RR)
CMS: 100-04,23,60.3

E0300 **Pediatric crib, hospital grade, fully enclosed, with or without top enclosure** Y ♿ (RR)
CMS: 100-04,23,60.3

E0301 **Hospital bed, heavy-duty, extra wide, with weight capacity greater than 350 pounds, but less than or equal to 600 pounds, with any type side rails, without mattress** Y ♿ (RR)
CMS: 100-04,23,60.3

E0302 **Hospital bed, extra heavy-duty, extra wide, with weight capacity greater than 600 pounds, with any type side rails, without mattress** Y ♿ (RR)
CMS: 100-04,23,60.3

E0303 **Hospital bed, heavy-duty, extra wide, with weight capacity greater than 350 pounds, but less than or equal to 600 pounds, with any type side rails, with mattress** Y ♿ (RR)
CMS: 100-04,23,60.3

E0304 **Hospital bed, extra heavy-duty, extra wide, with weight capacity greater than 600 pounds, with any type side rails, with mattress** Y ♿ (RR)
CMS: 100-04,23,60.3

E0305 **Bedside rails, half-length** Y ♿ (RR)
CMS: 100-04,23,60.3

E0310 **Bedside rails, full-length** Y ♿ (NU, RR, UE)
CMS: 100-04,23,60.3; 100-04,36,50.14

E0315 **Bed accessory: board, table, or support device, any type** E

E0316 **Safety enclosure frame/canopy for use with hospital bed, any type** Y ♿ (RR)
CMS: 100-04,23,60.3
AHA: 1Q, '02, 5

© 2019 Optum360, LLC

E0325 **Urinal; male, jug-type, any material** ♂ Y ♿ (NU, RR, UE)

E0326 **Urinal; female, jug-type, any material** A ♀ Y ♿ (NU, RR, UE)

E0328 **Hospital bed, pediatric, manual, 360 degree side enclosures, top of headboard, footboard and side rails up to 24 in above the spring, includes mattress** Y

E0329 **Hospital bed, pediatric, electric or semi-electric, 360 degree side enclosures, top of headboard, footboard and side rails up to 24 in above the spring, includes mattress** Y

E0350 **Control unit for electronic bowel irrigation/evacuation system** E

E0352 **Disposable pack (water reservoir bag, speculum, valving mechanism, and collection bag/box) for use with the electronic bowel irrigation/evacuation system** E

E0370 **Air pressure elevator for heel** E

E0371 **Nonpowered advanced pressure reducing overlay for mattress, standard mattress length and width** Y ♿ (RR)
CMS: 100-04,23,60.3

E0372 **Powered air overlay for mattress, standard mattress length and width** Y ♿ (RR)
CMS: 100-04,23,60.3

E0373 **Nonpowered advanced pressure reducing mattress** Y ♿ (RR)
CMS: 100-04,23,60.3

Oxygen and Related Respiratory Equipment

E0424 **Stationary compressed gaseous oxygen system, rental; includes container, contents, regulator, flowmeter, humidifier, nebulizer, cannula or mask, and tubing** Y ♿ (RR)
For the first claim filed for home oxygen equipment or therapy, submit a certificate of medical necessity that includes the oxygen flow rate, anticipated frequency and duration of oxygen therapy, and physician signature. Medicare accepts oxygen therapy as medically necessary in cases documenting any of the following: erythocythemia with a hematocrit greater than 56 percent; a P pulmonale on EKG; or dependent edema consistent with congestive heart failure.
CMS: 100-04,20,130.6; 100-04,20,30.6

E0425 **Stationary compressed gas system, purchase; includes regulator, flowmeter, humidifier, nebulizer, cannula or mask, and tubing** E

E0430 **Portable gaseous oxygen system, purchase; includes regulator, flowmeter, humidifier, cannula or mask, and tubing** E

E0431 **Portable gaseous oxygen system, rental; includes portable container, regulator, flowmeter, humidifier, cannula or mask, and tubing** Y ♿ (RR)
CMS: 100-04,20,130.6

E0433 **Portable liquid oxygen system, rental; home liquefier used to fill portable liquid oxygen containers, includes portable containers, regulator, flowmeter, humidifier, cannula or mask and tubing, with or without supply reservoir and contents gauge** Y ♿ (RR)
CMS: 100-04,20,130.6

E0434 **Portable liquid oxygen system, rental; includes portable container, supply reservoir, humidifier, flowmeter, refill adaptor, contents gauge, cannula or mask, and tubing** Y ♿ (RR)
CMS: 100-04,20,130.6

E0435 **Portable liquid oxygen system, purchase; includes portable container, supply reservoir, flowmeter, humidifier, contents gauge, cannula or mask, tubing and refill adaptor** E

E0439 **Stationary liquid oxygen system, rental; includes container, contents, regulator, flowmeter, humidifier, nebulizer, cannula or mask, & tubing** Y ♿ (RR)
CMS: 100-04,20,130.6

E0440 **Stationary liquid oxygen system, purchase; includes use of reservoir, contents indicator, regulator, flowmeter, humidifier, nebulizer, cannula or mask, and tubing** E

E0441 **Stationary oxygen contents, gaseous, 1 month's supply = 1 unit** Y ☑ ♿
CMS: 100-04,20,30.6

E0442 **Stationary oxygen contents, liquid, 1 month's supply = 1 unit** Y ☑ ♿

E0443 **Portable oxygen contents, gaseous, 1 month's supply = 1 unit** Y ☑ ♿
CMS: 100-04,20,30.6

E0444 **Portable oxygen contents, liquid, 1 month's supply = 1 unit** Y ☑ ♿

E0445 **Oximeter device for measuring blood oxygen levels noninvasively** N

E0446 **Topical oxygen delivery system, not otherwise specified, includes all supplies and accessories** A

E0447 **Portable oxygen contents, liquid, 1 month's supply = 1 unit, prescribed amount at rest or nighttime exceeds 4 liters per minute (LPM)**

E0455 **Oxygen tent, excluding croup or pediatric tents** Y

E0457 **Chest shell (cuirass)** E

E0459 **Chest wrap** E

E0462 **Rocking bed, with or without side rails** Y ♿ (RR)

E0465 **Home ventilator, any type, used with invasive interface, (e.g., tracheostomy tube)** Y ♿ (RR)

E0466 **Home ventilator, any type, used with noninvasive interface, (e.g., mask, chest shell)** Y ♿ (RR)

E0467 **Home ventilator, multi-function respiratory device, also performs any or all of the additional functions of oxygen concentration, drug nebulization, aspiration, and cough stimulation, includes all accessories, components and supplies for all functions** (RR)

E0470 **Respiratory assist device, bi-level pressure capability, without backup rate feature, used with noninvasive interface, e.g., nasal or facial mask (intermittent assist device with continuous positive airway pressure device)** Y ♿ (RR)
CMS: 100-03,240.4; 100-04,23,60.3

E0471 **Respiratory assist device, bi-level pressure capability, with back-up rate feature, used with noninvasive interface, e.g., nasal or facial mask (intermittent assist device with continuous positive airway pressure device)** Y ♿ (RR)
CMS: 100-03,240.4; 100-04,23,60.3

E0472 **Respiratory assist device, bi-level pressure capability, with backup rate feature, used with invasive interface, e.g., tracheostomy tube (intermittent assist device with continuous positive airway pressure device)** Y ♿ (RR)
CMS: 100-03,240.4; 100-04,23,60.3

E0480 **Percussor, electric or pneumatic, home model** Y ♿ (RR)

E0481 **Intrapulmonary percussive ventilation system and related accessories** E
AHA: 1Q, '02, 5

E0482 **Cough stimulating device, alternating positive and negative airway pressure** Y ♿ (RR)
AHA: 1Q, '02, 5

E0483 **High frequency chest wall oscillation system, includes all accessories and supplies, each** Y ☑ ♿ (RR)

© 2019 Optum360, LLC

E0484 **Oscillatory positive expiratory pressure device, nonelectric, any type, each** Y ☑ ♿ (NU, RR, UE)

E0485 **Oral device/appliance used to reduce upper airway collapsibility, adjustable or nonadjustable, prefabricated, includes fitting and adjustment** Y ♿ (NU, RR, UE)

E0486 **Oral device/appliance used to reduce upper airway collapsibility, adjustable or nonadjustable, custom fabricated, includes fitting and adjustment** Y ♿ (NU, RR, UE)

E0487 **Spirometer, electronic, includes all accessories** N

IPPB Machines

E0500 **IPPB machine, all types, with built-in nebulization; manual or automatic valves; internal or external power source** Y ♿ (RR)

Intermittent Positive Pressure Breathing (IPPB) devices

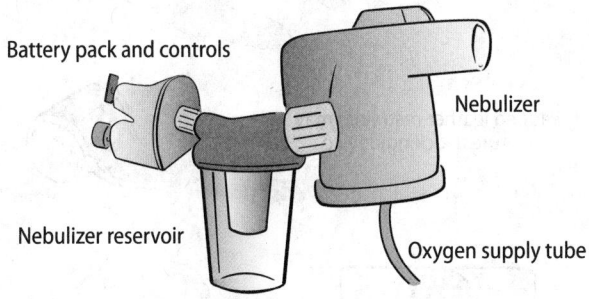

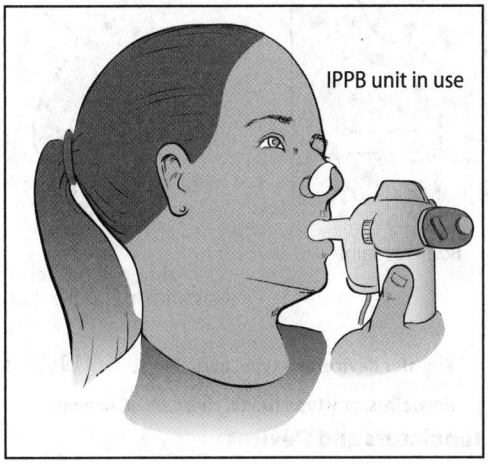

Humidifiers/Compressors/Nebulizers

E0550 **Humidifier, durable for extensive supplemental humidification during IPPB treatments or oxygen delivery** Y ♿ (RR)

E0555 **Humidifier, durable, glass or autoclavable plastic bottle type, for use with regulator or flowmeter** Y

E0560 **Humidifier, durable for supplemental humidification during IPPB treatment or oxygen delivery** Y ♿ (NU, RR, UE)
CMS: 100-04,23,60.3

E0561 **Humidifier, nonheated, used with positive airway pressure device** Y ♿ (NU, RR, UE)
CMS: 100-03,240.4; 100-04,23,60.3; 100-04,36,50.14

E0562 **Humidifier, heated, used with positive airway pressure device** Y ♿ (NU, RR, UE)
CMS: 100-03,240.4; 100-04,23,60.3; 100-04,36,50.14

E0565 **Compressor, air power source for equipment which is not self-contained or cylinder driven** Y ♿ (RR)

E0570 **Nebulizer, with compressor** Y ♿ (RR)

E0572 **Aerosol compressor, adjustable pressure, light duty for intermittent use** Y ♿ (RR)

E0574 **Ultrasonic/electronic aerosol generator with small volume nebulizer** Y ♿ (RR)

E0575 **Nebulizer, ultrasonic, large volume** Y ♿ (RR)

E0580 **Nebulizer, durable, glass or autoclavable plastic, bottle type, for use with regulator or flowmeter** Y ♿ (NU, RR, UE)
CMS: 100-04,23,60.3

E0585 **Nebulizer, with compressor and heater** Y ♿ (RR)

Pumps and Vaporizers

E0600 **Respiratory suction pump, home model, portable or stationary, electric** Y ♿ (RR)

E0601 **Continuous positive airway pressure (CPAP) device** Y ♿ (RR)
CMS: 100-03,240.4; 100-04,23,60.3

E0602 **Breast pump, manual, any type** M ♀ Y ♿ (NU, RR, UE)

E0603 **Breast pump, electric (AC and/or DC), any type** M ♀ N
AHA: 1Q, '02, 5

E0604 **Breast pump, hospital grade, electric (AC and/or DC), any type** M ♀ A
AHA: 1Q, '02, 5

E0605 **Vaporizer, room type** Y ♿ (NU, RR, UE)

E0606 **Postural drainage board** Y ♿ (RR)

Monitoring Devices

E0607 **Home blood glucose monitor** Y ♿ (NU, RR, UE)
Medicare covers home blood testing devices for diabetic patients when the devices are prescribed by the patients' physicians. Many commercial payers provide this coverage to noninsulin dependent diabetics as well.

E0610 **Pacemaker monitor, self-contained, (checks battery depletion, includes audible and visible check systems)** Y ♿ (NU, RR, UE)

E0615 **Pacemaker monitor, self-contained, checks battery depletion and other pacemaker components, includes digital/visible check systems** Y ♿ (NU, RR, UE)

E0616 **Implantable cardiac event recorder with memory, activator, and programmer** N

E0617 **External defibrillator with integrated electrocardiogram analysis** Y ♿ (RR)

E0618 **Apnea monitor, without recording feature** Y ♿ (RR)

E0619 **Apnea monitor, with recording feature** Y ♿ (RR)

E0620 **Skin piercing device for collection of capillary blood, laser, each** Y ♿ (RR)
AHA: 1Q, '02, 5

Patient Lifts

E0621 **Sling or seat, patient lift, canvas or nylon** Y ♿ (NU, RR, UE)

E0625 **Patient lift, bathroom or toilet, not otherwise classified** E

E0627 **Seat lift mechanism, electric, any type** Y ♿ (NU, RR, UE)
CMS: 100-04,20,100; 100-04,20,130.2; 100-04,20,130.3; 100-04,20,130.4; 100-04,20,130.5

E0629 **Seat lift mechanism, nonelectric, any type** Y ♿ (NU, RR, UE)
CMS: 100-04,20,100; 100-04,20,130.2; 100-04,20,130.3; 100-04,20,130.4; 100-04,20,130.5

E0630 **Patient lift, hydraulic or mechanical, includes any seat, sling, strap(s), or pad(s)** Y ♿ (RR)

E0635 **Patient lift, electric, with seat or sling** Y ♿ (RR)

E0636 **Multipositional patient support system, with integrated lift, patient accessible controls** Y ♿ (RR)

© 2019 Optum360, LLC

E0637 Combination sit-to-stand frame/table system, any size including pediatric, with seat lift feature, with or without wheels [E]

E0638 Standing frame/table system, one position (e.g., upright, supine or prone stander), any size including pediatric, with or without wheels [E]

E0639 Patient lift, moveable from room to room with disassembly and reassembly, includes all components/accessories [E] ♿ (RR)

E0640 Patient lift, fixed system, includes all components/accessories [E] ♿ (RR)

E0641 Standing frame/table system, multi-position (e.g., 3-way stander), any size including pediatric, with or without wheels [E]

E0642 Standing frame/table system, mobile (dynamic stander), any size including pediatric [E]

Compression Devices

E0650 Pneumatic compressor, nonsegmental home model [Y] ♿ (NU, RR, UE)

E0651 Pneumatic compressor, segmental home model without calibrated gradient pressure [Y] ♿ (NU, RR, UE)

E0652 Pneumatic compressor, segmental home model with calibrated gradient pressure [Y] ♿ (NU, RR, UE)

E0655 Nonsegmental pneumatic appliance for use with pneumatic compressor, half arm [Y] ♿ (NU, RR, UE)

E0656 Segmental pneumatic appliance for use with pneumatic compressor, trunk [Y] ♿ (RR)

E0657 Segmental pneumatic appliance for use with pneumatic compressor, chest [Y] ♿ (RR)

E0660 Nonsegmental pneumatic appliance for use with pneumatic compressor, full leg [Y] ♿ (NU, RR, UE)

E0665 Nonsegmental pneumatic appliance for use with pneumatic compressor, full arm [Y] ♿ (NU, RR, UE)

E0666 Nonsegmental pneumatic appliance for use with pneumatic compressor, half leg [Y] ♿ (NU, RR, UE)

E0667 Segmental pneumatic appliance for use with pneumatic compressor, full leg [Y] ♿ (NU, RR, UE)

E0668 Segmental pneumatic appliance for use with pneumatic compressor, full arm [Y] ♿ (NU, RR, UE)

E0669 Segmental pneumatic appliance for use with pneumatic compressor, half leg [Y] ♿ (NU, RR, UE)

E0670 Segmental pneumatic appliance for use with pneumatic compressor, integrated, two full legs and trunk [Y] ♿ (NU, RR, UE)

E0671 Segmental gradient pressure pneumatic appliance, full leg [Y] ♿ (NU, RR, UE)

E0672 Segmental gradient pressure pneumatic appliance, full arm [Y] ♿ (NU, RR, UE)

E0673 Segmental gradient pressure pneumatic appliance, half leg [Y] ♿ (NU, RR, UE)

E0675 Pneumatic compression device, high pressure, rapid inflation/deflation cycle, for arterial insufficiency (unilateral or bilateral system) [Y] ♿ (RR)

E0676 Intermittent limb compression device (includes all accessories), not otherwise specified [Y]

Ultraviolet Light

E0691 Ultraviolet light therapy system, includes bulbs/lamps, timer and eye protection; treatment area 2 sq ft or less [Y] ♿ (NU, RR, UE)

E0692 Ultraviolet light therapy system panel, includes bulbs/lamps, timer and eye protection, 4 ft panel [Y] ♿ (NU, RR, UE)

E0693 Ultraviolet light therapy system panel, includes bulbs/lamps, timer and eye protection, 6 ft panel [Y] ♿ (NU, RR, UE)

E0694 Ultraviolet multidirectional light therapy system in 6 ft cabinet, includes bulbs/lamps, timer, and eye protection [Y] ♿ (NU, RR, UE)

Safety Equipment

E0700 Safety equipment, device or accessory, any type [E]

Restraints (E0710)

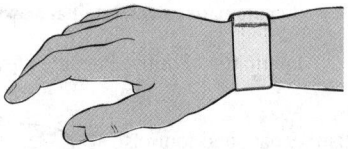

Fabric wrist restraint

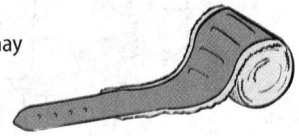

Padded leather restraints may feature a locking device

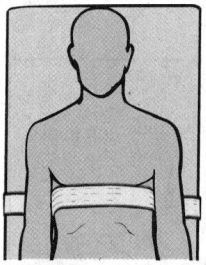

Body restraint

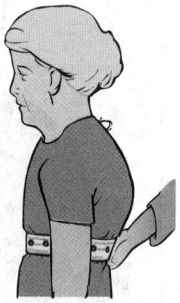

Fabric gait belt for assistance in walking (E0700)

E0705 Transfer device, any type, each [B] ☑ ♿ (NU, RR, UE)

E0710 Restraints, any type (body, chest, wrist, or ankle) [E]

Nerve Stimulators and Devices

E0720 Transcutaneous electrical nerve stimulation (TENS) device, two-lead, localized stimulation [Y] ♿ (NU)

A Certificate of Medical Necessity is required for the purchase of a TENS. It is not required for rentals.

CMS: 100-03,10.2; 100-03,160.27; 100-03,160.7.1; 100-04,20,30.1.2

E0730 Transcutaneous electrical nerve stimulation (TENS) device, four or more leads, for multiple nerve stimulation [Y] ♿ (NU)

A Certificate of Medical Necessity is required for the purchase of a TENS. It is not required for rentals.

CMS: 100-03,10.2; 100-03,160.27; 100-03,160.7.1; 100-04,20,30.1.2

E0731 Form-fitting conductive garment for delivery of TENS or NMES (with conductive fibers separated from the patient's skin by layers of fabric) [Y] ♿ (NU)

CMS: 100-03,10.2; 100-03,160.13

E0740 Nonimplanted pelvic floor electrical stimulator, complete system [Y] ♿ (RR)

E0744 Neuromuscular stimulator for scoliosis [Y] ♿ (RR)

E0745 Neuromuscular stimulator, electronic shock unit [Y] ♿ (RR)

© 2019 Optum360, LLC

E0746 **Electromyography (EMG), biofeedback device** N
Biofeedback therapy is covered by Medicare only for re-education of specific muscles or for treatment of incapacitating muscle spasm or weakness.

E0747 **Osteogenesis stimulator, electrical, noninvasive, other than spinal applications** Y (NU, RR, UE)
Medicare covers noninvasive osteogenic stimulation for nonunion of long bone fractures, failed fusion, or congenital pseudoarthroses.

E0748 **Osteogenesis stimulator, electrical, noninvasive, spinal applications** Y (NU, RR, UE)
Medicare covers noninvasive osteogenic stimulation as an adjunct to spinal fusion surgery for patients at high risk of pseudoarthroses due to previously failed spinal fusion, or for those undergoing fusion of three or more vertebrae.

E0749 **Osteogenesis stimulator, electrical, surgically implanted** N (RR)
Medicare covers invasive osteogenic stimulation for nonunion of long bone fractures or as an adjunct to spinal fusion surgery for patients at high risk of pseudoarthroses due to previously failed spinal fusion, or for those undergoing fusion of three or more vertebrae.
CMS: 100-04,4,190

E0755 **Electronic salivary reflex stimulator (intraoral/noninvasive)** E

E0760 **Osteogenesis stimulator, low intensity ultrasound, noninvasive** Y (NU, RR, UE)
CMS: 100-04,32,110.5

E0761 **Nonthermal pulsed high frequency radiowaves, high peak power electromagnetic energy treatment device** E

E0762 **Transcutaneous electrical joint stimulation device system, includes all accessories** B ♿ (RR)

E0764 **Functional neuromuscular stimulation, transcutaneous stimulation of sequential muscle groups of ambulation with computer control, used for walking by spinal cord injured, entire system, after completion of training program** Y (RR)

E0765 **FDA approved nerve stimulator, with replaceable batteries, for treatment of nausea and vomiting** Y ♿ (NU, RR, UE)

E0766 **Electrical stimulation device used for cancer treatment, includes all accessories, any type** Y (RR)

E0769 **Electrical stimulation or electromagnetic wound treatment device, not otherwise classified** B
CMS: 100-04,32,11.1

E0770 **Functional electrical stimulator, transcutaneous stimulation of nerve and/or muscle groups, any type, complete system, not otherwise specified** Y

Infusion Supplies

E0776 **IV pole** Y ♿ (NU, RR, UE)
CMS: 100-04,23,60.3

E0779 **Ambulatory infusion pump, mechanical, reusable, for infusion 8 hours or greater** Y ♿ (RR)

E0780 **Ambulatory infusion pump, mechanical, reusable, for infusion less than 8 hours** Y ♿ (NU)

E0781 **Ambulatory infusion pump, single or multiple channels, electric or battery operated, with administrative equipment, worn by patient** Y ♿ (RR)

E0782 **Infusion pump, implantable, nonprogrammable (includes all components, e.g., pump, catheter, connectors, etc.)** N (NU, RR, UE)
CMS: 100-04,4,190

E0783 **Infusion pump system, implantable, programmable (includes all components, e.g., pump, catheter, connectors, etc.)** N (NU, RR, UE)
CMS: 100-04,4,190

E0784 **External ambulatory infusion pump, insulin** Y ♿ (RR)
Covered by some commercial payers with preauthorization.

E0785 **Implantable intraspinal (epidural/intrathecal) catheter used with implantable infusion pump, replacement** N ♿ (KF)
CMS: 100-04,4,190

E0786 **Implantable programmable infusion pump, replacement (excludes implantable intraspinal catheter)** N (NU, RR, UE)

● **E0787** Jan **External ambulatory infusion pump, insulin, dosage rate adjustment using therapeutic continuous glucose sensing**

E0791 **Parenteral infusion pump, stationary, single, or multichannel** Y ♿ (RR)

Traction Equipment

E0830 **Ambulatory traction device, all types, each** N

E0840 **Traction frame, attached to headboard, cervical traction** Y ♿ (NU, RR, UE)

E0849 **Traction equipment, cervical, free-standing stand/frame, pneumatic, applying traction force to other than mandible** Y ♿ (RR)

E0850 **Traction stand, freestanding, cervical traction** Y ♿ (NU, RR, UE)

E0855 **Cervical traction equipment not requiring additional stand or frame** Y ♿ (RR)

E0856 **Cervical traction device, with inflatable air bladder(s)** Y ♿ (RR)

E0860 **Traction equipment, overdoor, cervical** Y ♿ (NU, RR, UE)

E0870 **Traction frame, attached to footboard, extremity traction (e.g., Buck's)** Y ♿ (NU, RR, UE)

E0880 **Traction stand, freestanding, extremity traction (e.g., Buck's)** Y ♿ (NU, RR, UE)

E0890 **Traction frame, attached to footboard, pelvic traction** Y ♿ (NU, RR, UE)

E0900 **Traction stand, freestanding, pelvic traction (e.g., Buck's)** Y ♿ (NU, RR, UE)

Orthopedic Devices

E0910 **Trapeze bars, also known as Patient Helper, attached to bed, with grab bar** Y ♿ (RR)
CMS: 100-04,23,60.3

E0911 **Trapeze bar, heavy-duty, for patient weight capacity greater than 250 pounds, attached to bed, with grab bar** Y ♿ (RR)
CMS: 100-04,23,60.3

E0912 **Trapeze bar, heavy-duty, for patient weight capacity greater than 250 pounds, freestanding, complete with grab bar** Y ♿ (RR)
CMS: 100-04,23,60.3

E0920 **Fracture frame, attached to bed, includes weights** Y ♿ (RR)

E0930 **Fracture frame, freestanding, includes weights** Y ♿ (RR)

E0935 **Continuous passive motion exercise device for use on knee only** Y ♿ (RR)

E0936 **Continuous passive motion exercise device for use other than knee** E

E0940 **Trapeze bar, freestanding, complete with grab bar** Y ♿ (RR)
CMS: 100-04,23,60.3

E0941 **Gravity assisted traction device, any type** Y ♿ (RR)

© 2019 Optum360, LLC

E0942 Cervical head harness/halter Y ♿ (NU, RR, UE)

E0944 Pelvic belt/harness/boot Y ♿ (NU, RR, UE)

E0945 Extremity belt/harness Y ♿ (NU, RR, UE)

E0946 Fracture, frame, dual with cross bars, attached to bed, (e.g., Balken, four-poster) Y ♿ (RR)

E0947 Fracture frame, attachments for complex pelvic traction Y ♿ (NU, RR, UE)

E0948 Fracture frame, attachments for complex cervical traction Y ♿ (NU, RR, UE)

Wheelchair Accessories

E0950 Wheelchair accessory, tray, each Y ☑ ♿ (NU, RR, UE)
CMS: 100-04,23,60.3

E0951 Heel loop/holder, any type, with or without ankle strap, each Y ☑ ♿ (NU, RR, UE)
CMS: 100-04,23,60.3

E0952 Toe loop/holder, any type, each Y ☑ ♿ (NU, RR, UE)
CMS: 100-04,23,60.3

E0953 Wheelchair accessory, lateral thigh or knee support, any type including fixed mounting hardware, each Y ♿ (NU, RR, UE)
CMS: 100-04,23,60.3

E0954 Wheelchair accessory, foot box, any type, includes attachment and mounting hardware, each foot Y ♿ (NU, RR, UE)
CMS: 100-04,23,60.3

E0955 Wheelchair accessory, headrest, cushioned, any type, including fixed mounting hardware, each Y ☑ ♿ (RR)
CMS: 100-04,23,60.3

E0956 Wheelchair accessory, lateral trunk or hip support, any type, including fixed mounting hardware, each Y ☑ ♿ (NU, RR, UE)
CMS: 100-04,23,60.3

E0957 Wheelchair accessory, medial thigh support, any type, including fixed mounting hardware, each Y ☑ ♿ (NU, RR, UE)
CMS: 100-04,23,60.3

E0958 Manual wheelchair accessory, one-arm drive attachment, each Y ☑ ♿ (RR)

E0959 Manual wheelchair accessory, adapter for amputee, each B ☑ ♿ (NU, RR, UE)

E0960 Wheelchair accessory, shoulder harness/straps or chest strap, including any type mounting hardware Y ♿ (NU, RR, UE)
CMS: 100-04,23,60.3

E0961 Manual wheelchair accessory, wheel lock brake extension (handle), each B ☑ ♿ (NU, RR, UE)

E0966 Manual wheelchair accessory, headrest extension, each B ☑ ♿ (NU, RR, UE)

E0967 Manual wheelchair accessory, hand rim with projections, any type, replacement only, each Y ☑ ♿ (NU, RR, UE)

E0968 Commode seat, wheelchair Y ♿ (RR)

E0969 Narrowing device, wheelchair Y ♿ (NU, RR, UE)

E0970 No. 2 footplates, except for elevating legrest E
See code(s): K0037, K0042

E0971 Manual wheelchair accessory, antitipping device, each B ☑ ♿ (NU, RR, UE)

E0973 Wheelchair accessory, adjustable height, detachable armrest, complete assembly, each B ☑ ♿ (NU, RR, UE)
CMS: 100-04,23,60.3

E0974 Manual wheelchair accessory, antirollback device, each B ☑ ♿ (NU, RR, UE)

E0978 Wheelchair accessory, positioning belt/safety belt/pelvic strap, each B ☑ ♿ (NU, RR, UE)
CMS: 100-04,23,60.3

E0980 Safety vest, wheelchair Y ♿ (NU, RR, UE)

E0981 Wheelchair accessory, seat upholstery, replacement only, each Y ☑ ♿ (NU, RR, UE)
CMS: 100-04,23,60.3

E0982 Wheelchair accessory, back upholstery, replacement only, each Y ☑ ♿ (NU, RR, UE)
CMS: 100-04,23,60.3

E0983 Manual wheelchair accessory, power add-on to convert manual wheelchair to motorized wheelchair, joystick control Y ♿ (RR)

E0984 Manual wheelchair accessory, power add-on to convert manual wheelchair to motorized wheelchair, tiller control Y ♿ (RR)

E0985 Wheelchair accessory, seat lift mechanism Y ♿ (RR)

E0986 Manual wheelchair accessory, push-rim activated power assist system Y ☑ ♿ (RR)

E0988 Manual wheelchair accessory, lever-activated, wheel drive, pair Y ☑ ♿ (RR)

E0990 Wheelchair accessory, elevating legrest, complete assembly, each B ☑ ♿ (NU, RR, UE)
CMS: 100-04,23,60.3

E0992 Manual wheelchair accessory, solid seat insert B ♿ (NU, RR, UE)

E0994 Armrest, each Y ☑ ♿ (NU, RR, UE)

E0995 Wheelchair accessory, calf rest/pad, replacement only, each B ☑ ♿ (NU, RR, UE)
CMS: 100-04,23,60.3

E1002 Wheelchair accessory, power seating system, tilt only Y ♿ (RR)
CMS: 100-04,23,60.3

E1003 Wheelchair accessory, power seating system, recline only, without shear reduction Y ♿ (RR)
CMS: 100-04,23,60.3

E1004 Wheelchair accessory, power seating system, recline only, with mechanical shear reduction Y ♿ (RR)
CMS: 100-04,23,60.3

E1005 Wheelchair accessory, power seating system, recline only, with power shear reduction Y ♿ (RR)
CMS: 100-04,23,60.3

E1006 Wheelchair accessory, power seating system, combination tilt and recline, without shear reduction Y ♿ (RR)
CMS: 100-04,23,60.3

E1007 Wheelchair accessory, power seating system, combination tilt and recline, with mechanical shear reduction Y ♿ (RR)
CMS: 100-04,23,60.3

E1008 Wheelchair accessory, power seating system, combination tilt and recline, with power shear reduction Y ♿ (RR)
CMS: 100-04,23,60.3

E1009 Wheelchair accessory, addition to power seating system, mechanically linked leg elevation system, including pushrod and legrest, each Y ☑ ♿ (NU, RR, UE)
CMS: 100-04,23,60.3

E1010 Wheelchair accessory, addition to power seating system, power leg elevation system, including legrest, pair Y ☑ ♿ (RR)
CMS: 100-04,23,60.3

© 2019 Optum360, LLC

E1011 Modification to pediatric size wheelchair, width adjustment package (not to be dispensed with initial chair) Y ♿ (NU, RR, UE)

E1012 Wheelchair accessory, addition to power seating system, center mount power elevating leg rest/platform, complete system, any type, each Y ♿ (RR)

E1014 Reclining back, addition to pediatric size wheelchair Y ♿ (RR)

E1015 Shock absorber for manual wheelchair, each Y ☑ ♿ (NU, RR, UE)

E1016 Shock absorber for power wheelchair, each Y ☑ ♿ (NU, RR, UE)
CMS: 100-04,23,60.3

E1017 Heavy-duty shock absorber for heavy-duty or extra heavy-duty manual wheelchair, each Y ☑ ♿ (NU, RR, UE)

E1018 Heavy-duty shock absorber for heavy-duty or extra heavy-duty power wheelchair, each Y ☑ ♿ (NU, RR, UE)

E1020 Residual limb support system for wheelchair, any type Y ♿ (RR)
CMS: 100-04,23,60.3

E1028 Wheelchair accessory, manual swingaway, retractable or removable mounting hardware for joystick, other control interface or positioning accessory Y ♿ (RR)
CMS: 100-04,23,60.3

E1029 Wheelchair accessory, ventilator tray, fixed Y ♿ (RR)
CMS: 100-04,23,60.3

E1030 Wheelchair accessory, ventilator tray, gimbaled Y ♿ (RR)
CMS: 100-04,23,60.3

E1031 Rollabout chair, any and all types with castors 5 in or greater Y ♿ (RR)

E1035 Multi-positional patient transfer system, with integrated seat, operated by care giver, patient weight capacity up to and including 300 lbs Y ♿ (RR)
CMS: 100-02,15,110

E1036 Multi-positional patient transfer system, extra-wide, with integrated seat, operated by caregiver, patient weight capacity greater than 300 lbs Y ♿ (RR)

E1037 Transport chair, pediatric size Y ♿ (RR)

E1038 Transport chair, adult size, patient weight capacity up to and including 300 pounds Y ♿ (RR)

E1039 Transport chair, adult size, heavy-duty, patient weight capacity greater than 300 pounds Y ♿ (RR)

Wheelchairs

E1050 Fully-reclining wheelchair, fixed full-length arms, swing-away detachable elevating legrests Y ♿ (RR)

E1060 Fully-reclining wheelchair, detachable arms, desk or full-length, swing-away detachable elevating legrests Y ♿ (RR)

E1070 Fully-reclining wheelchair, detachable arms (desk or full-length) swing-away detachable footrest Y ♿ (RR)

E1083 Hemi-wheelchair, fixed full-length arms, swing-away detachable elevating legrest Y ♿ (RR)

E1084 Hemi-wheelchair, detachable arms desk or full-length arms, swing-away detachable elevating legrests Y ♿ (RR)

E1085 Hemi-wheelchair, fixed full-length arms, swing-away detachable footrests E
See code(s): K0002

E1086 Hemi-wheelchair, detachable arms, desk or full-length, swing-away detachable footrests E
See code(s): K0002

E1087 High strength lightweight wheelchair, fixed full-length arms, swing-away detachable elevating legrests Y ♿ (RR)

E1088 High strength lightweight wheelchair, detachable arms desk or full-length, swing-away detachable elevating legrests Y ♿ (RR)

E1089 High-strength lightweight wheelchair, fixed-length arms, swing-away detachable footrest E
See code(s): K0004

E1090 High-strength lightweight wheelchair, detachable arms, desk or full-length, swing-away detachable footrests E
See code(s): K0004

E1092 Wide heavy-duty wheel chair, detachable arms (desk or full-length), swing-away detachable elevating legrests Y ♿ (RR)

E1093 Wide heavy-duty wheelchair, detachable arms, desk or full-length arms, swing-away detachable footrests Y ♿ (RR)

E1100 Semi-reclining wheelchair, fixed full-length arms, swing-away detachable elevating legrests Y ♿ (RR)

E1110 Semi-reclining wheelchair, detachable arms (desk or full-length) elevating legrest Y ♿ (RR)

E1130 Standard wheelchair, fixed full-length arms, fixed or swing-away detachable footrests E
See code(s): K0001

E1140 Wheelchair, detachable arms, desk or full-length, swing-away detachable footrests E
See code(s): K0001

E1150 Wheelchair, detachable arms, desk or full-length swing-away detachable elevating legrests Y ♿ (RR)

E1160 Wheelchair, fixed full-length arms, swing-away detachable elevating legrests Y ♿ (RR)

E1161 Manual adult size wheelchair, includes tilt in space Y ♿ (RR)

E1170 Amputee wheelchair, fixed full-length arms, swing-away detachable elevating legrests Y ♿ (RR)

E1171 Amputee wheelchair, fixed full-length arms, without footrests or legrest Y ♿ (RR)

E1172 Amputee wheelchair, detachable arms (desk or full-length) without footrests or legrest Y ♿ (RR)

E1180 Amputee wheelchair, detachable arms (desk or full-length) swing-away detachable footrests Y ♿ (RR)

E1190 Amputee wheelchair, detachable arms (desk or full-length) swing-away detachable elevating legrests Y ♿ (RR)

E1195 Heavy-duty wheelchair, fixed full-length arms, swing-away detachable elevating legrests Y ♿ (RR)

E1200 Amputee wheelchair, fixed full-length arms, swing-away detachable footrest Y ♿ (RR)

E1220 Wheelchair; specially sized or constructed, (indicate brand name, model number, if any) and justification Y

E1221 Wheelchair with fixed arm, footrests Y ♿ (RR)

E1222 Wheelchair with fixed arm, elevating legrests Y ♿ (RR)

E1223 Wheelchair with detachable arms, footrests Y ♿ (RR)

E1224 Wheelchair with detachable arms, elevating legrests Y ♿ (RR)

E1225 Wheelchair accessory, manual semi-reclining back, (recline greater than 15 degrees, but less than 80 degrees), each Y ☑ ♿ (RR)

© 2019 Optum360, LLC

E1226 **Wheelchair accessory, manual fully reclining back, (recline greater than 80 degrees), each** B ☑ ♿ (NU, RR, UE)
See also K0028

E1227 **Special height arms for wheelchair** Y ♿ (NU, RR, UE)

E1228 **Special back height for wheelchair** Y ♿ (RR)

E1229 **Wheelchair, pediatric size, not otherwise specified** Y

E1230 **Power operated vehicle (three- or four-wheel nonhighway), specify brand name and model number** Y ♿ (NU, RR, UE)
Prior authorization is required by Medicare for this item.

E1231 **Wheelchair, pediatric size, tilt-in-space, rigid, adjustable, with seating system** Y ♿ (NU, RR, UE)

E1232 **Wheelchair, pediatric size, tilt-in-space, folding, adjustable, with seating system** Y ♿ (RR)

E1233 **Wheelchair, pediatric size, tilt-in-space, rigid, adjustable, without seating system** Y ♿ (RR)

E1234 **Wheelchair, pediatric size, tilt-in-space, folding, adjustable, without seating system** Y ♿ (RR)

E1235 **Wheelchair, pediatric size, rigid, adjustable, with seating system** Y ♿ (RR)

E1236 **Wheelchair, pediatric size, folding, adjustable, with seating system** Y ♿ (RR)

E1237 **Wheelchair, pediatric size, rigid, adjustable, without seating system** Y ♿ (RR)

E1238 **Wheelchair, pediatric size, folding, adjustable, without seating system** Y ♿ (RR)

E1239 **Power wheelchair, pediatric size, not otherwise specified** Y

E1240 **Lightweight wheelchair, detachable arms, (desk or full-length) swing-away detachable, elevating legrest** Y ♿ (RR)

E1250 **Lightweight wheelchair, fixed full-length arms, swing-away detachable footrest** E
See code(s): K0003

E1260 **Lightweight wheelchair, detachable arms (desk or full-length) swing-away detachable footrest** E
See code(s): K0003

E1270 **Lightweight wheelchair, fixed full-length arms, swing-away detachable elevating legrests** Y ♿ (RR)

E1280 **Heavy-duty wheelchair, detachable arms (desk or full-length) elevating legrests** Y ♿ (RR)

E1285 **Heavy-duty wheelchair, fixed full-length arms, swing-away detachable footrest** E
See code(s): K0006

E1290 **Heavy-duty wheelchair, detachable arms (desk or full-length) swing-away detachable footrest** E
See code(s): K0006

E1295 **Heavy-duty wheelchair, fixed full-length arms, elevating legrest** Y ♿ (RR)

E1296 **Special wheelchair seat height from floor** Y ♿ (NU, RR, UE)

E1297 **Special wheelchair seat depth, by upholstery** Y ♿ (NU, RR, UE)

E1298 **Special wheelchair seat depth and/or width, by construction** Y ♿ (NU, RR, UE)

Whirlpool - Equipment

E1300 **Whirlpool, portable (overtub type)** E

E1310 **Whirlpool, nonportable (built-in type)** Y ♿ (NU, RR, UE)

Additional Oxygen Related Equipment

E1352 **Oxygen accessory, flow regulator capable of positive inspiratory pressure** Y

E1353 **Regulator** Y ♿
CMS: 100-04,23,60.3

E1354 **Oxygen accessory, wheeled cart for portable cylinder or portable concentrator, any type, replacement only, each** Y ☑

E1355 **Stand/rack** Y ♿
CMS: 100-04,23,60.3

E1356 **Oxygen accessory, battery pack/cartridge for portable concentrator, any type, replacement only, each** Y ☑

E1357 **Oxygen accessory, battery charger for portable concentrator, any type, replacement only, each** Y ☑

E1358 **Oxygen accessory, DC power adapter for portable concentrator, any type, replacement only, each** Y ☑

E1372 **Immersion external heater for nebulizer** Y ♿ (NU, RR, UE)

E1390 **Oxygen concentrator, single delivery port, capable of delivering 85 percent or greater oxygen concentration at the prescribed flow rate** Y ♿ (RR)
CMS: 100-04,20,130.6

E1391 **Oxygen concentrator, dual delivery port, capable of delivering 85 percent or greater oxygen concentration at the prescribed flow rate, each** Y ☑ ♿ (RR)
CMS: 100-04,20,130.6

E1392 **Portable oxygen concentrator, rental** Y ♿ (RR)
CMS: 100-04,20,130.6

E1399 **Durable medical equipment, miscellaneous** Y
CMS: 100-04,20,30.9; 100-04,32,110.5

E1405 **Oxygen and water vapor enriching system with heated delivery** Y ♿ (RR)
CMS: 100-04,20,20; 100-04,20,20.4

E1406 **Oxygen and water vapor enriching system without heated delivery** Y ♿ (RR)
CMS: 100-04,20,20; 100-04,20,20.4

Artificial Kidney Machines and Accessories

E1500 **Centrifuge, for dialysis** A ⊘
AHA: 1Q, '02, 5

E1510 **Kidney, dialysate delivery system kidney machine, pump recirculating, air removal system, flowrate meter, power off, heater and temperature control with alarm, IV poles, pressure gauge, concentrate container** A ⊘

E1520 **Heparin infusion pump for hemodialysis** A ⊘

E1530 **Air bubble detector for hemodialysis, each, replacement** A ☑ ⊘

E1540 **Pressure alarm for hemodialysis, each, replacement** A ☑ ⊘

E1550 **Bath conductivity meter for hemodialysis, each** A ☑ ⊘

E1560 **Blood leak detector for hemodialysis, each, replacement** A ☑ ⊘

E1570 **Adjustable chair, for ESRD patients** A ⊘

E1575 **Transducer protectors/fluid barriers, for hemodialysis, any size, per 10** A ☑ ⊘

E1580 **Unipuncture control system for hemodialysis** A ⊘

E1590 **Hemodialysis machine** A ⊘

E1592 **Automatic intermittent peritoneal dialysis system** A ⊘

E1594 **Cycler dialysis machine for peritoneal dialysis** A ⊘

© 2019 Optum360, LLC

E1600 Delivery and/or installation charges for hemodialysis equipment [A] ⊘

E1610 Reverse osmosis water purification system, for hemodialysis [A] ⊘

E1615 Deionizer water purification system, for hemodialysis [A] ⊘

E1620 Blood pump for hemodialysis, replacement [A] ⊘

E1625 Water softening system, for hemodialysis [A] ⊘

E1630 Reciprocating peritoneal dialysis system [A] ⊘

E1632 Wearable artificial kidney, each [A] ☑ ⊘

E1634 Peritoneal dialysis clamps, each [B] ☑

E1635 Compact (portable) travel hemodialyzer system [A] ⊘

E1636 Sorbent cartridges, for hemodialysis, per 10 [A] ☑ ⊘

E1637 Hemostats, each [A] ☑ ⊘
AHA: 1Q, '02, 5

E1639 Scale, each [A] ☑ ⊘
AHA: 1Q, '02, 5

E1699 Dialysis equipment, not otherwise specified [A] ⊘

Jaw Motion Rehabilitation System and Accessories

E1700 Jaw motion rehabilitation system [Y] ♿ (RR)
Medicare jurisdiction: local contractor.

E1701 Replacement cushions for jaw motion rehabilitation system, package of 6 [Y] ☑ ♿
Medicare jurisdiction: local contractor.

E1702 Replacement measuring scales for jaw motion rehabilitation system, package of 200 [Y] ☑ ♿
Medicare jurisdiction: local contractor.

Flexion/Extension Device

E1800 Dynamic adjustable elbow extension/flexion device, includes soft interface material [Y] ♿ (RR)

E1801 Static progressive stretch elbow device, extension and/or flexion, with or without range of motion adjustment, includes all components and accessories [Y] ♿ (RR)
AHA: 1Q, '02, 5

E1802 Dynamic adjustable forearm pronation/supination device, includes soft interface material [Y] ♿ (RR)

E1805 Dynamic adjustable wrist extension/flexion device, includes soft interface material [Y] ♿ (RR)

E1806 Static progressive stretch wrist device, flexion and/or extension, with or without range of motion adjustment, includes all components and accessories [Y] ♿ (RR)
AHA: 1Q, '02, 5

E1810 Dynamic adjustable knee extension/flexion device, includes soft interface material [Y] ♿ (RR)

E1811 Static progressive stretch knee device, extension and/or flexion, with or without range of motion adjustment, includes all components and accessories [Y] ♿ (RR)
AHA: 1Q, '02, 5

E1812 Dynamic knee, extension/flexion device with active resistance control [Y] ♿ (RR)

E1815 Dynamic adjustable ankle extension/flexion device, includes soft interface material [Y] ♿ (RR)

E1816 Static progressive stretch ankle device, flexion and/or extension, with or without range of motion adjustment, includes all components and accessories [Y] ♿ (RR)
AHA: 1Q, '02, 5

E1818 Static progressive stretch forearm pronation/supination device, with or without range of motion adjustment, includes all components and accessories [Y] ♿ (RR)
AHA: 1Q, '02, 5

E1820 Replacement soft interface material, dynamic adjustable extension/flexion device [Y] ♿ (NU, RR, UE)

E1821 Replacement soft interface material/cuffs for bi-directional static progressive stretch device [Y] ♿ (NU, RR, UE)
AHA: 1Q, '02, 5

E1825 Dynamic adjustable finger extension/flexion device, includes soft interface material [Y] ♿ (RR)

E1830 Dynamic adjustable toe extension/flexion device, includes soft interface material [Y] ♿ (RR)

E1831 Static progressive stretch toe device, extension and/or flexion, with or without range of motion adjustment, includes all components and accessories [Y] ♿ (RR)

E1840 Dynamic adjustable shoulder flexion/abduction/rotation device, includes soft interface material [Y] ♿ (RR)
AHA: 1Q, '02, 5

E1841 Static progressive stretch shoulder device, with or without range of motion adjustment, includes all components and accessories [Y] ♿ (RR)

Other Devices

E1902 Communication board, nonelectronic augmentative or alternative communication device [Y]
AHA: 1Q, '02, 5

E2000 Gastric suction pump, home model, portable or stationary, electric [Y] ♿ (RR)
AHA: 1Q, '02, 5

E2100 Blood glucose monitor with integrated voice synthesizer [Y] ♿ (NU, RR, UE)
AHA: 1Q, '02, 5

E2101 Blood glucose monitor with integrated lancing/blood sample [Y] ♿ (NU, RR, UE)
AHA: 1Q, '02, 5

E2120 Pulse generator system for tympanic treatment of inner ear endolymphatic fluid [Y] ♿ (RR)

DME Wheelchair Accessory

E2201 Manual wheelchair accessory, nonstandard seat frame, width greater than or equal to 20 in and less than 24 in [Y] ☑ ♿ (NU, RR, UE)

E2202 Manual wheelchair accessory, nonstandard seat frame width, 24-27 in [Y] ☑ ♿ (NU, RR, UE)

E2203 Manual wheelchair accessory, nonstandard seat frame depth, 20 to less than 22 in [Y] ☑ ♿ (NU, RR, UE)

E2204 Manual wheelchair accessory, nonstandard seat frame depth, 22 to 25 in [Y] ☑ ♿ (NU, RR, UE)

E2205 Manual wheelchair accessory, handrim without projections (includes ergonomic or contoured), any type, replacement only, each [Y] ☑ ♿ (NU, RR, UE)

E2206 Manual wheelchair accessory, wheel lock assembly, complete, replacement only, each [Y] ☑ ♿ (NU, RR, UE)

E2207 Wheelchair accessory, crutch and cane holder, each [Y] ☑ ♿ (NU, RR, UE)

E2208 Wheelchair accessory, cylinder tank carrier, each [Y] ☑ ♿ (NU, RR, UE)
CMS: 100-04,23,60.3

© 2019 Optum360, LLC

E2209 **Accessory, arm trough, with or without hand support, each** Y ☑ ♿ (NU, RR, UE)
CMS: 100-04,23,60.3

E2210 **Wheelchair accessory, bearings, any type, replacement only, each** Y ☑ ♿ (NU, RR, UE)
CMS: 100-04,23,60.3

E2211 **Manual wheelchair accessory, pneumatic propulsion tire, any size, each** Y ☑ ♿ (NU, RR, UE)

E2212 **Manual wheelchair accessory, tube for pneumatic propulsion tire, any size, each** Y ☑ ♿ (NU, RR, UE)

E2213 **Manual wheelchair accessory, insert for pneumatic propulsion tire (removable), any type, any size, each** Y ☑ ♿ (NU, RR, UE)

E2214 **Manual wheelchair accessory, pneumatic caster tire, any size, each** Y ☑ ♿ (NU, RR, UE)

E2215 **Manual wheelchair accessory, tube for pneumatic caster tire, any size, each** Y ☑ ♿ (NU, RR, UE)

E2216 **Manual wheelchair accessory, foam filled propulsion tire, any size, each** Y ☑ ♿ (NU, RR, UE)

E2217 **Manual wheelchair accessory, foam filled caster tire, any size, each** Y ☑ ♿ (NU, RR, UE)

E2218 **Manual wheelchair accessory, foam propulsion tire, any size, each** Y ☑ ♿ (NU, RR, UE)

E2219 **Manual wheelchair accessory, foam caster tire, any size, each** Y ☑ ♿ (NU, RR, UE)

E2220 **Manual wheelchair accessory, solid (rubber/plastic) propulsion tire, any size, replacement only, each** Y ☑ ♿ (NU, RR, UE)

E2221 **Manual wheelchair accessory, solid (rubber/plastic) caster tire (removable), any size, replacement only, each** Y ☑ ♿ (NU, RR, UE)

E2222 **Manual wheelchair accessory, solid (rubber/plastic) caster tire with integrated wheel, any size, replacement only, each** Y ☑ ♿ (NU, RR, UE)

E2224 **Manual wheelchair accessory, propulsion wheel excludes tire, any size, replacement only, each** Y ☑ ♿ (NU, RR, UE)

E2225 **Manual wheelchair accessory, caster wheel excludes tire, any size, replacement only, each** Y ☑ ♿ (NU, RR, UE)

E2226 **Manual wheelchair accessory, caster fork, any size, replacement only, each** Y ☑ ♿ (NU, RR, UE)

E2227 **Manual wheelchair accessory, gear reduction drive wheel, each** Y ☑ ♿ (RR)

E2228 **Manual wheelchair accessory, wheel braking system and lock, complete, each** Y ☑ ♿ (RR)

E2230 **Manual wheelchair accessory, manual standing system** Y

E2231 **Manual wheelchair accessory, solid seat support base (replaces sling seat), includes any type mounting hardware** Y ♿ (NU, RR, UE)

E2291 **Back, planar, for pediatric size wheelchair including fixed attaching hardware** Y

E2292 **Seat, planar, for pediatric size wheelchair including fixed attaching hardware** Y

E2293 **Back, contoured, for pediatric size wheelchair including fixed attaching hardware** Y

E2294 **Seat, contoured, for pediatric size wheelchair including fixed attaching hardware** Y

E2295 **Manual wheelchair accessory, for pediatric size wheelchair, dynamic seating frame, allows coordinated movement of multiple positioning features** Y

E2300 **Wheelchair accessory, power seat elevation system, any type** Y
CMS: 100-04,20,30.9

E2301 **Wheelchair accessory, power standing system, any type** Y

E2310 **Power wheelchair accessory, electronic connection between wheelchair controller and one power seating system motor, including all related electronics, indicator feature, mechanical function selection switch, and fixed mounting hardware** Y ♿ (RR)
CMS: 100-04,23,60.3

E2311 **Power wheelchair accessory, electronic connection between wheelchair controller and 2 or more power seating system motors, including all related electronics, indicator feature, mechanical function selection switch, and fixed mounting hardware** Y ♿ (RR)
CMS: 100-04,23,60.3

E2312 **Power wheelchair accessory, hand or chin control interface, mini-proportional remote joystick, proportional, including fixed mounting hardware** Y ♿ (RR)

E2313 **Power wheelchair accessory, harness for upgrade to expandable controller, including all fasteners, connectors and mounting hardware, each** Y ☑ ♿ (RR)

E2321 **Power wheelchair accessory, hand control interface, remote joystick, nonproportional, including all related electronics, mechanical stop switch, and fixed mounting hardware** Y ♿ (RR)
CMS: 100-04,23,60.3

E2322 **Power wheelchair accessory, hand control interface, multiple mechanical switches, nonproportional, including all related electronics, mechanical stop switch, and fixed mounting hardware** Y ♿ (RR)
CMS: 100-04,23,60.3

E2323 **Power wheelchair accessory, specialty joystick handle for hand control interface, prefabricated** Y ♿ (NU, RR, UE)
CMS: 100-04,23,60.3

E2324 **Power wheelchair accessory, chin cup for chin control interface** Y ♿ (NU, RR, UE)
CMS: 100-04,23,60.3

E2325 **Power wheelchair accessory, sip and puff interface, nonproportional, including all related electronics, mechanical stop switch, and manual swingaway mounting hardware** Y ♿ (RR)
CMS: 100-04,23,60.3

E2326 **Power wheelchair accessory, breath tube kit for sip and puff interface** Y ♿ (RR)
CMS: 100-04,23,60.3

E2327 **Power wheelchair accessory, head control interface, mechanical, proportional, including all related electronics, mechanical direction change switch, and fixed mounting hardware** Y ♿ (RR)
CMS: 100-04,23,60.3

E2328 **Power wheelchair accessory, head control or extremity control interface, electronic, proportional, including all related electronics and fixed mounting hardware** Y ♿ (RR)
CMS: 100-04,23,60.3

E2329 **Power wheelchair accessory, head control interface, contact switch mechanism, nonproportional, including all related electronics, mechanical stop switch, mechanical direction change switch, head array, and fixed mounting hardware** Y ♿ (RR)
CMS: 100-04,23,60.3

© 2019 Optum360, LLC

E2330 **Power wheelchair accessory, head control interface, proximity switch mechanism, nonproportional, including all related electronics, mechanical stop switch, mechanical direction change switch, head array, and fixed mounting hardware** Y ♿ (RR)
CMS: 100-04,23,60.3

E2331 **Power wheelchair accessory, attendant control, proportional, including all related electronics and fixed mounting hardware** Y

E2340 **Power wheelchair accessory, nonstandard seat frame width, 20-23 in** Y ☑ ♿ (NU, RR, UE)

E2341 **Power wheelchair accessory, nonstandard seat frame width, 24-27 in** Y ☑ ♿ (NU, RR, UE)

E2342 **Power wheelchair accessory, nonstandard seat frame depth, 20 or 21 in** Y ☑ ♿ (NU, RR, UE)

E2343 **Power wheelchair accessory, nonstandard seat frame depth, 22-25 in** Y ☑ ♿ (NU, RR, UE)

E2351 **Power wheelchair accessory, electronic interface to operate speech generating device using power wheelchair control interface** Y ♿ (NU, RR, UE)
CMS: 100-04,23,60.3

E2358 **Power wheelchair accessory, group 34 nonsealed lead acid battery, each** Y ☑

E2359 **Power wheelchair accessory, group 34 sealed lead acid battery, each (e.g., gel cell, absorbed glass mat)** Y ♿ (NU, RR, UE)

E2360 **Power wheelchair accessory, 22 NF nonsealed lead acid battery, each** Y ☑ ♿ (NU, RR, UE)

E2361 **Power wheelchair accessory, 22 NF sealed lead acid battery, each (e.g., gel cell, absorbed glassmat)** Y ☑ ♿ (NU, RR, UE)
CMS: 100-04,23,60.3

E2362 **Power wheelchair accessory, group 24 nonsealed lead acid battery, each** Y ☑ ♿ (NU, RR, UE)

E2363 **Power wheelchair accessory, group 24 sealed lead acid battery, each (e.g., gel cell, absorbed glassmat)** Y ☑ ♿ (NU, RR, UE)
CMS: 100-04,23,60.3

E2364 **Power wheelchair accessory, U-1 nonsealed lead acid battery, each** Y ☑ ♿ (NU, RR, UE)

E2365 **Power wheelchair accessory, U-1 sealed lead acid battery, each (e.g., gel cell, absorbed glassmat)** Y ☑ ♿ (NU, RR, UE)
CMS: 100-04,23,60.3

E2366 **Power wheelchair accessory, battery charger, single mode, for use with only one battery type, sealed or nonsealed, each** Y ☑ ♿ (NU, RR, UE)
CMS: 100-04,23,60.3

E2367 **Power wheelchair accessory, battery charger, dual mode, for use with either battery type, sealed or nonsealed, each** Y ☑ ♿ (NU, RR, UE)
CMS: 100-04,23,60.3

E2368 **Power wheelchair component, drive wheel motor, replacement only** Y ♿ (RR)
CMS: 100-04,23,60.3

E2369 **Power wheelchair component, drive wheel gear box, replacement only** Y ♿ (RR)
CMS: 100-04,23,60.3

E2370 **Power wheelchair component, integrated drive wheel motor and gear box combination, replacement only** Y ♿ (RR)
CMS: 100-04,23,60.3

E2371 **Power wheelchair accessory, group 27 sealed lead acid battery, (e.g., gel cell, absorbed glassmat), each** Y ☑ ♿ (NU, RR, UE)
CMS: 100-04,23,60.3

E2372 **Power wheelchair accessory, group 27 nonsealed lead acid battery, each** Y ☑ ♿ (NU, RR, UE)

E2373 **Power wheelchair accessory, hand or chin control interface, compact remote joystick, proportional, including fixed mounting hardware** Y ♿ (RR)
CMS: 100-04,23,60.3

E2374 **Power wheelchair accessory, hand or chin control interface, standard remote joystick (not including controller), proportional, including all related electronics and fixed mounting hardware, replacement only** Y ♿ (RR)
CMS: 100-04,23,60.3

E2375 **Power wheelchair accessory, nonexpandable controller, including all related electronics and mounting hardware, replacement only** Y ♿ (RR)
CMS: 100-04,23,60.3

E2376 **Power wheelchair accessory, expandable controller, including all related electronics and mounting hardware, replacement only** Y ♿ (RR)
CMS: 100-04,23,60.3

E2377 **Power wheelchair accessory, expandable controller, including all related electronics and mounting hardware, upgrade provided at initial issue** Y ♿ (RR)
CMS: 100-04,23,60.3

E2378 **Power wheelchair component, actuator, replacement only** Y ♿ (RR)
CMS: 100-04,23,60.3

E2381 **Power wheelchair accessory, pneumatic drive wheel tire, any size, replacement only, each** Y ☑ ♿ (NU, RR, UE)
CMS: 100-04,23,60.3

E2382 **Power wheelchair accessory, tube for pneumatic drive wheel tire, any size, replacement only, each** Y ☑ ♿ (NU, RR, UE)
CMS: 100-04,23,60.3

E2383 **Power wheelchair accessory, insert for pneumatic drive wheel tire (removable), any type, any size, replacement only, each** Y ☑ ♿ (NU, RR, UE)
CMS: 100-04,23,60.3

E2384 **Power wheelchair accessory, pneumatic caster tire, any size, replacement only, each** Y ☑ ♿ (NU, RR, UE)
CMS: 100-04,23,60.3

E2385 **Power wheelchair accessory, tube for pneumatic caster tire, any size, replacement only, each** Y ☑ ♿ (NU, RR, UE)
CMS: 100-04,23,60.3

E2386 **Power wheelchair accessory, foam filled drive wheel tire, any size, replacement only, each** Y ☑ ♿ (NU, RR, UE)
CMS: 100-04,23,60.3

E2387 **Power wheelchair accessory, foam filled caster tire, any size, replacement only, each** Y ☑ ♿ (NU, RR, UE)
CMS: 100-04,23,60.3

E2388 **Power wheelchair accessory, foam drive wheel tire, any size, replacement only, each** Y ☑ ♿ (NU, RR, UE)
CMS: 100-04,23,60.3

E2389 **Power wheelchair accessory, foam caster tire, any size, replacement only, each** Y ☑ ♿ (NU, RR, UE)
CMS: 100-04,23,60.3

E2390 **Power wheelchair accessory, solid (rubber/plastic) drive wheel tire, any size, replacement only, each** Y ☑ ♿ (NU, RR, UE)
CMS: 100-04,23,60.3

E2391 **Power wheelchair accessory, solid (rubber/plastic) caster tire (removable), any size, replacement only, each** Y ☑ ♿ (NU, RR, UE)
CMS: 100-04,23,60.3

© 2019 Optum360, LLC

E2392 Power wheelchair accessory, solid (rubber/plastic) caster tire with integrated wheel, any size, replacement only, each [Y] ☑ ♿ (NU, RR, UE)
CMS: 100-04,23,60.3

E2394 Power wheelchair accessory, drive wheel excludes tire, any size, replacement only, each [Y] ☑ ♿ (NU, RR, UE)
CMS: 100-04,23,60.3

E2395 Power wheelchair accessory, caster wheel excludes tire, any size, replacement only, each [Y] ☑ ♿ (NU, RR, UE)
CMS: 100-04,23,60.3

E2396 Power wheelchair accessory, caster fork, any size, replacement only, each [Y] ☑ ♿ (NU, RR, UE)
CMS: 100-04,23,60.3

E2397 Power wheelchair accessory, lithium-based battery, each [Y] ☑ ♿ (NU, RR, UE)

● **E2398** Jan Wheelchair accessory, dynamic positioning hardware for back

Wound Therapy

E2402 Negative pressure wound therapy electrical pump, stationary or portable [Y] ♿ (RR)
CMS: 100-02,7,40.1.2.8; 100-02,7,50.4.4; 100-04,23,60.3

Speech Generating Device

E2500 Speech generating device, digitized speech, using prerecorded messages, less than or equal to eight minutes recording time [Y] ☑ ♿ (NU, RR, UE)

E2502 Speech generating device, digitized speech, using prerecorded messages, greater than eight minutes but less than or equal to 20 minutes recording time [Y] ☑ ♿ (NU, RR, UE)

E2504 Speech generating device, digitized speech, using prerecorded messages, greater than 20 minutes but less than or equal to 40 minutes recording time [Y] ☑ ♿ (NU, RR, UE)

E2506 Speech generating device, digitized speech, using prerecorded messages, greater than 40 minutes recording time [Y] ☑ ♿ (NU, RR, UE)

E2508 Speech generating device, synthesized speech, requiring message formulation by spelling and access by physical contact with the device [Y] ♿ (NU, RR, UE)

E2510 Speech generating device, synthesized speech, permitting multiple methods of message formulation and multiple methods of device access [Y] ♿ (NU, RR, UE)

E2511 Speech generating software program, for personal computer or personal digital assistant [Y] ♿ (NU, RR, UE)

E2512 Accessory for speech generating device, mounting system [Y] ♿ (NU, RR, UE)

E2599 Accessory for speech generating device, not otherwise classified [Y]

Wheelchair Cushion

E2601 General use wheelchair seat cushion, width less than 22 in, any depth [Y] ♿ (NU, RR, UE)
CMS: 100-04,23,60.3

E2602 General use wheelchair seat cushion, width 22 in or greater, any depth [Y] ♿ (NU, RR, UE)
CMS: 100-04,23,60.3

E2603 Skin protection wheelchair seat cushion, width less than 22 in, any depth [Y] ♿ (NU, RR, UE)
CMS: 100-04,23,60.3

E2604 Skin protection wheelchair seat cushion, width 22 in or greater, any depth [Y] ♿ (NU, RR, UE)
CMS: 100-04,23,60.3

E2605 Positioning wheelchair seat cushion, width less than 22 in, any depth [Y] ♿ (NU, RR, UE)
CMS: 100-04,23,60.3

E2606 Positioning wheelchair seat cushion, width 22 in or greater, any depth [Y] ♿ (NU, RR, UE)
CMS: 100-04,23,60.3

E2607 Skin protection and positioning wheelchair seat cushion, width less than 22 in, any depth [Y] ♿ (NU, RR, UE)
CMS: 100-04,23,60.3

E2608 Skin protection and positioning wheelchair seat cushion, width 22 in or greater, any depth [Y] ♿ (NU, RR, UE)
CMS: 100-04,23,60.3

E2609 Custom fabricated wheelchair seat cushion, any size [Y]

E2610 Wheelchair seat cushion, powered [B]

E2611 General use wheelchair back cushion, width less than 22 in, any height, including any type mounting hardware [Y] ♿ (NU, RR, UE)
CMS: 100-04,23,60.3

E2612 General use wheelchair back cushion, width 22 in or greater, any height, including any type mounting hardware [Y] ♿ (NU, RR, UE)
CMS: 100-04,23,60.3

E2613 Positioning wheelchair back cushion, posterior, width less than 22 in, any height, including any type mounting hardware [Y] ♿ (NU, RR, UE)
CMS: 100-04,23,60.3

E2614 Positioning wheelchair back cushion, posterior, width 22 in or greater, any height, including any type mounting hardware [Y] ♿ (NU, RR, UE)
CMS: 100-04,23,60.3

E2615 Positioning wheelchair back cushion, posterior-lateral, width less than 22 in, any height, including any type mounting hardware [Y] ♿ (NU, RR, UE)
CMS: 100-04,23,60.3

E2616 Positioning wheelchair back cushion, posterior-lateral, width 22 in or greater, any height, including any type mounting hardware [Y] ♿ (NU, RR, UE)
CMS: 100-04,23,60.3

E2617 Custom fabricated wheelchair back cushion, any size, including any type mounting hardware [Y]

E2619 Replacement cover for wheelchair seat cushion or back cushion, each [Y] ☑ ♿ (NU, RR, UE)
CMS: 100-04,23,60.3

E2620 Positioning wheelchair back cushion, planar back with lateral supports, width less than 22 in, any height, including any type mounting hardware [Y] ♿ (NU, RR, UE)
CMS: 100-04,23,60.3

E2621 Positioning wheelchair back cushion, planar back with lateral supports, width 22 in or greater, any height, including any type mounting hardware [Y] ♿ (NU, RR, UE)
CMS: 100-04,23,60.3

E2622 Skin protection wheelchair seat cushion, adjustable, width less than 22 in, any depth [Y] ♿ (NU, RR, UE)

E2623 Skin protection wheelchair seat cushion, adjustable, width 22 in or greater, any depth [Y] ♿ (NU, RR, UE)

E2624 Skin protection and positioning wheelchair seat cushion, adjustable, width less than 22 in, any depth [Y] ♿ (NU, RR, UE)

E2625 Skin protection and positioning wheelchair seat cushion, adjustable, width 22 in or greater, any depth [Y] ♿ (NU, RR, UE)

© 2019 Optum360, LLC

Wheelchair Arm Support

E2626 Wheelchair accessory, shoulder elbow, mobile arm support attached to wheelchair, balanced, adjustable Y ♿ (NU, RR, UE)

E2627 Wheelchair accessory, shoulder elbow, mobile arm support attached to wheelchair, balanced, adjustable Rancho type Y ♿ (NU, RR, UE)

E2628 Wheelchair accessory, shoulder elbow, mobile arm support attached to wheelchair, balanced, reclining Y ♿ (NU, RR, UE)

E2629 Wheelchair accessory, shoulder elbow, mobile arm support attached to wheelchair, balanced, friction arm support (friction dampening to proximal and distal joints) Y ♿ (NU, RR, UE)

E2630 Wheelchair accessory, shoulder elbow, mobile arm support, monosuspension arm and hand support, overhead elbow forearm hand sling support, yoke type suspension support Y ♿ (NU, RR, UE)

E2631 Wheelchair accessory, addition to mobile arm support, elevating proximal arm Y ♿ (NU, RR, UE)

E2632 Wheelchair accessory, addition to mobile arm support, offset or lateral rocker arm with elastic balance control Y ♿ (NU, RR, UE)

E2633 Wheelchair accessory, addition to mobile arm support, supinator Y ♿ (NU, RR, UE)

Gait Trainer

E8000 Gait trainer, pediatric size, posterior support, includes all accessories and components E

E8001 Gait trainer, pediatric size, upright support, includes all accessories and components E

E8002 Gait trainer, pediatric size, anterior support, includes all accessories and components E

© 2019 Optum360, LLC

Procedures/Professional Services (Temporary) G0008-G9987

The G codes are used to identify professional health care procedures and services that would otherwise be coded in CPT but for which there are no CPT codes. Please refer to your CPT book for possible alternate code(s).

Immunization Administration

G0008 **Administration of influenza virus vaccine** [S]

CMS: 100-02,12,40.11; 100-02,13,220; 100-02,13,220.1; 100-02,13,220.3; 100-02,15,50.4.4.2; 100-04,18,10.2.1; 100-04,18,10.2.2.1; 100-04,18,10.2.5.2; 100-04,18,10.3.1.1; 100-04,18,10.4; 100-04,18,10.4.1; 100-04,18,10.4.2; 100-04,18,10.4.3; 1004-04,13,220.1

AHA: 4Q, '16, 1-3; 2Q, '09, 1; 2Q, '06, 5; 2Q, '03, 7

G0009 **Administration of pneumococcal vaccine** [S]

CMS: 100-02,12,40.11; 100-02,13,220; 100-02,13,220.1; 100-02,13,220.3; 100-02,15,50.4.4.2; 100-04,18,10.2.1; 100-04,18,10.2.2.1; 100-04,18,10.2.5.2; 100-04,18,10.3.1.1; 100-04,18,10.4; 100-04,18,10.4.1; 100-04,18,10.4.2; 100-04,18,10.4.3; 1004-04,13,220.1

AHA: 4Q, '16, 1-3; 2Q, '09, 1; 2Q, '03, 7

G0010 **Administration of hepatitis B vaccine** [S]

CMS: 100-02,12,40.11; 100-02,13,220; 100-02,13,220.1; 100-02,13,220.3; 100-02,15,50.4.4.2; 100-04,18,10.2.1; 100-04,18,10.2.2.1; 100-04,18,10.2.5.2; 100-04,18,10.3.1.1; 1004-04,13,220.1

AHA: 4Q, '16, 1-3

Semen Analysis

G0027 **Semen analysis; presence and/or motility of sperm excluding Huhner** ♂ [Q]

Professional Services

G0068 **Professional services for the administration of antiinfective, pain management, chelation, pulmonary hypertension, and/or inotropic infusion drug(s) for each infusion drug administration calendar day in the individual's home, each 15 minutes**

CMS: 100-04,20,180

G0069 **Professional services for the administration of subcutaneous immunotherapy for each infusion drug administration calendar day in the individual's home, each 15 minutes**

CMS: 100-04,20,180

G0070 **Professional services for the administration of chemotherapy for each infusion drug administration calendar day in the individual's home, each 15 minutes**

CMS: 100-04,20,180

G0071 **Payment for communication technology-based services for 5 minutes or more of a virtual (nonface-to-face) communication between a rural health clinic (RHC) or federally qualified health center (FQHC) practitioner and RHC or FQHC patient, or 5 minutes or more of remote evaluation of recorded video and/or images by an RHC or FQHC practitioner, occurring in lieu of an office visit; RHC or FQHC only**

G0076 **Brief (20 minutes) care management home visit for a new patient. For use only in a Medicare-approved CMMI model (services must be furnished within a beneficiary's home, domiciliary, rest home, assisted living and/or nursing facility)**

G0077 **Limited (30 minutes) care management home visit for a new patient. For use only in a Medicare-approved CMMI model (services must be furnished within a beneficiary's home, domiciliary, rest home, assisted living and/or nursing facility)**

G0078 **Moderate (45 minutes) care management home visit for a new patient. For use only in a Medicare-approved CMMI model (services must be furnished within a beneficiary's home, domiciliary, rest home, assisted living and/or nursing facility)**

G0079 **Comprehensive (60 minutes) care management home visit for a new patient. For use only in a Medicare-approved CMMI model (services must be furnished within a beneficiary's home, domiciliary, rest home, assisted living and/or nursing facility)**

G0080 **Extensive (75 minutes) care management home visit for a new patient. For use only in a Medicare-approved CMMI model (services must be furnished within a beneficiary's home, domiciliary, rest home, assisted living and/or nursing facility)**

G0081 **Brief (20 minutes) care management home visit for an existing patient. For use only in a Medicare-approved CMMI model (services must be furnished within a beneficiary's home, domiciliary, rest home, assisted living and/or nursing facility)**

G0082 **Limited (30 minutes) care management home visit for an existing patient. For use only in a Medicare-approved CMMI model (services must be furnished within a beneficiary's home, domiciliary, rest home, assisted living and/or nursing facility)**

G0083 **Moderate (45 minutes) care management home visit for an existing patient. For use only in a Medicare-approved CMMI model (services must be furnished within a beneficiary's home, domiciliary, rest home, assisted living and/or nursing facility)**

G0084 **Comprehensive (60 minutes) care management home visit for an existing patient. For use only in a Medicare-approved CMMI model (services must be furnished within a beneficiary's home, domiciliary, rest home, assisted living and/or nursing facility)**

G0085 **Extensive (75 minutes) care management home visit for an existing patient. For use only in a Medicare-approved CMMI model (services must be furnished within a beneficiary's home, domiciliary, rest home, assisted living and/or nursing facility)**

G0086 **Limited (30 minutes) care management home care plan oversight. For use only in a Medicare-approved CMMI model (services must be furnished within a beneficiary's home, domiciliary, rest home, assisted living and/or nursing facility)**

G0087 **Comprehensive (60 minutes) care management home care plan oversight. For use only in a Medicare-approved CMMI model (services must be furnished within a beneficiary's home, domiciliary, rest home, assisted living and/or nursing facility)**

Screening Services

G0101 **Cervical or vaginal cancer screening; pelvic and clinical breast examination** [A] ♀ [S] ⊘

G0101 can be reported with an E/M code when a separately identifiable E/M service was provided.

CMS: 100-02,13,220; 100-02,13,220.1; 100-03,210.2; 1004-04,13,220.1

AHA: 4Q, '02, 8; 3Q, '01, 6; 3Q, '01, 3

G0102 **Prostate cancer screening; digital rectal examination** ♂ [N] ⊘

CMS: 100-02,13,220; 100-02,13,220.1; 100-02,13,220.3

G0103 **Prostate cancer screening; prostate specific antigen test (PSA)** ♂ [A]

G0104 **Colorectal cancer screening; flexible sigmoidoscopy** [T] [A3] ⊘

Medicare covers colorectal screening for cancer via flexible sigmoidoscopy once every four years for patients 50 years or older.

CMS: 100-02,15,280.2.2; 100-04,18,60; 100-04,18,60.1; 100-04,18,60.1.1; 100-04,18,60.2; 100-04,18,60.2.1; 100-04,18,60.6; 100-04,18,60.7

AHA: 2Q, '09, 1

G0105 **Colorectal cancer screening; colonoscopy on individual at high risk** [T] [A2] ⊘

An individual with ulcerative enteritis or a history of a malignant neoplasm of the lower gastrointestinal tract is considered at high-risk for colorectal cancer, as defined by CMS.

CMS: 100-02,15,280.2.2; 100-04,12,30.1; 100-04,18,60; 100-04,18,60.1; 100-04,18,60.1.1; 100-04,18,60.2; 100-04,18,60.2.1; 100-04,18,60.6; 100-04,18,60.7; 100-04,18,60.8; 100-04,23,30.2; 100-04,4,250.18

AHA: 2Q, '09, 1

G0106 **Colorectal cancer screening; alternative to G0104, screening sigmoidoscopy, barium enema** [S]

CMS: 100-02,15,280.2.2; 100-04,18,60; 100-04,18,60.1; 100-04,18,60.1.1; 100-04,18,60.2; 100-04,18,60.2.1; 100-04,18,60.6; 100-04,18,60.7

AHA: 2Q, '09, 1

© 2019 Optum360, LLC

G0108 **Diabetes outpatient self-management training services, individual, per 30 minutes** A ☑ ⊘
CMS: 100-02,13,220.3; 100-02,15,300; 100-02,15,300.2; 100-02,15,300.3; 100-02,15,300.4; 100-04,12,190.3; 100-04,12,190.3.6; 100-04,12,190.6; 100-04,12,190.6.1; 100-04,12,190.7; 100-04,18,120.1; 100-04,4,300.6

G0109 **Diabetes outpatient self-management training services, group session (two or more), per 30 minutes** A ☑ ⊘
CMS: 100-02,15,300.2; 100-02,15,300.3; 100-04,12,190.3; 100-04,12,190.3.6; 100-04,12,190.6; 100-04,12,190.6.1; 100-04,12,190.7; 100-04,4,300.6

G0117 **Glaucoma screening for high risk patients furnished by an optometrist or ophthalmologist** S ⊘
CMS: 100-02,13,220; 100-02,13,220.1; 100-02,13,220.3; 100-02,15,280.1; 100-04,18,70.1.1; 1004-04,13,220.1
AHA: 1Q, '02, 5; 1Q, '02, 4; 3Q, '01, 12

G0118 **Glaucoma screening for high risk patient furnished under the direct supervision of an optometrist or ophthalmologist** S ⊘
CMS: 100-02,13,220; 100-02,13,220.1; 100-02,13,220.3; 100-02,15,280.1; 100-04,18,70.1.1; 1004-04,13,220.1
AHA: 1Q, '02, 5; 1Q, '02, 4; 3Q, '01, 12

G0120 **Colorectal cancer screening; alternative to G0105, screening colonoscopy, barium enema** S
CMS: 100-02,15,280.2.2; 100-04,18,60; 100-04,18,60.1; 100-04,18,60.1.1; 100-04,18,60.2; 100-04,18,60.2.1; 100-04,18,60.6; 100-04,18,60.7; 100-04,18,60.8

G0121 **Colorectal cancer screening; colonoscopy on individual not meeting criteria for high risk** T 42 ⊘
CMS: 100-02,15,280.2.2; 100-04,12,30.1; 100-04,18,60; 100-04,18,60.1; 100-04,18,60.1.1; 100-04,18,60.2; 100-04,18,60.2.1; 100-04,18,60.6; 100-04,23,30.2; 100-04,4,250.18
AHA: 3Q, '01, 12

G0122 **Colorectal cancer screening; barium enema** E
CMS: 100-04,18,60; 100-04,18,60.2; 100-04,18,60.2.1; 100-04,18,60.6; 100-04,18,60.7; 100-04,18,60.8

G0123 **Screening cytopathology, cervical or vaginal (any reporting system), collected in preservative fluid, automated thin layer preparation, screening by cytotechnologist under physician supervision** A ♀ A
See also P3000-P3001.
CMS: 100-03,210.2.1; 100-04,18,30.2.1; 100-04,18,30.5; 100-04,18,30.6

G0124 **Screening cytopathology, cervical or vaginal (any reporting system), collected in preservative fluid, automated thin layer preparation, requiring interpretation by physician** A ♀ B ⊘
See also P3000-P3001.
CMS: 100-03,210.2.1; 100-04,18,30.2.1; 100-04,18,30.5; 100-04,18,30.6

Miscellaneous Services

G0127 **Trimming of dystrophic nails, any number** 01 ⊘
CMS: 100-02,15,290

G0128 **Direct (face-to-face with patient) skilled nursing services of a registered nurse provided in a comprehensive outpatient rehabilitation facility, each 10 minutes beyond the first 5 minutes** B ☑ ⊘
CMS: 100-02,12,30.1; 100-02,12,40.8; 100-04,5,100.3; 100-04,5,20.4

G0129 **Occupational therapy services requiring the skills of a qualified occupational therapist, furnished as a component of a partial hospitalization treatment program, per session (45 minutes or more)** P ☑
CMS: 100-04,4,260.1; 100-04,4,260.1.1
AHA: 4Q, '12, 11-14

G0130 **Single energy x-ray absorptiometry (SEXA) bone density study, one or more sites; appendicular skeleton (peripheral) (e.g., radius, wrist, heel)** S 73

G0141 **Screening cytopathology smears, cervical or vaginal, performed by automated system, with manual rescreening, requiring interpretation by physician** A ♀ B ⊘
CMS: 100-03,210.2.1; 100-04,18,30.2.1; 100-04,18,30.5; 100-04,18,30.6

G0143 **Screening cytopathology, cervical or vaginal (any reporting system), collected in preservative fluid, automated thin layer preparation, with manual screening and rescreening by cytotechnologist under physician supervision** A ♀ A
CMS: 100-03,210.2.1; 100-04,18,30.2.1; 100-04,18,30.5; 100-04,18,30.6

G0144 **Screening cytopathology, cervical or vaginal (any reporting system), collected in preservative fluid, automated thin layer preparation, with screening by automated system, under physician supervision** A ♀ A
CMS: 100-03,210.2.1; 100-04,18,30.2.1; 100-04,18,30.5; 100-04,18,30.6

G0145 **Screening cytopathology, cervical or vaginal (any reporting system), collected in preservative fluid, automated thin layer preparation, with screening by automated system and manual rescreening under physician supervision** A ♀ A
CMS: 100-03,210.2.1; 100-04,18,30.2.1; 100-04,18,30.5; 100-04,18,30.6

G0147 **Screening cytopathology smears, cervical or vaginal, performed by automated system under physician supervision** A ♀ A
CMS: 100-03,210.2.1; 100-04,18,30.2.1; 100-04,18,30.5; 100-04,18,30.6

G0148 **Screening cytopathology smears, cervical or vaginal, performed by automated system with manual rescreening** A ♀ A
CMS: 100-03,210.2.1; 100-04,18,30.2.1; 100-04,18,30.5; 100-04,18,30.6

G0151 **Services performed by a qualified physical therapist in the home health or hospice setting, each 15 minutes** B ☑
CMS: 100-01,3,30.3; 100-04,10,40.2; 100-04,11,10; 100-04,11,30.3

G0152 **Services performed by a qualified occupational therapist in the home health or hospice setting, each 15 minutes** B ☑
CMS: 100-01,3,30.3; 100-04,10,40.2; 100-04,11,10; 100-04,11,30.3

G0153 **Services performed by a qualified speech-language pathologist in the home health or hospice setting, each 15 minutes** B ☑
CMS: 100-01,3,30.3; 100-04,10,40.2; 100-04,11,10; 100-04,11,30.3

G0155 **Services of clinical social worker in home health or hospice settings, each 15 minutes** B ☑
CMS: 100-01,3,30.3; 100-04,10,40.2; 100-04,11,10; 100-04,11,30.3

G0156 **Services of home health/hospice aide in home health or hospice settings, each 15 minutes** B ☑
CMS: 100-01,3,30.3; 100-04,10,40.2; 100-04,11,10; 100-04,11,30.3

G0157 **Services performed by a qualified physical therapist assistant in the home health or hospice setting, each 15 minutes** B ☑
CMS: 100-04,10,40.2; 100-04,11,10

G0158 **Services performed by a qualified occupational therapist assistant in the home health or hospice setting, each 15 minutes** B ☑
CMS: 100-04,10,40.2; 100-04,11,10

G0159 **Services performed by a qualified physical therapist, in the home health setting, in the establishment or delivery of a safe and effective physical therapy maintenance program, each 15 minutes** B ☑
CMS: 100-04,10,40.2

G0160 **Services performed by a qualified occupational therapist, in the home health setting, in the establishment or delivery of a safe and effective occupational therapy maintenance program, each 15 minutes** B ☑
CMS: 100-04,10,40.2

G0161 **Services performed by a qualified speech-language pathologist, in the home health setting, in the establishment or delivery of a safe and effective speech-language pathology maintenance program, each 15 minutes** B ☑
CMS: 100-04,10,40.2

© 2019 Optum360, LLC

G0162 **Skilled services by a registered nurse (RN) for management and evaluation of the plan of care; each 15 minutes (the patient's underlying condition or complication requires an RN to ensure that essential nonskilled care achieves its purpose in the home health or hospice setting)** B ☑
CMS: 100-04,10,40.2; 100-04,11,10

G0166 **External counterpulsation, per treatment session** Q1 ☑ ⊘
CMS: 100-04,32,130; 100-04,32,130.1

G0168 **Wound closure utilizing tissue adhesive(s) only** B ⊘
AHA: 1Q, '05, 5; 4Q, '01, 10; 3Q, '01, 13

G0175 **Scheduled interdisciplinary team conference (minimum of three exclusive of patient care nursing staff) with patient present** V
CMS: 100-04,4,160
AHA: 3Q, '01, 6; 3Q, '01, 3

G0176 **Activity therapy, such as music, dance, art or play therapies not for recreation, related to the care and treatment of patient's disabling mental health problems, per session (45 minutes or more)** P
CMS: 100-04,4,260.1; 100-04,4,260.1.1; 100-04,4,260.5
AHA: 4Q, '12, 11-14

G0177 **Training and educational services related to the care and treatment of patient's disabling mental health problems per session (45 minutes or more)** N
CMS: 100-04,4,260.1; 100-04,4,260.1.1
AHA: 4Q, '12, 11-14

G0179 **Physician re-certification for Medicare-covered home health services under a home health plan of care (patient not present), including contacts with home health agency and review of reports of patient status required by physicians to affirm the initial implementation of the plan of care that meets patient's needs, per re-certification period** M ⊘
CMS: 100-04,10,20.1.2; 100-04,12,180; 100-04,12,180.1

G0180 **Physician certification for Medicare-covered home health services under a home health plan of care (patient not present), including contacts with home health agency and review of reports of patient status required by physicians to affirm the initial implementation of the plan of care that meets patient's needs, per certification period** M ⊘
CMS: 100-04,10,20.1.2; 100-04,12,180; 100-04,12,180.1

G0181 **Physician supervision of a patient receiving Medicare-covered services provided by a participating home health agency (patient not present) requiring complex and multidisciplinary care modalities involving regular physician development and/or revision of care plans, review of subsequent reports of patient status, review of laboratory and other studies, communication (including telephone calls) with other health care professionals involved in the patient's care, integration of new information into the medical treatment plan and/or adjustment of medical therapy, within a calendar month, 30 minutes or more** M ⊘
CMS: 100-04,12,180; 100-04,12,180.1
AHA: 2Q, '15, 10

G0182 **Physician supervision of a patient under a Medicare-approved hospice (patient not present) requiring complex and multidisciplinary care modalities involving regular physician development and/or revision of care plans, review of subsequent reports of patient status, review of laboratory and other studies, communication (including telephone calls) with other health care professionals involved in the patient's care, integration of new information into the medical treatment plan and/or adjustment of medical therapy, within a calendar month, 30 minutes or more** M ⊘
CMS: 100-04,11,40.1.3.1; 100-04,12,180; 100-04,12,180.1
AHA: 2Q, '15, 10

G0186 **Destruction of localized lesion of choroid (for example, choroidal neovascularization); photocoagulation, feeder vessel technique (one or more sessions)** T A2 ⊘

G0219 **PET imaging whole body; melanoma for noncovered indications** E
CMS: 100-03,220.6.10; 100-03,220.6.12; 100-03,220.6.17; 100-03,220.6.3; 100-03,220.6.4; 100-03,220.6.6; 100-03,220.6.7; 100-04,13,60; 100-04,13,60.16
AHA: 1Q, '02, 5; 1Q, '02, 10; 2Q, '01, 5

G0235 **PET imaging, any site, not otherwise specified** E
CMS: 100-03,220.6.10; 100-03,220.6.12; 100-03,220.6.13; 100-03,220.6.17; 100-03,220.6.2; 100-03,220.6.3; 100-03,220.6.4; 100-03,220.6.5; 100-03,220.6.6; 100-03,220.6.7; 100-03,220.6.9; 100-04,13,60; 100-04,13,60.13; 100-04,13,60.14; 100-04,13,60.16; 100-04,13,60.17
AHA: 1Q, '07, 6

G0237 **Therapeutic procedures to increase strength or endurance of respiratory muscles, face-to-face, one-on-one, each 15 minutes (includes monitoring)** S ☑ ⊘
CMS: 100-02,12,30.1; 100-02,12,40.5
AHA: 1Q, '02, 5

G0238 **Therapeutic procedures to improve respiratory function, other than described by G0237, one-on-one, face-to-face, per 15 minutes (includes monitoring)** S ☑
CMS: 100-02,12,30.1; 100-02,12,40.5
AHA: 1Q, '02, 5

G0239 **Therapeutic procedures to improve respiratory function or increase strength or endurance of respiratory muscles, two or more individuals (includes monitoring)** S
CMS: 100-02,12,30.1; 100-02,12,40.5
AHA: 1Q, '02, 5

G0245 **Initial physician evaluation and management of a diabetic patient with diabetic sensory neuropathy resulting in a loss of protective sensation (LOPS) which must include: (1) the diagnosis of LOPS, (2) a patient history, (3) a physical examination that consists of at least the following elements: (a) visual inspection of the forefoot, hindfoot, and toe web spaces, (b) evaluation of a protective sensation, (c) evaluation of foot structure and biomechanics, (d) evaluation of vascular status and skin integrity, and (e) evaluation and recommendation of footwear, and (4) patient education** V ⊘
CMS: 100-04,32,80.2; 100-04,32,80.3; 100-04,32,80.6; 100-04,32,80.8
AHA: 4Q, '02, 9-10; 3Q, '02, 11

G0246 **Follow-up physician evaluation and management of a diabetic patient with diabetic sensory neuropathy resulting in a loss of protective sensation (LOPS) to include at least the following: (1) a patient history, (2) a physical examination that includes: (a) visual inspection of the forefoot, hindfoot, and toe web spaces, (b) evaluation of protective sensation, (c) evaluation of foot structure and biomechanics, (d) evaluation of vascular status and skin integrity, and (e) evaluation and recommendation of footwear, and (3) patient education** V ⊘
CMS: 100-03,70.2.1; 100-04,32,80; 100-04,32,80.2; 100-04,32,80.3; 100-04,32,80.6; 100-04,32,80.8
AHA: 4Q, '02, 9-10; 3Q, '02, 11

G0247 **Routine foot care by a physician of a diabetic patient with diabetic sensory neuropathy resulting in a loss of protective sensation (LOPS) to include the local care of superficial wounds (i.e., superficial to muscle and fascia) and at least the following, if present: (1) local care of superficial wounds, (2) debridement of corns and calluses, and (3) trimming and debridement of nails** Q1 ⊘
CMS: 100-03,70.2.1; 100-04,32,80; 100-04,32,80.2; 100-04,32,80.3; 100-04,32,80.6; 100-04,32,80.8
AHA: 4Q, '02, 9-10; 3Q, '02, 11

© 2019 Optum360, LLC

G0248 **Demonstration, prior to initiation of home INR monitoring, for patient with either mechanical heart valve(s), chronic atrial fibrillation, or venous thromboembolism who meets Medicare coverage criteria, under the direction of a physician; includes: face-to-face demonstration of use and care of the INR monitor, obtaining at least one blood sample, provision of instructions for reporting home INR test results, and documentation of patient's ability to perform testing and report results** V
CMS: 100-03,190.11; 100-04,32,60.4.1; 100-04,32,80
AHA: 4Q, '02, 9-10; 3Q, '02, 11

G0249 **Provision of test materials and equipment for home INR monitoring of patient with either mechanical heart valve(s), chronic atrial fibrillation, or venous thromboembolism who meets Medicare coverage criteria; includes: provision of materials for use in the home and reporting of test results to physician; testing not occurring more frequently than once a week; testing materials, billing units of service include four tests** V ☑
CMS: 100-03,190.11; 100-04,32,60.4.1
AHA: 4Q, '02, 9-10; 3Q, '02, 11

G0250 **Physician review, interpretation, and patient management of home INR testing for patient with either mechanical heart valve(s), chronic atrial fibrillation, or venous thromboembolism who meets Medicare coverage criteria; testing not occurring more frequently than once a week; billing units of service include four tests** M ☑ ⊘
CMS: 100-03,190.11; 100-04,32,60.4.1
AHA: 4Q, '02, 9-10; 3Q, '02, 11

G0252 **PET imaging, full and partial-ring PET scanners only, for initial diagnosis of breast cancer and/or surgical planning for breast cancer (e.g., initial staging of axillary lymph nodes)** E
CMS: 100-03,220.6.10; 100-03,220.6.3; 100-04,13,60; 100-04,13,60.16
AHA: 1Q, '07, 6; 4Q, '02, 9-10

G0255 **Current perception threshold/sensory nerve conduction test, (SNCT) per limb, any nerve** E
AHA: 4Q, '02, 9-10

G0257 **Unscheduled or emergency dialysis treatment for an ESRD patient in a hospital outpatient department that is not certified as an ESRD facility** S
CMS: 100-04,4,200.2; 100-04,8,60.4.7
AHA: 3Q, '14, 4; 1Q, '03, 7; 4Q, '02, 9-10

G0259 **Injection procedure for sacroiliac joint; arthrography** N
AHA: 4Q, '02, 9-10

G0260 **Injection procedure for sacroiliac joint; provision of anesthetic, steroid and/or other therapeutic agent, with or without arthrography** T A2
AHA: 4Q, '02, 9-10

G0268 **Removal of impacted cerumen (one or both ears) by physician on same date of service as audiologic function testing** N ⊘
AHA: 2Q, '16, 2-3; 1Q, '03, 11

G0269 **Placement of occlusive device into either a venous or arterial access site, postsurgical or interventional procedure (e.g., angioseal plug, vascular plug)** N ⊘
AHA: 4Q, '12, 10; 3Q, '11, 3; 4Q, '10, 6

G0270 **Medical nutrition therapy; reassessment and subsequent intervention(s) following second referral in same year for change in diagnosis, medical condition or treatment regimen (including additional hours needed for renal disease), individual, face-to-face with the patient, each 15 minutes** A ☑ ⊘
CMS: 100-04,12,190.3; 100-04,12,190.6; 100-04,12,190.6.1; 100-04,12,190.7

G0271 **Medical nutrition therapy, reassessment and subsequent intervention(s) following second referral in same year for change in diagnosis, medical condition, or treatment regimen (including additional hours needed for renal disease), group (two or more individuals), each 30 minutes** A ☑ ⊘

G0276 **Blinded procedure for lumbar stenosis, percutaneous image-guided lumbar decompression (PILD) or placebo-control, performed in an approved coverage with evidence development (CED) clinical trial** J B2
CMS: 100-03,150.13; 100-04,32,330.1; 100-04,32,330.2

G0277 **Hyperbaric oxygen under pressure, full body chamber, per 30 minute interval** S
AHA: 3Q, '15, 7

G0278 **Iliac and/or femoral artery angiography, nonselective, bilateral or ipsilateral to catheter insertion, performed at the same time as cardiac catheterization and/or coronary angiography, includes positioning or placement of the catheter in the distal aorta or ipsilateral femoral or iliac artery, injection of dye, production of permanent images, and radiologic supervision and interpretation (List separately in addition to primary procedure)** N ⊘
AHA: 3Q, '11, 3; 4Q, '06, 8

G0279 **Diagnostic digital breast tomosynthesis, unilateral or bilateral (list separately in addition to 77065 or 77066)** A
CMS: 100-04,18,20.2; 100-04,18,20.2.1; 100-04,18,20.2.2; 100-04,18,20.6

G0281 **Electrical stimulation, (unattended), to one or more areas, for chronic Stage III and Stage IV pressure ulcers, arterial ulcers, diabetic ulcers, and venous stasis ulcers not demonstrating measurable signs of healing after 30 days of conventional care, as part of a therapy plan of care** A
CMS: 100-02,15,220.4; 100-04,32,11.1; 100-04,5,10.3.2; 100-04,5,10.3.3
AHA: 2Q, '03, 7; 1Q, '03, 7

G0282 **Electrical stimulation, (unattended), to one or more areas, for wound care other than described in G0281** E
CMS: 100-04,32,11.1
AHA: 2Q, '03, 7; 1Q, '03, 7

G0283 **Electrical stimulation (unattended), to one or more areas for indication(s) other than wound care, as part of a therapy plan of care** A
CMS: 100-02,15,220.4; 100-04,5,10.3.2; 100-04,5,10.3.3
AHA: 2Q, '09, 1; 2Q, '03, 7; 1Q, '03, 7

G0288 **Reconstruction, computed tomographic angiography of aorta for surgical planning for vascular surgery** N

G0289 **Arthroscopy, knee, surgical, for removal of loose body, foreign body, debridement/shaving of articular cartilage (chondroplasty) at the time of other surgical knee arthroscopy in a different compartment of the same knee** N ⊘
AHA: 2Q, '03, 9

G0293 **Noncovered surgical procedure(s) using conscious sedation, regional, general, or spinal anesthesia in a Medicare qualifying clinical trial, per day** Q1 ☑
AHA: 4Q, '02, 9-10

G0294 **Noncovered procedure(s) using either no anesthesia or local anesthesia only, in a Medicare qualifying clinical trial, per day** Q1 ☑
AHA: 4Q, '02, 9-10

G0295 **Electromagnetic therapy, to one or more areas, for wound care other than described in G0329 or for other uses** E
AHA: 1Q, '03, 7

© 2019 Optum360, LLC

G0296 **Counseling visit to discuss need for lung cancer screening using low dose CT scan (LDCT) (service is for eligibility determination and shared decision making)** [S]
CMS: 100-02,13,220; 100-02,13,220.1; 100-02,13,220.3; 100-04,18,220; 100-04,18,220.1; 100-04,18,220.2; 100-04,18,220.3; 100-04,18,220.5; 1004-04,13,220.1

G0297 **Low dose CT scan (LDCT) for lung cancer screening** [S]
CMS: 100-04,18,220; 100-04,18,220.1; 100-04,18,220.2; 100-04,18,220.3; 100-04,18,220.5

G0299 **Direct skilled nursing services of a registered nurse (RN) in the home health or hospice setting, each 15 minutes** [B]
CMS: 100-01,3,30.3; 100-04,10,40.2; 100-04,11,30.3

G0300 **Direct skilled nursing services of a licensed practical nurse (LPN) in the home health or hospice setting, each 15 minutes** [B]
CMS: 100-01,3,30.3; 100-04,10,40.2; 100-04,11,30.3

G0302 **Preoperative pulmonary surgery services for preparation for LVRS, complete course of services, to include a minimum of 16 days of services** [S] ☑
G0303 **Preoperative pulmonary surgery services for preparation for LVRS, 10 to 15 days of services** [S] ☑
G0304 **Preoperative pulmonary surgery services for preparation for LVRS, 1 to 9 days of services** [S] ☑
G0305 **Postdischarge pulmonary surgery services after LVRS, minimum of 6 days of services** [S] ☑

G0306 **Complete CBC, automated (HgB, HCT, RBC, WBC, without platelet count) and automated WBC differential count** [Q]
CMS: 100-02,11,20.2

G0307 **Complete CBC, automated (HgB, HCT, RBC, WBC; without platelet count)** [Q]
CMS: 100-02,11,20.2

G0328 **Colorectal cancer screening; fecal occult blood test, immunoassay, one to three simultaneous determinations** [A]
CMS: 100-02,15,280.2.2; 100-04,16,70.8; 100-04,18,60; 100-04,18,60.1; 100-04,18,60.1.1; 100-04,18,60.2; 100-04,18,60.2.1; 100-04,18,60.6; 100-04,18,60.7
AHA: 2Q, '12, 9

G0329 **Electromagnetic therapy, to one or more areas for chronic Stage III and Stage IV pressure ulcers, arterial ulcers, diabetic ulcers and venous stasis ulcers not demonstrating measurable signs of healing after 30 days of conventional care as part of a therapy plan of care** [A]
CMS: 100-02,15,220.4; 100-04,32,11.2; 100-04,5,10.3.2; 100-04,5,10.3.3

G0333 **Pharmacy dispensing fee for inhalation drug(s); initial 30-day supply as a beneficiary** [M]

G0337 **Hospice evaluation and counseling services, preelection** [B]
CMS: 100-04,11,10

G0339 **Image guided robotic linear accelerator-based stereotactic radiosurgery, complete course of therapy in one session or first session of fractionated treatment** [B] ⊘
AHA: 4Q, '13, 8-10; 1Q, '04, 6

G0340 **Image guided robotic linear accelerator-based stereotactic radiosurgery, delivery including collimator changes and custom plugging, fractionated treatment, all lesions, per session, second through fifth sessions, maximum five sessions per course of treatment** [B] ⊘
AHA: 4Q, '13, 8-10; 1Q, '04, 6

G0341 **Percutaneous islet cell transplant, includes portal vein catheterization and infusion** [C] ⊘
CMS: 100-04,32,70

G0342 **Laparoscopy for islet cell transplant, includes portal vein catheterization and infusion** [C] ⊘
CMS: 100-04,32,70

G0343 **Laparotomy for islet cell transplant, includes portal vein catheterization and infusion** [C] ⊘
CMS: 100-04,32,70

~~**G0365**~~ Jan ~~**Vessel mapping of vessels for hemodialysis access (services for preoperative vessel mapping prior to creation of hemodialysis access using an autogenous hemodialysis conduit, including arterial inflow and venous outflow)**~~

G0372 **Physician service required to establish and document the need for a power mobility device** [M] ⊘
CMS: 100-04,12,30.6.15.4

Observation/Emergency Department Services

G0378 **Hospital observation service, per hour** [N]
CMS: 100-02,6,20.6; 100-04,01,50.3.2; 100-04,4,290.1; 100-04,4,290.2.2; 100-04,4,290.4.1; 100-04,4,290.4.2; 100-04,4,290.4.3; 100-04,4,290.5.1; 100-04,4,290.5.2; 100-04,4,290.5.3
AHA: 4Q, '05, 7, 9

G0379 **Direct admission of patient for hospital observation care** [J]
CMS: 100-02,6,20.6; 100-04,4,290.4.1; 100-04,4,290.4.2; 100-04,4,290.4.3; 100-04,4,290.5.1; 100-04,4,290.5.2; 100-04,4,290.5.3
AHA: 4Q, '05, 7, 9

G0380 **Level 1 hospital emergency department visit provided in a type B emergency department; (the ED must meet at least one of the following requirements: (1) it is licensed by the state in which it is located under applicable state law as an emergency room or emergency department; (2) it is held out to the public (by name, posted signs, advertising, or other means) as a place that provides care for emergency medical conditions on an urgent basis without requiring a previously scheduled appointment; or (3) during the calendar year immediately preceding the calendar year in which a determination under 42 CFR 489.24 is being made, based on a representative sample of patient visits that occurred during that calendar year, it provides at least one-third of all of its outpatient visits for the treatment of emergency medical conditions on an urgent basis without requiring a previously scheduled appointment)** [J]
CMS: 100-04,4,160
AHA: 4Q, '13, 7; 1Q, '09, 1; 4Q, '07, 1

G0381 **Level 2 hospital emergency department visit provided in a type B emergency department; (the ED must meet at least one of the following requirements: (1) it is licensed by the state in which it is located under applicable state law as an emergency room or emergency department; (2) it is held out to the public (by name, posted signs, advertising, or other means) as a place that provides care for emergency medical conditions on an urgent basis without requiring a previously scheduled appointment; or (3) during the calendar year immediately preceding the calendar year in which a determination under 42 CFR 489.24 is being made, based on a representative sample of patient visits that occurred during that calendar year, it provides at least one-third of all of its outpatient visits for the treatment of emergency medical conditions on an urgent basis without requiring a previously scheduled appointment)** [J]
CMS: 100-04,4,160
AHA: 4Q, '13, 7; 1Q, '09, 1; 4Q, '07, 1

© 2019 Optum360, LLC

G0382 **Level 3 hospital emergency department visit provided in a type B emergency department; (the ED must meet at least one of the following requirements: (1) it is licensed by the state in which it is located under applicable state law as an emergency room or emergency department; (2) it is held out to the public (by name, posted signs, advertising, or other means) as a place that provides care for emergency medical conditions on an urgent basis without requiring a previously scheduled appointment; or (3) during the calendar year immediately preceding the calendar year in which a determination under 42 CFR 489.24 is being made, based on a representative sample of patient visits that occurred during that calendar year, it provides at least one-third of all of its outpatient visits for the treatment of emergency medical conditions on an urgent basis without requiring a previously scheduled appointment)** J

CMS: 100-04,4,160

AHA: 4Q, '13, 7; 1Q, '09, 1; 4Q, '07, 1

G0383 **Level 4 hospital emergency department visit provided in a type B emergency department; (the ED must meet at least one of the following requirements: (1) it is licensed by the state in which it is located under applicable state law as an emergency room or emergency department; (2) it is held out to the public (by name, posted signs, advertising, or other means) as a place that provides care for emergency medical conditions on an urgent basis without requiring a previously scheduled appointment; or (3) during the calendar year immediately preceding the calendar year in which a determination under 42 CFR 489.24 is being made, based on a representative sample of patient visits that occurred during that calendar year, it provides at least one-third of all of its outpatient visits for the treatment of emergency medical conditions on an urgent basis without requiring a previously scheduled appointment)** J

CMS: 100-04,4,160

AHA: 4Q, '13, 7; 1Q, '09, 1; 4Q, '07, 1

G0384 **Level 5 hospital emergency department visit provided in a type B emergency department; (the ED must meet at least one of the following requirements: (1) it is licensed by the state in which it is located under applicable state law as an emergency room or emergency department; (2) it is held out to the public (by name, posted signs, advertising, or other means) as a place that provides care for emergency medical conditions on an urgent basis without requiring a previously scheduled appointment; or (3) during the calendar year immediately preceding the calendar year in which a determination under 42 CFR 489.24 is being made, based on a representative sample of patient visits that occurred during that calendar year, it provides at least one-third of all of its outpatient visits for the treatment of emergency medical conditions on an urgent basis without requiring a previously scheduled appointment)** J

CMS: 100-04,4,160; 100-04,4,290.5.1

AHA: 4Q, '13, 7; 1Q, '09, 1; 4Q, '07, 1

Other Services

G0390 **Trauma response team associated with hospital critical care service** S

CMS: 100-04,4,160.1

Alcohol or Substance Abuse

G0396 **Alcohol and/or substance (other than tobacco) abuse structured assessment (e.g., AUDIT, DAST), and brief intervention 15 to 30 minutes** S ☑ ⊘

CMS: 100-04,12,190.3; 100-04,12,190.6; 100-04,12,190.6.1; 100-04,12,190.7; 100-04,4,200.6

G0397 **Alcohol and/or substance (other than tobacco) abuse structured assessment (e.g., AUDIT, DAST), and intervention, greater than 30 minutes** S ☑ ⊘

CMS: 100-04,12,190.3; 100-04,12,190.6; 100-04,12,190.6.1; 100-04,12,190.7; 100-04,4,200.6

Home Sleep Study

G0398 **Home sleep study test (HST) with type II portable monitor, unattended; minimum of 7 channels: EEG, EOG, EMG, ECG/heart rate, airflow, respiratory effort and oxygen saturation** S

CMS: 100-03,240.4

AHA: 3Q, '08, 5

G0399 **Home sleep test (HST) with type III portable monitor, unattended; minimum of 4 channels: 2 respiratory movement/airflow, 1 ECG/heart rate and 1 oxygen saturation** S

CMS: 100-03,240.4

AHA: 3Q, '08, 5

G0400 **Home sleep test (HST) with type IV portable monitor, unattended; minimum of 3 channels** S

CMS: 100-03,240.4

AHA: 3Q, '08, 5

Initial Physical Exam

G0402 **Initial preventive physical examination; face-to-face visit, services limited to new beneficiary during the first 12 months of Medicare enrollment** V ⊘

CMS: 100-02,13,220; 100-02,13,220.1; 100-02,13,220.3; 100-04,12,100.1.1; 100-04,18,140.6; 100-04,18,80; 100-04,18,80.1; 100-04,18,80.2; 100-04,18,80.3.3; 100-04,18,80.4; 1004-04,13,220.1

AHA: 4Q, '09, 7

G0403 **Electrocardiogram, routine ECG with 12 leads; performed as a screening for the initial preventive physical examination with interpretation and report** M

CMS: 100-04,18,80; 100-04,18,80.1; 100-04,18,80.2

G0404 **Electrocardiogram, routine ECG with 12 leads; tracing only, without interpretation and report, performed as a screening for the initial preventive physical examination** S

CMS: 100-04,18,80; 100-04,18,80.1; 100-04,18,80.2; 100-04,18,80.3.3

G0405 **Electrocardiogram, routine ECG with 12 leads; interpretation and report only, performed as a screening for the initial preventive physical examination** B ⊘

CMS: 100-04,18,80; 100-04,18,80.1; 100-04,18,80.2

Follow-up Telehealth

G0406 **Follow-up inpatient consultation, limited, physicians typically spend 15 minutes communicating with the patient via telehealth** B ⊘

CMS: 100-04,12,190.3; 100-04,12,190.3.1; 100-04,12,190.3.3; 100-04,12,190.3.5; 100-04,12,190.6; 100-04,12,190.6.1; 100-04,12,190.7

G0407 **Follow-up inpatient consultation, intermediate, physicians typically spend 25 minutes communicating with the patient via telehealth** B ⊘

CMS: 100-04,12,190.3; 100-04,12,190.3.1; 100-04,12,190.3.3; 100-04,12,190.3.5; 100-04,12,190.6; 100-04,12,190.6.1; 100-04,12,190.7

G0408 **Follow-up inpatient consultation, complex, physicians typically spend 35 minutes communicating with the patient via telehealth** B ⊘

CMS: 100-04,12,190.3; 100-04,12,190.3.1; 100-04,12,190.3.3; 100-04,12,190.3.5; 100-04,12,190.6; 100-04,12,190.6.1; 100-04,12,190.7

Psychological Services

G0409 **Social work and psychological services, directly relating to and/or furthering the patient's rehabilitation goals, each 15 minutes, face-to-face; individual (services provided by a CORF qualified social worker or psychologist in a CORF)** B ☑

CMS: 100-02,12,30.1; 100-04,5,100.11; 100-04,5,100.4

© 2019 Optum360, LLC

G0410 **Group psychotherapy other than of a multiple-family group, in a partial hospitalization setting, approximately 45 to 50 minutes** P
CMS: 100-04,4,260.1; 100-04,4,260.1.1
AHA: 4Q, '12, 11-14; 4Q, '09, 9

G0411 **Interactive group psychotherapy, in a partial hospitalization setting, approximately 45 to 50 minutes** P
CMS: 100-04,4,260.1; 100-04,4,260.1.1
AHA: 4Q, '12, 11-14; 4Q, '09, 9

Fracture Care

G0412 **Open treatment of iliac spine(s), tuberosity avulsion, or iliac wing fracture(s), unilateral or bilateral for pelvic bone fracture patterns which do not disrupt the pelvic ring, includes internal fixation, when performed** C ⊘

G0413 **Percutaneous skeletal fixation of posterior pelvic bone fracture and/or dislocation, for fracture patterns which disrupt the pelvic ring, unilateral or bilateral, (includes ilium, sacroiliac joint and/or sacrum)** J ⊘

G0414 **Open treatment of anterior pelvic bone fracture and/or dislocation for fracture patterns which disrupt the pelvic ring, unilateral or bilateral, includes internal fixation when performed (includes pubic symphysis and/or superior/inferior rami)** C ⊘

G0415 **Open treatment of posterior pelvic bone fracture and/or dislocation, for fracture patterns which disrupt the pelvic ring, unilateral or bilateral, includes internal fixation, when performed (includes ilium, sacroiliac joint and/or sacrum)** C ⊘

Surgical Pathology

G0416 **Surgical pathology, gross and microscopic examinations, for prostate needle biopsy, any method** ♂ Q2
AHA: 2Q, '13, 6

Educational Services

G0420 **Face-to-face educational services related to the care of chronic kidney disease; individual, per session, per 1 hour** A ☑ ⊘
CMS: 100-02,15,200; 100-02,15,310; 100-02,15,310.1; 100-02,15,310.2; 100-02,15,310.4; 100-02,15,310.5; 100-04,12,190.3; 100-04,12,190.6; 100-04,12,190.6.1; 100-04,12,190.7

G0421 **Face-to-face educational services related to the care of chronic kidney disease; group, per session, per 1 hour** A ☑ ⊘
CMS: 100-02,15,200; 100-02,15,310; 100-02,15,310.1; 100-02,15,310.2; 100-02,15,310.4; 100-02,15,310.5; 100-04,12,190.3; 100-04,12,190.6; 100-04,12,190.6.1; 100-04,12,190.7

Cardiac and Pulmonary Rehabilitation

G0422 **Intensive cardiac rehabilitation; with or without continuous ECG monitoring with exercise, per session** S ☑ ⊘
CMS: 100-02,15,232; 100-04,32,140.2.2.1; 100-04,32,140.2.2.2; 100-04,32,140.3; 100-04,32,140.3.1; 100-08,15,4.2.8

G0423 **Intensive cardiac rehabilitation; with or without continuous ECG monitoring; without exercise, per session** S ☑ ⊘
CMS: 100-02,15,232; 100-04,32,140.2.2.1; 100-04,32,140.2.2.2; 100-04,32,140.3; 100-04,32,140.3.1; 100-08,15,4.2.8

G0424 **Pulmonary rehabilitation, including exercise (includes monitoring), 1 hour, per session, up to two sessions per day** S ☑ ⊘
CMS: 100-02,15,231; 100-04,32,140.4; 100-04,32,140.4.1

Inpatient Telehealth

G0425 **Telehealth consultation, emergency department or initial inpatient, typically 30 minutes communicating with the patient via telehealth** B ☑ ⊘
CMS: 100-04,12,190.3; 100-04,12,190.3.1; 100-04,12,190.3.2; 100-04,12,190.6; 100-04,12,190.6.1; 100-04,12,190.7

G0426 **Telehealth consultation, emergency department or initial inpatient, typically 50 minutes communicating with the patient via telehealth** B ☑ ⊘
CMS: 100-04,12,190.3; 100-04,12,190.3.1; 100-04,12,190.3.2; 100-04,12,190.6; 100-04,12,190.6.1; 100-04,12,190.7

G0427 **Telehealth consultation, emergency department or initial inpatient, typically 70 minutes or more communicating with the patient via telehealth** B ☑ ⊘
CMS: 100-04,12,190.3; 100-04,12,190.3.1; 100-04,12,190.3.2; 100-04,12,190.6; 100-04,12,190.6.1; 100-04,12,190.7

Defect Fillers

G0428 **Collagen meniscus implant procedure for filling meniscal defects (e.g., CMI, collagen scaffold, Menaflex)** E
CMS: 100-03,150.12

G0429 **Dermal filler injection(s) for the treatment of facial lipodystrophy syndrome (LDS) (e.g., as a result of highly active antiretroviral therapy)** T P3
CMS: 100-03,250.5; 100-04,32,260.1; 100-04,32,260.2.1; 100-04,32,260.2.2

Laboratory Services

G0432 **Infectious agent antibody detection by enzyme immunoassay (EIA) technique, HIV-1 and/or HIV-2, screening** A
CMS: 100-03,190.14; 100-03,190.9; 100-03,210.7; 100-04,18,130.1; 100-04,18,130.2; 100-04,18,130.3; 100-04,18,130.4; 100-04,18,130.5

G0433 **Infectious agent antibody detection by enzyme-linked immunosorbent assay (ELISA) technique, HIV-1 and/or HIV-2, screening** A
CMS: 100-03,190.14; 100-03,190.9; 100-03,210.7; 100-04,16,70.8; 100-04,18,130.1; 100-04,18,130.2; 100-04,18,130.3; 100-04,18,130.4; 100-04,18,130.5

G0435 **Infectious agent antibody detection by rapid antibody test, HIV-1 and/or HIV-2, screening** A
CMS: 100-03,190.14; 100-03,190.9; 100-03,210.7; 100-04,18,130.1; 100-04,18,130.2; 100-04,18,130.3; 100-04,18,130.4; 100-04,18,130.5

Counseling and Wellness Visit

G0438 **Annual wellness visit; includes a personalized prevention plan of service (PPS), initial visit** A
CMS: 100-02,13,220; 100-02,13,220.1; 100-02,13,220.3; 100-02,15,280.5; 100-02,15,280.5.1; 100-04,12,100.1.1; 100-04,18,140; 100-04,18,140.1; 100-04,18,140.5; 100-04,18,140.6; 100-04,18,140.8; 100-04,4,200.11; 1004-04,13,220.1

G0439 **Annual wellness visit, includes a personalized prevention plan of service (PPS), subsequent visit** A
CMS: 100-02,13,220; 100-02,13,220.1; 100-02,13,220.3; 100-02,15,280.5; 100-02,15,280.5.1; 100-04,12,100.1.1; 100-04,18,140; 100-04,18,140.1; 100-04,18,140.5; 100-04,18,140.6; 100-04,18,140.8; 100-04,4,200.11; 1004-04,13,220.1

Other Services

G0442 **Annual alcohol misuse screening, 15 minutes** S ☑
CMS: 100-03,210.8; 100-04,12,190.3; 100-04,12,190.6; 100-04,12,190.6.1; 100-04,12,190.7; 100-04,18,180; 100-04,18,180.1; 100-04,18,180.2; 100-04,18,180.3; 100-04,18,180.4; 100-04,18,180.5; 100-04,32,180.4; 100-04,32,180.5

G0443 **Brief face-to-face behavioral counseling for alcohol misuse, 15 minutes** S ☑
CMS: 100-03,210.8; 100-04,12,190.3; 100-04,12,190.6; 100-04,12,190.6.1; 100-04,12,190.7; 100-04,18,180; 100-04,18,180.1; 100-04,18,180.2; 100-04,18,180.3; 100-04,18,180.4; 100-04,18,180.5; 100-04,32,180.4; 100-04,32,180.5

G0444 **Annual depression screening, 15 minutes** S ☑
CMS: 100-04,12,190.3; 100-04,12,190.6; 100-04,12,190.6.1; 100-04,12,190.7; 100-04,18,190; 100-04,18,190.1; 100-04,18,190.2; 100-04,18,190.3

© 2019 Optum360, LLC

G0445 **Semiannual high intensity behavioral counseling to prevent STIs, individual, face-to-face, includes education skills training & guidance on how to change sexual behavior** S ☑
CMS: 100-03,210.10; 100-04,12,190.3; 100-04,12,190.6; 100-04,12,190.6.1; 100-04,12,190.7; 100-04,18,170.1; 100-04,18,170.2; 100-04,18,170.3; 100-04,18,170.4; 100-04,18,170.4.1; 100-04,18,170.5

G0446 **Annual, face-to-face intensive behavioral therapy for cardiovascular disease, individual, 15 minutes** S ☑
CMS: 100-03,210.11; 100-04,12,190.3; 100-04,12,190.6; 100-04,12,190.6.1; 100-04,12,190.7; 100-04,18,160; 100-04,18,160.1; 100-04,18,160.2.1; 100-04,18,160.2.2; 100-04,18,160.3; 100-04,18,160.4; 100-04,18,160.5
AHA: 2Q, '12, 8

G0447 **Face-to-face behavioral counseling for obesity, 15 minutes** S ☑
CMS: 100-03,210.12; 100-04,12,190.3; 100-04,12,190.6; 100-04,12,190.6.1; 100-04,12,190.7; 100-04,18,200; 100-04,18,200.1; 100-04,18,200.2; 100-04,18,200.3; 100-04,18,200.4; 100-04,18,200.5

G0448 **Insertion or replacement of a permanent pacing cardioverter-defibrillator system with transvenous lead(s), single or dual chamber with insertion of pacing electrode, cardiac venous system, for left ventricular pacing** B

G0451 **Development testing, with interpretation and report, per standardized instrument form** 03
CMS: 100-02,15,220.4; 100-04,5,10.3.2; 100-04,5,10.3.3

Molecular Pathology

G0452 **Molecular pathology procedure; physician interpretation and report** B

Neurophysiology Monitoring

G0453 **Continuous intraoperative neurophysiology monitoring, from outside the operating room (remote or nearby), per patient, (attention directed exclusively to one patient) each 15 minutes (list in addition to primary procedure)** N

Documentation and Preparation

G0454 **Physician documentation of face-to-face visit for durable medical equipment determination performed by nurse practitioner, physician assistant or clinical nurse specialist** B

G0455 **Preparation with instillation of fecal microbiota by any method, including assessment of donor specimen** 01
AHA: 3Q, '13, 8

Prostate Brachytherapy

G0458 **Low dose rate (LDR) prostate brachytherapy services, composite rate** ♂ B

Inpatient Telehealth Pharmacologic Management

G0459 **Inpatient telehealth pharmacologic management, including prescription, use, and review of medication with no more than minimal medical psychotherapy** B
CMS: 100-04,12,190.3; 100-04,12,190.6; 100-04,12,190.6.1; 100-04,12,190.7
AHA: 2Q, '13, 9

Other Wound/Ulcer Care

G0460 **Autologous platelet rich plasma for chronic wounds/ulcers, including phlebotomy, centrifugation, and all other preparatory procedures, administration and dressings, per treatment** T
CMS: 100-03,270.3; 100-04,32,11.3.1; 100-04,32,11.3.2; 100-04,32,11.3.3; 100-04,32,11.3.5; 100-04,32,11.3.6

Hospital Outpatient Visit

G0463 **Hospital outpatient clinic visit for assessment and management of a patient** J
CMS: 100-04,4,260.1; 100-04,4,260.1.1; 100-04,4,290.5.1; 100-04,4,290.5.3; 100-04,6,20.1.1.2
AHA: 4Q, '14, 2

Federally Qualified Health Center Visits

G0466 **Federally qualified health center (FQHC) visit, new patient** A

G0467 **Federally qualified health center (FQHC) visit, established patient** A

G0468 **Federally qualified health center (FQHC) visit, initial preventive physical exam (IPPE) or annual wellness visit (AWV)** A

G0469 **Federally qualified health center (FQHC) visit, mental health, new patient** A

G0470 **Federally qualified health center (FQHC) visit, mental health, established patient** A

HHA and SNF Specimen Collection

G0471 **Collection of venous blood by venipuncture or urine sample by catheterization from an individual in a skilled nursing facility (SNF) or by a laboratory on behalf of a home health agency (HHA)** A
CMS: 100-04,16,60.1.4

Hepatitis C Screening

G0472 **Hepatitis C antibody screening for individual at high risk and other covered indication(s)** A
CMS: 100-02,13,220; 100-02,13,220.1; 100-02,13,220.3; 100-03,210.13; 100-04,18,210; 100-04,18,210.2; 100-04,18,210.3; 100-04,18,210.4; 1004-04,13,220.1

Behavioral Counseling

G0473 **Face-to-face behavioral counseling for obesity, group (2-10), 30 minutes** S
CMS: 100-04,18,200.1; 100-04,18,200.2; 100-04,18,200.3; 100-04,18,200.4; 100-04,18,200.5

Screening Measures

G0475 **HIV antigen/antibody, combination assay, screening** A
CMS: 100-03,210.7; 100-04,18,130.1; 100-04,18,130.2; 100-04,18,130.3; 100-04,18,130.5

G0476 **Infectious agent detection by nucleic acid (DNA or RNA); human papillomavirus HPV), high-risk types (e.g., 16, 18, 31, 33, 35, 39, 45, 51, 52, 56, 58, 59, 68) for cervical cancer screening, must be performed in addition to pap test** ♀ A
CMS: 100-03,210.2.1; 100-04,18,30.2.1; 100-04,18,30.5; 100-04,18,30.6

Drug Testing

G0480 **Drug test(s), definitive, utilizing (1) drug identification methods able to identify individual drugs and distinguish between structural isomers (but not necessarily stereoisomers), including, but not limited to, GC/MS (any type, single or tandem) and LC/MS (any type, single or tandem and excluding immunoassays (e.g., IA, EIA, ELISA, EMIT, FPIA) and enzymatic methods (e.g., alcohol dehydrogenase)), (2) stable isotope or other universally recognized internal standards in all samples (e.g., to control for matrix effects, interferences and variations in signal strength), and (3) method or drug-specific calibration and matrix-matched quality control material (e.g., to control for instrument variations and mass spectral drift); qualitative or quantitative, all sources, includes specimen validity testing, per day; 1-7 drug class(es), including metabolite(s) if performed** Q

© 2019 Optum360, LLC

G0481 Drug test(s), definitive, utilizing (1) drug identification methods able to identify individual drugs and distinguish between structural isomers (but not necessarily stereoisomers), including, but not limited to, GC/MS (any type, single or tandem) and LC/MS (any type, single or tandem and excluding immunoassays (e.g., IA, EIA, ELISA, EMIT, FPIA) and enzymatic methods (e.g., alcohol dehydrogenase)), (2) stable isotope or other universally recognized internal standards in all samples (e.g., to control for matrix effects, interferences and variations in signal strength), and (3) method or drug-specific calibration and matrix-matched quality control material (e.g., to control for instrument variations and mass spectral drift); qualitative or quantitative, all sources, includes specimen validity testing, per day; 8-14 drug class(es), including metabolite(s) if performed Q

G0482 Drug test(s), definitive, utilizing (1) drug identification methods able to identify individual drugs and distinguish between structural isomers (but not necessarily stereoisomers), including, but not limited to, GC/MS (any type, single or tandem) and LC/MS (any type, single or tandem and excluding immunoassays (e.g., IA, EIA, ELISA, EMIT, FPIA) and enzymatic methods (e.g., alcohol dehydrogenase)), (2) stable isotope or other universally recognized internal standards in all samples (e.g., to control for matrix effects, interferences and variations in signal strength), and (3) method or drug-specific calibration and matrix-matched quality control material (e.g., to control for instrument variations and mass spectral drift); qualitative or quantitative, all sources, includes specimen validity testing, per day; 15-21 drug class(es), including metabolite(s) if performed Q

G0483 Drug test(s), definitive, utilizing (1) drug identification methods able to identify individual drugs and distinguish between structural isomers (but not necessarily stereoisomers), including, but not limited to, GC/MS (any type, single or tandem) and LC/MS (any type, single or tandem and excluding immunoassays (e.g., IA, EIA, ELISA, EMIT, FPIA) and enzymatic methods (e.g., alcohol dehydrogenase)), (2) stable isotope or other universally recognized internal standards in all samples (e.g., to control for matrix effects, interferences and variations in signal strength), and (3) method or drug-specific calibration and matrix-matched quality control material (e.g., to control for instrument variations and mass spectral drift); qualitative or quantitative, all sources, includes specimen validity testing, per day; 22 or more drug class(es), including metabolite(s) if performed Q

Home Health Nursing Visit

G0490 Face-to-face home health nursing visit by a rural health clinic (RHC) or federally qualified health center (FQHC) in an area with a shortage of home health agencies; (services limited to RN or LPN only) A

Dialysis Procedures

G0491 Dialysis procedure at a Medicare certified ESRD facility for acute kidney injury without ESRD B

G0492 Dialysis procedure with single evaluation by a physician or other qualified health care professional for acute kidney injury without ESRD B

Skilled Nursing Services

G0493 Skilled services of a registered nurse (RN) for the observation and assessment of the patient's condition, each 15 minutes (the change in the patient's condition requires skilled nursing personnel to identify and evaluate the patient's need for possible modification of treatment in the home health or hospice setting) B

G0494 Skilled services of a licensed practical nurse (LPN) for the observation and assessment of the patient's condition, each 15 minutes (the change in the patient's condition requires skilled nursing personnel to identify and evaluate the patient's need for possible modification of treatment in the home health or hospice setting) B

G0495 Skilled services of a registered nurse (RN), in the training and/or education of a patient or family member, in the home health or hospice setting, each 15 minutes B

G0496 Skilled services of a licensed practical nurse (LPN), in the training and/or education of a patient or family member, in the home health or hospice setting, each 15 minutes B

Chemotherapy Infusion

G0498 Chemotherapy administration, intravenous infusion technique; initiation of infusion in the office/clinic setting using office/clinic pump/supplies, with continuation of the infusion in the community setting (e.g., home, domiciliary, rest home or assisted living) using a portable pump provided by the office/clinic, includes follow up office/clinic visit at the conclusion of the infusion S

Hepatitis B Screening

G0499 Hepatitis B screening in nonpregnant, high-risk individual includes hepatitis B surface antigen (HBSAG), antibodies to HBSAG (anti-HBS) and antibodies to hepatitis B core antigen (anti-HBC), and is followed by a neutralizing confirmatory test, when performed, only for an initially reactive HBSAG result A

CMS: 100-03,1,210.6; 100-04,18,230; 100-04,18,230.1; 100-04,18,230.2; 100-04,18,230.3

Moderate Sedation

G0500 Moderate sedation services provided by the same physician or other qualified health care professional performing a gastrointestinal endoscopic service that sedation supports, requiring the presence of an independent trained observer to assist in the monitoring of the patient's level of consciousness and physiological status; initial 15 minutes of intra-service time; patient age 5 years or older (additional time may be reported with 99153, as appropriate) N

CMS: 100-04,18,60.1.1

Mobility-Assistive Technology

G0501 Resource-intensive services for patients for whom the use of specialized mobility-assistive technology (such as adjustable height chairs or tables, patient lift, and adjustable padded leg supports) is medically necessary and used during the provision of an office/outpatient, evaluation and management visit (list separately in addition to primary service) N

Care Management Services

G0506 Comprehensive assessment of and care planning for patients requiring chronic care management services (list separately in addition to primary monthly care management service) N

Telehealth Consultation

G0508 Telehealth consultation, critical care, initial, physicians typically spend 60 minutes communicating with the patient and providers via telehealth B

G0509 Telehealth consultation, critical care, subsequent, physicians typically spend 50 minutes communicating with the patient and providers via telehealth B

© 2019 Optum360, LLC

RHC or FQHC General Care Management

G0511 Rural health clinic or federally qualified health center (RHC or FQHC) only, general care management, 20 minutes or more of clinical staff time for chronic care management services or behavioral health integration services directed by an RHC or FQHC practitioner (physician, NP, PA, or CNM), per calendar month [A]

CMS: 100-02,13,230.2

G0512 Rural health clinic or federally qualified health center (RHC/FQHC) only, psychiatric collaborative care model (psychiatric COCM), 60 minutes or more of clinical staff time for psychiatric COCM services directed by an RHC or FQHC practitioner (physician, NP, PA, or CNM) and including services furnished by a behavioral health care manager and consultation with a psychiatric consultant, per calendar month [A]

CMS: 100-02,13,230.3

Prolonged Services

G0513 Prolonged preventive service(s) (beyond the typical service time of the primary procedure), in the office or other outpatient setting requiring direct patient contact beyond the usual service; first 30 minutes (list separately in addition to code for preventive service) [N]

G0514 Prolonged preventive service(s) (beyond the typical service time of the primary procedure), in the office or other outpatient setting requiring direct patient contact beyond the usual service; each additional 30 minutes (list separately in addition to code G0513 for additional 30 minutes of preventive service) [N]

Cognitive Skills

~~**G0515**~~ Jan ~~Development of cognitive skills to improve attention, memory, problem solving (includes compensatory training), direct (one-on-one) patient contact, each 15 minutes~~

Drug Delivery Implants

G0516 Insertion of nonbiodegradable drug delivery implants, four or more (services for subdermal rod implant) [Q1] [N1]

G0517 Removal of nonbiodegradable drug delivery implants, four or more (services for subdermal implants) [Q1] [N1]

G0518 Removal with reinsertion, nonbiodegradable drug delivery implants, four or more (services for subdermal implants) [Q1] [N1]

Drug Test(s)

G0659 Drug test(s), definitive, utilizing drug identification methods able to identify individual drugs and distinguish between structural isomers (but not necessarily stereoisomers), including but not limited to GC/MS (any type, single or tandem) and LC/MS (any type, single or tandem), excluding immunoassays (e.g., IA, EIA, ELISA, EMIT, FPIA) and enzymatic methods (e.g., alcohol dehydrogenase), performed without method or drug-specific calibration, without matrix-matched quality control material, or without use of stable isotope or other universally recognized internal standard(s) for each drug, drug metabolite or drug class per specimen; qualitative or quantitative, all sources, includes specimen validity testing, per day, any number of drug classes [Q]

Quality Measures

G0913 Improvement in visual function achieved within 90 days following cataract surgery [M]

G0914 Patient care survey was not completed by patient [M]

G0915 Improvement in visual function not achieved within 90 days following cataract surgery [M]

G0916 Satisfaction with care achieved within 90 days following cataract surgery [M]

G0917 Patient satisfaction survey was not completed by patient [M]

G0918 Satisfaction with care not achieved within 90 days following cataract surgery [M]

Clinical Decision Support Mechanism

● **G1000** Jan Clinical Decision Support Mechanism Applied Pathways, as defined by the Medicare Appropriate Use Criteria Program

● **G1001** Jan Clinical Decision Support Mechanism eviCore, as defined by the Medicare Appropriate Use Criteria Program

● **G1002** Jan Clinical Decision Support Mechanism MedCurrent, as defined by the Medicare Appropriate Use Criteria Program

● **G1003** Jan Clinical Decision Support Mechanism Medicalis, as defined by the Medicare Appropriate Use Criteria Program

● **G1004** Jan Clinical Decision Support Mechanism National Decision Support Company, as defined by the Medicare Appropriate Use Criteria Program

● **G1005** Jan Clinical Decision Support Mechanism National Imaging Associates, as defined by the Medicare Appropriate Use Criteria Program

● **G1006** Jan Clinical Decision Support Mechanism Test Appropriate, as defined by the Medicare Appropriate Use Criteria Program

● **G1007** Jan Clinical Decision Support Mechanism AIM Specialty Health, as defined by the Medicare Appropriate Use Criteria Program

● **G1008** Jan Clinical Decision Support Mechanism Cranberry Peak, as defined by the Medicare Appropriate Use Criteria Program

● **G1009** Jan Clinical Decision Support Mechanism Sage Health Management Solutions, as defined by the Medicare Appropriate Use Criteria Program

● **G1010** Jan Clinical Decision Support Mechanism Stanson, as defined by the Medicare Appropriate Use Criteria Program

● **G1011** Jan Clinical Decision Support Mechanism, qualified tool not otherwise specified, as defined by the Medicare Appropriate Use Criteria Program

Convulsive Therapy Procedure

G2000 Blinded administration of convulsive therapy procedure, either electroconvulsive therapy (ECT, current covered gold standard) or magnetic seizure therapy (MST, noncovered experimental therapy), performed in an approved IDE-based clinical trial, per treatment session

Assessments, Evaluations, and CMMI Home Visits

● **G2001** Jan Brief (20 minutes) in-home visit for a new patient postdischarge. For use only in a Medicare-approved CMMI model. (Services must be furnished within a beneficiary's home, domiciliary, rest home, assisted living and/or nursing facility within 90 days following discharge from an inpatient facility and no more than nine times.)

● **G2002** Jan Limited (30 minutes) in-home visit for a new patient postdischarge. For use only in a Medicare-approved CMMI model. (Services must be furnished within a beneficiary's home, domiciliary, rest home, assisted living and/or nursing facility within 90 days following discharge from an inpatient facility and no more than nine times.)

● **G2003** Jan Moderate (45 minutes) in-home visit for a new patient postdischarge. For use only in a Medicare-approved CMMI model. (Services must be furnished within a beneficiary's home, domiciliary, rest home, assisted living and/or nursing facility within 90 days following discharge from an inpatient facility and no more than nine times.)

© 2019 Optum360, LLC

● **G2004**[Jan] Comprehensive (60 minutes) in-home visit for a new patient postdischarge. For use only in a Medicare-approved CMMI model. (Services must be furnished within a beneficiary's home, domiciliary, rest home, assisted living and/or nursing facility within 90 days following discharge from an inpatient facility and no more than nine times.)

● **G2005**[Jan] Extensive (75 minutes) in-home visit for a new patient postdischarge. For use only in a Medicare-approved CMMI model. (Services must be furnished within a beneficiary's home, domiciliary, rest home, assisted living and/or nursing facility within 90 days following discharge from an inpatient facility and no more than nine times.)

● **G2006**[Jan] Brief (20 minutes) in-home visit for an existing patient postdischarge. For use only in a Medicare-approved CMMI model. (Services must be furnished within a beneficiary's home, domiciliary, rest home, assisted living and/or nursing facility within 90 days following discharge from an inpatient facility and no more than nine times.)

● **G2007**[Jan] Limited (30 minutes) in-home visit for an existing patient postdischarge. For use only in a Medicare-approved CMMI model. (Services must be furnished within a beneficiary's home, domiciliary, rest home, assisted living and/or nursing facility within 90 days following discharge from an inpatient facility and no more than nine times.)

● **G2008**[Jan] Moderate (45 minutes) in-home visit for an existing patient postdischarge. For use only in a Medicare-approved CMMI model. (Services must be furnished within a beneficiary's home, domiciliary, rest home, assisted living and/or nursing facility within 90 days following discharge from an inpatient facility and no more than nine times.)

● **G2009**[Jan] Comprehensive (60 minutes) in-home visit for an existing patient postdischarge. For use only in a Medicare-approved CMMI model. (Services must be furnished within a beneficiary's home, domiciliary, rest home, assisted living and/or nursing facility within 90 days following discharge from an inpatient facility and no more than nine times.)

G2010 Remote evaluation of recorded video and/or images submitted by an established patient (e.g., store and forward), including interpretation with follow-up with the patient within 24 business hours, not originating from a related E/M service provided within the previous 7 days nor leading to an E/M service or procedure within the next 24 hours or soonest available appointment

G2011 Alcohol and/or substance (other than tobacco) abuse structured assessment (e.g., audit, DAST), and brief intervention, 5-14 minutes

G2012 Brief communication technology-based service, e.g., virtual check-in, by a physician or other qualified health care professional who can report evaluation and management services, provided to an established patient, not originating from a related E/M service provided within the previous 7 days nor leading to an E/M service or procedure within the next 24 hours or soonest available appointment; 5-10 minutes of medical discussion

● **G2013**[Jan] Extensive (75 minutes) in-home visit for an existing patient postdischarge. For use only in a Medicare-approved CMMI model. (Services must be furnished within a beneficiary's home, domiciliary, rest home, assisted living and/or nursing facility within 90 days following discharge from an inpatient facility and no more than nine times.)

● **G2014**[Jan] Limited (30 minutes) care plan oversight. For use only in a Medicare-approved CMMI model. (Services must be furnished within a beneficiary's home, domiciliary, rest home, assisted living and/or nursing facility within 90 days following discharge from an inpatient facility and no more than nine times.)

● **G2015**[Jan] Comprehensive (60 minutes) home care plan oversight. For use only in a Medicare-approved CMMI model. (Services must be furnished within a beneficiary's home, domiciliary, rest home, assisted living and/or nursing facility within 90 days following discharge from an inpatient facility.)

Treatment in Place

● **G2021**[Jan] Health care practitioners rendering treatment in place (TIP)

● **G2022**[Jan] A model participant (ambulance supplier/provider), the beneficiary refuses services covered under the model (transport to an alternate destination/treatment in place)

Chronic Care Management

● **G2058**[Jan] Chronic care management services, each additional 20 minutes of clinical staff time directed by a physician or other qualified health care professional, per calendar month (list separately in addition to code for primary procedure). (Do not report G2058 for care management services of less than 20 minutes additional to the first 20 minutes of chronic care management services during a calendar month.) (Use G2058 in conjunction with 99490.) (Do not report 99490, G2058 in the same calendar month as 99487, 99489, 99491.)

Qualified Nonphysician Assessment

● **G2061**[Jan] Qualified nonphysician health care professional online assessment, for an established patient, for up to 7 days, cumulative time during the 7 days; 5-10 minutes

● **G2062**[Jan] Qualified nonphysician health care professional online assessment service, for an established patient, for up to 7 days, cumulative time during the 7 days; 11-20 minutes

● **G2063**[Jan] Qualified nonphysician qualified health care professional assessment service, for an established patient, for up to 7 days, cumulative time during the 7 days; 21 or more minutes

Comprehensive Care Management Service

● **G2064**[Jan] Comprehensive care management services for a single high risk disease, e.g., principal care management, at least 30 minutes of physician or other qualified health care professional time per calendar month with the following elements: one complex chronic condition lasting at least 3 months, which is the focus of the care plan, the condition is of sufficient severity to place patient at risk of hospitalization or have been the cause of a recent hospitalization, the condition requires development or revision of disease specific care plan, the condition requires frequent adjustments in the medication regimen, and/or the management of the condition is unusually complex due to comorbidities

● **G2065**[Jan] Comprehensive care management for a single high risk disease services, e.g., principal care management, at least 30 minutes of clinical staff time directed by a physician or other qualified health care professional, per calendar month with the following elements: one complex chronic condition lasting at least 3 months, which is the focus of the care plan, the condition is of sufficient severity to place patient at risk of hospitalization or have been cause of a recent hospitalization, the condition requires development or revision of disease-specific care plan, the condition requires frequent adjustments in the medication regimen, and/or the management of the condition is unusually complex due to comorbidities

Device Evaluation/Interrogation

● **G2066**[Jan] Interrogation device evaluation(s), (remote) up to 30 days; implantable cardiovascular physiologic monitor system, implantable loop recorder system, or subcutaneous cardiac rhythm monitor system, remote data acquisition(s), receipt of transmissions and technician review, technical support and distribution of results

© 2019 Optum360, LLC

Medication Assisted Treatment and Other Services

● **G2067**[Jan] **Medication assisted treatment, methadone; weekly bundle including dispensing and/or administration, substance use counseling, individual and group therapy, and toxicology testing, if performed (provision of the services by a Medicare-enrolled opioid treatment program)**

● **G2068**[Jan] **Medication assisted treatment, buprenorphine (oral); weekly bundle including dispensing and/or administration, substance use counseling, individual and group therapy, and toxicology testing if performed (provision of the services by a Medicare-enrolled opioid treatment program)**

● **G2069**[Jan] **Medication assisted treatment, buprenorphine (injectable); weekly bundle including dispensing and/or administration, substance use counseling, individual and group therapy, and toxicology testing if performed (provision of the services by a Medicare-enrolled opioid treatment program)**

● **G2070**[Jan] **Medication assisted treatment, buprenorphine (implant insertion); weekly bundle including dispensing and/or administration, substance use counseling, individual and group therapy, and toxicology testing if performed (provision of the services by a Medicare-enrolled opioid treatment program)**

● **G2071**[Jan] **Medication assisted treatment, buprenorphine (implant removal); weekly bundle including dispensing and/or administration, substance use counseling, individual and group therapy, and toxicology testing if performed (provision of the services by a Medicare-enrolled opioid treatment program)**

● **G2072**[Jan] **Medication assisted treatment, buprenorphine (implant insertion and removal); weekly bundle including dispensing and/or administration, substance use counseling, individual and group therapy, and toxicology testing if performed (provision of the services by a Medicare-enrolled opioid treatment program)**

● **G2073**[Jan] **Medication assisted treatment, naltrexone; weekly bundle including dispensing and/or administration, substance use counseling, individual and group therapy, and toxicology testing if performed (provision of the services by a Medicare-enrolled opioid treatment program)**

● **G2074**[Jan] **Medication assisted treatment, weekly bundle not including the drug, including substance use counseling, individual and group therapy, and toxicology testing if performed (provision of the services by a Medicare-enrolled opioid treatment program)**

● **G2075**[Jan] **Medication assisted treatment, medication not otherwise specified; weekly bundle including dispensing and/or administration, substance use counseling, individual and group therapy, and toxicology testing, if performed (provision of the services by a Medicare-enrolled opioid treatment program)**

● **G2076**[Jan] **Intake activities, including initial medical examination that is a complete, fully documented physical evaluation and initial assessment by a program physician or a primary care physician, or an authorized health care professional under the supervision of a program physician qualified personnel that includes preparation of a treatment plan that includes the patient's short-term goals and the tasks the patient must perform to complete the short-term goals; the patient's requirements for education, vocational rehabilitation, and employment; and the medical, psycho-social, economic, legal, or other supportive services that a patient needs, conducted by qualified personnel (provision of the services by a Medicare-enrolled opioid treatment program); list separately in addition to code for primary procedure**

● **G2077**[Jan] **Periodic assessment; assessing periodically by qualified personnel to determine the most appropriate combination of services and treatment (provision of the services by a Medicare-enrolled opioid treatment program); list separately in addition to code for primary procedure**

● **G2078**[Jan] **Take home supply of methadone; up to 7 additional day supply (provision of the services by a Medicare-enrolled opioid treatment program); list separately in addition to code for primary procedure**

● **G2079**[Jan] **Take home supply of buprenorphine (oral); up to 7 additional day supply (provision of the services by a Medicare-enrolled opioid treatment program); list separately in addition to code for primary procedure**

● **G2080**[Jan] **Each additional 30 minutes of counseling in a week of medication assisted treatment, (provision of the services by a Medicare-enrolled opioid treatment program); list separately in addition to code for primary procedure**

● **G2081**[Jan] **Patients age 66 and older in institutional special needs plans (SNP) or residing in long-term care with a POS code 32, 33, 34, 54 or 56 for more than 90 days during the measurement period**

● **G2082**[Jan] **Office or other outpatient visit for the evaluation and management of an established patient that requires the supervision of a physician or other qualified health care professional and provision of up to 56 mg of esketamine nasal self administration, includes 2 hours post administration observation**

● **G2083**[Jan] **Office or other outpatient visit for the evaluation and management of an established patient that requires the supervision of a physician or other qualified health care professional and provision of greater than 56 mg esketamine nasal self administration, includes 2 hours post administration observation**

● **G2086**[Jan] **Office-based treatment for opioid use disorder, including development of the treatment plan, care coordination, individual therapy and group therapy and counseling; at least 70 minutes in the first calendar month**

● **G2087**[Jan] **Office-based treatment for opioid use disorder, including care coordination, individual therapy and group therapy and counseling; at least 60 minutes in a subsequent calendar month**

● **G2088**[Jan] **Office-based treatment for opioid use disorder, including care coordination, individual therapy and group therapy and counseling; each additional 30 minutes beyond the first 120 minutes (list separately in addition to code for primary procedure)**

● **G2089**[Jan] **Most recent hemoglobin A1c (HbA1c) level 7.0% to 9.0%**

● **G2090**[Jan] **Patients 66 years of age and older with at least one claim/encounter for frailty during the measurement period and a dispensed medication for dementia during the measurement period or the year prior to the measurement period**

● **G2091**[Jan] **Patients 66 years of age and older with at least one claim/encounter for frailty during the measurement period and either one acute inpatient encounter with a diagnosis of advanced illness or two outpatient, observation, ED or nonacute inpatient encounters on different dates of service with an advanced illness diagnosis during the measurement period or the year prior to the measurement period**

● **G2092**[Jan] **Angiotensin converting enzyme (ACE) inhibitor or angiotensin receptor blocker (ARB) or angiotensin receptor-neprilysin inhibitor (ARNI) therapy prescribed or currently being taken**

● **G2093**[Jan] **Documentation of medical reason(s) for not prescribing ACE inhibitor or ARB or ARNI therapy (e.g., hypotensive patients who are at immediate risk of cardiogenic shock, hospitalized patients who have experienced marked azotemia, allergy, intolerance, other medical reasons)**

● **G2094**[Jan] **Documentation of patient reason(s) for not prescribing ACE inhibitor or ARB or ARNI therapy (e.g., patient declined, other patient reasons)**

© 2019 Optum360, LLC

● **G2095**[Jan] Documentation of system reason(s) for not prescribing ACE inhibitor or ARB or ARNI therapy (e.g., other system reasons)

● **G2096**[Jan] Angiotensin converting enzyme (ACE) inhibitor or angiotensin receptor blocker (ARB) or angiotensin receptor-neprilysin inhibitor (ARNI) therapy was not prescribed, reason not given

● **G2097**[Jan] Children with a competing diagnosis for upper respiratory infection within 3 days of diagnosis of pharyngitis (e.g., intestinal infection, pertussis, bacterial infection, Lyme disease, otitis media, acute sinusitis, acute pharyngitis, acute tonsillitis, chronic sinusitis, infection of the pharynx/larynx/tonsils/adenoids, prostatitis, cellulitis, mastoiditis, or bone infections, acute lymphadenitis, impetigo, skin staph infections, pneumonia/gonococcal infections, venereal disease (syphilis, chlamydia, inflammatory diseases [female reproductive organs]), infections of the kidney, cystitis or UTI

● **G2098**[Jan] Patients 66 years of age and older with at least one claim/encounter for frailty during the measurement period and a dispensed medication for dementia during the measurement period or the year prior to the measurement period

● **G2099**[Jan] Patients 66 years of age and older with at least one claim/encounter for frailty during the measurement period and either one acute inpatient encounter with a diagnosis of advanced illness or two outpatient, observation, ED or nonacute inpatient encounters on different dates of service with an advanced illness diagnosis during the measurement period or the year prior to the measurement period

● **G2100**[Jan] Patients 66 years of age and older with at least one claim/encounter for frailty during the measurement period and a dispensed medication for dementia during the measurement period or the year prior to the measurement period

● **G2101**[Jan] Patients 66 years of age and older with at least one claim/encounter for frailty during the measurement period and either one acute inpatient encounter with a diagnosis of advanced illness or two outpatient, observation, ED or nonacute inpatient encounters on different dates of service with an advanced illness diagnosis during the measurement period or the year prior to the measurement period

● **G2102**[Jan] Dilated retinal eye exam with interpretation by an ophthalmologist or optometrist documented and reviewed

● **G2103**[Jan] Seven standard field stereoscopic photos with interpretation by an ophthalmologist or optometrist documented and reviewed

● **G2104**[Jan] Eye imaging validated to match diagnosis from seven standard field stereoscopic photos results documented and reviewed

● **G2105**[Jan] Patients age 66 or older in institutional special needs plans (SNP) or residing in long-term care with POS code 32, 33, 34, 54 or 56 for more than 90 days during the measurement period

● **G2106**[Jan] Patients 66 years of age and older with at least one claim/encounter for frailty during the measurement period and a dispensed medication for dementia during the measurement period or the year prior to the measurement period

● **G2107**[Jan] Patients 66 years of age and older with at least one claim/encounter for frailty during the measurement period and either one acute inpatient encounter with a diagnosis of advanced illness or two outpatient, observation, ED or nonacute inpatient encounters on different dates of service with an advanced illness diagnosis during the measurement period or the year prior to the measurement period

● **G2108**[Jan] Patients age 66 or older in institutional special needs plans (SNP) or residing in long-term care with POS code 32, 33, 34, 54 or 56 for more than 90 days during the measurement period

● **G2109**[Jan] Patients 66 years of age and older with at least one claim/encounter for frailty during the measurement period and a dispensed medication for dementia during the measurement period or the year prior to the measurement period

● **G2110**[Jan] Patients 66 years of age and older with at least one claim/encounter for frailty during the measurement period and either one acute inpatient encounter with a diagnosis of advanced illness or two outpatient, observation, ED or nonacute inpatient encounters on different dates of service with an advanced illness diagnosis during the measurement period or the year prior to the measurement period

● **G2112**[Jan] Patient receiving <=5 mg daily prednisone (or equivalent), or RA activity is worsening, or glucocorticoid use is for less than 6 months

● **G2113**[Jan] Patient receiving >5 mg daily prednisone (or equivalent) for longer than 6 months, and improvement or no change in disease activity

● **G2114**[Jan] Patients 66-80 years of age with at least one claim/encounter for frailty during the measurement period and a dispensed medication for dementia during the measurement period or the year prior to the measurement period

● **G2115**[Jan] Patients 66 years of age and older with at least one claim/encounter for frailty during the measurement period and a dispensed medication for dementia during the measurement period or the year prior to the measurement period

● **G2116**[Jan] Patients 66 years of age and older with at least one claim/encounter for frailty during the measurement period and either one acute inpatient encounter with a diagnosis of advanced illness or two outpatient, observation, ED or nonacute inpatient encounters on different dates of service with an advanced illness diagnosis during the measurement period or the year prior to the measurement period

● **G2117**[Jan] Patients 66-80 years of age with at least one claim/encounter for frailty during the measurement period and either one acute inpatient encounter with a diagnosis of advanced illness or two outpatient, observation, ED or nonacute inpatient encounters on different dates of service with an advanced illness diagnosis during the measurement period or the year prior to the measurement period

● **G2118**[Jan] Patients 81 years of age and older with evidence of frailty during the measurement period

● **G2119**[Jan] Within the past 2 years, calcium and/or vitamin D optimization has been ordered or performed

● **G2120**[Jan] Within the past 2 years, calcium and/or vitamin D optimization has not been ordered or performed

● **G2121**[Jan] Psychosis, depression, anxiety, apathy, and impulse control disorder assessed

● **G2122**[Jan] Psychosis, depression, anxiety, apathy, and impulse control disorder not assessed

● **G2123**[Jan] Patients 66-80 years of age and had at least one claim/encounter for frailty during the measurement period and either one acute inpatient encounter with a diagnosis of advanced illness or two outpatient, observation, ED or nonacute inpatient encounters on different dates of service with an advanced illness diagnosis during the measurement period or the year prior to the measurement period

● **G2124**[Jan] Patients 66-80 years of age and had at least one claim/encounter for frailty during the measurement period and a dispensed dementia medication

● **G2125**[Jan] Patients 81 years of age and older with evidence of frailty during the measurement period

© 2019 Optum360, LLC

● **G2126**[Jan] Patients 66 years of age or older and had at least one claim/encounter for frailty during the measurement period and either one acute inpatient encounter with a diagnosis of advanced illness or two outpatient, observation, ED or nonacute inpatient encounters on different dates of service with an advanced illness diagnosis during the measurement period or the year prior to the measurement period

● **G2127**[Jan] Patients 66 years of age or older and had at least one claim/encounter for frailty during the measurement period and a dispensed dementia medication

● **G2128**[Jan] Documentation of medical reason(s) for not on a daily aspirin or other antiplatelet (e.g., history of gastrointestinal bleed, intracranial bleed, blood disorders, idiopathic thrombocytopenic purpura (ITP), gastric bypass or documentation of active anticoagulant use during the measurement period)

● **G2129**[Jan] Procedure related BP's not taken during an outpatient visit. Examples include same day surgery, ambulatory service center, GI, lab, dialysis, infusion center, chemotherapy

● **G2130**[Jan] Patients age 66 or older in institutional special needs plans (SNP) or residing in long-term care with POS code 32, 33, 34, 54 or 56 for more than 90 days during the measurement period

● **G2131**[Jan] Patients 81 years and older with a diagnosis of frailty

● **G2132**[Jan] Patients 66-80 years of age with at least one claim/encounter for frailty during the measurement period and a dispensed medication for dementia during the measurement period or the year prior to the measurement period

● **G2133**[Jan] Patients 66-80 years of age with at least one claim/encounter for frailty during the measurement period and either one acute inpatient encounter with a diagnosis of advanced illness or two outpatient, observation, ED or nonacute inpatient encounters on different dates of service with an advanced illness diagnosis during the measurement period or the year prior to the measurement period

● **G2134**[Jan] Patients 66 years of age or older with at least one claim/encounter for frailty during the measurement period and a dispensed medication for dementia during the measurement period or the year prior to the measurement period

● **G2135**[Jan] Patients 66 years of age or older with at least one claim/encounter for frailty during the measurement period and either one acute inpatient encounter with a diagnosis of advanced illness or two outpatient, observation, ED or nonacute inpatient encounters on different dates of service with an advanced illness diagnosis during the measurement period or the year prior to the measurement period

● **G2136**[Jan] Back pain measured by the visual analog scale (VAS) at 3 months (6 to 20 weeks) postoperatively was less than or equal to 3.0 or back pain measured by the visual analog scale (VAS) within 3 months preoperatively and at 3 months (6 to 20 weeks) postoperatively demonstrated an improvement of 5.0 points or greater

● **G2137**[Jan] Back pain measured by the visual analog scale (VAS) at 3 months (6 to 20 weeks) postoperatively was greater than 3.0 and back pain measured by the visual analog scale (VAS) within 3 months preoperatively and at 3 months (6 to 20 weeks) postoperatively demonstrated a change of less than an improvement of 5.0 points

● **G2138**[Jan] Back pain as measured by the visual analog scale (VAS) at 1 year (9 to 15 months) postoperatively was less than or equal to 3.0 or back pain measured by the visual analog scale (VAS) within 3 months preoperatively and at 1 year (9 to 15 months) postoperatively demonstrated a change of 5.0 points or greater

● **G2139**[Jan] Back pain measured by the visual analog scale (VAS) pain at 1 year (9 to 15 months) postoperatively was greater than 3.0 and back pain measured by the visual analog scale (VAS) within 3 months preoperatively and at 1 year (9 to 15 months) postoperatively demonstrated a change of less than 5.0

● **G2140**[Jan] Leg pain measured by the visual analog scale (VAS) at 3 months (6 to 20 weeks) postoperatively was less than or equal to 3.0 or leg pain measured by the visual analog scale (VAS) within 3 months preoperatively and at 3 months (6 to 20 weeks) postoperatively demonstrated an improvement of 5.0 points or greater

● **G2141**[Jan] Leg pain measured by the visual analog scale (VAS) at 3 months (6 to 20 weeks) postoperatively was greater than 3.0 and leg pain measured by the visual analog scale (VAS) within 3 months preoperatively and at 3 months (6 to 20 weeks) postoperatively demonstrated less than an improvement of 5.0 points

● **G2142**[Jan] Functional status measured by the Oswestry Disability Index (ODI version 2.1a) at 1 year (9 to 15 months) postoperatively was less than or equal to 22 or functional status measured by the ODI version 2.1a within 3 months preoperatively and at 1 year (9 to 15 months) postoperatively demonstrated a change of 30 points or greater

● **G2143**[Jan] Functional status measured by the Oswestry Disability Index (ODI version 2.1a) at 1 year (9 to 15 months) postoperatively was greater than 22 and functional status measured by the ODI version 2.1a within 3 months preoperatively and at 1 year (9 to 15 months) postoperatively demonstrated a change of less than 30 points

● **G2144**[Jan] Functional status measured by the Oswestry Disability Index (ODI version 2.1a) at 3 months (6 to 20 weeks) postoperatively was less than or equal to 22 or functional status measured by the ODI version 2.1a within 3 months preoperatively and at 3 months (6 to 20 weeks) postoperatively demonstrated a change of 30 points or greater

● **G2145**[Jan] Functional status measured by the Oswestry Disability Index (ODI version 2.1a) at 3 months (6 to 20 weeks) postoperatively was greater than 22 and functional status measured by the ODI version 2.1a within 3 months preoperatively and at 3 months (6 to 20 weeks) postoperatively demonstrated a change of less than 30 points

● **G2146**[Jan] Leg pain as measured by the visual analog scale (VAS) at 1 year (9 to 15 months) postoperatively was less than or equal to 3.0 or leg pain measured by the visual analog scale (VAS) within 3 months preoperatively and at 1 year (9 to 15 months) postoperatively demonstrated an improvement of 5.0 points or greater

● **G2147**[Jan] Leg pain measured by the visual analog scale (VAS) at 1 year (9 to 15 months) postoperatively was greater than 3.0 and leg pain measured by the visual analog scale (VAS) within 3 months preoperatively and at 1 year (9 to 15 months) postoperatively demonstrated less than an improvement of 5.0 points

● **G2148**[Jan] Performance met: multimodal pain management was used

● **G2149**[Jan] Documentation of medical reason(s) for not using multimodal pain management (e.g., allergy to multiple classes of analgesics, intubated patient, hepatic failure, patient reports no pain during PACU stay, other medical reason(s))

● **G2150**[Jan] Performance not met: multimodal pain management was not used

● **G2151**[Jan] Patients with diagnosis of a degenerative neurological condition such as ALS, MS, Parkinson's diagnosed at any time before or during the episode of care

● **G2152**[Jan] Performance met: the residual change score is equal to or greater than 0

© 2019 Optum360, LLC

● G2153 Jan In hospice or using hospice services during the measurement period

● G2154 Jan Patient received at least one Td vaccine or one Tdap vaccine between nine years prior to the start of the measurement period and the end of the measurement period

● G2155 Jan Patient had history of at least one of the following contraindications any time during or before the measurement period: anaphylaxis due to Tdap vaccine, anaphylaxis due to Td vaccine or its components; encephalopathy due to Tdap or Td vaccination (post tetanus vaccination encephalitis, post diphtheria vaccination encephalitis or post pertussis vaccination encephalitis)

● G2156 Jan Patient did not receive at least one Td vaccine or one Tdap vaccine between nine years prior to the start of the measurement period and the end of the measurement period; or have history of at least one of the following contraindications any time during or before the measurement period: anaphylaxis due to Tdap vaccine, anaphylaxis due to Td vaccine or its components; encephalopathy due to Tdap or Td vaccination (post tetanus vaccination encephalitis, post diphtheria vaccination encephalitis or post pertussis vaccination encephalitis)

● G2157 Jan Patients received both the 13-valent pneumococcal conjugate vaccine and the 23-valent pneumococcal polysaccharide vaccine at least 12 months apart, with the first occurrence after the age of 60 before or during the measurement period

● G2158 Jan Patient had prior pneumococcal vaccine adverse reaction any time during or before the measurement period

● G2159 Jan Patient did not receive both the 13-valent pneumococcal conjugate vaccine and the 23-valent pneumococcal polysaccharide vaccine at least 12 months apart, with the first occurrence after the age of 60 before or during measurement period; or have prior pneumococcal vaccine adverse reaction any time during or before the measurement period

● G2160 Jan Patient received at least one dose of the herpes zoster live vaccine or two doses of the herpes zoster recombinant vaccine (at least 28 days apart) anytime on or after the patient's 50th birthday before or during the measurement period

● G2161 Jan Patient had prior adverse reaction caused by zoster vaccine or its components any time during or before the measurement period

● G2162 Jan Patient did not receive at least one dose of the herpes zoster live vaccine or two doses of the herpes zoster recombinant vaccine (at least 28 days apart) anytime on or after the patient's 50th birthday before or during the measurement period; or have prior adverse reaction caused by zoster vaccine or its components any time during or before the measurement period

● G2163 Jan Patient received an influenza vaccine on or between July 1 of the year prior to the measurement period and June 30 of the measurement period

● G2164 Jan Patient had a prior influenza virus vaccine adverse reaction any time before or during the measurement period

● G2165 Jan Patient did not receive an influenza vaccine on or between July 1 of the year prior to the measurement period and June 30 of the measurement period; or did not have a prior influenza virus vaccine adverse reaction any time before or during the measurement period

● G2166 Jan Patient refused to participate at admission and/or discharge; patient unable to complete the neck FS PROM at admission or discharge due to cognitive deficit, visual deficit, motor deficit, language barrier, or low reading level, and a suitable proxy/recorder is not available; patient self discharged early; medical reason

● G2167 Jan Performance not met: the residual change score is less than 0

Radiation Therapy

G6001 Ultrasonic guidance for placement of radiation therapy fields B

G6002 Stereoscopic x-ray guidance for localization of target volume for the delivery of radiation therapy B

G6003 Radiation treatment delivery, single treatment area, single port or parallel opposed ports, simple blocks or no blocks: up to 5 mev B

G6004 Radiation treatment delivery, single treatment area, single port or parallel opposed ports, simple blocks or no blocks: 6-10 mev B

G6005 Radiation treatment delivery, single treatment area, single port or parallel opposed ports, simple blocks or no blocks: 11-19 mev B

G6006 Radiation treatment delivery, single treatment area, single port or parallel opposed ports, simple blocks or no blocks: 20 mev or greater B

G6007 Radiation treatment delivery, two separate treatment areas, three or more ports on a single treatment area, use of multiple blocks: up to 5 mev B

G6008 Radiation treatment delivery, two separate treatment areas, three or more ports on a single treatment area, use of multiple blocks: 6-10 mev B

G6009 Radiation treatment delivery, two separate treatment areas, three or more ports on a single treatment area, use of multiple blocks: 11-19 mev B

G6010 Radiation treatment delivery, two separate treatment areas, three or more ports on a single treatment area, use of multiple blocks: 20 mev or greater B

G6011 Radiation treatment delivery, three or more separate treatment areas, custom blocking, tangential ports, wedges, rotational beam, compensators, electron beam; up to 5 mev B

G6012 Radiation treatment delivery, three or more separate treatment areas, custom blocking, tangential ports, wedges, rotational beam, compensators, electron beam; 6-10 mev B

G6013 Radiation treatment delivery, three or more separate treatment areas, custom blocking, tangential ports, wedges, rotational beam, compensators, electron beam; 11-19 mev B

G6014 Radiation treatment delivery, three or more separate treatment areas, custom blocking, tangential ports, wedges, rotational beam, compensators, electron beam; 20 mev or greater B

G6015 Intensity modulated treatment delivery, single or multiple fields/arcs,via narrow spatially and temporally modulated beams, binary, dynamic MLC, per treatment session B

G6016 Compensator-based beam modulation treatment delivery of inverse planned treatment using three or more high resolution (milled or cast) compensator, convergent beam modulated fields, per treatment session B

G6017 Intra-fraction localization and tracking of target or patient motion during delivery of radiation therapy (e.g., 3D positional tracking, gating, 3D surface tracking), each fraction of treatment B

Quality Measures

G8395 Left ventricular ejection fraction (LVEF) ≥ 40% or documentation as normal or mildly depressed left ventricular systolic function M

G8396 Left ventricular ejection fraction (LVEF) not performed or documented M

© 2019 Optum360, LLC

G8397 Dilated macular or fundus exam performed, including documentation of the presence or absence of macular edema and level of severity of retinopathy M

G8398 Dilated macular or fundus exam not performed M

G8399 Patient with documented results of a central dual-energy x-ray absorptiometry (DXA) ever being performed M

G8400 Patient with central dual-energy x-ray absorptiometry (DXA) results not documented, reason not given M

G8404 Lower extremity neurological exam performed and documented M

G8405 Lower extremity neurological exam not performed M

G8410 Footwear evaluation performed and documented M

G8415 Footwear evaluation was not performed M

G8416 Clinician documented that patient was not an eligible candidate for footwear evaluation measure M

G8417 BMI is documented above normal parameters and a follow-up plan is documented M

G8418 BMI is documented below normal parameters and a follow-up plan is documented M

G8419 BMI documented outside normal parameters, no follow-up plan documented, no reason given M

G8420 BMI is documented within normal parameters and no follow-up plan is required M

G8421 BMI not documented and no reason is given M

G8422 BMI not documented, documentation the patient is not eligible for BMI calculation M

G8427 Eligible clinician attests to documenting in the medical record they obtained, updated, or reviewed the patient's current medications M

G8428 Current list of medications not documented as obtained, updated, or reviewed by the eligible clinician, reason not given M

G8430 Eligible clinician attests to documenting in the medical record the patient is not eligible for a current list of medications being obtained, updated, or reviewed by the eligible clinician M

G8431 Screening for depression is documented as being positive and a follow-up plan is documented M

G8432 Depression screening not documented, reason not given M

G8433 Screening for depression not completed, documented reason M

G8442 Pain assessment not documented as being performed, documentation the patient is not eligible for a pain assessment using a standardized tool at the time of the encounter M

G8450 Beta-blocker therapy prescribed M

G8451 Beta-blocker therapy for LVEF < 40% not prescribed for reasons documented by the clinician (e.g., low blood pressure, fluid overload, asthma, patients recently treated with an intravenous positive inotropic agent, allergy, intolerance, other medical reasons, patient declined, other patient reasons, or other reasons attributable to the health care system) M

G8452 Beta-blocker therapy not prescribed M

G8465 High or very high risk of recurrence of prostate cancer M

G8473 Angiotensin converting enzyme (ACE) inhibitor or angiotensin receptor blocker (ARB) therapy prescribed M

G8474 Angiotensin converting enzyme (ACE) inhibitor or angiotensin receptor blocker (ARB) therapy not prescribed for reasons documented by the clinician (e.g., allergy, intolerance, pregnancy, renal failure due to ACE inhibitor, diseases of the aortic or mitral valve, other medical reasons) or (e.g., patient declined, other patient reasons) or (e.g., lack of drug availability, other reasons attributable to the health care system) M

G8475 Angiotensin converting enzyme (ACE) inhibitor or angiotensin receptor blocker (ARB) therapy not prescribed, reason not given M

G8476 Most recent blood pressure has a systolic measurement of < 140 mm Hg and a diastolic measurement of < 90 mm Hg M

G8477 Most recent blood pressure has a systolic measurement of >=140 mm Hg and/or a diastolic measurement of >=90 mm Hg M

G8478 Blood pressure measurement not performed or documented, reason not given M

G8482 Influenza immunization administered or previously received M

G8483 Influenza immunization was not administered for reasons documented by clinician (e.g., patient allergy or other medical reasons, patient declined or other patient reasons, vaccine not available or other system reasons) M

G8484 Influenza immunization was not administered, reason not given M

G8506 Patient receiving angiotensin converting enzyme (ACE) inhibitor or angiotensin receptor blocker (ARB) therapy M

G8509 Pain assessment documented as positive using a standardized tool, follow-up plan not documented, reason not given M

G8510 Screening for depression is documented as negative, a follow-up plan is not required M

G8511 Screening for depression documented as positive, follow-up plan not documented, reason not given M

G8535 Elder maltreatment screen not documented; documentation that patient is not eligible for the elder maltreatment screen at the time of the encounter M

G8536 No documentation of an elder maltreatment screen, reason not given M

G8539 Functional outcome assessment documented as positive using a standardized tool and a care plan based on identified deficiencies on the date of functional outcome assessment, is documented M

G8540 Functional outcome assessment not documented as being performed, documentation the patient is not eligible for a functional outcome assessment using a standardized tool at the time of the encounter M

G8541 Functional outcome assessment using a standardized tool, not documented, reason not given M

G8542 Functional outcome assessment using a standardized tool is documented; no functional deficiencies identified, care plan not required M

G8543 Documentation of a positive functional outcome assessment using a standardized tool; care plan not documented, reason not given M

G8559 Patient referred to a physician (preferably a physician with training in disorders of the ear) for an otologic evaluation M

G8560 Patient has a history of active drainage from the ear within the previous 90 days M

G8561 Patient is not eligible for the referral for otologic evaluation for patients with a history of active drainage measure M

© 2019 Optum360, LLC

G8562 Patient does not have a history of active drainage from the ear within the previous 90 days M

G8563 Patient not referred to a physician (preferably a physician with training in disorders of the ear) for an otologic evaluation, reason not given M

G8564 Patient was referred to a physician (preferably a physician with training in disorders of the ear) for an otologic evaluation, reason not specified) M

G8565 Verification and documentation of sudden or rapidly progressive hearing loss M

G8566 Patient is not eligible for the "referral for otologic evaluation for sudden or rapidly progressive hearing loss" measure M

G8567 Patient does not have verification and documentation of sudden or rapidly progressive hearing loss M

G8568 Patient was not referred to a physician (preferably a physician with training in disorders of the ear) for an otologic evaluation, reason not given M

G8569 Prolonged postoperative intubation (> 24 hrs) required M

G8570 Prolonged postoperative intubation (> 24 hrs) not required M

G8571 Development of deep sternal wound infection/mediastinitis within 30 days postoperatively M

G8572 No deep sternal wound infection/mediastinitis M

G8573 Stroke following isolated CABG surgery M

G8574 No stroke following isolated CABG surgery M

G8575 Developed postoperative renal failure or required dialysis M

G8576 No postoperative renal failure/dialysis not required M

G8577 Re-exploration required due to mediastinal bleeding with or without tamponade, graft occlusion, valve dysfunction or other cardiac reason M

G8578 Re-exploration not required due to mediastinal bleeding with or without tamponade, graft occlusion, valve dysfunction or other cardiac reason M

G8598 Aspirin or another antiplatelet therapy used M

G8599 Aspirin or another antiplatelet therapy not used, reason not given M

G8600 IV tPA initiated within 3 hours (≤ 180 minutes) of time last known well M

G8601 IV tPA not initiated within 3 hours (≤ 180 minutes) of time last known well for reasons documented by clinician M

G8602 IV tPA not initiated within 3 hours (≤ 180 minutes) of time last known well, reason not given M

G8627 Surgical procedure performed within 30 days following cataract surgery for major complications (e.g., retained nuclear fragments, endophthalmitis, dislocated or wrong power iol, retinal detachment, or wound dehiscence) M

G8628 Surgical procedure not performed within 30 days following cataract surgery for major complications (e.g., retained nuclear fragments, endophthalmitis, dislocated or wrong power iol, retinal detachment, or wound dehiscence) M

G8633 Pharmacologic therapy (other than minerals/vitamins) for osteoporosis prescribed M

G8635 Pharmacologic therapy for osteoporosis was not prescribed, reason not given M

G8647 Risk-adjusted functional status change residual score for the knee impairment successfully calculated and the score was equal to zero (0) or greater than zero (> 0) M ☑

G8648 Risk-adjusted functional status change residual score for the knee impairment successfully calculated and the score was less than zero (< 0) M ☑

~~**G8649**~~ Jan ~~Risk-adjusted functional status change residual score for the knee impairment not measured because the patient did not complete the FS status survey near discharge, patient not appropriate~~

▲ **G8650** Jan Risk adjusted functional status change residual score for the knee impairment not measured because the patient did not complete the knee FS PROM at initial evaluation and/or near discharge, reason not given M

G8651 Risk-adjusted functional status change residual score for the hip impairment successfully calculated and the score was equal to zero (0) or greater than zero (> 0) M ☑

G8652 Risk-adjusted functional status change residual score for the hip impairment successfully calculated and the score was less than zero (< 0) M ☑

~~**G8653**~~ Jan ~~Risk-adjusted functional status change residual scores for the hip impairment not measured because the patient did not complete the FS status survey near discharge, patient not appropriate~~

G8654 Risk-adjusted functional status change residual score for the hip impairment not measured because the patient did not complete the FS intake survey on admission and/or follow up FS status survey near discharge, reason not given M

G8655 Risk-adjusted functional status change residual score for the foot or ankle successfully calculated and the score was equal to zero (0) or greater than zero (> 0) M ☑

G8656 Risk-adjusted functional status change residual score for the lower leg, foot or ankle impairment successfully calculated and the score was less than zero (< 0) M ☑

~~**G8657**~~ Jan ~~Risk-adjusted functional status change residual score for the lower leg, foot or ankle impairment not measured because the patient did not complete the FS status survey near discharge, patient not appropriate~~

G8658 Risk-adjusted functional status change residual score for the lower leg, foot or ankle impairment not measured because the patient did not complete the FS intake survey on admission and/or follow up FS status survey near discharge, reason not given M

G8659 Risk-adjusted functional status change residual score for the low back impairment successfully calculated and the score was equal to zero (0) or greater than zero (> 0) M ☑

G8660 Risk-adjusted functional status change residual score for the low back impairment successfully calculated and the score was less than zero (< 0) M ☑

G8661 Risk-adjusted functional status change residual score for the low back impairment not measured because the patient did not complete the FS status survey near discharge, patient not appropriate M

▲ **G8662** Jan Risk- adjusted functional status change residual score for the low back impairment not measured because the patient did not complete the low back FS PROM at initial evaluation and/or near discharge, reason not given M

G8663 Risk-adjusted functional status change residual score for the shoulder impairment successfully calculated and the score was equal to zero (0) or greater than zero (> 0) M ☑

G8664 Risk-adjusted functional status change residual score for the shoulder impairment successfully calculated and the score was less than zero (< 0) M ☑

© 2019 Optum360, LLC

~~G8665 Jan Risk-adjusted functional status change residual score for the shoulder impairment not measured because the patient did not complete the FS status survey near discharge, patient not appropriate~~

▲ G8666 Jan Risk adjusted functional status change residual score for the shoulder impairment not measured because the patient did not complete the shoulder FS PROM at initial evaluation and/or near discharge, reason not given M

G8667 Risk-adjusted functional status change residual score for the elbow, wrist or hand impairment successfully calculated and the score was equal to zero (0) or greater than zero (> 0) M ☑

G8668 Risk-adjusted functional status change residual score for the elbow, wrist or hand impairment successfully calculated and the score was less than zero (< 0) M ☑

~~G8669 Jan Risk-adjusted functional status change residual score for the elbow, wrist or hand impairment not measured because the patient did not complete the FS status survey near discharge, patient not appropriate~~

▲ G8670 Jan Risk adjusted functional status change residual score for the elbow, wrist or hand impairment not measured because the patient did not complete the elbow/wrist/hand FS PROM at initial evaluation and/or near discharge, reason not given M

G8671 Risk-adjusted functional status change residual score for the neck, cranium, mandible, thoracic spine, ribs or other general orthopedic impairment successfully calculated and the score was equal to zero (0) or greater than zero (> 0) M ☑

G8672 Risk-adjusted functional status change residual score for the neck, cranium, mandible, thoracic spine, ribs or other general orthopedic impairment successfully calculated and the score was less than zero (< 0) M ☑

~~G8673 Jan Risk-adjusted functional status change residual score for the neck, cranium, mandible, thoracic spine, ribs or other general orthopedic impairment not measured because the patient did not complete the FS status survey near discharge, patient not appropriate~~

▲ G8674 Jan Risk adjusted functional status change residual score for the neck, cranium, mandible, thoracic spine, ribs or other general orthopedic impairment not measured because the patient did not complete the general orthopedic FS PROM at initial evaluation and/or near discharge, reason not given M

G8694 Left ventricular ejection fraction (LVEF) < 40% M ☑

G8708 Patient not prescribed or dispensed antibiotic M

G8709 Patient prescribed or dispensed antibiotic for documented medical reason(s) within three days after the initial diagnosis of URI (e.g., intestinal infection, pertussis, bacterial infection, lyme disease, otitis media, acute sinusitis, acute pharyngitis, acute tonsillitis, chronic sinusitis, infection of the pharynx/larynx/tonsils/adenoids, prostatitis, cellulitis, mastoiditis, or bone infections, acute lymphadenitis, impetigo, skin staph infections, pneumonia/gonococcal infections, venereal disease (syphilis, chlamydia, inflammatory diseases (female reproductive organs)), infections of the kidney, cystitis or UTI, and acne) M

G8710 Patient prescribed or dispensed antibiotic M

G8711 Prescribed or dispensed antibiotic M

G8712 Antibiotic not prescribed or dispensed M

G8721 PT category (primary tumor), PN category (regional lymph nodes), and histologic grade were documented in pathology report M

G8722 Documentation of medical reason(s) for not including the PT category, the PN category or the histologic grade in the pathology report (e.g., re-excision without residual tumor; noncarcinomasanal canal) M

G8723 Specimen site is other than anatomic location of primary tumor M

G8724 PT category, PN category and histologic grade were not documented in the pathology report, reason not given M

G8730 Pain assessment documented as positive using a standardized tool and a follow-up plan is documented M

G8731 Pain assessment using a standardized tool is documented as negative, no follow-up plan required M

G8732 No documentation of pain assessment, reason not given M

G8733 Elder maltreatment screen documented as positive and a follow-up plan is documented M

G8734 Elder maltreatment screen documented as negative, no follow-up required M

G8735 Elder maltreatment screen documented as positive, follow-up plan not documented, reason not given M

G8749 Absence of signs of melanoma (tenderness, jaundice, localized neurologic signs such as weakness, or any other sign suggesting systemic spread) or absence of symptoms of melanoma (cough, dyspnea, pain, paresthesia, or any other symptom suggesting the possibility of systemic spread of melanoma) M

G8752 Most recent systolic blood pressure < 140 mm Hg M ☑

G8753 Most recent systolic blood pressure ≥ 140 mm Hg M ☑

G8754 Most recent diastolic blood pressure < 90 mm Hg M ☑

G8755 Most recent diastolic blood pressure ≥ 90 mm Hg M ☑

G8756 No documentation of blood pressure measurement, reason not given M

G8783 Normal blood pressure reading documented, follow-up not required M

G8785 Blood pressure reading not documented, reason not given M

G8797 Specimen site other than anatomic location of esophagus M

G8798 Specimen site other than anatomic location of prostate M

G8806 Performance of trans-abdominal or trans-vaginal ultrasound and pregnancy location documented A ♀ M

G8807 Transabdominal or transvaginal ultrasound not performed for reasons documented by clinician (e.g., patient has visited the ED multiple times within 72 hours, patient has a documented intrauterine pregnancy (IUP)) A ♀ M

G8808 Transabdominal or transvaginal ultrasound not performed, reason not given A ♀ M

G8809 Rh immune globulin (RhoGAM) ordered M ♀ M

G8810 Rh-immunoglobulin (RhoGAM) not ordered for reasons documented by clinician (e.g., patient had prior documented receipt of RhoGAM within 12 weeks, patient refusal) M ♀ M

G8811 Documentation Rh immunoglobulin (RhoGAM) was not ordered, reason not given M ♀ M

G8815 Documented reason in the medical records for why the statin therapy was not prescribed (i.e., lower extremity bypass was for a patient with nonartherosclerotic disease) M

G8816 Statin medication prescribed at discharge M

G8817 Statin therapy not prescribed at discharge, reason not given M

© 2019 Optum360, LLC

G8818 Patient discharge to home no later than postoperative day #7 M

G8825 Patient not discharged to home by postoperative day #7 M

G8826 Patient discharged to home no later than postoperative day #2 following EVAR M

G8833 Patient not discharged to home by postoperative day #2 following EVAR M

G8834 Patient discharged to home no later than postoperative day #2 following CEA M

G8838 Patient not discharged to home by postoperative day #2 following CEA M

G8839 Sleep apnea symptoms assessed, including presence or absence of snoring and daytime sleepiness M

G8840 Documentation of reason(s) for not documenting an assessment of sleep symptoms (e.g., patient didn't have initial daytime sleepiness, patient visited between initial testing and initiation of therapy) M

G8841 Sleep apnea symptoms not assessed, reason not given M

G8842 Apnea hypopnea index (AHI) or respiratory disturbance index (RDI) measured at the time of initial diagnosis M

G8843 Documentation of reason(s) for not measuring an apnea hypopnea index (AHI) or a respiratory disturbance index (RDI) at the time of initial diagnosis (e.g., psychiatric disease, dementia, patient declined, financial, insurance coverage, test ordered but not yet completed) M

G8844 Apnea hypopna index (AHI) or respiratory disturbance index (RDI) not measured at the time of initial diagnosis, reason not given M

G8845 Positive airway pressure therapy prescribed M

G8846 Moderate or severe obstructive sleep apnea (apnea hypopnea index (AHI) or respiratory disturbance index (RDI) of 15 or greater) M ☑

G8849 Documentation of reason(s) for not prescribing positive airway pressure therapy (e.g., patient unable to tolerate, alternative therapies use, patient declined, financial, insurance coverage) M

G8850 Positive airway pressure therapy not prescribed, reason not given M

G8851 Objective measurement of adherence to positive airway pressure therapy, documented M

G8852 Positive airway pressure therapy prescribed M

G8854 Documentation of reason(s) for not objectively measuring adherence to positive airway pressure therapy (e.g., patient did not bring data from continuous positive airway pressure (CPAP), therapy not yet initiated, not available on machine) M

G8855 Objective measurement of adherence to positive airway pressure therapy not performed, reason not given M

G8856 Referral to a physician for an otologic evaluation performed M

G8857 Patient is not eligible for the referral for otologic evaluation measure (e.g., patients who are already under the care of a physician for acute or chronic dizziness) M

G8858 Referral to a physician for an otologic evaluation not performed, reason not given M

~~**G8861**~~ Jan ~~Within the past 2 years, central dual-energy x-ray absorptiometry (DXA) ordered and documented, review of systems and medication history or pharmacologic therapy (other than minerals/vitamins) for osteoporosis prescribed~~

G8863 Patients not assessed for risk of bone loss, reason not given M

G8864 Pneumococcal vaccine administered or previously received M

G8865 Documentation of medical reason(s) for not administering or previously receiving pneumococcal vaccine (e.g., patient allergic reaction, potential adverse drug reaction) M

G8866 Documentation of patient reason(s) for not administering or previously receiving pneumococcal vaccine (e.g., patient refusal) M

G8867 Pneumococcal vaccine not administered or previously received, reason not given M

G8869 Patient has documented immunity to hepatitis B and initiating anti-TNF therapy M

G8872 Excised tissue evaluated by imaging intraoperatively to confirm successful inclusion of targeted lesion M

G8873 Patients with needle localization specimens which are not amenable to intraoperative imaging such as MRI needle wire localization, or targets which are tentatively identified on mammogram or ultrasound which do not contain a biopsy marker but which can be verified on intraoperative inspection or pathology (e.g., needle biopsy site where the biopsy marker is remote from the actual biopsy site) M

G8874 Excised tissue not evaluated by imaging intraoperatively to confirm successful inclusion of targeted lesion M

G8875 Clinician diagnosed breast cancer preoperatively by a minimally invasive biopsy method M

G8876 Documentation of reason(s) for not performing minimally invasive biopsy to diagnose breast cancer preoperatively (e.g., lesion too close to skin, implant, chest wall, etc., lesion could not be adequately visualized for needle biopsy, patient condition prevents needle biopsy [weight, breast thickness, etc.], duct excision without imaging abnormality, prophylactic mastectomy, reduction mammoplasty, excisional biopsy performed by another physician) M

G8877 Clinician did not attempt to achieve the diagnosis of breast cancer preoperatively by a minimally invasive biopsy method, reason not given M

G8878 Sentinel lymph node biopsy procedure performed M

G8880 Documentation of reason(s) sentinel lymph node biopsy not performed (e.g., reasons could include but not limited to: noninvasive cancer, incidental discovery of breast cancer on prophylactic mastectomy, incidental discovery of breast cancer on reduction mammoplasty, preoperative biopsy proven lymph node (LN) metastases, inflammatory carcinoma, Stage III locally advanced cancer, recurrent invasive breast cancer, clinically node positive after neoadjuvant systemic therapy, patient refusal after informed consent, patient with significant age, comorbidities, or limited life expectancy and favorable tumor; adjuvant systemic therapy unlikely to change) M

G8881 Stage of breast cancer is greater than T1N0M0 or T2N0M0 M

G8882 Sentinel lymph node biopsy procedure not performed, reason not given M

G8883 Biopsy results reviewed, communicated, tracked and documented M

G8884 Clinician documented reason that patient's biopsy results were not reviewed M

G8885 Biopsy results not reviewed, communicated, tracked or documented M

© 2019 Optum360, LLC

G8907 Patient documented not to have experienced any of the following events: a burn prior to discharge; a fall within the facility; wrong site/side/patient/procedure/implant event; or a hospital transfer or hospital admission upon discharge from the facility M

G8908 Patient documented to have received a burn prior to discharge M

G8909 Patient documented not to have received a burn prior to discharge M

G8910 Patient documented to have experienced a fall within ASC M

G8911 Patient documented not to have experienced a fall within ASC M

G8912 Patient documented to have experienced a wrong site, wrong side, wrong patient, wrong procedure or wrong implant event M

G8913 Patient documented not to have experienced a wrong site, wrong side, wrong patient, wrong procedure or wrong implant event M

G8914 Patient documented to have experienced a hospital transfer or hospital admission upon discharge from ASC M

G8915 Patient documented not to have experienced a hospital transfer or hospital admission upon discharge from ASC M

G8916 Patient with preoperative order for IV antibiotic surgical site infection (SSI) prophylaxis, antibiotic initiated on time M

G8917 Patient with preoperative order for IV antibiotic surgical site infection (SSI) prophylaxis, antibiotic not initiated on time M

G8918 Patient without preoperative order for IV antibiotic surgical site infection (SSI) prophylaxis M

G8923 Left ventricular ejection fraction (LVEF) < 40% or documentation of moderately or severely depressed left ventricular systolic function M

G8924 Spirometry test results demonstrate FEV1/FVC < 70%, FEV < 60% predicted and patient has COPD symptoms (e.g., dyspnea, cough/sputum, wheezing) M

G8925 Spirometry test results demonstrate FEV1 >= 60%, FEV1/FVC >= 70%, predicted or patient does not have COPD symptoms M

G8926 Spirometry test not performed or documented, reason not given M

G8934 Left ventricular ejection fraction (LVEF) < 40% or documentation of moderately or severely depressed left ventricular systolic function M

G8935 Clinician prescribed angiotensin converting enzyme (ACE) inhibitor or angiotensin receptor blocker (ARB) therapy M

G8936 Clinician documented that patient was not an eligible candidate for angiotensin converting enzyme (ACE) inhibitor or angiotensin receptor blocker (ARB) therapy (e.g., allergy, intolerance, pregnancy, renal failure due to ACE inhibitor, diseases of the aortic or mitral valve, other medical reasons) or (e.g., patient declined, other patient reasons) or (e.g., lack of drug availability, other reasons attributable to the health care system) M

G8937 Clinician did not prescribe angiotensin converting enzyme (ACE) inhibitor or angiotensin receptor blocker (ARB) therapy, reason not given M

G8938 BMI is documented as being outside of normal limits, follow-up plan is not documented, documentation the patient is not eligible M

G8939 Pain assessment documented as positive, follow-up plan not documented, documentation the patient is not eligible at the time of the encounter M

G8941 Elder maltreatment screen documented as positive, follow-up plan not documented, documentation the patient is not eligible for follow-up plan at the time of the encounter M

G8942 Functional outcomes assessment using a standardized tool is documented within the previous 30 days and care plan, based on identified deficiencies on the date of the functional outcome assessment, is documented M

G8944 AJCC melanoma cancer stage 0 through IIC melanoma M

G8946 Minimally invasive biopsy method attempted but not diagnostic of breast cancer (e.g., high risk lesion of breast such as atypical ductal hyperplasia, lobular neoplasia, atypical lobular hyperplasia, lobular carcinoma in situ, atypical columnar hyperplasia, flat epithelial atypia, radial scar, complex sclerosing lesion, papillary lesion, or any lesion with spindle cells) M

G8950 Prehypertensive or hypertensive blood pressure reading documented, and the indicated follow-up is documented M

G8952 Prehypertensive or hypertensive blood pressure reading documented, indicated follow-up not documented, reason not given M

G8955 Most recent assessment of adequacy of volume management documented M

G8956 Patient receiving maintenance hemodialysis in an outpatient dialysis facility M

G8958 Assessment of adequacy of volume management not documented, reason not given M

G8959 Clinician treating major depressive disorder communicates to clinician treating comorbid condition M

G8960 Clinician treating major depressive disorder did not communicate to clinician treating comorbid condition, reason not given M

G8961 Cardiac stress imaging test primarily performed on low-risk surgery patient for preoperative evaluation within 30 days preceding this surgery M

G8962 Cardiac stress imaging test performed on patient for any reason including those who did not have low risk surgery or test that was performed more than 30 days preceding low risk surgery M

G8963 Cardiac stress imaging performed primarily for monitoring of asymptomatic patient who had PCI wihin 2 years M

G8964 Cardiac stress imaging test performed primarily for any other reason than monitoring of asymptomatic patient who had PCI wthin 2 years (e.g., symptomatic patient, patient greater than 2 years since PCI, initial evaluation, etc.) M

G8965 Cardiac stress imaging test primarily performed on low CHD risk patient for initial detection and risk assessment M

G8966 Cardiac stress imaging test performed on symptomatic or higher than low CHD risk patient or for any reason other than initial detection and risk assessment M

G8967 Warfarin or another FDA-approved oral anticoagulant is prescribed M

G8968 Documentation of medical reason(s) for not prescribing warfarin or another FDA-approved anticoagulant (e.g., atrial appendage device in place) M

G8969 Documentation of patient reason(s) for not prescribing warfarin or another FDA-approved oral anticoagulant that is FDA approved for the prevention of thromboembolism (e.g., patient choice of having atrial appendage device placed) M

© 2019 Optum360, LLC

G8970 No risk factors or one moderate risk factor for thromboembolism M

G8973 Most recent hemoglobin (HgB) level < 10 g/dl M

G8974 Hemoglobin level measurement not documented, reason not given M

G8975 Documentation of medical reason(s) for patient having a hemoglobin level < 10 g/dl (e.g., patients who have nonrenal etiologies of anemia [e.g., sickle cell anemia or other hemoglobinopathies, hypersplenism, primary bone marrow disease, anemia related to chemotherapy for diagnosis of malignancy, postoperative bleeding, active bloodstream or peritoneal infection], other medical reasons) M

G8976 Most recent hemoglobin (HgB) level >= 10 g/dl M

Functional Limitation

G8978 Jan ~~Mobility: walking and moving around functional limitation, current status, at therapy episode outset and at reporting intervals~~

G8979 Jan ~~Mobility: walking and moving around functional limitation, projected goal status, at therapy episode outset, at reporting intervals, and at discharge or to end reporting~~

G8980 Jan ~~Mobility: walking and moving around functional limitation, discharge status, at discharge from therapy or to end reporting~~

G8981 Jan ~~Changing and maintaining body position functional limitation, current status, at therapy episode outset and at reporting intervals~~

G8982 Jan ~~Changing and maintaining body position functional limitation, projected goal status, at therapy episode outset, at reporting intervals, and at discharge or to end reporting~~

G8983 Jan ~~Changing and maintaining body position functional limitation, discharge status, at discharge from therapy or to end reporting~~

G8984 Jan ~~Carrying, moving and handling objects functional limitation, current status, at therapy episode outset and at reporting intervals~~

G8985 Jan ~~Carrying, moving and handling objects, projected goal status, at therapy episode outset, at reporting intervals, and at discharge or to end reporting~~

G8986 Jan ~~Carrying, moving and handling objects functional limitation, discharge status, at discharge from therapy or to end reporting~~

G8987 Jan ~~Self care functional limitation, current status, at therapy episode outset and at reporting intervals~~

G8988 Jan ~~Self care functional limitation, projected goal status, at therapy episode outset, at reporting intervals, and at discharge or to end reporting~~

G8989 Jan ~~Self care functional limitation, discharge status, at discharge from therapy or to end reporting~~

G8990 Jan ~~Other physical or occupational therapy primary functional limitation, current status, at therapy episode outset and at reporting intervals~~

G8991 Jan ~~Other physical or occupational therapy primary functional limitation, projected goal status, at therapy episode outset, at reporting intervals, and at discharge or to end reporting~~

G8992 Jan ~~Other physical or occupational therapy primary functional limitation, discharge status, at discharge from therapy or to end reporting~~

G8993 Jan ~~Other physical or occupational therapy subsequent functional limitation, current status, at therapy episode outset and at reporting intervals~~

G8994 Jan ~~Other physical or occupational therapy subsequent functional limitation, projected goal status, at therapy episode outset, at reporting intervals, and at discharge or to end reporting~~

G8995 Jan ~~Other physical or occupational therapy subsequent functional limitation, discharge status, at discharge from therapy or to end reporting~~

G8996 Jan ~~Swallowing functional limitation, current status at therapy episode outset and at reporting intervals~~

G8997 Jan ~~Swallowing functional limitation, projected goal status, at therapy episode outset, at reporting intervals, and at discharge or to end reporting~~

G8998 Jan ~~Swallowing functional limitation, discharge status, at discharge from therapy or to end reporting~~

G8999 Jan ~~Motor speech functional limitation, current status at therapy episode outset and at reporting intervals~~

Coordinated Care

G9001 Coordinated care fee, initial rate B

G9002 Coordinated care fee B

G9003 Coordinated care fee, risk adjusted high, initial B

G9004 Coordinated care fee, risk adjusted low, initial B

G9005 Coordinated care fee risk adjusted maintenance B

G9006 Coordinated care fee, home monitoring B

G9007 Coordinated care fee, scheduled team conference B

G9008 Coordinated care fee, physician coordinated care oversight services B

G9009 Coordinated care fee, risk adjusted maintenance, Level 3 B

G9010 Coordinated care fee, risk adjusted maintenance, Level 4 B

G9011 Coordinated care fee, risk adjusted maintenance, Level 5 B

G9012 Other specified case management service not elsewhere classified B

Demonstration Project

G9013 ESRD demo basic bundle Level I E

G9014 ESRD demo expanded bundle including venous access and related services E

G9016 Smoking cessation counseling, individual, in the absence of or in addition to any other evaluation and management service, per session (6-10 minutes) [demo project code only] E ☑
CMS: 100-03,210.4.1

G9017 Jan ~~Amantadine HCl, oral, per 100 mg (for use in a Medicare-approved demonstration project)~~

G9018 Jan ~~Zanamivir, inhalation powder, administered through inhaler, per 10 mg (for use in a Medicare-approved demonstration project)~~

G9019 Jan ~~Oseltamivir phosphate, oral, per 75 mg (for use in a Medicare-approved demonstration project)~~

G9020 Jan ~~Rimantadine HCl, oral, per 100 mg (for use in a Medicare-approved demonstration project)~~

G9033 Jan ~~Amantadine HCl, oral brand, per 100 mg (for use in a Medicare-approved demonstration project)~~

G9034 Jan ~~Zanamivir, inhalation powder, administered through inhaler, brand, per 10 mg (for use in a Medicare-approved demonstration project)~~

G9035 Jan ~~Oseltamivir phosphate, oral, brand, per 75 mg (for use in a Medicare-approved demonstration project)~~

G9036 Jan ~~Rimantadine HCl, oral, brand, per 100 mg (for use in a Medicare-approved demonstration project)~~

© 2019 Optum360, LLC

G9050 Oncology; primary focus of visit; work-up, evaluation, or staging at the time of cancer diagnosis or recurrence (for use in a Medicare-approved demonstration project) E

G9051 Oncology; primary focus of visit; treatment decision-making after disease is staged or restaged, discussion of treatment options, supervising/coordinating active cancer-directed therapy or managing consequences of cancer-directed therapy (for use in a Medicare-approved demonstration project) E

G9052 Oncology; primary focus of visit; surveillance for disease recurrence for patient who has completed definitive cancer-directed therapy and currently lacks evidence of recurrent disease; cancer-directed therapy might be considered in the future (for use in a Medicare-approved demonstration project) E

G9053 Oncology; primary focus of visit; expectant management of patient with evidence of cancer for whom no cancer-directed therapy is being administered or arranged at present; cancer-directed therapy might be considered in the future (for use in a Medicare-approved demonstration project) E

G9054 Oncology; primary focus of visit; supervising, coordinating or managing care of patient with terminal cancer or for whom other medical illness prevents further cancer treatment; includes symptom management, end-of-life care planning, management of palliative therapies (for use in a Medicare-approved demonstration project) E

G9055 Oncology; primary focus of visit; other, unspecified service not otherwise listed (for use in a Medicare-approved demonstration project) E

G9056 Oncology; practice guidelines; management adheres to guidelines (for use in a Medicare-approved demonstration project) E

G9057 Oncology; practice guidelines; management differs from guidelines as a result of patient enrollment in an institutional review board-approved clinical trial (for use in a Medicare-approved demonstration project) E

G9058 Oncology; practice guidelines; management differs from guidelines because the treating physician disagrees with guideline recommendations (for use in a Medicare-approved demonstration project) E

G9059 Oncology; practice guidelines; management differs from guidelines because the patient, after being offered treatment consistent with guidelines, has opted for alternative treatment or management, including no treatment (for use in a Medicare-approved demonstration project) E

G9060 Oncology; practice guidelines; management differs from guidelines for reason(s) associated with patient comorbid illness or performance status not factored into guidelines (for use in a Medicare-approved demonstration project) E

G9061 Oncology; practice guidelines; patient's condition not addressed by available guidelines (for use in a Medicare-approved demonstration project) E

G9062 Oncology; practice guidelines; management differs from guidelines for other reason(s) not listed (for use in a Medicare-approved demonstration project) E

G9063 Oncology; disease status; limited to nonsmall cell lung cancer; extent of disease initially established as Stage I (prior to neoadjuvant therapy, if any) with no evidence of disease progression, recurrence, or metastases (for use in a Medicare-approved demonstration project) M

G9064 Oncology; disease status; limited to nonsmall cell lung cancer; extent of disease initially established as Stage II (prior to neoadjuvant therapy, if any) with no evidence of disease progression, recurrence, or metastases (for use in a Medicare-approved demonstration project) M

G9065 Oncology; disease status; limited to nonsmall cell lung cancer; extent of disease initially established as Stage III a (prior to neoadjuvant therapy, if any) with no evidence of disease progression, recurrence, or metastases (for use in a Medicare-approved demonstration project) M

G9066 Oncology; disease status; limited to nonsmall cell lung cancer; Stage III B-IV at diagnosis, metastatic, locally recurrent, or progressive (for use in a Medicare-approved demonstration project) M

G9067 Oncology; disease status; limited to nonsmall cell lung cancer; extent of disease unknown, staging in progress, or not listed (for use in a Medicare-approved demonstration project) M

G9068 Oncology; disease status; limited to small cell and combined small cell/nonsmall cell; extent of disease initially established as limited with no evidence of disease progression, recurrence, or metastases (for use in a Medicare-approved demonstration project) M

G9069 Oncology; disease status; small cell lung cancer, limited to small cell and combined small cell/nonsmall cell; extensive Stage at diagnosis, metastatic, locally recurrent, or progressive (for use in a Medicare-approved demonstration project) M

G9070 Oncology; disease status; small cell lung cancer, limited to small cell and combined small cell/nonsmall; extent of disease unknown, staging in progress, or not listed (for use in a Medicare-approved demonstration project) M

G9071 Oncology; disease status; invasive female breast cancer (does not include ductal carcinoma in situ); adenocarcinoma as predominant cell type; Stage I or Stage IIA-IIB; or T3, N1, M0; and ER and/or PR positive; with no evidence of disease progression, recurrence, or metastases (for use in a Medicare-approved demonstration project) ♀ M

G9072 Oncology; disease status; invasive female breast cancer (does not include ductal carcinoma in situ); adenocarcinoma as predominant cell type; Stage I, or Stage IIA-IIB; or T3, N1, M0; and ER and PR negative; with no evidence of disease progression, recurrence, or metastases (for use in a Medicare-approved demonstration project) ♀ M

G9073 Oncology; disease status; invasive female breast cancer (does not include ductal carcinoma in situ); adenocarcinoma as predominant cell type; Stage IIIA-IIIB; and not T3, N1, M0; and ER and/or PR positive; with no evidence of disease progression, recurrence, or metastases (for use in a Medicare-approved demonstration project) ♀ M

G9074 Oncology; disease status; invasive female breast cancer (does not include ductal carcinoma in situ); adenocarcinoma as predominant cell type; Stage IIIA-IIIB; and not T3, N1, M0; and ER and PR negative; with no evidence of disease progression, recurrence, or metastases (for use in a Medicare-approved demonstration project) ♀ M

G9075 Oncology; disease status; invasive female breast cancer (does not include ductal carcinoma in situ); adenocarcinoma as predominant cell type; M1 at diagnosis, metastatic, locally recurrent, or progressive (for use in a Medicare-approved demonstration project) ♀ M

G9077 Oncology; disease status; prostate cancer, limited to adenocarcinoma as predominant cell type; T1-T2c and Gleason 2-7 and PSA < or equal to 20 at diagnosis with no evidence of disease progression, recurrence, or metastases (for use in a Medicare-approved demonstration project) ♂ M

© 2019 Optum360, LLC

G9078 Oncology; disease status; prostate cancer, limited to adenocarcinoma as predominant cell type; T2 or T3a Gleason 8-10 or PSA > 20 at diagnosis with no evidence of disease progression, recurrence, or metastases (for use in a Medicare-approved demonstration project) ♂ M

G9079 Oncology; disease status; prostate cancer, limited to adenocarcinoma as predominant cell type; T3b-T4, any N; any T, N1 at diagnosis with no evidence of disease progression, recurrence, or metastases (for use in a Medicare-approved demonstration project) ♂ M

G9080 Oncology; disease status; prostate cancer, limited to adenocarcinoma; after initial treatment with rising PSA or failure of PSA decline (for use in a Medicare-approved demonstration project) ♂ M

G9083 Oncology; disease status; prostate cancer, limited to adenocarcinoma; extent of disease unknown, staging in progress, or not listed (for use in a Medicare-approved demonstration project) ♂ M

G9084 Oncology; disease status; colon cancer, limited to invasive cancer, adenocarcinoma as predominant cell type; extent of disease initially established as T1-3, N0, M0 with no evidence of disease progression, recurrence or metastases (for use in a Medicare-approved demonstration project) M

G9085 Oncology; disease status; colon cancer, limited to invasive cancer, adenocarcinoma as predominant cell type; extent of disease initially established as T4, N0, M0 with no evidence of disease progression, recurrence, or metastases (for use in a Medicare-approved demonstration project) M

G9086 Oncology; disease status; colon cancer, limited to invasive cancer, adenocarcinoma as predominant cell type; extent of disease initially established as T1-4, N1-2, M0 with no evidence of disease progression, recurrence, or metastases (for use in a Medicare-approved demonstration project) M

G9087 Oncology; disease status; colon cancer, limited to invasive cancer, adenocarcinoma as predominant cell type; M1 at diagnosis, metastatic, locally recurrent, or progressive with current clinical, radiologic, or biochemical evidence of disease (for use in a Medicare-approved demonstration project) M

G9088 Oncology; disease status; colon cancer, limited to invasive cancer, adenocarcinoma as predominant cell type; M1 at diagnosis, metastatic, locally recurrent, or progressive without current clinical, radiologic, or biochemical evidence of disease (for use in a Medicare-approved demonstration project) M

G9089 Oncology; disease status; colon cancer, limited to invasive cancer, adenocarcinoma as predominant cell type; extent of disease unknown, staging in progress or not listed (for use in a Medicare-approved demonstration project) M

G9090 Oncology; disease status; rectal cancer, limited to invasive cancer, adenocarcinoma as predominant cell type; extent of disease initially established as T1-2, N0, M0 (prior to neoadjuvant therapy, if any) with no evidence of disease progression, recurrence, or metastases (for use in a Medicare-approved demonstration project) M

G9091 Oncology; disease status; rectal cancer, limited to invasive cancer, adenocarcinoma as predominant cell type; extent of disease initially established as T3, N0, M0 (prior to neoadjuvant therapy, if any) with no evidence of disease progression, recurrence, or metastases (for use in a Medicare-approved demonstration project) M

G9092 Oncology; disease status; rectal cancer, limited to invasive cancer, adenocarcinoma as predominant cell type; extent of disease initially established as T1-3, N1-2, M0 (prior to neoadjuvant therapy, if any) with no evidence of disease progression, recurrence or metastases (for use in a Medicare-approved demonstration project) M

G9093 Oncology; disease status; rectal cancer, limited to invasive cancer, adenocarcinoma as predominant cell type; extent of disease initially established as T4, any N, M0 (prior to neoadjuvant therapy, if any) with no evidence of disease progression, recurrence, or metastases (for use in a Medicare-approved demonstration project) M

G9094 Oncology; disease status; rectal cancer, limited to invasive cancer, adenocarcinoma as predominant cell type; M1 at diagnosis, metastatic, locally recurrent, or progressive (for use in a Medicare-approved demonstration project) M

G9095 Oncology; disease status; rectal cancer, limited to invasive cancer, adenocarcinoma as predominant cell type; extent of disease unknown, staging in progress or not listed (for use in a Medicare-approved demonstration project) M

G9096 Oncology; disease status; esophageal cancer, limited to adenocarcinoma or squamous cell carcinoma as predominant cell type; extent of disease initially established as T1-T3, N0-N1 or NX (prior to neoadjuvant therapy, if any) with no evidence of disease progression, recurrence, or metastases (for use in a Medicare-approved demonstration project) M

G9097 Oncology; disease status; esophageal cancer, limited to adenocarcinoma or squamous cell carcinoma as predominant cell type; extent of disease initially established as T4, any N, M0 (prior to neoadjuvant therapy, if any) with no evidence of disease progression, recurrence, or metastases (for use in a Medicare-approved demonstration project) M

G9098 Oncology; disease status; esophageal cancer, limited to adenocarcinoma or squamous cell carcinoma as predominant cell type; M1 at diagnosis, metastatic, locally recurrent, or progressive (for use in a Medicare-approved demonstration project) M

G9099 Oncology; disease status; esophageal cancer, limited to adenocarcinoma or squamous cell carcinoma as predominant cell type; extent of disease unknown, staging in progress, or not listed (for use in a Medicare-approved demonstration project) M

G9100 Oncology; disease status; gastric cancer, limited to adenocarcinoma as predominant cell type; post R0 resection (with or without neoadjuvant therapy) with no evidence of disease recurrence, progression, or metastases (for use in a Medicare-approved demonstration project) M

G9101 Oncology; disease status; gastric cancer, limited to adenocarcinoma as predominant cell type; post R1 or R2 resection (with or without neoadjuvant therapy) with no evidence of disease progression, or metastases (for use in a Medicare-approved demonstration project) M

G9102 Oncology; disease status; gastric cancer, limited to adenocarcinoma as predominant cell type; clinical or pathologic M0, unresectable with no evidence of disease progression, or metastases (for use in a Medicare-approved demonstration project) M

G9103 Oncology; disease status; gastric cancer, limited to adenocarcinoma as predominant cell type; clinical or pathologic M1 at diagnosis, metastatic, locally recurrent, or progressive (for use in a Medicare-approved demonstration project) M

© 2019 Optum360, LLC

G9104 Oncology; disease status; gastric cancer, limited to adenocarcinoma as predominant cell type; extent of disease unknown, staging in progress, or not listed (for use in a Medicare-approved demonstration project) M

G9105 Oncology; disease status; pancreatic cancer, limited to adenocarcinoma as predominant cell type; post R0 resection without evidence of disease progression, recurrence, or metastases (for use in a Medicare-approved demonstration project) M

G9106 Oncology; disease status; pancreatic cancer, limited to adenocarcinoma; post R1 or R2 resection with no evidence of disease progression, or metastases (for use in a Medicare-approved demonstration project) M

G9107 Oncology; disease status; pancreatic cancer, limited to adenocarcinoma; unresectable at diagnosis, M1 at diagnosis, metastatic, locally recurrent, or progressive (for use in a Medicare-approved demonstration project) M

G9108 Oncology; disease status; pancreatic cancer, limited to adenocarcinoma; extent of disease unknown, staging in progress, or not listed (for use in a Medicare-approved demonstration project) M

G9109 Oncology; disease status; head and neck cancer, limited to cancers of oral cavity, pharynx and larynx with squamous cell as predominant cell type; extent of disease initially established as T1-T2 and N0, M0 (prior to neoadjuvant therapy, if any) with no evidence of disease progression, recurrence, or metastases (for use in a Medicare-approved demonstration project) M

G9110 Oncology; disease status; head and neck cancer, limited to cancers of oral cavity, pharynx and larynx with squamous cell as predominant cell type; extent of disease initially established as T3-4 and/or N1-3, M0 (prior to neoadjuvant therapy, if any) with no evidence of disease progression, recurrence, or metastases (for use in a Medicare-approved demonstration project) M

G9111 Oncology; disease status; head and neck cancer, limited to cancers of oral cavity, pharynx and larynx with squamous cell as predominant cell type; M1 at diagnosis, metastatic, locally recurrent, or progressive (for use in a Medicare-approved demonstration project) M

G9112 Oncology; disease status; head and neck cancer, limited to cancers of oral cavity, pharynx and larynx with squamous cell as predominant cell type; extent of disease unknown, staging in progress, or not listed (for use in a Medicare-approved demonstration project) M

G9113 Oncology; disease status; ovarian cancer, limited to epithelial cancer; pathologic Stage IA-B (Grade 1) without evidence of disease progression, recurrence, or metastases (for use in a Medicare-approved demonstration project) ♀ M

G9114 Oncology; disease status; ovarian cancer, limited to epithelial cancer; pathologic Stage IA-B (Grade 2-3); or Stage IC (all grades); or Stage II; without evidence of disease progression, recurrence, or metastases (for use in a Medicare-approved demonstration project) ♀ M

G9115 Oncology; disease status; ovarian cancer, limited to epithelial cancer; pathologic Stage III-IV; without evidence of progression, recurrence, or metastases (for use in a Medicare-approved demonstration project) ♀ M

G9116 Oncology; disease status; ovarian cancer, limited to epithelial cancer; evidence of disease progression, or recurrence, and/or platinum resistance (for use in a Medicare-approved demonstration project) ♀ M

G9117 Oncology; disease status; ovarian cancer, limited to epithelial cancer; extent of disease unknown, staging in progress, or not listed (for use in a Medicare-approved demonstration project) ♀ M

G9123 Oncology; disease status; chronic myelogenous leukemia, limited to Philadelphia chromosome positive and/or BCR-ABL positive; chronic phase not in hematologic, cytogenetic, or molecular remission (for use in a Medicare-approved demonstration project) M

G9124 Oncology; disease status; chronic myelogenous leukemia, limited to Philadelphia chromosome positive and /or BCR-ABL positive; accelerated phase not in hematologic cytogenetic, or molecular remission (for use in a Medicare-approved demonstration project) M

G9125 Oncology; disease status; chronic myelogenous leukemia, limited to Philadelphia chromosome positive and/or BCR-ABL positive; blast phase not in hematologic, cytogenetic, or molecular remission (for use in a Medicare-approved demonstration project) M

G9126 Oncology; disease status; chronic myelogenous leukemia, limited to Philadelphia chromosome positive and/or BCR-ABL positive; in hematologic, cytogenetic, or molecular remission (for use in a Medicare-approved demonstration project) M

G9128 Oncology; disease status; limited to multiple myeloma, systemic disease; smoldering, Stage I (for use in a Medicare-approved demonstration project) M

G9129 Oncology; disease status; limited to multiple myeloma, systemic disease; Stage II or higher (for use in a Medicare-approved demonstration project) M

G9130 Oncology; disease status; limited to multiple myeloma, systemic disease; extent of disease unknown, staging in progress, or not listed (for use in a Medicare-approved demonstration project) M

G9131 Oncology; disease status; invasive female breast cancer (does not include ductal carcinoma in situ); adenocarcinoma as predominant cell type; extent of disease unknown, staging in progress, or not listed (for use in a Medicare-approved demonstration project) ♀ M

G9132 Oncology; disease status; prostate cancer, limited to adenocarcinoma; hormone-refractory/androgen-independent (e.g., rising PSA on antiandrogen therapy or postorchiectomy); clinical metastases (for use in a Medicare-approved demonstration project) ♂ M

G9133 Oncology; disease status; prostate cancer, limited to adenocarcinoma; hormone-responsive; clinical metastases or M1 at diagnosis (for use in a Medicare-approved demonstration project) ♂ M

G9134 Oncology; disease status; non-Hodgkin's lymphoma, any cellular classification; Stage I, II at diagnosis, not relapsed, not refractory (for use in a Medicare-approved demonstration project) M

G9135 Oncology; disease status; non-Hodgkin's lymphoma, any cellular classification; Stage III, IV, not relapsed, not refractory (for use in a Medicare-approved demonstration project) M

G9136 Oncology; disease status; non-Hodgkin's lymphoma, transformed from original cellular diagnosis to a second cellular classification (for use in a Medicare-approved demonstration project) M

G9137 Oncology; disease status; non-Hodgkin's lymphoma, any cellular classification; relapsed/refractory (for use in a Medicare-approved demonstration project) M

© 2019 Optum360, LLC

G9138 Oncology; disease status; non-Hodgkin's lymphoma, any cellular classification; diagnostic evaluation, stage not determined, evaluation of possible relapse or nonresponse to therapy, or not listed (for use in a Medicare-approved demonstration project) M

G9139 Oncology; disease status; chronic myelogenous leukemia, limited to Philadelphia chromosome positive and/or BCR-ABL positive; extent of disease unknown, staging in progress, not listed (for use in a Medicare-approved demonstration project) M

G9140 Frontier Extended Stay Clinic demonstration; for a patient stay in a clinic approved for the CMS demonstration project; the following measures should be present: the stay must be equal to or greater than 4 hours; weather or other conditions must prevent transfer or the case falls into a category of monitoring and observation cases that are permitted by the rules of the demonstration; there is a maximum Frontier Extended Stay Clinic (FESC) visit of 48 hours, except in the case when weather or other conditions prevent transfer; payment is made on each period up to 4 hours, after the first 4 hours A ☑

Warfarin Testing

G9143 Warfarin responsiveness testing by genetic technique using any method, any number of specimen(s) N
CMS: 100-03,90.1; 100-04,32,250.1; 100-04,32,250.2

Outpatient IV Insulin TX

G9147 Outpatient Intravenous Insulin Treatment (OIVIT) either pulsatile or continuous, by any means, guided by the results of measurements for: respiratory quotient; and/or, urine urea nitrogen (UUN); and/or, arterial, venous or capillary glucose; and/or potassium concentration E
CMS: 100-03,40.7; 100-04,4,320.1; 100-04,4,320.2

Quality Assurance

G9148 National Committee for Quality Assurance-Level 1 Medical Home M

G9149 National Committee for Quality Assurance-Level 2 Medical Home M

G9150 National Committee for Quality Assurance-Level 3 Medical Home M

G9151 MAPCP Demonstration-state provided services M

G9152 MAPCP Demonstration-Community Health Teams M

G9153 MAPCP Demonstration-Physician Incentive Pool M

Wheelchair Evaluation

G9156 Evaluation for wheelchair requiring face-to-face visit with physician M

Monitor

G9157 Transesophageal Doppler used for cardiac monitoring B
CMS: 100-04,32,310; 100-04,32,310.2; 100-04,32,310.3

Functional Limitation

~~**G9158**~~ Jan ~~Motor speech functional limitation, discharge status, at discharge from therapy or to end reporting~~

~~**G9159**~~ Jan ~~Spoken language comprehension functional limitation, current status at therapy episode outset and at reporting intervals~~

~~**G9160**~~ Jan ~~Spoken language comprehension functional limitation, projected goal status at therapy episode outset, at reporting intervals, and at discharge or to end reporting~~

~~**G9161**~~ Jan ~~Spoken language comprehension functional limitation, discharge status, at discharge from therapy or to end reporting~~

~~**G9162**~~ Jan ~~Spoken language expression functional limitation, current status at therapy episode outset and at reporting intervals~~

~~**G9163**~~ Jan ~~Spoken language expression functional limitation, projected goal status at therapy episode outset, at reporting intervals, and at discharge or to end reporting~~

~~**G9164**~~ Jan ~~Spoken language expression functional limitation, discharge status at discharge from therapy or to end reporting~~

~~**G9165**~~ Jan ~~Attention functional limitation, current status at therapy episode outset and at reporting intervals~~

~~**G9166**~~ Jan ~~Attention functional limitation, projected goal status at therapy episode outset, at reporting intervals, and at discharge or to end reporting~~

~~**G9167**~~ Jan ~~Attention functional limitation, discharge status at discharge from therapy or to end reporting~~

~~**G9168**~~ Jan ~~Memory functional limitation, current status at therapy episode outset and at reporting intervals~~

~~**G9169**~~ Jan ~~Memory functional limitation, projected goal status at therapy episode outset, at reporting intervals, and at discharge or to end reporting~~

~~**G9170**~~ Jan ~~Memory functional limitation, discharge status at discharge from therapy or to end reporting~~

~~**G9171**~~ Jan ~~Voice functional limitation, current status at therapy episode outset and at reporting intervals~~

~~**G9172**~~ Jan ~~Voice functional limitation, projected goal status at therapy episode outset, at reporting intervals, and at discharge or to end reporting~~

~~**G9173**~~ Jan ~~Voice functional limitation, discharge status at discharge from therapy or to end reporting~~

~~**G9174**~~ Jan ~~Other speech language pathology functional limitation, current status at therapy episode outset and at reporting intervals~~

~~**G9175**~~ Jan ~~Other speech language pathology functional limitation, projected goal status at therapy episode outset, at reporting intervals, and at discharge or to end reporting~~

~~**G9176**~~ Jan ~~Other speech language pathology functional limitation, discharge status at discharge from therapy or to end reporting~~

~~**G9186**~~ Jan ~~Motor speech functional limitation, projected goal status at therapy episode outset, at reporting intervals, and at discharge or to end reporting~~

BPCI Services

G9187 Bundled payments for care improvement initiative home visit for patient assessment performed by a qualified health care professional for individuals not considered homebound including, but not limited to, assessment of safety, falls, clinical status, fluid status, medication reconciliation/management, patient compliance with orders/plan of care, performance of activities of daily living, appropriateness of care setting; (for use only in the Medicare-approved bundled payments for care improvement initiative); may not be billed for a 30-day period covered by a transitional care management code E

Miscellaneous Quality Measures

G9188 Beta-blocker therapy not prescribed, reason not given M

G9189 Beta-blocker therapy prescribed or currently being taken M

G9190 Documentation of medical reason(s) for not prescribing beta-blocker therapy (e.g., allergy, intolerance, other medical reasons) M

G9191 Documentation of patient reason(s) for not prescribing beta-blocker therapy (e.g., patient declined, other patient reasons) M

G9192 Documentation of system reason(s) for not prescribing beta-blocker therapy (e.g., other reasons attributable to the health care system) M

© 2019 Optum360, LLC

G9196 Documentation of medical reason(s) for not ordering a first or second generation cephalosporin for antimicrobial prophylaxis (e.g., patients enrolled in clinical trials, patients with documented infection prior to surgical procedure of interest, patients who were receiving antibiotics more than 24 hours prior to surgery [except colon surgery patients taking oral prophylactic antibiotics], patients who were receiving antibiotics within 24 hours prior to arrival [except colon surgery patients taking oral prophylactic antibiotics], other medical reason(s)) M

G9197 Documentation of order for first or second generation cephalosporin for antimicrobial prophylaxis M

G9198 Order for first or second generation cephalosporin for antimicrobial prophylaxis was not documented, reason not given M

G9212 DSM-IVTM criteria for major depressive disorder documented at the initial evaluation M

G9213 DSM-IV-TR criteria for major depressive disorder not documented at the initial evaluation, reason not otherwise specified M

G9223 Pneumocystis jiroveci pneumonia prophylaxis prescribed within 3 months of low CD4+ cell count below 500 cells/mm3 or a CD4 percentage below 15% M

G9225 Foot exam was not performed, reason not given M

G9226 Foot examination performed (includes examination through visual inspection, sensory exam with 10-g monofilament plus testing any one of the following: vibration using 128-Hz tuning fork, pinprick sensation, ankle reflexes, or vibration perception threshold, and pulse exam; report when all of the three components are completed) M

G9227 Functional outcome assessment documented, care plan not documented, documentation the patient is not eligible for a care plan at the time of the encounter M

G9228 Chlamydia, gonorrhea and syphilis screening results documented (report when results are present for all of the three screenings) M

G9229 Chlamydia, gonorrhea, and syphilis screening results not documented (patient refusal is the only allowed exception) M

G9230 Chlamydia, gonorrhea, and syphilis not screened, reason not given M

G9231 Documentation of end stage renal disease (ESRD), dialysis, renal transplant before or during the measurement period or pregnancy during the measurement period M

G9232 Clinician treating major depressive disorder did not communicate to clinician treating comorbid condition for specified patient reason (e.g., patient is unable to communicate the diagnosis of a comorbid condition; the patient is unwilling to communicate the diagnosis of a comorbid condition; or the patient is unaware of the comorbid condition, or any other specified patient reason) M

▲ **G9239**[Jan] Documentation of reasons for patient initiating maintenance hemodialysis with a catheter as the mode of vascular access (e.g., patient has a maturing arteriovenous fistula (AVF)/arteriovenous graft (AVG), time limited trial of hemodialysis, other medical reasons, patient declined AVF/AVG, other patient reasons, patient followed by reporting nephrologist for fewer than 90 days, other system reasons) M

G9240 Patient whose mode of vascular access is a catheter at the time maintenance hemodialysis is initiated M

G9241 Patient whose mode of vascular access is not a catheter at the time maintenance hemodialysis is initiated M

G9242 Documentation of viral load equal to or greater than 200 copies/ml or viral load not performed M

G9243 Documentation of viral load less than 200 copies/ml M

G9246 Patient did not have at least one medical visit in each 6 month period of the 24 month measurement period, with a minimum of 60 days between medical visits M

G9247 Patient had at least one medical visit in each 6 month period of the 24 month measurement period, with a minimum of 60 days between medical visits M

G9250 Documentation of patient pain brought to a comfortable level within 48 hours from initial assessment M

G9251 Documentation of patient with pain not brought to a comfortable level within 48 hours from initial assessment M

G9254 Documentation of patient discharged to home later than post-operative day 2 following CAS M

G9255 Documentation of patient discharged to home no later than post operative day 2 following CAS M

G9256 Documentation of patient death following CAS M

G9257 Documentation of patient stroke following CAS M

G9258 Documentation of patient stroke following CEA M

G9259 Documentation of patient survival and absence of stroke following CAS M

G9260 Documentation of patient death following CEA M

G9261 Documentation of patient survival and absence of stroke following CEA M

G9262 Documentation of patient death in the hospital following endovascular AAA repair M

G9263 Documentation of patient discharged alive following endovascular AAA repair M

▲ **G9264**[Jan] Documentation of patient receiving maintenance hemodialysis for greater than or equal to 90 days with a catheter for documented reasons (e.g., other medical reasons, patient declined arteriovenous fistula (AVF)/arteriovenous graft (AVG), other patient reasons) M

G9265 Patient receiving maintenance hemodialysis for greater than or equal to 90 days with a catheter as the mode of vascular access M

G9266 Patient receiving maintenance hemodialysis for greater than or equal to 90 days without a catheter as the mode of vascular access M

G9267 Documentation of patient with one or more complications or mortality within 30 days M

G9268 Documentation of patient with one or more complications within 90 days M

G9269 Documentation of patient without one or more complications and without mortality within 30 days M

G9270 Documentation of patient without one or more complications within 90 days M

G9273 Blood pressure has a systolic value of < 140 and a diastolic value of < 90 M

G9274 Blood pressure has a systolic value of = 140 and a diastolic value of = 90 or systolic value < 140 and diastolic value = 90 or systolic value = 140 and diastolic value < 90 M

G9275 Documentation that patient is a current nontobacco user M

G9276 Documentation that patient is a current tobacco user M

© 2019 Optum360, LLC

G9277 Documentation that the patient is on daily aspirin or antiplatelet or has documentation of a valid contraindication or exception to aspirin/antiplatelet; contraindications/exceptions include anticoagulant use, allergy to aspirin or antiplatelets, history of gastrointestinal bleed and bleeding disorder. Additionally, the following exceptions documented by the physician as a reason for not taking daily aspirin or antiplatelet are acceptable (use of nonsteroidal anti-inflammatory agents, documented risk for drug interaction, uncontrolled hypertension defined as > 180 systolic or > 110 diastolic or gastroesophageal reflux) M

G9278 Documentation that the patient is not on daily aspirin or antiplatelet regimen M

G9279 Pneumococcal screening performed and documentation of vaccination received prior to discharge M

G9280 Pneumococcal vaccination not administered prior to discharge, reason not specified M

G9281 Screening performed and documentation that vaccination not indicated/patient refusal M

G9282 Documentation of medical reason(s) for not reporting the histological type or NSCLC-NOS classification with an explanation (e.g., biopsy taken for other purposes in a patient with a history of nonsmall cell lung cancer or other documented medical reasons) M

G9283 Nonsmall cell lung cancer biopsy and cytology specimen report documents classification into specific histologic type or classified as NSCLC-NOS with an explanation M

G9284 Nonsmall cell lung cancer biopsy and cytology specimen report does not document classification into specific histologic type or classified as NSCLC-NOS with an explanation M

G9285 Specimen site other than anatomic location of lung or is not classified as nonsmall cell lung cancer M

G9286 Antibiotic regimen prescribed within 10 days after onset of symptoms M

G9287 Antibiotic regimen not prescribed within 10 days after onset of symptoms M

G9288 Documentation of medical reason(s) for not reporting the histological type or NSCLC-NOS classification with an explanation (e.g., a solitary fibrous tumor in a person with a history of nonsmall cell carcinoma or other documented medical reasons) M

G9289 Nonsmall cell lung cancer biopsy and cytology specimen report documents classification into specific histologic type or classified as NSCLC-NOS with an explanation M

G9290 Nonsmall cell lung cancer biopsy and cytology specimen report does not document classification into specific histologic type or classified as NSCLC-NOS with an explanation M

G9291 Specimen site other than anatomic location of lung, is not classified as nonsmall cell lung cancer or classified as NSCLC-NOS M

G9292 Documentation of medical reason(s) for not reporting PT category and a statement on thickness and ulceration and for PT1, mitotic rate (e.g., negative skin biopsies in a patient with a history of melanoma or other documented medical reasons) M

G9293 Pathology report does not include the PT category and a statement on thickness and ulceration and for PT1, mitotic rate M

G9294 Pathology report includes the PT category and a statement on thickness and ulceration and for PT1, mitotic rate M

G9295 Specimen site other than anatomic cutaneous location M

G9296 Patients with documented shared decision-making including discussion of conservative (nonsurgical) therapy (e.g., NSAIDs, analgesics, weight loss, exercise, injections) prior to the procedure M

G9297 Shared decision-making including discussion of conservative (nonsurgical) therapy (e.g., NSAIDs, analgesics, weight loss, exercise, injections) prior to the procedure, not documented, reason not given M

G9298 Patients who are evaluated for venous thromboembolic and cardiovascular risk factors within 30 days prior to the procedure (e.g., history of DVT, PE, MI, arrhythmia and stroke) M

G9299 Patients who are not evaluated for venous thromboembolic and cardiovascular risk factors within 30 days prior to the procedure including (e.g., history of DVT, PE, MI, arrhythmia and stroke, reason not given) M

G9300 Documentation of medical reason(s) for not completely infusing the prophylactic antibiotic prior to the inflation of the proximal tourniquet (e.g., a tourniquet was not used) M

G9301 Patients who had the prophylactic antibiotic completely infused prior to the inflation of the proximal tourniquet M

G9302 Prophylactic antibiotic not completely infused prior to the inflation of the proximal tourniquet, reason not given M

G9303 Operative report does not identify the prosthetic implant specifications including the prosthetic implant manufacturer, the brand name of the prosthetic implant and the size of each prosthetic implant, reason not given M

G9304 Operative report identifies the prosthetic implant specifications including the prosthetic implant manufacturer, the brand name of the prosthetic implant and the size of each prosthetic implant M

G9305 Intervention for presence of leak of endoluminal contents through an anastomosis not required M

G9306 Intervention for presence of leak of endoluminal contents through an anastomosis required M

G9307 No return to the operating room for a surgical procedure, for complications of the principal operative procedure, within 30 days of the principal operative procedure M

G9308 Unplanned return to the operating room for a surgical procedure, for complications of the principal operative procedure, within 30 days of the principal operative procedure M

G9309 No unplanned hospital readmission within 30 days of principal procedure M

G9310 Unplanned hospital readmission within 30 days of principal procedure M

G9311 No surgical site infection M

G9312 Surgical site infection M

G9313 Amoxicillin, with or without clavulanate, not prescribed as first line antibiotic at the time of diagnosis for documented reason M

G9314 Amoxicillin, with or without clavulanate, not prescribed as first line antibiotic at the time of diagnosis, reason not given M

G9315 Documentation amoxicillin, with or without clavulanate, prescribed as a first line antibiotic at the time of diagnosis M

G9316 Documentation of patient-specific risk assessment with a risk calculator based on multi-institutional clinical data, the specific risk calculator used, and communication of risk assessment from risk calculator with the patient or family M

© 2019 Optum360, LLC

G9317 Documentation of patient-specific risk assessment with a risk calculator based on multi-institutional clinical data, the specific risk calculator used, and communication of risk assessment from risk calculator with the patient or family not completed M

G9318 Imaging study named according to standardized nomenclature M

G9319 Imaging study not named according to standardized nomenclature, reason not given M

G9321 Count of previous CT (any type of CT) and cardiac nuclear medicine (myocardial perfusion) studies documented in the 12-month period prior to the current study M

G9322 Count of previous CT and cardiac nuclear medicine (myocardial perfusion) studies not documented in the 12-month period prior to the current study, reason not given M

G9326 CT studies performed not reported to a radiation dose index registry that is capable of collecting at a minimum all necessary data elements, reason not given M

G9327 CT studies performed reported to a radiation dose index registry that is capable of collecting at a minimum all necessary data elements M

G9329 DICOM format image data available to nonaffiliated external health care facilities or entities on a secure, media free, reciprocally searchable basis with patient authorization for at least a 12-month period after the study not documented in final report, reason not given M

G9344 Due to system reasons search not conducted for DICOM format images for prior patient CT imaging studies completed at nonaffiliated external health care facilities or entities within the past 12 months that are available through a secure, authorized, media-free, shared archive (e.g., nonaffiliated external health care facilities or entities does not have archival abilities through a shared archival system) M

G9345 Follow-up recommendations documented according to recommended guidelines for incidentally detected pulmonary nodules (e.g., follow-up CT imaging studies needed or that no follow-up is needed) based at a minimum on nodule size and patient risk factors M

G9347 Follow-up recommendations not documented according to recommended guidelines for incidentally detected pulmonary nodules, reason not given M

G9348 CT scan of the paranasal sinuses ordered at the time of diagnosis for documented reasons M

▲ **G9349** Jan CT scan of the paranasal sinuses ordered at the time of diagnosis or received within 28 days after date of diagnosis M

G9350 CT scan of the paranasal sinuses not ordered at the time of diagnosis or received within 28 days after date of diagnosis M

G9351 More than one CT scan of the paranasal sinuses ordered or received within 90 days after diagnosis M

G9352 More than one CT scan of the paranasal sinuses ordered or received within 90 days after the date of diagnosis, reason not given M

G9353 More than one CT scan of the paranasal sinuses ordered or received within 90 days after the date of diagnosis for documented reasons (e.g., patients with complications, second CT obtained prior to surgery, other medical reasons) M

G9354 One CT scan or no CT scan of the paranasal sinuses ordered within 90 days after the date of diagnosis M

▲ **G9355** Jan Early elective delivery or early induction not performed (less than 39 weeks gestation) M

▲ **G9356** Jan Early elective delivery or early induction performed (less than 39 week gestation) M

G9357 Post-partum screenings, evaluations and education performed M

G9358 Post-partum screenings, evaluations and education not performed M

▲ **G9359** Jan Documentation of negative or managed positive TB screen with further evidence that TB is not active prior to the treatment with a biologic immune response modifier M

G9360 No documentation of negative or managed positive TB screen M

G9361 Medical indication for induction (documentation of reason(s) for elective delivery [C-section] or early induction [e.g., hemorrhage and placental complications, hypertension, preeclampsia and eclampsia, rupture of membranes-premature or prolonged, maternal conditions complicating pregnancy/delivery, fetal conditions complicating pregnancy/delivery, late pregnancy, prior uterine surgery, or participation in clinical trial]) M

G9364 Sinusitis caused by, or presumed to be caused by, bacterial infection M

G9365 One high-risk medication ordered M

G9366 One high-risk medication not ordered M

G9367 At least two orders for the same high-risk medication M

G9368 At least two orders for the same high-risk medications not ordered M

G9380 Patient offered assistance with end of life issues during the measurement period M

G9382 Patient not offered assistance with end of life issues during the measurement period M

G9383 Patient received screening for HCV infection within the 12 month reporting period M

G9384 Documentation of medical reason(s) for not receiving annual screening for HCV infection (e.g., decompensated cirrhosis indicating advanced disease [i.e., ascites, esophageal variceal bleeding, hepatic encephalopathy], hepatocellular carcinoma, waitlist for organ transplant, limited life expectancy, other medical reasons) M

G9385 Documentation of patient reason(s) for not receiving annual screening for HCV infection (e.g., patient declined, other patient reasons) M

G9386 Screening for HCV infection not received within the twelve-month reporting period, reason not given M

G9389 Unplanned rupture of the posterior capsule requiring vitrectomy during cataract surgery M

G9390 No unplanned rupture of the posterior capsule requiring vitrectomy during cataract surgery M

G9393 Patient with an initial PHQ-9 score greater than nine who achieves remission at twelve months as demonstrated by a twelve-month (+/- 30 days) PHQ-9 score of less than five M

G9394 Patient who had a diagnosis of bipolar disorder or personality disorder, death, permanent nursing home resident or receiving hospice or palliative care any time during the measurement or assessment period M

G9395 Patient with an initial PHQ-9 score greater than nine who did not achieve remission at twelve months as demonstrated by a twelve-month (+/- 30 days) PHQ-9 score greater than or equal to five M

© 2019 Optum360, LLC

G9396 Patient with an initial PHQ-9 score greater than nine who was not assessed for remission at twelve months (+/- 30 days) M

G9399 Documentation in the patient record of a discussion between the physician/clinician and the patient that includes all of the following: treatment choices appropriate to genotype, risks and benefits, evidence of effectiveness, and patient preferences toward the outcome of the treatment M

G9400 Documentation of medical or patient reason(s) for not discussing treatment options; medical reasons: patient is not a candidate for treatment due to advanced physical or mental health comorbidity (including active substance use); currently receiving antiviral treatment; successful antiviral treatment (with sustained virologic response) prior to reporting period; other documented medical reasons; patient reasons: patient unable or unwilling to participate in the discussion or other patient reasons M

G9401 No documentation in the patient record of a discussion between the physician or other qualified health care professional and the patient that includes all of the following: treatment choices appropriate to genotype, risks and benefits, evidence of effectiveness, and patient preferences toward treatment M

G9402 Patient received follow-up on the date of discharge or within 30 days after discharge M

G9403 Clinician documented reason patient was not able to complete 30-day follow-up from acute inpatient setting discharge (e.g., patient death prior to follow-up visit, patient noncompliant for visit follow-up) M

G9404 Patient did not receive follow-up on the date of discharge or within 30 days after discharge M

▲ **G9405**[Jan] Patient received follow up within 7 days after discharge M

G9406 Clinician documented reason patient was not able to complete 7-day follow-up from acute inpatient setting discharge (i.e., patient death prior to follow-up visit, patient noncompliance for visit follow-up) M

G9407 Patient did not receive follow-up on or within 7 days after discharge M

G9408 Patients with cardiac tamponade and/or pericardiocentesis occurring within 30 days M

G9409 Patients without cardiac tamponade and/or pericardiocentesis occurring within 30 days M

G9410 Patient admitted within 180 days, status post CIED implantation, replacement, or revision with an infection requiring device removal or surgical revision M

G9411 Patient not admitted within 180 days, status post CIED implantation, replacement, or revision with an infection requiring device removal or surgical revision M

G9412 Patient admitted within 180 days, status post CIED implantation, replacement, or revision with an infection requiring device removal or surgical revision M

G9413 Patient not admitted within 180 days, status post CIED implantation, replacement, or revision with an infection requiring device removal or surgical revision M

▲ **G9414**[Jan] Patient had one dose of meningococcal vaccine (serogroups A, C, W, Y) on or between the patient's 11th and 13th birthdays M

G9415 Patient did not have one dose of meningococcal vaccine on or between the patient's 11th and 13th birthdays M

G9416 Patient had one tetanus, diphtheria toxoids and acellular pertussis vaccine (TDaP) on or between the patient's 10th and 13th birthdays M

G9417 Patient did not have one tetanus, diphtheria toxoids and acellular pertussis vaccine (TDaP) on or between the patient's 10th and 13th birthdays M

G9418 Primary nonsmall cell lung cancer biopsy and cytology specimen report documents classification into specific histologic type or classified as NSCLC-NOS with an explanation M

G9419 Documentation of medical reason(s) for not including the histological type or NSCLC-NOS classification with an explanation (e.g., biopsy taken for other purposes in a patient with a history of primary nonsmall cell lung cancer or other documented medical reasons) M

G9420 Specimen site other than anatomic location of lung or is not classified as primary nonsmall cell lung cancer M

G9421 Primary nonsmall cell lung cancer biopsy and cytology specimen report does not document classification into specific histologic type or classified as NSCLC-NOS with an explanation M

G9422 Primary lung carcinoma resection report documents PT category, PN category and for nonsmall cell lung cancer, histologic type (squamous cell carcinoma, adenocarcinoma and not NSCLC-NOS) M

G9423 Documentation of medical reason for not including PT category, PN category and histologic type (for patient with appropriate exclusion criteria [e.g., metastatic disease, benign tumors, malignant tumors other than carcinomas, inadequate surgical specimens]) M

G9424 Specimen site other than anatomic location of lung, or classified as NSCLC-NOS M

G9425 Primary lung carcinoma resection report does not document PT category, PN category and for nonsmall cell lung cancer, histologic type (squamous cell carcinoma, adenocarcinoma) M

G9426 Improvement in median time from ED arrival to initial ED oral or parenteral pain medication administration performed for ED admitted patients M

G9427 Improvement in median time from ED arrival to initial ED oral or parenteral pain medication administration not performed for ED admitted patients M

G9428 Pathology report includes the PT category and a statement on thickness, ulceration and mitotic rate M

G9429 Documentation of medical reason(s) for not including PT category and a statement on thickness, ulceration and mitotic rate (e.g., negative skin biopsies in a patient with a history of melanoma or other documented medical reasons) M

G9430 Specimen site other than anatomic cutaneous location M

G9431 Pathology report does not include the PT category and a statement on thickness, ulceration and mitotic rate M

G9432 Asthma well-controlled based on the ACT, C-ACT, ACQ, or ATAQ score and results documented M

G9434 Asthma not well-controlled based on the ACT, C-ACT, ACQ, or ATAQ score, or specified asthma control tool not used, reason not given M

G9448 Patients who were born in the years 1945-1965 M

G9449 History of receiving blood transfusions prior to 1992 A M

G9450 History of injection drug use M

G9451 Patient received one-time screening for HCV infection M

© 2019 Optum360, LLC

G9452 Documentation of medical reason(s) for not receiving one-time screening for HCV infection (e.g., decompensated cirrhosis indicating advanced disease [i.e., ascites, esophageal variceal bleeding, hepatic encephalopathy], hepatocellular carcinoma, waitlist for organ transplant, limited life expectancy, other medical reasons) M

G9453 Documentation of patient reason(s) for not receiving one-time screening for HCV infection (e.g., patient declined, other patient reasons) M

G9454 One-time screening for HCV infection not received within 12-month reporting period and no documentation of prior screening for HCV infection, reason not given M

G9455 Patient underwent abdominal imaging with ultrasound, contrast enhanced CT or contrast MRI for HCC M

G9456 Documentation of medical or patient reason(s) for not ordering or performing screening for HCC. Medical reason: comorbid medical conditions with expected survival < 5 years, hepatic decompensation and not a candidate for liver transplantation, or other medical reasons; patient reasons: patient declined or other patient reasons (e.g., cost of tests, time related to accessing testing equipment) M

G9457 Patient did not undergo abdominal imaging and did not have a documented reason for not undergoing abdominal imaging in the submission period M

G9458 Patient documented as tobacco user and received tobacco cessation intervention (must include at least one of the following: advice given to quit smoking or tobacco use, counseling on the benefits of quitting smoking or tobacco use, assistance with or referral to external smoking or tobacco cessation support programs, or current enrollment in smoking or tobacco use cessation program) if identified as a tobacco user M

G9459 Currently a tobacco nonuser M

G9460 Tobacco assessment or tobacco cessation intervention not performed, reason not given M

G9468 Patient not receiving corticosteroids greater than or equal to 10 mg/day of prednisone equivalents for 60 or greater consecutive days or a single prescription equating to 600 mg prednisone or greater for all fills M

▲ **G9469**Jan Patients who have received or are receiving corticosteroids greater than or equal to 10 mg/day of prednisone equivalents for 90 or greater consecutive days or a single prescription equating to 900 mg prednisone or greater for all fills M

G9470 Patients not receiving corticosteroids greater than or equal to 10 mg/day of prednisone equivalents for 60 or greater consecutive days or a single prescription equating to 600 mg prednisone or greater for all fills M

G9471 Within the past 2 years, central dual-energy x-ray absorptiometry (DXA) not ordered or documented M

G9472 Jan ~~Within the past 2 years, central dual-energy x-ray absorptiometry (DXA) not ordered and documented, no review of systems and no medication history or pharmacologic therapy (other than minerals/vitamins) for osteoporosis prescribed~~

Hospice Services

G9473 Services performed by chaplain in the hospice setting, each 15 minutes B

G9474 Services performed by dietary counselor in the hospice setting, each 15 minutes B

G9475 Services performed by other counselor in the hospice setting, each 15 minutes B

G9476 Services performed by volunteer in the hospice setting, each 15 minutes B

G9477 Services performed by care coordinator in the hospice setting, each 15 minutes B

G9478 Services performed by other qualified therapist in the hospice setting, each 15 minutes B

G9479 Services performed by qualified pharmacist in the hospice setting, each 15 minutes B

Medicare Care Choice Model Program

G9480 Admission to Medicare Care Choice Model Program (MCCM) B

CMS Innovation Center Demonstration Project

G9481 Remote in-home visit for the evaluation and management of a new patient for use only in a Medicare-approved CMS Innovation Center Demonstration Project, which requires these three key components: a problem focused history; a problem focused examination; straightforward medical decision making, furnished in real time using interactive audio and video technology. Counseling and coordination of care with other physicians, other qualified health care professionals or agencies are provided consistent with the nature of the problem(s) and the needs of the patient or the family or both. Usually, the presenting problem(s) are self limited or minor. Typically, 10 minutes are spent with the patient or family or both via real time, audio and video intercommunications technology B

G9482 Remote in-home visit for the evaluation and management of a new patient for use only in a Medicare-approved CMS Innovation Center Demonstration Project, which requires these three key components: an expanded problem focused history; an expanded problem focused examination; straightforward medical decision making, furnished in real time using interactive audio and video technology. Counseling and coordination of care with other physicians, other qualified health care professionals or agencies are provided consistent with the nature of the problem(s) and the needs of the patient or the family or both. Usually, the presenting problem(s) are of low to moderate severity. Typically, 20 minutes are spent with the patient or family or both via real time, audio and video intercommunications technology B

G9483 Remote in-home visit for the evaluation and management of a new patient for use only in a Medicare-approved CMS Innovation Center Demonstration Project, which requires these three key components: a detailed history; a detailed examination; medical decision making of low complexity, furnished in real time using interactive audio and video technology. Counseling and coordination of care with other physicians, other qualified health care professionals or agencies are provided consistent with the nature of the problem(s) and the needs of the patient or the family or both. Usually, the presenting problem(s) are of moderate severity. Typically, 30 minutes are spent with the patient or family or both via real time, audio and video intercommunications technology B

G9484 Remote in-home visit for the evaluation and management of a new patient for use only in a Medicare-approved CMS Innovation Center Demonstration Project, which requires these three key components: a comprehensive history; a comprehensive examination; medical decision making of moderate complexity, furnished in real time using interactive audio and video technology. Counseling and coordination of care with other physicians, other qualified health care professionals or agencies are provided consistent with the nature of the problem(s) and the needs of the patient or the family or both. Usually, the presenting problem(s) are of moderate to high severity. Typically, 45 minutes are spent with the patient or family or both via real time, audio and video intercommunications technology B

© 2019 Optum360, LLC

G9485 Remote in-home visit for the evaluation and management of a new patient for use only in a Medicare-approved CMS Innovation Center Demonstration Project, which requires these three key components: a comprehensive history; a comprehensive examination; medical decision making of high complexity, furnished in real time using interactive audio and video technology. Counseling and coordination of care with other physicians, other qualified health care professionals or agencies are provided consistent with the nature of the problem(s) and the needs of the patient or the family or both. Usually, the presenting problem(s) are of moderate to high severity. Typically, 60 minutes are spent with the patient or family or both via real time, audio and video intercommunications technology [B]

G9486 Remote in-home visit for the evaluation and management of an established patient for use only in a Medicare-approved CMS Innovation Center Demonstration Project, which requires at least two of the following three key components: a problem focused history; a problem focused examination; straightforward medical decision making, furnished in real time using interactive audio and video technology. Counseling and coordination of care with other physicians, other qualified health care professionals or agencies are provided consistent with the nature of the problem(s) and the needs of the patient or the family or both. Usually, the presenting problem(s) are self limited or minor. Typically, 10 minutes are spent with the patient or family or both via real time, audio and video intercommunications technology [B]

G9487 Remote in-home visit for the evaluation and management of an established patient for use only in a Medicare-approved CMS Innovation Center Demonstration Project, which requires at least two of the following three key components: an expanded problem focused history; an expanded problem focused examination; medical decision making of low complexity, furnished in real time using interactive audio and video technology. Counseling and coordination of care with other physicians, other qualified health care professionals or agencies are provided consistent with the nature of the problem(s) and the needs of the patient or the family or both. Usually, the presenting problem(s) are of low to moderate severity. Typically, 15 minutes are spent with the patient or family or both via real time, audio and video intercommunications technology [B]

G9488 Remote in-home visit for the evaluation and management of an established patient for use only in a Medicare-approved CMS Innovation Center Demonstration Project, which requires at least two of the following three key components: a detailed history; a detailed examination; medical decision making of moderate complexity, furnished in real time using interactive audio and video technology. Counseling and coordination of care with other physicians, other qualified health care professionals or agencies are provided consistent with the nature of the problem(s) and the needs of the patient or the family or both. Usually, the presenting problem(s) are of moderate to high severity. Typically, 25 minutes are spent with the patient or family or both via real time, audio and video intercommunications technology [B]

G9489 Remote in-home visit for the evaluation and management of an established patient for use only in a Medicare-approved CMS Innovation Center Demonstration Project, which requires at least two of the following three key components: a comprehensive history; a comprehensive examination; medical decision making of high complexity, furnished in real time using interactive audio and video technology. Counseling and coordination of care with other physicians, other qualified health care professionals or agencies are provided consistent with the nature of the problem(s) and the needs of the patient or the family or both. Usually, the presenting problem(s) are of moderate to high severity. Typically, 40 minutes are spent with the patient or family or both via real time, audio and video intercommunications technology [B]

G9490 CMS Innovation Center Models, home visit for patient assessment performed by clinical staff for an individual not considered homebound, including, but not necessarily limited to patient assessment of clinical status, safety/fall prevention, functional status/ambulation, medication reconciliation/management, compliance with orders/plan of care, performance of activities of daily living, and ensuring beneficiary connections to community and other services. (For use only in Medicare-approved CMS Innovation Center Models); may not be billed for a 30 day period covered by a transitional care management code [B]

Quality Measures

G9497 Received instruction from the anesthesiologist or proxy prior to the day of surgery to abstain from smoking on the day of surgery [M]

G9498 Antibiotic regimen prescribed [M]

G9500 Radiation exposure indices, or exposure time and number of fluorographic images in final report for procedures using fluoroscopy, documented [M]

G9501 Radiation exposure indices, or exposure time and number of fluorographic images not documented in final report for procedure using fluoroscopy, reason not given [M]

G9502 Documentation of medical reason for not performing foot exam (i.e., patients who have had either a bilateral amputation above or below the knee, or both a left and right amputation above or below the knee before or during the measurement period) [M]

G9503 Patient taking tamsulosin HCl ♂ [M]

G9504 Documented reason for not assessing hepatitis B virus (HBV) status (e.g., patient not initiating anti-TNF therapy, patient declined) prior to initiating anti-TNF therapy [M]

G9505 Antibiotic regimen prescribed within 10 days after onset of symptoms for documented medical reason [M]

G9506 Biologic immune response modifier prescribed [M]

G9507 Documentation that the patient is on a statin medication or has documentation of a valid contraindication or exception to statin medications; contraindications/exceptions that can be defined by diagnosis codes include pregnancy during the measurement period, active liver disease, rhabdomyolysis, end stage renal disease on dialysis and heart failure; provider documented contraindications/exceptions include breastfeeding during the measurement period, woman of child-bearing age not actively taking birth control, allergy to statin, drug interaction (HIV protease inhibitors, nefazodone, cyclosporine, gemfibrozil, and danazol) and intolerance (with supporting documentation of trying a statin at least once within the last 5 years or diagnosis codes for myostitis or toxic myopathy related to drugs) [M]

G9508 Documentation that the patient is not on a statin medication [M]

© 2019 Optum360, LLC

G9509 Adult patients 18 years of age or older with major depression or dysthymia who reached remission at twelve months as demonstrated by a twelve-month (+/-60 days) PHQ-9 or PHQ-9M score of less than 5 M

▲ **G9510** Jan Adult patients 18 years of age or older with major depression or dysthymia who did not reach remission at 12 months as demonstrated by a 12 month (+/-60 days) PHQ-9 or PHQ-9M score of less than 5. Either PHQ-9 or PHQ-9M score was not assessed or is greater than or equal to 5 M

G9511 Index PHQ-9 or PHQ-9M score greater than 9 documented during the twelve-month denominator identification period M

G9512 Individual had a PDC of 0.8 or greater M

G9513 Individual did not have a PDC of 0.8 or greater M

G9514 Patient required a return to the operating room within 90 days of surgery M

G9515 Patient did not require a return to the operating room within 90 days of surgery M

G9516 Patient achieved an improvement in visual acuity, from their preoperative level, within 90 days of surgery M

G9517 Patient did not achieve an improvement in visual acuity, from their preoperative level, within 90 days of surgery, reason not given M

G9518 Documentation of active injection drug use M

▲ **G9519** Jan Patient achieves final refraction (spherical equivalent) +/- 1.0 diopters of their planned refraction within 90 days of surgery M

▲ **G9520** Jan Patient does not achieve final refraction (spherical equivalent) +/- 1.0 diopters of their planned refraction within 90 days of surgery M

G9521 Total number of emergency department visits and inpatient hospitalizations less than two in the past 12 months M

G9522 Total number of emergency department visits and inpatient hospitalizations equal to or greater than two in the past 12 months or patient not screened, reason not given M

G9523 Patient discontinued from hemodialysis or peritoneal dialysis M

Hospice Care

G9524 Patient was referred to hospice care M

G9525 Documentation of patient reason(s) for not referring to hospice care (e.g., patient declined, other patient reasons) M

G9526 Patient was not referred to hospice care, reason not given M

Blunt Head Trauma

G9529 Patient with minor blunt head trauma had an appropriate indication(s) for a head CT M

G9530 Patient presented with a minor blunt head trauma and had a head CT ordered for trauma by an emergency care provider M

▲ **G9531** Jan Patient has documentation of ventricular shunt, brain tumor, multisystem trauma, or is currently taking an antiplatelet medication including: abciximab, anagrelide, cangrelor, cilostazol, clopidogrel, dipyridamole, eptifibatide, prasugrel, ticlopidine, ticagrelor, tirofiban, or vorapaxar M

G9532 Patient had a head CT for trauma ordered by someone other than an emergency care provider or was ordered for a reason other than trauma M

G9533 Patient with minor blunt head trauma did not have an appropriate indication(s) for a head CT M

Miscellaneous Quality Measures

G9539 Intent for potential removal at time of placement M

G9540 Patient alive 3 months post procedure M

G9541 Filter removed within 3 months of placement M

G9542 Documented reassessment for the appropriateness of filter removal within 3 months of placement M

G9543 Documentation of at least two attempts to reach the patient to arrange a clinical reassessment for the appropriateness of filter removal within 3 months of placement M

G9544 Patients that do not have the filter removed, documented reassessment for the appropriateness of filter removal, or documentation of at least two attempts to reach the patient to arrange a clinical reassessment for the appropriateness of filter removal within 3 months of placement M

▲ **G9547** Jan Cystic renal lesion that is simple appearing (Bosniak I or II), or adrenal lesion less than or equal to 1.0 cm or adrenal lesion greater than 1.0 cm but less than or equal to 4.0 cm classified as likely benign by unenhanced CT or washout protocol CT, or MRI with in- and opposed-phase sequences or other equivalent institutional imaging protocols M

▲ **G9548** Jan Final reports for imaging studies stating no follow up imaging is recommended M

▲ **G9549** Jan Documentation of medical reason(s) that follow up imaging is indicated (e.g., patient has lymphadenopathy, signs of metastasis or an active diagnosis or history of cancer, and other medical reason(s)) M

▲ **G9550** Jan Final reports for imaging studies with follow up imaging recommended M

▲ **G9551** Jan Final reports for imaging studies without an incidentally found lesion noted M

G9552 Incidental thyroid nodule < 1.0 cm noted in report M

G9553 Prior thyroid disease diagnosis M

G9554 Final reports for CT, CTA, MRI or MRA of the chest or neck or ultrasound of the neck with follow-up imaging recommended M

G9555 Documentation of medical reason(s) for recommending follow up imaging (e.g., patient has multiple endocrine neoplasia, patient has cervical lymphadenopathy, other medical reason(s)) M

G9556 Final reports for CT, CTA, MRI or MRA of the chest or neck or ultrasound of the neck with follow-up imaging not recommended M

G9557 Final reports for CT, CTA, MRI or MRA studies of the chest or neck or ultrasound of the neck without an incidentally found thyroid nodule < 1.0 cm noted or no nodule found M

G9558 Patient treated with a beta-lactam antibiotic as definitive therapy M

G9559 Documentation of medical reason(s) for not prescribing a beta-lactam antibiotic (e.g., allergy, intolerance to beta-lactam antibiotics) M

G9560 Patient not treated with a beta-lactam antibiotic as definitive therapy, reason not given M

Opiate Therapy

G9561 Patients prescribed opiates for longer than six weeks M

G9562 Patients who had a follow-up evaluation conducted at least every three months during opioid therapy M

© 2019 Optum360, LLC

G9563 Patients who did not have a follow-up evaluation conducted at least every three months during opioid therapy M

G9573 Adult patients 18 years of age or older with major depression or dysthymia who did not reach remission at six months as demonstrated by a six-month (+/-60 days) PHQ-9 or PHQ-9M score of less than five M

G9574 Adult patients 18 years of age or older with major depression or dysthymia who did not reach remission at six months as demonstrated by a six-month (+/-60 days) PHQ-9 or PHQ-9M score of less than five; either PHQ-9 or PHQ-9M score was not assessed or is greater than or equal to five M

G9577 Patients prescribed opiates for longer than six weeks M

G9578 Documentation of signed opioid treatment agreement at least once during opioid therapy M

G9579 No documentation of a signed opioid treatment agreement at least once during opioid therapy M

Stroke Therapy

G9580 Door to puncture time of less than 2 hours M

G9582 Door to puncture time of greater than 2 hours, no reason given M

Opiate Therapy

G9583 Patients prescribed opiates for longer than six weeks M

G9584 Patient evaluated for risk of misuse of opiates by using a brief validated instrument (e.g., opioid risk tool, SOAPP-R) or patient interviewed at least once during opioid therapy M

G9585 Patient not evaluated for risk of misuse of opiates by using a brief validated instrument (e.g., opioid risk tool, SOAAP-R) or patient not interviewed at least once during opioid therapy M

Blunt Head Trauma

G9593 Pediatric patient with minor blunt head trauma classified as low risk according to the PECARN prediction rules M

G9594 Patient presented with a minor blunt head trauma and had a head CT ordered for trauma by an emergency care provider M

▲ G9595 Jan Patient has documentation of ventricular shunt, brain tumor, or coagulopathy M

G9596 Pediatric patient had a head CT for trauma ordered by someone other than an emergency care provider or was ordered for a reason other than trauma M

G9597 Pediatric patient with minor blunt head trauma not classified as low risk according to the PECARN prediction rules M

Aortic Aneurysm

G9598 Aortic aneurysm 5.5-5.9 cm maximum diameter on centerline formatted CT or minor diameter on axial formatted CT M

G9599 Aortic aneurysm 6.0 cm or greater maximum diameter on centerline formatted CT or minor diameter on axial formatted CT M

G9600 Symptomatic AAAS that required urgent/emergent (nonelective) repair M

Discharge to Home

G9601 Patient discharge to home no later than postoperative day #7 M

G9602 Patient not discharged to home by postoperative day #7 M

Patient Survey

G9603 Patient survey score improved from baseline following treatment M

G9604 Patient survey results not available M

G9605 Patient survey score did not improve from baseline following treatment M

Intraoperative Cystoscopy

G9606 Intraoperative cystoscopy performed to evaluate for lower tract injury M

G9607 Documented medical reasons for not performing intraoperative cystoscopy (e.g., urethral pathology precluding cystoscopy, any patient who has a congenital or acquired absence of the urethra) or in the case of patient death M

G9608 Intraoperative cystoscopy not performed to evaluate for lower tract injury M

Aspirin/Antiplatelet Therapy

G9609 Documentation of an order for antiplatelet agents M

G9610 Documentation of medical reason(s) in the patient's record for not ordering antiplatelet agents M

G9611 Order for antiplatelet agents was not documented in the patient's record, reason not given M

Colonoscopy Documentation

G9612 Photodocumentation of two or more cecal landmarks to establish a complete examination M

G9613 Documentation of postsurgical anatomy (e.g., right hemicolectomy, ileocecal resection, etc.) M

G9614 Photodocumentation of less than two cecal landmarks (i.e., no cecal landmarks or only one cecal landmark) to establish a complete examination M

Preoperative Assessment

G9615 Preoperative assessment documented M

G9616 Documentation of reason(s) for not documenting a preoperative assessment (e.g., patient with a gynecologic or other pelvic malignancy noted at the time of surgery) M

G9617 Preoperative assessment not documented, reason not given M

Uterine Malignancy Screening

G9618 Documentation of screening for uterine malignancy or those that had an ultrasound and/or endometrial sampling of any kind ♀M

G9620 Patient not screened for uterine malignancy, or those that have not had an ultrasound and/or endometrial sampling of any kind, reason not given ♀M

Alcohol Use

G9621 Patient identified as an unhealthy alcohol user when screened for unhealthy alcohol use using a systematic screening method and received brief counseling M

G9622 Patient not identified as an unhealthy alcohol user when screened for unhealthy alcohol use using a systematic screening method M

G9623 Documentation of medical reason(s) for not screening for unhealthy alcohol use (e.g., limited life expectancy, other medical reasons) M

G9624 Patient not screened for unhealthy alcohol use using a systematic screening method or patient did not receive brief counseling if identified as an unhealthy alcohol user, reason not given M

© 2019 Optum360, LLC

Bladder/Ureter Injury

G9625 Patient sustained bladder injury at the time of surgery or discovered subsequently up to 30 days post-surgery M

G9626 Documented medical reason for not reporting bladder injury (e.g., gynecologic or other pelvic malignancy documented, concurrent surgery involving bladder pathology, injury that occurs during urinary incontinence procedure, patient death from nonmedical causes not related to surgery, patient died during procedure without evidence of bladder injury) M

G9627 Patient did not sustain bladder injury at the time of surgery nor discovered subsequently up to 30 days post-surgery M

G9628 Patient sustained bowel injury at the time of surgery or discovered subsequently up to 30 days post-surgery M

G9629 Documented medical reasons for not reporting bowel injury (e.g., gynecologic or other pelvic malignancy documented, planned (e.g., not due to an unexpected bowel injury) resection and/or re-anastomosis of bowel, or patient death from nonmedical causes not related to surgery, patient died during procedure without evidence of bowel injury) M

G9630 Patient did not sustain a bowel injury at the time of surgery nor discovered subsequently up to 30 days post-surgery M

G9631 Patient sustained ureter injury at the time of surgery or discovered subsequently up to 30 days postsurgery M

G9632 Documented medical reasons for not reporting ureter injury (e.g., gynecologic or other pelvic malignancy documented, concurrent surgery involving bladder pathology, injury that occurs during a urinary incontinence procedure, patient death from nonmedical causes not related to surgery, patient died during procedure without evidence of ureter injury) M

G9633 Patient did not sustain ureter injury at the time of surgery nor discovered subsequently up to 30 days postsurgery M

Health-Related Quality of Life

G9634 Health-related quality of life assessed with tool during at least two visits and quality of life score remained the same or improved M

G9635 Health-related quality of life not assessed with tool for documented reason(s) (e.g., patient has a cognitive or neuropsychiatric impairment that impairs his/her ability to complete the HRQOL survey, patient has the inability to read and/or write in order to complete the HRQOL questionnaire) M

G9636 Health-related quality of life not assessed with tool during at least two visits or quality of life score declined M

Quality Measures

G9637 Final reports with documentation of one or more dose reduction techniques (e.g., automated exposure control, adjustment of the mA and/or kV according to patient size, use of iterative reconstruction technique) M

G9638 Final reports without documentation of one or more dose reduction techniques (e.g., automated exposure control, adjustment of the mA and/or kV according to patient size, use of iterative reconstruction technique) M

G9639 Major amputation or open surgical bypass not required within 48 hours of the index endovascular lower extremity revascularization procedure M

G9640 Documentation of planned hybrid or staged procedure M

G9641 Major amputation or open surgical bypass required within 48 hours of the index endovascular lower extremity revascularization procedure M

G9642 Current smokers (e.g., cigarette, cigar, pipe, e-cigarette or marijuana) M

G9643 Elective surgery M

G9644 Patients who abstained from smoking prior to anesthesia on the day of surgery or procedure M

G9645 Patients who did not abstain from smoking prior to anesthesia on the day of surgery or procedure M

G9646 Patients with 90 day MRS score of 0 to 2 M

G9647 Patients in whom MRS score could not be obtained at 90 day follow-up M

G9648 Patients with 90 day MRS score greater than 2 M

Psoriasis Therapy

G9649 Psoriasis assessment tool documented meeting any one of the specified benchmarks (e.g., (PGA; 5-point or 6-point scale), body surface area (BSA), psoriasis area and severity index (PASI) and/or dermatology life quality index (DLQI)) M

G9651 Psoriasis assessment tool documented not meeting any one of the specified benchmarks (e.g., (PGA; 5-point or 6-point scale), body surface area (BSA), psoriasis area and severity index (PASI) and/or dermatology life quality index (DLQI)) or psoriasis assessment tool not documented M

Anesthesia Services

G9654 Monitored anesthesia care (MAC) M

G9655 A transfer of care protocol or handoff tool/checklist that includes the required key handoff elements is used M

G9656 Patient transferred directly from anesthetizing location to PACU or other non-ICU location M

G9658 A transfer of care protocol or handoff tool/checklist that includes the required key handoff elements is not used M

Reason for Colonoscopy

G9659 Patients greater than 85 years of age who did not have a history of colorectal cancer or valid medical reason for the colonoscopy, including: iron deficiency anemia, lower gastrointestinal bleeding, Crohn's disease (i.e., regional enteritis), familial adenomatous polyposis, Lynch syndrome (i.e., hereditary nonpolyposis colorectal cancer), inflammatory bowel disease, ulcerative colitis, abnormal finding of gastrointestinal tract, or changes in bowel habits M

G9660 Documentation of medical reason(s) for a colonoscopy performed on a patient greater than 85 years of age (e.g., last colonoscopy incomplete, last colonoscopy had inadequate prep, iron deficiency anemia, lower gastrointestinal bleeding, Crohn's disease (i.e., regional enteritis), familial history of adenomatous polyposis, Lynch syndrome (i.e., hereditary nonpolyposis colorectal cancer), inflammatory bowel disease, ulcerative colitis, abnormal finding of gastrointestinal tract, or changes in bowel habits) M

G9661 Patients greater than 85 years of age who received a routine colonoscopy for a reason other than the following: an assessment of signs/symptoms of GI tract illness, and/or the patient is considered high risk, and/or to follow-up on previously diagnosed advance lesions M

Statin Therapy

G9662 Previously diagnosed or have an active diagnosis of clinical ASCVD M

▲ **G9663** Jan Any fasting or direct LDL-C laboratory test result <= 190 mg/dl M

G9664 Patients who are currently statin therapy users or received an order (prescription) for statin therapy M

© 2019 Optum360, LLC

G9665 Patients who are not currently statin therapy users or did not receive an order (prescription) for statin therapy M

G9666 The highest fasting or direct LDL-C laboratory test result of 70/189 mg/dl in the measurement period or two years prior to the beginning of the measurement period M

Cardiovascular Measures

G9674 Patients with clinical ASCVD diagnosis M

G9675 Patients who have ever had a fasting or direct laboratory result of LDL-C = 190 mg/dl M

G9676 Patients aged 40 to 75 years at the beginning of the measurement period with type 1 or type 2 diabetes and with an LDL-C result of 70/189 mg/dl recorded as the highest fasting or direct laboratory test result in the measurement year or during the two years prior to the beginning of the measurement period M

Oncology Demonstration Project

G9678 Oncology Care Model (OCM) Monthly Enhanced Oncology Services (MEOS) payment for OCM-enhanced services. G9678 payments may only be made to OCM practitioners for OCM beneficiaries for the furnishment of enhanced services as defined in the OCM participation agreement B

G9678 may only be billed for OCM beneficiaries by OCM practitioners.

Nursing Facility Care

G9679 Onsite acute care treatment of a nursing facility resident with pneumonia. May only be billed once per day per beneficiary B

G9680 Onsite acute care treatment of a nursing facility resident with CHF. May only be billed once per day per beneficiary B

G9681 Onsite acute care treatment of a nursing facility resident with COPD or asthma. May only be billed once per day per beneficiary B

G9682 Onsite acute care treatment of a nursing facility resident with a skin infection. May only be billed once per day per beneficiary B

G9683 Facility service(s) for the onsite acute care treatment of a nursing facility resident with fluid or electrolyte disorder. (May only be billed once per day per beneficiary.) This service is for a demonstration project B

G9684 Onsite acute care treatment of a nursing facility resident for a UTI. May only be billed once per day per beneficiary B

G9685 Physician service or other qualified health care professional for the evaluation and management of a beneficiary's acute change in condition in a nursing facility. This service is for a demonstration project M

Other Quality Measures

G9687 Hospice services provided to patient any time during the measurement period M

G9688 Patients using hospice services any time during the measurement period M

G9689 Patient admitted for performance of elective carotid intervention M

G9690 Patient receiving hospice services any time during the measurement period M

G9691 Patient had hospice services any time during the measurement period M

G9692 Hospice services received by patient any time during the measurement period M

G9693 Patient use of hospice services any time during the measurement period M

G9694 Hospice services utilized by patient any time during the measurement period M

G9695 Long-acting inhaled bronchodilator prescribed M

G9696 Documentation of medical reason(s) for not prescribing a long-acting inhaled bronchodilator M

G9697 Documentation of patient reason(s) for not prescribing a long-acting inhaled bronchodilator M

G9698 Documentation of system reason(s) for not prescribing a long-acting inhaled bronchodilator M

G9699 Long-acting inhaled bronchodilator not prescribed, reason not otherwise specified M

G9700 Patients who use hospice services any time during the measurement period M

G9701 Children who are taking antibiotics in the 30 days prior to the date of the encounter during which the diagnosis was established M

G9702 Patients who use hospice services any time during the measurement period M

G9703 Children who are taking antibiotics in the 30 days prior to the diagnosis of pharyngitis M

G9704 AJCC breast cancer Stage I: T1 mic or T1a documented M

G9705 AJCC breast cancer Stage I: T1b (tumor > 0.5 cm but <= 1 cm in greatest dimension) documented M

G9706 Low (or very low) risk of recurrence, prostate cancer M

G9707 Patient received hospice services any time during the measurement period M

G9708 Women who had a bilateral mastectomy or who have a history of a bilateral mastectomy or for whom there is evidence of a right and a left unilateral mastectomy M

G9709 Hospice services used by patient any time during the measurement period M

G9710 Patient was provided hospice services any time during the measurement period M

G9711 Patients with a diagnosis or past history of total colectomy or colorectal cancer M

G9712 Documentation of medical reason(s) for prescribing or dispensing antibiotic (e.g., intestinal infection, pertussis, bacterial infection, lyme disease, otitis media, acute sinusitis, acute pharyngitis, acute tonsillitis, chronic sinusitis, infection of the pharynx/larynx/tonsils/adenoids, prostatitis, cellulitis/mastoiditis/bone infections, acute lymphadenitis, impetigo, skin staph infections, pneumonia, gonococcal infections/venereal disease (syphilis, chlamydia, inflammatory diseases [female reproductive organs]), infections of the kidney, cystitis/UTI, acne, HIV disease/asymptomatic HIV, cystic fibrosis, disorders of the immune system, malignancy neoplasms, chronic bronchitis, emphysema, bronchiectasis, extrinsic allergic alveolitis, chronic airway obstruction, chronic obstructive asthma, pneumoconiosis and other lung disease due to external agents, other diseases of the respiratory system, and tuberculosis M

G9713 Patients who use hospice services any time during the measurement period M

G9714 Patient is using hospice services any time during the measurement period M

© 2019 Optum360, LLC

G9715 Patients who use hospice services any time during the measurement period M

G9716 BMI is documented as being outside of normal limits, follow-up plan is not completed for documented reason M

G9717 Documentation stating the patient has an active diagnosis of depression or has diagnosed bipolar disorder, therefore screening or follow-up not required M

G9718 Hospice services for patient provided any time during the measurement period M

G9719 Patient is not ambulatory, bed ridden, immobile, confined to chair, wheelchair bound, dependent on helper pushing wheelchair, independent in wheelchair or minimal help in wheelchair M

G9720 Hospice services for patient occurred any time during the measurement period M

G9721 Patient not ambulatory, bed ridden, immobile, confined to chair, wheelchair bound, dependent on helper pushing wheelchair, independent in wheelchair or minimal help in wheelchair M

G9722 Documented history of renal failure or baseline serum creatinine = 4.0 mg/dl; renal transplant recipients are not considered to have preoperative renal failure, unless, since transplantation the CR has been or is 4.0 or higher M

G9723 Hospice services for patient received any time during the measurement period M

G9724 Patients who had documentation of use of anticoagulant medications overlapping the measurement year M

G9725 Patients who use hospice services any time during the measurement period M

G9726 Patient refused to participate M

▲ **G9727**Jan Patient unable to complete the knee FS PROM at initial evaluation and/or discharge due to blindness, illiteracy, severe mental incapacity or language incompatibility and an adequate proxy is not available M

G9728 Patient refused to participate M

▲ **G9729**Jan Patient unable to complete the hip FS PROM at initial evaluation and discharge due to blindness, illiteracy, severe mental incapacity or language incompatibility and an adequate proxy is not available M

G9730 Patient refused to participate M

▲ **G9731**Jan Patient unable to complete the ankle/foot FS PROM at initial evaluation and/or discharge due to blindness, illiteracy, severe mental incapacity or language incompatibility and an adequate proxy is not available M

G9732 Patient refused to participate M

▲ **G9733**Jan Patient unable to complete the low back FS PROM at initial evaluation and/or discharge due to blindness, illiteracy, severe mental incapacity or language incompatibility and an adequate proxy is not available M

G9734 Patient refused to participate M

▲ **G9735**Jan Patient unable to complete the shoulder FS PROM at initial evaluation and/or discharge due to blindness, illiteracy, severe mental incapacity or language incompatibility and an adequate proxy is not available M

G9736 Patient refused to participate M

▲ **G9737**Jan Patient unable to complete the elbow/wrist/hand FS PROM at initial evaluation and/or discharge due to blindness, illiteracy, severe mental incapacity or language incompatibility and an adequate proxy is not available M

G9738 Patient refused to participate M

▲ **G9739**Jan Patient unable to complete the general orthopedic FS PROM at initial evaluation and/or discharge due to blindness, illiteracy, severe mental incapacity or language incompatibility and an adequate proxy is not available M

G9740 Hospice services given to patient any time during the measurement period M

G9741 Patients who use hospice services any time during the measurement period M

~~**G9742**Jan Psychiatric symptoms assessed~~

~~**G9743**Jan Psychiatric symptoms not assessed, reason not otherwise specified~~

G9744 Patient not eligible due to active diagnosis of hypertension M

G9745 Documented reason for not screening or recommending a follow-up for high blood pressure M

G9746 Patient has mitral stenosis or prosthetic heart valves or patient has transient or reversible cause of AF (e.g., pneumonia, hyperthyroidism, pregnancy, cardiac surgery) M

G9747 Patient is undergoing palliative dialysis with a catheter M

G9748 Patient approved by a qualified transplant program and scheduled to receive a living donor kidney transplant M

G9749 Patient is undergoing palliative dialysis with a catheter M

G9750 Patient approved by a qualified transplant program and scheduled to receive a living donor kidney transplant M

G9751 Patient died at any time during the 24-month measurement period M

G9752 Emergency surgery M

G9753 Documentation of medical reason for not conducting a search for DICOM format images for prior patient CT imaging studies completed at nonaffiliated external healthcare facilities or entities within the past 12 months that are available through a secure, authorized, media-free, shared archive (e.g., trauma, acute myocardial infarction, stroke, aortic aneurysm where time is of the essence) M

G9754 A finding of an incidental pulmonary nodule M

G9755 Documentation of medical reason(s) for not including a recommended interval and modality for follow-up or for no follow-up, and source of recommendations (e.g., patients with unexplained fever, immunocompromised patients who are at risk for infection) M

G9756 Surgical procedures that included the use of silicone oil M

G9757 Surgical procedures that included the use of silicone oil M

G9758 Patient in hospice at any time during the measurement period M

G9759 History of preoperative posterior capsule rupture M

G9760 Patients who use hospice services any time during the measurement period M

G9761 Patients who use hospice services any time during the measurement period M

G9762 Patient had at least two HPV vaccines (with at least 146 days between the two) or three HPV vaccines on or between the patient's 9th and 13th birthdays M

G9763 Patient did not have at least two HPV vaccines (with at least 146 days between the two) or three HPV vaccines on or between the patient's 9th and 13th birthdays M

G9764 Patient has been treated with a systemic medication for psoriasis vulgaris M

© 2019 Optum360, LLC

G9765 Documentation that the patient declined change in medication or alternative therapies were unavailable, has documented contraindications, or has not been treated with a systemic medication for at least six consecutive months (e.g., experienced adverse effects or lack of efficacy with all other therapy options) in order to achieve better disease control as measured by PGA, BSA, PASI, or DLQI M

G9766 Patients who are transferred from one institution to another with a known diagnosis of CVA for endovascular stroke treatment M

G9767 Hospitalized patients with newly diagnosed CVA considered for endovascular stroke treatment M

G9768 Patients who utilize hospice services any time during the measurement period M

G9769 Patient had a bone mineral density test in the past two years or received osteoporosis medication or therapy in the past 12 months M

G9770 Peripheral nerve block (PNB) M

G9771 At least one body temperature measurement equal to or greater than 35.5 degrees celsius (or 95.9 degrees fahrenheit) achieved within the 30 minutes immediately before or the 15 minutes immediately after anesthesia end time M

▲ G9772 Jan Documentation of medical reason(s) for not achieving at least one body temperature measurement equal to or greater than 35.5 degrees Celsius (or 95.9 degrees Fahrenheit) within the 30 minutes immediately before or the 15 minutes immediately after anesthesia end time (e.g., emergency cases, intentional hypothermia, etc.) M

G9773 At least one body temperature measurement equal to or greater than 35.5 degrees celsius (or 95.9 degrees fahrenheit) not achieved within the 30 minutes immediately before or the 15 minutes immediately after anesthesia end time, reason not given M

G9774 Patients who have had a hysterectomy M

G9775 Patient received at least two prophylactic pharmacologic antiemetic agents of different classes preoperatively and/or intraoperatively M

G9776 Documentation of medical reason for not receiving at least two prophylactic pharmacologic antiemetic agents of different classes preoperatively and/or intraoperatively (e.g., intolerance or other medical reason) M

G9777 Patient did not receive at least two prophylactic pharmacologic antiemetic agents of different classes preoperatively and/or intraoperatively M

G9778 Patients who have a diagnosis of pregnancy M

G9779 Patients who are breastfeeding M

G9780 Patients who have a diagnosis of rhabdomyolysis M

▲ G9781 Jan Documentation of medical reason(s) for not currently being a statin therapy user or receive an order (prescription) for statin therapy (e.g., patient with adverse effect, allergy or intolerance to statin medication therapy, patients who are receiving palliative or hospice care, patients with active liver disease or hepatic disease or insufficiency, and patients with end stage renal disease (ESRD)) M

G9782 History of or active diagnosis of familial or pure hypercholesterolemia M

G9783 Documentation of patients with diabetes who have a most recent fasting or direct LDL- C laboratory test result < 70 mg/dl and are not taking statin therapy M

G9784 Pathologists/dermatopathologists providing a second opinion on a biopsy M

▲ G9785 Jan Pathology report diagnosing cutaneous basal cell carcinoma, squamous cell carcinoma, or melanoma (to include in situ disease) sent from the pathologist/dermatopathologist to the biopsying clinician for review within 7 days from the time when the tissue specimen was received by the pathologist M

▲ G9786 Jan Pathology report diagnosing cutaneous basal cell carcinoma, squamous cell carcinoma, or melanoma (to include in situ disease) was not sent from the pathologist/dermatopathologist to the biopsying clinician for review within 7 days from the time when the tissue specimen was received by the pathologist M

G9787 Patient alive as of the last day of the measurement year M

G9788 Most recent BP is less than or equal to 140/90 mm Hg M

G9789 Blood pressure recorded during inpatient stays, emergency room visits, urgent care visits, and patient self-reported BP's (home and health fair BP results) M

G9790 Most recent BP is greater than 140/90 mm Hg, or blood pressure not documented M

G9791 Most recent tobacco status is tobacco free M

G9792 Most recent tobacco status is not tobacco free M

G9793 Patient is currently on a daily aspirin or other antiplatelet M

G9794 Documentation of medical reason(s) for not on a daily aspirin or other antiplatelet (e.g., history of gastrointestinal bleed, intracranial bleed, idiopathic thrombocytopenic purpura (ITP), gastric bypass or documentation of active anticoagulant use during the measurement period) M

G9795 Patient is not currently on a daily aspirin or other antiplatelet M

G9796 Patient is currently on a statin therapy M

G9797 Patient is not on a statin therapy M

▲ G9798 Jan Discharge(s) for AMI between July 1 of the year prior measurement period to June 30 of the measurement period M

G9799 Patients with a medication dispensing event indicator of a history of asthma any time during the patient's history through the end of the measure period M

G9800 Patients who are identified as having an intolerance or allergy to beta-blocker therapy M

G9801 Hospitalizations in which the patient was transferred directly to a nonacute care facility for any diagnosis M

G9802 Patients who use hospice services any time during the measurement period M

G9803 Patient prescribed at least a 135-day treatment within the 180-day measurement interval with beta-blockers postdischarge for AMI M

G9804 Patient was not prescribed at least a 135-day treatment within the 180-day measurement interval with beta-blockers postdischarge for AMI M

G9805 Patients who use hospice services any time during the measurement period M

G9806 Patients who received cervical cytology or an HPV test M

G9807 Patients who did not receive cervical cytology or an HPV test M

G9808 Any patients who had no asthma controller medications dispensed during the measurement year M

© 2019 Optum360, LLC

G9809 Patients who use hospice services any time during the measurement period [M]

G9810 Patient achieved a PDC of at least 75% for their asthma controller medication [M]

G9811 Patient did not achieve a PDC of at least 75% for their asthma controller medication [M]

G9812 Patient died including all deaths occurring during the hospitalization in which the operation was performed, even if after 30 days, and those deaths occurring after discharge from the hospital, but within 30 days of the procedure [M]

G9813 Patient did not die within 30 days of the procedure or during the index hospitalization [M]

G9814 Death occurring during the index acute care hospitalization [M]

G9815 Death did not occur during the index acute care hospitalization [M]

G9816 Death occurring after discharge from the hospital but within 30 days post procedure [M]

G9817 Death did not occur after discharge from the hospital within 30 days post procedure [M]

G9818 Documentation of sexual activity [M]

G9819 Patients who use hospice services any time during the measurement period [M]

G9820 Documentation of a chlamydia screening test with proper follow-up [M]

G9821 No documentation of a chlamydia screening test with proper follow-up [M]

G9822 Women who had an endometrial ablation procedure during the year prior to the index date (exclusive of the index date) [M]

G9823 Endometrial sampling or hysteroscopy with biopsy and results documented [M]

G9824 Endometrial sampling or hysteroscopy with biopsy and results not documented [M]

G9825 HER2/neu negative or undocumented/unknown [M]

G9826 Patient transferred to practice after initiation of chemotherapy [M]

G9827 HER2-targeted therapies not administered during the initial course of treatment [M]

G9828 HER2-targeted therapies administered during the initial course of treatment [M]

G9829 Breast adjuvant chemotherapy administered [M]

G9830 HER2/neu positive [M]

G9831 AJCC Stage at breast cancer diagnosis = II or III [M]

G9832 AJCC Stage at breast cancer diagnosis = I (Ia or Ib) and T-Stage at breast cancer diagnosis does not equal = T1, T1a, T1b [M]

G9833 Patient transfer to practice after initiation of chemotherapy [M]

G9834 Patient has metastatic disease at diagnosis [M]

G9835 Trastuzumab administered within 12 months of diagnosis [M]

G9836 Reason for not administering trastuzumab documented (e.g., patient declined, patient died, patient transferred, contraindication or other clinical exclusion, neoadjuvant chemotherapy or radiation not complete) [M]

G9837 Trastuzumab not administered within 12 months of diagnosis [M]

G9838 Patient has metastatic disease at diagnosis [M]

G9839 Anti-EGFR monoclonal antibody therapy [M]

G9840 RAS (KRAS and NRAS) gene mutation testing performed before initiation of anti-EGFR MoAb [M]

G9841 RAS (KRAS and NRAS) gene mutation testing not performed before initiation of anti-EGFR MoAb [M]

G9842 Patient has metastatic disease at diagnosis [M]

G9843 RAS (KRAS or NRAS) gene mutation [M]

G9844 Patient did not receive anti-EGFR monoclonal antibody therapy [M]

G9845 Patient received anti-EGFR monoclonal antibody therapy [M]

G9846 Patients who died from cancer [M]

G9847 Patient received chemotherapy in the last 14 days of life [M]

G9848 Patient did not receive chemotherapy in the last 14 days of life [M]

G9849 Patients who died from cancer [M]

G9850 Patient had more than one emergency department visit in the last 30 days of life [M]

G9851 Patient had one or less emergency department visits in the last 30 days of life [M]

G9852 Patients who died from cancer [M]

G9853 Patient admitted to the ICU in the last 30 days of life [M]

G9854 Patient was not admitted to the ICU in the last 30 days of life [M]

G9855 Patients who died from cancer [M]

G9856 Patient was not admitted to hospice [M]

G9857 Patient admitted to hospice [M]

G9858 Patient enrolled in hospice [M]

G9859 Patients who died from cancer [M]

G9860 Patient spent less than three days in hospice care [M]

G9861 Patient spent greater than or equal to three days in hospice care [M]

G9862 Documentation of medical reason(s) for not recommending at least a 10 year follow-up interval (e.g., inadequate prep, familial or personal history of colonic polyps, patient had no adenoma and age is = 66 years old, or life expectancy < 10 years old, other medical reasons) [M]

G9868 Receipt and analysis of remote, asynchronous images for dermatologic and/or ophthalmologic evaluation, for use under the Next Generation ACO model, less than 10 minutes [B]

G9869 Receipt and analysis of remote, asynchronous images for dermatologic and/or ophthalmologic evaluation, for use under the Next Generation ACO model, 10-20 minutes [B]

G9870 Receipt and analysis of remote, asynchronous images for dermatologic and/or ophthalmologic evaluation, for use under the Next Generation ACO model, 20 or more minutes [B]

G9873 First Medicare Diabetes Prevention Program (MDPP) core session was attended by an MDPP beneficiary under the MDPP Expanded Model (EM). A core session is an MDPP service that: (1) is furnished by an MDPP supplier during months 1 through 6 of the MDPP services period; (2) is approximately 1 hour in length; and (3) adheres to a CDC-approved DPP curriculum for core sessions [M]

© 2019 Optum360, LLC

G9874 Four total Medicare Diabetes Prevention Program (MDPP) core sessions were attended by an MDPP beneficiary under the MDPP Expanded Model (EM). A core session is an MDPP service that: (1) is furnished by an MDPP supplier during months 1 through 6 of the MDPP services period; (2) is approximately 1 hour in length; and (3) adheres to a CDC-approved DPP curriculum for core sessions M

G9875 Nine total Medicare Diabetes Prevention Program (MDPP) core sessions were attended by an MDPP beneficiary under the MDPP Expanded Model (EM). A core session is an MDPP service that: (1) is furnished by an MDPP supplier during months 1 through 6 of the MDPP services period; (2) is approximately 1 hour in length; and (3) adheres to a CDC-approved DPP curriculum for core sessions M

G9876 Two Medicare Diabetes Prevention Program (MDPP) core maintenance sessions (MS) were attended by an MDPP beneficiary in months (mo) 7-9 under the MDPP Expanded Model (EM). A core maintenance session is an MDPP service that: (1) is furnished by an MDPP supplier during months 7 through 12 of the MDPP services period; (2) is approximately 1 hour in length; and (3) adheres to a CDC-approved DPP curriculum for maintenance sessions. The beneficiary did not achieve at least 5% weight loss (WL) from his/her baseline weight, as measured by at least one in-person weight measurement at a core maintenance session in months 7-9 M

G9877 Two Medicare Diabetes Prevention Program (MDPP) core maintenance sessions (MS) were attended by an MDPP beneficiary in months (mo) 10-12 under the MDPP Expanded Model (EM). A core maintenance session is an MDPP service that: (1) is furnished by an MDPP supplier during months 7 through 12 of the MDPP services period; (2) is approximately 1 hour in length; and (3) adheres to a CDC-approved DPP curriculum for maintenance sessions. The beneficiary did not achieve at least 5% weight loss (WL) from his/her baseline weight, as measured by at least one in-person weight measurement at a core maintenance session in months 10-12 M

G9878 Two Medicare Diabetes Prevention Program (MDPP) core maintenance sessions (MS) were attended by an MDPP beneficiary in months (mo) 7-9 under the MDPP Expanded Model (EM). A core maintenance session is an MDPP service that: (1) is furnished by an MDPP supplier during months 7 through 12 of the MDPP services period; (2) is approximately 1 hour in length; and (3) adheres to a CDC-approved DPP curriculum for maintenance sessions. The beneficiary achieved at least 5% weight loss (WL) from his/her baseline weight, as measured by at least one in-person weight measurement at a core maintenance session in months 7-9 M

G9879 Two Medicare Diabetes Prevention Program (MDPP) core maintenance sessions (MS) were attended by an MDPP beneficiary in months (mo) 10-12 under the MDPP Expanded Model (EM). A core maintenance session is an MDPP service that: (1) is furnished by an MDPP supplier during months 7 through 12 of the MDPP services period; (2) is approximately 1 hour in length; and (3) adheres to a CDC-approved DPP curriculum for maintenance sessions. The beneficiary achieved at least 5% weight loss (WL) from his/her baseline weight, as measured by at least one in-person weight measurement at a core maintenance session in months 10-12 M

G9880 The MDPP beneficiary achieved at least 5% weight loss (WL) from his/her baseline weight in months 1-12 of the MDPP services period under the MDPP Expanded Model (EM). This is a one-time payment available when a beneficiary first achieves at least 5% weight loss from baseline as measured by an in-person weight measurement at a core session or core maintenance session M

G9881 The MDPP beneficiary achieved at least 9% weight loss (WL) from his/her baseline weight in months 1-24 under the MDPP Expanded Model (EM). This is a one-time payment available when a beneficiary first achieves at least 9% weight loss from baseline as measured by an in-person weight measurement at a core session, core maintenance session, or ongoing maintenance session M

G9882 Two Medicare Diabetes Prevention Program (MDPP) ongoing maintenance sessions (MS) were attended by an MDPP beneficiary in months (mo) 13-15 under the MDPP Expanded Model (EM). An ongoing maintenance session is an MDPP service that: (1) is furnished by an MDPP supplier during months 13 through 24 of the MDPP services period; (2) is approximately 1 hour in length; and (3) adheres to a CDC-approved DPP curriculum for maintenance sessions. The beneficiary maintained at least 5% weight loss (WL) from his/her baseline weight, as measured by at least one in-person weight measurement at an ongoing maintenance session in months 13-15 M

G9883 Two Medicare Diabetes Prevention Program (MDPP) ongoing maintenance sessions (MS) were attended by an MDPP beneficiary in months (mo) 16-18 under the MDPP Expanded Model (EM). An ongoing maintenance session is an MDPP service that: (1) is furnished by an MDPP supplier during months 13 through 24 of the MDPP services period; (2) is approximately 1 hour in length; and (3) adheres to a CDC-approved DPP curriculum for maintenance sessions. The beneficiary maintained at least 5% weight loss (WL) from his/her baseline weight, as measured by at least one in-person weight measurement at an ongoing maintenance session in months 16-18 M

G9884 Two Medicare Diabetes Prevention Program (MDPP) ongoing maintenance sessions (MS) were attended by an MDPP beneficiary in months (mo) 19-21 under the MDPP Expanded Model (EM). An ongoing maintenance session is an MDPP service that: (1) is furnished by an MDPP supplier during months 13 through 24 of the MDPP services period; (2) is approximately 1 hour in length; and (3) adheres to a CDC-approved DPP curriculum for maintenance sessions. The beneficiary maintained at least 5% weight loss (WL) from his/her baseline weight, as measured by at least one in-person weight measurement at an ongoing maintenance session in months 19-21 M

G9885 Two Medicare Diabetes Prevention Program (MDPP) ongoing maintenance sessions (MS) were attended by an MDPP beneficiary in months (mo) 22-24 under the MDPP Expanded Model (EM). An ongoing maintenance session is an MDPP service that: (1) is furnished by an MDPP supplier during months 13 through 24 of the MDPP services period; (2) is approximately 1 hour in length; and (3) adheres to a CDC-approved DPP curriculum for maintenance sessions. The beneficiary maintained at least 5% weight loss (WL) from his/her baseline weight, as measured by at least one in-person weight measurement at an ongoing maintenance session in months 22-24 M

G9890 Bridge Payment: A one-time payment for the first Medicare Diabetes Prevention Program (MDPP) core session, core maintenance session, or ongoing maintenance session furnished by an MDPP supplier to an MDPP beneficiary during months 1-24 of the MDPP Expanded Model (EM) who has previously received MDPP services from a different MDPP supplier under the MDPP Expanded Model. A supplier may only receive one bridge payment per MDPP beneficiary M

G9891 MDPP session reported as a line-item on a claim for a payable MDPP Expanded Model (EM) HCPCS code for a session furnished by the billing supplier under the MDPP Expanded Model and counting toward achievement of the attendance performance goal for the payable MDPP Expanded Model HCPCS code. (This code is for reporting purposes only) M

© 2019 Optum360, LLC

G9892 Documentation of patient reason(s) for not performing a dilated macular examination M

G9893 Dilated macular exam was not performed, reason not otherwise specified M

G9894 Androgen deprivation therapy prescribed/administered in combination with external beam radiotherapy to the prostate M

G9895 Documentation of medical reason(s) for not prescribing/administering androgen deprivation therapy in combination with external beam radiotherapy to the prostate (e.g., salvage therapy) M

G9896 Documentation of patient reason(s) for not prescribing/administering androgen deprivation therapy in combination with external beam radiotherapy to the prostate M

G9897 Patients who were not prescribed/administered androgen deprivation therapy in combination with external beam radiotherapy to the prostate, reason not given M

▲ **G9898**[Jan] Patient age 65 or older in institutional special needs plans (SNP) or residing in long-term care with POS code 32, 33, 34, 54, or 56 for more than 90 days during the measurement period M

G9899 Screening, diagnostic, film, digital or digital breast tomosynthesis (3D) mammography results documented and reviewed M

G9900 Screening, diagnostic, film, digital or digital breast tomosynthesis (3D) mammography results were not documented and reviewed, reason not otherwise specified M

▲ **G9901**[Jan] Patient age 65 or older in institutional special needs plans (SNP) or residing in long-term care with POS code 32, 33, 34, 54, or 56 for more than 90 days during the measurement period M

G9902 Patient screened for tobacco use and identified as a tobacco user M

G9903 Patient screened for tobacco use and identified as a tobacco nonuser M

G9904 Documentation of medical reason(s) for not screening for tobacco use (e.g., limited life expectancy, other medical reason) M

G9905 Patient not screened for tobacco use, reason not given M

G9906 Patient identified as a tobacco user received tobacco cessation intervention (counseling and/or pharmacotherapy) M

G9907 Documentation of medical reason(s) for not providing tobacco cessation intervention (e.g., limited life expectancy, other medical reason) M

G9908 Patient identified as tobacco user did not receive tobacco cessation intervention (counseling and/or pharmacotherapy), reason not given M

G9909 Documentation of medical reason(s) for not providing tobacco cessation intervention if identified as a tobacco user (e.g., limited life expectancy, other medical reason) M

▲ **G9910**[Jan] Patients age 66 or older in institutional special needs plans (SNP) or residing in long-term care with POS code 32, 33, 34, 54 or 56 for more than 90 days during the measurement period M

G9911 Clinically node negative (T1N0M0 or T2N0M0) invasive breast cancer before or after neoadjuvant systemic therapy M

G9912 Hepatitis B virus (HBV) status assessed and results interpreted prior to initiating anti-TNF (tumor necrosis factor) therapy M

G9913 Hepatitis B virus (HBV) status not assessed and results interpreted prior to initiating anti-TNF (tumor necrosis factor) therapy, reason not given M

G9914 Patient receiving an anti-TNF agent M

G9915 No record of HBV results documented M

G9916 Functional status performed once in the last 12 months M

▲ **G9917**[Jan] Documentation of advanced stage dementia and caregiver knowledge is limited M

G9918 Functional status not performed, reason not otherwise specified M

G9919 Screening performed and positive and provision of recommendations M

G9920 Screening performed and negative M

G9921 No screening performed, partial screening performed or positive screen without recommendations and reason is not given or otherwise specified M

G9922 Safety concerns screen provided and if positive then documented mitigation recommendations M

G9923 Safety concerns screen provided and negative M

G9924 Documentation of medical reason(s) for not providing safety concerns screen or for not providing recommendations, orders or referrals for positive screen (e.g., patient in palliative care, other medical reason) M

G9925 Safety concerns screening not provided, reason not otherwise specified M

G9926 Safety concerns screening positive screen is without provision of mitigation recommendations, including but not limited to referral to other resources M

G9927 Documentation of system reason(s) for not prescribing warfarin or another FDA-approved anticoagulation due to patient being currently enrolled in a clinical trial related to AF/atrial flutter treatment M

G9928 Warfarin or another FDA-approved anticoagulant not prescribed, reason not given M

G9929 Patient with transient or reversible cause of AF (e.g., pneumonia, hyperthyroidism, pregnancy, cardiac surgery) M

G9930 Patients who are receiving comfort care only M

G9931 Documentation of CHA2DS2-VASc risk score of 0 or 1 M

G9932 Documentation of patient reason(s) for not having records of negative or managed positive TB screen (e.g., patient does not return for Mantoux (PPD) skin test evaluation) M

G9933 Adenoma(s) or colorectal cancer detected during screening colonoscopy M

G9934 Documentation that neoplasm detected is only diagnosed as traditional serrated adenoma, sessile serrated polyp, or sessile serrated adenoma M

G9935 Adenoma(s) or colorectal cancer not detected during screening colonoscopy M

G9936 Surveillance colonoscopy - personal history of colonic polyps, colon cancer, or other malignant neoplasm of rectum, rectosigmoid junction, and anus M

G9937 Diagnostic colonoscopy M

▲ **G9938**[Jan] Patients age 66 or older in institutional special needs plans (SNP) or residing in long-term care with POS code 32, 33, 34, 54, or 56 for more than 90 days during the measurement period M

G9939 Pathologist(s)/dermatopathologist(s) is the same clinician who performed the biopsy M

© 2019 Optum360, LLC

G9940 Documentation of medical reason(s) for not on a statin (e.g., pregnancy, in vitro fertilization, clomiphene Rx, ESRD, cirrhosis, muscular pain and disease during the measurement period or prior year) M

G9941[Jan] ~~Back pain was measured by the visual analog scale (VAS) within three months preoperatively and at three months (6 - 20 weeks) postoperatively~~

▲ **G9942**[Jan] Patient had any additional spine procedures performed on the same date as the lumbar discectomy/laminectomy M

G9943 Back pain was not measured by the visual analog scale (VAS) within three months preoperatively and at three months (6 - 20 weeks) postoperatively M

G9944[Jan] ~~Back pain was measured by the visual analog scale (VAS) within three months preoperatively and at one year (9 - 15 months) postoperatively~~

G9945 Patient had cancer, fracture or infection related to the lumbar spine or patient had idiopathic or congenital scoliosis M

G9946 Back pain was not measured by the visual analog scale (VAS) within three months preoperatively and at one year (9 - 15 months) postoperatively M

G9947[Jan] ~~Leg pain was measured by the visual analog scale (VAS) within three months preoperatively and at three months (6 - 20 weeks) postoperatively~~

▲ **G9948**[Jan] Patient had any additional spine procedures performed on the same date as the lumbar discectomy/laminectomy M

▲ **G9949**[Jan] Leg pain was not measured by the visual analog scale (VAS) at 3 months (6 to 20 weeks) postoperatively M

G9954 Patient exhibits 2 or more risk factors for postoperative vomiting M

G9955 Cases in which an inhalational anesthetic is used only for induction M

G9956 Patient received combination therapy consisting of at least two prophylactic pharmacologic antiemetic agents of different classes preoperatively and/or intraoperatively M

G9957 Documentation of medical reason for not receiving combination therapy consisting of at least two prophylactic pharmacologic antiemetic agents of different classes preoperatively and/or intraoperatively (e.g., intolerance or other medical reason) M

G9958 Patient did not receive combination therapy consisting of at least two prophylactic pharmacologic antiemetic agents of different classes preoperatively and/or intraoperatively M

G9959 Systemic antimicrobials not prescribed M

G9960 Documentation of medical reason(s) for prescribing systemic antimicrobials M

G9961 Systemic antimicrobials prescribed M

G9962 Embolization endpoints are documented separately for each embolized vessel and ovarian artery angiography or embolization performed in the presence of variant uterine artery anatomy M

G9963 Embolization endpoints are not documented separately for each embolized vessel or ovarian artery angiography or embolization not performed in the presence of variant uterine artery anatomy M

G9964 Patient received at least one well-child visit with a PCP during the performance period M

G9965 Patient did not receive at least one well-child visit with PCP during the performance period M

G9966 Children who were screened for risk of developmental, behavioral and social delays using a standardized tool with interpretation and report M

G9967 Children who were not screened for risk of developmental, behavioral and social delays using a standardized tool with interpretation and report M

G9968 Patient was referred to another provider or specialist during the performance period M

G9969 Provider who referred the patient to another provider received a report from the provider to whom the patient was referred M

G9970 Provider who referred the patient to another provider did not receive a report from the provider to whom the patient was referred M

G9974 Dilated macular exam performed, including documentation of the presence or absence of macular thickening or geographic atrophy or hemorrhage and the level of macular degeneration severity M

G9975 Documentation of medical reason(s) for not performing a dilated macular examination M

G9976 Documentation of patient reason(s) for not performing a dilated macular examination

G9977 Dilated macular exam was not performed, reason not otherwise specified

G9978 Remote in-home visit for the evaluation and management of a new patient for use only in a Medicare-approved Bundled Payments for Care Improvement Advanced (BPCI Advanced) model episode of care, which requires these three key components: a problem focused history; a problem focused examination; straightforward medical decision making, furnished in real time using interactive audio and video technology. Counseling and coordination of care with other physicians, other qualified health care professionals or agencies are provided consistent with the nature of the problem(s) and the needs of the patient or the family or both. Usually, the presenting problem(s) are self limited or minor. Typically, 10 minutes are spent with the patient or family or both via real time, audio and video intercommunications technology

G9979 Remote in-home visit for the evaluation and management of a new patient for use only in a Medicare-approved Bundled Payments for Care Improvement Advanced (BPCI Advanced) model episode of care, which requires these three key components: an expanded problem focused history; an expanded problem focused examination; straightforward medical decision making, furnished in real time using interactive audio and video technology. Counseling and coordination of care with other physicians, other qualified health care professionals or agencies are provided consistent with the nature of the problem(s) and the needs of the patient or the family or both. Usually, the presenting problem(s) are of low to moderate severity. Typically, 20 minutes are spent with the patient or family or both via real time, audio and video intercommunications technology

© 2019 Optum360, LLC

G9980 Remote in-home visit for the evaluation and management of a new patient for use only in a Medicare-approved Bundled Payments for Care Improvement Advanced (BPCI Advanced) model episode of care, which requires these three key components: a detailed history; a detailed examination; medical decision making of low complexity, furnished in real time using interactive audio and video technology. Counseling and coordination of care with other physicians, other qualified health care professionals or agencies are provided consistent with the nature of the problem(s) and the needs of the patient or the family or both. Usually, the presenting problem(s) are of moderate severity. Typically, 30 minutes are spent with the patient or family or both via real time, audio and video intercommunications technology

G9981 Remote in-home visit for the evaluation and management of a new patient for use only in a Medicare-approved Bundled Payments for Care Improvement Advanced (BPCI Advanced) model episode of care, which requires these three key components: a comprehensive history; a comprehensive examination; medical decision making of moderate complexity, furnished in real time using interactive audio and video technology. Counseling and coordination of care with other physicians, other qualified health care professionals or agencies are provided consistent with the nature of the problem(s) and the needs of the patient or the family or both. Usually, the presenting problem(s) are of moderate to high severity. Typically, 45 minutes are spent with the patient or family or both via real time, audio and video intercommunications technology

G9982 Remote in-home visit for the evaluation and management of a new patient for use only in a Medicare-approved Bundled Payments for Care Improvement Advanced (BPCI Advanced) model episode of care, which requires these three key components: a comprehensive history; a comprehensive examination; medical decision making of high complexity, furnished in real time using interactive audio and video technology. Counseling and coordination of care with other physicians, other qualified health care professionals or agencies are provided consistent with the nature of the problem(s) and the needs of the patient or the family or both. Usually, the presenting problem(s) are of moderate to high severity. Typically, 60 minutes are spent with the patient or family or both via real time, audio and video intercommunications technology

G9983 Remote in-home visit for the evaluation and management of an established patient for use only in a Medicare-approved Bundled Payments for Care Improvement Advanced (BPCI Advanced) model episode of care, which requires at least two of the following three key components: a problem focused history; a problem focused examination; straightforward medical decision making, furnished in real time using interactive audio and video technology. Counseling and coordination of care with other physicians, other qualified health care professionals or agencies are provided consistent with the nature of the problem(s) and the needs of the patient or the family or both. Usually, the presenting problem(s) are self limited or minor. Typically, 10 minutes are spent with the patient or family or both via real time, audio and video intercommunications technology

G9984 Remote in-home visit for the evaluation and management of an established patient for use only in a Medicare-approved Bundled Payments for Care Improvement Advanced (BPCI Advanced) model episode of care, which requires at least two of the following three key components: an expanded problem focused history; an expanded problem focused examination; medical decision making of low complexity, furnished in real time using interactive audio and video technology. Counseling and coordination of care with other physicians, other qualified health care professionals or agencies are provided consistent with the nature of the problem(s) and the needs of the patient or the family or both. Usually, the presenting problem(s) are of low to moderate severity. Typically, 15 minutes are spent with the patient or family or both via real time, audio and video intercommunications technology

G9985 Remote in-home visit for the evaluation and management of an established patient for use only in a Medicare-approved Bundled Payments for Care Improvement Advanced (BPCI Advanced) model episode of care, which requires at least two of the following three key components: a detailed history; a detailed examination; medical decision making of moderate complexity, furnished in real time using interactive audio and video technology. Counseling and coordination of care with other physicians, other qualified health care professionals or agencies are provided consistent with the nature of the problem(s) and the needs of the patient or the family or both. Usually, the presenting problem(s) are of moderate to high severity. Typically, 25 minutes are spent with the patient or family or both via real time, audio and video intercommunications technology

G9986 Remote in-home visit for the evaluation and management of an established patient for use only in a Medicare-approved Bundled Payments for Care Improvement Advanced (BPCI Advanced) model episode of care, which requires at least two of the following three key components: a comprehensive history; a comprehensive examination; medical decision making of high complexity, furnished in real time using interactive audio and video technology. Counseling and coordination of care with other physicians, other qualified health care professionals or agencies are provided consistent with the nature of the problem(s) and the needs of the patient or the family or both. Usually, the presenting problem(s) are of moderate to high severity. Typically, 40 minutes are spent with the patient or family or both via real time, audio and video intercommunications technology

G9987 Bundled Payments for Care Improvement Advanced (BPCI Advanced) model home visit for patient assessment performed by clinical staff for an individual not considered homebound, including, but not necessarily limited to patient assessment of clinical status, safety/fall prevention, functional status/ambulation, medication reconciliation/management, compliance with orders/plan of care, performance of activities of daily living, and ensuring beneficiary connections to community and other services; for use only for a BPCI Advanced model episode of care; may not be billed for a 30-day period covered by a transitional care management code

© 2019 Optum360, LLC

Alcohol and Drug Abuse Treatment Services H0001-H2037

The H codes are used by those state Medicaid agencies that are mandated by state law to establish separate codes for identifying mental health services that include alcohol and drug treatment services.

H0001 Alcohol and/or drug assessment

H0002 Behavioral health screening to determine eligibility for admission to treatment program

H0003 Alcohol and/or drug screening; laboratory analysis of specimens for presence of alcohol and/or drugs

H0004 Behavioral health counseling and therapy, per 15 minutes ☑

H0005 Alcohol and/or drug services; group counseling by a clinician

H0006 Alcohol and/or drug services; case management

H0007 Alcohol and/or drug services; crisis intervention (outpatient)

H0008 Alcohol and/or drug services; subacute detoxification (hospital inpatient)

H0009 Alcohol and/or drug services; acute detoxification (hospital inpatient)

H0010 Alcohol and/or drug services; subacute detoxification (residential addiction program inpatient)

H0011 Alcohol and/or drug services; acute detoxification (residential addiction program inpatient)

H0012 Alcohol and/or drug services; subacute detoxification (residential addiction program outpatient)

H0013 Alcohol and/or drug services; acute detoxification (residential addiction program outpatient)

H0014 Alcohol and/or drug services; ambulatory detoxification

H0015 Alcohol and/or drug services; intensive outpatient (treatment program that operates at least 3 hours/day and at least 3 days/week and is based on an individualized treatment plan), including assessment, counseling; crisis intervention, and activity therapies or education

H0016 Alcohol and/or drug services; medical/somatic (medical intervention in ambulatory setting)

H0017 Behavioral health; residential (hospital residential treatment program), without room and board, per diem ☑

H0018 Behavioral health; short-term residential (nonhospital residential treatment program), without room and board, per diem ☑

H0019 Behavioral health; long-term residential (nonmedical, nonacute care in a residential treatment program where stay is typically longer than 30 days), without room and board, per diem ☑

H0020 Alcohol and/or drug services; methadone administration and/or service (provision of the drug by a licensed program)

H0021 Alcohol and/or drug training service (for staff and personnel not employed by providers)

H0022 Alcohol and/or drug intervention service (planned facilitation)

H0023 Behavioral health outreach service (planned approach to reach a targeted population)

H0024 Behavioral health prevention information dissemination service (one-way direct or nondirect contact with service audiences to affect knowledge and attitude)

H0025 Behavioral health prevention education service (delivery of services with target population to affect knowledge, attitude and/or behavior)

H0026 Alcohol and/or drug prevention process service, community-based (delivery of services to develop skills of impactors)

H0027 Alcohol and/or drug prevention environmental service (broad range of external activities geared toward modifying systems in order to mainstream prevention through policy and law)

H0028 Alcohol and/or drug prevention problem identification and referral service (e.g., student assistance and employee assistance programs), does not include assessment

H0029 Alcohol and/or drug prevention alternatives service (services for populations that exclude alcohol and other drug use e.g., alcohol free social events)

H0030 Behavioral health hotline service

H0031 Mental health assessment, by nonphysician

H0032 Mental health service plan development by nonphysician

H0033 Oral medication administration, direct observation

H0034 Medication training and support, per 15 minutes ☑

H0035 Mental health partial hospitalization, treatment, less than 24 hours ☑

H0036 Community psychiatric supportive treatment, face-to-face, per 15 minutes ☑

H0037 Community psychiatric supportive treatment program, per diem ☑

H0038 Self-help/peer services, per 15 minutes ☑

H0039 Assertive community treatment, face-to-face, per 15 minutes ☑

H0040 Assertive community treatment program, per diem ☑

H0041 Foster care, child, nontherapeutic, per diem A ☑

H0042 Foster care, child, nontherapeutic, per month A ☑

H0043 Supported housing, per diem ☑

H0044 Supported housing, per month ☑

H0045 Respite care services, not in the home, per diem ☑

H0046 Mental health services, not otherwise specified

H0047 Alcohol and/or other drug abuse services, not otherwise specified

H0048 Alcohol and/or other drug testing: collection and handling only, specimens other than blood

H0049 Alcohol and/or drug screening

H0050 Alcohol and/or drug services, brief intervention, per 15 minutes ☑

H1000 Prenatal care, at-risk assessment M ♀
AHA: 1Q, '02, 5

H1001 Prenatal care, at-risk enhanced service; antepartum management M ♀
AHA: 1Q, '02, 5

H1002 Prenatal care, at risk enhanced service; care coordination M ♀
AHA: 1Q, '02, 5

H1003 Prenatal care, at-risk enhanced service; education M ♀
AHA: 1Q, '02, 5

H1004 Prenatal care, at-risk enhanced service; follow-up home visit M ♀
AHA: 1Q, '02, 5

H1005 Prenatal care, at-risk enhanced service package (includes H1001-H1004) M ♀
AHA: 1Q, '02, 5

H1010 Nonmedical family planning education, per session ☑

© 2019 Optum360, LLC

H1011	Family assessment by licensed behavioral health professional for state defined purposes	
H2000	Comprehensive multidisciplinary evaluation	
H2001	Rehabilitation program, per 1/2 day	☑
H2010	Comprehensive medication services, per 15 minutes	☑
H2011	Crisis intervention service, per 15 minutes	☑
H2012	Behavioral health day treatment, per hour	☑
H2013	Psychiatric health facility service, per diem	☑
H2014	Skills training and development, per 15 minutes	☑
H2015	Comprehensive community support services, per 15 minutes	☑
H2016	Comprehensive community support services, per diem	☑
H2017	Psychosocial rehabilitation services, per 15 minutes	☑
H2018	Psychosocial rehabilitation services, per diem	☑
H2019	Therapeutic behavioral services, per 15 minutes	☑
H2020	Therapeutic behavioral services, per diem	☑
H2021	Community-based wrap-around services, per 15 minutes	☑
H2022	Community-based wrap-around services, per diem	☑
H2023	Supported employment, per 15 minutes	☑
H2024	Supported employment, per diem	☑
H2025	Ongoing support to maintain employment, per 15 minutes	☑
H2026	Ongoing support to maintain employment, per diem	☑
H2027	Psychoeducational service, per 15 minutes	☑
H2028	Sexual offender treatment service, per 15 minutes	☑
H2029	Sexual offender treatment service, per diem	☑
H2030	Mental health clubhouse services, per 15 minutes	☑
H2031	Mental health clubhouse services, per diem	☑
H2032	Activity therapy, per 15 minutes	☑
H2033	Multisystemic therapy for juveniles, per 15 minutes	☑
H2034	Alcohol and/or drug abuse halfway house services, per diem	☑
H2035	Alcohol and/or other drug treatment program, per hour	☑
H2036	Alcohol and/or other drug treatment program, per diem	☑
H2037	Developmental delay prevention activities, dependent child of client, per 15 minutes	A ☑

© 2019 Optum360, LLC

J Codes Drugs J0120-J8499

J codes include drugs that ordinarily cannot be self-administered, chemotherapy drugs, immunosuppressive drugs, inhalation solutions, and other miscellaneous drugs and solutions.

Miscellaneous Drugs

J0120 **Injection, tetracycline, up to 250 mg** N N1 ☑

● **J0121**Jan **Injection, omadacycline, 1 mg** K2
Use this code for Nuzyra.

● **J0122**Jan **Injection, eravacycline, 1 mg** K2
Use this code for Xerava.

J0129 **Injection, abatacept, 10 mg (code may be used for Medicare when drug administered under the direct supervision of a physician, not for use when drug is self-administered)** K K2 ☑
Use this code for Orencia.
CMS: 100-02,15,50.5

J0130 **Injection abciximab, 10 mg** N N1 ☑
Use this code for ReoPro.

J0131 **Injection, acetaminophen, 10 mg** N N1 ☑
Use this code for OFIRMEV.

J0132 **Injection, acetylcysteine, 100 mg** N N1 ☑
Use this code for Acetadote.

J0133 **Injection, acyclovir, 5 mg** N N1 ☑
Use this code for Zovirax.
CMS: 100-04,20,180

J0135 **Injection, adalimumab, 20 mg** K K2 ☑
Use this code for Humira.
CMS: 100-02,15,50.5
AHA: 3Q, '05, 7, 9; 2Q, '05, 11

J0153 **Injection, adenosine, 1 mg (not to be used to report any adenosine phosphate compounds)** N N1 ☑
Use this code for Adenocard, Adenoscan.
AHA: 1Q, '15, 6

J0171 **Injection, adrenalin, epinephrine, 0.1 mg** N N1 ☑

J0178 **Injection, aflibercept, 1 mg** K K2 ☑
Use this code for Eylea.

● **J0179**Jan **Injection, brolucizumab-dbll, 1 mg**
Use this code for Beovu.

J0180 **Injection, agalsidase beta, 1 mg** K K2 ☑
Use this code for Fabrazyme.
AHA: 2Q, '05, 11

J0185 **Injection, aprepitant, 1 mg** K2
Use this code for Cinvanti.

J0190 **Injection, biperiden lactate, per 5 mg** E ☑

J0200 **Injection, alatrofloxacin mesylate, 100 mg** E ☑

J0202 **Injection, alemtuzumab, 1 mg** K K2 ☑
Use this code for Lemtrada.
AHA: 1Q, '16, 6-8

J0205 **Injection, alglucerase, per 10 units** E ☑
Use this code for Ceredase.
AHA: 2Q, '05, 11

J0207 **Injection, amifostine, 500 mg** K K2 ☑
Use this code for Ethyol.

J0210 **Injection, methyldopate HCl, up to 250 mg** N N1 ☑
Use this code for Aldomet.

J0215 **Injection, alefacept, 0.5 mg** E ☑
Use this for Amevive.

J0220 **Injection, alglucosidase alfa, 10 mg, not otherwise specified** K K2 ☑
Use this code for Myozyme.
AHA: 2Q, '13, 5; 1Q, '08, 6

J0221 **Injection, alglucosidase alfa, (Lumizyme), 10 mg** K K2 ☑
AHA: 2Q, '13, 5

● **J0222**Jan **Injection, patisiran, 0.1 mg** K2
Use this code for Onpattro.

J0256 **Injection, alpha 1-proteinase inhibitor (human), not otherwise specified, 10 mg** K K2 ☑
Use this code for Aralast, Aralast NP, Prolastin C, Zemira.
AHA: 2Q, '13, 5; 2Q, '05, 11

J0257 **Injection, alpha 1 proteinase inhibitor (human), (GLASSIA), 10 mg** K K2 ☑

J0270 **Injection, alprostadil, 1.25 mcg (code may be used for Medicare when drug administered under the direct supervision of a physician, not for use when drug is self-administered)** B ☑
Use this code for Alprostadil, Caverject, Edex, Prostin VR Pediatric.

J0275 **Alprostadil urethral suppository (code may be used for Medicare when drug administered under the direct supervision of a physician, not for use when drug is self-administered)** B ☑
Use this code for Muse.

J0278 **Injection, amikacin sulfate, 100 mg** N N1 ☑
Use this code for Amikin.

J0280 **Injection, aminophyllin, up to 250 mg** N N1 ☑
AHA: 4Q, '05, 1-6

J0282 **Injection, amiodarone HCl, 30 mg** N N1 ☑
Use this code for Cordarone IV.

J0285 **Injection, amphotericin B, 50 mg** N N1 ☑
Use this for Amphocin, Fungizone.
CMS: 100-04,20,180

J0287 **Injection, amphotericin B lipid complex, 10 mg** K K2 ☑
Use this code for Abelcet.
CMS: 100-04,20,180

J0288 **Injection, amphotericin B cholesteryl sulfate complex, 10 mg** E ☑
Use this code for Amphotec.
CMS: 100-04,20,180

J0289 **Injection, amphotericin B liposome, 10 mg** K K2 ☑
Use this code for Ambisome.
CMS: 100-04,20,180

J0290 **Injection, ampicillin sodium, 500 mg** N N1 ☑

● **J0291**Jan **Injection, plazomicin, 5 mg** K2
Use this code for Zemdri.

J0295 **Injection, ampicillin sodium/sulbactam sodium, per 1.5 g** N N1 ☑
Use this code for Unasyn.

J0300 **Injection, amobarbital, up to 125 mg** K K2 ☑
Use this code for Amytal.

J0330 **Injection, succinylcholine chloride, up to 20 mg** N N1 ☑
Use this code for Anectine, Quelicin.

J0348 **Injection, anidulafungin, 1 mg** N N1 ☑
Use this code for Eraxis.

J0350 **Injection, anistreplase, per 30 units** E ☑
Use this code for Eminase.

J0360 **Injection, hydralazine HCl, up to 20 mg** N N1 ☑

© 2019 Optum360, LLC

J0364 **Injection, apomorphine HCl, 1 mg** E ☑
Use this code for Apokyn.
CMS: 100-02,15,50.5

J0365 **Injection, aprotinin, 10,000 kiu** E ☑
Use this code for Trasylol.

J0380 **Injection, metaraminol bitartrate, per 10 mg** N N1 ☑
Use this code for Aramine.

J0390 **Injection, chloroquine HCl, up to 250 mg** N N1 ☑
Use this code for Aralen.

J0395 **Injection, arbutamine HCl, 1 mg** E ☑

J0400 **Injection, aripiprazole, intramuscular, 0.25 mg** K N1 ☑
Use this code for Abilify.
AHA: 1Q, '08, 6

J0401 **Injection, aripiprazole, extended release, 1 mg** K K2 ☑
Use this code for the Abilify Maintena kit.
AHA: 1Q, '14, 6

J0456 **Injection, azithromycin, 500 mg** N N1 ☑
Use this code for Zithromax.

J0461 **Injection, atropine sulfate, 0.01 mg** N N1 ☑
Use this code for AtroPen.

J0470 **Injection, dimercaprol, per 100 mg** K N1 ☑
Use this code for BAL.

J0475 **Injection, baclofen, 10 mg** K K2 ☑
Use this code for Lioresal, Gablofen.

J0476 **Injection, baclofen, 50 mcg for intrathecal trial** K N1 ☑
Use this code for Lioresal, Gablofen.

J0480 **Injection, basiliximab, 20 mg** K K2 ☑
Use this code for Simulect.

J0485 **Injection, belatacept, 1 mg** K K2 ☑
Use this code for Nulojix.

J0490 **Injection, belimumab, 10 mg** K K2 ☑
Use this code for BENLYSTA.

J0500 **Injection, dicyclomine HCl, up to 20 mg** N N1 ☑
Use this code for Bentyl.

J0515 **Injection, benztropine mesylate, per 1 mg** N N1 ☑
Use this code for Cogentin.

J0517 **Injection, benralizumab, 1 mg** K2
Use this code for Fasenra.

J0520 **Injection, bethanechol chloride, Myotonachol or Urecholine, up to 5 mg** E ☑

J0558 **Injection, penicillin G benzathine and penicillin G procaine, 100,000 units** N K2 ☑
Use this code for Bicillin CR, Bicillin CR 900/300, Bicillin CR Tubex.

J0561 **Injection, penicillin G benzathine, 100,000 units** K K2 ☑
AHA: 2Q, '13, 5

J0565 **Injection, bezlotoxumab, 10 mg** G K2
Use this code for Zinplava.

J0567 **Injection, cerliponase alfa, 1 mg** K2
Use this code for Brineura.

J0570 **Buprenorphine implant, 74.2 mg** G K2 ☑
Use this code for Probuphine.
AHA: 1Q, '17, 9-10

J0571 **Buprenorphine, oral, 1 mg** E ☑
Use this code for Subutex.
AHA: 1Q, '15, 6

J0572 **Buprenorphine/naloxone, oral, less than or equal to 3 mg buprenorphine** E ☑
Use this code for Bunavail, Suboxone, Zubsolv.
AHA: 1Q, '15, 6

J0573 **Buprenorphine/naloxone, oral, greater than 3 mg, but less than or equal to 6 mg buprenorphine** E ☑
Use this code for Bunavail, Suboxone, Zubsolv.
AHA: 1Q, '16, 6-8; 1Q, '15, 6

J0574 **Buprenorphine/naloxone, oral, greater than 6 mg, but less than or equal to 10 mg buprenorphine** E ☑
Use this code for Bunavail, Suboxone.
AHA: 1Q, '16, 6-8; 1Q, '15, 6

J0575 **Buprenorphine/naloxone, oral, greater than 10 mg buprenorphine** E ☑
Use this code for Suboxone.
AHA: 1Q, '16, 6-8; 1Q, '15, 6

J0583 **Injection, bivalirudin, 1 mg** N N1 ☑
Use this code for Angiomax.

J0584 **Injection, burosumab-twza, 1 mg** K2
Use this code for Crysvita.
CMS: 100-04,4,260.1; 100-04,4,260.1.1

J0585 **Injection, onabotulinumtoxinA, 1 unit** K K2 ☑
Use this code for Botox, Botox Cosmetic.

J0586 **Injection, abobotulinumtoxinA, 5 units** K K2 ☑
Use this code for Dysport.

J0587 **Injection, rimabotulinumtoxinB, 100 units** K K2 ☑
Use this code for Myobloc.
AHA: 2Q, '02, 8-9; 1Q, '02, 5

J0588 **Injection, incobotulinumtoxinA, 1 unit** K K2 ☑
Use this code for XEOMIN.

J0592 **Injection, buprenorphine HCl, 0.1 mg** N N1 ☑
Use this code for Buprenex.

● **J0593**[Jan] **Injection, lanadelumab-flyo, 1 mg (code may be used for Medicare when drug administered under direct supervision of a physician, not for use when drug is self-administered)** K2
Use this code for Takhzyro.

J0594 **Injection, busulfan, 1 mg** K K2 ☑
Use this code for Busulfex.

J0595 **Injection, butorphanol tartrate, 1 mg** N N1 ☑
Use this code for Stadol.
AHA: 2Q, '05, 11

J0596 **Injection, C1 esterase inhibitor (recombinant), Ruconest, 10 units** K K2 ☑
CMS: 100-02,15,50.5

J0597 **Injection, C1 esterase inhibitor (human), Berinert, 10 units** K K2 ☑

J0598 **Injection, C1 esterase inhibitor (human), Cinryze, 10 units** K K2 ☑

J0599 **Injection, C1 esterase inhibitor (human), (Haegarda), 10 units** K2

J0600 **Injection, edetate calcium disodium, up to 1,000 mg** K K2 ☑
Use this code for Calcium Disodium Versenate, Calcium EDTA.

J0604 **Cinacalcet, oral, 1 mg, (for ESRD on dialysis)** B
Use this code for Sensipar.

J0606 **Injection, etelcalcetide, 0.1 mg** K K2
Use this code for Parsabiv.

J0610 **Injection, calcium gluconate, per 10 ml** N N1 ☑

© 2019 Optum360, LLC

J0620 **Injection, calcium glycerophosphate and calcium lactate, per 10 ml** N N1 ☑

J0630 **Injection, calcitonin salmon, up to 400 units** K K2 ☑
Use this code for Calcimar, Miacalcin.
CMS: 100-04,10,90.1

J0636 **Injection, calcitriol, 0.1 mcg** N N1 ☑
Use this code for Calcijex.

J0637 **Injection, caspofungin acetate, 5 mg** K K2 ☑
Use this code for Cancidas.

J0638 **Injection, canakinumab, 1 mg** K K2 ☑
Use this code for ILARIS.

J0640 **Injection, leucovorin calcium, per 50 mg** N N1 ☑
AHA: 1Q, '09, 10

▲ **J0641**Jan **Injection, levoleucovorin, not otherwise specified, 0.5 mg** K K2 ☑

● **J0642**Jan **Injection, levoleucovorin (Khapzory), 0.5 mg**

J0670 **Injection, mepivacaine HCl, per 10 ml** N N1 ☑
Use this code for Carbocaine, Polocaine, Isocaine HCl, Scandonest

J0690 **Injection, cefazolin sodium, 500 mg** N N1 ☑

J0692 **Injection, cefepime HCl, 500 mg** N N1 ☑
AHA: 1Q, '02, 5

J0694 **Injection, cefoxitin sodium, 1 g** N N1 ☑

J0695 **Injection, ceftolozane 50 mg and tazobactam 25 mg** K K2 ☑
Use this code for Zerbaxa.

J0696 **Injection, ceftriaxone sodium, per 250 mg** N N1 ☑

J0697 **Injection, sterile cefuroxime sodium, per 750 mg** N N1 ☑

J0698 **Injection, cefotaxime sodium, per g** N N1 ☑

J0702 **Injection, betamethasone acetate 3 mg and betamethasone sodium phosphate 3 mg** N N1 ☑

J0706 **Injection, caffeine citrate, 5 mg** N N1 ☑
AHA: 2Q, '02, 8-9; 1Q, '02, 5

J0710 **Injection, cephapirin sodium, up to 1 g** E ☑

J0712 **Injection, ceftaroline fosamil, 10 mg** K K2 ☑

J0713 **Injection, ceftazidime, per 500 mg** N N1 ☑

J0714 **Injection, ceftazidime and avibactam, 0.5 g/0.125 g** K K2 ☑
Use this code for Avycaz.
AHA: 1Q, '16, 6-8

J0715 **Injection, ceftizoxime sodium, per 500 mg** N N1 ☑

J0716 **Injection, Centruroides immune f(ab)2, up to 120 mg** K K2 ☑
Use this code for Anascorp.

J0717 **Injection, certolizumab pegol, 1 mg (code may be used for Medicare when drug administered under the direct supervision of a physician, not for use when drug is self-administered)** K K2 ☑
CMS: 100-02,15,50.5
AHA: 1Q, '14, 7

J0720 **Injection, chloramphenicol sodium succinate, up to 1 g** N N1 ☑

J0725 **Injection, chorionic gonadotropin, per 1,000 USP units** N K2 ☑
CMS: 100-02,15,50.5

J0735 **Injection, clonidine HCl, 1 mg** N N1 ☑

J0740 **Injection, cidofovir, 375 mg** K K2 ☑

J0743 **Injection, cilastatin sodium; imipenem, per 250 mg** N N1 ☑

J0744 **Injection, ciprofloxacin for intravenous infusion, 200 mg** N N1 ☑
AHA: 1Q, '02, 5

J0745 **Injection, codeine phosphate, per 30 mg** N N1 ☑

J0770 **Injection, colistimethate sodium, up to 150 mg** N N1 ☑

J0775 **Injection, collagenase, clostridium histolyticum, 0.01 mg** K K2 ☑

J0780 **Injection, prochlorperazine, up to 10 mg** N N1 ☑

J0795 **Injection, corticorelin ovine triflutate, 1 mcg** K K2 ☑

J0800 **Injection, corticotropin, up to 40 units** K N1 ☑
CMS: 100-02,15,50.5

J0834 **Injection, cosyntropin, 0.25 mg** N N1 ☑
Use this code for Cortrosyn.

J0840 **Injection, crotalidae polyvalent immune fab (ovine), up to 1 g** K K2 ☑

J0841 **Injection, crotalidae immune F(ab')2 (equine), 120 mg** K2
Use this code for Anavip.
CMS: 100-04,4,260.1; 100-04,4,260.1.1

J0850 **Injection, cytomegalovirus immune globulin intravenous (human), per vial** K K2 ☑

J0875 **Injection, dalbavancin, 5 mg** K K2 ☑
Use this code for Dalvance.

J0878 **Injection, daptomycin, 1 mg** K K2 ☑
Use this code for Cubicin.
AHA: 2Q, '05, 11

J0881 **Injection, darbepoetin alfa, 1 mcg (non-ESRD use)** K K2 ☑
Use this code for Aranesp.
CMS: 100-03,110.21; 100-04,17,80.12

J0882 **Injection, darbepoetin alfa, 1 mcg (for ESRD on dialysis)** K K2 ☑ ⊘
Use this code for Aranesp.
CMS: 100-04,8,60.4; 100-04,8,60.4.1; 100-04,8,60.4.2; 100-04,8,60.4.5.1; 100-04,8,60.4.6.3; 100-04,8,60.4.6.4; 100-04,8,60.4.6.5

J0883 **Injection, argatroban, 1 mg (for non-ESRD use)** K K2 ☑

J0884 **Injection, argatroban, 1 mg (for ESRD on dialysis)** K K2 ☑

J0885 **Injection, epoetin alfa, (for non-ESRD use), 1000 units** K K2 ☑
Use this code for Epogen/Procrit.
CMS: 100-03,110.21; 100-04,17,80.12
AHA: 2Q, '06, 4, 5

J0887 **Injection, epoetin beta, 1 mcg, (for ESRD on dialysis)** N N1 ☑
Use this code for Mircera.
AHA: 1Q, '15, 6

J0888 **Injection, epoetin beta, 1 mcg, (for non-ESRD use)** K N1 ☑
Use this code for Mircera.
AHA: 1Q, '15, 6

J0890 **Injection, peginesatide, 0.1 mg (for ESRD on dialysis)** E ☑
Use this code for Omontys.
CMS: 100-04,8,60.4; 100-04,8,60.4.1; 100-04,8,60.4.2; 100-04,8,60.4.5.1; 100-04,8,60.4.7

J0894 **Injection, decitabine, 1 mg** K K2 ☑ ⊘
Use this code for Dacogen.

J0895 **Injection, deferoxamine mesylate, 500 mg** N N1 ☑
Use this code for Desferal.
CMS: 100-04,20,180

J0897 **Injection, denosumab, 1 mg** K K2 ☑
Use this code for XGEVA, Prolia.
AHA: 1Q, '16, 5

© 2019 Optum360, LLC

J0945 **Injection, brompheniramine maleate, per 10 mg** N N1 ☑

J1000 **Injection, depo-estradiol cypionate, up to 5 mg** N N1 ☑
Use this code for depGynogen, Depogen, Estradiol Cypionate.

J1020 **Injection, methylprednisolone acetate, 20 mg** N N1 ☑
Use this code for Depo-Medrol.
AHA: 2Q, '09, 9; 3Q, '05, 10

J1030 **Injection, methylprednisolone acetate, 40 mg** N N1 ☑
Use this code for DepoMedalone40, Depo-Medrol, Sano-Drol.
AHA: 2Q, '09, 9; 3Q, '05, 10

J1040 **Injection, methylprednisolone acetate, 80 mg** N N1 ☑
Use this code for Cortimed, DepMedalone, DepoMedalone 80, Depo-Medrol, Duro Cort, Methylcotolone, Pri-Methylate, Sano-Drol.
AHA: 2Q, '09, 9

J1050 **Injection, medroxyprogesterone acetate, 1 mg** N N1 ☑

J1071 **Injection, testosterone cypionate, 1 mg** N N1 ☑
Use this code for Depo-testostrone.
AHA: 2Q, '15, 7; 1Q, '15, 6

J1094 **Injection, dexamethasone acetate, 1 mg** N N1 ☑
Use this code for Cortastat LA, Dalalone L.A., Dexamethasone Acetate Anhydrous, Dexone LA.

J1095 **Injection, dexamethasone 9%, intraocular, 1 mcg** K2

● **J1096**[Jan] **Dexamethasone, lacrimal ophthalmic insert, 0.1 mg** K2
Use this code for Dextenza.

● **J1097**[Jan] **Phenylephrine 10.16 mg/ml and ketorolac 2.88 mg/ml ophthalmic irrigation solution, 1 ml** K2
Use this code for Omidria.

J1100 **Injection, dexamethasone sodium phosphate, 1 mg** N N1 ☑
Use this code for Cortastat, Dalalone, Decaject, Dexone, Solurex, Adrenocort, Primethasone, Dexasone, Dexim, Medidex, Spectro-Dex.

J1110 **Injection, dihydroergotamine mesylate, per 1 mg** K N1 ☑
Use this code for D.H.E. 45.

J1120 **Injection, acetazolamide sodium, up to 500 mg** N N1 ☑
Use this code for Diamox.
AHA: 4Q, '05, 1-6; 3Q, '04, 1-10

J1130 **Injection, diclofenac sodium, 0.5 mg** K N1 ☑
Use this code for Dyloject.
AHA: 1Q, '17, 9-10

J1160 **Injection, digoxin, up to 0.5 mg** N N1 ☑
Use this code for Lanoxin.
AHA: 4Q, '05, 1-6

J1162 **Injection, digoxin immune fab (ovine), per vial** K K2 ☑
Use this code for Digibind, Digifab.

J1165 **Injection, phenytoin sodium, per 50 mg** N N1 ☑
Use this code for Dilantin.

J1170 **Injection, hydromorphone, up to 4 mg** N N1 ☑
Use this code for Dilaudid, Dilaudid-HP.
CMS: 100-04,20,180

J1180 **Injection, dyphylline, up to 500 mg** E ☑

J1190 **Injection, dexrazoxane HCl, per 250 mg** K K2 ☑
Use this code for Zinecard.

J1200 **Injection, diphenhydramine HCl, up to 50 mg** N N1 ☑
Use this code for Benadryl, Benahist 10, Benahist 50, Benoject-10, Benoject-50, Bena-D 10, Bena-D 50, Nordryl, Dihydrex, Dimine, Diphenacen-50, Hyrexin-50, Truxadryl, Wehdryl.
AHA: 1Q, '02, 1-2

J1205 **Injection, chlorothiazide sodium, per 500 mg** N N1 ☑
Use this code for Diuril Sodium.

J1212 **Injection, DMSO, dimethyl sulfoxide, 50%, 50 ml** K K2 ☑
Use this code for Rimso 50. DMSO is covered only as a treatment of interstitial cystitis.

J1230 **Injection, methadone HCl, up to 10 mg** N N1 ☑
Use this code for Dolophine HCl.

J1240 **Injection, dimenhydrinate, up to 50 mg** N N1 ☑
Use this code for Dramamine, Dinate, Dommanate, Dramanate, Dramilin, Dramocen, Dramoject, Dymenate, Hydrate, Marmine, Wehamine.

J1245 **Injection, dipyridamole, per 10 mg** N N1 ☑
Use this code for Persantine IV.
AHA: 4Q, '05, 1-6; 3Q, '04, 1-10

J1250 **Injection, dobutamine HCl, per 250 mg** N N1 ☑
CMS: 100-04,20,180
AHA: 4Q, '05, 1-6; 3Q, '04, 1-10

J1260 **Injection, dolasetron mesylate, 10 mg** N N1 ☑
Use this code for Anzemet.

J1265 **Injection, dopamine HCl, 40 mg** N N1 ☑
CMS: 100-04,20,180
AHA: 4Q, '05, 1-6

J1267 **Injection, doripenem, 10 mg** N N1 ☑
Use this code for Doribax.

J1270 **Injection, doxercalciferol, 1 mcg** N N1 ☑
Use this code for Hectorol.
AHA: 1Q, '02, 5

J1290 **Injection, ecallantide, 1 mg** K K2 ☑
Use this code for KALBITOR.

J1300 **Injection, eculizumab, 10 mg** K K2 ☑
Use this code for Soliris.
AHA: 1Q, '08, 6

J1301 **Injection, edaravone, 1 mg** K2
Use this code for Radicava.

● **J1303**[Jan] **Injection, ravulizumab-cwvz, 10 mg** K2
Use this code for Ultomiris.

J1320 **Injection, amitriptyline HCl, up to 20 mg** N N1 ☑
Use this code for Elavil.

J1322 **Injection, elosulfase alfa, 1 mg** K K2 ☑
Use this code for Vimizim.
AHA: 1Q, '15, 6

J1324 **Injection, enfuvirtide, 1 mg** E ☑
Use this code for Fuzeon.
CMS: 100-02,15,50.5

J1325 **Injection, epoprostenol, 0.5 mg** N N1 ☑
Use this code for Flolan and Veletri. See K0455 for infusion pump for epoprosterol.
CMS: 100-04,20,180

J1327 **Injection, eptifibatide, 5 mg** K K2 ☑
Use this code for Integrilin.

J1330 **Injection, ergonovine maleate, up to 0.2 mg** N ☑
Medicare jurisdiction: local contractor. Use this code for Ergotrate Maleate.

J1335 **Injection, ertapenem sodium, 500 mg** N N1 ☑
Use this code for Invanz.

J1364 **Injection, erythromycin lactobionate, per 500 mg** K K2 ☑

J1380 **Injection, estradiol valerate, up to 10 mg** N N1 ☑
Use this code for Delestrogen, Dioval, Dioval XX, Dioval 40, Duragen-10, Duragen-20, Duragen-40, Estradiol L.A., Estradiol L.A. 20, Estradiol L.A. 40, Gynogen L.A. 10, Gynogen L.A. 20, Gynogen L.A. 40, Valergen 10, Valergen 20, Valergen 40, Estra-L 20, Estra-L 40, L.A.E. 20.

© 2019 Optum360, LLC

J1410 **Injection, estrogen conjugated, per 25 mg** K K2 ☑
Use this code for Natural Estrogenic Substance, Premarin Intravenous, Primestrin Aqueous.

J1428 **Injection, eteplirsen, 10 mg** G K2
Use this code for Exondys 51.

J1430 **Injection, ethanolamine oleate, 100 mg** K K2 ☑
Use this code for Ethamiolin.

J1435 **Injection, estrone, per 1 mg** E ☑
Use this code for Estone Aqueous, Estragyn, Estro-A, Estrone, Estronol, Theelin Aqueous, Estone 5, Kestrone 5.

J1436 **Injection, etidronate disodium, per 300 mg** E ☑
Use this code for Didronel.

J1438 **Injection, etanercept, 25 mg (code may be used for Medicare when drug administered under the direct supervision of a physician, not for use when drug is self-administered)** K K2 ☑
Use this code for Enbrel.
CMS: 100-02,15,50.5

J1439 **Injection, ferric carboxymaltose, 1 mg** K K2 ☑
Use this code for Injectafer.
AHA: 1Q, '15, 6

J1442 **Injection, filgrastim (G-CSF), excludes biosimilars, 1 mcg** K K2 ☑
Use this code for Neupogen.
AHA: 1Q, '14, 7

J1443 **Injection, ferric pyrophosphate citrate solution, 0.1 mg of iron** N ☑
Use this code for Triferic solution.
AHA: 1Q, '16, 6-8

● **J1444**Jan **Injection, ferric pyrophosphate citrate powder, 0.1 mg of iron**
Use this code for Triferic powder.

J1447 **Injection, tbo-filgrastim, 1 mcg** K K2 ☑
Use this code for Granix.
AHA: 1Q, '16, 6-8

J1450 **Injection, fluconazole, 200 mg** N N1 ☑
Use this code for Diflucan.
CMS: 100-02,15,50.6

J1451 **Injection, fomepizole, 15 mg** K K2 ☑
Use this code for Antizol.
CMS: 100-02,15,50.6

J1452 **Injection, fomivirsen sodium, intraocular, 1.65 mg** E ☑
Use this code for Vitravene.
CMS: 100-02,15,50.4.2; 100-02,15,50.6

J1453 **Injection, fosaprepitant, 1 mg** K K2 ☑
Use this code for Emend.
CMS: 100-02,15,50.6

J1454 **Injection, fosnetupitant 235 mg and palonosetron 0.25 mg** K2
Use this code for Akynzeo.
CMS: 100-02,15,50.6

J1455 **Injection, foscarnet sodium, per 1,000 mg** K K2 ☑
Use this code for Foscavir.
CMS: 100-02,15,50.6; 100-04,20,180

J1457 **Injection, gallium nitrate, 1 mg** E ☑
Use this code for Ganite.
CMS: 100-02,15,50.6; 100-04,20,180
AHA: 2Q, '05, 11

J1458 **Injection, galsulfase, 1 mg** K K2 ☑
Use this code for Naglazyme.
CMS: 100-02,15,50.6

J1459 **Injection, immune globulin (Privigen), intravenous, nonlyophilized (e.g., liquid), 500 mg** K K2 ☑
CMS: 100-02,15,50.6

J1460 **Injection, gamma globulin, intramuscular, 1 cc** K K2 ☑
Use this code for GamaSTAN SD.
CMS: 100-02,15,50.6; 100-04,17,80.6

J1555 **Injection, immune globulin (Cuvitru), 100 mg** K K2
CMS: 100-02,15,50.6; 100-04,20,180

J1556 **Injection, immune globulin (Bivigam), 500 mg** K K2 ☑
CMS: 100-02,15,50.6

J1557 **Injection, immune globulin, (Gammaplex), intravenous, nonlyophilized (e.g., liquid), 500 mg** K K2 ☑
CMS: 100-02,15,50.6

J1559 **Injection, immune globulin (Hizentra), 100 mg** K K2 ☑
CMS: 100-02,15,50.6; 100-04,20,180

J1560 **Injection, gamma globulin, intramuscular, over 10 cc** K K2 ☑
Use this code for GamaSTAN SD.
CMS: 100-02,15,50.6; 100-04,17,80.6

J1561 **Injection, immune globulin, (Gamunex/Gamunex-C/Gammaked), nonlyophilized (e.g., liquid), 500 mg** K K2 ☑
CMS: 100-02,15,50.6; 100-04,20,180
AHA: 1Q, '08, 6

J1562 **Injection, immune globulin (Vivaglobin), 100 mg** E ☑
CMS: 100-02,15,50.6; 100-04,20,180

J1566 **Injection, immune globulin, intravenous, lyophilized (e.g., powder), not otherwise specified, 500 mg** K K2 ☑
Use this code for Carimune, Gammagard S/D.
CMS: 100-02,15,50.6
AHA: 2Q, '13, 5

J1568 **Injection, immune globulin, (Octagam), intravenous, nonlyophilized (e.g., liquid), 500 mg** K K2 ☑
CMS: 100-02,15,50.6
AHA: 1Q, '08, 6

J1569 **Injection, immune globulin, (Gammagard liquid), nonlyophilized, (e.g., liquid), 500 mg** K K2 ☑
CMS: 100-02,15,50.6; 100-04,20,180
AHA: 1Q, '08, 6

J1570 **Injection, ganciclovir sodium, 500 mg** N N1 ☑
Use this code for Cytovene.
CMS: 100-04,20,180

J1571 **Injection, hepatitis B immune globulin (Hepagam B), intramuscular, 0.5 ml** K K2 ☑
AHA: 3Q, '08, 7, 8; 1Q, '08, 6

J1572 **Injection, immune globulin, (Flebogamma/Flebogamma Dif), intravenous, nonlyophilized (e.g., liquid), 500 mg** K K2 ☑
AHA: 1Q, '08, 6

J1573 **Injection, hepatitis B immune globulin (Hepagam B), intravenous, 0.5 ml** K K2 ☑
AHA: 3Q, '08, 7, 8; 1Q, '08, 6

J1575 **Injection, immune globulin/hyaluronidase, 100 mg immuneglobulin** K K2 ☑
Use this code for HyQvia.
CMS: 100-04,20,180
AHA: 1Q, '16, 6-8

J1580 **Injection, garamycin, gentamicin, up to 80 mg** N N1 ☑
Use this code for Gentamicin Sulfate, Jenamicin.

J1595 **Injection, glatiramer acetate, 20 mg** K K2 ☑
Use this code for Copaxone.
CMS: 100-02,15,50.5

© 2019 Optum360, LLC

J1599 **Injection, immune globulin, intravenous, nonlyophilized (e.g., liquid), not otherwise specified, 500 mg** N N1 ☑
AHA: 2Q, '13, 5

J1600 **Injection, gold sodium thiomalate, up to 50 mg** E ☑
Use this code for Myochrysine.
CMS: 100-04,4,20.6.4

J1602 **Injection, golimumab, 1 mg, for intravenous use** K K2 ☑
Use this code for Simponi.
AHA: 1Q, '14, 6

J1610 **Injection, glucagon HCl, per 1 mg** K K2 ☑
Use this code for Glucagen.
AHA: 4Q, '05, 1-6

J1620 **Injection, gonadorelin HCl, per 100 mcg** E ☑
Use this code for Factrel, Lutrepulse.

J1626 **Injection, granisetron HCl, 100 mcg** N N1 ☑
Use this code for Kytril.
CMS: 100-04,4,20.6.4

J1627 **Injection, granisetron, extended-release, 0.1 mg** G K2
Use this code for Sustol.

J1628 **Injection, guselkumab, 1 mg** K2
Use this code for Tremfya.

J1630 **Injection, haloperidol, up to 5 mg** N N1 ☑
Use this code for Haldol.
CMS: 100-04,4,20.6.4

J1631 **Injection, haloperidol decanoate, per 50 mg** N N1 ☑
Use this code for Haldol Decanoate-50.
CMS: 100-04,4,20.6.4

J1640 **Injection, hemin, 1 mg** K K2 ☑
Use this code for Panhematin.

J1642 **Injection, heparin sodium, (heparin lock flush), per 10 units** N N1 ☑
Use this code for Hep-Lock, Hep-Lock U/P, Hep-Pak, Lok-Pak.
CMS: 100-04,4,20.6.4
AHA: 4Q, '05, 1-6

J1644 **Injection, Heparin sodium, per 1000 units** N N1 ☑
Use this code for Heparin Sodium, Liquaemin Sodium.
CMS: 100-04,4,20.6.4

J1645 **Injection, dalteparin sodium, per 2500 IU** N N1 ☑
Use this code for Fragmin.
CMS: 100-02,15,50.5; 100-04,4,20.6.4

J1650 **Injection, enoxaparin sodium, 10 mg** N N1 ☑
Use this code for Lovenox.
CMS: 100-02,15,50.5; 100-04,4,20.6.4

J1652 **Injection, fondaparinux sodium, 0.5 mg** N N1 ☑
Use this code for Atrixtra.
CMS: 100-02,15,50.5

J1655 **Injection, tinzaparin sodium, 1000 IU** N N1 ☑
Use this code for Innohep.
CMS: 100-02,15,50.5; 100-04,4,20.6.4
AHA: 1Q, '02, 5

J1670 **Injection, tetanus immune globulin, human, up to 250 units** K K2 ☑
Use this code for HyperTET SD.

J1675 **Injection, histrelin acetate, 10 mcg** B ☑
Use this code for Supprelin LA.

J1700 **Injection, hydrocortisone acetate, up to 25 mg** N N1 ☑
Use this code for Hydrocortone Acetate.
CMS: 100-04,4,20.6.4

J1710 **Injection, hydrocortisone sodium phosphate, up to 50 mg** N N1 ☑
Use this code for Hydrocortone Phosphate.
CMS: 100-04,4,20.6.4

J1720 **Injection, hydrocortisone sodium succinate, up to 100 mg** N N1 ☑
Use this code for Solu-Cortef, A-Hydrocort.
CMS: 100-04,4,20.6.4

J1726 **Injection, hydroxyprogesterone caproate, (Makena), 10 mg** K K2

J1729 **Injection, hydroxyprogesterone caproate, not otherwise specified, 10 mg** N N1

J1730 **Injection, diazoxide, up to 300 mg** E ☑

J1740 **Injection, ibandronate sodium, 1 mg** K K2 ☑
Use this code for Boniva.

J1741 **Injection, ibuprofen, 100 mg** N N1 ☑
Use this code for Caldolor.

J1742 **Injection, ibutilide fumarate, 1 mg** K K2 ☑
Use this code for Corvert.

J1743 **Injection, idursulfase, 1 mg** K K2 ☑
Use this code for Elaprase.

J1744 **Injection, icatibant, 1 mg** K K2 ☑
Use this code for Firazyr.
CMS: 100-02,15,50.5

J1745 **Injection, infliximab, excludes biosimilar, 10 mg** K K2 ☑
Use this code for Remicade.

J1746 **Injection, ibalizumab-uiyk, 10 mg** K2
Use this code for Trogarzo.
CMS: 100-04,4,260.1; 100-04,4,260.1.1

J1750 **Injection, iron dextran, 50 mg** K K2 ☑
Use this code for INFeD.

J1756 **Injection, iron sucrose, 1 mg** N N1 ☑
Use this code for Venofer.
CMS: 100-04,8,60.2.4; 100-04,8,60.2.4.2

J1786 **Injection, imiglucerase, 10 units** K K2 ☑
Use this code for Cerezyme.

J1790 **Injection, droperidol, up to 5 mg** N N1 ☑
Use this code for Inapsine.
CMS: 100-04,4,20.6.4

J1800 **Injection, propranolol HCl, up to 1 mg** N N1 ☑
Use this code for Inderal.
CMS: 100-04,4,20.6.4
AHA: 4Q, '05, 1-6

J1810 **Injection, droperidol and fentanyl citrate, up to 2 ml ampule** E ☑
AHA: 2Q, '02, 8-9

J1815 **Injection, insulin, per 5 units** N N1 ☑
Use this code for Humalog, Humulin, Iletin, Insulin Lispo, Lantus, Levemir, NPH, Pork insulin, Regular insulin, Ultralente, Velosulin, Humulin R, Iletin II Regular Pork, Insulin Purified Pork, Relion, Lente Iletin I, Novolin R, Humulin R U-500.
CMS: 100-04,4,20.6.4
AHA: 4Q, '05, 1-6

J1817 **Insulin for administration through DME (i.e., insulin pump) per 50 units** N N1 ☑
Use this code for Humalog, Humulin, Vesolin BR, Iletin II NPH Pork, Lispro-PFC, Novolin, Novolog, Novolog Flexpen, Novolog Mix, Relion Novolin.
AHA: 4Q, '05, 1-6

© 2019 Optum360, LLC

J1826 **Injection, interferon beta-1a, 30 mcg** K K2 ☑
Use this code for AVONEX, Rebif.
AHA: 4Q, '14, 6; 2Q, '11, 9

J1830 **Injection interferon beta-1b, 0.25 mg (code may be used for Medicare when drug administered under the direct supervision of a physician, not for use when drug is self-administered)** K K2 ☑
Use this code for Betaseron.
CMS: 100-02,15,50.5

J1833 **Injection, isavuconazonium, 1 mg** K K2 ☑
Use this code for Cresemba.

J1835 **Injection, itraconazole, 50 mg** E ☑
Use this code for Sporonox IV.
CMS: 100-04,4,20.6.4
AHA: 1Q, '02, 5

J1840 **Injection, kanamycin sulfate, up to 500 mg** N N1 ☑
Use this code for Kantrex.
CMS: 100-04,4,20.6.4

J1850 **Injection, kanamycin sulfate, up to 75 mg** N N1 ☑
Use this code for Kantrex.
CMS: 100-04,4,20.6.4
AHA: 2Q, '13, 5

J1885 **Injection, ketorolac tromethamine, per 15 mg** N N1 ☑
Use this code for Toradol.
CMS: 100-04,4,20.6.4

J1890 **Injection, cephalothin sodium, up to 1 g** N N1 ☑
CMS: 100-04,4,20.6.4

J1930 **Injection, lanreotide, 1 mg** K K2 ☑
Use this code for Somatuline.

J1931 **Injection, laronidase, 0.1 mg** K K2 ☑
Use this code for Aldurazyme.
AHA: 2Q, '05, 11; 1Q, '05, 7, 9-10

J1940 **Injection, furosemide, up to 20 mg** N N1 ☑
Use this code for Lasix.
CMS: 100-04,4,20.6.4
AHA: 4Q, '05, 1-6; 3Q, '04, 1-10

~~**J1942**~~ Jan ~~**Injection, aripiprazole lauroxil, 1 mg**~~
To report, see ~J1943-J1944

● **J1943** Jan **Injection, aripiprazole lauroxil, (Aristada Initio), 1 mg** K2

● **J1944** Jan **Injection, aripiprazole lauroxil, (Aristada), 1 mg** K2

J1945 **Injection, lepirudin, 50 mg** E ☑
Use this code for Refludan.
This drug is used for patients with heparin-induced thrombocytopenia.

J1950 **Injection, leuprolide acetate (for depot suspension), per 3.75 mg** K K2 ☑
Use this code for Lupron Depot-Pedi.

J1953 **Injection, levetiracetam, 10 mg** N N1 ☑
Use this code for Keppra.

J1955 **Injection, levocarnitine, per 1 g** B ☑
Use this code for Carnitor.

J1956 **Injection, levofloxacin, 250 mg** N N1 ☑
Use this code for Levaquin.
CMS: 100-04,4,20.6.4

J1960 **Injection, levorphanol tartrate, up to 2 mg** N N1 ☑
Use this code for Levo-Dromoran.
CMS: 100-04,4,20.6.4

J1980 **Injection, hyoscyamine sulfate, up to 0.25 mg** N N1 ☑
Use this code for Levsin.
CMS: 100-04,4,20.6.4

J1990 **Injection, chlordiazepoxide HCl, up to 100 mg** N N1 ☑
Use this code for Librium.
CMS: 100-04,4,20.6.4

J2001 **Injection, lidocaine HCl for intravenous infusion, 10 mg** N N1 ☑
Use this code for Xylocaine.
CMS: 100-04,4,20.6.4

J2010 **Injection, lincomycin HCl, up to 300 mg** N N1 ☑
Use this code for Lincocin.
CMS: 100-04,4,20.6.4

J2020 **Injection, linezolid, 200 mg** N N1 ☑
Use this code for Zyvok.
AHA: 2Q, '02, 8-9; 1Q, '02, 5

J2060 **Injection, lorazepam, 2 mg** N N1 ☑
Use this code for Ativan.
CMS: 100-04,4,20.6.4

J2062 **Loxapine for inhalation, 1 mg** K2
Use this code for Adasuve.

J2150 **Injection, mannitol, 25% in 50 ml** N N1 ☑
Use this code for Osmitrol.
CMS: 100-04,4,20.6.4

J2170 **Injection, mecasermin, 1 mg** N N1 ☑
Use this code for Iplex, Increlex.
CMS: 100-02,15,50.5; 100-04,4,20.6.4

J2175 **Injection, meperidine HCl, per 100 mg** N N1 ☑
Use this code for Demerol.
CMS: 100-04,20,180; 100-04,4,20.6.4

J2180 **Injection, meperidine and promethazine HCl, up to 50 mg** N N1 ☑
Use this code for Mepergan Injection.
CMS: 100-04,4,20.6.4

J2182 **Injection, mepolizumab, 1 mg** G K2 ☑
Use this code for Nucala.

J2185 **Injection, meropenem, 100 mg** N N1 ☑
Use this code for Merrem.
CMS: 100-04,4,20.6.4
AHA: 2Q, '05, 11

J2186 **Injection, meropenem, vaborbactam, 10 mg/10 mg, (20 mg)** K2
Use this code for Vabomere.
CMS: 100-04,4,260.1; 100-04,4,260.1.1

J2210 **Injection, methylergonovine maleate, up to 0.2 mg** N N1 ☑
Use this code for Methergine.
CMS: 100-04,4,20.6.4

J2212 **Injection, methylnaltrexone, 0.1 mg** N N1 ☑
Use this code for Relistor.
CMS: 100-02,15,50.5

J2248 **Injection, micafungin sodium, 1 mg** N N1 ☑
Use this code for Mycamine.

J2250 **Injection, midazolam HCl, per 1 mg** N N1 ☑
Use this code for Versed.
CMS: 100-04,4,20.6.4

J2260 **Injection, milrinone lactate, 5 mg** N N1 ☑
Use this code for Primacor.
CMS: 100-04,20,180; 100-04,4,20.6.4

J2265 **Injection, minocycline HCl, 1 mg** K K2 ☑
Use this code for MINOCIN.

© 2019 Optum360, LLC

J2270 **Injection, morphine sulfate, up to 10 mg** N N1 ☑
Use this code for Depodur, Infumorph.
CMS: 100-04,20,180; 100-04,4,20.6.4
AHA: 2Q, '13, 5; 4Q, '05, 1-6; 3Q, '04, 1-10

J2274 **Injection, morphine sulfate, preservative free for epidural or intrathecal use, 10 mg** N N1 ☑
Use this code for DepoDur, Astromorph PF, Durarmorph PF.
CMS: 100-04,20,180
AHA: 1Q, '15, 6

J2278 **Injection, ziconotide, 1 mcg** K K2 ☑
Use this code for Prialt.
CMS: 100-04,20,180

J2280 **Injection, moxifloxacin, 100 mg** N N1 ☑
Use this code for Avelox.
CMS: 100-04,4,20.6.4
AHA: 2Q, '05, 11

J2300 **Injection, nalbuphine HCl, per 10 mg** N N1 ☑
Use this code for Nubain.
CMS: 100-04,4,20.6.4

J2310 **Injection, naloxone HCl, per 1 mg** N N1 ☑
Use this code for Narcan.

J2315 **Injection, naltrexone, depot form, 1 mg** K K2 ☑
Use this code for Vivitrol.

J2320 **Injection, nandrolone decanoate, up to 50 mg** K K2 ☑

J2323 **Injection, natalizumab, 1 mg** K K2 ☑
Use this code for Tysabri.
AHA: 1Q, '08, 6

J2325 **Injection, nesiritide, 0.1 mg** K K2 ☑
Use this code for Natrecor.
CMS: 100-03,200.1

J2326 **Injection, nusinersen, 0.1 mg** G K2
Use this code for Spinraza.

J2350 **Injection, ocrelizumab, 1 mg** G K2
Use this code for Ocrevus.

J2353 **Injection, octreotide, depot form for intramuscular injection, 1 mg** K K2 ☑
Use this code for Sandostatin LAR.

J2354 **Injection, octreotide, nondepot form for subcutaneous or intravenous injection, 25 mcg** N N1 ☑
Use this code for Sandostatin.
CMS: 100-02,15,50.5

J2355 **Injection, oprelvekin, 5 mg** K K2 ☑
Use this code for Neumega.
AHA: 2Q, '05, 11

J2357 **Injection, omalizumab, 5 mg** K K2 ☑
Use this code for Xolair.
AHA: 2Q, '05, 11

J2358 **Injection, olanzapine, long-acting, 1 mg** N N1 ☑
Use this code for ZYPREXA RELPREVV.

J2360 **Injection, orphenadrine citrate, up to 60 mg** N N1 ☑
Use this code for Norflex.

J2370 **Injection, phenylephrine HCl, up to 1 ml** N N1 ☑

J2400 **Injection, chloroprocaine HCl, per 30 ml** N N1 ☑
Use this code for Nesacaine, Nesacaine-MPF.

J2405 **Injection, ondansetron HCl, per 1 mg** N N1 ☑
Use this code for Zofran.

J2407 **Injection, oritavancin, 10 mg** K K2 ☑
Use this code for Orbactiv.

J2410 **Injection, oxymorphone HCl, up to 1 mg** N N1 ☑
Use this code for Numorphan, Oxymorphone HCl.

J2425 **Injection, palifermin, 50 mcg** K K2 ☑
Use this code for Kepivance.

J2426 **Injection, paliperidone palmitate extended release, 1 mg** K K2 ☑
Use this code for INVEGA SUSTENNA.

J2430 **Injection, pamidronate disodium, per 30 mg** N N1 ☑
Use this code for Aredia.

J2440 **Injection, papaverine HCl, up to 60 mg** N N1 ☑

J2460 **Injection, oxytetracycline HCl, up to 50 mg** E ☑
Use this code for Terramycin IM.

J2469 **Injection, palonosetron HCl, 25 mcg** K K2 ☑
Use this code for Aloxi.
AHA: 2Q, '05, 11; 1Q, '05, 7, 9-10

J2501 **Injection, paricalcitol, 1 mcg** N N1 ☑
Use this code For Zemplar.

J2502 **Injection, pasireotide long acting, 1 mg** K K2 ☑
Use this code for Signifor LAR.

J2503 **Injection, pegaptanib sodium, 0.3 mg** K N1 ☑
Use this code for Macugen.

J2504 **Injection, pegademase bovine, 25 IU** K K2 ☑
Use this code for Adagen.

J2505 **Injection, pegfilgrastim, 6 mg** K K2 ☑
Use this code for Neulasta.

J2507 **Injection, pegloticase, 1 mg** K K2 ☑
Use this code for KRYSTEXXA.

J2510 **Injection, penicillin G procaine, aqueous, up to 600,000 units** N N1 ☑
Use this code for Wycillin, Duracillin A.S., Pfizerpen A.S., Crysticillin 300 A.S., Crysticillin 600 A.S.

J2513 **Injection, pentastarch, 10% solution, 100 ml** E ☑

J2515 **Injection, pentobarbital sodium, per 50 mg** K K2 ☑
Use this code for Nembutal Sodium Solution.

J2540 **Injection, penicillin G potassium, up to 600,000 units** N N1 ☑
Use this code for Pfizerpen.

J2543 **Injection, piperacillin sodium/tazobactam sodium, 1 g/0.125 g (1.125 g)** N N1 ☑
Use this code for Zosyn.

J2545 **Pentamidine isethionate, inhalation solution, FDA-approved final product, noncompounded, administered through DME, unit dose form, per 300 mg** B ☑
Use this code for Nebupent, Pentam 300.

J2547 **Injection, peramivir, 1 mg** K K2 ☑
Use this code for Rapivab.

J2550 **Injection, promethazine HCl, up to 50 mg** N N1 ☑
Use this code for Phenergan.

J2560 **Injection, phenobarbital sodium, up to 120 mg** N N1 ☑

J2562 **Injection, plerixafor, 1 mg** K K2 ☑
Use this code for Mozobil.

J2590 **Injection, oxytocin, up to 10 units** N N1 ☑
Use this code for Pitocin, Syntocinon.

J2597 **Injection, desmopressin acetate, per 1 mcg** K K2 ☑
Use this code for DDAVP.

J2650 **Injection, prednisolone acetate, up to 1 ml** N N1 ☑

J2670 **Injection, tolazoline HCl, up to 25 mg** N ☑

© 2019 Optum360, LLC

J2675 **Injection, progesterone, per 50 mg** N N1 ☑
Use this code for Gesterone, Gestrin.

J2680 **Injection, fluphenazine decanoate, up to 25 mg** N N1 ☑

J2690 **Injection, procainamide HCl, up to 1 g** N N1 ☑
Use this code for Pronestyl.

J2700 **Injection, oxacillin sodium, up to 250 mg** N N1 ☑
Use this code for Bactocill

J2704 **Injection, propofol, 10 mg** N N1 ☑
Use this code for Diprivan.
AHA: 1Q, '15, 6

J2710 **Injection, neostigmine methylsulfate, up to 0.5 mg** N N1 ☑
Use this code for Prostigmin.

J2720 **Injection, protamine sulfate, per 10 mg** N N1 ☑

J2724 **Injection, protein C concentrate, intravenous, human, 10 IU** K K2 ☑

J2725 **Injection, protirelin, per 250 mcg** E ☑
Use this code for Thyrel TRH.

J2730 **Injection, pralidoxime chloride, up to 1 g** N N1 ☑
Use this code for Protopam Chloride.

J2760 **Injection, phentolamine mesylate, up to 5 mg** K K2 ☑
Use this code for Regitine.

J2765 **Injection, metoclopramide HCl, up to 10 mg** N N1 ☑
Use this code for Reglan.

J2770 **Injection, quinupristin/dalfopristin, 500 mg (150/350)** K K2 ☑
Use this code for Synercid.

J2778 **Injection, ranibizumab, 0.1 mg** K K2 ☑
Use this code for Lucentis.
AHA: 1Q, '08, 6

J2780 **Injection, ranitidine HCl, 25 mg** N N1 ☑
Use this code for Zantac.

J2783 **Injection, rasburicase, 0.5 mg** K K2 ☑
Use this code for Elitek.
AHA: 2Q, '05, 11; 2Q, '04, 8

J2785 **Injection, regadenoson, 0.1 mg** N N1 ☑
Use this code for Lexiscan.

J2786 **Injection, reslizumab, 1 mg** G K2 ☑
Use this code for Cinqair.

J2787 **Riboflavin 5'-phosphate, ophthalmic solution, up to 3 ml**
Use this code for Photrexa Viscous.
CMS: 100-04,4,260.1; 100-04,4,260.1.1

J2788 **Injection, Rho D immune globulin, human, minidose, 50 mcg (250 IU)** N N1 ☑
Use this code for RhoGam, MiCRhoGAM.

J2790 **Injection, Rho D immune globulin, human, full dose, 300 mcg (1500 IU)** N N1 ☑
Use this code for RhoGam, HypRho SD.

J2791 **Injection, Rho D immune globulin (human), (Rhophylac), intramuscular or intravenous, 100 IU** N N1 ☑
Use this for Rhophylac.
AHA: 1Q, '08, 6

J2792 **Injection, Rho D immune globulin, intravenous, human, solvent detergent, 100 IU** K K2 ☑
Use this code for WINRho SDF.

J2793 **Injection, rilonacept, 1 mg** K N1 ☑
Use this code for Arcalyst.
CMS: 100-02,15,50.5

▲ **J2794**[Jan] **Injection, risperidone (RISPERDAL CONSTA), 0.5 mg** K K2 ☑
AHA: 2Q, '05, 11; 1Q, '05, 7, 9-10

J2795 **Injection, ropivacaine HCl, 1 mg** N N1 ☑
Use this code for Naropin.

J2796 **Injection, romiplostim, 10 mcg** K K2 ☑
Use this code for Nplate.

J2797 **Injection, rolapitant, 0.5 mg** K2
Use this code for Varubi.

● **J2798**[Jan] **Injection, risperidone, (Perseris), 0.5 mg** K2

J2800 **Injection, methocarbamol, up to 10 ml** N N1 ☑
Use this code for Robaxin.

J2805 **Injection, sincalide, 5 mcg** N N1 ☑
Use this code for Kinevac.
AHA: 4Q, '05, 1-6

J2810 **Injection, theophylline, per 40 mg** N N1 ☑

J2820 **Injection, sargramostim (GM-CSF), 50 mcg** K K2 ☑
Use this code for Leukine.

J2840 **Injection, sebelipase alfa, 1 mg** G K2 ☑
Use this code for Kanuma.

J2850 **Injection, secretin, synthetic, human, 1 mcg** K K2 ☑

J2860 **Injection, siltuximab, 10 mg** K K2 ☑
Use this code for Sylvant.

J2910 **Injection, aurothioglucose, up to 50 mg** E ☑
Use this code for Solganal.

J2916 **Injection, sodium ferric gluconate complex in sucrose injection, 12.5 mg** N N1 ☑
CMS: 100-03,110.10

J2920 **Injection, methylprednisolone sodium succinate, up to 40 mg** N N1 ☑
Use this code for Solu-Medrol, A-methaPred.

J2930 **Injection, methylprednisolone sodium succinate, up to 125 mg** N N1 ☑
Use this code for Solu-Medrol, A-methaPred.

J2940 **Injection, somatrem, 1 mg** E ☑
Use this code for Protropin.
AHA: 2Q, '02, 8-9; 1Q, '02, 5

J2941 **Injection, somatropin, 1 mg** K N1 ☑
Use this code for Humatrope, Genotropin Nutropin, Biotropin, Genotropin, Genotropin Miniquick, Norditropin, Nutropin, Nutropin AQ, Saizen, Saizen Somatropin RDNA Origin, Serostim, Serostim RDNA Origin, Zorbtive.
CMS: 100-02,15,50.5
AHA: 2Q, '02, 8-9; 1Q, '02, 5

J2950 **Injection, promazine HCl, up to 25 mg** N N1 ☑
Use this code for Sparine, Prozine-50.

J2993 **Injection, reteplase, 18.1 mg** K K2 ☑
Use this code for Retavase.

J2995 **Injection, streptokinase, per 250,000 IU** N ☑
Use this code for Streptase.

J2997 **Injection, alteplase recombinant, 1 mg** K K2 ☑
Use this code for Activase, Cathflo.
AHA: 1Q, '14, 4

J3000 **Injection, streptomycin, up to 1 g** N N1 ☑
Use this code for Streptomycin Sulfate.

J3010 **Injection, fentanyl citrate, 0.1 mg** N N1 ☑
Use this code for Sublimaze.
CMS: 100-04,20,180

© 2019 Optum360, LLC

J3030 **Injection, sumatriptan succinate, 6 mg (code may be used for Medicare when drug administered under the direct supervision of a physician, not for use when drug is self-administered)** N N1 ☑
Use this code for Imitrex.
CMS: 100-02,15,50.5

● **J3031**Jan **Injection, fremanezumab-vfrm, 1 mg (code may be used for Medicare when drug administered under the direct supervision of a physician, not for use when drug is self-administered)** K2
Use this code for Ajovy.

J3060 **Injection, taliglucerase alfa, 10 units** K K2 ☑
Use this code for Elelyso.

J3070 **Injection, pentazocine, 30 mg** K N1 ☑
Use this code for Talwin.

J3090 **Injection, tedizolid phosphate, 1 mg** K K2 ☑
Use this code for Sivextro.

J3095 **Injection, telavancin, 10 mg** K K2 ☑
Use this code for VIBATIV.

J3101 **Injection, tenecteplase, 1 mg** K K2 ☑
Use this code for TNKase.

J3105 **Injection, terbutaline sulfate, up to 1 mg** N N1 ☑
For terbutaline in inhalation solution, see K0525 and K0526.

J3110 **Injection, teriparatide, 10 mcg** B ☑
Use this code for Forteo.
CMS: 100-02,15,50.5; 100-04,10,90.1

● **J3111**Jan **Injection, romosozumab-aqqg, 1 mg** K2
Use this code for Evenity.

J3121 **Injection, testosterone enanthate, 1 mg** N N1 ☑
Use this code for Delatstryl.
AHA: 1Q, '15, 6

J3145 **Injection, testosterone undecanoate, 1 mg** K K2 ☑
Use this code for Aveed.
AHA: 1Q, '15, 6

J3230 **Injection, chlorpromazine HCl, up to 50 mg** N N1 ☑
Use this code for Thorazine.

J3240 **Injection, thyrotropin alpha, 0.9 mg, provided in 1.1 mg vial** K K2 ☑
Use this code for Thyrogen.
AHA: 4Q, '05, 1-6; 2Q, '05, 11; 3Q, '04, 1-10

J3243 **Injection, tigecycline, 1 mg** K K2 ☑
Use this code for Tygacil.

J3245 **Injection, tildrakizumab, 1 mg** K2
Use this code for Ilumya.

J3246 **Injection, tirofiban HCl, 0.25 mg** K K2 ☑
Use this code for Aggrastat.
AHA: 1Q, '05, 7, 9-10

J3250 **Injection, trimethobenzamide HCl, up to 200 mg** N N1 ☑
Use this code for Tigan, Tiject-20, Arrestin.

J3260 **Injection, tobramycin sulfate, up to 80 mg** N N1 ☑
Use this code for Nebcin.

J3262 **Injection, tocilizumab, 1 mg** K K2 ☑
Use this code for ACTEMRA.

J3265 **Injection, torsemide, 10 mg/ml** N N1 ☑
Use this code for Demadex, Torsemide.

J3280 **Injection, thiethylperazine maleate, up to 10 mg** E ☑

J3285 **Injection, treprostinil, 1 mg** K K2 ☑
Use this code for Remodulin.
CMS: 100-04,20,180

J3300 **Injection, triamcinolone acetonide, preservative free, 1 mg** K K2 ☑
Use this code for TRIVARIS, TRIESENCE.

J3301 **Injection, triamcinolone acetonide, not otherwise specified, 10 mg** N N1 ☑
Use this code for Kenalog-10, Kenalog-40, Tri-Kort, Kenaject-40, Cenacort A-40, Triam-A, Trilog.
AHA: 2Q, '13, 5

J3302 **Injection, triamcinolone diacetate, per 5 mg** N N1 ☑
Use this code for Aristocort, Aristocort Intralesional, Aristocort Forte, Amcort, Trilone, Cenacort Forte.

J3303 **Injection, triamcinolone hexacetonide, per 5 mg** N N1 ☑
Use this code for Aristospan Intralesional, Aristospan Intra-articular.

J3304 **Injection, triamcinolone acetonide, preservative-free, extended-release, microsphere formulation, 1 mg** K2
Use this code for Zilretta.

J3305 **Injection, trimetrexate glucuronate, per 25 mg** E ☑
Use this code for Neutrexin.

J3310 **Injection, perphenazine, up to 5 mg** N N1 ☑
Use this code for Trilafon.

J3315 **Injection, triptorelin pamoate, 3.75 mg** ♂ K K2 ☑
Use this code for Trelstar Depot, Trelstar Depot Plus Debioclip Kit, Trelstar LA.

J3316 **Injection, triptorelin, extended-release, 3.75 mg** K2
Use this code for Triptodur.

J3320 **Injection, spectinomycin dihydrochloride, up to 2 g** E ☑
Use this code for Trobicin.

J3350 **Injection, urea, up to 40 g** N N1 ☑

J3355 **Injection, urofollitropin, 75 IU** E ☑
Use this code for Metrodin, Bravelle, Fertinex.
CMS: 100-02,15,50.5

J3357 **Ustekinumab, for subcutaneous injection, 1 mg** K K2 ☑
Use this code for STELARA.
CMS: 100-02,15,50.5
AHA: 1Q, '17, 1-3; 4Q, '16, 10

J3358 **Ustekinumab, for intravenous injection, 1 mg** G K2
Use this code for Stelara.

J3360 **Injection, diazepam, up to 5 mg** N N1 ☑
Use this code for Diastat, Dizac, Valium.
AHA: 2Q, '07, 6

J3364 **Injection, urokinase, 5,000 IU vial** N N1 ☑
Use this code for Kinlytic.

J3365 **Injection, IV, urokinase, 250,000 IU vial** E ☑
Use this code for Kinlytic.

J3370 **Injection, vancomycin HCl, 500 mg** N N1 ☑
Use this code for Vancocin.

J3380 **Injection, vedolizumab, 1 mg** K K2 ☑
Use this code for Entyvio.

J3385 **Injection, velaglucerase alfa, 100 units** K K2 ☑
Use this code for VPRIV.

J3396 **Injection, verteporfin, 0.1 mg** K K2 ☑
Use this code for Visudyne.
CMS: 100-03,80.2; 100-03,80.2.1; 100-03,80.3; 100-03,80.3.1; 100-04,32,300; 100-04,32,300.1; 100-04,32,300.2
AHA: 1Q, '05, 7, 9-10

J3397 **Injection, vestronidase alfa-vjbk, 1 mg** K2
Use this code for Mepsevii.
CMS: 100-04,4,260.1; 100-04,4,260.1.1

© 2019 Optum360, LLC

J3398 **Injection, voretigene neparvovec-rzyl, 1 billion vector genomes** K2
Use this code for Luxturna.

J3400 **Injection, triflupromazine HCl, up to 20 mg** E ☑

J3410 **Injection, hydroxyzine HCl, up to 25 mg** N N1 ☑
Use this code for Vistaril, Vistaject-25, Hyzine, Hyzine-50.

J3411 **Injection, thiamine HCl, 100 mg** N N1 ☑
AHA: 2Q, '05, 11

J3415 **Injection, pyridoxine HCl, 100 mg** N N1 ☑
AHA: 2Q, '05, 11

J3420 **Injection, vitamin B-12 cyanocobalamin, up to 1,000 mcg** N N1 ☑
Use this code for Sytobex, Redisol, Rubramin PC, Betalin 12, Berubigen, Cobex, Cobal, Crystal B12, Cyano, Cyanocobalamin, Hydroxocobalamin, Hydroxycobal, Nutri-Twelve.

J3430 **Injection, phytonadione (vitamin K), per 1 mg** N N1 ☑
Use this code for AquaMephyton, Konakion, Menadione, Phytonadione.

J3465 **Injection, voriconazole, 10 mg** K N1 ☑
AHA: 2Q, '05, 11

J3470 **Injection, hyaluronidase, up to 150 units** N N1 ☑

J3471 **Injection, hyaluronidase, ovine, preservative free, per 1 USP unit (up to 999 USP units)** N N1 ☑

J3472 **Injection, hyaluronidase, ovine, preservative free, per 1,000 USP units** N N1 ☑

J3473 **Injection, hyaluronidase, recombinant, 1 USP unit** N N1 ☑

J3475 **Injection, magnesium sulfate, per 500 mg** N N1 ☑
Use this code for Mag Sul, Sulfa Mag.

J3480 **Injection, potassium chloride, per 2 mEq** N N1 ☑

J3485 **Injection, zidovudine, 10 mg** N N1 ☑
Use this code for Retrovir, Zidovudine.

J3486 **Injection, ziprasidone mesylate, 10 mg** N N1 ☑
Use this code for Geodon.
AHA: 2Q, '05, 11

J3489 **Injection, zoledronic acid, 1 mg** N N1 ☑
Use this code for Reclast and Zometa.

J3490 **Unclassified drugs** N N1 ☑
CMS: 100-02,15,50.5; 100-03,1,110.22; 100-03,110.22; 100-04,10,90.1; 100-04,32,280.1; 100-04,32,280.2; 100-04,4,260.1; 100-04,4,260.1.1; 100-04,8,60.2.1.1
AHA: 1Q, '17, 8; 1Q, '17, 1-3; 3Q, '15, 7; 4Q, '14, 5; 2Q, '14, 8; 2Q, '13, 5; 1Q, '13, 9; 4Q, '12, 9; 2Q, '09, 1; 1Q, '08, 6; 4Q, '05, 1-6; 3Q, '04, 1-10

J3520 **Edetate disodium, per 150 mg** E ☑
Use this code for Endrate, Disotate, Meritate, Chealamide, E.D.T.A. This drug is used in chelation therapy, a treatment for atherosclerosis that is not covered by Medicare.

J3530 **Nasal vaccine inhalation** N N1 ☑

J3535 **Drug administered through a metered dose inhaler** E ☑

J3570 **Laetrile, amygdalin, vitamin B-17** E ☑
The FDA has found Laetrile to have no safe or effective therapeutic purpose.

J3590 **Unclassified biologics** N N1 ☑
CMS: 100-02,15,50.5; 100-03,1,110.22; 100-03,110.22; 100-04,32,280.1; 100-04,32,280.2
AHA: 1Q, '17, 1-3; 4Q, '16, 10; 3Q, '15, 7; 4Q, '12, 9

J3591 **Unclassified drug or biological used for ESRD on dialysis**
CMS: 100-04,4,260.1; 100-04,4,260.1.1

J7030 **Infusion, normal saline solution, 1,000 cc** N N1 ☑

J7040 **Infusion, normal saline solution, sterile (500 ml=1 unit)** N N1 ☑

J7042 **5% dextrose/normal saline (500 ml = 1 unit)** N N1 ☑

J7050 **Infusion, normal saline solution, 250 cc** N N1 ☑

J7060 **5% dextrose/water (500 ml = 1 unit)** N N1 ☑

J7070 **Infusion, D-5-W, 1,000 cc** N N1 ☑

J7100 **Infusion, dextran 40, 500 ml** N N1 ☑
Use this code for Gentran, 10% LMD, Rheomacrodex.

J7110 **Infusion, dextran 75, 500 ml** N N1 ☑
Use this code for Gentran 75.

J7120 **Ringers lactate infusion, up to 1,000 cc** N N1 ☑

J7121 **5% dextrose in lactated ringers infusion, up to 1000 cc** N N1 ☑
AHA: 1Q, '16, 6-8

J7131 **Hypertonic saline solution, 1 ml** N N1 ☑

J7170 **Injection, emicizumab-kxwh, 0.5 mg** K2
Use this code for Hemlibra.

J7175 **Injection, Factor X, (human), 1 IU** K K2 ☑
Use this code for Coagadex.
AHA: 1Q, '17, 9-10

J7177 **Injection, human fibrinogen concentrate (Fibryga), 1 mg** K2
CMS: 100-04,4,260.1; 100-04,4,260.1.1

J7178 **Injection, human fibrinogen concentrate, not otherwise specified, 1 mg** K K2 ☑
Use this code for RiaSTAP.

J7179 **Injection, von Willebrand factor (recombinant), (Vonvendi), 1 IU VWF:RCo** G K2 ☑
AHA: 1Q, '17, 9-10

J7180 **Injection, Factor XIII (antihemophilic factor, human), 1 IU** K K2 ☑
Use this code for Corifact.

J7181 **Injection, Factor XIII A-subunit, (recombinant), per IU** K K2 ☑
AHA: 1Q, '15, 6

J7182 **Injection, Factor VIII, (antihemophilic factor, recombinant), (NovoEight), per IU** K K2 ☑
AHA: 1Q, '15, 6

J7183 **Injection, von Willebrand factor complex (human), Wilate, 1 IU VWF:RCO** K K2 ☑

J7185 **Injection, Factor VIII (antihemophilic factor, recombinant) (Xyntha), per IU** K K2 ☑

J7186 **Injection, antihemophilic Factor VIII/von Willebrand factor complex (human), per Factor VIII IU** K K2 ☑
Use this code for Alphanate.
CMS: 100-04,17,80.4.1

J7187 **Injection, von Willebrand factor complex (Humate-P), per IU VWF:RCO** K K2 ☑
CMS: 100-04,17,80.4.1

J7188 **Injection, Factor VIII (antihemophilic factor, recombinant), per IU** K K2 ☑
Use this code for Obizur.
AHA: 1Q, '16, 6-8

J7189 **Factor VIIa (antihemophilic factor, recombinant), per 1 mcg** K K2 ☑
CMS: 100-04,17,80.4.1

J7190 **Factor VIII (antihemophilic factor, human) per IU** K K2 ☑
Use this code for Koate-DVI, Monarc-M, Monoclate-P.
CMS: 100-04,17,80.4; 100-04,17,80.4.1

© 2019 Optum360, LLC

J7191 **Factor VIII (antihemophilic factor (porcine)), per IU** E ☑
CMS: 100-04,17,80.4; 100-04,17,80.4.1

J7192 **Factor VIII (antihemophilic factor, recombinant) per IU, not otherwise specified** K K2 ☑
Use this code for Recombinate, Kogenate FS, Helixate FX, Advate rAHF-PFM, Antihemophilic Factor Human Method M Monoclonal Purified, Refacto.
CMS: 100-04,17,80.4; 100-04,17,80.4.1
AHA: 2Q, '13, 5

J7193 **Factor IX (antihemophilic factor, purified, nonrecombinant) per IU** K K2 ☑
Use this code for AlphaNine SD, Mononine.
CMS: 100-04,17,80.4; 100-04,17,80.4.1
AHA: 2Q, '02, 8-9

J7194 **Factor IX complex, per IU** K K2 ☑
Use this code for Konyne-80, Profilnine SD, Proplex T, Proplex T, Bebulin VH, factor IX+ complex, Profilnine SD.
CMS: 100-04,17,80.4; 100-04,17,80.4.1

J7195 **Injection, Factor IX (antihemophilic factor, recombinant) per IU, not otherwise specified** K K2 ☑
Use this code for Benefix.
CMS: 100-04,17,80.4; 100-04,17,80.4.1
AHA: 2Q, '02, 8-9; 1Q, '02, 5

J7196 **Injection, antithrombin recombinant, 50 IU** E ☑
Use this code for ATryn.

J7197 **Antithrombin III (human), per IU** K K2 ☑
Use this code for Thrombate III, ATnativ.
CMS: 100-04,17,80.4.1

J7198 **Antiinhibitor, per IU** K K2 ☑
Medicare jurisdiction: local contractor. Use this code for Autoplex T, Feiba VH AICC.
CMS: 100-03,110.3; 100-04,17,80.4; 100-04,17,80.4.1

J7199 **Hemophilia clotting factor, not otherwise classified** B ☑
Medicare jurisdiction: local contractor.
CMS: 100-04,17,80.4; 100-04,17,80.4.1
AHA: 2Q, '13, 5

J7200 **Injection, Factor IX, (antihemophilic factor, recombinant), Rixubis, per IU** K K2 ☑
AHA: 1Q, '15, 6

J7201 **Injection, Factor IX, Fc fusion protein, (recombinant), Alprolix, 1 IU** K K2 ☑
AHA: 1Q, '15, 6

J7202 **Injection, Factor IX, albumin fusion protein, (recombinant), Idelvion, 1 IU** G K2 ☑

J7203 **Injection Factor IX, (antihemophilic factor, recombinant), glycoPEGylated, (Rebinyn), 1 IU** K2

J7205 **Injection, Factor VIII Fc fusion protein (recombinant), per IU** K K2 ☑
Use this code for Eloctate.

J7207 **Injection, Factor VIII, (antihemophilic factor, recombinant), PEGylated, 1 IU** G K2 ☑
Use this code for Adynovate.

● **J7208**[Jan] **Injection, Factor VIII, (antihemophilic factor, recombinant), PEGylated-aucl, (Jivi), 1 IU** K2

J7209 **Injection, Factor VIII, (antihemophilic factor, recombinant), (Nuwiq), 1 IU** G K2 ☑

J7210 **Injection, Factor VIII, (antihemophilic factor, recombinant), (Afstyla), 1 IU** G K2

J7211 **Injection, Factor VIII, (antihemophilic factor, recombinant), (Kovaltry), 1 IU** K K2

J7296 **Levonorgestrel-releasing intrauterine contraceptive system, (Kyleena), 19.5 mg** ♀ E

J7297 **Levonorgestrel-releasing intrauterine contraceptive system (Liletta), 52 mg** M ♀ E ☑
AHA: 1Q, '16, 6-8

J7298 **Levonorgestrel-releasing intrauterine contraceptive system (Mirena), 52 mg** M ♀ E ☑
AHA: 1Q, '16, 6-8

J7300 **Intrauterine copper contraceptive** E ☑
Use this code for Paragard T380A.

J7301 **Levonorgestrel-releasing intrauterine contraceptive system (Skyla), 13.5 mg** M ♀ E ☑
AHA: 4Q, '14, 6

J7303 **Contraceptive supply, hormone containing vaginal ring, each** ♀ E ☑
Use this code for Nuvaring Vaginal Ring.

J7304 **Contraceptive supply, hormone containing patch, each** E ☑

J7306 **Levonorgestrel (contraceptive) implant system, including implants and supplies** E ☑

J7307 **Etonogestrel (contraceptive) implant system, including implant and supplies** E ☑
Use this code for Implanon and Nexplanon.

J7308 **Aminolevulinic acid HCl for topical administration, 20%, single unit dosage form (354 mg)** K K2 ☑
Use this code for Levulan Kerastick.
AHA: 2Q, '05, 11; 1Q, '02, 5

J7309 **Methyl aminolevulinate (MAL) for topical administration, 16.8%, 1 g** N ☑
Use this code for Metvixia.

J7310 **Ganciclovir, 4.5 mg, long-acting implant** E ☑
Use this code for Vitrasert.

▲ **J7311**[Jan] **Injection, fluocinolone acetonide, intravitreal implant (Retisert), 0.01 mg** K K2 ☑

J7312 **Injection, dexamethasone, intravitreal implant, 0.1 mg** K K2 ☑
Use this code for OZURDEX.

▲ **J7313**[Jan] **Injection, fluocinolone acetonide, intravitreal implant (Iluvien), 0.01 mg** K K2 ☑

● **J7314**[Jan] **Injection, fluocinolone acetonide, intravitreal implant (Yutiq), 0.01 mg** K2

J7315 **Mitomycin, opthalmic, 0.2 mg** N M1 ☑
Use this code for Mitosol.
AHA: 4Q, '16, 8; 2Q, '14, 8; 2Q, '13, 9

J7316 **Injection, ocriplasmin, 0.125 mg** K K2 ☑
Use this code for Jetrea.

J7318 **Hyaluronan or derivative, Durolane, for intra-articular injection, 1 mg** K2

J7320 **Hyaluronan or derivative, GenVisc 850, for intra-articular injection, 1 mg** K K2 ☑

J7321 **Hyaluronan or derivative, Hyalgan, Supartz or Visco-3, for intra-articular injection, per dose** K K2 ☑
AHA: 4Q, '12, 9; 1Q, '08, 6

J7322 **Hyaluronan or derivative, Hymovis, for intra-articular injection, 1 mg** G K2 ☑

J7323 **Hyaluronan or derivative, Euflexxa, for intra-articular injection, per dose** K K2 ☑
AHA: 4Q, '12, 9; 1Q, '08, 6

© 2019 Optum360, LLC

J7324 **Hyaluronan or derivative, Orthovisc, for intra-articular injection, per dose** K K2 ☑
AHA: 4Q, '12, 9; 1Q, '08, 6

J7325 **Hyaluronan or derivative, Synvisc or Synvisc-One, for intra-articular injection, 1 mg** K K2 ☑
AHA: 4Q, '12, 9

J7326 **Hyaluronan or derivative, Gel-One, for intra-articular injection, per dose** K K2 ☑
AHA: 4Q, '12, 9

J7327 **Hyaluronan or derivative, Monovisc, for intra-articular injection, per dose** K K2 ☑
AHA: 1Q, '15, 6

J7328 **Hyaluronan or derivative, GELSYN-3, for intra-articular injection, 0.1 mg** G K2 ☑
AHA: 1Q, '16, 6-8

J7329 **Hyaluronan or derivative, Trivisc, for intra-articular injection, 1 mg** K2
CMS: 100-04,4,260.1; 100-04,4,260.1.1

J7330 **Autologous cultured chondrocytes, implant** B ☑
Medicare jurisdiction: local contractor. Use this code for Carticel.
AHA: 4Q, '10, 1

● **J7331**[Jan] **Hyaluronan or derivative, SYNOJOYNT, for intra-articular injection, 1 mg**

● **J7332**[Jan] **Hyaluronan or derivative, Triluron, for intra-articular injection, 1 mg**

J7336 **Capsaicin 8% patch, per sq cm** K K2 ☑
Use this code for Qutenza.
AHA: 1Q, '15, 6

J7340 **Carbidopa 5 mg/levodopa 20 mg enteral suspension, 100 ml** K N1 ☑
Use this code for Duopa.
AHA: 1Q, '16, 6-8

J7342 **Instillation, ciprofloxacin otic suspension, 6 mg** G K2 ☑
Use this code for Otipro.

J7345 **Aminolevulinic acid HCl for topical administration, 10% gel, 10 mg** G K2
Use this code for Ameluz.

● **J7401**[Jan] **Mometasone furoate sinus implant, 10 mcg**
Use this code for Sinuva.

J7500 **Azathioprine, oral, 50 mg** N N1 ☑
Use this code for Azasan, Imuran.
CMS: 100-04,17,80.3

J7501 **Azathioprine, parenteral, 100 mg** K K2 ☑
CMS: 100-04,17,80.3

J7502 **Cyclosporine, oral, 100 mg** N N1 ☑
Use this code for Neoral, Sandimmune, Gengraf, Sangcya.
CMS: 100-04,17,80.3

J7503 **Tacrolimus, extended release, (Envarsus XR), oral, 0.25 mg** G N1 ☑
AHA: 1Q, '16, 6-8

J7504 **Lymphocyte immune globulin, antithymocyte globulin, equine, parenteral, 250 mg** K K2 ☑
Use this code for Atgam.
CMS: 100-03,260.7; 100-04,17,80.3

J7505 **Muromonab-CD3, parenteral, 5 mg** K N1 ☑
Use this code for Orthoclone OKT3.
CMS: 100-04,17,80.3

J7507 **Tacrolimus, immediate release, oral, 1 mg** N N1 ☑
Use this code for Prograf.
CMS: 100-04,17,80.3

J7508 **Tacrolimus, extended release, (Astagraf XL), oral, 0.1 mg** N N1 ☑
AHA: 1Q, '16, 6-8; 1Q, '14, 6

J7509 **Methylprednisolone, oral, per 4 mg** N N1 ☑
Use this code for Medrol, Methylpred.
CMS: 100-04,17,80.3

J7510 **Prednisolone, oral, per 5 mg** N N1 ☑
Use this code for Delta-Cortef, Cotolone, Pediapred, Prednoral, Prelone.
CMS: 100-04,17,80.3

J7511 **Lymphocyte immune globulin, antithymocyte globulin, rabbit, parenteral, 25 mg** K K2 ☑
Use this code for Thymoglobulin.
CMS: 100-04,17,80.3
AHA: 2Q, '02, 8-9; 1Q, '02, 5

J7512 **Prednisone, immediate release or delayed release, oral, 1 mg** N N1 ☑
AHA: 1Q, '16, 6-8

J7513 **Daclizumab, parenteral, 25 mg** E ☑
Use this code for Zenapax.
CMS: 100-04,17,80.3
AHA: 2Q, '05, 11

J7515 **Cyclosporine, oral, 25 mg** N N1 ☑
Use this code for Neoral, Sandimmune, Gengraf, Sangcya.
CMS: 100-04,17,80.3

J7516 **Cyclosporine, parenteral, 250 mg** N N1 ☑
Use this code for Neoral, Sandimmune, Gengraf, Sangcya.
CMS: 100-04,17,80.3

J7517 **Mycophenolate mofetil, oral, 250 mg** N N1 ☑
Use this code for CellCept.
CMS: 100-04,17,80.3

J7518 **Mycophenolic acid, oral, 180 mg** N N1 ☑
Use this code for Myfortic Delayed Release.
CMS: 100-04,17,80.3.1
AHA: 2Q, '05, 11

J7520 **Sirolimus, oral, 1 mg** N N1 ☑
Use this code for Rapamune.
CMS: 100-04,17,80.3

J7525 **Tacrolimus, parenteral, 5 mg** K K2 ☑
Use this code for Prograf.
CMS: 100-04,17,80.3

J7527 **Everolimus, oral, 0.25 mg** N N1 ☑
Use this code for Zortress, Afinitor.

J7599 **Immunosuppressive drug, not otherwise classified** N N1 ☑
Determine if an alternative HCPCS Level II or a CPT code better describes the service being reported. This code should be used only if a more specific code is unavailable.
CMS: 100-04,17,80.3
AHA: 2Q, '13, 5

Inhalation Drugs

J7604 **Acetylcysteine, inhalation solution, compounded product, administered through DME, unit dose form, per g** M ☑

J7605 **Arformoterol, inhalation solution, FDA-approved final product, noncompounded, administered through DME, unit dose form, 15 mcg** M ☑
CMS: 100-02,15,50.5

© 2019 Optum360, LLC

J7606 **Formoterol fumarate, inhalation solution, FDA-approved final product, noncompounded, administered through DME, unit dose form, 20 mcg** M ☑
Use this code for PERFOROMIST.
CMS: 100-02,15,50.5

J7607 **Levalbuterol, inhalation solution, compounded product, administered through DME, concentrated form, 0.5 mg** M ☑
CMS: 100-03,200.2

J7608 **Acetylcysteine, inhalation solution, FDA-approved final product, noncompounded, administered through DME, unit dose form, per g** M ☑
Use this code for Acetadote, Mucomyst, Mucosil.

J7609 **Albuterol, inhalation solution, compounded product, administered through DME, unit dose, 1 mg** M ☑

J7610 **Albuterol, inhalation solution, compounded product, administered through DME, concentrated form, 1 mg** M ☑

J7611 **Albuterol, inhalation solution, FDA-approved final product, noncompounded, administered through DME, concentrated form, 1 mg** M ☑
Use this code for Accuneb, Proventil, Respirol, Ventolin.
AHA: 2Q, '08, 10

J7612 **Levalbuterol, inhalation solution, FDA-approved final product, noncompounded, administered through DME, concentrated form, 0.5 mg** M ☑
Use this code for Xopenex HFA.
CMS: 100-03,200.2
AHA: 2Q, '08, 10

J7613 **Albuterol, inhalation solution, FDA-approved final product, noncompounded, administered through DME, unit dose, 1 mg** M ☑
Use this code for Accuneb, Proventil, Respirol, Ventolin.
AHA: 2Q, '08, 10

J7614 **Levalbuterol, inhalation solution, FDA-approved final product, noncompounded, administered through DME, unit dose, 0.5 mg** M ☑
Use this code for Xopenex.
CMS: 100-03,200.2
AHA: 2Q, '08, 10

J7615 **Levalbuterol, inhalation solution, compounded product, administered through DME, unit dose, 0.5 mg** M ☑
CMS: 100-03,200.2

J7620 **Albuterol, up to 2.5 mg and ipratropium bromide, up to 0.5 mg, FDA-approved final product, noncompounded, administered through DME** M ☑

J7622 **Beclomethasone, inhalation solution, compounded product, administered through DME, unit dose form, per mg** M ☑
Use this code for Beclovent, Beconase.
AHA: 1Q, '02, 5

J7624 **Betamethasone, inhalation solution, compounded product, administered through DME, unit dose form, per mg** M ☑
AHA: 1Q, '02, 5

J7626 **Budesonide, inhalation solution, FDA-approved final product, noncompounded, administered through DME, unit dose form, up to 0.5 mg** M ☑
Use this code for Pulmicort, Pulmicort Flexhaler, Pulmicort Respules, Vanceril.
AHA: 1Q, '02, 5

J7627 **Budesonide, inhalation solution, compounded product, administered through DME, unit dose form, up to 0.5 mg** M ☑

J7628 **Bitolterol mesylate, inhalation solution, compounded product, administered through DME, concentrated form, per mg** M ☑

J7629 **Bitolterol mesylate, inhalation solution, compounded product, administered through DME, unit dose form, per mg** M ☑

J7631 **Cromolyn sodium, inhalation solution, FDA-approved final product, noncompounded, administered through DME, unit dose form, per 10 mg** M ☑
Use this code for Intal, Nasalcrom.

J7632 **Cromolyn sodium, inhalation solution, compounded product, administered through DME, unit dose form, per 10 mg** M ☑

J7633 **Budesonide, inhalation solution, FDA-approved final product, noncompounded, administered through DME, concentrated form, per 0.25 mg** M ☑
Use this code for Pulmicort, Pulmicort Flexhaler, Pulmicort Respules, Vanceril.

J7634 **Budesonide, inhalation solution, compounded product, administered through DME, concentrated form, per 0.25 mg** M ☑

J7635 **Atropine, inhalation solution, compounded product, administered through DME, concentrated form, per mg** M ☑

J7636 **Atropine, inhalation solution, compounded product, administered through DME, unit dose form, per mg** M ☑

J7637 **Dexamethasone, inhalation solution, compounded product, administered through DME, concentrated form, per mg** M ☑

J7638 **Dexamethasone, inhalation solution, compounded product, administered through DME, unit dose form, per mg** M ☑

J7639 **Dornase alfa, inhalation solution, FDA-approved final product, noncompounded, administered through DME, unit dose form, per mg** M ☑
Use this code for Pulmozyme.
CMS: 100-02,15,50.5

J7640 **Formoterol, inhalation solution, compounded product, administered through DME, unit dose form, 12 mcg** E ☑

J7641 **Flunisolide, inhalation solution, compounded product, administered through DME, unit dose, per mg** M ☑
Use this code for Aerobid, Flunisolide.
AHA: 1Q, '02, 5

J7642 **Glycopyrrolate, inhalation solution, compounded product, administered through DME, concentrated form, per mg** M ☑

J7643 **Glycopyrrolate, inhalation solution, compounded product, administered through DME, unit dose form, per mg** M ☑

J7644 **Ipratropium bromide, inhalation solution, FDA-approved final product, noncompounded, administered through DME, unit dose form, per mg** M ☑
Use this code for Atrovent.

J7645 **Ipratropium bromide, inhalation solution, compounded product, administered through DME, unit dose form, per mg** M ☑

J7647 **Isoetharine HCl, inhalation solution, compounded product, administered through DME, concentrated form, per mg** M ☑

J7648 **Isoetharine HCl, inhalation solution, FDA-approved final product, noncompounded, administered through DME, concentrated form, per mg** M ☑
Use this code for Beta-2.

J7649 **Isoetharine HCl, inhalation solution, FDA-approved final product, noncompounded, administered through DME, unit dose form, per mg** M ☑

J7650 **Isoetharine HCl, inhalation solution, compounded product, administered through DME, unit dose form, per mg** M ☑

J7657 **Isoproterenol HCl, inhalation solution, compounded product, administered through DME, concentrated form, per mg** M ☑

© 2019 Optum360, LLC

J7658 **Isoproterenol HCl, inhalation solution, FDA-approved final product, noncompounded, administered through DME, concentrated form, per mg** M ☑
Use this code for Isuprel HCl.

J7659 **Isoproterenol HCl, inhalation solution, FDA-approved final product, noncompounded, administered through DME, unit dose form, per mg** M ☑
Use this code for Isuprel HCl.

J7660 **Isoproterenol HCl, inhalation solution, compounded product, administered through DME, unit dose form, per mg** M ☑

J7665 **Mannitol, administered through an inhaler, 5 mg** N N1 ☑
Use this code for ARIDOL.

J7667 **Metaproterenol sulfate, inhalation solution, compounded product, concentrated form, per 10 mg** M ☑

J7668 **Metaproterenol sulfate, inhalation solution, FDA-approved final product, noncompounded, administered through DME, concentrated form, per 10 mg** M ☑
Use this code for Alupent.

J7669 **Metaproterenol sulfate, inhalation solution, FDA-approved final product, noncompounded, administered through DME, unit dose form, per 10 mg** M ☑
Use this code for Alupent.

J7670 **Metaproterenol sulfate, inhalation solution, compounded product, administered through DME, unit dose form, per 10 mg** M ☑

J7674 **Methacholine chloride administered as inhalation solution through a nebulizer, per 1 mg** N N1 ☑
AHA: 2Q, '05, 11

J7676 **Pentamidine isethionate, inhalation solution, compounded product, administered through DME, unit dose form, per 300 mg** M ☑

● **J7677**[Jan] **Revefenacin inhalation solution, FDA-approved final product, noncompounded, administered through DME, 1 mcg**
Use this code for Yupelri.

J7680 **Terbutaline sulfate, inhalation solution, compounded product, administered through DME, concentrated form, per mg** M ☑
Use this code for Brethine.

J7681 **Terbutaline sulfate, inhalation solution, compounded product, administered through DME, unit dose form, per mg** M ☑
Use this code for Brethine.

J7682 **Tobramycin, inhalation solution, FDA-approved final product, noncompounded, unit dose form, administered through DME, per 300 mg** M ☑
Use this code for Tobi.
CMS: 100-02,15,50.5

J7683 **Triamcinolone, inhalation solution, compounded product, administered through DME, concentrated form, per mg** M ☑
Use this code for Azmacort.

J7684 **Triamcinolone, inhalation solution, compounded product, administered through DME, unit dose form, per mg** M ☑
Use this code for Azmacort.

J7685 **Tobramycin, inhalation solution, compounded product, administered through DME, unit dose form, per 300 mg** M ☑

J7686 **Treprostinil, inhalation solution, FDA-approved final product, noncompounded, administered through DME, unit dose form, 1.74 mg** M ☑
Use this code for Tyvaso.
CMS: 100-02,15,50.5

J7699 **NOC drugs, inhalation solution administered through DME** M ☑
CMS: 100-02,15,50.5

J7799 **NOC drugs, other than inhalation drugs, administered through DME** N N1 ☑
CMS: 100-04,20,180
AHA: 3Q, '15, 7

J7999 **Compounded drug, not otherwise classified** N N1 ☑
CMS: 100-04,20,180
AHA: 1Q, '17, 1-3; 4Q, '16, 8; 1Q, '16, 6-8

J8498 **Antiemetic drug, rectal/suppository, not otherwise specified** B ☑
AHA: 2Q, '13, 5

J8499 **Prescription drug, oral, nonchemotherapeutic, NOS** E ☑
CMS: 100-02,15,50.5
AHA: 2Q, '13, 5

J Codes Chemotherapy Drugs J8501-J9999

Oral Chemotherapy Drugs

J8501 **Aprepitant, oral, 5 mg** K N1 ☑
Use this code for Emend.
CMS: 100-02,15,50.5.4; 100-03,110.18; 100-04,17,80.2.1; 100-04,17,80.2.4
AHA: 3Q, '05, 7, 9

J8510 **Busulfan, oral, 2 mg** N N1 ☑
Use this code for Busulfex, Myleran.
CMS: 100-04,17,80.1.1

J8515 **Cabergoline, oral, 0.25 mg** E ☑
Use this code for Dostinex.

J8520 **Capecitabine, oral, 150 mg** N N1 ☑
Use this code for Xeloda.
CMS: 100-04,17,80.1.1

J8521 **Capecitabine, oral, 500 mg** N N1 ☑
Use this code for Xeloda.
CMS: 100-04,17,80.1.1

J8530 **Cyclophosphamide, oral, 25 mg** N N1 ☑
Use this code for Cytoxan.
CMS: 100-04,17,80.1.1
AHA: 1Q, '02, 1-2

J8540 **Dexamethasone, oral, 0.25 mg** N N1 ☑
Use this code for Decadron.

J8560 **Etoposide, oral, 50 mg** K K2 ☑
Use this code for VePesid.
CMS: 100-04,17,80.1.1

J8562 **Fludarabine phosphate, oral, 10 mg** E ☑
Use this code for Oforta.

J8565 **Gefitinib, oral, 250 mg** E ☑
Use this code for Iressa.
CMS: 100-04,17,80.1.1
AHA: 4Q, '14, 6

J8597 **Antiemetic drug, oral, not otherwise specified** N N1 ☑
AHA: 2Q, '13, 5

J8600 **Melphalan, oral, 2 mg** N K2 ☑
Use this code for Alkeran.
CMS: 100-04,17,80.1.1

J8610 **Methotrexate, oral, 2.5 mg** N N1 ☑
Use this code for Trexall, RHEUMATREX.
CMS: 100-04,17,80.1.1

J8650 **Nabilone, oral, 1 mg** E ☑
Use this code for Cesamet.

© 2019 Optum360, LLC

J8655 **Netupitant 300 mg and palonosetron 0.5 mg, oral** K K2 ☑
Use this code for Akynzeo.

J8670 **Rolapitant, oral, 1 mg** K K2 ☑
Use this code for Varubi.

J8700 **Temozolomide, oral, 5 mg** N N1 ☑
Use this code for Temodar.

J8705 **Topotecan, oral, 0.25 mg** K N1 ☑
Use this code for Hycamtin.

J8999 **Prescription drug, oral, chemotherapeutic, NOS** B ☑
Determine if an alternative HCPCS Level II or a CPT code better describes the service being reported. This code should be used only if a more specific code is unavailable.
CMS: 100-04,17,80.1.1; 100-04,17,80.1.2
AHA: 2Q, '13, 5

Injectable Chemotherapy Drugs

These codes cover the cost of the chemotherapy drug only, not the administration.

J9000 **Injection, doxorubicin HCl, 10 mg** N N1 ☑ ⊘
Use this code for Adriamycin PFS, Adriamycin RDF, Rubex.
CMS: 100-04,20,180
AHA: 4Q, '07, 5

J9015 **Injection, aldesleukin, per single use vial** K K2 ☑ ⊘
Use this code for Proleukin, IL-2, Interleukin.
AHA: 2Q, '05, 11

J9017 **Injection, arsenic trioxide, 1 mg** K K2 ☑ ⊘
Use this code for Trisenox.
AHA: 2Q, '05, 11; 2Q, '02, 8-9; 1Q, '02, 5

J9019 **Injection, asparaginase (Erwinaze), 1,000 IU** K K2 ☑

J9020 **Injection, asparaginase, not otherwise specified, 10,000 units** N ☑ ⊘
Use this code for Elspar.
AHA: 2Q, '13, 5

J9022 **Injection, atezolizumab, 10 mg** G K2
Use this code for Tecentriq.

J9023 **Injection, avelumab, 10 mg** G K2
Use this code for Bavencio.

J9025 **Injection, azacitidine, 1 mg** K K2 ☑ ⊘
Use this code for Vidaza.

J9027 **Injection, clofarabine, 1 mg** K K2 ☑ ⊘
Use this code for Clolar.

○ **J9030**Jan **BCG live intravesical instillation, 1 mg** K2
Use this code for Pacis, TICE BCG.

~~**J9031**Jan **BCG (intravesical) per instillation**~~

J9032 **Injection, belinostat, 10 mg** K K2 ☑
Use this code for Beleodaq.

J9033 **Injection, bendamustine HCl (Treanda), 1 mg** K K2 ☑ ⊘

J9034 **Injection, bendamustine HCl (Bendeka), 1 mg** G K2 ☑
AHA: 1Q, '17, 9-10

J9035 **Injection, bevacizumab, 10 mg** K K2 ☑ ⊘
Use this code for Avastin.
CMS: 100-03,110.17
AHA: 3Q, '13, 9; 2Q, '13; 2Q, '05, 11

● **J9036**Jan **Injection, bendamustine hydrochloride, (Belrapzo/bendamustine), 1 mg** K2

J9039 **Injection, blinatumomab, 1 mcg** K K2 ☑
Use this code for Blincyto.
CMS: 100-04,20,180

J9040 **Injection, bleomycin sulfate, 15 units** N N1 ☑ ⊘
Use this code for Blenoxane.
CMS: 100-04,20,180

J9041 **Injection, bortezomib (Velcade), 0.1 mg** K K2 ☑ ⊘
AHA: 2Q, '05, 11; 1Q, '05, 7, 9-10

J9042 **Injection, brentuximab vedotin, 1 mg** K K2 ☑
Use this code for Adcentris.

J9043 **Injection, cabazitaxel, 1 mg** K K2 ☑
Use this code for Jevtana.

J9044 **Injection, bortezomib, not otherwise specified, 0.1 mg** K2
CMS: 100-04,4,260.1; 100-04,4,260.1.1

J9045 **Injection, carboplatin, 50 mg** N N1 ☑ ⊘
Use this code for Paraplatin.

J9047 **Injection, carfilzomib, 1 mg** K K2 ☑
Use this code for Kyprolis.

J9050 **Injection, carmustine, 100 mg** K K2 ☑ ⊘
Use this code for BiCNU.

J9055 **Injection, cetuximab, 10 mg** K K2 ☑ ⊘
Use this code for Erbitux.
CMS: 100-03,110.17
AHA: 2Q, '05, 11

J9057 **Injection, copanlisib, 1 mg** K2
Use this code for Aliqopa.

J9060 **Injection, cisplatin, powder or solution, 10 mg** N N1 ☑ ⊘
Use this code for Plantinol AQ.
AHA: 2Q, '13, 6

J9065 **Injection, cladribine, per 1 mg** K K2 ☑ ⊘
Use this code for Leustatin.
CMS: 100-04,20,180

J9070 **Cyclophosphamide, 100 mg** K K2 ☑ ⊘
Use this code for Endoxan-Asta.

J9098 **Injection, cytarabine liposome, 10 mg** K K2 ☑ ⊘
Use this code for Depocyt.

J9100 **Injection, cytarabine, 100 mg** N N1 ☑ ⊘
Use this code for Cytosar-U, Ara-C, Tarabin CFS.
CMS: 100-04,20,180

● **J9118**Jan **Injection, calaspargase pegol-mknl, 10 units**
Use this code for Asparla.

● **J9119**Jan **Injection, cemiplimab-rwlc, 1 mg** K2
Use this code for Libtayo.

J9120 **Injection, dactinomycin, 0.5 mg** K K2 ☑ ⊘
Use this code for Cosmegen.

J9130 **Dacarbazine, 100 mg** N N1 ☑ ⊘
Use this code for DTIC-Dome.
AHA: 1Q, '08, 6

J9145 **Injection, daratumumab, 10 mg** G K2 ☑
Use this code for Darzalex.

J9150 **Injection, daunorubicin, 10 mg** K K2 ☑ ⊘
Use this code for Cerubidine.

J9151 **Injection, daunorubicin citrate, liposomal formulation, 10 mg** E ☑ ⊘
Use this code for Daunoxome.

J9153 **Injection, liposomal, 1 mg daunorubicin and 2.27 mg cytarabine** K2
Use this code for Vyxeos.

J9155 **Injection, degarelix, 1 mg** K K2 ☑
CMS: 100-02,15,50.5

© 2019 Optum360, LLC

J9160 **Injection, denileukin diftitox, 300 mcg** E ☑ ⊘
Use this code for Ontak.
AHA: 2Q, '05, 11

J9165 **Injection, diethylstilbestrol diphosphate, 250 mg** E ☑

J9171 **Injection, docetaxel, 1 mg** K K2 ☑ ⊘
Use this code for Taxotere.

J9173 **Injection, durvalumab, 10 mg** K2
Use this code for Imfinzi.

J9175 **Injection, Elliotts' B solution, 1 ml** N N1 ☑

J9176 **Injection, elotuzumab, 1 mg** G K2 ☑
Use this code for Empliciti.

J9178 **Injection, epirubicin HCl, 2 mg** N N1 ☑ ⊘
Use this code for Ellence.

J9179 **Injection, eribulin mesylate, 0.1 mg** K K2 ☑
Use this code for Halaven.

J9181 **Injection, etoposide, 10 mg** N N1 ☑ ⊘
Use this code for VePesid, Toposar.

J9185 **Injection, fludarabine phosphate, 50 mg** K N1 ☑ ⊘
Use this code for Fludara.

J9190 **Injection, fluorouracil, 500 mg** N N1 ☑
Use this code for Adrucil.
CMS: 100-04,20,180

● **J9199**[Jan] **Injection, gemcitabine HCl (Infugem), 200 mg**

J9200 **Injection, floxuridine, 500 mg** N N1 ☑ ⊘
Use this code for FUDR.
CMS: 100-04,20,180

▲ **J9201**[Jan] **Injection, gemcitabine HCl, not otherwise specified, 200 mg** N N1 ☑ ⊘
Use this code for Gemzar.

J9202 **Goserelin acetate implant, per 3.6 mg** K K2 ☑
Use this code for Zoladex.

J9203 **Injection, gemtuzumab ozogamicin, 0.1 mg** G K2
Use this code for Mylotarg.

● **J9204**[Jan] **Injection, mogamulizumab-kpkc, 1 mg** K2
Use this code for Poteligeo.

J9205 **Injection, irinotecan liposome, 1 mg** G K2 ☑
Use this code for Onivyde.

J9206 **Injection, irinotecan, 20 mg** N N1 ☑ ⊘
Use this code for Camptosar.
CMS: 100-03,110.17

J9207 **Injection, ixabepilone, 1 mg** K K2 ☑ ⊘
Use this code for IXEMPRA.

J9208 **Injection, ifosfamide, 1 g** N N1 ☑ ⊘
Use this code for IFEX, Mitoxana.

J9209 **Injection, mesna, 200 mg** N N1 ☑
Use this code for Mesnex.

● **J9210**[Jan] **Injection, emapalumab-lzsg, 1 mg** K2
Use this code for Gamifant.

J9211 **Injection, idarubicin HCl, 5 mg** K N1 ☑ ⊘
Use this code for Idamycin.

J9212 **Injection, interferon alfacon-1, recombinant, 1 mcg** N ☑
Use this code for Infergen.

J9213 **Injection, interferon, alfa-2a, recombinant, 3 million units** N K2 ☑
Use this code for Roferon-A.

J9214 **Injection, interferon, alfa-2b, recombinant, 1 million units** K K2 ☑
Use this code for Intron A, Rebetron Kit.
CMS: 100-02,15,50.5

J9215 **Injection, interferon, alfa-N3, (human leukocyte derived), 250,000 IU** E ☑
Use this code for Alferon N.

J9216 **Injection, interferon, gamma 1-b, 3 million units** K ☑
Use this code for Actimmune.
CMS: 100-02,15,50.5
AHA: 2Q, '05, 11

J9217 **Leuprolide acetate (for depot suspension), 7.5 mg** K K2 ☑
Use this code for Lupron Depot, Eligard.
AHA: 3Q, '15, 3

J9218 **Leuprolide acetate, per 1 mg** K N1 ☑
Use this code for Lupron.
CMS: 100-02,15,50.5
AHA: 3Q, '15, 3

J9219 **Leuprolide acetate implant, 65 mg** E ☑
Use this code for Lupron Implant, Viadur.
AHA: 4Q, '01, 5

J9225 **Histrelin implant (Vantas), 50 mg** K K2 ☑ ⊘

J9226 **Histrelin implant (Supprelin LA), 50 mg** K K2 ☑
AHA: 1Q, '08, 6

J9228 **Injection, ipilimumab, 1 mg** K K2 ☑
Use this code for YERVOY.

J9229 **Injection, inotuzumab ozogamicin, 0.1 mg** K2
Use this code for Besponsa.

J9230 **Injection, mechlorethamine HCl, (nitrogen mustard), 10 mg** K K2 ☑ ⊘
Use this code for Mustargen.

J9245 **Injection, melphalan HCl, 50 mg** K K2 ☑ ⊘
Use this code for Alkeran, L-phenylalanine mustard.

J9250 **Methotrexate sodium, 5 mg** N N1 ☑
Use this code for Folex, Folex PFS, Methotrexate LPF.

J9260 **Methotrexate sodium, 50 mg** N N1 ☑
Use this code for Folex, Folex PFS, Methotrexate LPF.

J9261 **Injection, nelarabine, 50 mg** K K2 ☑ ⊘
Use this code for Arranon.

J9262 **Injection, omacetaxine mepesuccinate, 0.01 mg** K K2 ☑
Use this code for Synribo.
CMS: 100-02,15,50.5

J9263 **Injection, oxaliplatin, 0.5 mg** N N1 ☑ ⊘
Use this code for Eloxatin.
AHA: 1Q, '09, 10

J9264 **Injection, paclitaxel protein-bound particles, 1 mg** K K2 ☑ ⊘
Use this code for Abraxane.

J9266 **Injection, pegaspargase, per single dose vial** K K2 ☑ ⊘
Use this code for Oncaspar.
AHA: 2Q, '02, 8-9

J9267 **Injection, paclitaxel, 1 mg** N N1 ☑
Use this code for Taxol.
AHA: 1Q, '15, 6

J9268 **Injection, pentostatin, 10 mg** K K2 ☑ ⊘
Use this code for Nipent.

● **J9269**[Jan] **Injection, tagraxofusp-erzs, 10 mcg** K2
Use this code for Elzonris.

© 2019 Optum360, LLC

J9270 **Injection, plicamycin, 2.5 mg** N K2 ☑ ⊘
Use this code for Mithacin.

J9271 **Injection, pembrolizumab, 1 mg** K K2 ☑
Use this code for Keytruda.

J9280 **Injection, mitomycin, 5 mg** K K2 ☑ ⊘
Use this code for Mutamycin.
AHA: 4Q, '16, 8; 2Q, '14, 8

J9285 **Injection, olaratumab, 10 mg** G K2
Use this code for Lartruvo.

J9293 **Injection, mitoxantrone HCl, per 5 mg** K K2 ☑ ⊘
Use this code for Navantrone.

J9295 **Injection, necitumumab, 1 mg** G K2 ☑
Use this code for Portrazza.

J9299 **Injection, nivolumab, 1 mg** K K2 ☑
Use this code for Opdivo.

J9301 **Injection, obinutuzumab, 10 mg** K K2 ☑
Use this code for Gazyva.
AHA: 1Q, '15, 6

J9302 **Injection, ofatumumab, 10 mg** K K2 ☑
Use this code for Arzerra.

J9303 **Injection, panitumumab, 10 mg** K K2 ☑ ⊘
Use this code for Vectibix.
AHA: 1Q, '08, 6

J9305 **Injection, pemetrexed, 10 mg** K K2 ☑ ⊘
Use this code for Alimta.
AHA: 2Q, '05, 11

J9306 **Injection, pertuzumab, 1 mg** K K2 ☑
Use this code for Perjeta.

J9307 **Injection, pralatrexate, 1 mg** K K2 ☑
Use this code for FOLOTYN.

J9308 **Injection, ramucirumab, 5 mg** K K2 ☑
Use this code for Cyramza.

● **J9309**[Jan] **Injection, polatuzumab vedotin-piiq, 1 mg**
Use this code for Polivy.

J9311 **Injection, rituximab 10 mg and hyaluronidase** K2
Use this code for Rituxin Hycela.

J9312 **Injection, rituximab, 10 mg** K2
Use this code for Rituxin.

● **J9313**[Jan] **Injection, moxetumomab pasudotox-tdfk, 0.01 mg** K2
Use this code for Lumoxiti.

J9315 **Injection, romidepsin, 1 mg** K K2 ☑
Use this code for ISTODAX.

J9320 **Injection, streptozocin, 1 g** K K2 ☑ ⊘
Use this code for Zanosar.

J9325 **Injection, talimogene laherparepvec, per 1 million plaque forming units** G K2 ☑
Use this code for Imlygic.

J9328 **Injection, temozolomide, 1 mg** K K2 ☑ ⊘
Use this code for Temodar.

J9330 **Injection, temsirolimus, 1 mg** K K2 ☑ ⊘
Use this code for TORISEL.

J9340 **Injection, thiotepa, 15 mg** K K2 ☑ ⊘
Use this code for Thioplex.

J9351 **Injection, topotecan, 0.1 mg** N N1 ☑
Use this code for Hycamtin.

J9352 **Injection, trabectedin, 0.1 mg** G K2 ☑
Use this code for Yondelis.

J9354 **Injection, ado-trastuzumab emtansine, 1 mg** K K2 ☑
Use this code for Kadcyla.

▲ **J9355**[Jan] **Injection, trastuzumab, excludes biosimilar, 10 mg** K K2 ☑ ⊘
Use this code for Herceptin.

● **J9356**[Jan] **Injection, trastuzumab, 10 mg and hyaluronidase-oysk** K2
Use this code for Herceptin Hylecta.

J9357 **Injection, valrubicin, intravesical, 200 mg** K K2 ☑ ⊘
Use this code for Valstar.

J9360 **Injection, vinblastine sulfate, 1 mg** N N1 ☑ ⊘
Use this code for Velban.
CMS: 100-04,20,180

J9370 **Vincristine sulfate, 1 mg** N N1 ☑ ⊘
Use this code for Oncovin, Vincasar PFS.
CMS: 100-04,20,180

J9371 **Injection, vincristine sulfate liposome, 1 mg** K K2 ☑
Use this code for Marqibo kit.
AHA: 1Q, '14, 6

J9390 **Injection, vinorelbine tartrate, 10 mg** N N1 ☑ ⊘
Use this code for Navelbine.
AHA: 2Q, '05, 8

J9395 **Injection, fulvestrant, 25 mg** K K2 ☑ ⊘
Use this code for Faslodex.

J9400 **Injection, ziv-aflibercept, 1 mg** K K2 ☑
Use this code for Zaltrap.

J9600 **Injection, porfimer sodium, 75 mg** K K2 ☑ ⊘
Use this code for Photofrin.

J9999 **Not otherwise classified, antineoplastic drugs** N N1 ☑
Determine if an alternative HCPCS Level II or a CPT code better describes the service being reported. This code should be used only if a more specific code is unavailable.
CMS: 100-02,15,50.5; 100-04,4,260.1; 100-04,4,260.1.1
AHA: 1Q, '17, 1-3; 3Q, '15, 7; 2Q, '13, 5; 1Q, '13, 9; 4Q, '12, 9; 1Q, '08, 6; 1Q, '02, 1-2

© 2019 Optum360, LLC

Temporary Codes K0001-K1005

The K codes were established for use by the DME Medicare Administrative Contractors (DME MACs). The K codes are developed when the currently existing permanent national codes for supplies and certain product categories do not include the codes needed to implement a DME MAC medical review policy.

Wheelchairs and Accessories

K0001 **Standard wheelchair** Y ♿ (RR)

K0002 **Standard hemi (low seat) wheelchair** Y ♿ (RR)

K0003 **Lightweight wheelchair** Y ♿ (RR)

K0004 **High strength, lightweight wheelchair** Y ♿ (RR)

K0005 **Ultralightweight wheelchair** Y ♿ (NU, RR, UE)

K0006 **Heavy-duty wheelchair** Y ♿ (RR)

K0007 **Extra heavy-duty wheelchair** Y ♿ (RR)

K0008 **Custom manual wheelchair/base** Y

K0009 **Other manual wheelchair/base** Y ♿ (RR)

K0010 **Standard-weight frame motorized/power wheelchair** Y ♿ (RR)

K0011 **Standard-weight frame motorized/power wheelchair with programmable control parameters for speed adjustment, tremor dampening, acceleration control and braking** Y ♿ (RR)
CMS: 100-04,20,30.9

K0012 **Lightweight portable motorized/power wheelchair** Y ♿ (RR)

K0013 **Custom motorized/power wheelchair base** Y

K0014 **Other motorized/power wheelchair base** Y

K0015 **Detachable, nonadjustable height armrest, each** Y ☑ ♿ (RR)
CMS: 100-04,23,60.3

K0017 **Detachable, adjustable height armrest, base, replacement only, each** Y ☑ ♿ (NU, RR, UE)
CMS: 100-04,23,60.3

K0018 **Detachable, adjustable height armrest, upper portion, replacement only, each** Y ☑ ♿ (NU, RR, UE)
CMS: 100-04,23,60.3

K0019 **Arm pad, replacement only, each** Y ☑ ♿ (NU, RR, UE)
CMS: 100-04,23,60.3

K0020 **Fixed, adjustable height armrest, pair** Y ☑ ♿ (NU, RR, UE)
CMS: 100-04,23,60.3

K0037 **High mount flip-up footrest, each** Y ☑ ♿ (NU, RR, UE)
CMS: 100-04,23,60.3

K0038 **Leg strap, each** Y ☑ ♿ (NU, RR, UE)
CMS: 100-04,23,60.3

K0039 **Leg strap, H style, each** Y ☑ ♿ (NU, RR, UE)
CMS: 100-04,23,60.3

K0040 **Adjustable angle footplate, each** Y ☑ ♿ (NU, RR, UE)
CMS: 100-04,23,60.3

K0041 **Large size footplate, each** Y ☑ ♿ (NU, RR, UE)
CMS: 100-04,23,60.3

K0042 **Standard size footplate, replacement only, each** Y ☑ ♿ (NU, RR, UE)
CMS: 100-04,23,60.3

K0043 **Footrest, lower extension tube, replacement only, each** Y ☑ ♿ (NU, RR, UE)
CMS: 100-04,23,60.3

K0044 **Footrest, upper hanger bracket, replacement only, each** Y ☑ ♿ (NU, RR, UE)
CMS: 100-04,23,60.3

K0045 **Footrest, complete assembly, replacement only, each** Y ♿ (NU, RR, UE)
CMS: 100-04,23,60.3

K0046 **Elevating legrest, lower extension tube, replacement only, each** Y ☑ ♿ (NU, RR, UE)
CMS: 100-04,23,60.3

K0047 **Elevating legrest, upper hanger bracket, replacement only, each** Y ☑ ♿ (NU, RR, UE)
CMS: 100-04,23,60.3

K0050 **Ratchet assembly, replacement only** Y ♿ (NU, RR, UE)
CMS: 100-04,23,60.3

K0051 **Cam release assembly, footrest or legrest, replacement only, each** Y ☑ ♿ (NU, RR, UE)
CMS: 100-04,23,60.3

K0052 **Swingaway, detachable footrests, replacement only, each** Y ☑ ♿ (NU, RR, UE)
CMS: 100-04,23,60.3

K0053 **Elevating footrests, articulating (telescoping), each** Y ☑ ♿ (NU, RR, UE)
CMS: 100-04,23,60.3

K0056 **Seat height less than 17 in or equal to or greater than 21 in for a high-strength, lightweight, or ultralightweight wheelchair** Y ☑ ♿ (NU, RR, UE)

K0065 **Spoke protectors, each** Y ☑ ♿ (NU, RR, UE)

K0069 **Rear wheel assembly, complete, with solid tire, spokes or molded, replacement only, each** Y ☑ ♿ (NU, RR, UE)

K0070 **Rear wheel assembly, complete, with pneumatic tire, spokes or molded, replacement only, each** Y ☑ ♿ (RR)

K0071 **Front caster assembly, complete, with pneumatic tire, replacement only, each** Y ☑ ♿ (NU, RR, UE)

K0072 **Front caster assembly, complete, with semi-pneumatic tire, replacement only, each** Y ☑ ♿ (NU, RR, UE)

K0073 **Caster pin lock, each** Y ☑ ♿ (NU, RR, UE)

K0077 **Front caster assembly, complete, with solid tire, replacement only, each** Y ☑ ♿ (NU, RR, UE)

K0098 **Drive belt for power wheelchair, replacement only** Y ♿ (NU, RR, UE)
CMS: 100-04,23,60.3

K0105 **IV hanger, each** Y ☑ ♿ (NU, RR, UE)

K0108 **Wheelchair component or accessory, not otherwise specified** Y

K0195 **Elevating legrests, pair (for use with capped rental wheelchair base)** Y ♿ (RR)
CMS: 100-04,23,60.3

Equipment, Replacement, Repair, Rental

K0455 **Infusion pump used for uninterrupted parenteral administration of medication, (e.g., epoprostenol or treprostinol)** Y ♿ (RR)

K0462 **Temporary replacement for patient-owned equipment being repaired, any type** Y
CMS: 100-04,20,40.1

K0552 **Supplies for external noninsulin drug infusion pump, syringe type cartridge, sterile, each** Y ☑ ♿

K0553 **Supply allowance for therapeutic continuous glucose monitor (CGM), includes all supplies and accessories, 1 month supply = 1 unit of service** Y ♿ (KF)

K0554 **Receiver (monitor), dedicated, for use with therapeutic glucose continuous monitor system** Y ♿ (NU, RR, UE)

© 2019 Optum360, LLC

K0601 Replacement battery for external infusion pump owned by patient, silver oxide, 1.5 volt, each Y ☑ ♿ (NU)
AHA: 2Q, '03, 7

K0602 Replacement battery for external infusion pump owned by patient, silver oxide, 3 volt, each Y ☑ ♿ (NU)
AHA: 2Q, '03, 7

K0603 Replacement battery for external infusion pump owned by patient, alkaline, 1.5 volt, each Y ☑ ♿ (NU)
AHA: 2Q, '03, 7

K0604 Replacement battery for external infusion pump owned by patient, lithium, 3.6 volt, each Y ☑ ♿ (NU)
AHA: 2Q, '03, 7

K0605 Replacement battery for external infusion pump owned by patient, lithium, 4.5 volt, each Y ☑ ♿ (NU)
AHA: 2Q, '03, 7

K0606 Automatic external defibrillator, with integrated electrocardiogram analysis, garment type Y (RR)
AHA: 4Q, '03, 4-5

K0607 Replacement battery for automated external defibrillator, garment type only, each Y ☑ ♿ (RR)
AHA: 4Q, '03, 4-5

K0608 Replacement garment for use with automated external defibrillator, each Y ☑ ♿ (NU, RR, UE)
AHA: 4Q, '03, 4-5

K0609 Replacement electrodes for use with automated external defibrillator, garment type only, each Y ☑ ♿ (KF)
AHA: 4Q, '03, 4-5

K0669 Wheelchair accessory, wheelchair seat or back cushion, does not meet specific code criteria or no written coding verification from DME PDAC Y

K0672 Addition to lower extremity orthotic, removable soft interface, all components, replacement only, each A ☑ ♿

K0730 Controlled dose inhalation drug delivery system Y ♿ (RR)

K0733 Power wheelchair accessory, 12 to 24 amp hour sealed lead acid battery, each (e.g., gel cell, absorbed glassmat) Y ♿ (NU, RR, UE)
CMS: 100-04,23,60.3

K0738 Portable gaseous oxygen system, rental; home compressor used to fill portable oxygen cylinders; includes portable containers, regulator, flowmeter, humidifier, cannula or mask, and tubing Y ♿ (RR)
CMS: 100-04,20,130.6

K0739 Repair or nonroutine service for durable medical equipment other than oxygen equipment requiring the skill of a technician, labor component, per 15 minutes Y ☑

K0740 Repair or nonroutine service for oxygen equipment requiring the skill of a technician, labor component, per 15 minutes E ☑

K0743 Suction pump, home model, portable, for use on wounds Y

K0744 Absorptive wound dressing for use with suction pump, home model, portable, pad size 16 sq in or less A ☑

K0745 Absorptive wound dressing for use with suction pump, home model, portable, pad size more than 16 sq in but less than or equal to 48 sq in A ☑

K0746 Absorptive wound dressing for use with suction pump, home model, portable, pad size greater than 48 sq in A

Power Operated Vehicle and Accessories

K0800 Power operated vehicle, group 1 standard, patient weight capacity up to and including 300 pounds Y ♿ (NU, RR, UE)
CMS: 100-04,12,30.6.15.4; 100-04,23,60.3

K0801 Power operated vehicle, group 1 heavy-duty, patient weight capacity 301 to 450 pounds Y ♿ (NU, RR, UE)
CMS: 100-04,12,30.6.15.4; 100-04,23,60.3

K0802 Power operated vehicle, group 1 very heavy-duty, patient weight capacity 451 to 600 pounds Y ♿ (NU, RR, UE)
CMS: 100-04,12,30.6.15.4; 100-04,23,60.3

K0806 Power operated vehicle, group 2 standard, patient weight capacity up to and including 300 pounds Y ♿ (NU, RR, UE)
CMS: 100-04,12,30.6.15.4; 100-04,23,60.3

K0807 Power operated vehicle, group 2 heavy-duty, patient weight capacity 301 to 450 pounds Y ♿ (NU, RR, UE)
CMS: 100-04,12,30.6.15.4; 100-04,23,60.3

K0808 Power operated vehicle, group 2 very heavy-duty, patient weight capacity 451 to 600 pounds Y ♿ (NU, RR, UE)
CMS: 100-04,12,30.6.15.4; 100-04,23,60.3

K0812 Power operated vehicle, not otherwise classified Y
CMS: 100-04,12,30.6.15.4

Power Wheelchairs

K0813 Power wheelchair, group 1 standard, portable, sling/solid seat and back, patient weight capacity up to and including 300 pounds Y ♿ (RR)
CMS: 100-04,23,60.3

K0814 Power wheelchair, group 1 standard, portable, captain's chair, patient weight capacity up to and including 300 pounds Y ♿ (RR)
CMS: 100-04,23,60.3

K0815 Power wheelchair, group 1 standard, sling/solid seat and back, patient weight capacity up to and including 300 pounds Y ♿ (RR)
CMS: 100-04,23,60.3

K0816 Power wheelchair, group 1 standard, captain's chair, patient weight capacity up to and including 300 pounds Y ♿ (RR)
CMS: 100-04,23,60.3

K0820 Power wheelchair, group 2 standard, portable, sling/solid seat/back, patient weight capacity up to and including 300 pounds Y ♿ (RR)
CMS: 100-04,23,60.3

K0821 Power wheelchair, group 2 standard, portable, captain's chair, patient weight capacity up to and including 300 pounds Y ♿ (RR)
CMS: 100-04,23,60.3

K0822 Power wheelchair, group 2 standard, sling/solid seat/back, patient weight capacity up to and including 300 pounds Y ♿ (RR)
CMS: 100-04,23,60.3

K0823 Power wheelchair, group 2 standard, captain's chair, patient weight capacity up to and including 300 pounds Y ♿ (RR)
CMS: 100-04,23,60.3

K0824 Power wheelchair, group 2 heavy-duty, sling/solid seat/back, patient weight capacity 301 to 450 pounds Y ♿ (RR)
CMS: 100-04,23,60.3

K0825 Power wheelchair, group 2 heavy-duty, captain's chair, patient weight capacity 301 to 450 pounds Y ♿ (RR)
CMS: 100-04,23,60.3

© 2019 Optum360, LLC

K0826 **Power wheelchair, group 2 very heavy-duty, sling/solid seat/back, patient weight capacity 451 to 600 pounds** Y ♿ (RR)
CMS: 100-04,23,60.3

K0827 **Power wheelchair, group 2 very heavy-duty, captain's chair, patient weight capacity 451 to 600 pounds** Y ♿ (RR)
CMS: 100-04,23,60.3

K0828 **Power wheelchair, group 2 extra heavy-duty, sling/solid seat/back, patient weight capacity 601 pounds or more** Y ♿ (RR)
CMS: 100-04,23,60.3

K0829 **Power wheelchair, group 2 extra heavy-duty, captain's chair, patient weight 601 pounds or more** Y ♿ (RR)
CMS: 100-04,23,60.3

K0830 **Power wheelchair, group 2 standard, seat elevator, sling/solid seat/back, patient weight capacity up to and including 300 pounds** Y

K0831 **Power wheelchair, group 2 standard, seat elevator, captain's chair, patient weight capacity up to and including 300 pounds** Y

K0835 **Power wheelchair, group 2 standard, single power option, sling/solid seat/back, patient weight capacity up to and including 300 pounds** Y ♿ (RR)
CMS: 100-04,23,60.3

K0836 **Power wheelchair, group 2 standard, single power option, captain's chair, patient weight capacity up to and including 300 pounds** Y ♿ (RR)
CMS: 100-04,23,60.3

K0837 **Power wheelchair, group 2 heavy-duty, single power option, sling/solid seat/back, patient weight capacity 301 to 450 pounds** Y ♿ (RR)
CMS: 100-04,23,60.3

K0838 **Power wheelchair, group 2 heavy-duty, single power option, captain's chair, patient weight capacity 301 to 450 pounds** Y ♿ (RR)
CMS: 100-04,23,60.3

K0839 **Power wheelchair, group 2 very heavy-duty, single power option sling/solid seat/back, patient weight capacity 451 to 600 pounds** Y ♿ (RR)
CMS: 100-04,23,60.3

K0840 **Power wheelchair, group 2 extra heavy-duty, single power option, sling/solid seat/back, patient weight capacity 601 pounds or more** Y ♿ (RR)
CMS: 100-04,23,60.3

K0841 **Power wheelchair, group 2 standard, multiple power option, sling/solid seat/back, patient weight capacity up to and including 300 pounds** Y ♿ (RR)
CMS: 100-04,23,60.3

K0842 **Power wheelchair, group 2 standard, multiple power option, captain's chair, patient weight capacity up to and including 300 pounds** Y ♿ (RR)
CMS: 100-04,23,60.3

K0843 **Power wheelchair, group 2 heavy-duty, multiple power option, sling/solid seat/back, patient weight capacity 301 to 450 pounds** Y ♿ (RR)
CMS: 100-04,23,60.3

K0848 **Power wheelchair, group 3 standard, sling/solid seat/back, patient weight capacity up to and including 300 pounds** Y ♿ (RR)
CMS: 100-04,20,30.9; 100-04,23,60.3

K0849 **Power wheelchair, group 3 standard, captain's chair, patient weight capacity up to and including 300 pounds** Y ♿ (RR)
CMS: 100-04,20,30.9; 100-04,23,60.3

K0850 **Power wheelchair, group 3 heavy-duty, sling/solid seat/back, patient weight capacity 301 to 450 pounds** Y ♿ (RR)
CMS: 100-04,20,30.9; 100-04,23,60.3

K0851 **Power wheelchair, group 3 heavy-duty, captain's chair, patient weight capacity 301 to 450 pounds** Y ♿ (RR)
CMS: 100-04,20,30.9; 100-04,23,60.3

K0852 **Power wheelchair, group 3 very heavy-duty, sling/solid seat/back, patient weight capacity 451 to 600 pounds** Y ♿ (RR)
CMS: 100-04,20,30.9; 100-04,23,60.3

K0853 **Power wheelchair, group 3 very heavy-duty, captain's chair, patient weight capacity 451 to 600 pounds** Y ♿ (RR)
CMS: 100-04,20,30.9; 100-04,23,60.3

K0854 **Power wheelchair, group 3 extra heavy-duty, sling/solid seat/back, patient weight capacity 601 pounds or more** Y ♿ (RR)
CMS: 100-04,20,30.9; 100-04,23,60.3

K0855 **Power wheelchair, group 3 extra heavy-duty, captain's chair, patient weight capacity 601 pounds or more** Y ♿ (RR)
CMS: 100-04,20,30.9; 100-04,23,60.3

K0856 **Power wheelchair, group 3 standard, single power option, sling/solid seat/back, patient weight capacity up to and including 300 pounds** Y ♿ (RR)
CMS: 100-04,20,30.9; 100-04,23,60.3

K0857 **Power wheelchair, group 3 standard, single power option, captain's chair, patient weight capacity up to and including 300 pounds** Y ♿ (RR)
CMS: 100-04,20,30.9; 100-04,23,60.3

K0858 **Power wheelchair, group 3 heavy-duty, single power option, sling/solid seat/back, patient weight 301 to 450 pounds** Y ♿ (RR)
CMS: 100-04,20,30.9; 100-04,23,60.3

K0859 **Power wheelchair, group 3 heavy-duty, single power option, captain's chair, patient weight capacity 301 to 450 pounds** Y ♿ (RR)
CMS: 100-04,20,30.9; 100-04,23,60.3

K0860 **Power wheelchair, group 3 very heavy-duty, single power option, sling/solid seat/back, patient weight capacity 451 to 600 pounds** Y ♿ (RR)
CMS: 100-04,20,30.9; 100-04,23,60.3

K0861 **Power wheelchair, group 3 standard, multiple power option, sling/solid seat/back, patient weight capacity up to and including 300 pounds** Y ♿ (RR)
CMS: 100-04,20,30.9; 100-04,23,60.3

K0862 **Power wheelchair, group 3 heavy-duty, multiple power option, sling/solid seat/back, patient weight capacity 301 to 450 pounds** Y ♿ (RR)
CMS: 100-04,20,30.9; 100-04,23,60.3

K0863 **Power wheelchair, group 3 very heavy-duty, multiple power option, sling/solid seat/back, patient weight capacity 451 to 600 pounds** Y ♿ (RR)
CMS: 100-04,20,30.9; 100-04,23,60.3

K0864 **Power wheelchair, group 3 extra heavy-duty, multiple power option, sling/solid seat/back, patient weight capacity 601 pounds or more** Y ♿ (RR)
CMS: 100-04,20,30.9; 100-04,23,60.3

K0868 **Power wheelchair, group 4 standard, sling/solid seat/back, patient weight capacity up to and including 300 pounds** Y

© 2019 Optum360, LLC

K0869 Power wheelchair, group 4 standard, captain's chair, patient weight capacity up to and including 300 pounds [Y]

K0870 Power wheelchair, group 4 heavy-duty, sling/solid seat/back, patient weight capacity 301 to 450 pounds [Y]

K0871 Power wheelchair, group 4 very heavy-duty, sling/solid seat/back, patient weight capacity 451 to 600 pounds [Y]

K0877 Power wheelchair, group 4 standard, single power option, sling/solid seat/back, patient weight capacity up to and including 300 pounds [Y]

K0878 Power wheelchair, group 4 standard, single power option, captain's chair, patient weight capacity up to and including 300 pounds [Y]

K0879 Power wheelchair, group 4 heavy-duty, single power option, sling/solid seat/back, patient weight capacity 301 to 450 pounds [Y]

K0880 Power wheelchair, group 4 very heavy-duty, single power option, sling/solid seat/back, patient weight 451 to 600 pounds [Y]

K0884 Power wheelchair, group 4 standard, multiple power option, sling/solid seat/back, patient weight capacity up to and including 300 pounds [Y]

K0885 Power wheelchair, group 4 standard, multiple power option, captain's chair, patient weight capacity up to and including 300 pounds [Y]

K0886 Power wheelchair, group 4 heavy-duty, multiple power option, sling/solid seat/back, patient weight capacity 301 to 450 pounds [Y]

K0890 Power wheelchair, group 5 pediatric, single power option, sling/solid seat/back, patient weight capacity up to and including 125 pounds [Y]

K0891 Power wheelchair, group 5 pediatric, multiple power option, sling/solid seat/back, patient weight capacity up to and including 125 pounds [Y]

K0898 Power wheelchair, not otherwise classified [Y]

K0899 Power mobility device, not coded by DME PDAC or does not meet criteria [Y]

CMS: 100-04,12,30.6.15.4

Other DME

K0900 Customized durable medical equipment, other than wheelchair [Y]

● **K1001**[Jan] Electronic positional obstructive sleep apnea treatment, with sensor, includes all components and accessories, any type

● **K1002**[Jan] Cranial electrotherapy stimulation (CES) system, includes all supplies and accessories, any type

● **K1003**[Jan] Whirlpool tub, walk in, portable

● **K1004**[Jan] Low frequency ultrasonic diathermy treatment device for home use, includes all components and accessories

● **K1005**[Jan] Disposable collection and storage bag for breast milk, any size, any type, each

© 2019 Optum360, LLC

Orthotic Procedures and Devices L0112-L4631

L codes include orthotic and prosthetic procedures and devices, as well as scoliosis equipment, orthopedic shoes, and prosthetic implants.

Cervical

L0112 **Cranial cervical orthosis, congenital torticollis type, with or without soft interface material, adjustable range of motion joint, custom fabricated** A ♿

L0113 **Cranial cervical orthosis, torticollis type, with or without joint, with or without soft interface material, prefabricated, includes fitting and adjustment** A ♿

L0120 **Cervical, flexible, nonadjustable, prefabricated, off-the-shelf (foam collar)** A ♿

L0130 **Cervical, flexible, thermoplastic collar, molded to patient** A ♿

L0140 **Cervical, semi-rigid, adjustable (plastic collar)** A ♿

L0150 **Cervical, semi-rigid, adjustable molded chin cup (plastic collar with mandibular/occipital piece)** A ♿

L0160 **Cervical, semi-rigid, wire frame occipital/mandibular support, prefabricated, off-the-shelf** A ♿

L0170 **Cervical, collar, molded to patient model** A ♿

L0172 **Cervical, collar, semi-rigid thermoplastic foam, two piece, prefabricated, off-the-shelf** A ♿

L0174 **Cervical, collar, semi-rigid, thermoplastic foam, two piece with thoracic extension, prefabricated, off-the-shelf** A ♿

Multiple Post Collar

L0180 **Cervical, multiple post collar, occipital/mandibular supports, adjustable** A ♿

L0190 **Cervical, multiple post collar, occipital/mandibular supports, adjustable cervical bars (SOMI, Guilford, Taylor types)** A ♿

L0200 **Cervical, multiple post collar, occipital/mandibular supports, adjustable cervical bars, and thoracic extension** A ♿

Thoracic

L0220 **Thoracic, rib belt, custom fabricated** A ♿

L0450 **Thoracic-lumbar-sacral orthosis (TLSO), flexible, provides trunk support, upper thoracic region, produces intracavitary pressure to reduce load on the intervertebral disks with rigid stays or panel(s), includes shoulder straps and closures, prefabricated, off-the-shelf** A ♿

TLSO brace with adjustable straps and pads (L0450). The model at right and similar devices such as the Boston brace are molded polymer over foam and may be bivalve (front and back components)

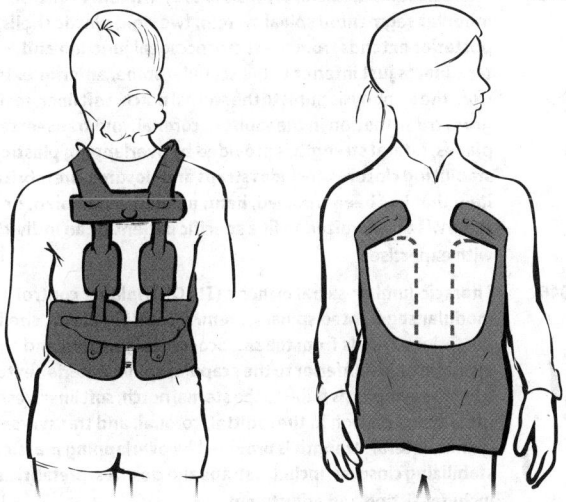

Thoracic lumbar sacral othosis (TLSO)

L0452 **Thoracic-lumbar-sacral orthosis (TLSO), flexible, provides trunk support, upper thoracic region, produces intracavitary pressure to reduce load on the intervertebral disks with rigid stays or panel(s), includes shoulder straps and closures, custom fabricated** A ♿

L0454 **Thoracic-lumbar-sacral orthosis (TLSO), flexible, provides trunk support, extends from sacrococcygeal junction to above T-9 vertebra, restricts gross trunk motion in the sagittal plane, produces intracavitary pressure to reduce load on the intervertebral disks with rigid stays or panel(s), includes shoulder straps and closures, prefabricated item that has been trimmed, bent, molded, assembled, or otherwise customized to fit a specific patient by an individual with expertise** A ♿

L0455 **Thoracic-lumbar-sacral orthosis (TLSO), flexible, provides trunk support, extends from sacrococcygeal junction to above T-9 vertebra, restricts gross trunk motion in the sagittal plane, produces intracavitary pressure to reduce load on the intervertebral disks with rigid stays or panel(s), includes shoulder straps and closures, prefabricated, off-the-shelf** A ♿

L0456 **Thoracic-lumbar-sacral orthosis (TLSO), flexible, provides trunk support, thoracic region, rigid posterior panel and soft anterior apron, extends from the sacrococcygeal junction and terminates just inferior to the scapular spine, restricts gross trunk motion in the sagittal plane, produces intracavitary pressure to reduce load on the intervertebral disks, includes straps and closures, prefabricated item that has been trimmed, bent, molded, assembled, or otherwise customized to fit a specific patient by an individual with expertise** A ♿

L0457 **Thoracic-lumbar-sacral orthosis (TLSO), flexible, provides trunk support, thoracic region, rigid posterior panel and soft anterior apron, extends from the sacrococcygeal junction and terminates just inferior to the scapular spine, restricts gross trunk motion in the sagittal plane, produces intracavitary pressure to reduce load on the intervertebral disks, includes straps and closures, prefabricated, off-the-shelf** A ♿

© 2019 Optum360, LLC

L0458 Thoracic-lumbar-sacral orthosis (TLSO), triplanar control, modular segmented spinal system, two rigid plastic shells, posterior extends from the sacrococcygeal junction and terminates just inferior to the scapular spine, anterior extends from the symphysis pubis to the xiphoid, soft liner, restricts gross trunk motion in the sagittal, coronal, and transverse planes, lateral strength is provided by overlapping plastic and stabilizing closures, includes straps and closures, prefabricated, includes fitting and adjustment A ♿

L0460 Thoracic-lumbar-sacral orthosis (TLSO), triplanar control, modular segmented spinal system, two rigid plastic shells, posterior extends from the sacrococcygeal junction and terminates just inferior to the scapular spine, anterior extends from the symphysis pubis to the sternal notch, soft liner, restricts gross trunk motion in the sagittal, coronal, and transverse planes, lateral strength is provided by overlapping plastic and stabilizing closures, includes straps and closures, prefabricated item that has been trimmed, bent, molded, assembled, or otherwise customized to fit a specific patient by an individual with expertise A ♿

L0462 Thoracic-lumbar-sacral orthosis (TLSO), triplanar control, modular segmented spinal system, three rigid plastic shells, posterior extends from the sacrococcygeal junction and terminates just inferior to the scapular spine, anterior extends from the symphysis pubis to the sternal notch, soft liner, restricts gross trunk motion in the sagittal, coronal, and transverse planes, lateral strength is provided by overlapping plastic and stabilizing closures, includes straps and closures, prefabricated, includes fitting and adjustment A ♿

L0464 Thoracic-lumbar-sacral orthosis (TLSO), triplanar control, modular segmented spinal system, four rigid plastic shells, posterior extends from sacrococcygeal junction and terminates just inferior to scapular spine, anterior extends from symphysis pubis to the sternal notch, soft liner, restricts gross trunk motion in sagittal, coronal, and transverse planes, lateral strength is provided by overlapping plastic and stabilizing closures, includes straps and closures, prefabricated, includes fitting and adjustment A ♿

L0466 Thoracic-lumbar-sacral orthosis (TLSO), sagittal control, rigid posterior frame and flexible soft anterior apron with straps, closures and padding, restricts gross trunk motion in sagittal plane, produces intracavitary pressure to reduce load on intervertebral disks, prefabricated item that has been trimmed, bent, molded, assembled, or otherwise customized to fit a specific patient by an individual with expertise A ♿

L0467 Thoracic-lumbar-sacral orthosis (TLSO), sagittal control, rigid posterior frame and flexible soft anterior apron with straps, closures and padding, restricts gross trunk motion in sagittal plane, produces intracavitary pressure to reduce load on intervertebral disks, prefabricated, off-the-shelf A ♿

L0468 Thoracic-lumbar-sacral orthosis (TLSO), sagittal-coronal control, rigid posterior frame and flexible soft anterior apron with straps, closures and padding, extends from sacrococcygeal junction over scapulae, lateral strength provided by pelvic, thoracic, and lateral frame pieces, restricts gross trunk motion in sagittal, and coronal planes, produces intracavitary pressure to reduce load on intervertebral disks, prefabricated item that has been trimmed, bent, molded, assembled, or otherwise customized to fit a specific patient by an individual with expertise A ♿

L0469 Thoracic-lumbar-sacral orthosis (TLSO), sagittal-coronal control, rigid posterior frame and flexible soft anterior apron with straps, closures and padding, extends from sacrococcygeal junction over scapulae, lateral strength provided by pelvic, thoracic, and lateral frame pieces, restricts gross trunk motion in sagittal and coronal planes, produces intracavitary pressure to reduce load on intervertebral disks, prefabricated, off-the-shelf A ♿

L0470 Thoracic-lumbar-sacral orthosis (TLSO), triplanar control, rigid posterior frame and flexible soft anterior apron with straps, closures and padding extends from sacrococcygeal junction to scapula, lateral strength provided by pelvic, thoracic, and lateral frame pieces, rotational strength provided by subclavicular extensions, restricts gross trunk motion in sagittal, coronal, and transverse planes, provides intracavitary pressure to reduce load on the intervertebral disks, includes fitting and shaping the frame, prefabricated, includes fitting and adjustment A ♿

L0472 Thoracic-lumbar-sacral orthosis (TLSO), triplanar control, hyperextension, rigid anterior and lateral frame extends from symphysis pubis to sternal notch with two anterior components (one pubic and one sternal), posterior and lateral pads with straps and closures, limits spinal flexion, restricts gross trunk motion in sagittal, coronal, and transverse planes, includes fitting and shaping the frame, prefabricated, includes fitting and adjustment A ♿

L0480 Thoracic-lumbar-sacral orthosis (TLSO), triplanar control, one-piece rigid plastic shell without interface liner, with multiple straps and closures, posterior extends from sacrococcygeal junction and terminates just inferior to scapular spine, anterior extends from symphysis pubis to sternal notch, anterior or posterior opening, restricts gross trunk motion in sagittal, coronal, and transverse planes, includes a carved plaster or CAD-CAM model, custom fabricated A ♿

L0482 Thoracic-lumbar-sacral orthosis (TLSO), triplanar control, one-piece rigid plastic shell with interface liner, multiple straps and closures, posterior extends from sacrococcygeal junction and terminates just inferior to scapular spine, anterior extends from symphysis pubis to sternal notch, anterior or posterior opening, restricts gross trunk motion in sagittal, coronal, and transverse planes, includes a carved plaster or CAD-CAM model, custom fabricated A ♿

L0484 Thoracic-lumbar-sacral orthosis (TLSO), triplanar control, two-piece rigid plastic shell without interface liner, with multiple straps and closures, posterior extends from sacrococcygeal junction and terminates just inferior to scapular spine, anterior extends from symphysis pubis to sternal notch, lateral strength is enhanced by overlapping plastic, restricts gross trunk motion in the sagittal, coronal, and transverse planes, includes a carved plaster or CAD-CAM model, custom fabricated A ♿

L0486 Thoracic-lumbar-sacral orthosis (TLSO), triplanar control, two-piece rigid plastic shell with interface liner, multiple straps and closures, posterior extends from sacrococcygeal junction and terminates just inferior to scapular spine, anterior extends from symphysis pubis to sternal notch, lateral strength is enhanced by overlapping plastic, restricts gross trunk motion in the sagittal, coronal, and transverse planes, includes a carved plaster or CAD-CAM model, custom fabricated A ♿

L0488 Thoracic-lumbar-sacral orthosis (TLSO), triplanar control, one-piece rigid plastic shell with interface liner, multiple straps and closures, posterior extends from sacrococcygeal junction and terminates just inferior to scapular spine, anterior extends from symphysis pubis to sternal notch, anterior or posterior opening, restricts gross trunk motion in sagittal, coronal, and transverse planes, prefabricated, includes fitting and adjustment A ♿

L0490 Thoracic-lumbar-sacral orthosis (TLSO), sagittal-coronal control, one-piece rigid plastic shell, with overlapping reinforced anterior, with multiple straps and closures, posterior extends from sacrococcygeal junction and terminates at or before the T-9 vertebra, anterior extends from symphysis pubis to xiphoid, anterior opening, restricts gross trunk motion in sagittal and coronal planes, prefabricated, includes fitting and adjustment A ♿

© 2019 Optum360, LLC

L0491 Thoracic-lumbar-sacral orthosis (TLSO), sagittal-coronal control, modular segmented spinal system, two rigid plastic shells, posterior extends from the sacrococcygeal junction and terminates just inferior to the scapular spine, anterior extends from the symphysis pubis to the xiphoid, soft liner, restricts gross trunk motion in the sagittal and coronal planes, lateral strength is provided by overlapping plastic and stabilizing closures, includes straps and closures, prefabricated, includes fitting and adjustment A ♿

L0492 Thoracic-lumbar-sacral orthosis (TLSO), sagittal-coronal control, modular segmented spinal system, three rigid plastic shells, posterior extends from the sacrococcygeal junction and terminates just inferior to the scapular spine, anterior extends from the symphysis pubis to the xiphoid, soft liner, restricts gross trunk motion in the sagittal and coronal planes, lateral strength is provided by overlapping plastic and stabilizing closures, includes straps and closures, prefabricated, includes fitting and adjustment A ♿

Cervical-Thoracic-Lumbar-Sacral Orthoses

L0621 Sacroiliac orthosis, flexible, provides pelvic-sacral support, reduces motion about the sacroiliac joint, includes straps, closures, may include pendulous abdomen design, prefabricated, off-the-shelf A ♿

L0622 Sacroiliac orthosis, flexible, provides pelvic-sacral support, reduces motion about the sacroiliac joint, includes straps, closures, may include pendulous abdomen design, custom fabricated A ♿

L0623 Sacroiliac orthosis, provides pelvic-sacral support, with rigid or semi-rigid panels over the sacrum and abdomen, reduces motion about the sacroiliac joint, includes straps, closures, may include pendulous abdomen design, prefabricated, off-the-shelf A ♿

L0624 Sacroiliac orthosis, provides pelvic-sacral support, with rigid or semi-rigid panels placed over the sacrum and abdomen, reduces motion about the sacroiliac joint, includes straps, closures, may include pendulous abdomen design, custom fabricated A ♿

L0625 Lumbar orthosis, flexible, provides lumbar support, posterior extends from L-1 to below L-5 vertebra, produces intracavitary pressure to reduce load on the intervertebral discs, includes straps, closures, may include pendulous abdomen design, shoulder straps, stays, prefabricated, off-the-shelf A ♿

L0626 Lumbar orthosis, sagittal control, with rigid posterior panel(s), posterior extends from L-1 to below L-5 vertebra, produces intracavitary pressure to reduce load on the intervertebral discs, includes straps, closures, may include padding, stays, shoulder straps, pendulous abdomen design, prefabricated item that has been trimmed, bent, molded, assembled, or otherwise customized to fit a specific patient by an individual with expertise A ♿

L0627 Lumbar orthosis, sagittal control, with rigid anterior and posterior panels, posterior extends from L-1 to below L-5 vertebra, produces intracavitary pressure to reduce load on the intervertebral discs, includes straps, closures, may include padding, shoulder straps, pendulous abdomen design, prefabricated item that has been trimmed, bent, molded, assembled, or otherwise customized to fit a specific patient by an individual with expertise A ♿

L0628 Lumbar-sacral orthosis (LSO), flexible, provides lumbo-sacral support, posterior extends from sacrococcygeal junction to T-9 vertebra, produces intracavitary pressure to reduce load on the intervertebral discs, includes straps, closures, may include stays, shoulder straps, pendulous abdomen design, prefabricated, off-the-shelf A ♿

L0629 Lumbar-sacral orthosis (LSO), flexible, provides lumbo-sacral support, posterior extends from sacrococcygeal junction to T-9 vertebra, produces intracavitary pressure to reduce load on the intervertebral discs, includes straps, closures, may include stays, shoulder straps, pendulous abdomen design, custom fabricated A ♿

L0630 Lumbar-sacral orthosis (LSO), sagittal control, with rigid posterior panel(s), posterior extends from sacrococcygeal junction to T-9 vertebra, produces intracavitary pressure to reduce load on the intervertebral discs, includes straps, closures, may include padding, stays, shoulder straps, pendulous abdomen design, prefabricated item that has been trimmed, bent, molded, assembled, or otherwise customized to fit a specific patient by an individual with expertise A ♿

L0631 Lumbar-sacral orthosis (LSO), sagittal control, with rigid anterior and posterior panels, posterior extends from sacrococcygeal junction to T-9 vertebra, produces intracavitary pressure to reduce load on the intervertebral discs, includes straps, closures, may include padding, shoulder straps, pendulous abdomen design, prefabricated item that has been trimmed, bent, molded, assembled, or otherwise customized to fit a specific patient by an individual with expertise A ♿

L0632 Lumbar-sacral orthosis (LSO), sagittal control, with rigid anterior and posterior panels, posterior extends from sacrococcygeal junction to T-9 vertebra, produces intracavitary pressure to reduce load on the intervertebral discs, includes straps, closures, may include padding, shoulder straps, pendulous abdomen design, custom fabricated A ♿

L0633 Lumbar-sacral orthosis (LSO), sagittal-coronal control, with rigid posterior frame/panel(s), posterior extends from sacrococcygeal junction to T-9 vertebra, lateral strength provided by rigid lateral frame/panels, produces intracavitary pressure to reduce load on intervertebral discs, includes straps, closures, may include padding, stays, shoulder straps, pendulous abdomen design, prefabricated item that has been trimmed, bent, molded, assembled, or otherwise customized to fit a specific patient by an individual with expertise A ♿

L0634 Lumbar-sacral orthosis (LSO), sagittal-coronal control, with rigid posterior frame/panel(s), posterior extends from sacrococcygeal junction to T-9 vertebra, lateral strength provided by rigid lateral frame/panel(s), produces intracavitary pressure to reduce load on intervertebral discs, includes straps, closures, may include padding, stays, shoulder straps, pendulous abdomen design, custom fabricated A ♿

L0635 Lumbar-sacral orthosis (LSO), sagittal-coronal control, lumbar flexion, rigid posterior frame/panel(s), lateral articulating design to flex the lumbar spine, posterior extends from sacrococcygeal junction to T-9 vertebra, lateral strength provided by rigid lateral frame/panel(s), produces intracavitary pressure to reduce load on intervertebral discs, includes straps, closures, may include padding, anterior panel, pendulous abdomen design, prefabricated, includes fitting and adjustment A ♿

L0636 Lumbar-sacral orthosis (LSO), sagittal-coronal control, lumbar flexion, rigid posterior frame/panels, lateral articulating design to flex the lumbar spine, posterior extends from sacrococcygeal junction to T-9 vertebra, lateral strength provided by rigid lateral frame/panels, produces intracavitary pressure to reduce load on intervertebral discs, includes straps, closures, may include padding, anterior panel, pendulous abdomen design, custom fabricated A ♿

© 2019 Optum360, LLC

L0637 Lumbar-sacral orthosis (LSO), sagittal-coronal control, with rigid anterior and posterior frame/panels, posterior extends from sacrococcygeal junction to T-9 vertebra, lateral strength provided by rigid lateral frame/panels, produces intracavitary pressure to reduce load on intervertebral discs, includes straps, closures, may include padding, shoulder straps, pendulous abdomen design, prefabricated item that has been trimmed, bent, molded, assembled, or otherwise customized to fit a specific patient by an individual with expertise A

L0638 Lumbar-sacral orthosis (LSO), sagittal-coronal control, with rigid anterior and posterior frame/panels, posterior extends from sacrococcygeal junction to T-9 vertebra, lateral strength provided by rigid lateral frame/panels, produces intracavitary pressure to reduce load on intervertebral discs, includes straps, closures, may include padding, shoulder straps, pendulous abdomen design, custom fabricated A

L0639 Lumbar-sacral orthosis (LSO), sagittal-coronal control, rigid shell(s)/panel(s), posterior extends from sacrococcygeal junction to T-9 vertebra, anterior extends from symphysis pubis to xyphoid, produces intracavitary pressure to reduce load on the intervertebral discs, overall strength is provided by overlapping rigid material and stabilizing closures, includes straps, closures, may include soft interface, pendulous abdomen design, prefabricated item that has been trimmed, bent, molded, assembled, or otherwise customized to fit a specific patient by an individual with expertise A

L0640 Lumbar-sacral orthosis (LSO), sagittal-coronal control, rigid shell(s)/panel(s), posterior extends from sacrococcygeal junction to T-9 vertebra, anterior extends from symphysis pubis to xyphoid, produces intracavitary pressure to reduce load on the intervertebral discs, overall strength is provided by overlapping rigid material and stabilizing closures, includes straps, closures, may include soft interface, pendulous abdomen design, custom fabricated A

L0641 Lumbar orthosis, sagittal control, with rigid posterior panel(s), posterior extends from L-1 to below L-5 vertebra, produces intracavitary pressure to reduce load on the intervertebral discs, includes straps, closures, may include padding, stays, shoulder straps, pendulous abdomen design, prefabricated, off-the-shelf A

L0642 Lumbar orthosis, sagittal control, with rigid anterior and posterior panels, posterior extends from L-1 to below L-5 vertebra, produces intracavitary pressure to reduce load on the intervertebral discs, includes straps, closures, may include padding, shoulder straps, pendulous abdomen design, prefabricated, off-the-shelf A

L0643 Lumbar-sacral orthosis (LSO), sagittal control, with rigid posterior panel(s), posterior extends from sacrococcygeal junction to T-9 vertebra, produces intracavitary pressure to reduce load on the intervertebral discs, includes straps, closures, may include padding, stays, shoulder straps, pendulous abdomen design, prefabricated, off-the-shelf A

L0648 Lumbar-sacral orthosis (LSO), sagittal control, with rigid anterior and posterior panels, posterior extends from sacrococcygeal junction to T-9 vertebra, produces intracavitary pressure to reduce load on the intervertebral discs, includes straps, closures, may include padding, shoulder straps, pendulous abdomen design, prefabricated, off-the-shelf A

L0649 Lumbar-sacral orthosis (LSO), sagittal-coronal control, with rigid posterior frame/panel(s), posterior extends from sacrococcygeal junction to T-9 vertebra, lateral strength provided by rigid lateral frame/panels, produces intracavitary pressure to reduce load on intervertebral discs, includes straps, closures, may include padding, stays, shoulder straps, pendulous abdomen design, prefabricated, off-the-shelf A

L0650 Lumbar-sacral orthosis (LSO), sagittal-coronal control, with rigid anterior and posterior frame/panel(s), posterior extends from sacrococcygeal junction to T-9 vertebra, lateral strength provided by rigid lateral frame/panel(s), produces intracavitary pressure to reduce load on intervertebral discs, includes straps, closures, may include padding, shoulder straps, pendulous abdomen design, prefabricated, off-the-shelf A

L0651 Lumbar-sacral orthosis (LSO), sagittal-coronal control, rigid shell(s)/panel(s), posterior extends from sacrococcygeal junction to T-9 vertebra, anterior extends from symphysis pubis to xyphoid, produces intracavitary pressure to reduce load on the intervertebral discs, overall strength is provided by overlapping rigid material and stabilizing closures, includes straps, closures, may include soft interface, pendulous abdomen design, prefabricated, off-the-shelf A

L0700 Cervical-thoracic-lumbar-sacral orthosis (CTLSO), anterior-posterior-lateral control, molded to patient model, (Minerva type) A

L0710 Cervical-thoracic-lumbar-sacral orthosis (CTLSO), anterior-posterior-lateral control, molded to patient model, with interface material, (Minerva type) A

Halo Procedure

L0810 Halo procedure, cervical halo incorporated into jacket vest A

L0820 Halo procedure, cervical halo incorporated into plaster body jacket A

L0830 Halo procedure, cervical halo incorporated into Milwaukee type orthotic A

L0859 Addition to halo procedure, magnetic resonance image compatible systems, rings and pins, any material A

L0861 Addition to halo procedure, replacement liner/interface material A

Additions to Spinal Orthoses

L0970 Thoracic-lumbar-sacral orthosis (TLSO), corset front A

L0972 Lumbar-sacral orthosis (LSO), corset front A

L0974 Thoracic-lumbar-sacral orthosis (TLSO), full corset A

L0976 Lumbar-sacral orthosis (LSO), full corset A

L0978 Axillary crutch extension A

L0980 Peroneal straps, prefabricated, off-the-shelf, pair A ☑

L0982 Stocking supporter grips, prefabricated, off-the-shelf, set of four (4) A ☑

L0984 Protective body sock, prefabricated, off-the-shelf, each A ☑

L0999 Addition to spinal orthosis, not otherwise specified A

Determine if an alternative HCPCS Level II or a CPT code better describes the service being reported. This code should be used only if a more specific code is unavailable.

Orthotic Devices - Scoliosis Procedures

The orthotic care of scoliosis differs from other orthotic care in that the treatment is more dynamic in nature and uses continual modification of the orthosis to the patient's changing condition. This coding structure uses the proper names - or eponyms - of the procedures because they have historic and universal acceptance in the profession. It should be recognized that variations to the basic procedures described by the founders/developers are accepted in various medical and orthotic practices throughout the country. All procedures include model of patient when indicated.

© 2019 Optum360, LLC

L1000 **Cervical-thoracic-lumbar-sacral orthosis (CTLSO) (Milwaukee), inclusive of furnishing initial orthotic, including model** A

A variety of configurations are available for the Milwaukee brace (L1000)

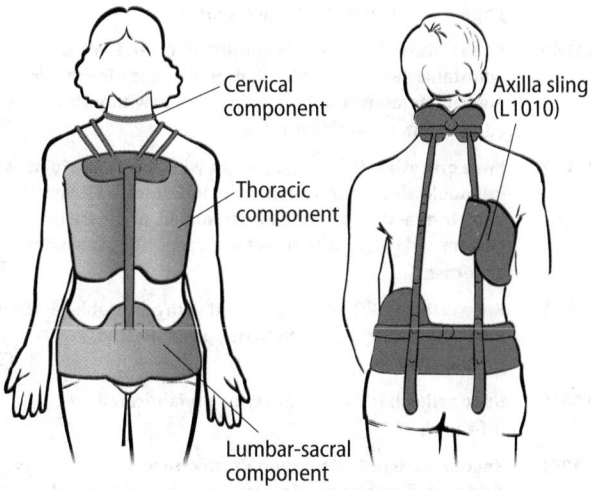

Milwaukee-style braces, cervical thoracic lumbar sacral orthosis (CTSLO)

L1001 **Cervical-thoracic-lumbar-sacral orthosis (CTLSO), immobilizer, infant size, prefabricated, includes fitting and adjustment** A A

L1005 **Tension based scoliosis orthosis and accessory pads, includes fitting and adjustment** A
AHA: 1Q, '02, 5

L1010 **Addition to cervical-thoracic-lumbar-sacral orthosis (CTLSO) or scoliosis orthosis, axilla sling** A

L1020 **Addition to cervical-thoracic-lumbar-sacral orthosis (CTLSO) or scoliosis orthosis, kyphosis pad** A

L1025 **Addition to cervical-thoracic-lumbar-sacral orthosis (CTLSO) or scoliosis orthosis, kyphosis pad, floating** A

L1030 **Addition to cervical-thoracic-lumbar-sacral orthosis (CTLSO) or scoliosis orthosis, lumbar bolster pad** A

L1040 **Addition to cervical-thoracic-lumbar-sacral orthosis (CTLSO) or scoliosis orthosis, lumbar or lumbar rib pad** A

L1050 **Addition to cervical-thoracic-lumbar-sacral orthosis (CTLSO) or scoliosis orthosis, sternal pad** A

L1060 **Addition to cervical-thoracic-lumbar-sacral orthosis (CTLSO) or scoliosis orthosis, thoracic pad** A

L1070 **Addition to cervical-thoracic-lumbar-sacral orthosis (CTLSO) or scoliosis orthosis, trapezius sling** A

L1080 **Addition to cervical-thoracic-lumbar-sacral orthosis (CTLSO) or scoliosis orthosis, outrigger** A

L1085 **Addition to cervical-thoracic-lumbar-sacral orthosis (CTLSO) or scoliosis orthosis, outrigger, bilateral with vertical extensions** A

L1090 **Addition to cervical-thoracic-lumbar-sacral orthosis (CTLSO) or scoliosis orthosis, lumbar sling** A

L1100 **Addition to cervical-thoracic-lumbar-sacral orthosis (CTLSO) or scoliosis orthosis, ring flange, plastic or leather** A

L1110 **Addition to cervical-thoracic-lumbar-sacral orthosis (CTLSO) or scoliosis orthosis, ring flange, plastic or leather, molded to patient model** A

L1120 **Addition to cervical-thoracic-lumbar-sacral orthosis (CTLSO), scoliosis orthosis, cover for upright, each** A ☑

Thoracic-Lumbar-Sacral Orthosis (TLSO) (Low Profile)

L1200 **Thoracic-lumbar-sacral orthosis (TLSO), inclusive of furnishing initial orthosis only** A

L1210 **Addition to thoracic-lumbar-sacral orthosis (TLSO), (low profile), lateral thoracic extension** A

L1220 **Addition to thoracic-lumbar-sacral orthosis (TLSO), (low profile), anterior thoracic extension** A

L1230 **Addition to thoracic-lumbar-sacral orthosis (TLSO), (low profile), Milwaukee type superstructure** A

L1240 **Addition to thoracic-lumbar-sacral orthosis (TLSO), (low profile), lumbar derotation pad** A

L1250 **Addition to thoracic-lumbar-sacral orthosis (TLSO), (low profile), anterior ASIS pad** A

L1260 **Addition to thoracic-lumbar-sacral orthosis (TLSO), (low profile), anterior thoracic derotation pad** A

L1270 **Addition to thoracic-lumbar-sacral orthosis (TLSO), (low profile), abdominal pad** A

L1280 **Addition to thoracic-lumbar-sacral orthosis (TLSO), (low profile), rib gusset (elastic), each** A ☑

L1290 **Addition to thoracic-lumbar-sacral orthosis (TLSO), (low profile), lateral trochanteric pad** A

Other Scoliosis Procedures

L1300 **Other scoliosis procedure, body jacket molded to patient model** A

L1310 **Other scoliosis procedure, postoperative body jacket** A

L1499 **Spinal orthosis, not otherwise specified** A

Determine if an alternative HCPCS Level II or a CPT code better describes the service being reported. This code should be used only if a more specific code is unavailable.

Hip Orthoses (HO) - Flexible

L1600 **Hip orthosis (HO), abduction control of hip joints, flexible, Frejka type with cover, prefabricated item that has been trimmed, bent, molded, assembled, or otherwise customized to fit a specific patient by an individual with expertise** A

L1610 **Hip orthosis (HO), abduction control of hip joints, flexible, (Frejka cover only), prefabricated item that has been trimmed, bent, molded, assembled, or otherwise customized to fit a specific patient by an individual with expertise** A

L1620 **Hip orthosis (HO), abduction control of hip joints, flexible, (Pavlik harness), prefabricated item that has been trimmed, bent, molded, assembled, or otherwise customized to fit a specific patient by an individual with expertise** A

L1630 **Hip orthosis (HO), abduction control of hip joints, semi-flexible (Von Rosen type), custom fabricated** A

L1640 **Hip orthosis (HO), abduction control of hip joints, static, pelvic band or spreader bar, thigh cuffs, custom fabricated** A

L1650 **Hip orthosis (HO), abduction control of hip joints, static, adjustable, (Ilfled type), prefabricated, includes fitting and adjustment** A

L1652 **Hip orthosis (HO), bilateral thigh cuffs with adjustable abductor spreader bar, adult size, prefabricated, includes fitting and adjustment, any type** A

L1660 **Hip orthosis (HO), abduction control of hip joints, static, plastic, prefabricated, includes fitting and adjustment** A

© 2019 Optum360, LLC

L1680 Hip orthosis (HO), abduction control of hip joints, dynamic, pelvic control, adjustable hip motion control, thigh cuffs (Rancho hip action type), custom fabricated A

L1685 Hip orthosis (HO), abduction control of hip joint, postoperative hip abduction type, custom fabricated A

L1686 Hip orthosis (HO), abduction control of hip joint, postoperative hip abduction type, prefabricated, includes fitting and adjustment A

L1690 Combination, bilateral, lumbo-sacral, hip, femur orthosis providing adduction and internal rotation control, prefabricated, includes fitting and adjustment A

Legg Perthes

L1700 Legg Perthes orthosis, (Toronto type), custom fabricated A

L1710 Legg Perthes orthosis, (Newington type), custom fabricated A

L1720 Legg Perthes orthosis, trilateral, (Tachdijan type), custom fabricated A

L1730 Legg Perthes orthosis, (Scottish Rite type), custom fabricated A

L1755 Legg Perthes orthosis, (Patten bottom type), custom fabricated A

Knee Orthosis

L1810 Knee orthosis (KO), elastic with joints, prefabricated item that has been trimmed, bent, molded, assembled, or otherwise customized to fit a specific patient by an individual with expertise A

L1812 Knee orthosis (KO), elastic with joints, prefabricated, off-the-shelf A

L1820 Knee orthosis (KO), elastic with condylar pads and joints, with or without patellar control, prefabricated, includes fitting and adjustment A

L1830 Knee orthosis (KO), immobilizer, canvas longitudinal, prefabricated, off-the-shelf A

L1831 Knee orthosis (KO), locking knee joint(s), positional orthosis, prefabricated, includes fitting and adjustment A

L1832 Knee orthosis (KO), adjustable knee joints (unicentric or polycentric), positional orthosis, rigid support, prefabricated item that has been trimmed, bent, molded, assembled, or otherwise customized to fit a specific patient by an individual with expertise A

L1833 Knee orthosis (KO), adjustable knee joints (unicentric or polycentric), positional orthosis, rigid support, prefabricated, off-the shelf A

L1834 Knee orthosis (KO), without knee joint, rigid, custom fabricated A

L1836 Knee orthosis (KO), rigid, without joint(s), includes soft interface material, prefabricated, off-the-shelf A

L1840 Knee orthosis (KO), derotation, medial-lateral, anterior cruciate ligament, custom fabricated A

L1843 Knee orthosis (KO), single upright, thigh and calf, with adjustable flexion and extension joint (unicentric or polycentric), medial-lateral and rotation control, with or without varus/valgus adjustment, prefabricated item that has been trimmed, bent, molded, assembled, or otherwise customized to fit a specific patient by an individual with expertise A

L1844 Knee orthosis (KO), single upright, thigh and calf, with adjustable flexion and extension joint (unicentric or polycentric), medial-lateral and rotation control, with or without varus/valgus adjustment, custom fabricated A

L1845 Knee orthosis (KO), double upright, thigh and calf, with adjustable flexion and extension joint (unicentric or polycentric), medial-lateral and rotation control, with or without varus/valgus adjustment, prefabricated item that has been trimmed, bent, molded, assembled, or otherwise customized to fit a specific patient by an individual with expertise A

L1846 Knee orthosis (KO), double upright, thigh and calf, with adjustable flexion and extension joint (unicentric or polycentric), medial-lateral and rotation control, with or without varus/valgus adjustment, custom fabricated A

L1847 Knee orthosis (KO), double upright with adjustable joint, with inflatable air support chamber(s), prefabricated item that has been trimmed, bent, molded, assembled, or otherwise customized to fit a specific patient by an individual with expertise A

L1848 Knee orthosis (KO), double upright with adjustable joint, with inflatable air support chamber(s), prefabricated, off-the-shelf A

L1850 Knee orthosis (KO), Swedish type, prefabricated, off-the-shelf A

L1851 Knee orthosis (KO), single upright, thigh and calf, with adjustable flexion and extension joint (unicentric or polycentric), medial-lateral and rotation control, with or without varus/valgus adjustment, prefabricated, off-the-shelf A

L1852 Knee orthosis (KO), double upright, thigh and calf, with adjustable flexion and extension joint (unicentric or polycentric), medial-lateral and rotation control, with or without varus/valgus adjustment, prefabricated, off-the-shelf A

L1860 Knee orthosis (KO), modification of supracondylar prosthetic socket, custom fabricated (SK) A

Ankle-Foot Orthosis (AFO)

L1900 Ankle-foot orthosis (AFO), spring wire, dorsiflexion assist calf band, custom fabricated A

L1902 Ankle orthosis (AO), ankle gauntlet or similar, with or without joints, prefabricated, off-the-shelf A

L1904 Ankle orthosis (AO), ankle gauntlet or similar, with or without joints, custom fabricated A

L1906 Ankle foot orthosis (AFO), multiligamentous ankle support, prefabricated, off-the-shelf A

L1907 Ankle orthosis (AO), supramalleolar with straps, with or without interface/pads, custom fabricated A

L1910 Ankle-foot orthosis (AFO), posterior, single bar, clasp attachment to shoe counter, prefabricated, includes fitting and adjustment A

L1920 Ankle-foot orthosis (AFO), single upright with static or adjustable stop (Phelps or Perlstein type), custom fabricated A

L1930 Ankle-foot orthosis (AFO), plastic or other material, prefabricated, includes fitting and adjustment A

L1932 Ankle-foot orthosis (AFO), rigid anterior tibial section, total carbon fiber or equal material, prefabricated, includes fitting and adjustment A

L1940 Ankle-foot orthosis (AFO), plastic or other material, custom fabricated A

© 2019 Optum360, LLC

L1945 Ankle-foot orthosis (AFO), plastic, rigid anterior tibial section (floor reaction), custom fabricated A ♿

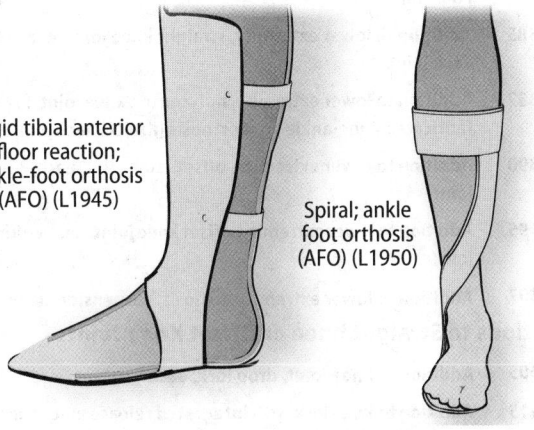

L1950 Ankle-foot orthosis (AFO), spiral, (Institute of Rehabilitative Medicine type), plastic, custom fabricated A ♿

L1951 Ankle-foot orthosis (AFO), spiral, (Institute of rehabilitative Medicine type), plastic or other material, prefabricated, includes fitting and adjustment A ♿

L1960 Ankle-foot orthosis (AFO), posterior solid ankle, plastic, custom fabricated A ♿

L1970 Ankle-foot orthosis (AFO), plastic with ankle joint, custom fabricated A ♿

L1971 Ankle-foot orthosis (AFO), plastic or other material with ankle joint, prefabricated, includes fitting and adjustment A ♿

L1980 Ankle-foot orthosis (AFO), single upright free plantar dorsiflexion, solid stirrup, calf band/cuff (single bar 'BK' orthosis), custom fabricated A ♿

L1990 Ankle-foot orthosis (AFO), double upright free plantar dorsiflexion, solid stirrup, calf band/cuff (double bar 'BK' orthosis), custom fabricated A ♿

Knee-Ankle-Foot Orthosis (KAFO) - Or Any Combination

L2000 Knee-ankle-foot orthosis (KAFO), single upright, free knee, free ankle, solid stirrup, thigh and calf bands/cuffs (single bar 'AK' orthosis), custom fabricated A ♿

L2005 Knee-ankle-foot orthosis (KAFO), any material, single or double upright, stance control, automatic lock and swing phase release, any type activation, includes ankle joint, any type, custom fabricated A ♿

● **L2006**[Jan] Knee-ankle-foot (KAF) device, any material, single or double upright, swing and/or stance phase microprocessor control with adjustability, includes all components (e.g., sensors, batteries, charger), any type activation, with or without ankle joint(s), custom fabricated

L2010 Knee-ankle-foot orthosis (KAFO), single upright, free ankle, solid stirrup, thigh and calf bands/cuffs (single bar 'AK' orthosis), without knee joint, custom fabricated A ♿

L2020 Knee-ankle-foot orthosis (KAFO), double upright, free ankle, solid stirrup, thigh and calf bands/cuffs (double bar 'AK' orthosis), custom fabricated A ♿

L2030 Knee-ankle-foot orthosis (KAFO), double upright, free ankle, solid stirrup, thigh and calf bands/cuffs, (double bar 'AK' orthosis), without knee joint, custom fabricated A ♿

L2034 Knee-ankle-foot orthosis (KAFO), full plastic, single upright, with or without free motion knee, medial-lateral rotation control, with or without free motion ankle, custom fabricated A ♿

L2035 Knee-ankle-foot orthosis (KAFO), full plastic, static (pediatric size), without free motion ankle, prefabricated, includes fitting and adjustment A ♿

L2036 Knee-ankle-foot orthosis (KAFO), full plastic, double upright, with or without free motion knee, with or without free motion ankle, custom fabricated A ♿

L2037 Knee-ankle-foot orthosis (KAFO), full plastic, single upright, with or without free motion knee, with or without free motion ankle, custom fabricated A ♿

L2038 Knee-ankle-foot orthosis (KAFO), full plastic, with or without free motion knee, multi-axis ankle, custom fabricated A ♿

Torsion Control: Hip-Knee-Ankle-Foot Orthosis (HKAFO)

L2040 Hip-knee-ankle-foot orthosis (HKAFO), torsion control, bilateral rotation straps, pelvic band/belt, custom fabricated A ♿

L2050 Hip-knee-ankle-foot orthosis (HKAFO), torsion control, bilateral torsion cables, hip joint, pelvic band/belt, custom fabricated A ♿

L2060 Hip-knee-ankle-foot orthosis (HKAFO), torsion control, bilateral torsion cables, ball bearing hip joint, pelvic band/ belt, custom fabricated A ♿

L2070 Hip-knee-ankle-foot orthosis (HKAFO), torsion control, unilateral rotation straps, pelvic band/belt, custom fabricated A ♿

L2080 Hip-knee-ankle-foot orthosis (HKAFO), torsion control, unilateral torsion cable, hip joint, pelvic band/belt, custom fabricated A ♿

L2090 Hip-knee-ankle-foot orthosis (HKAFO), torsion control, unilateral torsion cable, ball bearing hip joint, pelvic band/ belt, custom fabricated A ♿

L2106 Ankle-foot orthosis (AFO), fracture orthosis, tibial fracture cast orthosis, thermoplastic type casting material, custom fabricated A ♿

L2108 Ankle-foot orthosis (AFO), fracture orthosis, tibial fracture cast orthosis, custom fabricated A ♿

L2112 Ankle-foot orthosis (AFO), fracture orthosis, tibial fracture orthosis, soft, prefabricated, includes fitting and adjustment A ♿

L2114 Ankle-foot orthosis (AFO), fracture orthosis, tibial fracture orthosis, semi-rigid, prefabricated, includes fitting and adjustment A ♿

L2116 Ankle-foot orthosis (AFO), fracture orthosis, tibial fracture orthosis, rigid, prefabricated, includes fitting and adjustment A ♿

L2126 Knee-ankle-foot orthosis (KAFO), fracture orthosis, femoral fracture cast orthosis, thermoplastic type casting material, custom fabricated A ♿

L2128 Knee-ankle-foot orthosis (KAFO), fracture orthosis, femoral fracture cast orthosis, custom fabricated A ♿

L2132 Knee-ankle-foot orthosis (KAFO), fracture orthosis, femoral fracture cast orthosis, soft, prefabricated, includes fitting and adjustment A ♿

L2134 Knee-ankle-foot orthosis (KAFO), fracture orthosis, femoral fracture cast orthosis, semi-rigid, prefabricated, includes fitting and adjustment A ♿

L2136 Knee-ankle-foot orthosis (KAFO), fracture orthosis, femoral fracture cast orthosis, rigid, prefabricated, includes fitting and adjustment A ♿

© 2019 Optum360, LLC

Additions to Fracture Orthosis

L2180 Addition to lower extremity fracture orthosis, plastic shoe insert with ankle joints

L2182 Addition to lower extremity fracture orthosis, drop lock knee joint

L2184 Addition to lower extremity fracture orthosis, limited motion knee joint

L2186 Addition to lower extremity fracture orthosis, adjustable motion knee joint, Lerman type

L2188 Addition to lower extremity fracture orthosis, quadrilateral brim

L2190 Addition to lower extremity fracture orthosis, waist belt

L2192 Addition to lower extremity fracture orthosis, hip joint, pelvic band, thigh flange, and pelvic belt

Additions to Lower Extremity Orthosis: Shoe-Ankle-Shin-Knee

L2200 Addition to lower extremity, limited ankle motion, each joint

L2210 Addition to lower extremity, dorsiflexion assist (plantar flexion resist), each joint

L2220 Addition to lower extremity, dorsiflexion and plantar flexion assist/resist, each joint

L2230 Addition to lower extremity, split flat caliper stirrups and plate attachment

L2232 Addition to lower extremity orthosisis, rocker bottom for total contact ankle-foot orthos (AFO), for custom fabricated orthosis only

L2240 Addition to lower extremity, round caliper and plate attachment

L2250 Addition to lower extremity, foot plate, molded to patient model, stirrup attachment

L2260 Addition to lower extremity, reinforced solid stirrup (Scott-Craig type)

L2265 Addition to lower extremity, long tongue stirrup

L2270 Addition to lower extremity, varus/valgus correction (T) strap, padded/lined or malleolus pad

L2275 Addition to lower extremity, varus/valgus correction, plastic modification, padded/lined

L2280 Addition to lower extremity, molded inner boot

L2300 Addition to lower extremity, abduction bar (bilateral hip involvement), jointed, adjustable

L2310 Addition to lower extremity, abduction bar, straight

L2320 Addition to lower extremity, nonmolded lacer, for custom fabricated orthosis only

L2330 Addition to lower extremity, lacer molded to patient model, for custom fabricated orthosis only

L2335 Addition to lower extremity, anterior swing band

L2340 Addition to lower extremity, pretibial shell, molded to patient model

L2350 Addition to lower extremity, prosthetic type, (BK) socket, molded to patient model, (used for PTB, AFO orthoses)

L2360 Addition to lower extremity, extended steel shank

L2370 Addition to lower extremity, Patten bottom

L2375 Addition to lower extremity, torsion control, ankle joint and half solid stirrup

L2380 Addition to lower extremity, torsion control, straight knee joint, each joint

L2385 Addition to lower extremity, straight knee joint, heavy-duty, each joint

L2387 Addition to lower extremity, polycentric knee joint, for custom fabricated knee-ankle-foot orthosis (KAFO), each joint

L2390 Addition to lower extremity, offset knee joint, each joint

L2395 Addition to lower extremity, offset knee joint, heavy-duty, each joint

L2397 Addition to lower extremity orthosis, suspension sleeve

Additions to Straight Knee or Offset Knee Joints

L2405 Addition to knee joint, drop lock, each

L2415 Addition to knee lock with integrated release mechanism (bail, cable, or equal), any material, each joint

L2425 Addition to knee joint, disc or dial lock for adjustable knee flexion, each joint

L2430 Addition to knee joint, ratchet lock for active and progressive knee extension, each joint

L2492 Addition to knee joint, lift loop for drop lock ring

Additions: Thigh/Weight Bearing - Gluteal/Ischial Weight Bearing

L2500 Addition to lower extremity, thigh/weight bearing, gluteal/ischial weight bearing, ring

L2510 Addition to lower extremity, thigh/weight bearing, quadri-lateral brim, molded to patient model

L2520 Addition to lower extremity, thigh/weight bearing, quadri-lateral brim, custom fitted

L2525 Addition to lower extremity, thigh/weight bearing, ischial containment/narrow M-L brim molded to patient model

L2526 Addition to lower extremity, thigh/weight bearing, ischial containment/narrow M-L brim, custom fitted

L2530 Addition to lower extremity, thigh/weight bearing, lacer, nonmolded

L2540 Addition to lower extremity, thigh/weight bearing, lacer, molded to patient model

L2550 Addition to lower extremity, thigh/weight bearing, high roll cuff

Additions: Pelvic and Thoracic Control

L2570 Addition to lower extremity, pelvic control, hip joint, Clevis type two-position joint, each

L2580 Addition to lower extremity, pelvic control, pelvic sling

L2600 Addition to lower extremity, pelvic control, hip joint, Clevis type, or thrust bearing, free, each

L2610 Addition to lower extremity, pelvic control, hip joint, Clevis or thrust bearing, lock, each

L2620 Addition to lower extremity, pelvic control, hip joint, heavy-duty, each

L2622 Addition to lower extremity, pelvic control, hip joint, adjustable flexion, each

L2624 Addition to lower extremity, pelvic control, hip joint, adjustable flexion, extension, abduction control, each

© 2019 Optum360, LLC

L2627 Addition to lower extremity, pelvic control, plastic, molded to patient model, reciprocating hip joint and cables

L2628 Addition to lower extremity, pelvic control, metal frame, reciprocating hip joint and cables

L2630 Addition to lower extremity, pelvic control, band and belt, unilateral

L2640 Addition to lower extremity, pelvic control, band and belt, bilateral

L2650 Addition to lower extremity, pelvic and thoracic control, gluteal pad, each

L2660 Addition to lower extremity, thoracic control, thoracic band

L2670 Addition to lower extremity, thoracic control, paraspinal uprights

L2680 Addition to lower extremity, thoracic control, lateral support uprights

Additions: General

L2750 Addition to lower extremity orthosis, plating chrome or nickel, per bar

L2755 Addition to lower extremity orthosis, high strength, lightweight material, all hybrid lamination/prepreg composite, per segment, for custom fabricated orthosis only

L2760 Addition to lower extremity orthosis, extension, per extension, per bar (for lineal adjustment for growth)

L2768 Orthotic side bar disconnect device, per bar

AHA: 1Q, '02, 5

L2780 Addition to lower extremity orthosis, noncorrosive finish, per bar

L2785 Addition to lower extremity orthosis, drop lock retainer, each

L2795 Addition to lower extremity orthosis, knee control, full kneecap

L2800 Addition to lower extremity orthosis, knee control, knee cap, medial or lateral pull, for use with custom fabricated orthosis only

L2810 Addition to lower extremity orthosis, knee control, condylar pad

L2820 Addition to lower extremity orthosis, soft interface for molded plastic, below knee section

L2830 Addition to lower extremity orthosis, soft interface for molded plastic, above knee section

L2840 Addition to lower extremity orthosis, tibial length sock, fracture or equal, each

L2850 Addition to lower extremity orthosis, femoral length sock, fracture or equal, each

L2861 Addition to lower extremity joint, knee or ankle, concentric adjustable torsion style mechanism for custom fabricated orthotics only, each

L2999 Lower extremity orthoses, not otherwise specified

Determine if an alternative HCPCS Level II or a CPT code better describes the service being reported. This code should be used only if a more specific code is unavailable.

Orthopedic Footwear

Inserts

L3000 Foot insert, removable, molded to patient model, UCB type, Berkeley shell, each

L3001 Foot, insert, removable, molded to patient model, Spenco, each

L3002 Foot insert, removable, molded to patient model, Plastazote or equal, each

L3003 Foot insert, removable, molded to patient model, silicone gel, each

L3010 Foot insert, removable, molded to patient model, longitudinal arch support, each

L3020 Foot insert, removable, molded to patient model, longitudinal/metatarsal support, each

L3030 Foot insert, removable, formed to patient foot, each

L3031 Foot, insert/plate, removable, addition to lower extremity orthosis, high strength, lightweight material, all hybrid lamination/prepreg composite, each

Arch Support, Removable, Premolded

L3040 Foot, arch support, removable, premolded, longitudinal, each

L3050 Foot, arch support, removable, premolded, metatarsal, each

L3060 Foot, arch support, removable, premolded, longitudinal/metatarsal, each

Arch Support, Nonremovable, Attached to Shoe

L3070 Foot, arch support, nonremovable, attached to shoe, longitudinal, each

L3080 Foot, arch support, nonremovable, attached to shoe, metatarsal, each

L3090 Foot, arch support, nonremovable, attached to shoe, longitudinal/metatarsal, each

L3100 Hallus-valgus night dynamic splint, prefabricated, off-the-shelf

Abduction and Rotation Bars

L3140 Foot, abduction rotation bar, including shoes

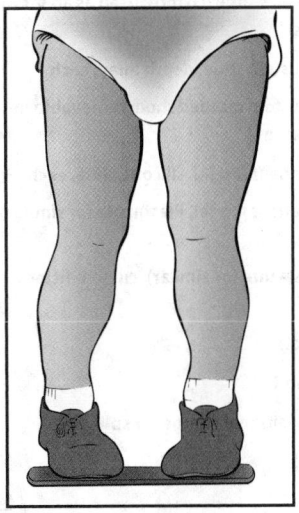

A Denis-Browne style splint is a bar that can be applied by a strap or mounted on a shoe. This type of splint generally corrects congenital conditions such as genu varus

The angle may be adjusted on a plate on the sole of the shoe

Denis-Browne splint

L3150 Foot, abduction rotation bar, without shoes

L3160 Foot, adjustable shoe-styled positioning device

L3170 Foot, plastic, silicone or equal, heel stabilizer, prefabricated, off-the-shelf, each

© 2019 Optum360, LLC

Orthopedic Shoes and Boots

L3201	Orthopedic shoe, Oxford with supinator or pronator, infant	A A
L3202	Orthopedic shoe, Oxford with supinator or pronator, child	A A
L3203	Orthopedic shoe, Oxford with supinator or pronator, junior	A A
L3204	Orthopedic shoe, hightop with supinator or pronator, infant	A A
L3206	Orthopedic shoe, hightop with supinator or pronator, child	A A
L3207	Orthopedic shoe, hightop with supinator or pronator, junior	A A
L3208	Surgical boot, each, infant	A A ☑
L3209	Surgical boot, each, child	A A ☑
L3211	Surgical boot, each, junior	A A ☑
L3212	Benesch boot, pair, infant	A A ☑
L3213	Benesch boot, pair, child	A A ☑
L3214	Benesch boot, pair, junior	A A ☑
L3215	Orthopedic footwear, ladies shoe, Oxford, each	A ♀ E ☑
L3216	Orthopedic footwear, ladies shoe, depth inlay, each	A ♀ E ☑
L3217	Orthopedic footwear, ladies shoe, hightop, depth inlay, each	A ♀ E ☑
L3219	Orthopedic footwear, mens shoe, Oxford, each	A ♂ E ☑
L3221	Orthopedic footwear, mens shoe, depth inlay, each	A ♂ E ☑
L3222	Orthopedic footwear, mens shoe, hightop, depth inlay, each	A ♂ E ☑
L3224	Orthopedic footwear, woman's shoe, Oxford, used as an integral part of a brace (orthosis)	♀ A ♿
L3225	Orthopedic footwear, man's shoe, Oxford, used as an integral part of a brace (orthosis)	♂ A ♿
L3230	Orthopedic footwear, custom shoe, depth inlay, each	A ☑
L3250	Orthopedic footwear, custom molded shoe, removable inner mold, prosthetic shoe, each	A ☑
L3251	Foot, shoe molded to patient model, silicone shoe, each	A ☑
L3252	Foot, shoe molded to patient model, Plastazote (or similar), custom fabricated, each	A ☑
L3253	Foot, molded shoe, Plastazote (or similar), custom fitted, each	A ☑
L3254	Nonstandard size or width	A
L3255	Nonstandard size or length	A
L3257	Orthopedic footwear, additional charge for split size	A
L3260	Surgical boot/shoe, each	E ☑
L3265	Plastazote sandal, each	A ☑

Shoe Modification - Lifts

L3300	Lift, elevation, heel, tapered to metatarsals, per in	A ☑ ♿
L3310	Lift, elevation, heel and sole, neoprene, per in	A ☑ ♿
L3320	Lift, elevation, heel and sole, cork, per in	A ☑
L3330	Lift, elevation, metal extension (skate)	A ♿
L3332	Lift, elevation, inside shoe, tapered, up to one-half in	A ☑ ♿
L3334	Lift, elevation, heel, per in	A ☑ ♿

Shoe Modification - Wedges

L3340	Heel wedge, SACH	A ♿
L3350	Heel wedge	A ♿
L3360	Sole wedge, outside sole	A ♿
L3370	Sole wedge, between sole	A ♿
L3380	Clubfoot wedge	A ♿
L3390	Outflare wedge	A ♿
L3400	Metatarsal bar wedge, rocker	A ♿
L3410	Metatarsal bar wedge, between sole	A ♿
L3420	Full sole and heel wedge, between sole	A ♿

Shoe Modifications - Heels

L3430	Heel, counter, plastic reinforced	A ♿
L3440	Heel, counter, leather reinforced	A ♿
L3450	Heel, SACH cushion type	A ♿
L3455	Heel, new leather, standard	A ♿
L3460	Heel, new rubber, standard	A ♿
L3465	Heel, Thomas with wedge	A ♿
L3470	Heel, Thomas extended to ball	A ♿
L3480	Heel, pad and depression for spur	A ♿
L3485	Heel, pad, removable for spur	A

Miscellaneous Shoe Additions

L3500	Orthopedic shoe addition, insole, leather	A ♿
L3510	Orthopedic shoe addition, insole, rubber	A ♿
L3520	Orthopedic shoe addition, insole, felt covered with leather	A ♿
L3530	Orthopedic shoe addition, sole, half	A ♿
L3540	Orthopedic shoe addition, sole, full	A ♿
L3550	Orthopedic shoe addition, toe tap, standard	A ♿
L3560	Orthopedic shoe addition, toe tap, horseshoe	A ♿
L3570	Orthopedic shoe addition, special extension to instep (leather with eyelets)	A ♿
L3580	Orthopedic shoe addition, convert instep to Velcro closure	A ♿
L3590	Orthopedic shoe addition, convert firm shoe counter to soft counter	A ♿
L3595	Orthopedic shoe addition, March bar	A ♿

Transfer or Replacement

L3600	Transfer of an orthosis from one shoe to another, caliper plate, existing	A ♿
L3610	Transfer of an orthosis from one shoe to another, caliper plate, new	A ♿
L3620	Transfer of an orthosis from one shoe to another, solid stirrup, existing	A ♿
L3630	Transfer of an orthosis from one shoe to another, solid stirrup, new	A ♿
L3640	Transfer of an orthosis from one shoe to another, Dennis Browne splint (Riveton), both shoes	A ♿

© 2019 Optum360, LLC

L3649 Orthopedic shoe, modification, addition or transfer, not otherwise specified [A]

Determine if an alternative HCPCS Level II or a CPT code better describes the service being reported. This code should be used only if a more specific code is unavailable.

Shoulder Orthosis (SO)

L3650 Shoulder orthosis (SO), figure of eight design abduction restrainer, prefabricated, off-the-shelf [A]

L3660 Shoulder orthosis (SO), figure of eight design abduction restrainer, canvas and webbing, prefabricated, off-the-shelf [A]

L3670 Shoulder orthosis (SO), acromio/clavicular (canvas and webbing type), prefabricated, off-the-shelf [A]

L3671 Shoulder orthosis (SO), shoulder joint design, without joints, may include soft interface, straps, custom fabricated, includes fitting and adjustment [A]

L3674 Shoulder orthosis (SO), abduction positioning (airplane design), thoracic component and support bar, with or without nontorsion joint/turnbuckle, may include soft interface, straps, custom fabricated, includes fitting and adjustment [A]

L3675 Shoulder orthosis (SO), vest type abduction restrainer, canvas webbing type or equal, prefabricated, off-the-shelf [A]

L3677 Shoulder orthosis (SO), shoulder joint design, without joints, may include soft interface, straps, prefabricated item that has been trimmed, bent, molded, assembled, or otherwise customized to fit a specific patient by an individual with expertise [A]

AHA: 1Q, '02, 5

L3678 Shoulder orthosis (SO), shoulder joint design, without joints, may include soft interface, straps, prefabricated, off-the-shelf [A]

Elbow Orthosis (EO)

L3702 Elbow orthosis (EO), without joints, may include soft interface, straps, custom fabricated, includes fitting and adjustment [A]

L3710 Elbow orthosis (EO), elastic with metal joints, prefabricated, off-the-shelf [A]

L3720 Elbow orthosis (EO), double upright with forearm/arm cuffs, free motion, custom fabricated [A]

L3730 Elbow orthosis (EO), double upright with forearm/arm cuffs, extension/ flexion assist, custom fabricated [A]

L3740 Elbow orthosis (EO), double upright with forearm/arm cuffs, adjustable position lock with active control, custom fabricated [A]

L3760 Elbow orthosis (EO), with adjustable position locking joint(s), prefabricated, item that has been trimmed, bent, molded, assembled, or otherwise customized to fit a specific patient by an individual with expertise [A]

L3761 Elbow orthosis (EO), with adjustable position locking joint(s), prefabricated, off-the-shelf [A]

L3762 Elbow orthosis (EO), rigid, without joints, includes soft interface material, prefabricated, off-the-shelf [A]

L3763 Elbow-wrist-hand orthosis (EWHO), rigid, without joints, may include soft interface, straps, custom fabricated, includes fitting and adjustment [A]

L3764 Elbow-wrist-hand orthosis (EWHO), includes one or more nontorsion joints, elastic bands, turnbuckles, may include soft interface, straps, custom fabricated, includes fitting and adjustment [A]

L3765 Elbow-wrist-hand-finger orthosis (EWHFO), rigid, without joints, may include soft interface, straps, custom fabricated, includes fitting and adjustment [A]

L3766 Elbow-wrist-hand-finger orthosis (EWHFO), includes one or more nontorsion joints, elastic bands, turnbuckles, may include soft interface, straps, custom fabricated, includes fitting and adjustment [A]

Wrist-Hand-Finger Orthosis (WHFO)

L3806 Wrist-hand-finger orthosis (WHFO), includes one or more nontorsion joint(s), turnbuckles, elastic bands/springs, may include soft interface material, straps, custom fabricated, includes fitting and adjustment [A]

L3807 Wrist-hand-finger orthosis (WHFO), without joint(s), prefabricated item that has been trimmed, bent, molded, assembled, or otherwise customized to fit a specific patient by an individual with expertise [A]

L3808 Wrist-hand-finger orthosis (WHFO), rigid without joints, may include soft interface material; straps, custom fabricated, includes fitting and adjustment [A]

L3809 Wrist-hand-finger orthosis (WHFO), without joint(s), prefabricated, off-the-shelf, any type [A]

Additions to Upper Extremity Orthosis

L3891 Addition to upper extremity joint, wrist or elbow, concentric adjustable torsion style mechanism for custom fabricated orthotics only, each [E] ☑

Dynamic Flexor Hinge, Reciprocal Wrist Extension/Flexion, Finger Flexion/Extension

L3900 Wrist-hand-finger orthosis (WHFO), dynamic flexor hinge, reciprocal wrist extension/ flexion, finger flexion/extension, wrist or finger driven, custom fabricated [A]

L3901 Wrist-hand-finger orthosis (WHFO), dynamic flexor hinge, reciprocal wrist extension/ flexion, finger flexion/extension, cable driven, custom fabricated [A]

External Power

L3904 Wrist-hand-finger orthosis (WHFO), external powered, electric, custom fabricated [A]

Other Upper Extremity Orthoses

L3905 Wrist-hand orthosis (WHO), includes one or more nontorsion joints, elastic bands, turnbuckles, may include soft interface, straps, custom fabricated, includes fitting and adjustment [A]

L3906 Wrist-hand orthosis (WHO), without joints, may include soft interface, straps, custom fabricated, includes fitting and adjustment [A]

L3908 Wrist-hand orthosis (WHO), wrist extension control cock-up, nonmolded, prefabricated, off-the-shelf [A]

L3912 Hand-finger orthosis (HFO), flexion glove with elastic finger control, prefabricated, off-the-shelf [A]

L3913 Hand-finger orthosis (HFO), without joints, may include soft interface, straps, custom fabricated, includes fitting and adjustment [A]

L3915 Wrist-hand orthosis (WHO), includes one or more nontorsion joint(s), elastic bands, turnbuckles, may include soft interface, straps, prefabricated item that has been trimmed, bent, molded, assembled, or otherwise customized to fit a specific patient by an individual with expertise [A]

L3916 Wrist-hand orthosis (WHO), includes one or more nontorsion joint(s), elastic bands, turnbuckles, may include soft interface, straps, prefabricated, off-the-shelf [A]

© 2019 Optum360, LLC

L3917 Hand orthosis (HO), metacarpal fracture orthosis, prefabricated item that has been trimmed, bent, molded, assembled, or otherwise customized to fit a specific patient by an individual with expertise A

L3918 Hand orthosis (HO), metacarpal fracture orthosis, prefabricated, off-the-shelf A

L3919 Hand orthosis (HO), without joints, may include soft interface, straps, custom fabricated, includes fitting and adjustment A

L3921 Hand-finger orthosis (HFO), includes one or more nontorsion joints, elastic bands, turnbuckles, may include soft interface, straps, custom fabricated, includes fitting and adjustment A

L3923 Hand-finger orthosis (HFO), without joints, may include soft interface, straps, prefabricated item that has been trimmed, bent, molded, assembled, or otherwise customized to fit a specific patient by an individual with expertise A

L3924 Hand-finger orthosis (HFO), without joints, may include soft interface, straps, prefabricated, off-the-shelf A

L3925 Finger orthosis (FO), proximal interphalangeal (PIP)/distal interphalangeal (DIP), nontorsion joint/spring, extension/flexion, may include soft interface material, prefabricated, off-the-shelf A

L3927 Finger orthosis (FO), proximal interphalangeal (PIP)/distal interphalangeal (DIP), without joint/spring, extension/flexion (e.g., static or ring type), may include soft interface material, prefabricated, off-the-shelf A

L3929 Hand-finger orthosis (HFO), includes one or more nontorsion joint(s), turnbuckles, elastic bands/springs, may include soft interface material, straps, prefabricated item that has been trimmed, bent, molded, assembled, or otherwise customized to fit a specific patient by an individual with expertise A

L3930 Hand-finger orthosis (HFO), includes one or more nontorsion joint(s), turnbuckles, elastic bands/springs, may include soft interface material, straps, prefabricated, off-the-shelf A

L3931 Wrist-hand-finger orthosis (WHFO), includes one or more nontorsion joint(s), turnbuckles, elastic bands/springs, may include soft interface material, straps, prefabricated, includes fitting and adjustment A

L3933 Finger orthosis (FO), without joints, may include soft interface, custom fabricated, includes fitting and adjustment A

L3935 Finger orthosis (FO), nontorsion joint, may include soft interface, custom fabricated, includes fitting and adjustment A

L3956 Addition of joint to upper extremity orthosis, any material; per joint A ☑

Shoulder, Elbow, Wrist, Hand Orthosis

L3960 Shoulder-elbow-wrist-hand orthosis (SEWHO), abduction positioning, airplane design, prefabricated, includes fitting and adjustment A

L3961 Shoulder-elbow-wrist-hand orthosis (SEWHO), shoulder cap design, without joints, may include soft interface, straps, custom fabricated, includes fitting and adjustment A

L3962 Shoulder-elbow-wrist-hand orthosis (SEWHO), abduction positioning, Erb's palsy design, prefabricated, includes fitting and adjustment A

L3967 Shoulder-elbow-wrist-hand orthosis (SEWHO), abduction positioning (airplane design), thoracic component and support bar, without joints, may include soft interface, straps, custom fabricated, includes fitting and adjustment A

Additions to Mobile Arm Supports

L3971 Shoulder-elbow-wrist-hand orthotic (SEWHO), shoulder cap design, includes one or more nontorsion joints, elastic bands, turnbuckles, may include soft interface, straps, custom fabricated, includes fitting and adjustment A

L3973 Shoulder-elbow-wrist-hand orthosis (SEWHO), abduction positioning (airplane design), thoracic component and support bar, includes one or more nontorsion joints, elastic bands, turnbuckles, may include soft interface, straps, custom fabricated, includes fitting and adjustment A

L3975 Shoulder-elbow-wrist-hand-finger orthosis (SEWHO), shoulder cap design, without joints, may include soft interface, straps, custom fabricated, includes fitting and adjustment A

L3976 Shoulder-elbow-wrist-hand-finger orthosis (SEWHO), abduction positioning (airplane design), thoracic component and support bar, without joints, may include soft interface, straps, custom fabricated, includes fitting and adjustment A

L3977 Shoulder-elbow-wrist-hand-finger orthosis (SEWHO), shoulder cap design, includes one or more nontorsion joints, elastic bands, turnbuckles, may include soft interface, straps, custom fabricated, includes fitting and adjustment A

L3978 Shoulder-elbow-wrist-hand-finger orthosis (SEWHO), abduction positioning (airplane design), thoracic component and support bar, includes one or more nontorsion joints, elastic bands, turnbuckles, may include soft interface, straps, custom fabricated, includes fitting and adjustment A

Fracture Orthotic

L3980 Upper extremity fracture orthosis, humeral, prefabricated, includes fitting and adjustment A

L3981 Upper extremity fracture orthosis, humeral, prefabricated, includes shoulder cap design, with or without joints, forearm section, may include soft interface, straps, includes fitting and adjustments A

L3982 Upper extremity fracture orthosis, radius/ulnar, prefabricated, includes fitting and adjustment A

L3984 Upper extremity fracture orthosis, wrist, prefabricated, includes fitting and adjustment A

L3995 Addition to upper extremity orthosis, sock, fracture or equal, each A ☑

L3999 Upper limb orthosis, not otherwise specified A

Repairs

L4000 Replace girdle for spinal orthosis (cervical-thoracic-lumbar-sacral orthosis (CTLSO) or spinal orthosis SO) A

L4002 Replacement strap, any orthosis, includes all components, any length, any type A

L4010 Replace trilateral socket brim A

L4020 Replace quadrilateral socket brim, molded to patient model A

L4030 Replace quadrilateral socket brim, custom fitted A

L4040 Replace molded thigh lacer, for custom fabricated orthosis only A

L4045 Replace nonmolded thigh lacer, for custom fabricated orthosis only A

L4050 Replace molded calf lacer, for custom fabricated orthosis only A

L4055 Replace nonmolded calf lacer, for custom fabricated orthosis only A

© 2019 Optum360, LLC

L4060 Replace high roll cuff

L4070 Replace proximal and distal upright for KAFO

L4080 Replace metal bands KAFO, proximal thigh

L4090 Replace metal bands KAFO-AFO, calf or distal thigh

L4100 Replace leather cuff KAFO, proximal thigh

L4110 Replace leather cuff KAFO-AFO, calf or distal thigh

L4130 Replace pretibial shell

L4205 Repair of orthotic device, labor component, per 15 minutes

L4210 Repair of orthotic device, repair or replace minor parts

Miscellaneous Lower Limb Supports

L4350 Ankle control orthosis, stirrup style, rigid, includes any type interface (e.g., pneumatic, gel), prefabricated, off-the-shelf

L4360 Walking boot, pneumatic and/or vacuum, with or without joints, with or without interface material, prefabricated item that has been trimmed, bent, molded, assembled, or otherwise customized to fit a specific patient by an individual with expertise

L4361 Walking boot, pneumatic and/or vacuum, with or without joints, with or without interface material, prefabricated, off-the-shelf

L4370 Pneumatic full leg splint, prefabricated, off-the-shelf

L4386 Walking boot, nonpneumatic, with or without joints, with or without interface material, prefabricated item that has been trimmed, bent, molded, assembled, or otherwise customized to fit a specific patient by an individual with expertise

L4387 Walking boot, nonpneumatic, with or without joints, with or without interface material, prefabricated, off-the-shelf

L4392 Replacement, soft interface material, static AFO

L4394 Replace soft interface material, foot drop splint

L4396 Static or dynamic ankle foot orthosis, including soft interface material, adjustable for fit, for positioning, may be used for minimal ambulation, prefabricated item that has been trimmed, bent, molded, assembled, or otherwise customized to fit a specific patient by an individual with expertise

L4397 Static or dynamic ankle foot orthosis, including soft interface material, adjustable for fit, for positioning, may be used for minimal ambulation, prefabricated, off-the-shelf

L4398 Foot drop splint, recumbent positioning device, prefabricated, off-the-shelf

L4631 Ankle-foot orthosis (AFO), walking boot type, varus/valgus correction, rocker bottom, anterior tibial shell, soft interface, custom arch support, plastic or other material, includes straps and closures, custom fabricated

Prosthetic Procedures L5000-L9900

The codes in this section are considered as "base" or "basic procedures or prosthetics" and may be modified by listing items/procedures or special materials from the "additions" sections and adding them to the base procedure.

Partial Foot

L5000 Partial foot, shoe insert with longitudinal arch, toe filler

L5010 Partial foot, molded socket, ankle height, with toe filler

L5020 Partial foot, molded socket, tibial tubercle height, with toe filler

Ankle

L5050 Ankle, Symes, molded socket, SACH foot

L5060 Ankle, Symes, metal frame, molded leather socket, articulated ankle/foot

Below Knee

L5100 Below knee (BK), molded socket, shin, SACH foot

L5105 Below knee (BK), plastic socket, joints and thigh lacer, SACH foot

Knee Disarticulation

L5150 Knee disarticulation (or through knee), molded socket, external knee joints, shin, SACH foot

L5160 Knee disarticulation (or through knee), molded socket, bent knee configuration, external knee joints, shin, SACH foot

Above Knee

L5200 Above knee (AK), molded socket, single axis constant friction knee, shin, SACH foot

L5210 Above knee (AK), short prosthesis, no knee joint (stubbies), with foot blocks, no ankle joints, each

L5220 Above knee (AK), short prosthesis, no knee joint (stubbies), with articulated ankle/foot, dynamically aligned, each

L5230 Above knee (AK), for proximal femoral focal deficiency, constant friction knee, shin, SACH foot

Hip Disarticulation

L5250 Hip disarticulation, Canadian type; molded socket, hip joint, single axis constant friction knee, shin, SACH foot

L5270 Hip disarticulation, tilt table type; molded socket, locking hip joint, single axis constant friction knee, shin, SACH foot

Hemipelvectomy

L5280 Hemipelvectomy, Canadian type; molded socket, hip joint, single axis constant friction knee, shin, SACH foot

L5301 Below knee (BK), molded socket, shin, SACH foot, endoskeletal system
AHA: 1Q, '02, 5

L5312 Knee disarticulation (or through knee), molded socket, single axis knee, pylon, SACH foot, endoskeletal system

L5321 Above knee (AK), molded socket, open end, SACH foot, endoskeletal system, single axis knee
AHA: 1Q, '02, 5

L5331 Hip disarticulation, Canadian type, molded socket, endoskeletal system, hip joint, single axis knee, SACH foot
AHA: 1Q, '02, 5

L5341 Hemipelvectomy, Canadian type, molded socket, endoskeletal system, hip joint, single axis knee, SACH foot
AHA: 1Q, '02, 5

© 2019 Optum360, LLC

Immediate Postsurgical or Early Fitting Procedures

L5400 Immediate postsurgical or early fitting, application of initial rigid dressing, including fitting, alignment, suspension, and one cast change, below knee (BK)

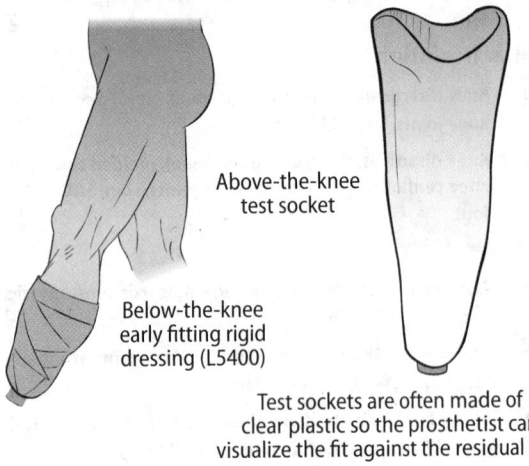

L5410 Immediate postsurgical or early fitting, application of initial rigid dressing, including fitting, alignment and suspension, below knee (BK), each additional cast change and realignment

L5420 Immediate postsurgical or early fitting, application of initial rigid dressing, including fitting, alignment and suspension and one cast change above knee (AK) or knee disarticulation

L5430 Immediate postsurgical or early fitting, application of initial rigid dressing, including fitting, alignment and suspension, above knee (AK) or knee disarticulation, each additional cast change and realignment

L5450 Immediate postsurgical or early fitting, application of nonweight bearing rigid dressing, below knee (BK)

L5460 Immediate postsurgical or early fitting, application of nonweight bearing rigid dressing, above knee (AK)

Initial Prosthesis

L5500 Initial, below knee (BK) PTB type socket, nonalignable system, pylon, no cover, SACH foot, plaster socket, direct formed

L5505 Initial, above knee (AK), knee disarticulation, ischial level socket, nonalignable system, pylon, no cover, SACH foot, plaster socket, direct formed

Preparatory Prosthesis

L5510 Preparatory, below knee (BK) PTB type socket, nonalignable system, pylon, no cover, SACH foot, plaster socket, molded to model

L5520 Preparatory, below knee (BK) PTB type socket, nonalignable system, pylon, no cover, SACH foot, thermoplastic or equal, direct formed

L5530 Preparatory, below knee (BK) PTB type socket, nonalignable system, pylon, no cover, SACH foot, thermoplastic or equal, molded to model

L5535 Preparatory, below knee (BK) PTB type socket, nonalignable system, no cover, SACH foot, prefabricated, adjustable open end socket

L5540 Preparatory, below knee (BK) PTB type socket, nonalignable system, pylon, no cover, SACH foot, laminated socket, molded to model

L5560 Preparatory, above knee (AK), knee disarticulation, ischial level socket, nonalignable system, pylon, no cover, SACH foot, plaster socket, molded to model

L5570 Preparatory, above knee (AK), knee disarticulation, ischial level socket, nonalignable system, pylon, no cover, SACH foot, thermoplastic or equal, direct formed

L5580 Preparatory, above knee (AK), knee disarticulation, ischial level socket, nonalignable system, pylon, no cover, SACH foot, thermoplastic or equal, molded to model

L5585 Preparatory, above knee (AK), knee disarticulation, ischial level socket, nonalignable system, pylon, no cover, SACH foot, prefabricated adjustable open end socket

L5590 Preparatory, above knee (AK), knee disarticulation, ischial level socket, nonalignable system, pylon, no cover, SACH foot, laminated socket, molded to model

L5595 Preparatory, hip disarticulation/hemipelvectomy, pylon, no cover, SACH foot, thermoplastic or equal, molded to patient model

L5600 Preparatory, hip disarticulation/hemipelvectomy, pylon, no cover, SACH foot, laminated socket, molded to patient model

Additions

Additions: Lower Extremity

L5610 Addition to lower extremity, endoskeletal system, above knee (AK), hydracadence system

L5611 Addition to lower extremity, endoskeletal system, above knee (AK), knee disarticulation, four-bar linkage, with friction swing phase control

L5613 Addition to lower extremity, endoskeletal system, above knee (AK), knee disarticulation, four-bar linkage, with hydraulic swing phase control

L5614 Addition to lower extremity, exoskeletal system, above knee (AK), knee disarticulation, four-bar linkage, with pneumatic swing phase control

L5616 Addition to lower extremity, endoskeletal system, above knee (AK), universal multiplex system, friction swing phase control

L5617 Addition to lower extremity, quick change self-aligning unit, above knee (AK) or below knee (BK), each

Additions: Test Sockets

L5618 Addition to lower extremity, test socket, Symes

L5620 Addition to lower extremity, test socket, below knee (BK)

L5622 Addition to lower extremity, test socket, knee disarticulation

L5624 Addition to lower extremity, test socket, above knee (AK)

L5626 Addition to lower extremity, test socket, hip disarticulation

L5628 Addition to lower extremity, test socket, hemipelvectomy

L5629 Addition to lower extremity, below knee, acrylic socket

© 2019 Optum360, LLC

Additions: Socket Variations

L5630 Addition to lower extremity, Symes type, expandable wall socket

L5631 Addition to lower extremity, above knee (AK) or knee disarticulation, acrylic socket

L5632 Addition to lower extremity, Symes type, PTB brim design socket

L5634 Addition to lower extremity, Symes type, posterior opening (Canadian) socket

L5636 Addition to lower extremity, Symes type, medial opening socket

L5637 Addition to lower extremity, below knee (BK), total contact

L5638 Addition to lower extremity, below knee (BK), leather socket

L5639 Addition to lower extremity, below knee (BK), wood socket

L5640 Addition to lower extremity, knee disarticulation, leather socket

L5642 Addition to lower extremity, above knee (AK), leather socket

L5643 Addition to lower extremity, hip disarticulation, flexible inner socket, external frame

L5644 Addition to lower extremity, above knee (AK), wood socket

L5645 Addition to lower extremity, below knee (BK), flexible inner socket, external frame

L5646 Addition to lower extremity, below knee (BK), air, fluid, gel or equal, cushion socket

L5647 Addition to lower extremity, below knee (BK), suction socket

L5648 Addition to lower extremity, above knee (AK), air, fluid, gel or equal, cushion socket

L5649 Addition to lower extremity, ischial containment/narrow M-L socket

L5650 Additions to lower extremity, total contact, above knee (AK) or knee disarticulation socket

L5651 Addition to lower extremity, above knee (AK), flexible inner socket, external frame

L5652 Addition to lower extremity, suction suspension, above knee (AK) or knee disarticulation socket

L5653 Addition to lower extremity, knee disarticulation, expandable wall socket

Additions: Socket Insert and Suspension

L5654 Addition to lower extremity, socket insert, Symes, (Kemblo, Pelite, Aliplast, Plastazote or equal)

L5655 Addition to lower extremity, socket insert, below knee (BK) (Kemblo, Pelite, Aliplast, Plastazote or equal)

L5656 Addition to lower extremity, socket insert, knee disarticulation (Kemblo, Pelite, Aliplast, Plastazote or equal)

L5658 Addition to lower extremity, socket insert, above knee (AK) (Kemblo, Pelite, Aliplast, Plastazote or equal)

L5661 Addition to lower extremity, socket insert, multidurometer Symes

L5665 Addition to lower extremity, socket insert, multidurometer, below knee (BK)

L5666 Addition to lower extremity, below knee (BK), cuff suspension

L5668 Addition to lower extremity, below knee (BK), molded distal cushion

L5670 Addition to lower extremity, below knee (BK), molded supracondylar suspension (PTS or similar)

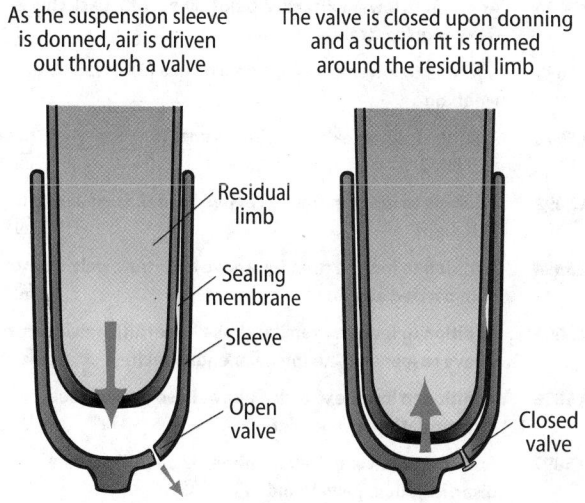

L5671 Addition to lower extremity, below knee (BK)/above knee (AK) suspension locking mechanism (shuttle, lanyard, or equal), excludes socket insert

AHA: 1Q, '02, 5

L5672 Addition to lower extremity, below knee (BK), removable medial brim suspension

L5673 Addition to lower extremity, below knee (BK)/above knee (AK), custom fabricated from existing mold or prefabricated, socket insert, silicone gel, elastomeric or equal, for use with locking mechanism

L5676 Additions to lower extremity, below knee (BK), knee joints, single axis, pair

L5677 Additions to lower extremity, below knee (BK), knee joints, polycentric, pair

L5678 Additions to lower extremity, below knee (BK), joint covers, pair

L5679 Addition to lower extremity, below knee (BK)/above knee (AK), custom fabricated from existing mold or prefabricated, socket insert, silicone gel, elastomeric or equal, not for use with locking mechanism

L5680 Addition to lower extremity, below knee (BK), thigh lacer, nonmolded

L5681 Addition to lower extremity, below knee (BK)/above knee (AK), custom fabricated socket insert for congenital or atypical traumatic amputee, silicone gel, elastomeric or equal, for use with or without locking mechanism, initial only (for other than initial, use code L5673 or L5679)

L5682 Addition to lower extremity, below knee (BK), thigh lacer, gluteal/ischial, molded

© 2019 Optum360, LLC

L5683 Addition to lower extremity, below knee (BK)/above knee (AK), custom fabricated socket insert for other than congenital or atypical traumatic amputee, silicone gel, elastomeric or equal, for use with or without locking mechanism, initial only (for other than initial, use code L5673 or L5679) A

L5684 Addition to lower extremity, below knee, fork strap A

L5685 Addition to lower extremity prosthesis, below knee, suspension/sealing sleeve, with or without valve, any material, each A

L5686 Addition to lower extremity, below knee (BK), back check (extension control) A

L5688 Addition to lower extremity, below knee (BK), waist belt, webbing A

L5690 Addition to lower extremity, below knee (BK), waist belt, padded and lined A

L5692 Addition to lower extremity, above knee (AK), pelvic control belt, light A

L5694 Addition to lower extremity, above knee (AK), pelvic control belt, padded and lined A

L5695 Addition to lower extremity, above knee (AK), pelvic control, sleeve suspension, neoprene or equal, each A ☑

L5696 Addition to lower extremity, above knee (AK) or knee disarticulation, pelvic joint A

L5697 Addition to lower extremity, above knee (AK) or knee disarticulation, pelvic band A

L5698 Addition to lower extremity, above knee (AK) or knee disarticulation, Silesian bandage A

L5699 All lower extremity prostheses, shoulder harness A

Replacements

L5700 Replacement, socket, below knee (BK), molded to patient model A

L5701 Replacement, socket, above knee (AK)/knee disarticulation, including attachment plate, molded to patient model A

L5702 Replacement, socket, hip disarticulation, including hip joint, molded to patient model A

L5703 Ankle, Symes, molded to patient model, socket without solid ankle cushion heel (SACH) foot, replacement only A

L5704 Custom shaped protective cover, below knee (BK) A

L5705 Custom shaped protective cover, above knee (AK) A

L5706 Custom shaped protective cover, knee disarticulation A

L5707 Custom shaped protective cover, hip disarticulation A

Additions: Exoskeletal Knee-Shin System

L5710 Addition, exoskeletal knee-shin system, single axis, manual lock A

L5711 Additions exoskeletal knee-shin system, single axis, manual lock, ultra-light material A

L5712 Addition, exoskeletal knee-shin system, single axis, friction swing and stance phase control (safety knee) A

L5714 Addition, exoskeletal knee-shin system, single axis, variable friction swing phase control A

L5716 Addition, exoskeletal knee-shin system, polycentric, mechanical stance phase lock A

L5718 Addition, exoskeletal knee-shin system, polycentric, friction swing and stance phase control A

L5722 Addition, exoskeletal knee-shin system, single axis, pneumatic swing, friction stance phase control A

L5724 Addition, exoskeletal knee-shin system, single axis, fluid swing phase control A

L5726 Addition, exoskeletal knee-shin system, single axis, external joints, fluid swing phase control A

L5728 Addition, exoskeletal knee-shin system, single axis, fluid swing and stance phase control A

L5780 Addition, exoskeletal knee-shin system, single axis, pneumatic/hydra pneumatic swing phase control A

L5781 Addition to lower limb prosthesis, vacuum pump, residual limb volume management and moisture evacuation system A

L5782 Addition to lower limb prosthesis, vacuum pump, residual limb volume management and moisture evacuation system, heavy-duty A

Component Modification

L5785 Addition, exoskeletal system, below knee (BK), ultra-light material (titanium, carbon fiber or equal) A

L5790 Addition, exoskeletal system, above knee (AK), ultra-light material (titanium, carbon fiber or equal) A

L5795 Addition, exoskeletal system, hip disarticulation, ultra-light material (titanium, carbon fiber or equal) A

Additions: Endoskeletal Knee-Shin System

L5810 Addition, endoskeletal knee-shin system, single axis, manual lock A

L5811 Addition, endoskeletal knee-shin system, single axis, manual lock, ultra-light material A

L5812 Addition, endoskeletal knee-shin system, single axis, friction swing and stance phase control (safety knee) A

L5814 Addition, endoskeletal knee-shin system, polycentric, hydraulic swing phase control, mechanical stance phase lock A

L5816 Addition, endoskeletal knee-shin system, polycentric, mechanical stance phase lock A

L5818 Addition, endoskeletal knee-shin system, polycentric, friction swing and stance phase control A

L5822 Addition, endoskeletal knee-shin system, single axis, pneumatic swing, friction stance phase control A

L5824 Addition, endoskeletal knee-shin system, single axis, fluid swing phase control A

L5826 Addition, endoskeletal knee-shin system, single axis, hydraulic swing phase control, with miniature high activity frame A

L5828 Addition, endoskeletal knee-shin system, single axis, fluid swing and stance phase control A

L5830 Addition, endoskeletal knee-shin system, single axis, pneumatic/swing phase control A

L5840 Addition, endoskeletal knee-shin system, four-bar linkage or multiaxial, pneumatic swing phase control A

L5845 Addition, endoskeletal knee-shin system, stance flexion feature, adjustable A

L5848 Addition to endoskeletal knee-shin system, fluid stance extension, dampening feature, with or without adjustability A

L5850 Addition, endoskeletal system, above knee (AK) or hip disarticulation, knee extension assist A

© 2019 Optum360, LLC

L5855 Addition, endoskeletal system, hip disarticulation, mechanical hip extension assist

L5856 Addition to lower extremity prosthesis, endoskeletal knee-shin system, microprocessor control feature, swing and stance phase, includes electronic sensor(s), any type

L5857 Addition to lower extremity prosthesis, endoskeletal knee-shin system, microprocessor control feature, swing phase only, includes electronic sensor(s), any type

L5858 Addition to lower extremity prosthesis, endoskeletal knee-shin system, microprocessor control feature, stance phase only, includes electronic sensor(s), any type

L5859 Addition to lower extremity prosthesis, endoskeletal knee-shin system, powered and programmable flexion/extension assist control, includes any type motor(s)

L5910 Addition, endoskeletal system, below knee (BK), alignable system

L5920 Addition, endoskeletal system, above knee (AK) or hip disarticulation, alignable system

L5925 Addition, endoskeletal system, above knee (AK), knee disarticulation or hip disarticulation, manual lock

L5930 Addition, endoskeletal system, high activity knee control frame

L5940 Addition, endoskeletal system, below knee (BK), ultra-light material (titanium, carbon fiber or equal)

L5950 Addition, endoskeletal system, above knee (AK), ultra-light material (titanium, carbon fiber or equal)

L5960 Addition, endoskeletal system, hip disarticulation, ultra-light material (titanium, carbon fiber or equal)

L5961 Addition, endoskeletal system, polycentric hip joint, pneumatic or hydraulic control, rotation control, with or without flexion and/or extension control

L5962 Addition, endoskeletal system, below knee (BK), flexible protective outer surface covering system

L5964 Addition, endoskeletal system, above knee (AK), flexible protective outer surface covering system

L5966 Addition, endoskeletal system, hip disarticulation, flexible protective outer surface covering system

L5968 Addition to lower limb prosthesis, multiaxial ankle with swing phase active dorsiflexion feature

L5969 Addition, endoskeletal ankle-foot or ankle system, power assist, includes any type motor(s)

L5970 All lower extremity prostheses, foot, external keel, SACH foot

L5971 All lower extremity prostheses, solid ankle cushion heel (SACH) foot, replacement only

L5972 All lower extremity prostheses, foot, flexible keel

L5973 Endoskeletal ankle foot system, microprocessor controlled feature, dorsiflexion and/or plantar flexion control, includes power source

L5974 All lower extremity prostheses, foot, single axis ankle/foot

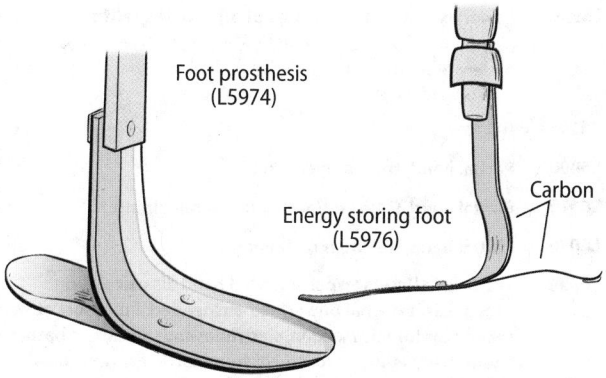

L5975 All lower extremity prostheses, combination single axis ankle and flexible keel foot

L5976 All lower extremity prostheses, energy storing foot (Seattle Carbon Copy II or equal)

L5978 All lower extremity prostheses, foot, multiaxial ankle/foot

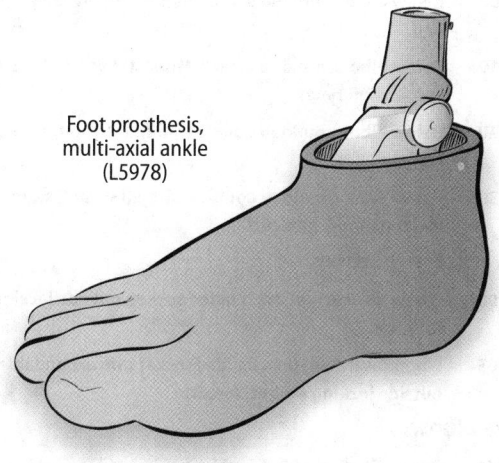

L5979 All lower extremity prostheses, multiaxial ankle, dynamic response foot, one-piece system

L5980 All lower extremity prostheses, flex-foot system

L5981 All lower extremity prostheses, flex-walk system or equal

L5982 All exoskeletal lower extremity prostheses, axial rotation unit

L5984 All endoskeletal lower extremity prostheses, axial rotation unit, with or without adjustability

L5985 All endoskeletal lower extremity prostheses, dynamic prosthetic pylon

L5986 All lower extremity prostheses, multiaxial rotation unit (MCP or equal)

L5987 All lower extremity prostheses, shank foot system with vertical loading pylon

L5988 Addition to lower limb prosthesis, vertical shock reducing pylon feature

© 2019 Optum360, LLC

L5990 Addition to lower extremity prosthesis, user adjustable heel height A
AHA: 1Q, '02, 5

L5999 Lower extremity prosthesis, not otherwise specified A
Determine if an alternative HCPCS Level II or a CPT code better describes the service being reported. This code should be used only if a more specific code is unavailable.

Partial Hand

L6000 Partial hand, thumb remaining A

L6010 Partial hand, little and/or ring finger remaining A

L6020 Partial hand, no finger remaining A

L6026 Transcarpal/metacarpal or partial hand disarticulation prosthesis, external power, self-suspended, inner socket with removable forearm section, electrodes and cables, two batteries, charger, myoelectric control of terminal device, excludes terminal device(s) A

Wrist Disarticulation

L6050 Wrist disarticulation, molded socket, flexible elbow hinges, triceps pad A

L6055 Wrist disarticulation, molded socket with expandable interface, flexible elbow hinges, triceps pad A

Below Elbow

L6100 Below elbow, molded socket, flexible elbow hinge, triceps pad A

L6110 Below elbow, molded socket (Muenster or Northwestern suspension types) A

L6120 Below elbow, molded double wall split socket, step-up hinges, half cuff A

L6130 Below elbow, molded double wall split socket, stump activated locking hinge, half cuff A

Elbow Disarticulation

L6200 Elbow disarticulation, molded socket, outside locking hinge, forearm A

L6205 Elbow disarticulation, molded socket with expandable interface, outside locking hinges, forearm A

Above Elbow

L6250 Above elbow, molded double wall socket, internal locking elbow, forearm A

Shoulder Disarticulation

L6300 Shoulder disarticulation, molded socket, shoulder bulkhead, humeral section, internal locking elbow, forearm A

L6310 Shoulder disarticulation, passive restoration (complete prosthesis) A

L6320 Shoulder disarticulation, passive restoration (shoulder cap only) A

Interscapular Thoracic

L6350 Interscapular thoracic, molded socket, shoulder bulkhead, humeral section, internal locking elbow, forearm A

L6360 Interscapular thoracic, passive restoration (complete prosthesis) A

L6370 Interscapular thoracic, passive restoration (shoulder cap only) A

Immediate and Early Postsurgical Procedures

L6380 Immediate postsurgical or early fitting, application of initial rigid dressing, including fitting alignment and suspension of components, and one cast change, wrist disarticulation or below elbow A

L6382 Immediate postsurgical or early fitting, application of initial rigid dressing including fitting alignment and suspension of components, and one cast change, elbow disarticulation or above elbow A ☑

L6384 Immediate postsurgical or early fitting, application of initial rigid dressing including fitting alignment and suspension of components, and one cast change, shoulder disarticulation or interscapular thoracic A ☑

L6386 Immediate postsurgical or early fitting, each additional cast change and realignment A ☑

L6388 Immediate postsurgical or early fitting, application of rigid dressing only A

Molded Socket

L6400 Below elbow, molded socket, endoskeletal system, including soft prosthetic tissue shaping A

L6450 Elbow disarticulation, molded socket, endoskeletal system, including soft prosthetic tissue shaping A

L6500 Above elbow, molded socket, endoskeletal system, including soft prosthetic tissue shaping A

L6550 Shoulder disarticulation, molded socket, endoskeletal system, including soft prosthetic tissue shaping A

L6570 Interscapular thoracic, molded socket, endoskeletal system, including soft prosthetic tissue shaping A

Preparatory Socket

L6580 Preparatory, wrist disarticulation or below elbow, single wall plastic socket, friction wrist, flexible elbow hinges, figure of eight harness, humeral cuff, Bowden cable control, USMC or equal pylon, no cover, molded to patient model A

L6582 Preparatory, wrist disarticulation or below elbow, single wall socket, friction wrist, flexible elbow hinges, figure of eight harness, humeral cuff, Bowden cable control, USMC or equal pylon, no cover, direct formed A

L6584 Preparatory, elbow disarticulation or above elbow, single wall plastic socket, friction wrist, locking elbow, figure of eight harness, fair lead cable control, USMC or equal pylon, no cover, molded to patient model A

L6586 Preparatory, elbow disarticulation or above elbow, single wall socket, friction wrist, locking elbow, figure of eight harness, fair lead cable control, USMC or equal pylon, no cover, direct formed A

L6588 Preparatory, shoulder disarticulation or interscapular thoracic, single wall plastic socket, shoulder joint, locking elbow, friction wrist, chest strap, fair lead cable control, USMC or equal pylon, no cover, molded to patient model A

L6590 Preparatory, shoulder disarticulation or interscapular thoracic, single wall socket, shoulder joint, locking elbow, friction wrist, chest strap, fair lead cable control, USMC or equal pylon, no cover, direct formed A

Additions: Upper Limb

The following procedures/modifications/components may be added to other base procedures. The items in this section should reflect the additional complexity of each modification procedure, in addition to the base procedure, at the time of the original order.

L6600 Upper extremity additions, polycentric hinge, pair A ☑

© 2019 Optum360, LLC

L6605 Upper extremity additions, single pivot hinge, pair

L6610 Upper extremity additions, flexible metal hinge, pair

L6611 Addition to upper extremity prosthesis, external powered, additional switch, any type

L6615 Upper extremity addition, disconnect locking wrist unit

L6616 Upper extremity addition, additional disconnect insert for locking wrist unit, each

L6620 Upper extremity addition, flexion/extension wrist unit, with or without friction

L6621 Upper extremity prosthesis addition, flexion/extension wrist with or without friction, for use with external powered terminal device

L6623 Upper extremity addition, spring assisted rotational wrist unit with latch release

L6624 Upper extremity addition, flexion/extension and rotation wrist unit

L6625 Upper extremity addition, rotation wrist unit with cable lock

L6628 Upper extremity addition, quick disconnect hook adapter, Otto Bock or equal

L6629 Upper extremity addition, quick disconnect lamination collar with coupling piece, Otto Bock or equal

L6630 Upper extremity addition, stainless steel, any wrist

L6632 Upper extremity addition, latex suspension sleeve, each

L6635 Upper extremity addition, lift assist for elbow

L6637 Upper extremity addition, nudge control elbow lock

L6638 Upper extremity addition to prosthesis, electric locking feature, only for use with manually powered elbow

L6640 Upper extremity additions, shoulder abduction joint, pair

L6641 Upper extremity addition, excursion amplifier, pulley type

L6642 Upper extremity addition, excursion amplifier, lever type

L6645 Upper extremity addition, shoulder flexion-abduction joint, each

L6646 Upper extremity addition, shoulder joint, multipositional locking, flexion, adjustable abduction friction control, for use with body powered or external powered system

L6647 Upper extremity addition, shoulder lock mechanism, body powered actuator

L6648 Upper extremity addition, shoulder lock mechanism, external powered actuator

L6650 Upper extremity addition, shoulder universal joint, each

L6655 Upper extremity addition, standard control cable, extra

L6660 Upper extremity addition, heavy-duty control cable

L6665 Upper extremity addition, Teflon, or equal, cable lining

L6670 Upper extremity addition, hook to hand, cable adapter

L6672 Upper extremity addition, harness, chest or shoulder, saddle type

L6675 Upper extremity addition, harness, (e.g., figure of eight type), single cable design

L6676 Upper extremity addition, harness, (e.g., figure of eight type), dual cable design

L6677 Upper extremity addition, harness, triple control, simultaneous operation of terminal device and elbow

L6680 Upper extremity addition, test socket, wrist disarticulation or below elbow

L6682 Upper extremity addition, test socket, elbow disarticulation or above elbow

L6684 Upper extremity addition, test socket, shoulder disarticulation or interscapular thoracic

L6686 Upper extremity addition, suction socket

L6687 Upper extremity addition, frame type socket, below elbow or wrist disarticulation

L6688 Upper extremity addition, frame type socket, above elbow or elbow disarticulation

L6689 Upper extremity addition, frame type socket, shoulder disarticulation

L6690 Upper extremity addition, frame type socket, interscapular-thoracic

L6691 Upper extremity addition, removable insert, each

L6692 Upper extremity addition, silicone gel insert or equal, each

L6693 Upper extremity addition, locking elbow, forearm counterbalance

L6694 Addition to upper extremity prosthesis, below elbow/above elbow, custom fabricated from existing mold or prefabricated, socket insert, silicone gel, elastomeric or equal, for use with locking mechanism

L6695 Addition to upper extremity prosthesis, below elbow/above elbow, custom fabricated from existing mold or prefabricated, socket insert, silicone gel, elastomeric or equal, not for use with locking mechanism

L6696 Addition to upper extremity prosthesis, below elbow/above elbow, custom fabricated socket insert for congenital or atypical traumatic amputee, silicone gel, elastomeric or equal, for use with or without locking mechanism, initial only (for other than initial, use code L6694 or L6695)

L6697 Addition to upper extremity prosthesis, below elbow/above elbow, custom fabricated socket insert for other than congenital or atypical traumatic amputee, silicone gel, elastomeric or equal, for use with or without locking mechanism, initial only (for other than initial, use code L6694 or L6695)

L6698 Addition to upper extremity prosthesis, below elbow/above elbow, lock mechanism, excludes socket insert

Terminal Device

L6703 Terminal device, passive hand/mitt, any material, any size

L6704 Terminal device, sport/recreational/work attachment, any material, any size

L6706 Terminal device, hook, mechanical, voluntary opening, any material, any size, lined or unlined

L6707 Terminal device, hook, mechanical, voluntary closing, any material, any size, lined or unlined

© 2019 Optum360, LLC

L6708 Terminal device, hand, mechanical, voluntary opening, any material, any size

L6709 Terminal device, hand, mechanical, voluntary closing, any material, any size

L6711 Terminal device, hook, mechanical, voluntary opening, any material, any size, lined or unlined, pediatric

L6712 Terminal device, hook, mechanical, voluntary closing, any material, any size, lined or unlined, pediatric

L6713 Terminal device, hand, mechanical, voluntary opening, any material, any size, pediatric

L6714 Terminal device, hand, mechanical, voluntary closing, any material, any size, pediatric

L6715 Terminal device, multiple articulating digit, includes motor(s), initial issue or replacement

L6721 Terminal device, hook or hand, heavy-duty, mechanical, voluntary opening, any material, any size, lined or unlined

L6722 Terminal device, hook or hand, heavy-duty, mechanical, voluntary closing, any material, any size, lined or unlined

Addition to Terminal Device

L6805 Addition to terminal device, modifier wrist unit

L6810 Addition to terminal device, precision pinch device

L6880 Electric hand, switch or myoelectric controlled, independently articulating digits, any grasp pattern or combination of grasp patterns, includes motor(s)

L6881 Automatic grasp feature, addition to upper limb electric prosthetic terminal device
AHA: 1Q, '02, 5

L6882 Microprocessor control feature, addition to upper limb prosthetic terminal device
AHA: 1Q, '02, 5

Replacement Socket

L6883 Replacement socket, below elbow/wrist disarticulation, molded to patient model, for use with or without external power

L6884 Replacement socket, above elbow/elbow disarticulation, molded to patient model, for use with or without external power

L6885 Replacement socket, shoulder disarticulation/interscapular thoracic, molded to patient model, for use with or without external power

Hand Restoration

L6890 Addition to upper extremity prosthesis, glove for terminal device, any material, prefabricated, includes fitting and adjustment

L6895 Addition to upper extremity prosthesis, glove for terminal device, any material, custom fabricated

L6900 Hand restoration (casts, shading and measurements included), partial hand, with glove, thumb or one finger remaining

L6905 Hand restoration (casts, shading and measurements included), partial hand, with glove, multiple fingers remaining

L6910 Hand restoration (casts, shading and measurements included), partial hand, with glove, no fingers remaining

L6915 Hand restoration (shading and measurements included), replacement glove for above

External Power

L6920 Wrist disarticulation, external power, self-suspended inner socket, removable forearm shell, Otto Bock or equal switch, cables, two batteries and one charger, switch control of terminal device

L6925 Wrist disarticulation, external power, self-suspended inner socket, removable forearm shell, Otto Bock or equal electrodes, cables, two batteries and one charger, myoelectronic control of terminal device

L6930 Below elbow, external power, self-suspended inner socket, removable forearm shell, Otto Bock or equal switch, cables, two batteries and one charger, switch control of terminal device

L6935 Below elbow, external power, self-suspended inner socket, removable forearm shell, Otto Bock or equal electrodes, cables, two batteries and one charger, myoelectronic control of terminal device

L6940 Elbow disarticulation, external power, molded inner socket, removable humeral shell, outside locking hinges, forearm, Otto Bock or equal switch, cables, two batteries and one charger, switch control of terminal device

L6945 Elbow disarticulation, external power, molded inner socket, removable humeral shell, outside locking hinges, forearm, Otto Bock or equal electrodes, cables, two batteries and one charger, myoelectronic control of terminal device

L6950 Above elbow, external power, molded inner socket, removable humeral shell, internal locking elbow, forearm, Otto Bock or equal switch, cables, two batteries and one charger, switch control of terminal device

L6955 Above elbow, external power, molded inner socket, removable humeral shell, internal locking elbow, forearm, Otto Bock or equal electrodes, cables, two batteries and one charger, myoelectronic control of terminal device

L6960 Shoulder disarticulation, external power, molded inner socket, removable shoulder shell, shoulder bulkhead, humeral section, mechanical elbow, forearm, Otto Bock or equal switch, cables, two batteries and one charger, switch control of terminal device

L6965 Shoulder disarticulation, external power, molded inner socket, removable shoulder shell, shoulder bulkhead, humeral section, mechanical elbow, forearm, Otto Bock or equal electrodes, cables, two batteries and one charger, myoelectronic control of terminal device

L6970 Interscapular-thoracic, external power, molded inner socket, removable shoulder shell, shoulder bulkhead, humeral section, mechanical elbow, forearm, Otto Bock or equal switch, cables, two batteries and one charger, switch control of terminal device

L6975 Interscapular-thoracic, external power, molded inner socket, removable shoulder shell, shoulder bulkhead, humeral section, mechanical elbow, forearm, Otto Bock or equal electrodes, cables, two batteries and one charger, myoelectronic control of terminal device

Electric Hand and Accessories

L7007 Electric hand, switch or myoelectric controlled, adult

L7008 Electric hand, switch or myoelectric, controlled, pediatric

L7009 Electric hook, switch or myoelectric controlled, adult

L7040 Prehensile actuator, switch controlled

© 2019 Optum360, LLC

L7045 Electric hook, switch or myoelectric controlled, pediatric [A] ⊘ ♿

Electronic Elbow and Accessories

L7170 Electronic elbow, Hosmer or equal, switch controlled [A] ⊘ ♿

L7180 Electronic elbow, microprocessor sequential control of elbow and terminal device [A] ⊘ ♿

L7181 Electronic elbow, microprocessor simultaneous control of elbow and terminal device [A] ⊘ ♿

L7185 Electronic elbow, adolescent, Variety Village or equal, switch controlled [A] ⊘ ♿

L7186 Electronic elbow, child, Variety Village or equal, switch controlled [A] ⊘ ♿

L7190 Electronic elbow, adolescent, Variety Village or equal, myoelectronically controlled [A] ⊘ ♿

L7191 Electronic elbow, child, Variety Village or equal, myoelectronically controlled [A] ⊘ ♿

Electronic Wrist and Accessories

L7259 Electronic wrist rotator, any type [A] ♿

Battery Components

L7360 Six volt battery, each [A] ☑ ♿

L7362 Battery charger, six volt, each [A] ☑ ⊘ ♿

L7364 Twelve volt battery, each [A] ☑ ⊘ ♿

L7366 Battery charger, 12 volt, each [A] ☑ ⊘ ♿

L7367 Lithium ion battery, rechargeable, replacement [A] ⊘ ♿

L7368 Lithium ion battery charger, replacement only [A] ⊘ ♿

Additions to Upper Extremity Prosthesis

L7400 Addition to upper extremity prosthesis, below elbow/wrist disarticulation, ultra-light material (titanium, carbon fiber or equal) [A] ⊘ ♿

L7401 Addition to upper extremity prosthesis, above elbow disarticulation, ultra-light material (titanium, carbon fiber or equal) [A] ⊘ ♿

L7402 Addition to upper extremity prosthesis, shoulder disarticulation/interscapular thoracic, ultra-light material (titanium, carbon fiber or equal) [A] ⊘ ♿

L7403 Addition to upper extremity prosthesis, below elbow/wrist disarticulation, acrylic material [A] ⊘ ♿

L7404 Addition to upper extremity prosthesis, above elbow disarticulation, acrylic material [A] ⊘ ♿

L7405 Addition to upper extremity prosthesis, shoulder disarticulation/interscapular thoracic, acrylic material [A] ⊘ ♿

L7499 Upper extremity prosthesis, not otherwise specified [A]

Repairs

L7510 Repair of prosthetic device, repair or replace minor parts [A]
Medicare jurisdiction: local contractor if repair of implanted prosthetic device.

L7520 Repair prosthetic device, labor component, per 15 minutes [A] ☑
Medicare jurisdiction: local contractor if repair of implanted prosthetic device.

Prosthesis Supplies

L7600 Prosthetic donning sleeve, any material, each [E] ☑

L7700 Gasket or seal, for use with prosthetic socket insert, any type, each [A] ♿

Male Prosthetic

L7900 Male vacuum erection system ♂ [E]

L7902 Tension ring, for vacuum erection device, any type, replacement only, each ♂ [E]

Breast Prosthesis

L8000 Breast prosthesis, mastectomy bra, without integrated breast prosthesis form, any size, any type ♀ [A] ♿

L8001 Breast prosthesis, mastectomy bra, with integrated breast prosthesis form, unilateral, any size, any type ♀ [A] ♿
AHA: 1Q, '02, 5

L8002 Breast prosthesis, mastectomy bra, with integrated breast prosthesis form, bilateral, any size, any type ♀ [A] ♿
AHA: 1Q, '02, 5

L8010 Breast prosthesis, mastectomy sleeve ♀ [A]

L8015 External breast prosthesis garment, with mastectomy form, post mastectomy ♀ [A] ♿

L8020 Breast prosthesis, mastectomy form ♀ [A] ♿

L8030 Breast prosthesis, silicone or equal, without integral adhesive ♀ [A] ♿

L8031 Breast prosthesis, silicone or equal, with integral adhesive [A] ♿

▲ **L8032**[Jan] Nipple prosthesis, prefabricated, reusable, any type, each [A] ☑ ♿

● **L8033**[Jan] Nipple prosthesis, custom fabricated, reusable, any material, any type, each

L8035 Custom breast prosthesis, post mastectomy, molded to patient model ♀ [A] ♿

L8039 Breast prosthesis, not otherwise specified ♀ [A]

Face and Ear Prosthesis

L8040 Nasal prosthesis, provided by a nonphysician [A] ♿ (KM, KN)
CMS: 100-04,20,30.9

Nasal prosthesis (L8040)

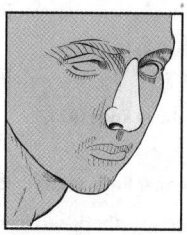

Orbital and midfacial prosthesis (L8041-L8042)

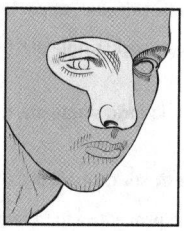

Prosthesis ▭

Facial prosthetics are typically custom manufactured from polymers and carefully matched to the original features. The maxilla, zygoma, frontal, and nasal bones are often involved, either singly or in combination (L8040-L8044)

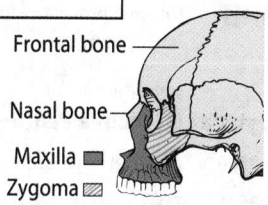

(L8043–L8044)

L8041 Midfacial prosthesis, provided by a nonphysician [A] ♿ (KM, KN)
CMS: 100-04,20,30.9

L8042 Orbital prosthesis, provided by a nonphysician [A] ♿ (KM, KN)
CMS: 100-04,20,30.9

L8043 Upper facial prosthesis, provided by a nonphysician [A] ♿ (KM, KN)
CMS: 100-04,20,30.9

© 2019 Optum360, LLC

L8044 **Hemi-facial prosthesis, provided by a nonphysician** A ♿ (KM, KN)
CMS: 100-04,20,30.9

L8045 **Auricular prosthesis, provided by a nonphysician** A ♿ (KM, KN)
CMS: 100-04,20,30.9

L8046 **Partial facial prosthesis, provided by a nonphysician** A ♿ (KM, KN)
CMS: 100-04,20,30.9

L8047 **Nasal septal prosthesis, provided by a nonphysician** A ♿ (KM, KN)
CMS: 100-04,20,30.9

L8048 **Unspecified maxillofacial prosthesis, by report, provided by a nonphysician** A

L8049 **Repair or modification of maxillofacial prosthesis, labor component, 15 minute increments, provided by a nonphysician** A

Trusses

L8300 **Truss, single with standard pad** A ♿

L8310 **Truss, double with standard pads** A ♿

L8320 **Truss, addition to standard pad, water pad** A ♿

L8330 **Truss, addition to standard pad, scrotal pad** ♂ A ♿

Prosthetic Socks

L8400 **Prosthetic sheath, below knee, each** A ☑ ♿

L8410 **Prosthetic sheath, above knee, each** A ☑ ♿

L8415 **Prosthetic sheath, upper limb, each** A ☑ ♿

L8417 **Prosthetic sheath/sock, including a gel cushion layer, below knee (BK) or above knee (AK), each** A ☑ ♿

L8420 **Prosthetic sock, multiple ply, below knee (BK), each** A ☑ ♿

L8430 **Prosthetic sock, multiple ply, above knee (AK), each** A ☑ ♿

L8435 **Prosthetic sock, multiple ply, upper limb, each** A ☑ ♿

L8440 **Prosthetic shrinker, below knee (BK), each** A ☑ ♿

L8460 **Prosthetic shrinker, above knee (AK), each** A ☑ ♿

L8465 **Prosthetic shrinker, upper limb, each** A ☑ ♿

L8470 **Prosthetic sock, single ply, fitting, below knee (BK), each** A ☑ ♿

L8480 **Prosthetic sock, single ply, fitting, above knee (AK), each** A ☑ ♿

L8485 **Prosthetic sock, single ply, fitting, upper limb, each** A ☑ ♿

L8499 **Unlisted procedure for miscellaneous prosthetic services** A
Determine if an alternative HCPCS Level II or a CPT code better describes the service being reported. This code should be used only if a more specific code is unavailable.

Larynx and Trachea Prothetics and Accessories

L8500 **Artificial larynx, any type** A ♿

L8501 **Tracheostomy speaking valve** A ♿

L8505 **Artificial larynx replacement battery/accessory, any type** A
AHA: 1Q, '02, 5

L8507 **Tracheo-esophageal voice prosthesis, patient inserted, any type, each** A ☑ ♿
AHA: 1Q, '02, 5

L8509 **Tracheo-esophageal voice prosthesis, inserted by a licensed health care provider, any type** A ♿
AHA: 1Q, '02, 5

L8510 **Voice amplifier** A ♿
AHA: 1Q, '02, 5

L8511 **Insert for indwelling tracheo-esophageal prosthesis, with or without valve, replacement only, each** A ☑ ♿

L8512 **Gelatin capsules or equivalent, for use with tracheo-esophageal voice prosthesis, replacement only, per 10** A ☑ ♿

L8513 **Cleaning device used with tracheoesophageal voice prosthesis, pipet, brush, or equal, replacement only, each** A ☑ ♿

L8514 **Tracheo-esophageal puncture dilator, replacement only, each** A ☑ ♿

L8515 **Gelatin capsule, application device for use with tracheo-esophageal voice prosthesis, each** A ☑ ♿

Breast Implant

L8600 **Implantable breast prosthesis, silicone or equal** ♀ N NI ♿
Medicare covers implants inserted in post-mastectomy reconstruction in a breast cancer patient. Always report concurrent to the implant procedure.
CMS: 100-04,4,190

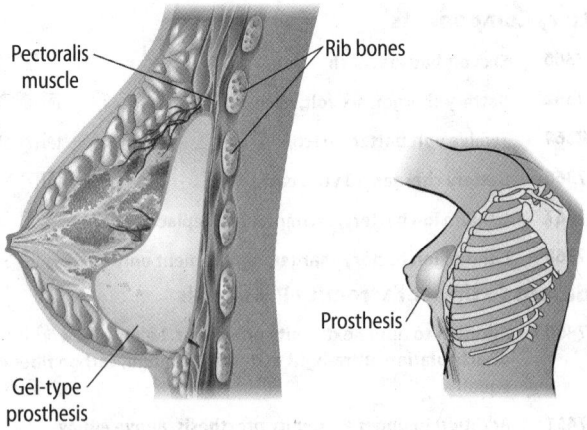

Bulking Agents

L8603 **Injectable bulking agent, collagen implant, urinary tract, 2.5 ml syringe, includes shipping and necessary supplies** N NI ☑ ♿
CMS: 100-04,4,190

L8604 **Injectable bulking agent, dextranomer/hyaluronic acid copolymer implant, urinary tract, 1 ml, includes shipping and necessary supplies** N NI ☑

L8605 **Injectable bulking agent, dextranomer/hyaluronic acid copolymer implant, anal canal, 1 ml, includes shipping and necessary supplies** N NI ♿

L8606 **Injectable bulking agent, synthetic implant, urinary tract, 1 ml syringe, includes shipping and necessary supplies** N NI ☑ ♿

L8607 **Injectable bulking agent for vocal cord medialization, 0.1 ml, includes shipping and necessary supplies** N NI ♿

Eye and Ear Implants and Accessories

L8608 **Miscellaneous external component, supply or accessory for use with the Argus II Retinal Prosthesis System**

L8609 **Artificial cornea** N NI ♿

L8610 **Ocular implant** N NI ♿
CMS: 100-04,4,190

L8612 **Aqueous shunt** N NI ♿
CMS: 100-04,4,190

© 2019 Optum360, LLC

L8613 **Ossicula implant**
CMS: 100-04,4,190

L8614 **Cochlear device, includes all internal and external components**
A cochlear implant is covered by Medicare when the patient has bilateral sensorineural deafness.
CMS: 100-04,14,40.8; 100-04,4,190
AHA: 3Q, '16, 10-15; 4Q, '03, 8; 3Q, '02, 4-5; 1Q, '01, 6

L8615 **Headset/headpiece for use with cochlear implant device, replacement**

L8616 **Microphone for use with cochlear implant device, replacement**

L8617 **Transmitting coil for use with cochlear implant device, replacement**

L8618 **Transmitter cable for use with cochlear implant device or auditory osseointegrated device, replacement**

L8619 **Cochlear implant, external speech processor and controller, integrated system, replacement**
Medicare jurisdiction: local contractor.

L8621 **Zinc air battery for use with cochlear implant device and auditory osseointegrated sound processors, replacement, each**

L8622 **Alkaline battery for use with cochlear implant device, any size, replacement, each**

L8623 **Lithium ion battery for use with cochlear implant device speech processor, other than ear level, replacement, each**

L8624 **Lithium ion battery for use with cochlear implant or auditory osseointegrated device speech processor, ear level, replacement, each**

L8625 **External recharging system for battery for use with cochlear implant or auditory osseointegrated device, replacement only, each**

L8627 **Cochlear implant, external speech processor, component, replacement**

L8628 **Cochlear implant, external controller component, replacement**

L8629 **Transmitting coil and cable, integrated, for use with cochlear implant device, replacement**

Upper Extremity Implants

L8630 **Metacarpophalangeal joint implant**
CMS: 100-04,4,190

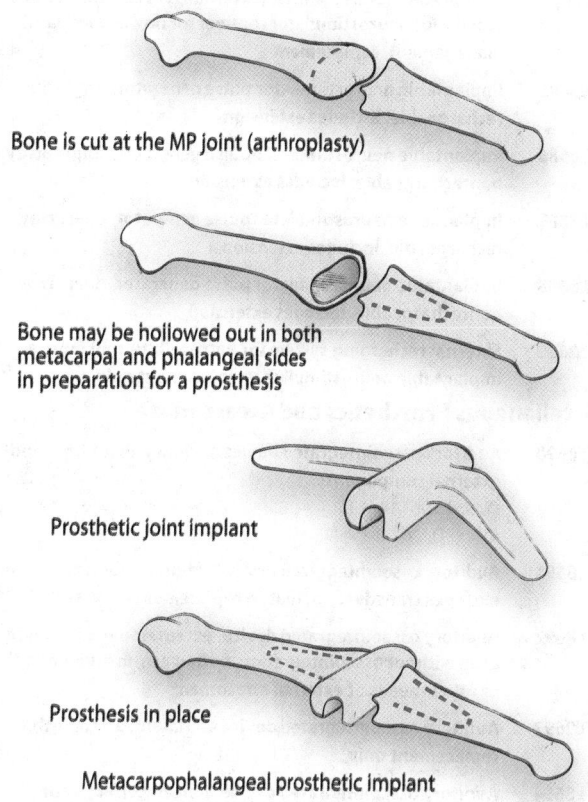

L8631 **Metacarpal phalangeal joint replacement, two or more pieces, metal (e.g., stainless steel or cobalt chrome), ceramic-like material (e.g., pyrocarbon), for surgical implantation (all sizes, includes entire system)**

Lower Extremity Implants

L8641 **Metatarsal joint implant**
CMS: 100-04,4,190

L8642 **Hallux implant**
CMS: 100-04,4,190

Interphalangeal Implants

L8658 **Interphalangeal joint spacer, silicone or equal, each**
CMS: 100-04,4,190

L8659 **Interphalangeal finger joint replacement, two or more pieces, metal (e.g., stainless steel or cobalt chrome), ceramic-like material (e.g., pyrocarbon) for surgical implantation, any size**

Cardiovascular Implant

L8670 **Vascular graft material, synthetic, implant**
CMS: 100-04,4,190

Neurostimulator and Accessories

L8679 **Implantable neurostimulator, pulse generator, any type**

L8680 **Implantable neurostimulator electrode, each**

L8681 **Patient programmer (external) for use with implantable programmable neurostimulator pulse generator, replacement only**

© 2019 Optum360, LLC

L8682 **Implantable neurostimulator radiofrequency receiver** N N1 ♿

L8683 **Radiofrequency transmitter (external) for use with implantable neurostimulator radiofrequency receiver** A ♿

L8684 **Radiofrequency transmitter (external) for use with implantable sacral root neurostimulator receiver for bowel and bladder management, replacement** A ♿

L8685 **Implantable neurostimulator pulse generator, single array, rechargeable, includes extension** E

L8686 **Implantable neurostimulator pulse generator, single array, nonrechargeable, includes extension** E

L8687 **Implantable neurostimulator pulse generator, dual array, rechargeable, includes extension** E

L8688 **Implantable neurostimulator pulse generator, dual array, nonrechargeable, includes extension** E

L8689 **External recharging system for battery (internal) for use with implantable neurostimulator, replacement only** A ♿

Miscellaneous Prosthetics and Accessories

L8690 **Auditory osseointegrated device, includes all internal and external components** N N1 ♿

CMS: 100-04,14,40.8
AHA: 3Q, '16, 10-15

L8691 **Auditory osseointegrated device, external sound processor, excludes transducer/actuator, replacement only, each** A ♿

L8692 **Auditory osseointegrated device, external sound processor, used without osseointegration, body worn, includes headband or other means of external attachment** E

L8693 **Auditory osseointegrated device abutment, any length, replacement only** A ♿

L8694 **Auditory osseointegrated device, transducer/actuator, replacement only, each** A ♿

L8695 **External recharging system for battery (external) for use with implantable neurostimulator, replacement only** A ♿

L8696 **Antenna (external) for use with implantable diaphragmatic/phrenic nerve stimulation device, replacement, each** A ♿

L8698 **Miscellaneous component, supply or accessory for use with total artificial heart system**

L8699 **Prosthetic implant, not otherwise specified** N N1

Determine if an alternative HCPCS Level II or a CPT code better describes the service being reported. This code should be used only if a more specific code is unavailable.

CMS: 100-04,4,190
AHA: 3Q, '15, 2

L8701 **Powered upper extremity range of motion assist device, elbow, wrist, hand with single or double upright(s), includes microprocessor, sensors, all components and accessories, custom fabricated**

L8702 **Powered upper extremity range of motion assist device, elbow, wrist, hand, finger, single or double upright(s), includes microprocessor, sensors, all components and accessories, custom fabricated**

L9900 **Orthotic and prosthetic supply, accessory, and/or service component of another HCPCS L code** N N1

© 2019 Optum360, LLC

Medical Services M0075-M0301

Other Medical Services

M codes include office services, cellular therapy, prolotherapy, intragastric hypothermia, IV chelation therapy, and fabric wrapping of an abdominal aneurysm.

M0075 **Cellular therapy** E

The therapeutic efficacy of injecting foreign proteins has not been established.

M0076 **Prolotherapy** E

The therapeutic efficacy of prolotherapy and joint sclerotherapy has not been established.

M0100 **Intragastric hypothermia using gastric freezing** E

Code with caution: This procedure is considered obsolete.

Cardiovascular Services

M0300 **IV chelation therapy (chemical endarterectomy)** E

Chelation therapy is considered experimental in the United States.

CMS: 100-03*; 100-03,20.22

M0301 **Fabric wrapping of abdominal aneurysm** E

Code with caution: This procedure has largely been replaced with more effective treatment modalities. Submit documentation.

Quality Measures M1000-M1144

Quality Measures

~~**M1000**~~ Jan ~~**Pain screened as moderate to severe**~~

~~**M1001**~~ Jan ~~**Plan of care to address moderate to severe pain documented on or before the date of the second visit with a clinician**~~

~~**M1002**~~ Jan ~~**Plan of care for moderate to severe pain not documented on or before the date of the second visit with a clinician, reason not given**~~

M1003 **TB screening performed and results interpreted within 12 months prior to initiation of first-time biologic disease modifying antirheumatic drug therapy for RA**

M1004 **Documentation of medical reason for not screening for TB or interpreting results (i.e., patient positive for TB and documentation of past treatment; patient who has recently completed a course of anti-TB therapy)**

M1005 **TB screening not performed or results not interpreted, reason not given**

M1006 **Disease activity not assessed, reason not given**

M1007 **>=50% of total number of a patient's outpatient RA encounters assessed**

M1008 **<50% of total number of a patient's outpatient RA encounters assessed**

▲ **M1009** Jan **Discharge/discontinuation of the episode of care documented in the medical record**

▲ **M1010** Jan **Discharge/discontinuation of the episode of care documented in the medical record**

▲ **M1011** Jan **Discharge/discontinuation of the episode of care documented in the medical record**

▲ **M1012** Jan **Discharge/discontinuation of the episode of care documented in the medical record**

▲ **M1013** Jan **Discharge/discontinuation of the episode of care documented in the medical record**

▲ **M1014** Jan **Discharge/discontinuation of the episode of care documented in the medical record**

▲ **M1015** Jan **Discharge/discontinuation of the episode of care documented in the medical record**

M1016 **Female patients unable to bear children**

M1017 **Patient admitted to palliative care services**

M1018 **Patients with an active diagnosis or history of cancer (except basal cell and squamous cell skin carcinoma), patients who are heavy tobacco smokers, lung cancer screening patients**

M1019 **Adolescent patients 12 to 17 years of age with major depression or dysthymia who reached remission at 12 months as demonstrated by a 12 month (+/-60 days) PHQ-9 or PHQ-9M score of less than 5**

M1020 **Adolescent patients 12 to 17 years of age with major depression or dysthymia who did not reach remission at 12 months as demonstrated by a 12 month (+/-60 days) PHQ-9 or PHQ-9M score of less than 5. Either PHQ-9 or PHQ-9M score was not assessed or is greater than or equal to 5**

M1021 **Patient had only urgent care visits during the performance period**

M1022 **Patients who were in hospice at any time during the performance period**

M1023 **Adolescent patients 12 to 17 years of age with major depression or dysthymia who reached remission at six months as demonstrated by a six month (+/-60 days) PHQ-9 or PHQ-9M score of less than 5**

M1024 **Adolescent patients 12 to 17 years of age with major depression or dysthymia who did not reach remission at six months as demonstrated by a six month (+/-60 days) PHQ-9 or PHQ-9M score of less than five. Either PHQ-9 or PHQ-9M score was not assessed or is greater than or equal to 5**

M1025 **Patients who were in hospice at any time during the performance period**

M1026 **Patients who were in hospice at any time during the performance period**

M1027 **Imaging of the head (CT or MRI) was obtained**

M1028 **Documentation of patients with primary headache diagnosis and imaging other than CT or MRI obtained**

M1029 **Imaging of the head (CT or MRI) was not obtained, reason not given**

~~**M1030**~~ Jan ~~**Patients with clinical indications for imaging of the head**~~

M1031 **Patients with no clinical indications for imaging of the head**

M1032 **Adults currently taking pharmacotherapy for OUD**

M1033 **Pharmacotherapy for OUD initiated after June 30th of performance period**

M1034 **Adults who have at least 180 days of continuous pharmacotherapy with a medication prescribed for OUD without a gap of more than seven days**

M1035 **Adults who are deliberately phased out of medication assisted treatment (MAT) prior to 180 days of continuous treatment**

M1036 **Adults who have not had at least 180 days of continuous pharmacotherapy with a medication prescribed for OUD without a gap of more than seven days**

M1037 **Patients with a diagnosis of lumbar spine region cancer at the time of the procedure**

M1038 **Patients with a diagnosis of lumbar spine region fracture at the time of the procedure**

M1039 **Patients with a diagnosis of lumbar spine region infection at the time of the procedure**

M1040 **Patients with a diagnosis of lumbar idiopathic or congenital scoliosis**

M1041 **Patient had cancer, fracture or infection related to the lumbar spine or patient had idiopathic or congenital scoliosis**

© 2019 Optum360, LLC

~~M1042~~ Jan ~~Functional status measurement with score was obtained utilizing the Oswestry Disability Index (ODI version 2.1a) patient reported outcome tool within three months preoperatively and at one year (9 to 15 months) postoperatively~~

▲ M1043 Jan Functional status was not measured by the Oswestry Disability Index (ODI version 2.1a) at 1 year (9 to 15 months) postoperatively

~~M1044~~ Jan ~~Functional status was measured by the Oswestry Disability Index (ODI version 2.1a) patient reported outcome tool within three months preoperatively and at one year (9 to 15 months) postoperatively~~

▲ M1045 Jan Functional status measured by the Oxford Knee Score (OKS) at 1 year (9 to 15 months) postoperatively was greater than or equal to 37

▲ M1046 Jan Functional status measured by the Oxford Knee Score (OKS) at 1 year (9 to 15 months) postoperatively was less than 37

~~M1047~~ Jan ~~Functional status was measured by the Oxford Knee Score (OKS) patient reported outcome tool within three months preoperatively and at one year (9 to 15 months) postoperatively~~

~~M1048~~ Jan ~~Functional status measurement with score was obtained utilizing the Oswestry Disability Index (ODI version 2.1a) patient reported outcome tool within three months preoperatively and at three months (6 to 20 weeks) postoperatively~~

▲ M1049 Jan Functional status was not measured by the Oswestry Disability Index (ODI version 2.1a) at 3 months (6 to 20 weeks) postoperatively

~~M1050~~ Jan ~~Functional status was measured by the Oswestry Disability Index (ODI version 2.1a) patient reported outcome tool within three months preoperatively and at three months (6 to 20 weeks) postoperatively~~

M1051 Patient had cancer, fracture or infection related to the lumbar spine or patient had idiopathic or congenital scoliosis

▲ M1052 Jan Leg pain was not measured by the visual analog scale (VAS) at 1 year (9 to 15 months) postoperatively

~~M1053~~ Jan ~~Leg pain was measured by the Visual Analog Scale (VAS) within three months preoperatively and at one year (9 to 15 months) postoperatively~~

M1054 Patient had only urgent care visits during the performance period

M1055 Aspirin or another antiplatelet therapy used

M1056 Prescribed anticoagulant medication during the performance period, history of GI bleeding, history of intracranial bleeding, bleeding disorder and specific provider documented reasons: allergy to aspirin or antiplatelets, use of nonsteroidal antiinflammatory agents, drug-drug interaction, uncontrolled hypertension > 180/110 mm Hg or gastroesophageal reflux disease

M1057 Aspirin or another antiplatelet therapy not used, reason not given

M1058 Patient was a permanent nursing home resident at any time during the performance period

M1059 Patient was in hospice or receiving palliative care at any time during the performance period

M1060 Patient died prior to the end of the performance period

M1061 Patient pregnancy

M1062 Patient immunocompromised

M1063 Patients receiving high doses of immunosuppressive therapy

M1064 Shingrix vaccine documented as administered or previously received

M1065 Shingrix vaccine was not administered for reasons documented by clinician (e.g., patient administered vaccine other than Shingrix, patient allergy or other medical reasons, patient declined or other patient reasons, vaccine not available or other system reasons)

M1066 Shingrix vaccine not documented as administered, reason not given

M1067 Hospice services for patient provided any time during the measurement period

M1068 Adults who are not ambulatory

M1069 Patient screened for future fall risk

M1070 Patient not screened for future fall risk, reason not given

M1071 Patient had any additional spine procedures performed on the same date as the lumbar discectomy/laminotomy

● M1106 Jan The start of an episode of care documented in the medical record

● M1107 Jan Documentation stating patient has a diagnosis of a degenerative neurological condition such as ALS, MS, or Parkinson's diagnosed at any time before or during the episode of care

● M1108 Jan Ongoing care not indicated, patient seen only one to two visits (e.g., home program only, referred to another provider or facility, consultation only)

● M1109 Jan Ongoing care not indicated, patient discharged after only one to two visits due to specific medical events, documented in the medical record that make the treatment episode impossible such as the patient becomes hospitalized or scheduled for surgery or hospitalized

● M1110 Jan Ongoing care not indicated, patient self-discharged early and seen only one to two visits (e.g., financial or insurance reasons, transportation problems, or reason unknown)

● M1111 Jan The start of an episode of care documented in the medical record

● M1112 Jan Documentation stating patient has a diagnosis of a degenerative neurological condition such as ALS, MS, or Parkinson's diagnosed at any time before or during the episode of care

● M1113 Jan Ongoing care not indicated, patient seen only one to two visits (e.g., home program only, referred to another provider or facility, consultation only)

● M1114 Jan Ongoing care not indicated, patient discharged after only one to two visits due to specific medical events, documented in the medical record that make the treatment episode impossible such as the patient becomes hospitalized or scheduled for surgery or hospitalized

● M1115 Jan Ongoing care not indicated, patient self-discharged early and seen only one to two visits (e.g., financial or insurance reasons, transportation problems, or reason unknown)

● M1116 Jan The start of an episode of care documented in the medical record

● M1117 Jan Documentation stating patient has a diagnosis of a degenerative neurological condition such as ALS, MS, or Parkinson's diagnosed at any time before or during the episode of care

● M1118 Jan Ongoing care not indicated, patient seen only one to two visits (e.g., home program only, referred to another provider or facility, consultation only)

● M1119 Jan Ongoing care not indicated, patient discharged after only one to two visits due to specific medical events, documented in the medical record that make the treatment episode impossible such as the patient becomes hospitalized or scheduled for surgery or hospitalized

● M1120 Jan Ongoing care not indicated, patient self-discharged early and seen only one to two visits (e.g., financial or insurance reasons, transportation problems, or reason unknown)

© 2019 Optum360, LLC

● **M1121**[Jan] **The start of an episode of care documented in the medical record**

● **M1122**[Jan] **Documentation stating patient has a diagnosis of a degenerative neurological condition such as ALS, MS, or Parkinson's diagnosed at any time before or during the episode of care**

● **M1123**[Jan] **Ongoing care not indicated, patient seen only one to two visits (e.g., home program only, referred to another provider or facility, consultation only)**

● **M1124**[Jan] **Ongoing care not indicated, patient discharged after only one to two visits due to specific medical events, documented in the medical record that make the treatment episode impossible such as the patient becomes hospitalized or scheduled for surgery**

● **M1125**[Jan] **Ongoing care not indicated, patient self-discharged early and seen only one to two visits (e.g., financial or insurance reasons, transportation problems, or reason unknown)**

● **M1126**[Jan] **The start of an episode of care documented in the medical record**

● **M1127**[Jan] **Documentation stating patient has a diagnosis of a degenerative neurological condition such as ALS, MS, or Parkinson's diagnosed at any time before or during the episode of care**

● **M1128**[Jan] **Ongoing care not indicated, patient seen only one to two visits (e.g., home program only, referred to another provider or facility, consultation only)**

● **M1129**[Jan] **Ongoing care not indicated, patient discharged after only one to two visits due to specific medical events, documented in the medical record that make the treatment episode impossible such as the patient becomes hospitalized or scheduled for surgery**

● **M1130**[Jan] **Ongoing care not indicated, patient self-discharged early and seen only one to two visits (e.g., financial or insurance reasons, transportation problems, or reason unknown)**

● **M1131**[Jan] **Documentation stating patient has a diagnosis of a degenerative neurological condition such as ALS, MS, or Parkinson's diagnosed at any time before or during the episode of care**

● **M1132**[Jan] **Ongoing care not indicated, patient seen only one to two visits (e.g., home program only, referred to another provider or facility, consultation only)**

● **M1133**[Jan] **Ongoing care not indicated, patient discharged after only one to two visits due to specific medical events, documented in the medical record that make the treatment episode impossible such as the patient becomes hospitalized or scheduled for surgery**

● **M1134**[Jan] **Ongoing care not indicated, patient self-discharged early and seen only one to two visits (e.g., financial or insurance reasons, transportation problems, or reason unknown**

● **M1135**[Jan] **The start of an episode of care documented in the medical record**

● **M1136**[Jan] **The start of an episode of care documented in the medical record**

● **M1137**[Jan] **Documentation stating patient has a diagnosis of a degenerative neurological condition such as ALS, MS, or Parkinson's diagnosed at any time before or during the episode of care**

● **M1138**[Jan] **Ongoing care not indicated, patient seen only one to two visits (e.g., home program only, referred to another provider or facility, consultation only)**

● **M1139**[Jan] **Ongoing care not indicated, patient self-discharged early and seen only one to two visits (e.g., financial or insurance reasons, transportation problems, or reason unknown)**

● **M1140**[Jan] **Ongoing care not indicated, patient discharged after only one to two visits due to specific medical events, documented in the medical record that make the treatment episode impossible such as the patient becomes hospitalized or scheduled for surgery or hospitalized**

● **M1141**[Jan] **Functional status was not measured by the Oxford Knee Score (OKS) at 1 year (9 to 15 months) postoperatively**

● **M1142**[Jan] **Emergent cases**

● **M1143**[Jan] **Initiated episode of rehabilitation therapy, medical, or chiropractic care for neck impairment**

● **M1144**[Jan] **Ongoing care not indicated, patient seen only one to two visits (e.g., home program only, referred to another provider or facility, consultation only**

© 2019 Optum360, LLC

Pathology and Laboratory Services P2028-P9615

P codes include chemistry, toxicology, and microbiology tests, screening Papanicolaou procedures, and various blood products.

Chemistry and Toxicology Tests

P2028 **Cephalin floculation, blood** A
Code with caution: This test is considered obsolete. Submit documentation.

P2029 **Congo red, blood** A
Code with caution: This test is considered obsolete. Submit documentation.

P2031 **Hair analysis (excluding arsenic)** E

P2033 **Thymol turbidity, blood** A
Code with caution: This test is considered obsolete. Submit documentation.

P2038 **Mucoprotein, blood (seromucoid) (medical necessity procedure)** A
Code with caution: This test is considered obsolete. Submit documentation.

Pathology Screening Tests

P3000 **Screening Papanicolaou smear, cervical or vaginal, up to three smears, by technician under physician supervision** A ♀A
One Pap test is covered by Medicare every two years, unless the physician suspects cervical abnormalities and shortens the interval. See also G0123-G0124.
CMS: 100-02,15,280.4; 100-03,210.2.1; 100-04,18,30.2.1; 100-04,18,30.5; 100-04,18,30.6

P3001 **Screening Papanicolaou smear, cervical or vaginal, up to three smears, requiring interpretation by physician** A ♀B ⊘
One Pap test is covered by Medicare every two years, unless the physician suspects cervical abnormalities and shortens the interval. See also G0123-G0124.
CMS: 100-02,15,280.4; 100-03,210.2.1; 100-04,18,30.2.1; 100-04,18,30.5; 100-04,18,30.6

Microbiology Tests

P7001 **Culture, bacterial, urine; quantitative, sensitivity study** E

Miscellaneous

P9010 **Blood (whole), for transfusion, per unit** R ☑
CMS: 100-01,3,20.5; 100-01,3,20.5.2; 100-01,3,20.5.3; 100-02,1,10; 100-04,3,40.2.2
AHA: 3Q, '04, 11-13

P9011 **Blood, split unit** R ☑
CMS: 100-01,3,20.5; 100-01,3,20.5.2; 100-01,3,20.5.3; 100-02,1,10; 100-04,3,40.2.2; 100-04,4,231.4
AHA: 2Q, '05, 1-3; 3Q, '04, 11-13

P9012 **Cryoprecipitate, each unit** R ☑
CMS: 100-02,1,10; 100-04,3,40.2.2
AHA: 3Q, '04, 11-13

P9016 **Red blood cells, leukocytes reduced, each unit** R ☑
CMS: 100-02,1,10; 100-04,3,40.2.2
AHA: 4Q, '04, 2; 3Q, '04, 11-13

P9017 **Fresh frozen plasma (single donor), frozen within 8 hours of collection, each unit** R ☑
CMS: 100-02,1,10; 100-04,3,40.2.2
AHA: 3Q, '04, 11-13

P9019 **Platelets, each unit** R ☑
CMS: 100-02,1,10; 100-04,3,40.2.2
AHA: 3Q, '04, 11-13

P9020 **Platelet rich plasma, each unit** R ☑
CMS: 100-04,3,40.2.2
AHA: 3Q, '04, 11-13

P9021 **Red blood cells, each unit** R ☑
CMS: 100-01,3,20.5; 100-01,3,20.5.2; 100-01,3,20.5.3; 100-02,1,10; 100-04,3,40.2.2
AHA: 4Q, '04, 2; 3Q, '04, 11-13

P9022 **Red blood cells, washed, each unit** R ☑
CMS: 100-01,3,20.5; 100-01,3,20.5.2; 100-01,3,20.5.3; 100-02,1,10; 100-04,3,40.2.2
AHA: 3Q, '04, 11-13

P9023 **Plasma, pooled multiple donor, solvent/detergent treated, frozen, each unit** R ☑
CMS: 100-02,1,10; 100-04,3,40.2.2
AHA: 3Q, '04, 11-13

P9031 **Platelets, leukocytes reduced, each unit** R ☑
CMS: 100-02,1,10; 100-04,3,40.2.2
AHA: 3Q, '04, 11-13

P9032 **Platelets, irradiated, each unit** R ☑
CMS: 100-02,1,10; 100-04,3,40.2.2
AHA: 2Q, '05, 1-3; 3Q, '04, 11-13

P9033 **Platelets, leukocytes reduced, irradiated, each unit** R ☑
CMS: 100-02,1,10; 100-04,3,40.2.2
AHA: 2Q, '05, 1-3; 3Q, '04, 11-13

P9034 **Platelets, pheresis, each unit** R ☑
CMS: 100-02,1,10; 100-04,3,40.2.2
AHA: 3Q, '04, 11-13

P9035 **Platelets, pheresis, leukocytes reduced, each unit** R ☑
CMS: 100-02,1,10; 100-04,3,40.2.2
AHA: 3Q, '04, 11-13

P9036 **Platelets, pheresis, irradiated, each unit** R ☑
CMS: 100-02,1,10; 100-04,3,40.2.2
AHA: 2Q, '05, 1-3; 3Q, '04, 11-13

P9037 **Platelets, pheresis, leukocytes reduced, irradiated, each unit** R ☑
CMS: 100-02,1,10; 100-04,3,40.2.2
AHA: 2Q, '05, 1-3; 3Q, '04, 11-13

P9038 **Red blood cells, irradiated, each unit** R ☑
CMS: 100-01,3,20.5; 100-01,3,20.5.2; 100-01,3,20.5.3; 100-02,1,10; 100-04,3,40.2.2
AHA: 2Q, '05, 1-3; 3Q, '04, 11-13

P9039 **Red blood cells, deglycerolized, each unit** R ☑
CMS: 100-02,1,10; 100-04,3,40.2.2
AHA: 3Q, '04, 11-13

P9040 **Red blood cells, leukocytes reduced, irradiated, each unit** R ☑
CMS: 100-02,1,10; 100-04,3,40.2.2
AHA: 2Q, '05, 1-3; 3Q, '04, 11-13

P9041 **Infusion, albumin (human), 5%, 50 ml** K K2 ☑
CMS: 100-02,1,10; 100-04,3,40.2.2
AHA: 3Q, '04, 11-13

P9043 **Infusion, plasma protein fraction (human), 5%, 50 ml** R ☑
CMS: 100-02,1,10; 100-04,3,40.2.2
AHA: 3Q, '04, 11-13

P9044 **Plasma, cryoprecipitate reduced, each unit** R ☑
CMS: 100-02,1,10; 100-04,3,40.2.2
AHA: 3Q, '04, 11-13

P9045 **Infusion, albumin (human), 5%, 250 ml** K K2 ☑
CMS: 100-02,1,10; 100-04,3,40.2.2
AHA: 3Q, '04, 11-13; 1Q, '02, 5

P9046 **Infusion, albumin (human), 25%, 20 ml** K K2 ☑
CMS: 100-02,1,10; 100-04,3,40.2.2
AHA: 3Q, '04, 11-13; 1Q, '02, 5

© 2019 Optum360, LLC

P9047 **Infusion, albumin (human), 25%, 50 ml** K A2 ☑
CMS: 100-02,1,10; 100-04,3,40.2.2
AHA: 3Q, '04, 11-13; 1Q, '02, 5

P9048 **Infusion, plasma protein fraction (human), 5%, 250 ml** R ☑
CMS: 100-02,1,10; 100-04,3,40.2.2
AHA: 3Q, '04, 11-13; 1Q, '02, 5

P9050 **Granulocytes, pheresis, each unit** E ☑
CMS: 100-02,1,10; 100-03,110.5; 100-04,3,40.2.2
AHA: 3Q, '04, 11-13; 1Q, '02, 5

P9051 **Whole blood or red blood cells, leukocytes reduced, CMV-negative, each unit** R ☑
CMS: 100-02,1,10; 100-04,3,40.2.2
AHA: 3Q, '04, 11-13

P9052 **Platelets, HLA-matched leukocytes reduced, apheresis/pheresis, each unit** R ☑
CMS: 100-02,1,10; 100-04,3,40.2.2
AHA: 3Q, '04, 11-13

P9053 **Platelets, pheresis, leukocytes reduced, CMV-negative, irradiated, each unit** R ☑
CMS: 100-02,1,10; 100-04,3,40.2.2
AHA: 2Q, '05, 1-3; 3Q, '04, 11-13

P9054 **Whole blood or red blood cells, leukocytes reduced, frozen, deglycerol, washed, each unit** R ☑
CMS: 100-02,1,10; 100-04,3,40.2.2
AHA: 3Q, '04, 11-13

P9055 **Platelets, leukocytes reduced, CMV-negative, apheresis/pheresis, each unit** R ☑
CMS: 100-02,1,10; 100-04,3,40.2.2
AHA: 3Q, '04, 11-13

P9056 **Whole blood, leukocytes reduced, irradiated, each unit** R ☑
CMS: 100-02,1,10; 100-04,3,40.2.2
AHA: 2Q, '05, 1-3; 3Q, '04, 11-13

P9057 **Red blood cells, frozen/deglycerolized/washed, leukocytes reduced, irradiated, each unit** R ☑
CMS: 100-02,1,10; 100-04,3,40.2.2
AHA: 2Q, '05, 1-3; 3Q, '04, 11-13

P9058 **Red blood cells, leukocytes reduced, CMV-negative, irradiated, each unit** R ☑
CMS: 100-02,1,10; 100-04,3,40.2.2
AHA: 2Q, '05, 1-3; 3Q, '04, 11-13

P9059 **Fresh frozen plasma between 8-24 hours of collection, each unit** R ☑
CMS: 100-02,1,10; 100-04,3,40.2.2
AHA: 3Q, '04, 11-13

P9060 **Fresh frozen plasma, donor retested, each unit** R ☑
CMS: 100-02,1,10; 100-04,3,40.2.2
AHA: 3Q, '04, 11-13

P9070 **Plasma, pooled multiple donor, pathogen reduced, frozen, each unit** R
AHA: 1Q, '16, 7

P9071 **Plasma (single donor), pathogen reduced, frozen, each unit** R
AHA: 1Q, '16, 7

P9073 **Platelets, pheresis, pathogen-reduced, each unit** R

● **P9099** Jan **Blood component or product not otherwise classified**

P9100 **Pathogen(s) test for platelets** S

P9603 **Travel allowance, one way in connection with medically necessary laboratory specimen collection drawn from homebound or nursing homebound patient; prorated miles actually travelled** A ☑
CMS: 100-04,16,60; 100-04,16,60.2

P9604 **Travel allowance, one way in connection with medically necessary laboratory specimen collection drawn from homebound or nursing homebound patient; prorated trip charge** A ☑
CMS: 100-04,16,60; 100-04,16,60.2

P9612 **Catheterization for collection of specimen, single patient, all places of service** A
CMS: 100-04,16,60
AHA: 2Q, '09, 1; 3Q, '07, 5

P9615 **Catheterization for collection of specimen(s) (multiple patients)** N
CMS: 100-04,16,60; 100-04,16,60.1.4

© 2019 Optum360, LLC

Q Codes (Temporary) Q0035-Q9992

Temporary Q codes are used to pay health care providers for supplies, drugs, and biologicals to which no permanent code has been assigned.

Q0035 **Cardiokymography** [01]

Covered only in conjunction with electrocardiographic stress testing in male patients with atypical angina or nonischemic chest pain, or female patients with angina.

Q0081 **Infusion therapy, using other than chemotherapeutic drugs, per visit** [B] ☑

AHA: 1Q, '05, 7, 9-10; 4Q, '04, 6; 2Q, '04, 11; 1Q, '04, 4-5; 4Q, '02, 6-7; 2Q, '02, 8-9; 2Q, '02; 1Q, '02, 7

Q0083 **Chemotherapy administration by other than infusion technique only (e.g., subcutaneous, intramuscular, push), per visit** [B] ☑

AHA: 1Q, '05, 7, 9-10; 4Q, '04, 6; 1Q, '04, 4-5; 1Q, '02, 7; 1Q, '02, 1-2

Q0084 **Chemotherapy administration by infusion technique only, per visit** [B] ☑

AHA: 1Q, '05, 7, 9-10; 4Q, '04, 6; 2Q, '04, 11; 1Q, '04, 4-5; 1Q, '02, 7; 1Q, '02, 1-2

Q0085 **Chemotherapy administration by both infusion technique and other technique(s) (e.g. subcutaneous, intramuscular, push), per visit** [B] ☑

AHA: 4Q, '04, 6; 1Q, '04, 4-5; 1Q, '02, 7; 1Q, '02, 1-2

Q0091 **Screening Papanicolaou smear; obtaining, preparing and conveyance of cervical or vaginal smear to laboratory** [A] ♀ [S] ⊘

One pap test is covered by Medicare every two years for low risk patients and every one year for high risk patients. Q0091 can be reported with an E/M code when a separately identifiable E/M service is provided.

CMS: 100-02,13,220; 100-02,13,220.1; 100-02,13,220.3; 100-02,15,280.4; 100-03,210.2.1; 100-04,18,30.2.1; 100-04,18,30.5; 100-04,18,30.6; 1004-04,13,220.1

AHA: 4Q, '08, 3; 4Q, '02, 8

Q0092 **Set-up portable x-ray equipment** [N]

CMS: 100-04,13,90.4

Q0111 **Wet mounts, including preparations of vaginal, cervical or skin specimens** [A]

Q0112 **All potassium hydroxide (KOH) preparations** [A]

Q0113 **Pinworm examinations** [A]

Q0114 **Fern test** ♀ [A]

Q0115 **Postcoital direct, qualitative examinations of vaginal or cervical mucous** [A] ♀ [A]

Q0138 **Injection, ferumoxytol, for treatment of iron deficiency anemia, 1 mg (non-ESRD use)** [K] [K2] ☑

Use this code for Feraheme.

Q0139 **Injection, ferumoxytol, for treatment of iron deficiency anemia, 1 mg (for ESRD on dialysis)** [K] [K2] ☑

Use this code for Feraheme.

Q0144 **Azithromycin dihydrate, oral, capsules/powder, 1 g** [E] ☑

Use this code for Zithromax, Zithromax Z-PAK.

Q0161 **Chlorpromazine HCl, 5 mg, oral, FDA-approved prescription antiemetic, for use as a complete therapeutic substitute for an IV antiemetic at the time of chemotherapy treatment, not to exceed a 48-hour dosage regimen** [N] [N1] ☑

CMS: 100-02,15,50.5.4; 100-03,110.18; 100-04,17,80.2.1

AHA: 1Q, '14, 7

Q0162 **Ondansetron 1 mg, oral, FDA-approved prescription antiemetic, for use as a complete therapeutic substitute for an IV antiemetic at the time of chemotherapy treatment, not to exceed a 48-hour dosage regimen** [N] [N1] ☑

Use this code for Zofran, Zuplenz.

CMS: 100-02,15,50.5.4; 100-03,110.18; 100-04,17,80.2.1

Q0163 **Diphenhydramine HCl, 50 mg, oral, FDA-approved prescription antiemetic, for use as a complete therapeutic substitute for an IV antiemetic at time of chemotherapy treatment not to exceed a 48-hour dosage regimen** [N] [N1] ☑

See also J1200. Medicare covers at the time of chemotherapy if regimen doesn't exceed 48 hours. Submit on the same claim as the chemotherapy. Use this code for Truxadryl.

CMS: 100-02,15,50.5.4; 100-03,110.18; 100-04,17,80.2.1

AHA: 2Q, '12, 9; 1Q, '08, 1; 1Q, '02, 1-2

Q0164 **Prochlorperazine maleate, 5 mg, oral, FDA-approved prescription antiemetic, for use as a complete therapeutic substitute for an IV antiemetic at the time of chemotherapy treatment, not to exceed a 48-hour dosage regimen** [N] [N1] ☑

Medicare covers at the time of chemotherapy if regimen doesn't exceed 48 hours. Submit on the same claim as the chemotherapy. Use this code for Compazine.

CMS: 100-02,15,50.5.4; 100-03,110.18; 100-04,17,80.2.1

AHA: 1Q, '08, 1

Q0166 **Granisetron HCl, 1 mg, oral, FDA-approved prescription antiemetic, for use as a complete therapeutic substitute for an IV antiemetic at the time of chemotherapy treatment, not to exceed a 24-hour dosage regimen** [N] [N1] ☑

Medicare covers at the time of chemotherapy if regimen doesn't exceed 48 hours. Submit on the same claim as the chemotherapy. Use this code for Kytril.

CMS: 100-02,15,50.5.4; 100-03,110.18; 100-04,17,80.2.1

AHA: 1Q, '08, 1

Q0167 **Dronabinol, 2.5 mg, oral, FDA-approved prescription antiemetic, for use as a complete therapeutic substitute for an IV antiemetic at the time of chemotherapy treatment, not to exceed a 48-hour dosage regimen** [N] [N1] ☑

Medicare covers at the time of chemotherapy if regimen doesn't exceed 48 hours. Submit on the same claim as the chemotherapy. Use this code for Marinol.

CMS: 100-02,15,50.5.4; 100-03,110.18; 100-04,17,80.2.1

AHA: 1Q, '08, 1

Q0169 **Promethazine HCl, 12.5 mg, oral, FDA-approved prescription antiemetic, for use as a complete therapeutic substitute for an IV antiemetic at the time of chemotherapy treatment, not to exceed a 48-hour dosage regimen** [N] [N1] ☑

Medicare covers at the time of chemotherapy if regimen doesn't exceed 48 hours. Submit on the same claim as the chemotherapy. Use this code for Phenergan, Amergan.

CMS: 100-02,15,50.5.4; 100-03,110.18; 100-04,17,80.2.1

AHA: 1Q, '08, 1

Q0173 **Trimethobenzamide HCl, 250 mg, oral, FDA-approved prescription antiemetic, for use as a complete therapeutic substitute for an IV antiemetic at the time of chemotherapy treatment, not to exceed a 48-hour dosage regimen** [N] [N1] ☑

Medicare covers at the time of chemotherapy if regimen doesn't exceed 48 hours. Submit on the same claim as the chemotherapy. Use this code for Tebamide, T-Gen, Ticon, Tigan, Triban, Thimazide.

CMS: 100-02,15,50.5.4; 100-03,110.18; 100-04,17,80.2.1

AHA: 1Q, '08, 1

Q0174 **Thiethylperazine maleate, 10 mg, oral, FDA-approved prescription antiemetic, for use as a complete therapeutic substitute for an IV antiemetic at the time of chemotherapy treatment, not to exceed a 48-hour dosage regimen** [E] ☑

Medicare covers at the time of chemotherapy if regimen doesn't exceed 48 hours. Submit on the same claim as the chemotherapy.

CMS: 100-02,15,50.5.4; 100-03,110.18; 100-04,17,80.2.1

AHA: 1Q, '08, 1

© 2019 Optum360, LLC

Q0175 **Perphenazine, 4 mg, oral, FDA-approved prescription antiemetic, for use as a complete therapeutic substitute for an IV antiemetic at the time of chemotherapy treatment, not to exceed a 48-hour dosage regimen** N N1 ☑

Medicare covers at the time of chemotherapy if regimen doesn't exceed 48 hours. Submit on the same claim as the chemotherapy. Use this code for Trilifon.

CMS: 100-02,15,50.5.4; 100-03,110.18; 100-04,17,80.2.1

AHA: 1Q, '08, 1

Q0177 **Hydroxyzine pamoate, 25 mg, oral, FDA-approved prescription antiemetic, for use as a complete therapeutic substitute for an IV antiemetic at the time of chemotherapy treatment, not to exceed a 48-hour dosage regimen** N N1 ☑

Medicare covers at the time of chemotherapy if regimen doesn't exceed 48 hours. Submit on the same claim as the chemotherapy. Use this code for Vistaril.

CMS: 100-02,15,50.5.4; 100-03,110.18; 100-04,17,80.2.1

AHA: 1Q, '08, 1

Q0180 **Dolasetron mesylate, 100 mg, oral, FDA-approved prescription antiemetic, for use as a complete therapeutic substitute for an IV antiemetic at the time of chemotherapy treatment, not to exceed a 24-hour dosage regimen** N N1 ☑

Medicare covers at the time of chemotherapy if regimen doesn't exceed 24 hours. Submit on the same claim as the chemotherapy. Use this code for Anzemet.

CMS: 100-02,15,50.5.4; 100-03,110.18; 100-04,17,80.2.1

AHA: 1Q, '08, 1

Q0181 **Unspecified oral dosage form, FDA-approved prescription antiemetic, for use as a complete therapeutic substitute for an IV antiemetic at the time of chemotherapy treatment, not to exceed a 48-hour dosage regimen** N N1 ☑

Medicare covers at the time of chemotherapy if regimen doesn't exceed 48-hours. Submit on the same claim as the chemotherapy.

CMS: 100-02,15,50.5.4; 100-03,110.18; 100-04,17,80.2.1

AHA: 2Q, '12, 9; 1Q, '08, 1

Q0477 **Power module patient cable for use with electric or electric/pneumatic ventricular assist device, replacement only** A ♿

Q0478 **Power adapter for use with electric or electric/pneumatic ventricular assist device, vehicle type** A ♿

Q0479 **Power module for use with electric or electric/pneumatic ventricular assist device, replacement only** A ♿

Q0480 **Driver for use with pneumatic ventricular assist device, replacement only** A ♿

AHA: 3Q, '05, 1-2

Q0481 **Microprocessor control unit for use with electric ventricular assist device, replacement only** A ♿

AHA: 3Q, '05, 1-2

Q0482 **Microprocessor control unit for use with electric/pneumatic combination ventricular assist device, replacement only** A ♿

AHA: 3Q, '05, 1-2

Q0483 **Monitor/display module for use with electric ventricular assist device, replacement only** A ♿

AHA: 3Q, '05, 1-2

Q0484 **Monitor/display module for use with electric or electric/pneumatic ventricular assist device, replacement only** A ♿

AHA: 3Q, '05, 1-2

Q0485 **Monitor control cable for use with electric ventricular assist device, replacement only** A ♿

AHA: 3Q, '05, 1-2

Q0486 **Monitor control cable for use with electric/pneumatic ventricular assist device, replacement only** A ♿

AHA: 3Q, '05, 1-2

Q0487 **Leads (pneumatic/electrical) for use with any type electric/pneumatic ventricular assist device, replacement only** A ♿

AHA: 3Q, '05, 1-2

Q0488 **Power pack base for use with electric ventricular assist device, replacement only** A

AHA: 3Q, '05, 1-2

Q0489 **Power pack base for use with electric/pneumatic ventricular assist device, replacement only** A ♿

AHA: 3Q, '05, 1-2

Q0490 **Emergency power source for use with electric ventricular assist device, replacement only** A ♿

AHA: 3Q, '05, 1-2

Q0491 **Emergency power source for use with electric/pneumatic ventricular assist device, replacement only** A ♿

AHA: 3Q, '05, 1-2

Q0492 **Emergency power supply cable for use with electric ventricular assist device, replacement only** A ♿

AHA: 3Q, '05, 1-2

Q0493 **Emergency power supply cable for use with electric/pneumatic ventricular assist device, replacement only** A ♿

AHA: 3Q, '05, 1-2

Q0494 **Emergency hand pump for use with electric or electric/pneumatic ventricular assist device, replacement only** A ♿

AHA: 3Q, '05, 1-2

Q0495 **Battery/power pack charger for use with electric or electric/pneumatic ventricular assist device, replacement only** A ♿

AHA: 3Q, '05, 1-2

Q0496 **Battery, other than lithium-ion, for use with electric or electric/pneumatic ventricular assist device, replacement only** A ♿

AHA: 3Q, '05, 1-2

Q0497 **Battery clips for use with electric or electric/pneumatic ventricular assist device, replacement only** A ♿

AHA: 3Q, '05, 1-2

Q0498 **Holster for use with electric or electric/pneumatic ventricular assist device, replacement only** A ♿

AHA: 3Q, '05, 1-2

Q0499 **Belt/vest/bag for use to carry external peripheral components of any type ventricular assist device, replacement only** A ♿

AHA: 3Q, '05, 1-2

Q0500 **Filters for use with electric or electric/pneumatic ventricular assist device, replacement only** A ☑ ♿

The base unit for this code is for each filter.

AHA: 3Q, '05, 1-2

Q0501 **Shower cover for use with electric or electric/pneumatic ventricular assist device, replacement only** A ♿

AHA: 3Q, '05, 1-2

Q0502 **Mobility cart for pneumatic ventricular assist device, replacement only** A ♿

AHA: 3Q, '05, 1-2

Q0503 **Battery for pneumatic ventricular assist device, replacement only, each** A ☑ ♿

AHA: 3Q, '05, 1-2

© 2019 Optum360, LLC

Q0504 **Power adapter for pneumatic ventricular assist device, replacement only, vehicle type** A ♿
AHA: 3Q, '05, 1-2

Q0506 **Battery, lithium-ion, for use with electric or electric/pneumatic ventricular assist device, replacement only** A ♿

Q0507 **Miscellaneous supply or accessory for use with an external ventricular assist device** A
CMS: 100-04,32,320.3.5

Q0508 **Miscellaneous supply or accessory for use with an implanted ventricular assist device** A
CMS: 100-04,32,320.3.5

Q0509 **Miscellaneous supply or accessory for use with any implanted ventricular assist device for which payment was not made under Medicare Part A** A
CMS: 100-04,32,320.3.5

Q0510 **Pharmacy supply fee for initial immunosuppressive drug(s), first month following transplant** B ☑

Q0511 **Pharmacy supply fee for oral anticancer, oral antiemetic, or immunosuppressive drug(s); for the first prescription in a 30-day period** B ☑

Q0512 **Pharmacy supply fee for oral anticancer, oral antiemetic, or immunosuppressive drug(s); for a subsequent prescription in a 30-day period** B ☑

Q0513 **Pharmacy dispensing fee for inhalation drug(s); per 30 days** B ☑

Q0514 **Pharmacy dispensing fee for inhalation drug(s); per 90 days** B ☑

Q0515 **Injection, sermorelin acetate, 1 mcg** E ☑

Q1004 **New technology, intraocular lens, category 4 as defined in Federal Register notice** E

Q1005 **New technology, intraocular lens, category 5 as defined in Federal Register notice** E

Q2004 **Irrigation solution for treatment of bladder calculi, for example renacidin, per 500 ml** N N1 ☑

Q2009 **Injection, fosphenytoin, 50 mg phenytoin equivalent** K N1 ☑
Use this code for Cerebyx.

Q2017 **Injection, teniposide, 50 mg** K K2 ☑
Use this code for Vumon.

Q2026 **Injection, Radiesse, 0.1 ml** E ☑
CMS: 100-03,250.5; 100-04,32,260.1; 100-04,32,260.2.1; 100-04,32,260.2.2

Q2028 **Injection, sculptra, 0.5 mg** E ☑
CMS: 100-04,32,260.2.2
AHA: 1Q, '14, 7

Q2034 **Influenza virus vaccine, split virus, for intramuscular use (Agriflu)** L L1 ☑
CMS: 100-04,18,10.1.2
AHA: 3Q, '12, 10

Q2035 **Influenza virus vaccine, split virus, when administered to individuals 3 years of age and older, for intramuscular use (AFLURIA)** A L L1 ☑
CMS: 100-02,15,50.4.4.2; 100-04,18,10.1.2

Q2036 **Influenza virus vaccine, split virus, when administered to individuals 3 years of age and older, for intramuscular use (FLULAVAL)** A L L1 ☑
CMS: 100-02,15,50.4.4.2; 100-04,18,10.1.2

Q2037 **Influenza virus vaccine, split virus, when administered to individuals 3 years of age and older, for intramuscular use (FLUVIRIN)** A L L1 ☑
CMS: 100-02,15,50.4.4.2; 100-04,18,10.1.2

Q2038 **Influenza virus vaccine, split virus, when administered to individuals 3 years of age and older, for intramuscular use (Fluzone)** A L L1 ☑
CMS: 100-02,15,50.4.4.2; 100-04,18,10.1.2

Q2039 **Influenza virus vaccine, not otherwise specified** A L L1 ☑
CMS: 100-02,15,50.4.4.2; 100-04,18,10.1.2

Q2041 **Axicabtagene ciloleucel, up to 200 million autologous anti-CD19 CAR positive T cells, including leukapheresis and dose preparation procedures, per therapeutic dose** G
Use this code for Yescarta.

Q2042 **Tisagenlecleucel, up to 600 million CAR-positive viable T cells, including leukapheresis and dose preparation procedures, per therapeutic dose**
Use this code for Kymriah.

Q2043 **Sipuleucel-T, minimum of 50 million autologous CD54+ cells activated with PAP-GM-CSF, including leukapheresis and all other preparatory procedures, per infusion** ♂ K K2 ☑
Use this code for PROVENGE.
CMS: 100-03,1,110.22; 100-03,110.22; 100-04,32,280.1; 100-04,32,280.2; 100-04,32,280.4; 100-04,32,280.5
AHA: 2Q, '12, 7; 3Q, '11, 9

Q2049 **Injection, doxorubicin HCl, liposomal, imported Lipodox, 10 mg** K K2 ☑
AHA: 3Q, '12, 10

Q2050 **Injection, doxorubicin HCl, liposomal, not otherwise specified, 10 mg** K K2 ☑ ⊘
AHA: 4Q, '13, 8-10; 3Q, '13, 10

Q2052 **Services, supplies and accessories used in the home under the Medicare intravenous immune globulin (IVIG) demonstration** E ☑
AHA: 2Q, '14, 8

Q3001 **Radioelements for brachytherapy, any type, each** B ☑ ⊘

Q3014 **Telehealth originating site facility fee** A ⊘
CMS: 100-04,12,190.5; 100-04,12,190.6

Q3027 **Injection, interferon beta-1a, 1 mcg for intramuscular use** K K2 ☑
Use this code for Avonex.
CMS: 100-02,15,50.5
AHA: 1Q, '14, 7

Q3028 **Injection, interferon beta-1a, 1 mcg for subcutaneous use** E ☑
Use this code for Rebif.
CMS: 100-02,15,50.5

Q3031 **Collagen skin test** N N1

Q4001 **Casting supplies, body cast adult, with or without head, plaster** A B ♿
CMS: 100-04,20,170
AHA: 2Q, '02, 1-3

Q4002 **Cast supplies, body cast adult, with or without head, fiberglass** A B ♿
CMS: 100-04,20,170
AHA: 2Q, '02, 1-3

Q4003 **Cast supplies, shoulder cast, adult (11 years +), plaster** A B ♿
CMS: 100-04,20,170
AHA: 2Q, '02, 1-3

Q4004 **Cast supplies, shoulder cast, adult (11 years +), fiberglass** A B ♿
CMS: 100-04,20,170
AHA: 2Q, '02, 1-3

© 2019 Optum360, LLC

Q4005 **Cast supplies, long arm cast, adult (11 years +), plaster** A B ♿
CMS: 100-04,20,170
AHA: 2Q, '02, 1-3

Q4006 **Cast supplies, long arm cast, adult (11 years +), fiberglass** A B ♿
CMS: 100-04,20,170
AHA: 2Q, '02, 1-3

Q4007 **Cast supplies, long arm cast, pediatric (0-10 years), plaster** A B ♿
CMS: 100-04,20,170
AHA: 2Q, '02, 1-3

Q4008 **Cast supplies, long arm cast, pediatric (0-10 years), fiberglass** A B ♿
CMS: 100-04,20,170
AHA: 2Q, '02, 1-3

Q4009 **Cast supplies, short arm cast, adult (11 years +), plaster** A B ♿
CMS: 100-04,20,170
AHA: 2Q, '02, 1-3

Q4010 **Cast supplies, short arm cast, adult (11 years +), fiberglass** A B ♿
CMS: 100-04,20,170
AHA: 2Q, '02, 1-3

Q4011 **Cast supplies, short arm cast, pediatric (0-10 years), plaster** A B ♿
CMS: 100-04,20,170
AHA: 2Q, '02, 1-3

Q4012 **Cast supplies, short arm cast, pediatric (0-10 years), fiberglass** A B ♿
CMS: 100-04,20,170
AHA: 2Q, '02, 1-3

Q4013 **Cast supplies, gauntlet cast (includes lower forearm and hand), adult (11 years +), plaster** A B ♿
CMS: 100-04,20,170
AHA: 2Q, '02, 1-3

Q4014 **Cast supplies, gauntlet cast (includes lower forearm and hand), adult (11 years +), fiberglass** A B ♿
CMS: 100-04,20,170
AHA: 2Q, '02, 1-3

Q4015 **Cast supplies, gauntlet cast (includes lower forearm and hand), pediatric (0-10 years), plaster** A B ♿
CMS: 100-04,20,170
AHA: 2Q, '02, 1-3

Q4016 **Cast supplies, gauntlet cast (includes lower forearm and hand), pediatric (0-10 years), fiberglass** A B ♿
CMS: 100-04,20,170
AHA: 2Q, '02, 1-3

Q4017 **Cast supplies, long arm splint, adult (11 years +), plaster** A B ♿
CMS: 100-04,20,170
AHA: 2Q, '02, 1-3

Q4018 **Cast supplies, long arm splint, adult (11 years +), fiberglass** A B ♿
CMS: 100-04,20,170
AHA: 2Q, '02, 1-3

Q4019 **Cast supplies, long arm splint, pediatric (0-10 years), plaster** A B ♿
CMS: 100-04,20,170
AHA: 2Q, '02, 1-3

Q4020 **Cast supplies, long arm splint, pediatric (0-10 years), fiberglass** A B ♿
CMS: 100-04,20,170
AHA: 2Q, '02, 1-3

Q4021 **Cast supplies, short arm splint, adult (11 years +), plaster** A B ♿
CMS: 100-04,20,170
AHA: 2Q, '02, 1-3

Q4022 **Cast supplies, short arm splint, adult (11 years +), fiberglass** A B ♿
CMS: 100-04,20,170
AHA: 2Q, '02, 1-3

Q4023 **Cast supplies, short arm splint, pediatric (0-10 years), plaster** A B ♿
CMS: 100-04,20,170
AHA: 2Q, '02, 1-3

Q4024 **Cast supplies, short arm splint, pediatric (0-10 years), fiberglass** A B ♿
CMS: 100-04,20,170
AHA: 2Q, '02, 1-3

Q4025 **Cast supplies, hip spica (one or both legs), adult (11 years +), plaster** A B ♿
CMS: 100-04,20,170
AHA: 2Q, '02, 1-3

Q4026 **Cast supplies, hip spica (one or both legs), adult (11 years +), fiberglass** A B ♿
CMS: 100-04,20,170
AHA: 2Q, '02, 1-3

Q4027 **Cast supplies, hip spica (one or both legs), pediatric (0-10 years), plaster** A B ♿
CMS: 100-04,20,170
AHA: 2Q, '02, 1-3

Q4028 **Cast supplies, hip spica (one or both legs), pediatric (0-10 years), fiberglass** A B ♿
CMS: 100-04,20,170
AHA: 2Q, '02, 1-3

Q4029 **Cast supplies, long leg cast, adult (11 years +), plaster** A B ♿
CMS: 100-04,20,170
AHA: 2Q, '02, 1-3

Q4030 **Cast supplies, long leg cast, adult (11 years +), fiberglass** A B ♿
CMS: 100-04,20,170
AHA: 2Q, '02, 1-3

Q4031 **Cast supplies, long leg cast, pediatric (0-10 years), plaster** A B ♿
CMS: 100-04,20,170
AHA: 2Q, '02, 1-3

Q4032 **Cast supplies, long leg cast, pediatric (0-10 years), fiberglass** A B ♿
CMS: 100-04,20,170
AHA: 2Q, '02, 1-3

Q4033 **Cast supplies, long leg cylinder cast, adult (11 years +), plaster** A B ♿
CMS: 100-04,20,170
AHA: 2Q, '02, 1-3

Q4034 **Cast supplies, long leg cylinder cast, adult (11 years +), fiberglass** A B ♿
CMS: 100-04,20,170
AHA: 2Q, '02, 1-3

© 2019 Optum360, LLC

Q4035 **Cast supplies, long leg cylinder cast, pediatric (0-10 years), plaster** A B ♿
CMS: 100-04,20,170
AHA: 2Q, '02, 1-3

Q4036 **Cast supplies, long leg cylinder cast, pediatric (0-10 years), fiberglass** A B ♿
CMS: 100-04,20,170
AHA: 2Q, '02, 1-3

Q4037 **Cast supplies, short leg cast, adult (11 years +), plaster** A B ♿
CMS: 100-04,20,170
AHA: 2Q, '02, 1-3

Q4038 **Cast supplies, short leg cast, adult (11 years +), fiberglass** A B ♿
CMS: 100-04,20,170
AHA: 2Q, '02, 1-3

Q4039 **Cast supplies, short leg cast, pediatric (0-10 years), plaster** A B ♿
CMS: 100-04,20,170
AHA: 2Q, '02, 1-3

Q4040 **Cast supplies, short leg cast, pediatric (0-10 years), fiberglass** A B ♿
CMS: 100-04,20,170
AHA: 2Q, '02, 1-3

Q4041 **Cast supplies, long leg splint, adult (11 years +), plaster** A B ♿
CMS: 100-04,20,170
AHA: 2Q, '02, 1-3

Q4042 **Cast supplies, long leg splint, adult (11 years +), fiberglass** A B ♿
CMS: 100-04,20,170
AHA: 2Q, '02, 1-3

Q4043 **Cast supplies, long leg splint, pediatric (0-10 years), plaster** A B ♿
CMS: 100-04,20,170
AHA: 2Q, '02, 1-3

Q4044 **Cast supplies, long leg splint, pediatric (0-10 years), fiberglass** A B ♿
CMS: 100-04,20,170
AHA: 2Q, '02, 1-3

Q4045 **Cast supplies, short leg splint, adult (11 years +), plaster** A B ♿
CMS: 100-04,20,170
AHA: 2Q, '02, 1-3

Q4046 **Cast supplies, short leg splint, adult (11 years +), fiberglass** A B ♿
CMS: 100-04,20,170
AHA: 2Q, '02, 1-3

Q4047 **Cast supplies, short leg splint, pediatric (0-10 years), plaster** A B ♿
CMS: 100-04,20,170
AHA: 2Q, '02, 1-3

Q4048 **Cast supplies, short leg splint, pediatric (0-10 years), fiberglass** A B ♿
CMS: 100-04,20,170
AHA: 2Q, '02, 1-3

Q4049 **Finger splint, static** B ♿
CMS: 100-04,20,170
AHA: 2Q, '07, 10; 2Q, '02, 1-3

Q4050 **Cast supplies, for unlisted types and materials of casts** B
CMS: 100-04,20,170
AHA: 2Q, '02, 1-3

Q4051 **Splint supplies, miscellaneous (includes thermoplastics, strapping, fasteners, padding and other supplies)** B
CMS: 100-04,20,170
AHA: 2Q, '02, 1-3

Q4074 **Iloprost, inhalation solution, FDA-approved final product, noncompounded, administered through DME, unit dose form, up to 20 mcg** Y ☑
CMS: 100-02,15,50.5

Q4081 **Injection, epoetin alfa, 100 units (for ESRD on dialysis)** N ☑
CMS: 100-04,8,60.4; 100-04,8,60.4.1; 100-04,8,60.4.2; 100-04,8,60.4.4; 100-04,8,60.4.4.1; 100-04,8,60.4.4.2; 100-04,8,60.4.5.1

Q4082 **Drug or biological, not otherwise classified, Part B drug competitive acquisition program (CAP)** B ☑

Q4100 **Skin substitute, not otherwise specified** N N1 ☑
CMS: 100-04,4,260.1; 100-04,4,260.1.1
AHA: 2Q, '12, 7; 2Q, '10, 2, 3

Q4101 **Apligraf, per sq cm** N N1 ☑
CMS: 100-04,4,260.1; 100-04,4,260.1.1
AHA: 2Q, '12, 7; 2Q, '10, 2, 3

Q4102 **Oasis wound matrix, per sq cm** N N1 ☑
CMS: 100-04,4,260.1; 100-04,4,260.1.1
AHA: 3Q, '12, 8; 2Q, '12, 7; 2Q, '10, 2, 3

Q4103 **Oasis burn matrix, per sq cm** N N1 ☑
CMS: 100-04,4,260.1; 100-04,4,260.1.1
AHA: 2Q, '12, 7; 2Q, '10, 2, 3

Q4104 **Integra bilayer matrix wound dressing (BMWD), per sq cm** N N1 ☑
CMS: 100-04,4,260.1; 100-04,4,260.1.1
AHA: 3Q, '14, 4; 2Q, '12, 7; 2Q, '10, 8; 2Q, '10, 2, 3

Q4105 **Integra dermal regeneration template (DRT) or Integra Omnigraft dermal regeneration matrix, per sq cm** N N1 ☑
CMS: 100-04,4,260.1; 100-04,4,260.1.1
AHA: 2Q, '12, 7; 2Q, '10, 8; 2Q, '10, 2, 3

Q4106 **Dermagraft, per sq cm** N N1 ☑
CMS: 100-04,4,260.1; 100-04,4,260.1.1
AHA: 2Q, '12, 7; 2Q, '10, 2, 3

Q4107 **GRAFTJACKET, per sq cm** N N1 ☑
CMS: 100-04,4,260.1; 100-04,4,260.1.1
AHA: 2Q, '12, 7; 2Q, '10, 2, 3

Q4108 **Integra matrix, per sq cm** N N1 ☑
CMS: 100-04,4,260.1; 100-04,4,260.1.1
AHA: 2Q, '12, 7; 2Q, '10, 8; 2Q, '10, 2, 3

Q4110 **PriMatrix, per sq cm** N N1 ☑
CMS: 100-04,4,260.1; 100-04,4,260.1.1
AHA: 2Q, '12, 7; 2Q, '10, 2, 3

Q4111 **GammaGraft, per sq cm** N N1 ☑
CMS: 100-04,4,260.1; 100-04,4,260.1.1
AHA: 2Q, '12, 7; 2Q, '10, 2, 3

Q4112 **Cymetra, injectable, 1 cc** N N1 ☑
AHA: 2Q, '12, 7; 2Q, '10, 2, 3

Q4113 **GRAFTJACKET XPRESS, injectable, 1 cc** N N1 ☑
AHA: 2Q, '12, 7; 2Q, '10, 2, 3

Q4114 **Integra flowable wound matrix, injectable, 1 cc** N N1 ☑
AHA: 2Q, '12, 7; 2Q, '10, 8; 2Q, '10, 2, 3

© 2019 Optum360, LLC

Q4115 **AlloSkin, per sq cm** N N1 ☑
CMS: 100-04,4,260.1; 100-04,4,260.1.1
AHA: 2Q, '12, 7; 2Q, '10, 2, 3

Q4116 **AlloDerm, per sq cm** N N1 ☑
CMS: 100-04,4,260.1; 100-04,4,260.1.1
AHA: 2Q, '12, 7; 2Q, '10, 2, 3

Q4117 **HYALOMATRIX, per sq cm** N N1 ☑
CMS: 100-04,4,260.1; 100-04,4,260.1.1

Q4118 **MatriStem micromatrix, 1 mg** N N1 ☑
AHA: 4Q, '13, 1-2; 2Q, '12, 7

Q4121 **TheraSkin, per sq cm** N N1 ☑
CMS: 100-04,4,260.1; 100-04,4,260.1.1
AHA: 2Q, '12, 7

▲ **Q4122** Jan **DermACELL, DermACELL AWM or DermACELL AWM Porous, per sq cm** N N1 ☑
CMS: 100-04,4,260.1; 100-04,4,260.1.1
AHA: 2Q, '12, 7

Q4123 **AlloSkin RT, per sq cm** N N1 ☑
CMS: 100-04,4,260.1; 100-04,4,260.1.1

Q4124 **OASIS ultra tri-layer wound matrix, per sq cm** N N1 ☑
CMS: 100-04,4,260.1; 100-04,4,260.1.1
AHA: 2Q, '12, 7

Q4125 **ArthroFlex, per sq cm** N N1 ☑

Q4126 **MemoDerm, DermaSpan, TranZgraft or IntegoPly, per sq cm** N N1 ☑
CMS: 100-04,4,260.1; 100-04,4,260.1.1

Q4127 **Talymed, per sq cm** N N1 ☑
CMS: 100-04,4,260.1; 100-04,4,260.1.1
AHA: 2Q, '13, 9

Q4128 **FlexHD, AllopatchHD, or Matrix HD, per sq cm** N N1 ☑
CMS: 100-04,4,260.1; 100-04,4,260.1.1

Q4130 **Strattice TM, per sq cm** N N1 ☑
AHA: 2Q, '12, 7

Q4132 **Grafix Core and GrafixPL Core, per sq cm** N N1 ☑
CMS: 100-04,4,260.1; 100-04,4,260.1.1

Q4133 **Grafix PRIME, GrafixPL PRIME, Stravix and StravixPL, per sq cm** N N1 ☑
CMS: 100-04,4,260.1; 100-04,4,260.1.1

Q4134 **HMatrix, per sq cm** N N1 ☑
CMS: 100-04,4,260.1; 100-04,4,260.1.1

Q4135 **Mediskin, per sq cm** N N1 ☑
CMS: 100-04,4,260.1; 100-04,4,260.1.1

Q4136 **E-Z Derm, per sq cm** N N1 ☑
CMS: 100-04,4,260.1; 100-04,4,260.1.1

Q4137 **AmnioExcel, AmnioExcel Plus or BioDExcel, per sq cm** N N1 ☑
CMS: 100-04,4,260.1; 100-04,4,260.1.1
AHA: 1Q, '14, 6

Q4138 **BioDFence DryFlex, per sq cm** N N1 ☑
CMS: 100-04,4,260.1; 100-04,4,260.1.1
AHA: 1Q, '14, 6

Q4139 **AmnioMatrix or BioDMatrix, injectable, 1 cc** N N1 ☑
AHA: 1Q, '14, 6

Q4140 **BioDFence, per sq cm** N N1 ☑
CMS: 100-04,4,260.1; 100-04,4,260.1.1
AHA: 1Q, '14, 6

Q4141 **AlloSkin AC, per sq cm** N N1 ☑
CMS: 100-04,4,260.1; 100-04,4,260.1.1
AHA: 1Q, '14, 6

Q4142 **XCM biologic tissue matrix, per sq cm** N N1 ☑
AHA: 1Q, '14, 6

Q4143 **Repriza, per sq cm** N N1 ☑
CMS: 100-04,4,260.1; 100-04,4,260.1.1
AHA: 1Q, '14, 6

Q4145 **EpiFix, injectable, 1 mg** N N1 ☑
AHA: 1Q, '14, 6

Q4146 **Tensix, per sq cm** N N1 ☑
CMS: 100-04,4,260.1; 100-04,4,260.1.1
AHA: 1Q, '14, 6

Q4147 **Architect, Architect PX, or Architect FX, extracellular matrix, per sq cm** N N1 ☑
CMS: 100-04,4,260.1; 100-04,4,260.1.1
AHA: 1Q, '14, 6

Q4148 **Neox Cord 1K, Neox Cord RT, or Clarix Cord 1K, per sq cm** N N1 ☑
CMS: 100-04,4,260.1; 100-04,4,260.1.1
AHA: 1Q, '14, 6

Q4149 **Excellagen, 0.1 cc** N N1 ☑
AHA: 1Q, '14, 6

Q4150 **AlloWrap DS or dry, per sq cm** N N1 ☑
CMS: 100-04,4,260.1; 100-04,4,260.1.1

Q4151 **AmnioBand or Guardian, per sq cm** N N1 ☑
CMS: 100-04,4,260.1; 100-04,4,260.1.1

Q4152 **DermaPure, per sq cm** N N1 ☑
CMS: 100-04,4,260.1; 100-04,4,260.1.1

Q4153 **Dermavest and Plurivest, per sq cm** N N1 ☑
CMS: 100-04,4,260.1; 100-04,4,260.1.1
AHA: 1Q, '16, 6-8

Q4154 **Biovance, per sq cm** N N1 ☑
CMS: 100-04,4,260.1; 100-04,4,260.1.1

Q4155 **Neox Flo or Clarix Flo 1 mg** N N1 ☑

Q4156 **Neox 100 or Clarix 100, per sq cm** N N1 ☑
CMS: 100-04,4,260.1; 100-04,4,260.1.1

Q4157 **Revitalon, per sq cm** N N1 ☑
CMS: 100-04,4,260.1; 100-04,4,260.1.1

Q4158 **Kerecis Omega3, per sq cm** N N1 ☑
CMS: 100-04,4,260.1; 100-04,4,260.1.1

Q4159 **Affinity, per sq cm** N N1 ☑
CMS: 100-04,4,260.1; 100-04,4,260.1.1

Q4160 **Nushield, per sq cm** N N1 ☑
CMS: 100-04,4,260.1; 100-04,4,260.1.1

Q4161 **bio-ConneKt wound matrix, per sq cm** N N1 ☑
CMS: 100-04,4,260.1; 100-04,4,260.1.1
AHA: 1Q, '16, 6-8

Q4162 **WoundEx Flow, BioSkin Flow, 0.5 cc** N N1 ☑
AHA: 1Q, '16, 6-8

Q4163 **WoundEx, BioSkin, per sq cm** N N1 ☑
CMS: 100-04,4,260.1; 100-04,4,260.1.1
AHA: 1Q, '16, 6-8

Q4164 **Helicoll, per sq cm** N N1 ☑
CMS: 100-04,4,260.1; 100-04,4,260.1.1
AHA: 1Q, '16, 6-8

© 2019 Optum360, LLC

▲ **Q4165** Jan **Keramatrix or Kerasorb, per sq cm** N N1 ☑
CMS: 100-04,4,260.1; 100-04,4,260.1.1
AHA: 1Q, '16, 6-8

Q4166 **Cytal, per sq cm** N N1 ☑
CMS: 100-04,4,260.1; 100-04,4,260.1.1
AHA: 1Q, '17, 9-10

Q4167 **Truskin, per sq cm** N N1 ☑
CMS: 100-04,4,260.1; 100-04,4,260.1.1
AHA: 1Q, '17, 9-10

Q4168 **AmnioBand, 1 mg** N N1 ☑
AHA: 1Q, '17, 9-10

Q4169 **Artacent wound, per sq cm** N N1 ☑
CMS: 100-04,4,260.1; 100-04,4,260.1.1
AHA: 1Q, '17, 9-10

Q4170 **Cygnus, per sq cm** N N1 ☑
CMS: 100-04,4,260.1; 100-04,4,260.1.1
AHA: 1Q, '17, 9-10

Q4171 **Interfyl, 1 mg** N N1 ☑
AHA: 1Q, '17, 9-10

Q4173 **PalinGen or PalinGen XPlus, per sq cm** N N1 ☑
CMS: 100-04,4,260.1; 100-04,4,260.1.1
AHA: 1Q, '17, 9-10

Q4174 **PalinGen or ProMatrX, 0.36 mg per 0.25 cc** N N1 ☑
AHA: 1Q, '17, 9-10

Q4175 **Miroderm, per sq cm** N N1 ☑
CMS: 100-04,4,260.1; 100-04,4,260.1.1
AHA: 1Q, '17, 9-10

Q4176 **NeoPatch, per sq cm** N N1
CMS: 100-04,4,260.1; 100-04,4,260.1.1

Q4177 **FlowerAmnioFlo, 0.1 cc** N N1

Q4178 **FlowerAmnioPatch, per sq cm** N N1
CMS: 100-04,4,260.1; 100-04,4,260.1.1

Q4179 **FlowerDerm, per sq cm** N N1
CMS: 100-04,4,260.1; 100-04,4,260.1.1

Q4180 **Revita, per sq cm** N N1
CMS: 100-04,4,260.1; 100-04,4,260.1.1

Q4181 **Amnio Wound, per sq cm** N N1
CMS: 100-04,4,260.1; 100-04,4,260.1.1

Q4182 **Transcyte, per sq cm** N N1
CMS: 100-04,4,260.1; 100-04,4,260.1.1

Q4183 **Surgigraft, per sq cm** N1
CMS: 100-04,4,260.1; 100-04,4,260.1.1

▲ **Q4184** Jan **Cellesta or Cellesta Duo, per sq cm** N1
CMS: 100-04,4,260.1; 100-04,4,260.1.1

Q4185 **Cellesta Flowable Amnion (25 mg per cc); per 0.5 cc** N1
CMS: 100-04,4,260.1; 100-04,4,260.1.1

Q4186 **Epifix, per sq cm** N1
CMS: 100-04,4,260.1; 100-04,4,260.1.1

Q4187 **Epicord, per sq cm** N1
CMS: 100-04,4,260.1; 100-04,4,260.1.1

Q4188 **AmnioArmor, per sq cm** N1
CMS: 100-04,4,260.1; 100-04,4,260.1.1

Q4189 **Artacent AC, 1 mg** N1
CMS: 100-04,4,260.1; 100-04,4,260.1.1

Q4190 **Artacent AC, per sq cm** N1
CMS: 100-04,4,260.1; 100-04,4,260.1.1

Q4191 **Restorigin, per sq cm** N1
CMS: 100-04,4,260.1; 100-04,4,260.1.1

Q4192 **Restorigin, 1 cc** N1
CMS: 100-04,4,260.1; 100-04,4,260.1.1

Q4193 **Coll-e-Derm, per sq cm** N1
CMS: 100-04,4,260.1; 100-04,4,260.1.1

Q4194 **Novachor, per sq cm** N1
CMS: 100-04,4,260.1; 100-04,4,260.1.1

Q4195 **PuraPly, per sq cm** K2
CMS: 100-04,4,260.1; 100-04,4,260.1.1

Q4196 **PuraPly AM, per sq cm** K2
CMS: 100-04,4,260.1; 100-04,4,260.1.1

Q4197 **PuraPly XT, per sq cm** N1
CMS: 100-04,4,260.1; 100-04,4,260.1.1

Q4198 **Genesis Amniotic Membrane, per sq cm** N1
CMS: 100-04,4,260.1; 100-04,4,260.1.1

Q4200 **SkinTE, per sq cm** N1
CMS: 100-04,4,260.1; 100-04,4,260.1.1

Q4201 **Matrion, per sq cm** N1
CMS: 100-04,4,260.1; 100-04,4,260.1.1

Q4202 **Keroxx (2.5 g/cc), 1 cc** N1
CMS: 100-04,4,260.1; 100-04,4,260.1.1

Q4203 **Derma-Gide, per sq cm** N1
CMS: 100-04,4,260.1; 100-04,4,260.1.1

Q4204 **XWRAP, per sq cm** N1
CMS: 100-04,4,260.1; 100-04,4,260.1.1

● **Q4205** Jan **Membrane Graft or Membrane Wrap, per sq cm**

● **Q4206** Jan **Fluid Flow or Fluid GF, 1 cc**

● **Q4208** Jan **Novafix, per sq cm**

● **Q4209** Jan **SurGraft, per sq cm**

● **Q4210** Jan **Axolotl Graft or Axolotl DualGraft, per sq cm**

● **Q4211** Jan **Amnion Bio or AxoBioMembrane, per sq cm**

● **Q4212** Jan **AlloGen, per cc**

● **Q4213** Jan **Ascent, 0.5 mg**

● **Q4214** Jan **Cellesta Cord, per sq cm**

● **Q4215** Jan **Axolotl Ambient or Axolotl Cryo, 0.1 mg**

● **Q4216** Jan **Artacent Cord, per sq cm**

● **Q4217** Jan **WoundFix, BioWound, WoundFix Plus, BioWound Plus, WoundFix Xplus or BioWound Xplus, per sq cm**

● **Q4218** Jan **SurgiCORD, per sq cm**

● **Q4219** Jan **SurgiGRAFT-DUAL, per sq cm**

● **Q4220** Jan **BellaCell HD or Surederm, per sq cm**

● **Q4221** Jan **Amnio Wrap2, per sq cm**

● **Q4222** Jan **ProgenaMatrix, per sq cm**

● **Q4226** Jan **MyOwn Skin, includes harvesting and preparation procedures, per sq cm**

Q5001 **Hospice or home health care provided in patient's home/residence** B
CMS: 100-01,3,30.3; 100-04,10,40.2; 100-04,11,10; 100-04,11,30.3

Q5002 **Hospice or home health care provided in assisted living facility** B
CMS: 100-01,3,30.3; 100-04,10,40.2; 100-04,11,10; 100-04,11,30.3

© 2019 Optum360, LLC

Q5003 **Hospice care provided in nursing long-term care facility (LTC) or nonskilled nursing facility (NF)** B
CMS: 100-01,3,30.3; 100-04,11,10; 100-04,11,30.3

Q5004 **Hospice care provided in skilled nursing facility (SNF)** B
CMS: 100-01,3,30.3; 100-04,11,10; 100-04,11,30.3

Q5005 **Hospice care provided in inpatient hospital** B
CMS: 100-01,3,30.3; 100-04,11,10; 100-04,11,30.3

Q5006 **Hospice care provided in inpatient hospice facility** B
CMS: 100-01,3,30.3; 100-04,11,10; 100-04,11,30.3

Q5007 **Hospice care provided in long-term care facility** B
CMS: 100-01,3,30.3; 100-04,11,10; 100-04,11,30.3

Q5008 **Hospice care provided in inpatient psychiatric facility** B
CMS: 100-01,3,30.3; 100-04,11,10; 100-04,11,30.3

Q5009 **Hospice or home health care provided in place not otherwise specified (NOS)** B
CMS: 100-01,3,30.3; 100-04,10,40.2; 100-04,11,10; 100-04,11,30.3

Q5010 **Hospice home care provided in a hospice facility** B
CMS: 100-01,3,30.3; 100-04,11,10; 100-04,11,30.3

Q5101 **Injection, filgrastim-sndz, biosimilar, (Zarxio), 1 mcg** G K2
AHA: 2Q, '16, 6-7; 4Q, '15, 4; 3Q, '15, 7

Q5103 **Injection, infliximab-dyyb, biosimilar, (Inflectra), 10 mg** G K2

Q5104 **Injection, infliximab-abda, biosimilar, (Renflexis), 10 mg** G K2

▲ **Q5105**[Jan] **Injection, epoetin alfa-epbx, biosimilar, (Retacrit) (for ESRD on dialysis), 100 units** K2
CMS: 100-04,8,60.4.2

▲ **Q5106**[Jan] **Injection, epoetin alfa-epbx, biosimilar, (Retacrit) (for non-ESRD use), 1000 units** K2

Q5107 **Injection, bevacizumab-awwb, biosimilar, (Mvasi), 10 mg** K2
CMS: 100-04,4,260.1; 100-04,4,260.1.1

Q5108 **Injection, pegfilgrastim-jmdb, biosimilar, (Fulphila), 0.5 mg** K2
CMS: 100-04,4,260.1; 100-04,4,260.1.1

Q5109 **Injection, infliximab-qbtx, biosimilar, (Ixifi), 10 mg**
CMS: 100-04,4,260.1; 100-04,4,260.1.1

Q5110 **Injection, filgrastim-aafi, biosimilar, (Nivestym), 1 mcg** K2
CMS: 100-04,4,260.1; 100-04,4,260.1.1

Q5111 **Injection, pegfilgrastim-cbqv, biosimilar, (Udenyca), 0.5 mg** K2
CMS: 100-04,4,260.1; 100-04,4,260.1.1

● **Q5112**[Jan] **Injection, trastuzumab-dttb, biosimilar, (Ontruzant), 10 mg**

● **Q5113**[Jan] **Injection, trastuzumab-pkrb, biosimilar, (Herzuma), 10 mg**

● **Q5114**[Jan] **Injection, Trastuzumab-dkst, biosimilar, (Ogivri), 10 mg**

● **Q5115**[Jan] **Injection, rituximab-abbs, biosimilar, (Truxima), 10 mg**

● **Q5116**[Jan] **Injection, trastuzumab-qyyp, biosimilar, (Trazimera), 10 mg**

● **Q5117**[Jan] **Injection, trastuzumab-anns, biosimilar, (Kanjinti), 10 mg** K2

● **Q5118**[Jan] **Injection, bevacizumab-bvcr, biosimilar, (Zirabev), 10 mg**

Q9950 **Injection, sulfur hexafluoride lipid microspheres, per ml** N K2
Use this code for Lumason.
CMS: 100-03,1,220.2
AHA: 4Q, '16, 9

Q9951 **Low osmolar contrast material, 400 or greater mg/ml iodine concentration, per ml** N N1 ☑
CMS: 100-03,1,220.2
AHA: 3Q, '12, 8

Q9953 **Injection, iron-based magnetic resonance contrast agent, per ml** N N1 ☑
CMS: 100-03,1,220.2
AHA: 3Q, '12, 8

Q9954 **Oral magnetic resonance contrast agent, per 100 ml** N N1 ☑
CMS: 100-03,1,220.2
AHA: 3Q, '12, 8

Q9955 **Injection, perflexane lipid microspheres, per ml** N N1 ☑
AHA: 3Q, '12, 8

Q9956 **Injection, octafluoropropane microspheres, per ml** N N1 ☑
Use this code for Optison.
AHA: 3Q, '12, 8

Q9957 **Injection, perflutren lipid microspheres, per ml** N N1 ☑
Use this code for Definity.
AHA: 3Q, '12, 8

Q9958 **High osmolar contrast material, up to 149 mg/ml iodine concentration, per ml** N N1 ☑
CMS: 100-03,1,220.2
AHA: 3Q, '12, 8; 4Q, '11, 6; 1Q, '07, 6; 3Q, '05, 7, 9

Q9959 **High osmolar contrast material, 150-199 mg/ml iodine concentration, per ml** N N1 ☑
CMS: 100-03,1,220.2
AHA: 3Q, '12, 8; 4Q, '11, 6; 3Q, '05, 7, 9

Q9960 **High osmolar contrast material, 200-249 mg/ml iodine concentration, per ml** N N1 ☑
CMS: 100-03,1,220.2
AHA: 3Q, '12, 8; 4Q, '11, 6; 1Q, '07, 6; 3Q, '05, 7, 9

Q9961 **High osmolar contrast material, 250-299 mg/ml iodine concentration, per ml** N N1 ☑
CMS: 100-03,1,220.2
AHA: 3Q, '12, 8; 4Q, '11, 6; 3Q, '05, 7, 9

Q9962 **High osmolar contrast material, 300-349 mg/ml iodine concentration, per ml** N N1 ☑
CMS: 100-03,1,220.2
AHA: 3Q, '12, 8; 4Q, '11, 6; 3Q, '05, 7, 9

Q9963 **High osmolar contrast material, 350-399 mg/ml iodine concentration, per ml** N N1 ☑
CMS: 100-03,1,220.2
AHA: 3Q, '12, 8; 4Q, '11, 6; 3Q, '05, 7, 9

Q9964 **High osmolar contrast material, 400 or greater mg/ml iodine concentration, per ml** N N1 ☑
CMS: 100-03,1,220.2
AHA: 3Q, '12, 8; 4Q, '11, 6; 3Q, '05, 7, 9

Q9965 **Low osmolar contrast material, 100-199 mg/ml iodine concentration, per ml** N N1 ☑
Use this code for Omnipaque 140, Omnipaque 180, Optiray 160, Optiray 140, ULTRAVIST 150.
CMS: 100-03,1,220.2
AHA: 3Q, '12, 8; 4Q, '11, 6; 1Q, '08, 6

Q9966 **Low osmolar contrast material, 200-299 mg/ml iodine concentration, per ml** N N1 ☑
Use this code for Omnipaque 240, Optiray 240, ULTRAVIST 240.
CMS: 100-03,1,220.2
AHA: 3Q, '12, 8; 4Q, '11, 6; 1Q, '08, 6

Q9967 **Low osmolar contrast material, 300-399 mg/ml iodine concentration, per ml** N N1 ☑
Use this code for Omnipaque 300, Omnipaque 350, Optiray, Optiray 300, Optiray 320, Oxilan 300, Oxilan 350, ULTRAVIST 300, ULTRAVIST 370.
CMS: 100-03,1,220.2
AHA: 3Q, '12, 8; 4Q, '11, 6; 1Q, '08, 6

© 2019 Optum360, LLC

Q9968 **Injection, nonradioactive, noncontrast, visualization adjunct (e.g., methylene blue, isosulfan blue), 1 mg** K K2 ☑

Q9969 **Tc-99m from nonhighly enriched uranium source, full cost recovery add-on, per study dose** K ☑

Q9982 **Flutemetamol F18, diagnostic, per study dose, up to 5 mCi** G N1

Use this code for Vizamyl.

Q9983 **Florbetaben F18, diagnostic, per study dose, up to 8.1 mCi** G N1

Use this code for Neuraceq.

Q9991 **Injection, buprenorphine extended-release (Sublocade), less than or equal to 100 mg** K2

Q9992 **Injection, buprenorphine extended-release (Sublocade), greater than 100 mg** K2

© 2019 Optum360, LLC

Diagnostic Radiology Services R0070-R0076

R codes are used for the transportation of portable x-ray and/or EKG equipment.

R0070 **Transportation of portable x-ray equipment and personnel to home or nursing home, per trip to facility or location, one patient seen** B ☑

Only a single, reasonable transportation charge is allowed for each trip the portable x-ray supplier makes to a location. When more than one patient is x-rayed at the same location, prorate the single allowable transport charge among all patients.

CMS: 100-04,13,90.3

R0075 **Transportation of portable x-ray equipment and personnel to home or nursing home, per trip to facility or location, more than one patient seen** B ☑

Only a single, reasonable transportation charge is allowed for each trip the portable x-ray supplier makes to a location. When more than one patient is x-rayed at the same location, prorate the single allowable transport charge among all patients.

CMS: 100-04,13,90.3

R0076 **Transportation of portable EKG to facility or location, per patient** B ☑

Only a single, reasonable transportation charge is allowed for each trip the portable EKG supplier makes to a location. When more than one patient is tested at the same location, prorate the single allowable transport charge among all patients.

CMS: 100-04,13,90.3

© 2019 Optum360, LLC

Temporary National Codes (Non-Medicare) S0012-S9999

The S codes are used by the Blue Cross/Blue Shield Association (BCBSA) and the Health Insurance Association of America (HIAA) to report drugs, services, and supplies for which there are no national codes but for which codes are needed by the private sector to implement policies, programs, or claims processing. They are for the purpose of meeting the particular needs of the private sector. These codes are also used by the Medicaid program, but they are not payable by Medicare.

S0012 **Butorphanol tartrate, nasal spray, 25 mg** ☑
Use this code for Stadol NS.

S0014 **Tacrine HCl, 10 mg** ☑
Use this code for Cognex.

S0017 **Injection, aminocaproic acid, 5 g** ☑
Use this code for Amicar.

S0020 **Injection, bupivicaine HCl, 30 ml** ☑
Use this code for Marcaine, Sensorcaine.

S0021 **Injection, cefoperazone sodium, 1 g** ☑
Use this code for Cefobid.

S0023 **Injection, cimetidine HCl, 300 mg** ☑
Use this code for Tagamet HCl.

S0028 **Injection, famotidine, 20 mg** ☑
Use this code for Pepcid.

S0030 **Injection, metronidazole, 500 mg** ☑
Use this code for Flagyl IV RTU.

S0032 **Injection, nafcillin sodium, 2 g** ☑
Use this code for Nallpen, Unipen.

S0034 **Injection, ofloxacin, 400 mg** ☑
Use this code for Floxin IV.

S0039 **Injection, sulfamethoxazole and trimethoprim, 10 ml** ☑
Use this code for Bactrim IV, Septra IV, SMZ-TMP, Sulfutrim.

S0040 **Injection, ticarcillin disodium and clavulanate potassium, 3.1 g** ☑
Use this code for Timentin.

S0073 **Injection, aztreonam, 500 mg** ☑
Use this code for Azactam.

S0074 **Injection, cefotetan disodium, 500 mg** ☑
Use this code for Cefotan.

S0077 **Injection, clindamycin phosphate, 300 mg** ☑
Use this code for Cleocin Phosphate.

S0078 **Injection, fosphenytoin sodium, 750 mg** ☑
Use this code for Cerebryx.

S0080 **Injection, pentamidine isethionate, 300 mg** ☑
Use this code for NebuPent, Pentam 300, Pentacarinat. See also code J2545.

S0081 **Injection, piperacillin sodium, 500 mg** ☑
Use this code for Pipracil.

S0088 **Imatinib, 100 mg** ☑
Use this code for Gleevec.

S0090 **Sildenafil citrate, 25 mg** A ☑
Use this code for Viagra.

S0091 **Granisetron HCl, 1 mg (for circumstances falling under the Medicare statute, use Q0166)** ☑
Use this code for Kytril.

S0092 **Injection, hydromorphone HCl, 250 mg (loading dose for infusion pump)** ☑
Use this code for Dilaudid, Hydromophone. See also J1170.

S0093 **Injection, morphine sulfate, 500 mg (loading dose for infusion pump)** ☑
Use this code for Duramorph, MS Contin, Morphine Sulfate. See also J2270, J2271, J2275.

S0104 **Zidovudine, oral, 100 mg** ☑
See also J3485 for Retrovir.

S0106 **Bupropion HCl sustained release tablet, 150 mg, per bottle of 60 tablets** ☑
Use this code for Wellbutrin SR tablets.

S0108 **Mercaptopurine, oral, 50 mg** ☑
Use this code for Purinethol oral.

S0109 **Methadone, oral, 5 mg** ☑
Use this code for Dolophine.

S0117 **Tretinoin, topical, 5 g** ☑

S0119 **Ondansetron, oral, 4 mg (for circumstances falling under the Medicare statute, use HCPCS Q code)** ☑
Use this code for Zofran, Zuplenz.

S0122 **Injection, menotropins, 75 IU** ☑
Use this code for Humegon, Pergonal, Repronex.
CMS: 100-02,15,50.5

S0126 **Injection, follitropin alfa, 75 IU** ☑
Use this code for Gonal-F.
CMS: 100-02,15,50.5

S0128 **Injection, follitropin beta, 75 IU** ♀☑
Use this code for Follistim.
CMS: 100-02,15,50.5

S0132 **Injection, ganirelix acetate, 250 mcg** ♀☑
Use this code for Antagon.
CMS: 100-02,15,50.5

S0136 **Clozapine, 25 mg** ☑
Use this code for Clozaril.

S0137 **Didanosine (ddI), 25 mg** ☑
Use this code for Videx.

S0138 **Finasteride, 5 mg** ♂☑
Use this code for Propecia (oral), Proscar (oral).

S0139 **Minoxidil, 10 mg** ☑

S0140 **Saquinavir, 200 mg** ☑
Use this code for Fortovase (oral), Invirase (oral).

S0142 **Colistimethate sodium, inhalation solution administered through DME, concentrated form, per mg** ☑

S0145 **Injection, PEGylated interferon alfa-2A, 180 mcg per ml** ☑
Use this code for Pegasys.
CMS: 100-02,15,50.5

S0148 **Injection, PEGylated interferon alfa-2B, 10 mcg** ☑
CMS: 100-02,15,50.5

S0155 **Sterile dilutant for epoprostenol, 50 ml** ☑
Use this code for Flolan.

S0156 **Exemestane, 25 mg** ☑
Use this code for Aromasin.

S0157 **Becaplermin gel 0.01%, 0.5 gm** ☑
Use this code for Regraex Gel.

S0160 **Dextroamphetamine sulfate, 5 mg** ☑

S0164 **Injection, pantoprazole sodium, 40 mg** ☑
Use this code for Protonix IV.

S0166 **Injection, olanzapine, 2.5 mg** ☑
Use this code for Zyprexa.

© 2019 Optum360, LLC

S0169 **Calcitrol, 0.25 mcg** ☑
Use this code for Calcijex.

S0170 **Anastrozole, oral, 1 mg** ☑
Use this code for Arimidex.

S0171 **Injection, bumetanide, 0.5 mg** ☑
Use this code for Bumex.

S0172 **Chlorambucil, oral, 2 mg** ☑
Use this code for Leukeran.

S0174 **Dolasetron mesylate, oral 50 mg (for circumstances falling under the Medicare statute, use Q0180)** ☑
Use this code for Anzemet.

S0175 **Flutamide, oral, 125 mg** ☑
Use this code for Eulexin.

S0176 **Hydroxyurea, oral, 500 mg** ☑
Use this code for Droxia, Hydrea, Mylocel.

S0177 **Levamisole HCl, oral, 50 mg** ☑
Use this code for Ergamisol.

S0178 **Lomustine, oral, 10 mg** ☑
Use this code for Ceenu.

S0179 **Megestrol acetate, oral, 20 mg** ☑
Use this code for Megace.

S0182 **Procarbazine HCl, oral, 50 mg** ☑
Use this code for Matulane.

S0183 **Prochlorperazine maleate, oral, 5 mg (for circumstances falling under the Medicare statute, use Q0164)** ☑
Use this code for Compazine.

S0187 **Tamoxifen citrate, oral, 10 mg** ☑
Use this code for Nolvadex.

S0189 **Testosterone pellet, 75 mg** ☑

S0190 **Mifepristone, oral, 200 mg** ♀☑
Use this code for Mifoprex 200 mg oral.

S0191 **Misoprostol, oral, 200 mcg** ☑

S0194 **Dialysis/stress vitamin supplement, oral, 100 capsules** ☑

S0197 **Prenatal vitamins, 30-day supply** ♀☑

S0199 **Medically induced abortion by oral ingestion of medication including all associated services and supplies (e.g., patient counseling, office visits, confirmation of pregnancy by HCG, ultrasound to confirm duration of pregnancy, ultrasound to confirm completion of abortion) except drugs** ♀

S0201 **Partial hospitalization services, less than 24 hours, per diem**

S0207 **Paramedic intercept, nonhospital-based ALS service (nonvoluntary), nontransport**

S0208 **Paramedic intercept, hospital-based ALS service (nonvoluntary), nontransport**

S0209 **Wheelchair van, mileage, per mile** ☑

S0215 **Nonemergency transportation; mileage, per mile** ☑
See also codes A0021-A0999 for transportation.

S0220 **Medical conference by a physician with interdisciplinary team of health professionals or representatives of community agencies to coordinate activities of patient care (patient is present); approximately 30 minutes** ☑

S0221 **Medical conference by a physician with interdisciplinary team of health professionals or representatives of community agencies to coordinate activities of patient care (patient is present); approximately 60 minutes** ☑

S0250 **Comprehensive geriatric assessment and treatment planning performed by assessment team** A

S0255 **Hospice referral visit (advising patient and family of care options) performed by nurse, social worker, or other designated staff**
CMS: 100-04,11,10

S0257 **Counseling and discussion regarding advance directives or end of life care planning and decisions, with patient and/or surrogate (list separately in addition to code for appropriate evaluation and management service)**

S0260 **History and physical (outpatient or office) related to surgical procedure (list separately in addition to code for appropriate evaluation and management service)**

S0265 **Genetic counseling, under physician supervision, each 15 minutes** ☑

S0270 **Physician management of patient home care, standard monthly case rate (per 30 days)** ☑

S0271 **Physician management of patient home care, hospice monthly case rate (per 30 days)** ☑

S0272 **Physician management of patient home care, episodic care monthly case rate (per 30 days)** ☑

S0273 **Physician visit at member's home, outside of a capitation arrangement**

S0274 **Nurse practitioner visit at member's home, outside of a capitation arrangement**

S0280 **Medical home program, comprehensive care coordination and planning, initial plan**

S0281 **Medical home program, comprehensive care coordination and planning, maintenance of plan**

S0285 **Colonoscopy consultation performed prior to a screening colonoscopy procedure**

S0302 **Completed early periodic screening diagnosis and treatment (EPSDT) service (list in addition to code for appropriate evaluation and management service)**

S0310 **Hospitalist services (list separately in addition to code for appropriate evaluation and management service)**

S0311 **Comprehensive management and care coordination for advanced illness, per calendar month**

S0315 **Disease management program; initial assessment and initiation of the program**

S0316 **Disease management program, follow-up/reassessment**

S0317 **Disease management program; per diem** ☑

S0320 **Telephone calls by a registered nurse to a disease management program member for monitoring purposes; per month**

S0340 **Lifestyle modification program for management of coronary artery disease, including all supportive services; first quarter/stage**

S0341 **Lifestyle modification program for management of coronary artery disease, including all supportive services; second or third quarter/stage**

S0342 **Lifestyle modification program for management of coronary artery disease, including all supportive services; fourth quarter/stage**

S0353 **Treatment planning and care coordination management for cancer initial treatment**

S0354 **Treatment planning and care coordination management for cancer established patient with a change of regimen**

S0390 **Routine foot care; removal and/or trimming of corns, calluses and/or nails and preventive maintenance in specific medical conditions (e.g., diabetes), per visit**

© 2019 Optum360, LLC

S0395 Impression casting of a foot performed by a practitioner other than the manufacturer of the orthotic

S0400 Global fee for extracorporeal shock wave lithotripsy treatment of kidney stone(s)

S0500 Disposable contact lens, per lens ☑

S0504 Single vision prescription lens (safety, athletic, or sunglass), per lens ☑

S0506 Bifocal vision prescription lens (safety, athletic, or sunglass), per lens ☑

S0508 Trifocal vision prescription lens (safety, athletic, or sunglass), per lens ☑

S0510 Nonprescription lens (safety, athletic, or sunglass), per lens ☑

S0512 Daily wear specialty contact lens, per lens ☑

S0514 Color contact lens, per lens ☑

S0515 Scleral lens, liquid bandage device, per lens

S0516 Safety eyeglass frames

S0518 Sunglasses frames

S0580 Polycarbonate lens (list this code in addition to the basic code for the lens)

S0581 Nonstandard lens (list this code in addition to the basic code for the lens)

S0590 Integral lens service, miscellaneous services reported separately

S0592 Comprehensive contact lens evaluation

S0595 Dispensing new spectacle lenses for patient supplied frame

S0596 Phakic intraocular lens for correction of refractive error ☑

S0601 Screening proctoscopy ♂

S0610 Annual gynecological examination, new patient A ♀

S0612 Annual gynecological examination, established patient A ♀

S0613 Annual gynecological examination; clinical breast examination without pelvic evaluation ♀

S0618 Audiometry for hearing aid evaluation to determine the level and degree of hearing loss

S0620 Routine ophthalmological examination including refraction; new patient

S0621 Routine ophthalmological examination including refraction; established patient

S0622 Physical exam for college, new or established patient (list separately in addition to appropriate evaluation and management code)

S0630 Removal of sutures; by a physician other than the physician who originally closed the wound

S0800 Laser in situ keratomileusis (LASIK)

S0810 Photorefractive keratectomy (PRK)

S0812 Phototherapeutic keratectomy (PTK)

S1001 Deluxe item, patient aware (list in addition to code for basic item)
CMS: 100-02,15,110

S1002 Customized item (list in addition to code for basic item)

S1015 IV tubing extension set

S1016 Non-PVC (polyvinyl chloride) intravenous administration set, for use with drugs that are not stable in PVC, e.g., Paclitaxel

S1030 Continuous noninvasive glucose monitoring device, purchase (for physician interpretation of data, use CPT code)

S1031 Continuous noninvasive glucose monitoring device, rental, including sensor, sensor replacement, and download to monitor (for physician interpretation of data, use CPT code)

S1034 Artificial pancreas device system (e.g., low glucose suspend [LGS] feature) including continuous glucose monitor, blood glucose device, insulin pump and computer algorithm that communicates with all of the devices

S1035 Sensor; invasive (e.g., subcutaneous), disposable, for use with artificial pancreas device system

S1036 Transmitter; external, for use with artificial pancreas device system

S1037 Receiver (monitor); external, for use with artificial pancreas device system

S1040 Cranial remolding orthotic, pediatric, rigid, with soft interface material, custom fabricated, includes fitting and adjustment(s)

~~**S1090**~~ Jan ~~**Mometasone furoate sinus implant, 370 micrograms**~~
To report, see ~J7401

S2053 Transplantation of small intestine and liver allografts

S2054 Transplantation of multivisceral organs

S2055 Harvesting of donor multivisceral organs, with preparation and maintenance of allografts; from cadaver donor

S2060 Lobar lung transplantation

S2061 Donor lobectomy (lung) for transplantation, living donor

S2065 Simultaneous pancreas kidney transplantation

S2066 Breast reconstruction with gluteal artery perforator (GAP) flap, including harvesting of the flap, microvascular transfer, closure of donor site and shaping the flap into a breast, unilateral

S2067 Breast reconstruction of a single breast with "stacked" deep inferior epigastric perforator (DIEP) flap(s) and/or gluteal artery perforator (GAP) flap(s), including harvesting of the flap(s), microvascular transfer, closure of donor site(s) and shaping the flap into a breast, unilateral

S2068 Breast reconstruction with deep inferior epigastric perforator (DIEP) flap or superficial inferior epigastric artery (SIEA) flap, including harvesting of the flap, microvascular transfer, closure of donor site and shaping the flap into a breast, unilateral

S2070 Cystourethroscopy, with ureteroscopy and/or pyeloscopy; with endoscopic laser treatment of ureteral calculi (includes ureteral catheterization)

S2079 Laparoscopic esophagomyotomy (Heller type)

S2080 Laser-assisted uvulopalatoplasty (LAUP)

S2083 Adjustment of gastric band diameter via subcutaneous port by injection or aspiration of saline

S2095 Transcatheter occlusion or embolization for tumor destruction, percutaneous, any method, using yttrium-90 microspheres

S2102 Islet cell tissue transplant from pancreas; allogeneic

S2103 Adrenal tissue transplant to brain

S2107 Adoptive immunotherapy i.e. development of specific antitumor reactivity (e.g., tumor-infiltrating lymphocyte therapy) per course of treatment

S2112 Arthroscopy, knee, surgical for harvesting of cartilage (chondrocyte cells)

S2115 Osteotomy, periacetabular, with internal fixation

S2117 Arthroereisis, subtalar

S2118 Metal-on-metal total hip resurfacing, including acetabular and femoral components

S2120 Low density lipoprotein (LDL) apheresis using heparin-induced extracorporeal LDL precipitation

© 2019 Optum360, LLC

S2140 Cord blood harvesting for transplantation, allogeneic

S2142 Cord blood-derived stem-cell transplantation, allogeneic

S2150 Bone marrow or blood-derived stem cells (peripheral or umbilical), allogeneic or autologous, harvesting, transplantation, and related complications; including: pheresis and cell preparation/storage; marrow ablative therapy; drugs, supplies, hospitalization with outpatient follow-up; medical/surgical, diagnostic, emergency, and rehabilitative services; and the number of days of pre- and posttransplant care in the global definition

S2152 Solid organ(s), complete or segmental, single organ or combination of organs; deceased or living donor(s), procurement, transplantation, and related complications; including: drugs; supplies; hospitalization with outpatient follow-up; medical/surgical, diagnostic, emergency, and rehabilitative services, and the number of days of pre- and posttransplant care in the global definition

S2202 Echosclerotherapy

S2205 Minimally invasive direct coronary artery bypass surgery involving mini-thoracotomy or mini-sternotomy surgery, performed under direct vision; using arterial graft(s), single coronary arterial graft

S2206 Minimally invasive direct coronary artery bypass surgery involving mini-thoracotomy or mini-sternotomy surgery, performed under direct vision; using arterial graft(s), two coronary arterial grafts

S2207 Minimally invasive direct coronary artery bypass surgery involving mini-thoracotomy or mini-sternotomy surgery, performed under direct vision; using venous graft only, single coronary venous graft

S2208 Minimally invasive direct coronary artery bypass surgery involving mini-thoracotomy or mini-sternotomy surgery, performed under direct vision; using single arterial and venous graft(s), single venous graft

S2209 Minimally invasive direct coronary artery bypass surgery involving mini-thoracotomy or mini-sternotomy surgery, performed under direct vision; using two arterial grafts and single venous graft

S2225 Myringotomy, laser-assisted

S2230 Implantation of magnetic component of semi-implantable hearing device on ossicles in middle ear

S2235 Implantation of auditory brain stem implant

S2260 Induced abortion, 17 to 24 weeks M ♀

S2265 Induced abortion, 25 to 28 weeks M ♀

S2266 Induced abortion, 29 to 31 weeks M ♀

S2267 Induced abortion, 32 weeks or greater M ♀

S2300 Arthroscopy, shoulder, surgical; with thermally-induced capsulorrhaphy

S2325 Hip core decompression

S2340 Chemodenervation of abductor muscle(s) of vocal cord

S2341 Chemodenervation of adductor muscle(s) of vocal cord

S2342 Nasal endoscopy for postoperative debridement following functional endoscopic sinus surgery, nasal and/or sinus cavity(s), unilateral or bilateral

S2348 Decompression procedure, percutaneous, of nucleus pulposus of intervertebral disc, using radiofrequency energy, single or multiple levels, lumbar

S2350 Diskectomy, anterior, with decompression of spinal cord and/or nerve root(s), including osteophytectomy; lumbar, single interspace

S2351 Diskectomy, anterior, with decompression of spinal cord and/or nerve root(s), including osteophytectomy; lumbar, each additional interspace (list separately in addition to code for primary procedure)

S2400 Repair, congenital diaphragmatic hernia in the fetus using temporary tracheal occlusion, procedure performed in utero M ♀

S2401 Repair, urinary tract obstruction in the fetus, procedure performed in utero M ♀

S2402 Repair, congenital cystic adenomatoid malformation in the fetus, procedure performed in utero M ♀

S2403 Repair, extralobar pulmonary sequestration in the fetus, procedure performed in utero M ♀

S2404 Repair, myelomeningocele in the fetus, procedure performed in utero M ♀

S2405 Repair of sacrococcygeal teratoma in the fetus, procedure performed in utero M ♀

S2409 Repair, congenital malformation of fetus, procedure performed in utero, not otherwise classified M ♀

S2411 Fetoscopic laser therapy for treatment of twin-to-twin transfusion syndrome M ♀

S2900 Surgical techniques requiring use of robotic surgical system (list separately in addition to code for primary procedure)
AHA: 2Q, '10, 6

S3000 Diabetic indicator; retinal eye exam, dilated, bilateral

S3005 Performance measurement, evaluation of patient self assessment, depression

S3600 STAT laboratory request (situations other than S3601)

S3601 Emergency STAT laboratory charge for patient who is homebound or residing in a nursing facility

S3620 Newborn metabolic screening panel, includes test kit, postage and the laboratory tests specified by the state for inclusion in this panel (e.g., galactose; hemoglobin, electrophoresis; hydroxyprogesterone, 17-d; phenylalanine (PKU); and thyroxine, total) A

S3630 Eosinophil count, blood, direct

S3645 HIV-1 antibody testing of oral mucosal transudate

S3650 Saliva test, hormone level; during menopause A ♀

S3652 Saliva test, hormone level; to assess preterm labor risk M ♀

S3655 Antisperm antibodies test (immunobead) M ♀

S3708 Gastrointestinal fat absorption study

S3722 Dose optimization by area under the curve (AUC) analysis, for infusional 5-fluorouracil

S3800 Genetic testing for amyotrophic lateral sclerosis (ALS)

S3840 DNA analysis for germline mutations of the RET proto-oncogene for susceptibility to multiple endocrine neoplasia type 2

S3841 Genetic testing for retinoblastoma

S3842 Genetic testing for Von Hippel-Lindau disease

S3844 DNA analysis of the connexin 26 gene (GJB2) for susceptibility to congenital, profound deafness

S3845 Genetic testing for alpha-thalassemia

S3846 Genetic testing for hemoglobin E beta-thalassemia

S3849 Genetic testing for Niemann-Pick disease

S3850 Genetic testing for sickle cell anemia

S3852 DNA analysis for APOE epsilon 4 allele for susceptibility to Alzheimer's disease

© 2019 Optum360, LLC

S3853 Genetic testing for myotonic muscular dystrophy

S3854 Gene expression profiling panel for use in the management of breast cancer treatment
AHA: 2Q, '16, 5

S3861 Genetic testing, sodium channel, voltage-gated, type V, alpha subunit (SCN5A) and variants for suspected Brugada Syndrome

S3865 Comprehensive gene sequence analysis for hypertrophic cardiomyopathy

S3866 Genetic analysis for a specific gene mutation for hypertrophic cardiomyopathy (HCM) in an individual with a known HCM mutation in the family

S3870 Comparative genomic hybridization (CGH) microarray testing for developmental delay, autism spectrum disorder and/or intellectual disability

S3900 Surface electromyography (EMG)

S3902 Ballistocardiogram

S3904 Masters two step

S4005 Interim labor facility global (labor occurring but not resulting in delivery) M ♀

S4011 In vitro fertilization; including but not limited to identification and incubation of mature oocytes, fertilization with sperm, incubation of embryo(s), and subsequent visualization for determination of development M ♀

S4013 Complete cycle, gamete intrafallopian transfer (GIFT), case rate M ♀

S4014 Complete cycle, zygote intrafallopian transfer (ZIFT), case rate M ♀

S4015 Complete in vitro fertilization cycle, not otherwise specified, case rate M ♀

S4016 Frozen in vitro fertilization cycle, case rate M ♀

S4017 Incomplete cycle, treatment cancelled prior to stimulation, case rate M ♀

S4018 Frozen embryo transfer procedure cancelled before transfer, case rate M ♀

S4020 In vitro fertilization procedure cancelled before aspiration, case rate M ♀

S4021 In vitro fertilization procedure cancelled after aspiration, case rate M ♀

S4022 Assisted oocyte fertilization, case rate M ♀

S4023 Donor egg cycle, incomplete, case rate M ♀

S4025 Donor services for in vitro fertilization (sperm or embryo), case rate A ♀

S4026 Procurement of donor sperm from sperm bank ♂

S4027 Storage of previously frozen embryos M ♀

S4028 Microsurgical epididymal sperm aspiration (MESA) A ♂

S4030 Sperm procurement and cryopreservation services; initial visit A ♂

S4031 Sperm procurement and cryopreservation services; subsequent visit A ♂

S4035 Stimulated intrauterine insemination (IUI), case rate M ♀

S4037 Cryopreserved embryo transfer, case rate M ♀

S4040 Monitoring and storage of cryopreserved embryos, per 30 days M ♀

S4042 Management of ovulation induction (interpretation of diagnostic tests and studies, nonface-to-face medical management of the patient), per cycle

S4981 Insertion of levonorgestrel-releasing intrauterine system ♀

S4989 Contraceptive intrauterine device (e.g., Progestacert IUD), including implants and supplies M ♀

S4990 Nicotine patches, legend ☑

S4991 Nicotine patches, nonlegend ☑

S4993 Contraceptive pills for birth control M ♀ ☑

S4995 Smoking cessation gum ☑

S5000 Prescription drug, generic ☑

S5001 Prescription drug, brand name ☑

S5010 5% dextrose and 0.45% normal saline, 1000 ml ☑

S5012 5% dextrose with potassium chloride, 1000 ml ☑

S5013 5% dextrose/0.45% normal saline with potassium chloride and magnesium sulfate, 1000 ml ☑

S5014 5% dextrose/0.45% normal saline with potassium chloride and magnesium sulfate, 1500 ml ☑

S5035 Home infusion therapy, routine service of infusion device (e.g., pump maintenance)

S5036 Home infusion therapy, repair of infusion device (e.g., pump repair)

S5100 Day care services, adult; per 15 minutes A ☑

S5101 Day care services, adult; per half day A ☑

S5102 Day care services, adult; per diem A ☑

S5105 Day care services, center-based; services not included in program fee, per diem ☑

S5108 Home care training to home care client, per 15 minutes ☑

S5109 Home care training to home care client, per session ☑

S5110 Home care training, family; per 15 minutes ☑

S5111 Home care training, family; per session

S5115 Home care training, nonfamily; per 15 minutes ☑

S5116 Home care training, nonfamily; per session ☑

S5120 Chore services; per 15 minutes ☑

S5121 Chore services; per diem ☑

S5125 Attendant care services; per 15 minutes ☑

S5126 Attendant care services; per diem ☑

S5130 Homemaker service, NOS; per 15 minutes ☑

S5131 Homemaker service, NOS; per diem ☑

S5135 Companion care, adult (e.g., IADL/ADL); per 15 minutes A ☑

S5136 Companion care, adult (e.g., IADL/ADL); per diem A ☑

S5140 Foster care, adult; per diem A ☑

S5141 Foster care, adult; per month A ☑

S5145 Foster care, therapeutic, child; per diem A ☑

S5146 Foster care, therapeutic, child; per month A ☑

S5150 Unskilled respite care, not hospice; per 15 minutes ☑

S5151 Unskilled respite care, not hospice; per diem ☑

S5160 Emergency response system; installation and testing

S5161 Emergency response system; service fee, per month (excludes installation and testing) ☑

© 2019 Optum360, LLC

S5162 Emergency response system; purchase only

S5165 Home modifications; per service

S5170 Home delivered meals, including preparation; per meal

S5175 Laundry service, external, professional; per order

S5180 Home health respiratory therapy, initial evaluation

S5181 Home health respiratory therapy, NOS, per diem

S5185 Medication reminder service, nonface-to-face; per month ☑

S5190 Wellness assessment, performed by nonphysician

S5199 Personal care item, NOS, each

S5497 Home infusion therapy, catheter care/maintenance, not otherwise classified; includes administrative services, professional pharmacy services, care coordination, and all necessary supplies and equipment (drugs and nursing visits coded separately), per diem ☑

S5498 Home infusion therapy, catheter care/maintenance, simple (single lumen), includes administrative services, professional pharmacy services, care coordination and all necessary supplies and equipment, (drugs and nursing visits coded separately), per diem ☑

S5501 Home infusion therapy, catheter care/maintenance, complex (more than one lumen), includes administrative services, professional pharmacy services, care coordination, and all necessary supplies and equipment (drugs and nursing visits coded separately), per diem ☑

S5502 Home infusion therapy, catheter care/maintenance, implanted access device, includes administrative services, professional pharmacy services, care coordination and all necessary supplies and equipment (drugs and nursing visits coded separately), per diem (use this code for interim maintenance of vascular access not currently in use) ☑

S5517 Home infusion therapy, all supplies necessary for restoration of catheter patency or declotting

S5518 Home infusion therapy, all supplies necessary for catheter repair

S5520 Home infusion therapy, all supplies (including catheter) necessary for a peripherally inserted central venous catheter (PICC) line insertion

S5521 Home infusion therapy, all supplies (including catheter) necessary for a midline catheter insertion

S5522 Home infusion therapy, insertion of peripherally inserted central venous catheter (PICC), nursing services only (no supplies or catheter included)

S5523 Home infusion therapy, insertion of midline venous catheter, nursing services only (no supplies or catheter included)

S5550 Insulin, rapid onset, 5 units ☑

S5551 Insulin, most rapid onset (Lispro or Aspart); 5 units ☑

S5552 Insulin, intermediate acting (NPH or LENTE); 5 units ☑

S5553 Insulin, long acting; 5 units ☑
CMS: 100-02,15,50.5

S5560 Insulin delivery device, reusable pen; 1.5 ml size ☑

S5561 Insulin delivery device, reusable pen; 3 ml size ☑

S5565 Insulin cartridge for use in insulin delivery device other than pump; 150 units ☑

S5566 Insulin cartridge for use in insulin delivery device other than pump; 300 units ☑

S5570 Insulin delivery device, disposable pen (including insulin); 1.5 ml size ☑
CMS: 100-02,15,50.5

S5571 Insulin delivery device, disposable pen (including insulin); 3 ml size ☑
CMS: 100-02,15,50.5

S8030 Scleral application of tantalum ring(s) for localization of lesions for proton beam therapy

S8035 Magnetic source imaging

S8037 Magnetic resonance cholangiopancreatography (MRCP)

S8040 Topographic brain mapping

S8042 Magnetic resonance imaging (MRI), low-field

S8055 Ultrasound guidance for multifetal pregnancy reduction(s), technical component (only to be used when the physician doing the reduction procedure does not perform the ultrasound, guidance is included in the CPT code for multifetal pregnancy reduction (59866) M ♀

S8080 Scintimammography (radioimmunoscintigraphy of the breast), unilateral, including supply of radiopharmaceutical

S8085 Fluorine-18 fluorodeoxyglucose (F-18 FDG) imaging using dual-head coincidence detection system (nondedicated PET scan)

S8092 Electron beam computed tomography (also known as ultrafast CT, cine CT)

S8096 Portable peak flow meter

S8097 Asthma kit (including but not limited to portable peak expiratory flow meter, instructional video, brochure, and/or spacer) ☑

S8100 Holding chamber or spacer for use with an inhaler or nebulizer; without mask

S8101 Holding chamber or spacer for use with an inhaler or nebulizer; with mask

S8110 Peak expiratory flow rate (physician services)

S8120 Oxygen contents, gaseous, 1 unit equals 1 cubic foot ☑

S8121 Oxygen contents, liquid, 1 unit equals 1 pound ☑

S8130 Interferential current stimulator, 2 channel

S8131 Interferential current stimulator, 4 channel

S8185 Flutter device

S8186 Swivel adaptor

S8189 Tracheostomy supply, not otherwise classified

S8210 Mucus trap

S8265 Haberman feeder for cleft lip/palate

S8270 Enuresis alarm, using auditory buzzer and/or vibration device

S8301 Infection control supplies, not otherwise specified

S8415 Supplies for home delivery of infant M ♀

S8420 Gradient pressure aid (sleeve and glove combination), custom made

S8421 Gradient pressure aid (sleeve and glove combination), ready made

S8422 Gradient pressure aid (sleeve), custom made, medium weight

S8423 Gradient pressure aid (sleeve), custom made, heavy weight

S8424 Gradient pressure aid (sleeve), ready made

S8425 Gradient pressure aid (glove), custom made, medium weight

S8426 Gradient pressure aid (glove), custom made, heavy weight

S8427 Gradient pressure aid (glove), ready made

© 2019 Optum360, LLC

S8428 Gradient pressure aid (gauntlet), ready made

S8429 Gradient pressure exterior wrap

S8430 Padding for compression bandage, roll ☑

S8431 Compression bandage, roll ☑

S8450 Splint, prefabricated, digit (specify digit by use of modifier) ☑

Various types of digit splints (S8450)

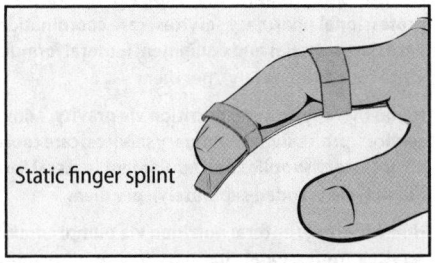

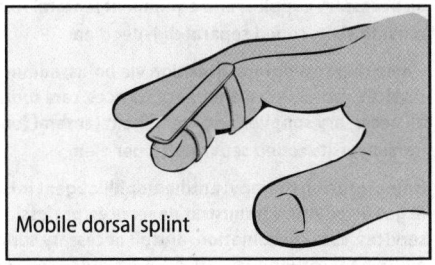

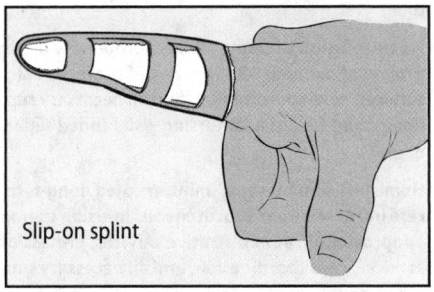

S8451 Splint, prefabricated, wrist or ankle ☑

S8452 Splint, prefabricated, elbow ☑

S8460 Camisole, postmastectomy

S8490 Insulin syringes (100 syringes, any size) ☑

S8930 Electrical stimulation of auricular acupuncture points; each 15 minutes of personal one-on-one contact with patient ☑

S8940 Equestrian/hippotherapy, per session

S8948 Application of a modality (requiring constant provider attendance) to one or more areas; low-level laser; each 15 minutes ☑

S8950 Complex lymphedema therapy, each 15 minutes ☑

S8990 Physical or manipulative therapy performed for maintenance rather than restoration

S8999 Resuscitation bag (for use by patient on artificial respiration during power failure or other catastrophic event)

S9001 Home uterine monitor with or without associated nursing services M ♀

S9007 Ultrafiltration monitor

S9024 Paranasal sinus ultrasound

S9025 Omnicardiogram/cardiointegram

S9034 Extracorporeal shockwave lithotripsy for gall stones (if performed with ERCP, use 43265)

S9055 Procuren or other growth factor preparation to promote wound healing

S9056 Coma stimulation per diem ☑

S9061 Home administration of aerosolized drug therapy (e.g., Pentamidine); administrative services, professional pharmacy services, care coordination, all necessary supplies and equipment (drugs and nursing visits coded separately), per diem ☑

S9083 Global fee urgent care centers

S9088 Services provided in an urgent care center (list in addition to code for service)

S9090 Vertebral axial decompression, per session ☑

S9097 Home visit for wound care

S9098 Home visit, phototherapy services (e.g., Bili-lite), including equipment rental, nursing services, blood draw, supplies, and other services, per diem ☑

S9110 Telemonitoring of patient in their home, including all necessary equipment; computer system, connections, and software; maintenance; patient education and support; per month

S9117 Back school, per visit ☑

S9122 Home health aide or certified nurse assistant, providing care in the home; per hour ☑

S9123 Nursing care, in the home; by registered nurse, per hour (use for general nursing care only, not to be used when CPT codes 99500-99602 can be used) ☑

S9124 Nursing care, in the home; by licensed practical nurse, per hour ☑

S9125 Respite care, in the home, per diem ☑

S9126 Hospice care, in the home, per diem ☑
CMS: 100-04,11,10

S9127 Social work visit, in the home, per diem ☑

S9128 Speech therapy, in the home, per diem ☑

S9129 Occupational therapy, in the home, per diem ☑

S9131 Physical therapy; in the home, per diem ☑

S9140 Diabetic management program, follow-up visit to non-MD provider ☑

S9141 Diabetic management program, follow-up visit to MD provider ☑

S9145 Insulin pump initiation, instruction in initial use of pump (pump not included)

S9150 Evaluation by ocularist

S9152 Speech therapy, re-evaluation

S9208 Home management of preterm labor, including administrative services, professional pharmacy services, care coordination, and all necessary supplies or equipment (drugs and nursing visits coded separately), per diem (do not use this code with any home infusion per diem code) M ♀☑

S9209 Home management of preterm premature rupture of membranes (PPROM), including administrative services, professional pharmacy services, care coordination, and all necessary supplies or equipment (drugs and nursing visits coded separately), per diem (do not use this code with any home infusion per diem code) M ♀☑

© 2019 Optum360, LLC

S9211 Home management of gestational hypertension, includes administrative services, professional pharmacy services, care coordination and all necessary supplies and equipment (drugs and nursing visits coded separately); per diem (do not use this code with any home infusion per diem code) M ♀ ☑

S9212 Home management of postpartum hypertension, includes administrative services, professional pharmacy services, care coordination, and all necessary supplies and equipment (drugs and nursing visits coded separately), per diem (do not use this code with any home infusion per diem code) ♀ ☑

S9213 Home management of preeclampsia, includes administrative services, professional pharmacy services, care coordination, and all necessary supplies and equipment (drugs and nursing services coded separately); per diem (do not use this code with any home infusion per diem code) M ♀ ☑

S9214 Home management of gestational diabetes, includes administrative services, professional pharmacy services, care coordination, and all necessary supplies and equipment (drugs and nursing visits coded separately); per diem (do not use this code with any home infusion per diem code) M ♀ ☑

S9325 Home infusion therapy, pain management infusion; administrative services, professional pharmacy services, care coordination, and all necessary supplies and equipment, (drugs and nursing visits coded separately), per diem (do not use this code with S9326, S9327 or S9328) ☑

S9326 Home infusion therapy, continuous (24 hours or more) pain management infusion; administrative services, professional pharmacy services, care coordination and all necessary supplies and equipment (drugs and nursing visits coded separately), per diem ☑

S9327 Home infusion therapy, intermittent (less than 24 hours) pain management infusion; administrative services, professional pharmacy services, care coordination, and all necessary supplies and equipment (drugs and nursing visits coded separately), per diem ☑

S9328 Home infusion therapy, implanted pump pain management infusion; administrative services, professional pharmacy services, care coordination, and all necessary supplies and equipment (drugs and nursing visits coded separately), per diem ☑

S9329 Home infusion therapy, chemotherapy infusion; administrative services, professional pharmacy services, care coordination, and all necessary supplies and equipment (drugs and nursing visits coded separately), per diem (do not use this code with S9330 or S9331) ☑

S9330 Home infusion therapy, continuous (24 hours or more) chemotherapy infusion; administrative services, professional pharmacy services, care coordination, and all necessary supplies and equipment (drugs and nursing visits coded separately), per diem ☑

S9331 Home infusion therapy, intermittent (less than 24 hours) chemotherapy infusion; administrative services, professional pharmacy services, care coordination, and all necessary supplies and equipment (drugs and nursing visits coded separately), per diem ☑

S9335 Home therapy, hemodialysis; administrative services, professional pharmacy services, care coordination, and all necessary supplies and equipment (drugs and nursing services coded separately), per diem ☑

S9336 Home infusion therapy, continuous anticoagulant infusion therapy (e.g., Heparin), administrative services, professional pharmacy services, care coordination and all necessary supplies and equipment (drugs and nursing visits coded separately), per diem ☑

S9338 Home infusion therapy, immunotherapy, administrative services, professional pharmacy services, care coordination, and all necessary supplies and equipment (drugs and nursing visits coded separately), per diem ☑

S9339 Home therapy; peritoneal dialysis, administrative services, professional pharmacy services, care coordination and all necessary supplies and equipment (drugs and nursing visits coded separately), per diem ☑

S9340 Home therapy; enteral nutrition; administrative services, professional pharmacy services, care coordination, and all necessary supplies and equipment (enteral formula and nursing visits coded separately), per diem ☑

S9341 Home therapy; enteral nutrition via gravity; administrative services, professional pharmacy services, care coordination, and all necessary supplies and equipment (enteral formula and nursing visits coded separately), per diem ☑

S9342 Home therapy; enteral nutrition via pump; administrative services, professional pharmacy services, care coordination, and all necessary supplies and equipment (enteral formula and nursing visits coded separately), per diem ☑

S9343 Home therapy; enteral nutrition via bolus; administrative services, professional pharmacy services, care coordination, and all necessary supplies and equipment (enteral formula and nursing visits coded separately), per diem ☑

S9345 Home infusion therapy, antihemophilic agent infusion therapy (e.g., Factor VIII); administrative services, professional pharmacy services, care coordination, and all necessary supplies and equipment (drugs and nursing visits coded separately), per diem ☑

S9346 Home infusion therapy, alpha-1-proteinase inhibitor (e.g., Prolastin); administrative services, professional pharmacy services, care coordination, and all necessary supplies and equipment (drugs and nursing visits coded separately), per diem ☑

S9347 Home infusion therapy, uninterrupted, long-term, controlled rate intravenous or subcutaneous infusion therapy (e.g., epoprostenol); administrative services, professional pharmacy services, care coordination, and all necessary supplies and equipment (drugs and nursing visits coded separately), per diem ☑

S9348 Home infusion therapy, sympathomimetic/inotropic agent infusion therapy (e.g., Dobutamine); administrative services, professional pharmacy services, care coordination, all necessary supplies and equipment (drugs and nursing visits coded separately), per diem ☑

S9349 Home infusion therapy, tocolytic infusion therapy; administrative services, professional pharmacy services, care coordination, and all necessary supplies and equipment (drugs and nursing visits coded separately), per diem M ♀ ☑

S9351 Home infusion therapy, continuous or intermittent antiemetic infusion therapy; administrative services, professional pharmacy services, care coordination, and all necessary supplies and equipment (drugs and visits coded separately), per diem ☑

S9353 Home infusion therapy, continuous insulin infusion therapy; administrative services, professional pharmacy services, care coordination, and all necessary supplies and equipment (drugs and nursing visits coded separately), per diem ☑

S9355 Home infusion therapy, chelation therapy; administrative services, professional pharmacy services, care coordination, and all necessary supplies and equipment (drugs and nursing visits coded separately), per diem ☑

© 2019 Optum360, LLC

S9357 Home infusion therapy, enzyme replacement intravenous therapy; (e.g., Imiglucerase); administrative services, professional pharmacy services, care coordination, and all necessary supplies and equipment (drugs and nursing visits coded separately), per diem ☑

S9359 Home infusion therapy, antitumor necrosis factor intravenous therapy; (e.g., Infliximab); administrative services, professional pharmacy services, care coordination, and all necessary supplies and equipment (drugs and nursing visits coded separately), per diem ☑

S9361 Home infusion therapy, diuretic intravenous therapy; administrative services, professional pharmacy services, care coordination, and all necessary supplies and equipment (drugs and nursing visits coded separately), per diem ☑

S9363 Home infusion therapy, antispasmotic therapy; administrative services, professional pharmacy services, care coordination, and all necessary supplies and equipment (drugs and nursing visits coded separately), per diem ☑

S9364 Home infusion therapy, total parenteral nutrition (TPN); administrative services, professional pharmacy services, care coordination, and all necessary supplies and equipment including standard TPN formula (lipids, specialty amino acid formulas, drugs other than in standard formula and nursing visits coded separately), per diem (do not use with home infusion codes S9365-S9368 using daily volume scales) ☑

S9365 Home infusion therapy, total parenteral nutrition (TPN); one liter per day, administrative services, professional pharmacy services, care coordination, and all necessary supplies and equipment including standard TPN formula (lipids, specialty amino acid formulas, drugs other than in standard formula and nursing visits coded separately), per diem ☑

S9366 Home infusion therapy, total parenteral nutrition (TPN); more than one liter but no more than two liters per day, administrative services, professional pharmacy services, care coordination, and all necessary supplies and equipment including standard TPN formula (lipids, specialty amino acid formulas, drugs other than in standard formula and nursing visits coded separately), per diem ☑

S9367 Home infusion therapy, total parenteral nutrition (TPN); more than two liters but no more than three liters per day, administrative services, professional pharmacy services, care coordination, and all necessary supplies and equipment including standard TPN formula (lipids, specialty amino acid formulas, drugs other than in standard formula and nursing visits coded separately), per diem ☑

S9368 Home infusion therapy, total parenteral nutrition (TPN); more than three liters per day, administrative services, professional pharmacy services, care coordination, and all necessary supplies and equipment including standard TPN formula (lipids, specialty amino acid formulas, drugs other than in standard formula and nursing visits coded separately), per diem ☑

S9370 Home therapy, intermittent antiemetic injection therapy; administrative services, professional pharmacy services, care coordination, and all necessary supplies and equipment (drugs and nursing visits coded separately), per diem ☑

S9372 Home therapy; intermittent anticoagulant injection therapy (e.g., Heparin); administrative services, professional pharmacy services, care coordination, and all necessary supplies and equipment (drugs and nursing visits coded separately), per diem (do not use this code for flushing of infusion devices with Heparin to maintain patency) ☑

S9373 Home infusion therapy, hydration therapy; administrative services, professional pharmacy services, care coordination, and all necessary supplies and equipment (drugs and nursing visits coded separately), per diem (do not use with hydration therapy codes S9374-S9377 using daily volume scales) ☑

S9374 Home infusion therapy, hydration therapy; 1 liter per day, administrative services, professional pharmacy services, care coordination, and all necessary supplies and equipment (drugs and nursing visits coded separately), per diem ☑

S9375 Home infusion therapy, hydration therapy; more than 1 liter but no more than 2 liters per day, administrative services, professional pharmacy services, care coordination, and all necessary supplies and equipment (drugs and nursing visits coded separately), per diem ☑

S9376 Home infusion therapy, hydration therapy; more than 2 liters but no more than 3 liters per day, administrative services, professional pharmacy services, care coordination, and all necessary supplies and equipment (drugs and nursing visits coded separately), per diem ☑

S9377 Home infusion therapy, hydration therapy; more than 3 liters per day, administrative services, professional pharmacy services, care coordination, and all necessary supplies (drugs and nursing visits coded separately), per diem ☑

S9379 Home infusion therapy, infusion therapy, not otherwise classified; administrative services, professional pharmacy services, care coordination, and all necessary supplies and equipment (drugs and nursing visits coded separately), per diem ☑

S9381 Delivery or service to high risk areas requiring escort or extra protection, per visit

S9401 Anticoagulation clinic, inclusive of all services except laboratory tests, per session

S9430 Pharmacy compounding and dispensing services

S9433 Medical food nutritionally complete, administered orally, providing 100% of nutritional intake

S9434 Modified solid food supplements for inborn errors of metabolism

S9435 Medical foods for inborn errors of metabolism

S9436 Childbirth preparation/Lamaze classes, nonphysician provider, per session M ♀☑

S9437 Childbirth refresher classes, nonphysician provider, per session M ♀

S9438 Cesarean birth classes, nonphysician provider, per session M ♀☑

S9439 VBAC (vaginal birth after cesarean) classes, nonphysician provider, per session M ♀☑

S9441 Asthma education, nonphysician provider, per session ☑

S9442 Birthing classes, nonphysician provider, per session M ♀☑

S9443 Lactation classes, nonphysician provider, per session M ♀☑

S9444 Parenting classes, nonphysician provider, per session ☑

S9445 Patient education, not otherwise classified, nonphysician provider, individual, per session ☑

S9446 Patient education, not otherwise classified, nonphysician provider, group, per session ☑

S9447 Infant safety (including CPR) classes, nonphysician provider, per session ☑

S9449 Weight management classes, nonphysician provider, per session ☑

© 2019 Optum360, LLC

S9451 Exercise classes, nonphysician provider, per session

S9452 Nutrition classes, nonphysician provider, per session

S9453 Smoking cessation classes, nonphysician provider, per session

S9454 Stress management classes, nonphysician provider, per session

S9455 Diabetic management program, group session

S9460 Diabetic management program, nurse visit

S9465 Diabetic management program, dietitian visit

S9470 Nutritional counseling, dietitian visit

S9472 Cardiac rehabilitation program, nonphysician provider, per diem

S9473 Pulmonary rehabilitation program, nonphysician provider, per diem

S9474 Enterostomal therapy by a registered nurse certified in enterostomal therapy, per diem

S9475 Ambulatory setting substance abuse treatment or detoxification services, per diem

S9476 Vestibular rehabilitation program, nonphysician provider, per diem

S9480 Intensive outpatient psychiatric services, per diem

S9482 Family stabilization services, per 15 minutes ☑

S9484 Crisis intervention mental health services, per hour ☑

S9485 Crisis intervention mental health services, per diem

S9490 Home infusion therapy, corticosteroid infusion; administrative services, professional pharmacy services, care coordination, and all necessary supplies and equipment (drugs and nursing visits coded separately), per diem ☑

S9494 Home infusion therapy, antibiotic, antiviral, or antifungal therapy; administrative services, professional pharmacy services, care coordination, and all necessary supplies and equipment (drugs and nursing visits coded separately), per diem (do not use this code with home infusion codes for hourly dosing schedules S9497-S9504) ☑

S9497 Home infusion therapy, antibiotic, antiviral, or antifungal therapy; once every 3 hours; administrative services, professional pharmacy services, care coordination, and all necessary supplies and equipment (drugs and nursing visits coded separately), per diem ☑

S9500 Home infusion therapy, antibiotic, antiviral, or antifungal therapy; once every 24 hours; administrative services, professional pharmacy services, care coordination, and all necessary supplies and equipment (drugs and nursing visits coded separately), per diem ☑

S9501 Home infusion therapy, antibiotic, antiviral, or antifungal therapy; once every 12 hours; administrative services, professional pharmacy services, care coordination, and all necessary supplies and equipment (drugs and nursing visits coded separately), per diem ☑

S9502 Home infusion therapy, antibiotic, antiviral, or antifungal therapy; once every 8 hours, administrative services, professional pharmacy services, care coordination, and all necessary supplies and equipment (drugs and nursing visits coded separately), per diem ☑

S9503 Home infusion therapy, antibiotic, antiviral, or antifungal; once every 6 hours; administrative services, professional pharmacy services, care coordination, and all necessary supplies and equipment (drugs and nursing visits coded separately), per diem ☑

S9504 Home infusion therapy, antibiotic, antiviral, or antifungal; once every 4 hours; administrative services, professional pharmacy services, care coordination, and all necessary supplies and equipment (drugs and nursing visits coded separately), per diem ☑

S9529 Routine venipuncture for collection of specimen(s), single homebound, nursing home, or skilled nursing facility patient ☑

S9537 Home therapy; hematopoietic hormone injection therapy (e.g., erythropoietin, G-CSF, GM-CSF); administrative services, professional pharmacy services, care coordination, and all necessary supplies and equipment (drugs and nursing visits coded separately), per diem ☑

S9538 Home transfusion of blood product(s); administrative services, professional pharmacy services, care coordination and all necessary supplies and equipment (blood products, drugs, and nursing visits coded separately), per diem ☑

S9542 Home injectable therapy, not otherwise classified, including administrative services, professional pharmacy services, care coordination, and all necessary supplies and equipment (drugs and nursing visits coded separately), per diem ☑

S9558 Home injectable therapy; growth hormone, including administrative services, professional pharmacy services, care coordination, and all necessary supplies and equipment (drugs and nursing visits coded separately), per diem ☑

S9559 Home injectable therapy, interferon, including administrative services, professional pharmacy services, care coordination, and all necessary supplies and equipment (drugs and nursing visits coded separately), per diem ☑

S9560 Home injectable therapy; hormonal therapy (e.g., leuprolide, goserelin), including administrative services, professional pharmacy services, care coordination, and all necessary supplies and equipment (drugs and nursing visits coded separately), per diem ☑

S9562 Home injectable therapy, palivizumab, including administrative services, professional pharmacy services, care coordination, and all necessary supplies and equipment (drugs and nursing visits coded separately), per diem ☑

S9590 Home therapy, irrigation therapy (e.g., sterile irrigation of an organ or anatomical cavity); including administrative services, professional pharmacy services, care coordination, and all necessary supplies and equipment (drugs and nursing visits coded separately), per diem ☑

S9810 Home therapy; professional pharmacy services for provision of infusion, specialty drug administration, and/or disease state management, not otherwise classified, per hour (do not use this code with any per diem code) ☑

S9900 Services by a Journal-listed Christian Science practitioner for the purpose of healing, per diem

S9901 Services by a Journal-listed Christian Science nurse, per hour

S9960 Ambulance service, conventional air services, nonemergency transport, one way (fixed wing)

S9961 Ambulance service, conventional air service, nonemergency transport, one way (rotary wing)

S9970 Health club membership, annual

S9975 Transplant related lodging, meals and transportation, per diem

S9976 Lodging, per diem, not otherwise classified

S9977 Meals, per diem, not otherwise specified

S9981 Medical records copying fee, administrative

S9982 Medical records copying fee, per page ☑

© 2019 Optum360, LLC

S9986	Not medically necessary service (patient is aware that service not medically necessary)
S9988	Services provided as part of a Phase I clinical trial
S9989	Services provided outside of the United States of America (list in addition to code(s) for services(s))
S9990	Services provided as part of a Phase II clinical trial
S9991	Services provided as part of a Phase III clinical trial
S9992	Transportation costs to and from trial location and local transportation costs (e.g., fares for taxicab or bus) for clinical trial participant and one caregiver/companion
S9994	Lodging costs (e.g., hotel charges) for clinical trial participant and one caregiver/companion
S9996	Meals for clinical trial participant and one caregiver/companion
S9999	Sales tax

© 2019 Optum360, LLC

National T Codes Established for State Medicaid Agencies T1000-T5999

The T codes are designed for use by Medicaid state agencies to establish codes for items for which there are no permanent national codes but for which codes are necessary to administer the Medicaid program (T codes are not accepted by Medicare but can be used by private insurers). This range of codes describes nursing and home health-related services, substance abuse treatment, and certain training-related procedures.

T1000 Private duty/independent nursing service(s), licensed, up to 15 minutes ☑

T1001 Nursing assessment/evaluation

T1002 RN services, up to 15 minutes ☑

T1003 LPN/LVN services, up to 15 minutes ☑

T1004 Services of a qualified nursing aide, up to 15 minutes ☑

T1005 Respite care services, up to 15 minutes ☑

T1006 Alcohol and/or substance abuse services, family/couple counseling

T1007 Alcohol and/or substance abuse services, treatment plan development and/or modification

T1009 Child sitting services for children of the individual receiving alcohol and/or substance abuse services

T1010 Meals for individuals receiving alcohol and/or substance abuse services (when meals not included in the program)

T1012 Alcohol and/or substance abuse services, skills development

T1013 Sign language or oral interpretive services, per 15 minutes ☑

T1014 Telehealth transmission, per minute, professional services bill separately

T1015 Clinic visit/encounter, all-inclusive
AHA: 1Q, '02, 5

T1016 Case management, each 15 minutes ☑

T1017 Targeted case management, each 15 minutes ☑

T1018 School-based individualized education program (IEP) services, bundled

T1019 Personal care services, per 15 minutes, not for an inpatient or resident of a hospital, nursing facility, ICF/MR or IMD, part of the individualized plan of treatment (code may not be used to identify services provided by home health aide or certified nurse assistant) ☑

T1020 Personal care services, per diem, not for an inpatient or resident of a hospital, nursing facility, ICF/MR or IMD, part of the individualized plan of treatment (code may not be used to identify services provided by home health aide or certified nurse assistant)

T1021 Home health aide or certified nurse assistant, per visit

T1022 Contracted home health agency services, all services provided under contract, per day

T1023 Screening to determine the appropriateness of consideration of an individual for participation in a specified program, project or treatment protocol, per encounter

T1024 Evaluation and treatment by an integrated, specialty team contracted to provide coordinated care to multiple or severely handicapped children, per encounter A

T1025 Intensive, extended multidisciplinary services provided in a clinic setting to children with complex medical, physical, mental and psychosocial impairments, per diem A

T1026 Intensive, extended multidisciplinary services provided in a clinic setting to children with complex medical, physical, medical and psychosocial impairments, per hour A

T1027 Family training and counseling for child development, per 15 minutes ☑

T1028 Assessment of home, physical and family environment, to determine suitability to meet patient's medical needs

T1029 Comprehensive environmental lead investigation, not including laboratory analysis, per dwelling

T1030 Nursing care, in the home, by registered nurse, per diem ☑

T1031 Nursing care, in the home, by licensed practical nurse, per diem ☑

T1040 Medicaid certified community behavioral health clinic services, per diem

T1041 Medicaid certified community behavioral health clinic services, per month

T1502 Administration of oral, intramuscular and/or subcutaneous medication by health care agency/professional, per visit ☑

T1503 Administration of medication, other than oral and/or injectable, by a health care agency/professional, per visit ☑

T1505 Electronic medication compliance management device, includes all components and accessories, not otherwise classified

T1999 Miscellaneous therapeutic items and supplies, retail purchases, not otherwise classified; identify product in "remarks"

T2001 Nonemergency transportation; patient attendant/escort

T2002 Nonemergency transportation; per diem ☑

T2003 Nonemergency transportation; encounter/trip

T2004 Nonemergency transport; commercial carrier, multipass

T2005 Nonemergency transportation; stretcher van

T2007 Transportation waiting time, air ambulance and nonemergency vehicle, one-half (1/2) hour increments ☑

T2010 Preadmission screening and resident review (PASRR) Level I identification screening, per screen ☑

T2011 Preadmission screening and resident review (PASRR) Level II evaluation, per evaluation

T2012 Habilitation, educational; waiver, per diem ☑

T2013 Habilitation, educational, waiver; per hour ☑

T2014 Habilitation, prevocational, waiver; per diem ☑

T2015 Habilitation, prevocational, waiver; per hour ☑

T2016 Habilitation, residential, waiver; per diem ☑

T2017 Habilitation, residential, waiver; 15 minutes ☑

T2018 Habilitation, supported employment, waiver; per diem ☑

T2019 Habilitation, supported employment, waiver; per 15 minutes ☑

T2020 Day habilitation, waiver; per diem ☑

T2021 Day habilitation, waiver; per 15 minutes ☑

T2022 Case management, per month ☑

T2023 Targeted case management; per month ☑

T2024 Service assessment/plan of care development, waiver

T2025 Waiver services; not otherwise specified (NOS)

T2026 Specialized childcare, waiver; per diem ☑

T2027 Specialized childcare, waiver; per 15 minutes ☑

T2028 Specialized supply, not otherwise specified, waiver

T2029 Specialized medical equipment, not otherwise specified, waiver

© 2019 Optum360, LLC

T2030 Assisted living, waiver; per month ☑

T2031 Assisted living; waiver, per diem ☑

T2032 Residential care, not otherwise specified (NOS), waiver; per month ☑

T2033 Residential care, not otherwise specified (NOS), waiver; per diem ☑

T2034 Crisis intervention, waiver; per diem ☑

T2035 Utility services to support medical equipment and assistive technology/devices, waiver

T2036 Therapeutic camping, overnight, waiver; each session ☑

T2037 Therapeutic camping, day, waiver; each session ☑

T2038 Community transition, waiver; per service ☑

T2039 Vehicle modifications, waiver; per service ☑

T2040 Financial management, self-directed, waiver; per 15 minutes ☑

T2041 Supports brokerage, self-directed, waiver; per 15 minutes ☑

T2042 Hospice routine home care; per diem ☑
CMS: 100-04,11,10

T2043 Hospice continuous home care; per hour ☑
CMS: 100-04,11,10

T2044 Hospice inpatient respite care; per diem ☑
CMS: 100-04,11,10

T2045 Hospice general inpatient care; per diem ☑
CMS: 100-04,11,10

T2046 Hospice long-term care, room and board only; per diem ☑
CMS: 100-04,11,10

T2048 Behavioral health; long-term care residential (nonacute care in a residential treatment program where stay is typically longer than 30 days), with room and board, per diem ☑

T2049 Nonemergency transportation; stretcher van, mileage; per mile ☑

T2101 Human breast milk processing, storage and distribution only ♀

T4521 Adult sized disposable incontinence product, brief/diaper, small, each ☑

T4522 Adult sized disposable incontinence product, brief/diaper, medium, each ☑

T4523 Adult sized disposable incontinence product, brief/diaper, large, each ☑

T4524 Adult sized disposable incontinence product, brief/diaper, extra large, each ☑

T4525 Adult sized disposable incontinence product, protective underwear/pull-on, small size, each ☑

T4526 Adult sized disposable incontinence product, protective underwear/pull-on, medium size, each ☑

T4527 Adult sized disposable incontinence product, protective underwear/pull-on, large size, each ☑

T4528 Adult sized disposable incontinence product, protective underwear/pull-on, extra large size, each ☑

T4529 Pediatric sized disposable incontinence product, brief/diaper, small/medium size, each ☑

T4530 Pediatric sized disposable incontinence product, brief/diaper, large size, each ☑

T4531 Pediatric sized disposable incontinence product, protective underwear/pull-on, small/medium size, each ☑

T4532 Pediatric sized disposable incontinence product, protective underwear/pull-on, large size, each ☑

T4533 Youth sized disposable incontinence product, brief/diaper, each ☑

T4534 Youth sized disposable incontinence product, protective underwear/pull-on, each ☑

T4535 Disposable liner/shield/guard/pad/undergarment, for incontinence, each ☑

T4536 Incontinence product, protective underwear/pull-on, reusable, any size, each ☑

T4537 Incontinence product, protective underpad, reusable, bed size, each ☑

T4538 Diaper service, reusable diaper, each diaper ☑

T4539 Incontinence product, diaper/brief, reusable, any size, each ☑

T4540 Incontinence product, protective underpad, reusable, chair size, each ☑

T4541 Incontinence product, disposable underpad, large, each ☑

T4542 Incontinence product, disposable underpad, small size, each ☑

T4543 Adult sized disposable incontinence product, protective brief/diaper, above extra large, each ☑

T4544 Adult sized disposable incontinence product, protective underwear/pull-on, above extra large, each

T4545 Incontinence product, disposable, penile wrap, each

T5001 Positioning seat for persons with special orthopedic needs

T5999 Supply, not otherwise specified

© 2019 Optum360, LLC

Vision Services V2020-V2799

These V codes include vision-related supplies, including spectacles, lenses, contact lenses, prostheses, intraocular lenses, and miscellaneous lenses.

Frames

V2020 **Frames, purchases** A ♿

V2025 **Deluxe frame** E
CMS: 100-04,1,30.3.5

Single Vision, Glass, or Plastic

V2100 **Sphere, single vision, plano to plus or minus 4.00, per lens** A ☑ ♿

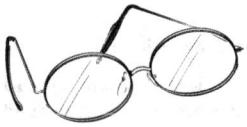

Monofocal spectacles (V2100–V2114)

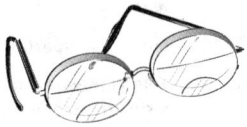

Trifocal spectacles (V2300–V2314)

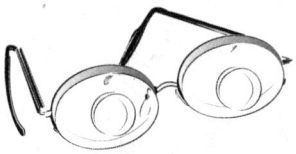

Low vision aids mounted to spectacles (V2610)

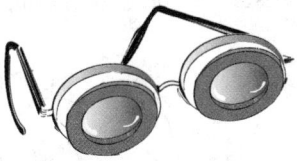

Telescopic or other compound lens fitted on spectacles as a low vision aid (V2615)

V2101 **Sphere, single vision, plus or minus 4.12 to plus or minus 7.00d, per lens** A ☑ ♿

V2102 **Sphere, single vision, plus or minus 7.12 to plus or minus 20.00d, per lens** A ☑ ♿

V2103 **Spherocylinder, single vision, plano to plus or minus 4.00d sphere, 0.12 to 2.00d cylinder, per lens** A ☑ ♿

V2104 **Spherocylinder, single vision, plano to plus or minus 4.00d sphere, 2.12 to 4.00d cylinder, per lens** A ☑ ♿

V2105 **Spherocylinder, single vision, plano to plus or minus 4.00d sphere, 4.25 to 6.00d cylinder, per lens** A ☑ ♿

V2106 **Spherocylinder, single vision, plano to plus or minus 4.00d sphere, over 6.00d cylinder, per lens** A ☑ ♿

V2107 **Spherocylinder, single vision, plus or minus 4.25 to plus or minus 7.00 sphere, 0.12 to 2.00d cylinder, per lens** A ☑ ♿

V2108 **Spherocylinder, single vision, plus or minus 4.25d to plus or minus 7.00d sphere, 2.12 to 4.00d cylinder, per lens** A ☑ ♿

V2109 **Spherocylinder, single vision, plus or minus 4.25 to plus or minus 7.00d sphere, 4.25 to 6.00d cylinder, per lens** A ☑ ♿

V2110 **Spherocylinder, single vision, plus or minus 4.25 to 7.00d sphere, over 6.00d cylinder, per lens** A ☑ ♿

V2111 **Spherocylinder, single vision, plus or minus 7.25 to plus or minus 12.00d sphere, 0.25 to 2.25d cylinder, per lens** A ☑ ♿

V2112 **Spherocylinder, single vision, plus or minus 7.25 to plus or minus 12.00d sphere, 2.25d to 4.00d cylinder, per lens** A ☑ ♿

V2113 **Spherocylinder, single vision, plus or minus 7.25 to plus or minus 12.00d sphere, 4.25 to 6.00d cylinder, per lens** A ☑ ♿

V2114 **Spherocylinder, single vision, sphere over plus or minus 12.00d, per lens** A ☑ ♿

V2115 **Lenticular (myodisc), per lens, single vision** A ☑ ♿

V2118 **Aniseikonic lens, single vision** A ♿

V2121 **Lenticular lens, per lens, single** A ☑ ♿

V2199 **Not otherwise classified, single vision lens** A

Bifocal, Glass, or Plastic

V2200 **Sphere, bifocal, plano to plus or minus 4.00d, per lens** A ☑ ♿

V2201 **Sphere, bifocal, plus or minus 4.12 to plus or minus 7.00d, per lens** A ☑ ♿

V2202 **Sphere, bifocal, plus or minus 7.12 to plus or minus 20.00d, per lens** A ☑ ♿

V2203 **Spherocylinder, bifocal, plano to plus or minus 4.00d sphere, 0.12 to 2.00d cylinder, per lens** A ☑ ♿

V2204 **Spherocylinder, bifocal, plano to plus or minus 4.00d sphere, 2.12 to 4.00d cylinder, per lens** A ☑ ♿

V2205 **Spherocylinder, bifocal, plano to plus or minus 4.00d sphere, 4.25 to 6.00d cylinder, per lens** A ☑ ♿

V2206 **Spherocylinder, bifocal, plano to plus or minus 4.00d sphere, over 6.00d cylinder, per lens** A ☑ ♿

V2207 **Spherocylinder, bifocal, plus or minus 4.25 to plus or minus 7.00d sphere, 0.12 to 2.00d cylinder, per lens** A ☑ ♿

V2208 **Spherocylinder, bifocal, plus or minus 4.25 to plus or minus 7.00d sphere, 2.12 to 4.00d cylinder, per lens** A ☑ ♿

V2209 **Spherocylinder, bifocal, plus or minus 4.25 to plus or minus 7.00d sphere, 4.25 to 6.00d cylinder, per lens** A ☑ ♿

V2210 **Spherocylinder, bifocal, plus or minus 4.25 to plus or minus 7.00d sphere, over 6.00d cylinder, per lens** A ☑ ♿

V2211 **Spherocylinder, bifocal, plus or minus 7.25 to plus or minus 12.00d sphere, 0.25 to 2.25d cylinder, per lens** A ☑ ♿

V2212 **Spherocylinder, bifocal, plus or minus 7.25 to plus or minus 12.00d sphere, 2.25 to 4.00d cylinder, per lens** A ☑ ♿

V2213 **Spherocylinder, bifocal, plus or minus 7.25 to plus or minus 12.00d sphere, 4.25 to 6.00d cylinder, per lens** A ☑ ♿

V2214 **Spherocylinder, bifocal, sphere over plus or minus 12.00d, per lens** A ☑ ♿

V2215 **Lenticular (myodisc), per lens, bifocal** A ☑ ♿

V2218 **Aniseikonic, per lens, bifocal** A ☑ ♿

V2219 **Bifocal seg width over 28mm** A ☑ ♿

V2220 **Bifocal add over 3.25d** A ☑ ♿

V2221 **Lenticular lens, per lens, bifocal** A ♿

V2299 **Specialty bifocal (by report)** A
Pertinent documentation to evaluate medical appropriateness should be included when this code is reported.

Trifocal, Glass, or Plastic

V2300 **Sphere, trifocal, plano to plus or minus 4.00d, per lens** A ☑ ♿

V2301 **Sphere, trifocal, plus or minus 4.12 to plus or minus 7.00d per lens** A ☑ ♿

V2302 **Sphere, trifocal, plus or minus 7.12 to plus or minus 20.00, per lens** A ☑ ♿

V2303 **Spherocylinder, trifocal, plano to plus or minus 4.00d sphere, 0.12 to 2.00d cylinder, per lens** A ☑ ♿

V2304 **Spherocylinder, trifocal, plano to plus or minus 4.00d sphere, 2.25 to 4.00d cylinder, per lens** A ☑ ♿

V2305 **Spherocylinder, trifocal, plano to plus or minus 4.00d sphere, 4.25 to 6.00 cylinder, per lens** A ☑ ♿

© 2019 Optum360, LLC

V2306 **Spherocylinder, trifocal, plano to plus or minus 4.00d sphere, over 6.00d cylinder, per lens** A ☑ ♿

V2307 **Spherocylinder, trifocal, plus or minus 4.25 to plus or minus 7.00d sphere, 0.12 to 2.00d cylinder, per lens** A ☑ ♿

V2308 **Spherocylinder, trifocal, plus or minus 4.25 to plus or minus 7.00d sphere, 2.12 to 4.00d cylinder, per lens** A ☑ ♿

V2309 **Spherocylinder, trifocal, plus or minus 4.25 to plus or minus 7.00d sphere, 4.25 to 6.00d cylinder, per lens** A ☑ ♿

V2310 **Spherocylinder, trifocal, plus or minus 4.25 to plus or minus 7.00d sphere, over 6.00d cylinder, per lens** A ☑ ♿

V2311 **Spherocylinder, trifocal, plus or minus 7.25 to plus or minus 12.00d sphere, 0.25 to 2.25d cylinder, per lens** A ☑ ♿

V2312 **Spherocylinder, trifocal, plus or minus 7.25 to plus or minus 12.00d sphere, 2.25 to 4.00d cylinder, per lens** A ☑ ♿

V2313 **Spherocylinder, trifocal, plus or minus 7.25 to plus or minus 12.00d sphere, 4.25 to 6.00d cylinder, per lens** A ☑ ♿

V2314 **Spherocylinder, trifocal, sphere over plus or minus 12.00d, per lens** A ☑ ♿

V2315 **Lenticular, (myodisc), per lens, trifocal** A ☑ ♿

V2318 **Aniseikonic lens, trifocal** A ♿

V2319 **Trifocal seg width over 28 mm** A ☑ ♿

V2320 **Trifocal add over 3.25d** A ☑ ♿

V2321 **Lenticular lens, per lens, trifocal** A ♿

V2399 **Specialty trifocal (by report)** A

Pertinent documentation to evaluate medical appropriateness should be included when this code is reported.

Variable Asphericity Lens, Glass, or Plastic

V2410 **Variable asphericity lens, single vision, full field, glass or plastic, per lens** A ☑ ♿

V2430 **Variable asphericity lens, bifocal, full field, glass or plastic, per lens** A ☑ ♿

V2499 **Variable sphericity lens, other type** A

Contact Lens

V2500 **Contact lens, PMMA, spherical, per lens** A ☑ ♿

V2501 **Contact lens, PMMA, toric or prism ballast, per lens** A ☑ ♿

V2502 **Contact lens PMMA, bifocal, per lens** A ☑ ♿

V2503 **Contact lens, PMMA, color vision deficiency, per lens** A ☑ ♿

V2510 **Contact lens, gas permeable, spherical, per lens** A ☑ ♿

V2511 **Contact lens, gas permeable, toric, prism ballast, per lens** A ☑ ♿

V2512 **Contact lens, gas permeable, bifocal, per lens** A ☑ ♿

V2513 **Contact lens, gas permeable, extended wear, per lens** A ☑ ♿

V2520 **Contact lens, hydrophilic, spherical, per lens** A ☑ ♿

Hydrophilic contact lenses are covered by Medicare only for aphakic patients. Local contractor if incident to physician services.

V2521 **Contact lens, hydrophilic, toric, or prism ballast, per lens** A ☑ ♿

Hydrophilic contact lenses are covered by Medicare only for aphakic patients. Local contractor if incident to physician services.

V2522 **Contact lens, hydrophilic, bifocal, per lens** A ☑ ♿

Hydrophilic contact lenses are covered by Medicare only for aphakic patients. Local contractor if incident to physician services.

V2523 **Contact lens, hydrophilic, extended wear, per lens** A ☑ ♿

Hydrophilic contact lenses are covered by Medicare only for aphakic patients.

V2530 **Contact lens, scleral, gas impermeable, per lens (for contact lens modification, see 92325)** A ☑ ♿

V2531 **Contact lens, scleral, gas permeable, per lens (for contact lens modification, see 92325)** A ☑ ♿

V2599 **Contact lens, other type** A

Local contractor if incident to physician services.

Vision Aids

V2600 **Hand held low vision aids and other nonspectacle mounted aids** A

V2610 **Single lens spectacle mounted low vision aids** A

V2615 **Telescopic and other compound lens system, including distance vision telescopic, near vision telescopes and compound microscopic lens system** A

Prosthetic Eye

V2623 **Prosthetic eye, plastic, custom** A ♿

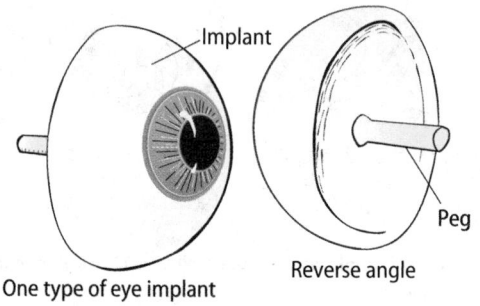

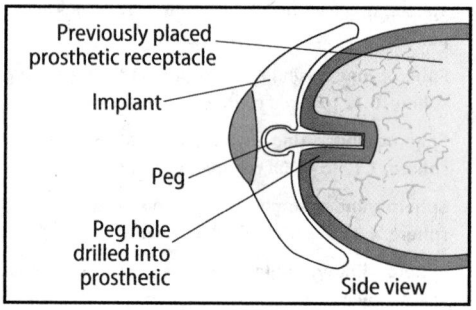

V2624 **Polishing/resurfacing of ocular prosthesis** A ♿

V2625 **Enlargement of ocular prosthesis** A ♿

V2626 **Reduction of ocular prosthesis** A ♿

V2627 **Scleral cover shell** A ♿

A scleral shell covers the cornea and the anterior sclera. Medicare covers a scleral shell when it is prescribed as an artificial support to a shrunken and sightless eye or as a barrier in the treatment of severe dry eye.

V2628 **Fabrication and fitting of ocular conformer** A ♿

V2629 **Prosthetic eye, other type** A

Intraocular Lenses

V2630 **Anterior chamber intraocular lens** N M ♿

The IOL must be FDA-approved for reimbursement. Medicare payment for an IOL is included in the payment for ASC facility services. Medicare jurisdiction: local contractor.

© 2019 Optum360, LLC

V2631 **Iris supported intraocular lens** N N1 ♿
The IOL must be FDA-approved for reimbursement. Medicare payment for an IOL is included in the payment for ASC facility services. Medicare jurisdiction: local contractor.

V2632 **Posterior chamber intraocular lens** N N1 ♿
The IOL must be FDA-approved for reimbursement. Medicare payment for an IOL is included in the payment for ASC facility services. Medicare jurisdiction: local contractor.
CMS: 100-04,32,120.2

Miscellaneous

V2700 **Balance lens, per lens** A ☑ ♿

V2702 **Deluxe lens feature** E

V2710 **Slab off prism, glass or plastic, per lens** A ☑ ♿

V2715 **Prism, per lens** A ☑ ♿

V2718 **Press-on lens, Fresnel prism, per lens** A ☑ ♿

V2730 **Special base curve, glass or plastic, per lens** A ☑ ♿

V2744 **Tint, photochromatic, per lens** A ☑ ♿

V2745 **Addition to lens; tint, any color, solid, gradient or equal, excludes photochromatic, any lens material, per lens** A ☑ ♿

V2750 **Antireflective coating, per lens** A ☑ ♿

V2755 **U-V lens, per lens** A ☑ ♿

V2756 **Eye glass case** E

V2760 **Scratch resistant coating, per lens** E ☑ ♿

V2761 **Mirror coating, any type, solid, gradient or equal, any lens material, per lens** B ☑

V2762 **Polarization, any lens material, per lens** E ☑ ♿

V2770 **Occluder lens, per lens** A ☑ ♿

V2780 **Oversize lens, per lens** A ☑ ♿

V2781 **Progressive lens, per lens** B ☑

V2782 **Lens, index 1.54 to 1.65 plastic or 1.60 to 1.79 glass, excludes polycarbonate, per lens** A ☑ ♿

V2783 **Lens, index greater than or equal to 1.66 plastic or greater than or equal to 1.80 glass, excludes polycarbonate, per lens** A ☑ ♿

V2784 **Lens, polycarbonate or equal, any index, per lens** A ☑ ♿

V2785 **Processing, preserving and transporting corneal tissue** F F4
Medicare jurisdiction: local contractor.
CMS: 100-04,4,200.1

V2786 **Specialty occupational multifocal lens, per lens** E ☑ ♿

V2787 **Astigmatism correcting function of intraocular lens** E
CMS: 100-04,32,120.1; 100-04,32,120.2

V2788 **Presbyopia correcting function of intraocular lens** E
CMS: 100-04,32,120.1; 100-04,32,120.2

V2790 **Amniotic membrane for surgical reconstruction, per procedure** N N1
Medicare jurisdiction: local contractor.
CMS: 100-04,4,200.4

V2797 **Vision supply, accessory and/or service component of another HCPCS vision code** E

V2799 **Vision item or service, miscellaneous** A
Determine if an alternative HCPCS Level II or a CPT code better describes the service being reported. This code should be used only if a more specific code is unavailable.

Hearing Services V5008-V5364

This range of codes describes hearing tests and related supplies and equipment, speech-language pathology screenings, and repair of augmentative communicative system.

Hearing Services

V5008 **Hearing screening** E

V5010 **Assessment for hearing aid** E

V5011 **Fitting/orientation/checking of hearing aid** E

V5014 **Repair/modification of a hearing aid** E

V5020 **Conformity evaluation** E

Monaural Hearing Aid

V5030 **Hearing aid, monaural, body worn, air conduction** E

V5040 **Hearing aid, monaural, body worn, bone conduction** E

V5050 **Hearing aid, monaural, in the ear** E

V5060 **Hearing aid, monaural, behind the ear** E

Other Hearing Services

V5070 **Glasses, air conduction** E

V5080 **Glasses, bone conduction** E

V5090 **Dispensing fee, unspecified hearing aid** E

V5095 **Semi-implantable middle ear hearing prosthesis** E

V5100 **Hearing aid, bilateral, body worn** E

V5110 **Dispensing fee, bilateral** E

Hearing Aids, Services, and Accessories

V5120 **Binaural, body** E

V5130 **Binaural, in the ear** E

V5140 **Binaural, behind the ear** E

V5150 **Binaural, glasses** E

V5160 **Dispensing fee, binaural** E

V5171 **Hearing aid, contralateral routing device, monaural, in the ear (ITE)**

V5172 **Hearing aid, contralateral routing device, monaural, in the canal (ITC)**

V5181 **Hearing aid, contralateral routing device, monaural, behind the ear (BTE)**

V5190 **Hearing aid, contralateral routing, monaural, glasses** E

V5200 **Dispensing fee, contralateral, monaural** E

V5211 **Hearing aid, contralateral routing system, binaural, ITE/ITE**

V5212 **Hearing aid, contralateral routing system, binaural, ITE/ITC**

V5213 **Hearing aid, contralateral routing system, binaural, ITE/BTE**

V5214 **Hearing aid, contralateral routing system, binaural, ITC/ITC**

V5215 **Hearing aid, contralateral routing system, binaural, ITC/BTE**

V5221 **Hearing aid, contralateral routing system, binaural, BTE/BTE**

V5230 **Hearing aid, contralateral routing system, binaural, glasses** E

V5240 **Dispensing fee, contralateral routing system, binaural** E

V5241 **Dispensing fee, monaural hearing aid, any type** E
AHA: 1Q, '02, 5

V5242 **Hearing aid, analog, monaural, CIC (completely in the ear canal)** E
AHA: 1Q, '02, 5

© 2019 Optum360, LLC

V5243 Hearing aid, analog, monaural, ITC (in the canal) E
AHA: 1Q, '02, 5

V5244 Hearing aid, digitally programmable analog, monaural, CIC E
AHA: 1Q, '02, 5

V5245 Hearing aid, digitally programmable, analog, monaural, ITC E
AHA: 1Q, '02, 5

V5246 Hearing aid, digitally programmable analog, monaural, ITE (in the ear) E
AHA: 1Q, '02, 5

V5247 Hearing aid, digitally programmable analog, monaural, BTE (behind the ear) E
AHA: 1Q, '02, 5

V5248 Hearing aid, analog, binaural, CIC E
AHA: 1Q, '02, 5

V5249 Hearing aid, analog, binaural, ITC E
AHA: 1Q, '02, 5

V5250 Hearing aid, digitally programmable analog, binaural, CIC E
AHA: 1Q, '02, 5

V5251 Hearing aid, digitally programmable analog, binaural, ITC E
AHA: 1Q, '02, 5

V5252 Hearing aid, digitally programmable, binaural, ITE E
AHA: 1Q, '02, 5

V5253 Hearing aid, digitally programmable, binaural, BTE E
AHA: 1Q, '02, 5

V5254 Hearing aid, digital, monaural, CIC E
AHA: 1Q, '02, 5

V5255 Hearing aid, digital, monaural, ITC E
AHA: 1Q, '02, 5

V5256 Hearing aid, digital, monaural, ITE E
AHA: 1Q, '02, 5

V5257 Hearing aid, digital, monaural, BTE E
AHA: 1Q, '02, 5

V5258 Hearing aid, digital, binaural, CIC E
AHA: 1Q, '02, 5

V5259 Hearing aid, digital, binaural, ITC E
AHA: 1Q, '02, 5

V5260 Hearing aid, digital, binaural, ITE E
AHA: 1Q, '02, 5

V5261 Hearing aid, digital, binaural, BTE E
AHA: 1Q, '02, 5

V5262 Hearing aid, disposable, any type, monaural E
AHA: 1Q, '02, 5

V5263 Hearing aid, disposable, any type, binaural E
AHA: 1Q, '02, 5

V5264 Ear mold/insert, not disposable, any type E
AHA: 1Q, '02, 5

V5265 Ear mold/insert, disposable, any type E
AHA: 1Q, '02, 5

V5266 Battery for use in hearing device E
AHA: 1Q, '02, 5

V5267 Hearing aid or assistive listening device/supplies/accessories, not otherwise specified E
AHA: 1Q, '02, 5

Assistive Listening Device

V5268 Assistive listening device, telephone amplifier, any type E
AHA: 1Q, '02, 5

V5269 Assistive listening device, alerting, any type E
AHA: 1Q, '02, 5

V5270 Assistive listening device, television amplifier, any type E
AHA: 1Q, '02, 5

V5271 Assistive listening device, television caption decoder E
AHA: 1Q, '02, 5

V5272 Assistive listening device, TDD E
AHA: 1Q, '02, 5

V5273 Assistive listening device, for use with cochlear implant E
AHA: 1Q, '02, 5

V5274 Assistive listening device, not otherwise specified E
AHA: 1Q, '02, 5

Miscellaneous Hearing Services

V5275 Ear impression, each E ☑
AHA: 1Q, '02, 5

V5281 Assistive listening device, personal FM/DM system, monaural (1 receiver, transmitter, microphone), any type E

V5282 Assistive listening device, personal FM/DM system, binaural (2 receivers, transmitter, microphone), any type E

V5283 Assistive listening device, personal FM/DM neck, loop induction receiver E

V5284 Assistive listening device, personal FM/DM, ear level receiver E

V5285 Assistive listening device, personal FM/DM, direct audio input receiver E

V5286 Assistive listening device, personal blue tooth FM/DM receiver E

V5287 Assistive listening device, personal FM/DM receiver, not otherwise specified E

V5288 Assistive listening device, personal FM/DM transmitter assistive listening device E

V5289 Assistive listening device, personal FM/DM adapter/boot coupling device for receiver, any type E

V5290 Assistive listening device, transmitter microphone, any type E

V5298 Hearing aid, not otherwise classified E

V5299 Hearing service, miscellaneous B ⊘
Determine if an alternative HCPCS Level II or a CPT code better describes the service being reported. This code should be used only if a more specific code is unavailable.

Speech-Language Pathology Services

V5336 Repair/modification of augmentative communicative system or device (excludes adaptive hearing aid) E
Medicare jurisdiction: DME regional contractor.

V5362 Speech screening E

V5363 Language screening E

V5364 Dysphagia screening E

© 2019 Optum360, LLC

Appendix 1 — Table of Drugs and Biologicals

INTRODUCTION AND DIRECTIONS

The HCPCS 2020 Table of Drugs and Biologicals is designed to quickly and easily direct the user to drug names and their corresponding codes. Both generic and brand or trade names are alphabetically listed in the "Drug Name" column of the table. The associated A, C, J, K, Q, or S code is given only for the generic name of the drug. While every effort is made to make the table comprehensive, it is not all-inclusive.

The "Unit Per" column lists the stated amount for the referenced generic drug as provided by CMS. "Up to" listings are inclusive of all quantities up to and including the listed amount. All other listings are for the amount of the drug as listed. The editors recognize that the availability of some drugs in the quantities listed is dependent on many variables beyond the control of the clinical ordering clerk. The availability in your area of regularly used drugs in the most cost-effective quantities should be relayed to your third-party payers.

The "Route of Administration" column addresses the most common methods of delivering the referenced generic drug as described in current pharmaceutical literature. The official definitions for Level II drug codes generally describe administration other than by oral method. Therefore, with a handful of exceptions, oral-delivered options for most drugs are omitted from the Route of Administration column.

Intravenous administration includes all methods, such as gravity infusion, injections, and timed pushes. When several routes of administration are listed, the first listing is simply the first, or most common, method as described in current reference literature. The "VAR" posting denotes various routes of administration and is used for drugs that are commonly administered into joints, cavities, tissues, or topical applications, in addition to other parenteral administrations. Listings posted with "OTH" alert the user to other administration methods, such as suppositories or catheter injections.

Please be reminded that the Table of Drugs and Biologicals, as well as all HCPCS Level II national definitions and listings, constitutes a post-treatment medical reference for billing purposes only. Although the editors have exercised all normal precautions to ensure the accuracy of the table and related material, the use of any of this information to select medical treatment is entirely inappropriate. Do not code directly from the table. Refer to the tabular section for complete information.

See Appendix 3 for abbreviations.

Drug Name	Unit Per	Route	Code
10% LMD	500 ML	IV	J7100
4-FACTOR PROTHROMBRIN COMPLEX CONCENTRATE	1 IU	IV	C9132
5% DEXTROSE AND .45% NORMAL SALINE	1000 ML	IV	S5010
5% DEXTROSE IN LACTATED RINGERS	1000 CC	IV	J7121
5% DEXTROSE WITH POTASSIUM CHLORIDE	1000 ML	IV	S5012
5% DEXTROSE/.45% NS WITH KCL AND MAG SULFATE	1000ML	IV	S5013
5% DEXTROSE/.45% NS WITH KCL AND MAG SULFATE	1500 ML	IV	S5014
5% DEXTROSE/NORMAL SALINE	5%	VAR	J7042
5% DEXTROSE/WATER	500 ML	IV	J7060
A-HYDROCORT	100 MG	IV, IM, SC	J1720
A-METHAPRED	125 MG	IM, IV	J2930
A-METHAPRED	40 MG	IM, IV	J2920
ABATACEPT	10 MG	IV	J0129
ABCIXIMAB	10 MG	IV	J0130
ABELCET	10 MG	IV	J0287
ABILIFY	0.25 MG	IM	J0400
ABILIFY MAINTENA KIT	1 MG	IM	J0401
ABLAVAR	1 ML	IV	A9583
ABOBOTULINUMTOXINA	5 UNITS	IM	J0586
ABRAXANE	1 MG	IV	J9264
ACCELULAR PERICARDIAL TISSUE MATRIX NONHUMAN	SQ CM	OTH	C9354
ACCUNEB NONCOMPOUNDED, CONCENTRATED	1 MG	INH	J7611
ACCUNEB NONCOMPOUNDED, UNIT DOSE	1 MG	INH	J7613
ACETADOTE	1 G	INH	J7608
ACETADOTE	100 MG	IV	J0132
ACETAMINOPHEN	10 MG	IV	J0131
ACETAZOLAMIDE SODIUM	500 MG	IM, IV	J1120
ACETYLCYSTEINE COMPOUNDED	PER G	INH	J7604
ACETYLCYSTEINE NONCOMPOUNDED	1 G	INH	J7608
ACTEMRA	1 MG	IV	J3262
ACTHREL	1 MCG	IV	J0795
ACTIMMUNE	3 MU	SC	J9216
ACTIVASE	1 MG	IV	J2997
ACUTECT	STUDY DOSE UP TO 20 MCI	IV	A9504
ACYCLOVIR	5 MG	IV	J0133
ADAGEN	25 IU	IM	J2504
ADALIMUMAB	20 MG	SC	J0135
ADASUVE	1 MG	INH	J2062
ADCETRIS	1 MG	IV	J9042
ADENOCARD	1 MG	IV	J0153
ADENOSINE	1 MG	IV	J0153
ADENSOSCAN	1 MG	IV	J0153
ADO-TRASTUZUMAB EMTANSINE	1 MG	IV	J9354
ADRENALIN	0.1 MG	IM, IV, SC	J0171
ADRENOCORT	1 MG	IM, IV, OTH	J1100
ADRIAMYCIN	10 MG	IV	J9000
ADRUCIL	500 MG	IV	J9190
ADYNOVATE	1 IU	IV	J7207
AEROBID	1 MG	INH	J7641
AFFINITY	SQ CM	OTH	Q4159
AFINITOR	0.25 MG	ORAL	J7527
AFLIBERCEPT	1 MG	OTH	J0178
AFLURIA	EA	IM	Q2035
AFSTYLA	1 I.U.	IV	J7210
AGALSIDASE BETA	1 MG	IV	J0180
AGGRASTAT	12.5 MG	IM, IV	J3246
AGRIFLU	UNKNOWN	IM	Q2034
~~AJOVY~~	~~1 MG~~	~~SC~~	~~C9040~~

© 2019 Optum360, LLC

Drug Name	Unit Per	Route	Code
AJOVY	1 MG	SC	J3031
AKYNZEO	235 MG/0.25 MG	IV	J1454
AKYNZEO	300 MG/0.5 MG	ORAL	J8655
ALATROFLOXACIN MESYLATE	100 MG	IV	J0200
ALBUTEROL AND IPRATROPIUM BROMIDE NONCOMPOUNDED	2.5MG/0.5 MG	INH	J7620
ALBUTEROL COMPOUNDED, CONCENTRATED	1 MG	INH	J7610
ALBUTEROL COMPOUNDED, UNIT DOSE	1 MG	INH	J7609
ALBUTEROL NONCOMPOUNDED, UNIT DOSE	1 MG	INH	J7613
ALBUTEROL, NONCOMPOUNDED, CONCENTRATED FORM	1 MG	INH	J7611
ALDESLEUKIN	1 VIAL	IV	J9015
ALDURAZYME	0.1 MG	IV	J1931
ALEFACEPT	0.5 MG	IV, IM	J0215
ALEMTUZUMAB	1 MG	IV	J0202
ALFERON N	250,000 IU	IM	J9215
ALGLUCERASE	10 U	IV	J0205
ALGLUCOSIDASE ALFA (LUMIZYME)	10 MG	IV	J0221
ALGLUCOSIDASE ALFA NOS	10 MG	IV	J0220
ALIMTA	10 MG	IV	J9305
ALIQOPA	1 MG	IV	J9057
ALKERAN	2 MG	ORAL	J8600
ALKERAN	50 MG	IV	J9245
ALLODERM	SQ CM	OTH	Q4116
ALLOGEN	1 CC	OTH	Q4212
ALLOGRAFT, CYMETRA	1 CC	INJ	Q4112
ALLOGRAFT, GRAFTJACKET EXPRESS	1 CC	INJ	Q4113
ALLOPATCHHD	SQ CM	OTH	Q4128
ALLOSKIN	SQ CM	OTH	Q4115
ALLOSKIN AC	SQ CM	OTH	Q4141
ALLOSKIN RT	SQ CM	OTH	Q4123
ALLOWRAP DS OR DRY	SQ CM	OTH	Q4150
ALOXI	25 MCG	IV	J2469
ALPHA 1 - PROTEINASE INHIBITOR (HUMAN) NOS	10 MG	IV	J0256
ALPHA 1-PROTENIASE INHIBITOR (HUMAN) (GLASSIA)	10 MG	IV	J0257
ALPHANATE	PER FACTOR VIII IU	IV	J7186
ALPHANINE SD	1 IU	IV	J7193
ALPROLIX	IU	IV	J7201
ALPROSTADIL	1.25 MCG	IV	J0270
ALPROSTADIL	EA	OTH	J0275
ALTEPLASE RECOMBINANT	1 MG	IV	J2997
ALUPENT, NONCOMPOUNDED, CONCENTRATED	10 MG	INH	J7668
ALUPENT, NONCOMPOUNDED, UNIT DOSE	10 MG	INH	J7669
AMANTADINE HCL (DEMONSTRATION PROJECT)	100 MG	ORAL	G9017
AMANTADINE HYDROCHLORIDE (BRAND NAME) (DEMONSTRTION PROJECT)	100 MG	ORAL	G9033
AMANTADINE HYDROCHLORIDE (GENERIC)	100 MG	ORAL	G9017
AMBISOME	10 MG	IV	J0289
AMCORT	5 MG	IM	J3302
AMELUZ	10 MG	OTH	J7345
AMERGAN	12.5 MG	ORAL	Q0169
AMEVIVE	0.5 MG	IV, IM	J0215
AMICAR	5 G	IV	S0017
AMIFOSTINE	500 MG	IV	J0207
AMIKACIN SULFATE	100 MG	IM, IV	J0278
AMINOCAPRIOC ACID	5 G	IV	S0017
AMINOLEVULINIC ACID HCL	10 MG	OTH	J7345
AMINOLEVULINIC ACID HCL	354 MG	OTH	J7308
AMINOPHYLLINE	250 MG	IV	J0280
AMIODARONE HCL	30 MG	IV	J0282
AMITRIPTYLINE HCL	20 MG	IM	J1320
AMMONIA N-13	STUDY DOSE UP TO 40 MCI	IV	A9526
AMNIOARMOR	SQ CM	OTH	Q4188
AMNIOBAND	1 MG	OTH	Q4168
AMNIOBAND	SQ CM	OTH	Q4151
AMNIOEXCEL	SQ CM	OTH	Q4137
AMNIOEXCEL PLUS	SQ CM	OTH	Q4137
AMNIOMATRIX	1 CC	OTH	Q4139
AMNION BIO	SQ CM	OTH	Q4211
AMNIOWOUND	SQ CM	OTH	Q4181
AMNIOWRAP2	SQ CM	OTH	Q4221
AMOBARBITAL	125 MG	IM, IV	J0300
AMPHOCIN	50 MG	IV	J0285
AMPHOTEC	10 MG	IV	J0287
AMPHOTERICIN B	50 MG	IV	J0285
AMPHOTERICIN B CHOLESTERYL SULFATE COMPLEX	10 MG	IV	J0288
AMPHOTERICIN B LIPID COMPLEX	10 MG	IV	J0287
AMPHOTERICIN B LIPOSOME	10 MG	IV	J0289
AMPICILLIN SODIUM	500 MG	IM, IV	J0290
AMPICILLIN SODIUM/SULBACTAM SODIUM	1.5 G	IM, IV	J0295
AMYGDALIN	VAR	INJ	J3570
AMYTAL	125 MG	IM, IV	J0300
AMYVID	UP TO 10 MILLICUIRES	IV	A9586
AN-DTPA DIAGNOSTIC	STUDY DOSE UP TO 25 MCI	IV	A9539
AN-DTPA THERAPEUTIC	STUDY DOSE UP TO 25 MCI	INH	A9567
ANASCORP	UP TO 120 MG	IV	J0716
ANASTROZOLE	1 MG	ORAL	S0170
ANAVIP	120 MG	IV	J0841
ANCEF	500 MG	IM, IV	J0690
ANDEXXA	10 MG	IV	C9041
ANECTINE	20 MG	IM, IV	J0330
ANGIOMAX	1 MG	IV	J0583

© 2019 Optum360, LLC

Drug Name	Unit Per	Route	Code
ANIDULAFUNGIN	1 MG	IV	J0348
ANISTREPLASE	30 U	IV	J0350
ANTAGON	250 MCG	SC	S0132
ANTI-INHIBITOR	1 IU	IV	J7198
ANTI-THYMOCYTE GLOBULIN,EQUINE	250 MG	OTH	J7504
ANTIEMETIC NOC	VAR	ORAL	Q0181
ANTIEMETIC DRUG NOC	VAR	OTH	J8498
ANTIEMETIC DRUG NOS	VAR	ORAL	J8597
ANTIHEMOPHILIC FACTOR HUMAN METHOD M MONOCLONAL PURIFIED	1 IU	IV	J7192
ANTIHEMOPHILIC FACTOR PORCINE	1 IU	IV	J7191
ANTIHEMOPHILIC FACTOR VIII, XYNTHA, RECOMBINANT	1 IU	IV	J7185
ANTIHEMOPHILIC FACTOR VIII/VON WILLEBRAND FACTOR COMPLEX, HUMAN	PER FACTOR VIII IU	IV	J7186
ANTITHROMBIN III	1 IU	IV	J7195
ANTITHROMBIN RECOMBINANT	50 IU	IV	J7196
ANTIZOL	15 MG	IV	J1451
ANZEMET	10 MG	IV	J1260
ANZEMET	100 MG	ORAL	Q0180
ANZEMET	50 MG	ORAL	S0174
APLIGRAF	SQ CM	OTH	Q4101
APOKYN	1 MG	SC	J0364
APOMORPHINE HYDROCHLORIDE	1 MG	SC	J0364
APREPITANT	1 MG	IV	J0185
APREPITANT	5 MG	ORAL	J8501
APROTININ	10,000 KIU	IV	J0365
AQUAMEPHYTON	1 MG	IM, SC, IV	J3430
ARA-C	100 MG	SC, IV	J9100
ARALEN	UP TO 250 MG	IM, IV	J0390
ARAMINE	10 MG	IV, IM, SC	J0380
ARANESP, ESRD USE	1 MCG	SC, IV	J0882
ARANESP, NON-ESRD USE	1 MCG	SC, IV	J0881
ARBUTAMINE HCL	1 MG	IV	J0395
ARCALYST	1 MG	SC	J2793
ARCHITECT EXTRACELLULAR MATRIX	SQ CM	OTH	Q4147
AREDIA	30 MG	IV	J2430
ARFORMOTEROL	15 MCG	INH	J7605
ARGATROBAN	1 MG	IV	J0883
ARGATROBAN	1 MG	IV	J0884
ARIDOL	5 MG	INH	J7665
ARIMIDEX	1 MG	ORAL	S0170
ARIPIPRAZOLE	0.25 MG	IM	J0400
~~ARIPIPRAZOLE LAUROXIL~~	~~1 MG~~	~~IM~~	~~C9035~~
~~ARIPIPRAZOLE LAUROXIL~~	~~1 MG~~	~~IM~~	~~J1942~~
ARIPIPRAZOLE LAUROXIL	1 MG	IM	J1943
ARIPIPRAZOLE LAUROXIL	1 MG	IM	J1944
ARIPIPRAZOLE, EXTENDED RELEASE	1 MG	IM	J0401
~~ARISTADA~~	~~1 MG~~	~~IM~~	~~J1942~~
ARISTADA	1 MG	IM	J1944

Drug Name	Unit Per	Route	Code
~~ARISTADA INITIO~~	~~1 MG~~	~~IM~~	~~C9035~~
ARISTADA INITIO	1 MG	IM	J1943
ARISTOCORT	5 MG	IM	J3302
ARISTOCORTE FORTE	5 MG	IM	J3302
ARISTOCORTE INTRALESIONAL	5 MG	OTH	J3302
ARISTOSPAN	5 MG	VAR	J3303
ARIXTRA	0.5 MG	SC	J1652
AROMASIN	25 MG	ORAL	S0156
ARRANON	50 MG	IV	J9261
ARRESTIN	200 MG	IM	J3250
ARSENIC TRIOXIDE	1 MG	IV	J9017
ARTACENT AC	1 MG	OTH	Q4189
ARTACENT AC	SQ CM	OTH	Q4190
ARTACENT CORD	SQ CM	OTH	Q4216
ARTACENT WOUND	SQ CM	OTH	Q4169
ARTHROFLEX	SQ CM	OTH	Q4125
ARTISS FIBRIN SEALANT	2 ML	OTH	C9250
ARZERRA	10 MG	IV	J9302
ASCENT	0.5 MG	OTH	Q4213
ASPARAGINASE	1,000 IU	IM,IV,SC	J9019
ASPARAGINASE	10,000 U	IM, IV, SC	J9020
ASPARLAS	10 UNITS	IV	J9118
ASTAGRAF XL	0.1 MG	ORAL	J7508
ASTRAMORPH PF	10 MG	OTH	J2274
ATEZOLIZUMAB	10 MG	INF	J9022
ATGAM	250 MG	OTH	J7504
ATIVAN	2 MG	IM, IV	J2060
ATOPICLAIR	ANY SIZE	OTH	A6250
ATROPEN	0.01 MG	IM	J0461
ATROPINE SULFATE	0.01 MG	IM, IV, SC	J0461
ATROPINE, COMPOUNDED, CONCENTRATED	I MG	INH	J7635
ATROPINE, COMPOUNDED, UNIT DOSE	1 MG	INH	J7636
ATROVENT, NONCOMPOUNDED, UNIT DOSE	1 MG	INH	J7644
ATRYN	50 IU	IV	J7196
AUROTHIOGLUCOSE	50 MG	IM	J2910
AUTOPLEX T	1 IU	IV	J7198
AVASTIN	0.25 MG	IV	C9257
AVASTIN	10 MG	IV	J9035
AVEED	1 MG	IM	J3145
AVELOX	100 MG	IV	J2280
AVELUMAB	10 MG	INF	J9023
AVONEX	1 MCG	IM	Q3027
AVONEX	30 MCG	IM	J1826
AVYCAZ	0.5 G/0.125 G	IV	J0714
AXICABTAGENE CILOLEUCEL	UP TO 200 MILLION CELLS	IV	Q2041
AXOBIOMEMBRANE	SQ CM	OTH	Q4211
AXOLOTL AMBIENT, AXOLOTL CRYO	0.1 MG	OTH	Q4215
AXOLOTL GRAFT, AXOLOTL DUALGRAFT	SQ CM	OTH	Q4210
AXUMIN	1 MCI	IV	A9588
AZACITIDINE	1 MG	SC	J9025

© 2019 Optum360, LLC

Drug Name	Unit Per	Route	Code
AZACTAM	500 MG	IV	S0073
AZASAN	50 MG	ORAL	J7500
AZATHIOPRINE	100 MG	OTH	J7501
AZATHIOPRINE	50 MG	ORAL	J7500
AZEDRA	1 MCI	IV	A9590
~~AZEDRA, DIAGNOSTIC~~	~~1 MCI~~	~~IV~~	~~C9407~~
~~AZEDRA, THERAPEUTIC~~	~~1 MCI~~	~~IV~~	~~C9408~~
AZITHROMYCIN	1 G	ORAL	Q0144
AZITHROMYCIN	500 MG	IV	J0456
AZMACORT	PER MG	INH	J7684
AZMACORT CONCENTRATED	PER MG	INH	J7683
AZTREONAM	500 MG	IV, IM	S0073
BACLOFEN	10 MG	IT	J0475
BACLOFEN	50 MCG	IT	J0476
BACTOCILL	250 MG	IM, IV	J2700
BACTRIM IV	10 ML	IV	S0039
BAL	100 MG	IM	J0470
BASILIXIMAB	20 MG	IV	J0480
BAVENCIO	10 MG	INF	J9023
BAXDELA	1 MG	ORAL, IV	C9462
~~BCG INTRAVESICLE~~	~~VIAL~~	~~OTH~~	~~J9031~~
BCG LIVE INTRAVESICAL	1 MG	OTH	J9030
BEBULIN VH	1 IU	IV	J7194
BECAPLERMIN GEL 0.01%	0.5 G	OTH	S0157
BECLOMETHASONE COMPOUNDED	1 MG	INH	J7622
BECLOVENT COMPOUNDED	1 MG	INH	J7622
BECONASE COMPOUNDED	1 MG	INH	J7622
BELATACEPT	1 MG	IV	J0485
BELEODAQ	10 MG	IV	J9032
BELIMUMAB	10 MG	IV	J0490
BELINOSTAT	10 MG	IV	J9032
BELLACELL HD	SQ CM	OTH	Q4220
~~BELRAPZO~~	~~1 MG~~	~~IV~~	~~C9042~~
BELRAPZO	1 MG	IV	J9036
BENA-D 10	50 MG	IV, IM	J1200
BENA-D 50	50 MG	IV, IM	J1200
BENADRYL	50 MG	IV, IM	J1200
BENAHIST 10	50 MG	IV, IM	J1200
BENAHIST 50	50 MG	IV, IM	J1200
~~BENDAMUSTINE HCL~~	~~1 MG~~	~~IV~~	~~C9042~~
BENDAMUSTINE HCL	1 MG	IV	J9033
BENDAMUSTINE HCL	1 MG	IV	J9034
BENDAMUSTINE HYDROCHLORIDE	1 MG	IV	J9036
BENDEKA	1 MG	IV	J9034
BENEFIX	1 IU	IV	J7195
BENLYSTA	10 MG	IV	J0490
BENOJECT-10	50 MG	IV, IM	J1200
BENOJECT-50	50 MG	IV, IM	J1200
BENRALIZUMAB	1 MG	SC	J0517
BENTYL	20 MG	IM	J0500
BENZTROPINE MESYLATE	1 MG	IM, IV	J0515
BEOVU	1 MG	INJ	J0179
BERINERT	10 U	IV	J0597
BERUBIGEN	1,000 MCG	SC, IM	J3420

Drug Name	Unit Per	Route	Code
BESPONSA	0.1 MG	IV	J9229
BETA-2	1 MG	INH	J7648
BETALIN 12	1,000 MCG	SC, IM	J3420
BETAMETHASONE ACETATE AND BETAMETHASONE SODIUM PHOSPHATE	3 MG, OF EACH	IM	J0702
BETAMETHASONE COMPOUNDED, UNIT DOSE	1 MG	INH	J7624
BETASERON	0.25 MG	SC	J1830
BETHANECHOL CHLORIDE, MYOTONACHOL OR URECHOLINE	5 MG	SC	J0520
BEVACIZUMAB	0.25 MG	IV	C9257
BEVACIZUMAB	10 MG	IV	J9035
BEVACIZUMAB-AWWB, BIOSIMILAR	10 MG	IV	Q5107
BEVACIZUMAB-BVCR, BIOSIMILAR	10 MG	IV	Q5118
BEZLOTOXUMAB	10 MG	INF	J0565
BICILLIN CR	100,000 UNITS	IM	J0558
BICILLIN CR 900/300	100,000 UNITS	IM	J0558
BICILLIN CR TUBEX	100,000 UNITS	IM	J0558
BICILLIN LA	100,000 U	IM	J0561
BICNU	100 MG	IV	J9050
BIO-CONNEKT	SQ CM	OTH	Q4161
BIOCLATE	1 IU	IV	J7192
BIODEXCEL	SQ CM	OTH	Q4137
BIODFENCE	SQ CM	OTH	Q4140
BIODFENCE DRYFLEX	SQ CM	OTH	Q4138
BIODMATRIX	1 CC	OTH	Q4139
BIOSKIN	SQ CM	OTH	Q4163
BIOSKIN FLOW	SQ CM	OTH	Q4162
BIOTROPIN	1 MG	SC	J2941
BIOVANCE	SQ CM	OTH	Q4154
BIOWOUND, BIOWOUND PLUS, BIOWOUND XPLUS	SQ CM	OTH	Q4217
BIPERIDEN LACTATE	5 MG	IM, IV	J0190
BITOLTEROL MESYLATE, COMPOUNDED CONCENTRATED	PER MG	INH	J7628
BITOLTEROL MESYLATE, COMPOUNDED UNIT DOSE	PER MG	INH	J7629
BIVALIRUDIN	1 MG	IV	J0583
BIVIGAM	500 MG	IV	J1556
BLENOXANE	15 U	IM, IV, SC	J9040
BLEOMYCIN LYOPHILLIZED	15 U	IM, IV, SC	J9040
BLEOMYCIN SULFATE	15 U	IM, IV, SC	J9040
BLINATUMOMAB	1 MCG	IV	J9039
BLINCYTO	1 MCG	IV	J9039
BONIVA	1 MG	IV	J1740
BORTEZOMIB	0.1 MG	IV, SC	J9041
BOTOX	1 UNIT	IM, OTH	J0585
BOTOX COSMETIC	1 UNIT	IM, OTH	J0585
BOTULINUM TOXIN TYPE A	1 UNIT	IM, OTH	J0585
BOTULINUM TOXIN TYPE B	100 U	OTH	J0587
BRAVELLE	75 IU	SC, IM	J3355
BRENTUXIMAB VENDOTIN	1 MG	IV	J9042

© 2019 Optum360, LLC

Drug Name	Unit Per	Route	Code
BRETHINE	PER MG	INH	J7681
BRETHINE CONCENTRATED	PER MG	INH	J7680
BREXANOLONE	1 MG	IV	C9055
BRICANYL	PER MG	INH	J7681
BRICANYL CONCENTRATED	PER MG	INH	J7680
BRINEURA	1 MG	OTH	J0567
BROLUCIZUMAB-DBLL	1 MG	INJ	J0179
BROM-A-COT	10 MG	IM, SC, IV	J0945
BROMPHENIRAMINE MALEATE	10 MG	IM, SC, IV	J0945
BUDESONIDE COMPOUNDED, CONCETRATED	0.25 MG	INH	J7634
BUDESONIDE, COMPOUNDED, UNIT DOSE	0.5 MG	INH	J7627
BUDESONIDE, NONCOMPOUNDED, CONCENTRATED	0.25 MG	INH	J7633
BUDESONIDE, NONCOMPOUNDED, UNIT DOSE	0.5 MG	INH	J7626
BUMETANIDE	0.5 MG	IM, IV	S0171
BUNAVAIL	2.1 MG	ORAL	J0572
BUNAVAIL	4.2 MG	ORAL	J0573
BUNAVAIL	6.3 MG	ORAL	J0574
BUPIVACAINE HCL	30 ML	VAR	S0020
BUPIVACAINE LIPOSOME	1 MG	VAR	C9290
BUPRENEX	0.1 MG	IM, IV	J0592
BUPRENORPHIN/NALOXONE	> 10 MG	ORAL	J0575
BUPRENORPHIN/NALOXONE	UP TO 3 MG	ORAL	J0572
BUPRENORPHINE EXTENDED-RELEASE	> 100 MG	SC	Q9992
BUPRENORPHINE EXTENDED-RELEASE	≤ 100 MG	SC	Q9991
BUPRENORPHINE HCL	0.1 MG	IM, IV	J0592
BUPRENORPHINE IMPLANT	74.2 MG	OTH	J0570
BUPRENORPHINE ORAL	1 MG	ORAL	J0571
BUPRENORPHINE/NALOXONE	3.1 TO 6 MG	ORAL	J0573
BUPRENORPHINE/NALOXONE	6.1 TO 10 MG	ORAL	J0574
BUPROPION HCL	150 MG	ORAL	S0106
BUROSUMAB-TWZA	1 MG	SC	J0584
BUSULFAN	1 MG	IV	J0594
BUSULFAN	2 MG	ORAL	J8510
BUSULFEX	2 MG	ORAL	J8510
BUTORPHANOL TARTRATE	2 MG	IM, IV	J0595
BUTORPHANOL TARTRATE	25 MG	OTH	S0012
C-1 ESTERASE INHIBITOR (HUMAN)	10 UNITS	SC	J0599
C1 ESTERASE INHIBITOR (HUMAN) (BERINERT)	10 UNITS	IV	J0597
C1 ESTERASE INHIBITOR (HUMAN) (CINRYZE)	10 UNITS	IV	J0598
C1 ESTERASE INHIBITOR (RECOMBINANT)	10 UNITS	IV	J0596
CABAZITAXEL	1 MG	IV	J9043
CABERGOLINE	0.25 MG	ORAL	J8515
CABLIVI	1 MG	IV, SC	C9047
CAFCIT	5 MG	IV	J0706
CAFFEINE CITRATE	5 MG	IV	J0706
CALASPARGASE PEGOL-MKNL	10 UNITS	IV	J9118

Drug Name	Unit Per	Route	Code
CALCIJEX	0.1 MCG	IM	J0636
CALCIJEX	0.25 MCG	INJ	S0169
CALCIMAR	UP TO 400 U	SC, IM	J0630
CALCITONIN SALMON	400 U	SC, IM	J0630
CALCITRIOL	0.1 MCG	IM	J0636
CALCITROL	0.25 MCG	IM	S0169
CALCIUM DISODIUM VERSENATE	1,000 MG	IV, SC, IM	J0600
CALCIUM GLUCONATE	10 ML	IV	J0610
CALCIUM GLYCEROPHOSPHATE AND CALCIUM LACTATE	10 ML	IM, SC	J0620
CALDOLOR	100 MG	IV	J1741
CAMPTOSAR	20 MG	IV	J9206
CANAKINUMAB	1 MG	SC	J0638
CANCIDAS	5 MG	IV	J0637
CAPECITABINE	150 MG	ORAL	J8520
CAPLACIZUMAB-YHDP	1 MG	IV, SC	C9047
CAPROMAB PENDETIDE	STUDY DOSE UP TO 10 MCI	IV	A9507
CAPSAICIN 8% PATCH	1 SQ CM	OTH	J7336
CARBIDOPA/LEVODOPA	5 MG/20 MG	ORAL	J7340
CARBOCAINE	10 ML	VAR	J0670
CARBOPLATIN	50 MG	IV	J9045
CARDIOGEN 82	STUDY DOSE UP TO 60 MCI	IV	A9555
CARDIOLITE	STUDY DOSE	IV	A9500
CARFILZOMIB	1 MG	IV	J9047
CARIMUNE	500 MG	IV	J1566
CARMUSTINE	100 MG	IV	J9050
CARNITOR	1 G	IV	J1955
CARTICEL		OTH	J7330
CASPOFUNGIN ACETATE	5 MG	IV	J0637
CATAPRES	1 MG	OTH	J0735
CATHFLO	1 MG	IV	J2997
CAVERJECT	1.25 MCG	VAR	J0270
CEA SCAN	STUDY DOSE UP TO 45 MCI	IV	A9568
CEENU	10 MG	ORAL	S0178
CEFAZOLIN SODIUM	500 MG	IM, IV	J0690
CEFEPIME HCL	500 MG	IV	J0692
CEFIZOX	500 MG	IV, IM	J0715
CEFOBID	1 G	IV	S0021
CEFOPERAZONE SODIUM	1 G	IV	S0021
CEFOTAN	500 MG	IM, IV	S0074
CEFOTAXIME SODIUM	1 GM	IV, IM	J0698
CEFOTETAN DISODIUM	500 MG	IM. IV	S0074
CEFOXITIN SODIUM	1 GM	IV, IM	J0694
CEFTAROLINE FOSAMIL	10 MG	IV	J0712
CEFTAZIDIME	500 MG	IM, IV	J0713
CEFTAZIDIME AND AVIBACTAM	0.5 G/0.125 G	IV	J0714
CEFTIZOXIME SODIUM	500 MG	IV, IM	J0715
CEFTOLOZANE AND TAZOBACTAM	50 MG/25 MG	IV	J0695
CEFTRIAXONE SODIUM	250 MG	IV, IM	J0696
CEFUROXIME	750 MG	IM, IV	J0697
CEFUROXIME SODIUM STERILE	750 MG	IM, IV	J0697
CELESTONE SOLUSPAN	3 MG	IM	J0702

© 2019 Optum360, LLC

Drug Name	Unit Per	Route	Code
CELLCEPT	250 MG	ORAL	J7517
CELLESTA CORD	SQ CM	OTH	Q4214
CELLESTA FLOWABLE AMNION	0.5 CC	OTH	Q4185
CELLESTA OR CELLESTA DUO	SQ CM	OTH	Q4184
~~CEMIPLIMAB-RWLC~~	~~1 MG~~	~~IV~~	~~C9044~~
CEMIPLIMAB-RWLC	1 MG	IV	J9119
CENACORT A-40	10 MG	IM	J3301
CENACORT FORTE	5 MG	IM	J3302
CENTRUROIDES (SCORPION) IMMUNE F(AB)2 (EQUINE)	UP TO 120 MG	IV	J0716
CEPHALOTHIN SODIUM	UP TO 1 G	INJ	J1890
CEPHAPIRIN SODIUM	1 G	IV	J0710
CEPTAZ	500 MG	IM, IV	J0713
CEREBRYX	50 MG	IM, IV	Q2009
CEREBRYX	750 MG	IM, IV	S0078
CEREDASE	10 U	IV	J0205
CERETEC	STUDY DOSE UP TO 25 MCI	IV	A9521
CEREZYME	10 U	IV	J1786
CERLIPONASE ALFA	1 MG	OTH	J0567
CERTOLIZUMAB PEGOL	1 MG	SC	J0717
CERUBIDINE	10 MG	IV	J9150
CESAMET	1 MG	ORAL	J8650
CETUXIMAB	10 MG	IV	J9055
CHEALAMIDE	150 MG	IV	J3520
CHLORAMBUCIL	2 MG	ORAL	S0172
CHLORAMPHENICOL SODIUM SUCCINATE	1 G	IV	J0720
CHLORDIAZEPOXIDE HCL	100 MG	IM, IV	J1990
CHLOROMYCETIN	1 G	IV	J0720
CHLOROPROCAINE HCL	30 ML	VAR	J2400
CHLOROQUINE HCL	UP TO 250 MG	IM, IV	J0390
CHLOROTHIAZIDE SODIUM	500 MG	IV	J1205
CHLORPROMAZINE HCL	5 MG	ORAL	Q0161
CHLORPROMAZINE HCL	50 MG	IM, IV	J3230
CHOLETEC	STUDY DOSE UP TO 15 MCI	IV	A9537
CHOLINE C 11, DIAGNOSTIC, PER STUDY DOSE	UP TO 20 MCI	IV	A9515
CHOREX	1000 USP	IM	J0725
CHORIONIC GONADOTROPIN	1,000 USP U	IM	J0725
CHROMIC PHOSPHATE P32 (THERAPEUTIC)	1 MCI	IV	A9564
CHROMITOPE SODIUM	STUDY DOSE UP TO 250 UCI	IV	A9553
CHROMIUM CR-51 SODIUM IOTHALAMATE, DIAGNOSTIC	STUDY DOSE UP TO 250 UCI	IV	A9553
CIDOFOVIR	375 MG	IV	J0740
CILASTATIN SODIUM	250 MG	IV, IM	J0743
CIMETIDINE HCL	300 MG	IM, IV	S0023
CIMZIA	1 MG	SC	J0717
CINACALCET	1 MG	ORAL	J0604
CINQUAIR	1 MG	IV	J2786
CINRZYE	10 UNITS	IV	J0598

Drug Name	Unit Per	Route	Code
CINVANTI	1 MG	IV	J0185
CIPRO	200 MG	IV	J0744
CIPROFLOXACIN FOR INTRAVENOUS INFUSION	200 MG	IV	J0744
CIPROFLOXACIN OTIC SUSPENSION	6 MG	OTIC	J7342
CIS-MDP	STUDY DOSE UP TO 30 MCI	IV	A9503
CIS-PYRO	STUDY DOSE UP TO 25 MCI	IV	A9538
CISPLATIN	10 MG	IV	J9060
CLADRIBINE	1 MG	IV	J9065
CLAFORAN	1 GM	IV, IM	J0698
CLARIX 100	SQ MC	OTH	Q4156
CLARIX CORD 1K	SQ CM	OTH	Q4148
CLARIXFLO	1 MG	OTH	Q4155
CLEOCIN PHOSPHATE	300 MG	IV	S0077
CLEVIDIPINE BUTYRATE	1 MG	IV	C9248
CLEVIPREX	1 MG	IV	C9248
CLINDAMYCIN PHOSPHATE	300 MG	IV	S0077
CLOFARABINE	1 MG	IV	J9027
CLOLAR	1 MG	IV	J9027
CLONIDINE HCL	1 MG	OTH	J0735
CLOZAPINE	25 MG	ORAL	S0136
CLOZARIL	25 MG	ORAL	S0136
COAGADEX	1 IU	IV	J7175
COAGULATION FACTOR XA	10 MG	IV	C9041
COBAL	1,000 MCG	IM, SC	J3420
COBALT CO-57 CYNOCOBALAMIN, DIAGNOSTIC	STUDY DOSE UP TO 1 UCI	ORAL	A9559
COBATOPE 57	STUDY DOSE UP TO 1 UCI	ORAL	A9559
COBEX	1,000 MCG	SC, IM	J3420
COCAINE HYDROCHLORIDE NASAL SOLUTION	1 MG	OTH	C9046
CODEINE PHOSPHATE	30 MG	IM, IV, SC	J0745
COGENTIN	1 MG	IM, IV	J0515
COGNEX	10 MG	ORAL	S0014
COLCHICINE	1 MG	IV	J0760
COLHIST	10 MG	IM, SC, IV	J0945
COLISTIMETHATE SODIUM	1 MG	INH	S0142
COLISTIMETHATE SODIUM	150 MG	IM, IV	J0770
COLL-E-DERM	SQ CM	OTH	Q4193
COLLAGEN BASED WOUND FILLER DRY FOAM	1 GM	OTH	A6010
COLLAGEN BASED WOUND FILLER, GEL/PASTE	1 GM	OTH	A6011
COLLAGEN MATRIX NERVE WRAP	0.5 CM	OTH	C9361
COLLAGEN NERVE CUFF	0.5 CM LENGTH	OTH	C9355
COLLAGEN WOUND DRESSING	SQ CM	OTH	Q4164
COLLAGENASE, CLOSTRIDIUM HISTOLYTICUM	0.01 MG	OTH	J0775
COLY-MYCIN M	150 MG	IM, IV	J0770
COMPAZINE	10 MG	IM, IV	J0780
COMPAZINE	5 MG	ORAL	Q0164
COMPAZINE	5 MG	ORAL	S0183

© 2019 Optum360, LLC

Drug Name	Unit Per	Route	Code
CONIVAPTAN HYDROCHLORIDE	1 MG	INJ	C9488
CONTRACEPTIVE SUPPLY, HORMONE CONTAINING PATCH	EACH	OTH	J7304
CONTRAST FOR ECHOCARDIOGRAM	STUDY	IV	A9700
COPANLISIB	1 MG	IV	J9057
COPAXONE	20 MG	SC	J1595
COPPER T MODEL TCU380A IUD COPPER WIRE/COPPER COLLAR	EA	OTH	J7300
CORDARONE	30 MG	IV	J0282
CORIFACT	1 IU	IV	J7180
CORTASTAT	1 MG	IM, IV, OTH	J1100
CORTASTAT LA	1 MG	IM	J1094
CORTICORELIN OVINE TRIFLUTATE	1 MCG	IV	J0795
CORTICOTROPIN	40 U	IV, IM, SC	J0800
CORTIMED	80 MG	IM	J1040
CORTROSYN	0.25 MG	IM, IV	J0834
CORVERT	1 MG	IV	J1742
COSMEGEN	0.5 MG	IV	J9120
COSYNTROPIN	0.25 MG	IM, IV	J0834
COTOLONE	5 MG	ORAL	J7510
CRESEMBA	1 MG	IV	J1833
CROFAB	UP TO 1 GM	IV	J0840
CROMOLYN SODIUM COMPOUNDED	PER 10 MG	INH	J7632
CROMOLYN SODIUM NONCOMPOUNDED	10 MG	INH	J7631
CROTALIDAE IMMUNE F(AB')2 (EQUINE)	120 MG	IV	J0841
CROTALIDAE POLYVALENT IMMUNE FAB (OVINE)	UP TO 1 GM	IV	J0840
CRYSTAL B12	1,000 MCG	IM, SC	J3420
CRYSTICILLIN 300 A.S.	600,000 UNITS	IM, IV	J2510
CRYSTICILLIN 600 A.S.	600,000 UNITS	IM, IV	J2510
CRYSVITA	1 MG	SC	J0584
CUBICIN	1 MG	IV	J0878
CUVITRU	100 MG	SC	J1555
CYANO	1,000 MCG	IM, SC	J3420
CYANOCOBALAMIN	1,000 MCG	IM, SC	J3420
CYANOCOBALAMIN COBALT 57/58	STUDY DOSE UP TO 1 UCI	IV	A9546
CYANOCOBALAMIN COBALT CO-57	STUDY DOSE UP TO 1 UCI	ORAL	A9559
CYCLOPHOSPHAMIDE	100 MG	IV	J9070
CYCLOPHOSPHAMIDE	25 MG	ORAL	J8530
CYCLOSPORINE	100 MG	ORAL	J7502
CYCLOSPORINE	25 MG	ORAL	J7515
CYCLOSPORINE	250 MG	IV	J7516
CYGNUS	SQ CM	OTH	Q4170
CYMETRA	1 CC	INJ	Q4112
CYRAMZA	5 MG	IV	J9308
CYSVIEW	STUDY DOSE	OTH	A9589
CYTAL	SQ CM	OTH	Q4166
CYTARABINE	100 MG	SC, IV	J9100
CYTARABINE LIPOSOME	10 MG	IT	J9098
CYTOGAM	VIAL	IV	J0850
CYTOMEGALOVIRUS IMMUNE GLOB	VIAL	IV	J0850
CYTOSAR-U	100 MG	SC, IV	J9100
CYTOTEC	200 MCG	ORAL	S0191
CYTOVENE	500 MG	IV	J1570
CYTOXAN	100 MG	IV	J9070
CYTOXAN	25 MG	ORAL	J8530
D.H.E. 45	1 MG	IM, IV	J1110
DACARBAZINE	100 MG	IV	J9130
DACLIZUMAB	25 MG	OTH	J7513
DACOGEN	1 MG	IV	J0894
DACTINOMYCIN	0.5 MG	IV	J9120
DALALONE	1 MG	IM, IV, OTH	J1100
DALALONE LA	1 MG	IM	J1094
DALBAVANCIN	5 MG	IV	J0875
DALTEPARIN SODIUM	2,500 IU	SC	J1645
DALVANCE	5 MG	IV	J0875
DAPTOMYCIN	1 MG	IV	J0878
DARATUMUMAB	10 MG	IV	J9145
DARBEPOETIN ALFA, ESRD USE	1 MCG	SC, IV	J0882
DARBEPOETIN ALFA, NON-ESRD USE	1 MCG	SC, IV	J0881
DARZALEX	10 MG	IV	J9145
DATSCAN	STUDY DOSE	IV	A9584
DAUNORUBICIN	10 MG	IV	J9150
DAUNORUBICIN CITRATE, LIPOOSOMAL FORMULATION	10 MG	IV	J9151
DAUNOXOME	10 MG	IV	J9151
DDAVP	1 MCG	IV, SC	J2597
DECADRON	0.25 MG	ORAL	J8540
DECAJECT	1 MG	IM, IV, OTH	J1100
DECITABINE	1 MG	IV	J0894
DECOLONE-50	50 MG	IM	J2320
DEFEROXAMINE MESYLATE	500 MG	IM, SC, IV	J0895
DEGARELIX	1 MG	SC	J9155
DELAFLOXACIN	1 MG	ORAL, IV	C9462
DELATESTRYL	1 MG	IM	J3121
DELESTROGEN	10 MG	IM	J1380
DELTA-CORTEF	5 MG	ORAL	J7510
DEMADEX	10 MG	IV	J3265
DEMEROL	100 MG	IM, IV, SC	J2175
DENILEUKIN DIFTITOX	300 MCG	IV	J9160
DENOSUMAB	1 MG	SC	J0897
DEPGYNOGEN	UP TO 5 MG	IM	J1000
DEPHENACEN-50	50 MG	IM, IV	J1200
DEPMEDALONE	40 MG	IM	J1030
DEPMEDALONE	80 MG	IM	J1040
DEPO-ESTRADIOL CYPIONATE	UP TO 5 MG	IM	J1000
DEPO-MEDROL	20 MG	IM, OTH	J1020
DEPO-MEDROL	40 MG	IM, OTH	J1030
DEPO-MEDROL	80 MG	IM, OTH	J1040
DEPO-TESTOSTERONE	1 MG	IM	J1071
DEPOCYT	10 MG	IT	J9098
DEPOGEN	UP TO 5 MG	IM	J1000
DERMA-GIDE	SQ CM	OTH	Q4203

© 2019 Optum360, LLC

Drug Name	Unit Per	Route	Code
DERMACELL, DERMACELL AWM OR DERMACELL AWM POROUS	SQ CM	OTH	Q4122
DERMAGRAFT	SQ CM	OTH	Q4106
DERMAL SUBSTITUTE, NATIVE, NONDENATURED COLLAGEN, FETAL	0.5 SQ CM	OTH	C9358
DERMAL SUBSTITUTE, NATIVE, NONDENATURED COLLAGEN, NEONATAL	0.5 SQ CM	OTH	C9360
DERMAPURE	SQ CM	OTH	Q4152
DERMAVEST AND PLURIVEST	SQ CM	OTH	Q4153
DESFERAL	500 MG	IM, SC, IV	J0895
DESMOPRESSIN ACETATE	1 MCG	IV, SC	J2597
DEXAMETHASONE	0.25 MG	ORAL	J8540
DEXAMETHASONE 9%	1 MCG	OTH	J1095
DEXAMETHASONE ACETATE	1 MG	IM	J1094
DEXAMETHASONE ACETATE ANHYDROUS	1 MG	IM	J1094
DEXAMETHASONE INTRAVITREAL IMPLANT	0.1 MG	OTH	J7312
DEXAMETHASONE SODIUM PHOSPHATE	1 MG	IM, IV, OTH	J1100
DEXAMETHASONE, COMPOUNDED, CONCENTRATED	1 MG	INH	J7637
DEXAMETHASONE, COMPOUNDED, UNIT DOSE	1 MG	INH	J7638
~~DEXAMETHASONE, LACRIMAL OPHTHALMIC INSERT~~	~~0.1 MG~~	~~OTH~~	~~C9048~~
DEXAMETHASONE, LACRIMAL OPHTHALMIC INSERT	0.1 MG	OTH	J1096
DEXASONE	1 MG	IM, IV, OTH	J1100
DEXEDRINE	5 MG	ORAL	S0160
DEXIM	1 MG	IM, IV, OTH	J1100
DEXONE	0.25 MG	ORAL	J8540
DEXONE	1 MG	IM, IV, OTH	J1100
DEXONE LA	1 MG	IM	J1094
DEXRAZOXANE HCL	250 MG	IV	J1190
~~DEXTENZA~~	~~0.1 MG~~	~~OTH~~	~~C9048~~
DEXTENZA	0.1 MG	OTH	J1096
DEXTRAN 40	500 ML	IV	J7100
DEXTROAMPHETAMINE SULFATE	5 MG	ORAL	S0160
DEXTROSE	500 ML	IV	J7060
DEXTROSE, STERILE WATER, AND/OR DEXTROSE DILUENT/FLUSH	10 ML	VAR	A4216
DEXTROSE/SODIUM CHLORIDE	5%	VAR	J7042
DEXTROSE/THEOPHYLLINE	40 MG	IV	J2810
DEXTROSTAT	5 MG	ORAL	S0160
DEXYCU	1 MCG	OTH	J1095
DI-SPAZ	UP TO 20 MG	IM	J0500
DIALYSIS/STRESS VITAMINS	100 CAPS	ORAL	S0194
DIAMOX	500 MG	IM, IV	J1120
DIASTAT	5 MG	IV, IM	J3360
DIAZEPAM	5 MG	IV, IM	J3360
DIAZOXIDE	300 MG	IV	J1730
DIBENT	UP TO 20 MG	IM	J0500
DICLOFENAC SODIUM	0.5 MG	OTH	J1130
DICYCLOMINE HCL	20 MG	IM	J0500

Drug Name	Unit Per	Route	Code
DIDANOSINE (DDI)	25 MG	ORAL	S0137
DIDRONEL	300 MG	IV	J1436
DIETHYLSTILBESTROL DIPHOSPHATE	250 MG	INJ	J9165
DIFLUCAN	200 MG	IV	J1450
DIGIBIND	VIAL	IV	J1162
DIGIFAB	VIAL	IV	J1162
DIGOXIN	0.5 MG	IM, IV	J1160
DIGOXIN IMMUNE FAB	VIAL	IV	J1162
DIHYDROERGOTAMINE MESYLATE	1 MG	IM, IV	J1110
DILANTIN	50 MG	IM, IV	J1165
DILAUDID	250 MG	OTH	S0092
DILAUDID	4 MG	SC, IM, IV	J1170
DIMENHYDRINATE	50 MG	IM, IV	J1240
DIMERCAPROL	100 MG	IM	J0470
DIMINE	50 MG	IV, IM	J1200
DINATE	50 MG	IM, IV	J1240
DIOVAL	10 MG	IM	J1380
DIOVAL 40	10 MG	IM	J1380
DIOVAL XX	10 MG	IM	J1380
DIPHENHYDRAMINE HCL	50 MG	IV, IM	J1200
DIPHENHYDRAMINE HCL	50 MG	ORAL	Q0163
DIPRIVAN	10 MG	IV	J2704
DIPYRIDAMOLE	10 MG	IV	J1245
DISOTATE	150 MG	IV	J3520
DIURIL	500 MG	IV	J1205
DIURIL SODIUM	500 MG	IV	J1205
DIZAC	5 MG	IV, IM	J3360
DMSO, DIMETHYL SULFOXIDE	50%, 50 ML	OTH	J1212
DOBUTAMINE HCL	250 MG	IV	J1250
DOBUTREX	250 MG	IV	J1250
DOCETAXEL	1 MG	IV	J9171
DOLASETRON MESYLATE	10 MG	IV	J1260
DOLASETRON MESYLATE	100 MG	ORAL	Q0180
DOLASETRON MESYLATE	50 MG	ORAL	S0174
DOLOPHINE	5 MG	ORAL	S0109
DOLOPHINE HCL	10 MG	IM, SC	J1230
DOMMANATE	50 MG	IM, IV	J1240
DOPAMINE HCL	40 MG	IV	J1265
DORIBAX	10 MG	IV	J1267
DORIPENEM	10 MG	IV	J1267
DORNASE ALPHA, NONCOMPOUNDED, UNIT DOSE	1 MG	INH	J7639
DOSTINEX	0.25 MG	ORAL	J8515
DOTAREM	0.1 ML	IV	A9575
DOXERCALCIFEROL	1 MG	IV	J1270
DOXORUBICIN HCL	10 MG	IV	J9000
DOXORUBICIN HYDROCHLORIDE, LIPOSOMAL, IMPORTED LIPODOX	10 MG	IV	Q2049
DOXORUBICIN HYDROCHLORIDE, LIPOSOMAL, NOT OTHERWISE SPECIFIED, 10 MG	10 MG	IV	Q2050
DRAMAMINE	50 MG	IM, IV	J1240
DRAMANATE	50 MG	IM, IV	J1240
DRAMILIN	50 MG	IM, IV	J1240
DRAMOCEN	50 MG	IM, IV	J1240

© 2019 Optum360, LLC

Drug Name	Unit Per	Route	Code
DRAMOJECT	50 MG	IM, IV	J1240
DRAXIMAGE MDP-10	STUDY DOSE UP TO 30 MCI	IV	A9503
DRAXIMAGE MDP-25	STUDY DOSE UP TO 30 MCI	IV	A9503
DRONABINAL	2.5 MG	ORAL	Q0167
DROPERIDOL	5 MG	IM, IV	J1790
DROPERIDOL AND FENTANYL CITRATE	2 ML	IM, IV	J1810
DROXIA	500 MG	ORAL	S0176
DTIC-DOME	100 MG	IV	J9130
DTPA	STUDY DOSE UP TO 25 MCI	INH	A9567
DTPA	STUDY DOSE UP TO 25 MCI	IV	A9539
DUOPA	5 MG/20 MG	ORAL	J7340
DURACILLIN A.S.	600,000 UNITS	IM, IV	J2510
DURACLON	1 MG	OTH	J0735
DURAGEN-10	10 MG	IM	J1380
DURAGEN-20	10 MG	IM	J1380
DURAGEN-40	10 MG	IM	J1380
DURAMORPH	500 MG	OTH	S0093
DURAMORPH PF	10 MG	OTH	J2274
DURO CORT	80 MG	IM	J1040
DUROLANE	1 MG	INJ	J7318
DURVALUMAB	10 MG	IV	J9173
DYLOJECT	0.5 MG	OTH	J1130
DYMENATE	50 MG	IM, IV	J1240
DYPHYLLINE	500 MG	IM	J1180
DYSPORT	5 UNITS	IM	J0586
E.D.T.A.	150 MG	IV	J3520
ECALLANTIDE	1 MG	SC	J1290
ECHOCARDIOGRAM IMAGE ENHANCER OCTAFLUOROPROPANE	1 ML	IV	Q9956
ECHOCARDIOGRAM IMAGE ENHANCER PERFLEXANE	1 ML	IV	Q9955
ECULIZUMAB	10 MG	IV	J1300
EDARAVONE	1 MG	IV	J1301
EDETATE CALCIUM DISODIUM	1,000 MG	IV, SC, IM	J0600
EDETATE DISODIUM	150 MG	IV	J3520
EDEX	1.25 MCG	VAR	J0270
ELAPRASE	1 MG	IV	J1743
ELAVIL	20 MG	IM	J1320
ELELYSO	10 U	IV	J3060
ELIGARD	7.5 MG	SC	J9217
ELITEK	0.5 MG	IM	J2783
ELLENCE	2 MG	IV	J9178
ELLIOTTS B SOLUTION	1 ML	IV, IT	J9175
ELOCTATE	IU	IV	J7205
ELOSULFASE ALFA	1 MG	IV	J1322
ELOTUZUMAB	1 MG	IV	J9176
ELOXATIN	0.5 MG	IV	J9263
ELSPAR	1,000 IU	IM,IV, SC	J9019
ELSPAR	10,000 U	IM, IV, SC	J9020
~~ELZONRIS~~	~~10 MCG~~	~~IV~~	~~C9049~~

Drug Name	Unit Per	Route	Code
ELZONRIS	10 MCG	IV	J9269
~~EMAPALUMAB-LZSG~~	~~1 MG~~	~~IV~~	~~C9050~~
EMAPALUMAB-LZSG	1 MG	IV	J9210
EMEND	1 MG	IV	J1453
EMEND	5 MG	ORAL	J8501
EMICIZUMAB-KXWH	0.5 MG	SC	J7170
EMINASE	30 U	IV	J0350
EMPLICITI	1 MG	IV	J9176
ENBREL	25 MG	IM, IV	J1438
ENDOXAN-ASTA	100 MG	IV	J9070
ENDRATE	150 MG	IV	J3520
ENFUVIRTIDE	1 MG	SC	J1324
ENOXAPARIN SODIUM	10 MG	SC	J1650
ENTYVIO	1 MG	IV	J3380
ENVARSUS XR	0.25 MG	ORAL	J7503
EOVIST	1 ML	IV	A9581
EPICORD	SQ CM	OTH	Q4187
EPIFIX	SQ CM	OTH	Q4186
EPIFIX, INJECTABLE	1 MG	OTH	Q4145
EPINEPHRINE	0.1 MG	IM, IV, SC	J0171
EPIRUBICIN HCL	2 MG	IV	J9178
EPOETIN ALFA FOR ESRD DIALYSIS	100 U	INJ	Q4081
EPOETIN ALFA, BIOSIMILAR	100 UNITS	INJ, IV	Q5105
EPOETIN ALFA, BIOSIMILAR	1000 UNITS	INJ, IV	Q5106
EPOETIN ALFA, NON-ESRD USE	1,000 U	SC, IV	J0885
EPOETIN BETA FOR ESRD ON DIALYSIS	1 MCG	IV	J0887
EPOETIN BETA FOR NON-ESRD	1 MCG	IV, SC	J0888
EPOGEN/NON-ESRD	1,000 U	SC, IV	J0885
EPOPROSTENOL	0.5 MG	IV	J1325
EPOPROSTENOL STERILE DILUTANT	50 ML	IV	S0155
EPTIFIBATIDE	5 MG	IM, IV	J1327
ERAVACYCLINE	1 MG	IV	J0122
ERAXIS	1 MG	IV	J0348
ERBITUX	10 MG	IV	J9055
ERGAMISOL	50 MG	ORAL	S0177
ERGONOVINE MALEATE	0.2 MG	IM, IV	J1330
ERIBULIN MESYLATE	0.1 MG	IV	J9179
ERTAPENEM SODIUM	500 MG	IM, IV	J1335
ERYTHROCIN LACTOBIONATE	500 MG	IV	J1364
ESTONE AQUEOUS	1 MG	IM, IV	J1435
ESTRA-L 20	10 MG	IM	J1380
ESTRA-L 40	10 MG	IM	J1380
ESTRADIOL CYPIONATE	UP TO 5 MG	IM	J1000
ESTRADIOL L.A.	10 MG	IM	J1380
ESTRADIOL L.A. 20	10 MG	IM	J1380
ESTRADIOL L.A. 40	10 MG	IM	J1380
ESTRADIOL VALERATE	10 MG	IM	J1380
ESTRAGYN	1 MG	IV, IM	J1435
ESTRO-A	1 MG	IV, IM	J1435
ESTROGEN CONJUGATED	25 MG	IV, IM	J1410
ESTRONE	1 MG	IV, IM	J1435
ESTRONOL	1 MG	IM, IV	J1435
ETANERCEPT	25 MG	IM, IV	J1438

© 2019 Optum360, LLC

Drug Name	Unit Per	Route	Code
ETELCALCETIDE	0.1 MG	IV	J0606
ETEPLIRSEN	10 MG	INF	J1428
ETHAMOLIN	100 MG	IV	J1430
ETHANOLAMINE OLEATE	100 MG	IV	J1430
ETHYOL	500 MG	IV	J0207
ETIDRONATE DISODIUM	300 MG	IV	J1436
ETONOGESTREL	IMPLANT	OTH	J7307
ETOPOSIDE	10 MG	IV	J9181
ETOPOSIDE	50 MG	ORAL	J8560
EUFLEXXA	DOSE	OTH	J7323
EULEXIN	125 MG	ORAL	S0175
EVENITY	1 MG	SC	J3111
EVEROLIMUS	0.25 MG	ORAL	J7527
EXAMETAZIME LABELED AUTOLOGOUS WHITE BLOOD CELLS, TECHNETIUM TC-99M	STUDY DOSE	IV	A9569
EXCELLAGEN	0.1 CC	OTH	Q4149
EXMESTANE	25 MG	ORAL	S0156
EXONDYS 51	10 MG	INF	J1428
EXPAREL	1 MG	VAR	C9290
EZ-DERM	SQ CM	OTH	Q4136
FABRAZYME	1 MG	IV	J0180
FACTOR IX (ANTIHEMOPHILIC FACTOR, RECOMBINANT), RIXIBUS, PER I.U.	IU	IV	J7200
FACTOR IX NON-RECOMBINANT	1 IU	IV	J7193
FACTOR IX RECOMBINANT	1 IU	IV	J7195
FACTOR IX+ COMPLEX	1 IU	IV	J7194
FACTOR IX, (ANTIHEMOPHILIC FACTOR, RECOMBINANT), GLYCOPEGYLATED	1 IU	IV	J7203
FACTOR IX, ALBUMIN FUSION PROTEIN, (RECOMBINANT)	1 IU	IV	J7202
FACTOR IX, FC FUSION PROTEIN (ANTIHEMOPHILIC FACTOR, RECOMBINANT), ALPROLIX	IU	IV	J7201
FACTOR VIIA RECOMBINANT	1 MCG	IV	J7189
FACTOR VIII (ANTIHEMOPHILIC FACTOR, RECOMBINANT)	1 IU	IV	J7209
FACTOR VIII (ANTIHEMOPHILIC FACTOR, RECOMBINANT)	IU	IV	J7188
FACTOR VIII (ANTIHEMOPHILIC FACTOR, RECOMBINANT) (NOVOEIGHT), PER IU	IU	IV	J7182
FACTOR VIII (ANTIHEMOPHILIC FACTOR, RECOMBINANT) PEGYLATED	1 IU	IV	J7207
FACTOR VIII FC FUSION (RECOMBINANT)	IU	IV	J7205
FACTOR VIII PORCINE	1 IU	IV	J7191
FACTOR VIII RECOMBINANT	1 IU	IV	J7192
FACTOR VIII, (ANTIHEMOPHILIC FACTOR, RECOMBINANT) (AFSTYLA)	1 I.U.	IV	J7210
FACTOR VIII, (ANTIHEMOPHILIC FACTOR, RECOMBINANT) (KOVALTRY)	1 I.U.	IV	J7211
~~FACTOR VIII, (ANTIHEMOPHILIC FACTOR, RECOMBINANT), PEGYLATED-AUCL~~	~~1 IU~~	~~IV~~	~~C9141~~
FACTOR VIII, (ANTIHEMOPHILIC FACTOR, RECOMBINANT), PEGYLATED-AUCL	1 IU	IV	J7208
FACTOR VIII, HUMAN	1 IU	IV	J7190
FACTOR X (HUMAN)	1 IU	IV	J7175
FACTOR XIII (ANTIHEMOPHILIC FACTOR, HUMAN)	1 IU	IV	J7180
FACTOR XIII A-SUBUNIT (RECOMBINANT)	10 IU	IV	J7181
FACTREL	100 MCG	SC, IV	J1620
FAMOTIDINE	20 MG	IV	S0028
FASENRA	1 MG	SC	J0517
FASLODEX	25 MG	IM	J9395
FDG	STUDY DOSE UP TO 45 MCI	IV	A9552
FEIBA-VH AICC	1 IU	IV	J7198
FENTANYL CITRATE	0.1 MG	IM, IV	J3010
FERAHEME (FOR ESRD)	1 MG	IV	Q0139
FERAHEME (NON-ESRD)	1 MG	IV	Q0138
FERIDEX IV	1 ML	IV	Q9953
FERRIC CARBOXYMALTOSE	1 MG	IV	J1439
FERRIC PYROPHOSPHATE CITRATE POWDER	0.1 MG	IV	J1444
FERRIC PYROPHOSPHATE CITRATE SOLUTION	0.1 MG	IV	J1443
FERRLECIT	12.5 MG	IV	J2916
FERTINEX	75 IU	SC	J3355
FERUMOXYTOL (FOR ESRD)	1 MG	IV	Q0139
FERUMOXYTOL (NON-ESRD)	1 MG	IV	Q0138
FIBRIN SEALANT (HUMAN)	2 ML	OTH	C9250
FIBRYGA	1 MG	IV	J7177
FILGRASTIM	1 MCG	SC, IV	J1442
FILGRASTIM-AAFI, BIOSIMILAR	1 MCG	INJ	Q5110
FILGRASTIM-SNDZ, BIOSIMILAR	1 MCG	IV, SC	Q5101
FINASTERIDE	5 MG	ORAL	S0138
FIRAZYR	1 MG	SC	J1744
FIRMAGON	1 MG	SC	J9155
FISH OIL TRIGLYCERIDES	10 G	IV	B4187
FLAGYL	500 MG	IV	S0030
FLEBOGAMMA	500 MG	IV	J1572
FLEXHD	SQ CM	OTH	Q4128
FLEXON	60 MG	IV, IM	J2360
FLOLAN	0.5 MG	IV	J1325
FLORBETABEN F18, DIAGNOSTIC	STUDY DOSE UP TO 8.1 MCI	IV	Q9983
FLOWERAMNIOFLO	SQ CM	OTH	Q4177
FLOWERAMNIOPATCH	SQ CM	OTH	Q4178
FLOWERDERM	SQ CM	OTH	Q4179
FLOXIN IV	400 MG	IV	S0034
FLOXURIDINE	500 MG	IV	J9200
FLUCICLOVINE F-18, DIAGNOSTIC	1 MCI	IV	A9588
FLUCONAZOLE	200 MG	IV	J1450
FLUDARA	50 MG	IV	J9185

© 2019 Optum360, LLC

Drug Name	Unit Per	Route	Code
FLUDARABINE PHOSPHATE	10 MG	ORAL	J8562
FLUDARABINE PHOSPHATE	50 MG	IV	J9185
FLUDEOXYGLUCOSE F18	STUDY DOSE UP TO 45 MCI	IV	A9552
FLUID FLOW, FLUID GF	1 CC	OTH	Q4206
FLULAVAL	EA	IM	Q2036
FLUMADINE (DEMONSTATION PROJECT)	100 MG	ORAL	G9036
FLUNISOLIDE, COMPOUNDED, UNIT DOSE	1 MG	INH	J7641
FLUOCINOLONE ACETONIDE INTRAVITREAL IMPLANT	IMPLANT	OTH	J7311
FLUOCINOLONE ACETONIDE, INTRAVITREAL IMPLANT	0.01 MG	OTH	J7313
FLUOCINOLONE ACETONIDE, INTRAVITREAL IMPLANT	0.01 MG	OTH	J7314
FLUORODEOXYGLUCOSE F-18 FDG, DIAGNOSTIC	STUDY DOSE UP TO 45 MCI	IV	A9552
FLUOROURACIL	500 MG	IV	J9190
FLUPHENAZINE DECANOATE	25 MG	SC, IM	J2680
FLUTAMIDE	125 MG	ORAL	S0175
FLUTEMETAMOL F18, DIAGNOSTIC	STUDY DOSE UP TO 5 MCI	IV	Q9982
FLUVIRIN	EA	IM	Q2037
FLUZONE	EA	IM	Q2038
FOLEX	5 MG	IV, IM, IT, IA	J9250
FOLEX	50 MG	IV, IM, IT, IA	J9260
FOLEX PFS	5 MG	IV, IM, IT, IA	J9250
FOLEX PFS	50 MG	IV, IM, IT, IA	J9260
FOLLISTIM	75 IU	SC, IM	S0128
FOLLITROPIN ALFA	75 IU	SC	S0126
FOLLITROPIN BETA	75 IU	SC, IM	S0128
FOLOTYN	1 MG	IV	J9307
FOMEPIZOLE	15 MG	IV	J1451
FOMIVIRSEN SODIUM	1.65 MG	OTH	J1452
FONDAPARINUX SODIUM	0.5 MG	SC	J1652
FORMOTEROL FUMERATE NONCOMPOUNDED UNIT DOSE FORM	20 MCG	INH	J7606
FORMOTEROL, COMPOUNDED, UNIT DOSE	12 MCG	INH	J7640
FORTAZ	500 MG	IM, IV	J0713
FORTEO	10 MCG	SC	J3110
FORTOVASE	200 MG	ORAL	S0140
FOSAPREPITANT	1 MG	IV	J1453
FOSCARNET SODIUM	1,000 MG	IV	J1455
FOSCAVIR	1,000 MG	IV	J1455
FOSNETUPITANT AND PALONOSETRON	235 MG/0.25 MG	IV	J1454
FOSPHENYTOIN	50 MG	IM, IV	Q2009
FOSPHENYTOIN SODIUM	750 MG	IM, IV	S0078
FRAGMIN	2,500 IU	SC	J1645
~~FREMANEZUMAB-VFRM~~	~~1 MG~~	~~SC~~	~~C9040~~
FREMANEZUMAB-VFRM	1 MG	SC	J3031
FUDR	500 MG	IV	J9200
FULPHILA	0.5 MG	SC	Q5108
FULVESTRANT	25 MG	IM	J9395
FUNGIZONE	50 MG	IV	J0285

Drug Name	Unit Per	Route	Code
FUROSEMIDE	20 MG	IM, IV	J1940
~~FUSILEV~~	~~1 MG~~	~~INJ, IV~~	~~C9043~~
FUZEON	1 MG	SC	J1324
GABLOFEN	10 MG	IT	J0475
GABLOFEN	50 MCG	IT	J0476
GADAVIST	0.1 ML	IV	A9585
GADOBENATE DIMEGLUMINE (MULTIHANCE MULTIPACK)	1 ML	IV	A9577
GADOBUTROL	0.1 ML	IV	A9585
GADOFOSVESET TRISODIUM	1 ML	IV	A9583
GADOLINIUM -BASED CONTRAST NOS	1 ML	IV	A9579
GADOTERATE MEGLUMINE	0.1 ML	IV	A9575
GADOTERIDOL (PROHANCE MULTIPACK)	1 ML	IV	A9576
GADOXETATE DISODIUM	1 ML	IV	A9581
GALLIUM GA-67	1 MCI	IV	A9556
GALLIUM GA-68, DOTATATE, DIAGNOSTIC	0.1 MCI	IV	A9587
GALLIUM NITRATE	1 MG	IV	J1457
GALSULFASE	1 MG	IV	J1458
GAMASTAN	1 CC	IM	J1460
GAMASTAN	OVER 10 CC	IM	J1560
GAMASTAN SD	1 CC	IM	J1460
GAMASTAN SD	OVER 10 CC	IM	J1560
~~GAMIFANT~~	~~1 MG~~	~~IV~~	~~C9050~~
GAMIFANT	1 MG	IV	J9210
GAMMA GLOBULIN	1 CC	IM	J1460
GAMMA GLOBULIN	OVER 10 CC	IM	J1560
GAMMAGARD	500 MG	IV	J1569
GAMMAGRAFT	SQ CM	OTH	Q4111
GAMMAKED	500 MG	IV, SC	J1561
GAMMAPLEX	500 MG	IV	J1557
GAMUNEX	500 MG	IV, SQ	J1561
GAMUNEX-C	500 MG	IV, SC	J1561
GANCICLOVIR	4.5 MG	OTH	J7310
GANCICLOVIR SODIUM	500 MG	IV	J1570
GANIRELIX ACETATE	250 MCG	SC	S0132
GANITE	1 MG	IV	J1457
GARAMYCIN	80 MG	IM, IV	J1580
GASTROCROM	10 MG	INH	J7631
GASTROMARK	1 ML	ORAL	Q9954
GATIFLOXACIN	10 MG	IV	J1590
GAZYVA	10 MG	IV	J9301
GEFITINIB	250 MG	ORAL	J8565
GEL-ONE	DOSE	OTH	J7326
GELSYN-3	0.1 MG	INJ	J7328
GEMCITABINE HCL	200 MG	IV	J9199
GEMCITABINE HCL	200 MG	IV	J9201
GEMTUZUMAB OZOGAMICIN	0.1 MG	INF	J9203
GEMZAR	200 MG	IV	J9201
GENESIS AMNIOTIC MEMBRANE	SQ CM	OTH	Q4198
GENGRAF	100 MG	ORAL	J7502
GENGRAF	25 MG	ORAL	J7515
GENOTROPIN	1 MG	SC	J2941
GENOTROPIN MINIQUICK	1 MG	SC	J2941

© 2019 Optum360, LLC

Drug Name	Unit Per	Route	Code
GENOTROPIN NUTROPIN	1 MG	SC	J2941
GENTAMICIN	80 MG	IM, IV	J1580
GENTRAN	500 ML	IV	J7100
GENTRAN 75	500 ML	IV	J7110
GENVISC 850	1 MG	OTH	J7320
GEODON	10 MG	IM	J3486
GEREF	1MCG	SC	Q0515
GLASSIA	10 MG	IV	J0257
GLATIRAMER ACETATE	20 MG	SC	J1595
GLEEVEC	100 MG	ORAL	S0088
GLOFIL-125	STUDY DOSE UP TO 10 UCI	IV	A9554
GLUCAGEN	1 MG	SC, IM, IV	J1610
GLUCAGON	1 MG	SC, IM, IV	J1610
GLUCOTOPE	STUDY DOSE UP TO 45 MCI	IV	A9552
GLYCOPYRROLATE, COMPOUNDED CONCENTRATED	PER MG	INH	J7642
GLYCOPYRROLATE, COMPOUNDED, UNIT DOSE	1 MG	INH	J7643
GOLD SODIUM THIOMALATE	50 MG	IM	J1600
GOLIMUMAB	1 MG	IV	J1602
GONADORELIN HCL	100 MCG	SC, IV	J1620
GONAL-F	75 IU	SC	S0126
GOPRELTO	1 MG	OTH	C9046
GOSERELIN ACETATE	3.6 MG	SC	J9202
GRAFIX CORE	SQ CM	OTH	Q4132
GRAFIX PRIME	SQ CM	OTH	Q4133
GRAFIXPL CORE	SQ CM	OTH	Q4132
GRAFIXPL PRIME	SQ CM	OTH	Q4133
GRAFTJACKET	SQ CM	OTH	Q4107
GRAFTJACKET EXPRESS	1 CC	INJ	Q4113
GRANISETRON HCL	1 MG	IV	S0091
GRANISETRON HCL	1 MG	ORAL	Q0166
GRANISETRON HCL	100 MCG	IV	J1626
GRANISETRON, EXTENDED-RELEASE	0.1 MG	SC	J1627
GRANIX	1 MCG	IV	J1447
GUARDIAN	SQ CM	OTH	Q4151
GUSELKUMAB	1 MG	SC	J1628
GYNOGEN L.A. 10	10 MG	IM	J1380
GYNOGEN L.A. 20	10 MG	IM	J1380
GYNOGEN L.A. 40	10 MG	IM	J1380
H.P. ACTHAR GEL	UP TO 40 UNITS	OTH	J0800
HAEGARDA	10 UNITS	SC	J0599
HALAVEN	0.1 MG	IV	J9179
HALDOL	5 MG	IM, IV	J1630
HALDOL DECANOATE	50 MG	IM	J1631
HALOPERIDOL	5 MG	IM, IV	J1630
HECTOROL	1 MG	IV	J1270
HELICOLL	SQ CM	OTH	Q4164
HELIXATE FS	1 IU	IV	J7192
HEMIN	1 MG	IV	J1640
HEMLIBRA	0.5 MG	SC	J7170
HEMOFIL	1 IU	IV	J7192
HEMOFIL-M	1 IU	IV	J7190
HEP LOCK	10 U	IV	J1642
HEP-PAK	10 UNITS	IV	J1642
HEPAGAM B	0.5 ML	IM	J1571
HEPAGAM B	0.5 ML	IV	J1573
HEPARIN SODIUM	1,000 U	IV, SC	J1644
HEPARIN SODIUM	10 U	IV	J1642
HEPATITIS B IMMUNE GLOBULIN	0.5 ML	IV	J1573
HEPATOLITE	STUDY DOSE UP TO 15 MCI	IV	A9510
HERCEPTIN HYLECTA	10 MG	SC	J9356
HERCEPTIN, EXCLUDES BIOSIMILAR	10 MG	IV	J9355
HERZUMA	10 MG	IV	Q5113
HEXADROL	0.25 MG	ORAL	J8540
HEXAMINOLEVULINATE HYDROCHLORIDE	STUDY DOSE	OTH	A9589
HIGH OSMOLAR CONTRAST MATERIAL, UP TO 149 MG/ML IODINE CONCENTRATION	1 ML	IV	Q9958
HIGH OSMOLAR CONTRAST MATERIAL, UP TO 150-199 MG/ML IODINE CONCENTRATION	1 ML	IV	Q9959
HIGH OSMOLAR CONTRAST MATERIAL, UP TO 200-249 MG/ML IODINE CONCENTRATION	1 ML	IV	Q9960
HIGH OSMOLAR CONTRAST MATERIAL, UP TO 250-299 MG/ML IODINE CONCENTRATION	1 ML	IV	Q9961
HIGH OSMOLAR CONTRAST MATERIAL, UP TO 300-349 MG/ML IODINE CONCENTRATION	1 ML	IV	Q9962
HIGH OSMOLAR CONTRAST MATERIAL, UP TO 350-399 MG/ML IODINE CONCENTRATION	1 ML	IV	Q9963
HIGH OSMOLAR CONTRAST MATERIAL, UP TO 400 OR GREATER MG/ML IODINE CONCENTRATION	1 ML	IV	Q9964
HISTERLIN IMPLANT (VANTAS)	50 MG	OTH	J9225
HISTRELIN ACETATE	10 MG	INJ	J1675
HISTRELIN IMPLANT (SUPPRELIN LA)	50 MG	OTH	J9226
HIZENTRA	100 MG	SC	J1559
HMATRIX	SQ CM	OTH	Q4134
HUMALOG	5 U	SC	J1815
HUMALOG	50 U	SC	J1817
HUMAN FIBRINOGEN CONCENTRATE	1 MG	IV	J7177
HUMAN FIBRINOGEN CONCENTRATE, NOT OTHERWISE SPECIFIED	1 MG	IV	J7178
HUMATE-P	1 IU	IV	J7187
HUMATROPE	1 MG	SC	J2941
HUMIRA	20 MG	SC	J0135
HUMULIN	5 U	SC	J1815
HUMULIN	50 U	SC	J1817
HUMULIN R	5 U	SC	J1815
HUMULIN R U-500	5 U	SC	J1815
HYALGAN	DOSE	OTH	J7321

© 2019 Optum360, LLC

Drug Name	Unit Per	Route	Code
HYALOMATRIX	SQ CM	OTH	Q4117
HYALURONAN	DOSE	OTH	J7321
HYALURONAN OR DERITIVE, GEL-ONE	DOSE	OTH	J7326
HYALURONAN OR DERIVATIVE	1 MG	INJ	J7331
HYALURONAN OR DERIVATIVE	1 MG	INJ	J7332
HYALURONAN OR DERIVATIVE, DUROLANE	1 MG	INJ	J7318
HYALURONAN OR DERIVATIVE, GEL-SYN-3, FOR INTRA-ARTICULAR INJECTION	0.1 MG	INJ	J7328
HYALURONAN OR DERIVATIVE, MONOVISC	DOSE	OTH	J7327
HYALURONAN OR DERIVATIVE, TRIVISC	1 MG	INJ	J7329
HYALURONAN OR DERIVITIVE FOR INTRA-ARTICULAR INJECTION	1 MG	OTH	J7320
HYALURONAN OR DERIVITIVE FOR INTRA-ARTICULAR INJECTION	1 MG	OTH	J7322
HYALURONAN, EUFLEXXA	DOSE	OTH	J7323
HYALURONAN, ORTHOVISC	DOSE	OTH	J7324
HYALURONAN, SYNVISC/SYNVISC-ONE	1 MG	OTH	J7325
HYALURONIDASE	150 UNITS	VAR	J3470
HYALURONIDASE RECOMBINANT	1 USP UNIT	SC	J3473
HYALURONIDASE, OVINE, PRESERVATIVE FREE	1 USP	OTH	J3471
HYALURONIDASE, OVINE, PRESERVATIVE FREE	1000 USP	OTH	J3472
HYCAMTIN	0.1 MG	IV	J9351
HYCAMTIN	0.25 MG	ORAL	J8705
HYDRALAZINE HCL	20 MG	IV, IM	J0360
HYDRATE	50 MG	IM, IV	J1240
HYDREA	500 MG	ORAL	S0176
HYDROCORTISONE ACETATE	25 MG	IV, IM, SC	J1700
HYDROCORTISONE SODIUM PHOSPHATE	50 MG	IV, IM, SC	J1710
HYDROCORTISONE SODIUM SUCCINATE	100 MG	IV, IM, SC	J1720
HYDROCORTONE PHOSPHATE	50 MG	SC, IM, IV	J1710
HYDROMORPHONE HCL	250 MG	OTH	S0092
HYDROMORPHONE HCL	4 MG	SC, IM, IV	J1170
HYDROXOCOBALAMIN	1,000 MCG	IM, SC	J3420
HYDROXYCOBAL	1,000 MCG	IM, SC	J3420
HYDROXYPROGESTERONE CAPROATE (MAKENA)	10 MG	IM	J1726
HYDROXYPROGESTERONE CAPROATE, NOT OTHERWISE SPECIFIED	10 MG	IM	J1729
HYDROXYUREA	500 MG	ORAL	S0176
HYDROXYZINE HCL	25 MG	IM	J3410
HYDROXYZINE PAMOATE	25 MG	ORAL	Q0177
HYMOVIS	1 MG	OTH	J7322
HYOSCYAMINE SULFATE	0.25 MG	SC, IM, IV	J1980
HYPERRHO S/D	300 MCG	IV	J2790
HYPERTET SD	UP TO 250 MG	IM	J1670
HYPERTONIC SALINE SOLUTION	1 ML	VAR	J7131
HYQVIA	100 MG	IV	J1575
HYREXIN	50 MG	IV, IM	J1200
HYZINE	25 MG	IM	J3410
HYZINE-50	25 MG	IM	J3410
IBALIZUMAB-UIYK	10 MG	IV	J1746
IBANDRONATE SODIUM	1 MG	IV	J1740
IBRITUMOMAB TUXETAN	STUDY DOSE UP TO 5 MCI	IV	A9542
IBUPROFEN	100 MG	IV	J1741
IBUTILIDE FUMARATE	1 MG	IV	J1742
ICATIBANT	1 MG	SC	J1744
IDAMYCIN	5 MG	IV	J9211
IDAMYCIN PFS	5 MG	IV	J9211
IDARUBICIN HCL	5 MG	IV	J9211
IDELVION	1 IU	IV	J7202
IDURSULFASE	1 MG	IV	J1743
IFEX	1 G	IV	J9208
IFOSFAMIDE	1 G	IV	J9208
IL-2	1 VIAL	IV	J9015
ILARIS	1 MG	SC	J0638
ILETIN	5 UNITS	SC	J1815
ILETIN II NPH PORK	50 U	SC	J1817
ILETIN II REGULAR PORK	5 U	SC	J1815
ILOPROST INHALATION SOLUTION	PER DOSE UP TO 20 MCG	INH	Q4074
ILUMYA	1 MG	SC	J3245
ILUVIEN	0.01 MG	OTH	J7313
IMAGENT	1 ML	IV	Q9955
IMATINIB	100 MG	ORAL	S0088
IMFINZI	10 MG	IV	J9173
IMIGLUCERASE	10 U	IV	J1786
IMITREX	6 MG	SC	J3030
IMLYGIC	1 MILLION	INTRALESIONAL	J9325
IMMUNE GLOBULIN (BIVIGAM)	500 MG	IV	J1556
IMMUNE GLOBULIN (CIVITRU)	100 MG	SC	J1555
IMMUNE GLOBULIN (FLEBOGAMMA, FLEBOGAMMA DIF)	500 MG	IV	J1572
IMMUNE GLOBULIN (GAMMAGARD LIQUID)	500 MG	IV	J1569
IMMUNE GLOBULIN (GAMMAPLEX)	500 MG	IV	J1557
IMMUNE GLOBULIN (GAMUNEX)	500 MG	IV	J1561
IMMUNE GLOBULIN (HIZENTRA)	100 MG	SC	J1559
IMMUNE GLOBULIN (OCTAGAM)	500 MG	IV	J1568
IMMUNE GLOBULIN (PRIVIGEN) NONLYOPHILIZED	500 MG	IV	J1459
IMMUNE GLOBULIN (RHOPHYLAC)	100 IU	IM, IV	J2791
IMMUNE GLOBULIN LYOPHILIZED	500 MG	IV	J1566
IMMUNE GLOBULIN SUBCUTANEOUS	100 MG	SC	J1562
IMMUNE GLOBULIN, NONLYOPHILIZED (NOS)	500 MG	IV	J1599
IMMUNE GLOBULIN/HYALURONIDASE	100 MG	IV	J1575

© 2019 Optum360, LLC

Drug Name	Unit Per	Route	Code
IMPLANON	IMPLANT	OTH	J7307
IMURAN	50 MG	ORAL	J7500
IN-111 SATUMOMAB PENDETIDE	STUDY DOSE UP TO MCI	IV	A4642
INAPSINE	5 MG	IM, IV	J1790
INCOBUTULINUMTOXINA	1 UNIT	IM	J0588
INDERAL	1 MG	IV	J1800
INDIUM IN-111 IBRITUMOMAB TIUXETAN, DIAGNOSTIC	STUDY DOSE UP TO 5 MCI	IV	A9542
INDIUM IN-111 LABELED AUTOLOGOUS PLATELETS	STUDY DOSAGE	IV	A9571
INDIUM IN-111 LABELED AUTOLOGOUS WHITE BLOOD CELLS	STUDY DOSE	IV	A9570
INDIUM IN-111 OXYQUINOLINE	0.5 MCI	IV	A9547
INDIUM IN-111 PENTETREOTIDE	STUDY DOSE UP TO 6 MCI	IV	A9572
INDURSALFASE	1 MG	IV	J1743
INFED	50 MG	IM, IV	J1750
INFERGEN	1 MCG	SC	J9212
~~INFLECTRA~~	~~10 MG~~	~~IV~~	~~Q5102~~
INFLECTRA	10 MG	IV	Q5103
INFLIXIMAB	10 MG	IV	J1745
~~INFLIXIMAB, BIOSIMILAR~~	~~10 MG~~	~~IV~~	~~Q5102~~
INFLIXIMAB-ABDA, BIOSIMILAR	10 MG	IV	Q5104
INFLIXIMAB-DYYB, BIOSIMILAR	10 MG	IV	Q5103
INFLIXIMAB-QBTX, BIOSIMILAR	10 MG	IV	Q5109
INFLUENZA VACCINE, AGRIFLU	UNKNOWN	IM	Q2034
INFLUENZA VIRUS VACCINE (AFLURIA)	EA	IM	Q2035
INFLUENZA VIRUS VACCINE (FLULAVAL)	EA	IM	Q2036
INFLUENZA VIRUS VACCINE (FLUVIRIN)	EA	IM	Q2037
INFLUENZA VIRUS VACCINE (FLUZONE)	EA	IM	Q2038
INFLUENZA VIRUS VACCINE, NOT OTHERWISE SPECIFIED	EA	IM	Q2039
INFUGEM	200 MG	IV	J9199
INFUMORPH	10 MG	IM, IV, SC	J2270
INJECTAFER	1 MG	IV	J1439
INNOHEP	1,000 IU	SC	J1655
INOTUZUMAB OZOGAMICIN	0.1 MG	IV	J9229
INSULIN	5 U	SC	J1815
INSULIN	50 U	SC	J1817
INSULIN LISPRO	5 U	SC	J1815
INSULIN LISPRO	5 U	SC	S5551
INSULIN PURIFIED REGULAR PORK	5 U	SC	J1815
INTAL	10 MG	INH	J7631
INTEGRA BILAYER MATRIX DRESSING	SQ CM	OTH	Q4104
INTEGRA DERMAL REGENERATION TEMPLATE	SQ CM	OTH	Q4105
INTEGRA FLOWABLE WOUND MATRIX	1 CC	INJ	Q4114
INTEGRA MATRIX	SQ CM	OTH	Q4108
INTEGRA MOZAIK OSTEOCONDUCTIVE SCAFFOLD PUTTY	0.5 CC	OTH	C9359
INTEGRA MOZAIK OSTEOCONDUCTIVE SCAFFOLD STRIP	0.5 CC	OTH	C9362
INTEGRA OMNIGRAFT DERMAL REGENERATION MATRIX	SQ CM	OTH	Q4105
INTEGRA OS OSTEOCONDUCTIVE SCAFFOLD PUTTY	0.5 CC	OTH	C9359
INTEGRILIN	5 MG	IM, IV	J1327
INTERFERON ALFA-2A	3,000,000 U	SC, IM	J9213
INTERFERON ALFA-2B	1,000,000 U	SC, IM	J9214
INTERFERON ALFA-N3	250,000 IU	IM	J9215
INTERFERON ALFACON-1	1 MCG	SC	J9212
INTERFERON BETA-1A	1 MCG	IM	Q3027
INTERFERON BETA-1A	1 MCG	SC	Q3028
INTERFERON BETA-1A	30 MCG	IM, SC	J1826
INTERFERON BETA-1B	0.25 MG	SC	J1830
INTERFERON, ALFA-2A, RECOMBINANT	3,000,000 U	SC, IM	J9213
INTERFERON, ALFA-2B, RECOMBINANT	1,000,000 U	SC, IM	J9214
INTERFERON, ALFA-N3, (HUMAN LEUKOCYTE DERIVED)	250,000 IU	IM	J9215
INTERFERON, GAMMA 1-B	3,000,000 U	SC	J9216
INTERFYL	1 MG	OTH	Q4171
INTERLUEKIN	1 VIAL	IV	J9015
INTRON A	1,000,000 U	SC, IM	J9214
INVANZ	500 MG	IM, IV	J1335
INVEGA SUSTENNA	1 MG	IM	J2426
INVIRASE	200 MG	ORAL	S0140
IOBENGUANE SULFATE I-131	0.5 MCI	IV	A9508
IOBENGUANE, I-123, DIAGNOSTIC	PER STUDY DOSE UP TO 15 MCI	IV	A9582
IODINE I-123 IOBENGUANE, DIAGNOSTIC	15 MCI	IV	A9582
IODINE I-123 IOFLUPANE	STUDY DOSE UP TO 5 MCI	IV	A9584
IODINE I-123 SODIUM IODIDE CAPSULE(S), DIAGNOSTIC	100-9999 UCI	ORAL	A9516
IODINE I-123 SODIUM IODIDE, DIAGNOSTIC	1 MCI	IV	A9509
IODINE I-125 SERUM ALBUMIN, DIAGNOSTIC	5 UCI	IV	A9532
IODINE I-125 SODIUM IOTHALAMATE, DIAGNOSTIC	STUDY DOSE UP TO 10 UCI	IV	A9554
IODINE I-125, SODIUM IODIDE SOLUTION, THERAPEUTIC	1 MCI	ORAL	A9527
IODINE I-131 IOBENGUANE SULFATE, DIAGNOSTIC	0.5 MCI	IV	A9508
~~IODINE I-131 IOBENGUANE, DIAGNOSTIC~~	~~1 MCI~~	~~IV~~	~~C9407~~
~~IODINE I-131 IOBENGUANE, THERAPEUTIC~~	~~1 MCI~~	~~IV~~	~~C9408~~
IODINE I-131 IODINATED SERUM ALBUMIN, DIAGNOSTIC	PER 5 UCI	IV	A9524
IODINE I-131 SODIUM IODIDE CAPSULE(S), DIAGNOSTIC	1 MCI	ORAL	A9528

© 2019 Optum360, LLC

Drug Name	Unit Per	Route	Code
IODINE I-131 SODIUM IODIDE CAPSULE(S), THERAPEUTIC	1 MCI	ORAL	A9517
IODINE I-131 SODIUM IODIDE SOLUTION, DIAGNOSTIC	1 MCI	ORAL	A9529
IODINE I-131 SODIUM IODIDE SOLUTION, THERAPEUTIC	1 MCI	ORAL	A9530
IODINE I-131 SODIUM IODIDE, DIAGNOSTIC	PER UCI UP TO 100 UCI	IV	A9531
IODINE I-131, IOBENGUANE	1 MCI	IV	A9590
IODOTOPE THERAPEUTIC CAPSULE(S)	1 MCI	ORAL	A9517
IODOTOPE THERAPEUTIC SOLUTION	1 MCI	ORAL	A9530
IOFLUPANE	STUDY DOSE UP TO 5 MCI	IV	A9584
ION-BASED MAGNETIC RESONANCE CONTRAST AGENT	1 ML	IV	Q9953
IOTHALAMATE SODIUM I-125	STUDY DOSE UP TO 10 UCI	IV	A9554
IPILIMUMAB	1 MG	IV	J9228
IPLEX	1 MG	SC	J2170
IPRATROPIUM BROMIDE, NONCOMPOUNDED, UNIT DOSE	1 MG	INH	J7644
IPTRATROPIUM BROMIDE COMPOUNDED, UNIT DOSE	1 MG	INH	J7645
IRESSA	250 MG	ORAL	J8565
IRINOTECAN	20 MG	IV	J9206
IRINOTECAN LIPOSOME	1 MG	IV	J9205
IRON DEXTRAN, 50 MG	50 MG	IM, IV	J1750
IRON SUCROSE	1 MG	IV	J1756
ISAVUCONAZONIUM	1 MG	IV	J1833
ISOCAINE	10 ML	VAR	J0670
ISOETHARINE HCL COMPOUNDED, CONCENTRATED	1 MG	INH	J7647
ISOETHARINE HCL COMPOUNDED, UNIT DOSE	1 MG	INH	J7650
ISOETHARINE HCL, NONCOMPOUNDED CONCENTRATED	PER MG	INH	J7648
ISOETHARINE HCL, NONCOMPOUNDED, UNIT DOSE	1 MG	INH	J7649
ISOJEX	5 UCI	IV	A9532
ISOPROTERENOL HCL COMPOUNDED, CONCENTRATED	1 MG	INH	J7657
ISOPROTERENOL HCL COMPOUNDED, UNIT DOSE	1 MG	INH	J7660
ISOPROTERENOL HCL, NONCOMPOUNDED CONCENTRATED	1 MG	INH	J7658
ISOPROTERNOL HCL, NONCOMPOUNDED, UNIT DOSE	1MG	INH	J7659
ISOSULFAN BLUE	1 MG	SC	Q9968
ISTODAX	1 MG	IV	J9315
ISUPREL	1 MG	INH	J7658
ISUPREL	1 MG	INH	J7659
ITRACONAZOLE	50 MG	IV	J1835
IVEEGAM	500 MG	IV	J1566
IXABEPILONE	1 MG	IV	J9207
IXEMPRA	1 MG	IV	J9207

Drug Name	Unit Per	Route	Code
IXIFI	10 MG	IV	Q5109
JETREA	0.125 MG	OTH	J7316
JEVTANA	1 MG	IV	J9043
~~JIVI~~	~~1 IU~~	~~IV~~	~~C9141~~
JIVI	1 IU	IV	J7208
KADCYLA	1 MG	IV	J9354
KALBITOR	1 MG	SC	J1290
KANAMYCIN	500 MG	IM, IV	J1840
KANAMYCIN	75 MG	IM, IV	J1850
KANJINTI	10 MG	IV	Q5117
KANTREX	500 MG	IM, IV	J1840
KANTREX	75 MG	IM, IV	J1850
KANUMA	1 MG	IV	J2840
KCENTRA	PER I.U.	IV	C9132
KEFZOL	500 MG	IM, IV	J0690
KENAJECT-40	10 MG	IM	J3301
KENALOG-10	10 MG	IM	J3301
KEPIVANCE	50 MCG	IV	J2425
KEPPRA	10 MG	IV	J1953
KERAMATRIX OR KERASORB	SQ CM	OTH	Q4165
KERECIS OMEGA3	SQ CM	OTH	Q4158
KEROXX	1 CC	OTH	Q4202
KESTRONE	1 MG	IV, IM	J1435
KETOROLAC TROMETHAMINE	15 MG	IM, IV	J1885
KEYTRUDA	1 MG	IV	J9271
KHAPZORY	0.5 MG	IV	J0642
KINEVAC	5 MCG	IV	J2805
KOATE-DVI	1 IU	IV	J7190
KOGENATE FS	1 IU	IV	J7192
KONAKION	1 MG	SC, IM, IV	J3430
KONYNE 80	1 IU	IV	J7194
KOVALTRY	1 I.U.	IV	J7211
KRYSTEXXA	1 MG	IV	J2507
KYLEENA	19.5 MG	OTH	J7296
KYMRIAH	UP TO 600 MILLION CELLS	IV	Q2042
KYPROLIS	1 MG	IV	J9047
KYTRIL	1 MG	IV	S0091
KYTRIL	1 MG	ORAL	Q0166
KYTRIL	100 MCG	IV	J1626
L-PHENYLALANINE MUSTARD	50 MG	IV	J9245
L.A.E. 20	10 MG	IM	J1380
LACOSAMIDE	1 MG	IV	C9254
LAETRILE	VAR	INJ	J3570
LANADELUMAB-FLYO	1 MG	SC	J0593
LANOXIN	0.5 MG	IM, IV	J1160
LANREOTIDE	1 MG	SC	J1930
LANTUS	5 U	SC	J1815
LARONIDASE	0.1 MG	IV	J1931
LARTRUVO	10 MG	INF	J9285
LASIX	20 MG	IM, IV	J1940
LEFAMULIN	1 MG	IV	C9054
LEMTRADA	1 MG	IV	J0202
LENTE ILETIN I	5 U	SC	J1815
LEPIRUDIN	50 MG	IV	J1945

© 2019 Optum360, LLC

Drug Name	Unit Per	Route	Code
LEUCOVORIN CALCIUM	50 MG	IM, IV	J0640
LEUKERAN	2 MG	ORAL	S0172
LEUKINE	50 MCG	IV	J2820
LEUPROLIDE ACETATE	1 MG	IM	J9218
LEUPROLIDE ACETATE	7.5 MG	SC	J9217
LEUPROLIDE ACETATE (FOR DEPOT SUSPENSION)	3.75 MG	IM	J1950
LEUPROLIDE ACETATE DEPOT	7.5 MG	SC	J9217
LEUPROLIDE ACETATE IMPLANT	65 MG	OTH	J9219
LEUSTATIN	1 MG	IV	J9065
LEVABUTEROL COMPOUNDED, UNIT DOSE	1 MG	INH	J7615
LEVABUTEROL, COMPOUNDED, CONCENTRATED	0.5 MG	INH	J7607
LEVALBUTEROL NONCOMPOUNDED, CONCENTRATED FORM	0.5 MG	INH	J7612
LEVALBUTEROL, NONCOMPOUNDED, UNIT DOSE	0.5 MG	INH	J7614
LEVAMISOLE HCL	50 MG	ORAL	S0177
LEVAQUIN	250 MG	IV	J1956
LEVEMIR	5 U	SC	J1815
LEVETIRACETAM	10 MG	IV	J1953
LEVO-DROMORAN	UP TO 2 MG	IV, IM	J1960
LEVOCARNITINE	1 G	IV	J1955
LEVOFLOXACIN	250 MG	IV	J1956
LEVOLEUCOVORIN	0.5 MG	IV	J0642
~~LEVOLEUCOVORIN~~	~~1 MG~~	~~INJ, IV~~	~~C9043~~
LEVOLEUCOVORIN, NOS	0.5 MG	IV	J0641
LEVONORGESTREL IMPLANT	IMPLANT	OTH	J7306
LEVONORGESTREL-RELEASING INTRAUTERINE CONTRACEPTIVE (MIRENA)	52 MG	OTH	J7298
LEVONORGESTREL-RELEASING INTRAUTERINE CONTRACEPTIVE (LILETTA)	52 MG	OTH	J7297
LEVONORGESTREL-RELEASING INTRAUTERINE CONTRACEPTIVE SYSTEM (KYLEENA)	19.5 MG	OTH	J7296
LEVONORGESTREL-RELEASING INTRAUTERINE CONTRACEPTIVE SYSTEM (SKYLA)	13.5 MG	OTH	J7301
LEVORPHANOL TARTRATE	2 MG	SC, IV, IM	J1960
LEVSIN	0.25 MG	SC, IM, IV	J1980
LEVULAN KERASTICK	354 MG	OTH	J7308
LEXISCAN	0.1 MG	IV	J2785
LIBRIUM	100 MG	IM, IV	J1990
~~LIBTAYO~~	~~1 MG~~	~~IV~~	~~C9044~~
LIBTAYO	1 MG	IV	J9119
LIDOCAINE 70 MG/TETRACAINE 70 MG	PATCH	OTH	C9285
LIDOCAINE HCL	10 MG	IV	J2001
LILETTA	52 MG	OTH	J7297
LINCOCIN HCL	300 MG	IV	J2010
LINCOMYCIN HCL	300 MG	IM, IV	J2010
LINEZOLID	200 MG	IV	J2020
LIORESAL	10 MG	IT	J0475
LIORESAL INTRATHECAL REFILL	50 MCG	IT	J0476

Drug Name	Unit Per	Route	Code
LIPODOX	10 MG	IV	Q2049
LIPOSOMAL, DAUNORUBICIN AND CYTARABINE	1 MG/2.27 MG	IV	J9153
LIQUAEMIN SODIUM	1,000 UNITS	SC, IV	J1644
LISPRO-PFC	50 U	SC	J1817
LOK-PAK	10 UNITS	IV	J1642
LOMUSTINE	10 MG	ORAL	S0178
LORAZEPAM	2 MG	IM, IV	J2060
LOVENOX	10 MG	SC	J1650
LOW OSMOLAR CONTRAST MATERIAL, 100-199 MG/ML IODINE CONCENTRATIONS	1 ML	IV	Q9965
LOW OSMOLAR CONTRAST MATERIAL, 200-299 MG/ML IODINE CONCENTRATION	1 ML	IV	Q9966
LOW OSMOLAR CONTRAST MATERIAL, 300-399 MG/ML IODINE CONCENTRATION	1 ML	IV	Q9967
LOW OSMOLAR CONTRAST MATERIAL, 400 OR GREATER MG/ML IODINE CONCENTRATION	1 ML	IV	Q9951
LOXAPINE	1 MG	INH	J2062
LUCENTIS	0.1 MG	IV	J2778
LUMASON	1 ML	IV	Q9950
LUMIZYME	10 MG	IV	J0221
~~LUMOXITI~~	~~0.01 MG~~	~~IV~~	~~C9045~~
LUMOXITI	0.01 MG	IV	J9313
LUPRON	1 MG	SC	J9218
LUPRON DEPOT	7.5 MG	SC	J9217
LUPRON DEPOT	PER 3.75 MG	IM	J1950
LUPRON IMPLANT	65 MG	OTH	J9219
LUTATHERA	1 MCI	IM	A9513
LUTETIUM LU 177, DOTATATE, THERAPEUTIC	1 MCI	IM	A9513
LUTREPULSE	100 MCG	SC, IV	J1620
LUXTURNA	1 BILLION VECTOR GENOMES	OTH	J3398
LYMPHAZURIN	1 MG	SC	Q9968
LYMPHOCYTE IMMUNE GLOBULIN, ANTITHYMOCYTE GLOBULIN, EQUINE	250 MG	OTH	J7504
LYMPHOCYTE IMMUNE GLOBULIN, ANTITHYMOCYTE GLOBULIN, RABBIT	25 MG	OTH	J7511
LYMPHOSEEK	0.5 MCI	SC, OTH	A9520
MACUGEN	0.3 MG	OTH	J2503
MAGNESIUM SULFATE	500 MG	IV	J3475
MAGNETIC RESONANCE CONTRAST AGENT	1 ML	ORAL	Q9954
MAGNEVIST	1 ML	IV	A9579
MAGROTEC	STUDY DOSE UP TO 10 MCI	IV	A9540
MAKENA	10 MG	IM	J1726
MANNITOL	25% IN 50 ML	IV	J2150
MANNITOL	5 MG	INH	J7665
MARCAINE HCL	30 ML	VAR	S0020
MARINOL	2.5 MG	ORAL	Q0167
MARMINE	50 MG	IM, IV	J1240

© 2019 Optum360, LLC

Drug Name	Unit Per	Route	Code
MARQIBO KIT	5 MG	IV	J9371
MATRION	SQ CM	OTH	Q4201
MATRISTEM MICROMATRIX	1 MG	OTH	Q4118
MATULANE	50 MG	ORAL	S0182
MAXIPIME	500 MG	IV	J0692
MDP-BRACCO	STUDY DOSE UP TO 30 MCI	IV	A9503
MECASERMIN	1 MG	SC	J2170
MECHLORETHAMINE HCL (NITROGEN MUSTARD)	10 MG	IV	J9230
MEDIDEX	1 MG	IM, IV, OTH	J1100
MEDISKIN	SQ CM	OTH	Q4135
MEDROL	4 MG	ORAL	J7509
MEDROXYPROGESTERONE ACETATE	1 MG	IM	J1050
MEFOXIN	1 G	IV	J0694
MEGACE	20 MG	ORAL	S0179
MEGESTROL ACETATE	20 MG	ORAL	S0179
MELPHALAN HCL	2 MG	ORAL	J8600
MELPHALAN HCL	50 MG	IV	J9245
MEMBRANE GRAFT OR MEMBRANE WRAP	SQ CM	OTH	Q4205
~~MEMETASONE SINUS IMPLANT~~	~~370 MCG~~	~~OTH~~	~~S1090~~
MEMODERM	SQ CM	OTH	Q4126
MENADIONE	1 MG	IM, SC, IV	J3430
MENOTROPINS	75 IU	SC, IM, IV	S0122
MEPERGAN	50 MG	IM, IV	J2180
MEPERIDINE AND PROMETHAZINE HCL	50 MG	IM, IV	J2180
MEPERIDINE HCL	100 MG	IM, IV, SC	J2175
MEPIVACAINE HCL	10 ML	VAR	J0670
MEPOLIZUMAB	100 MG	SQ	J2182
MEPSEVII	1 MG	IV	J3397
MERCAPTOPURINE	50 MG	ORAL	S0108
MERITATE	150 MG	IV	J3520
MEROPENEM	100 MG	IV	J2185
MEROPENEM, VABORBACTAM	10 MG/10 MG	IV	J2186
MERREM	100 MG	IV	J2185
MESNA	200 MG	IV	J9209
MESNEX	200 MG	IV	J9209
METAPROTERENOL SULFATE COMPOUNDED, UNIT DOSE	10 MG	INH	J7670
METAPROTERENOL SULFATE, NONCOMPOUNDED, CONCENTRATED	10 MG	INH	J7668
METAPROTERENOL SULFATE, NONCOMPOUNDED, UNIT DOSE	10 MG	INH	J7669
METARAMINOL BITARTRATE	10 MG	IV, IM, SC	J0380
METASTRON STRONTIUM 89 CHLORIDE	1 MCI	IV	A9600
METATRACE	STUDY DOSE UP TO 45 MCI	IV	A9552
METHACHOLINE CHLORIDE	1 MG	INH	J7674
METHADONE	5 MG	ORAL	S0109
METHADONE HCL	10 MG	IM, SC	J1230
METHAPREL, COMPOUNDED, UNIT DOSE	10 MG	INH	J7670
METHAPREL, NONCOMPOUNDED, CONCENTRATED	10 MG	INH	J7668
METHAPREL, NONCOMPOUNDED, UNIT DOSE	10 MG	INH	J7669
METHERGINE	0.2 MG	IM, IV	J2210
METHOTREXATE	2.5 MG	ORAL	J8610
METHOTREXATE	5 MG	IV, IM, IT, IA	J9250
METHOTREXATE	50 MG	IV, IM, IT, IA	J9260
METHOTREXATE LPF	5 MG	IV, IM, IT, IA	J9250
METHOTREXATE LPF	50 MG	IV, IM, IT, IA	J9260
METHYL AMINOLEVULINATE 16.8%	1 G	OTH	J7309
METHYLCOTOLONE	80 MG	IM	J1040
METHYLDOPA HCL	UP TO 250 MG	IV	J0210
METHYLDOPATE HCL	UP TO 250 MG	IV	J0210
METHYLENE BLUE	1 MG	SC	Q9968
METHYLERGONOVINE MALEATE	0.2 MG	IM, IV	J2210
METHYLNALTREXONE	0.1 MG	SC	J2212
METHYLPRED	4 MG	ORAL	J7509
METHYLPREDNISOLONE	125 MG	IM, IV	J2930
METHYLPREDNISOLONE	4 MG	ORAL	J7509
METHYLPREDNISOLONE	UP TO 40 MG	IM, IV	J2920
METHYLPREDNISOLONE ACETATE	20 MG	IM	J1020
METHYLPREDNISOLONE ACETATE	40 MG	IM	J1030
METHYLPREDNISOLONE ACETATE	80 MG	IM	J1040
METOCLOPRAMIDE	10 MG	IV	J2765
METRONIDAZOLE	500 MG	IV	S0030
METVIXIA 16.8%	1 G	OTH	J7309
MIACALCIN	400 U	SC, IM	J0630
MIBG	0.5 MCI	IV	A9508
MICAFUNGIN SODIUM	1 MG	IV	J2248
MICRHOGAM	50 MCG	IV	J2788
MICROPOROUS COLLAGEN IMPLANTABLE SLIT TUBE	1 CM LENGTH	OTH	C9353
MICROPOROUS COLLAGEN IMPLANTABLE TUBE	1 CM LENGTH	OTH	C9352
MIDAZOLAM HCI	1 MG	IM, IV	J2250
MIFEPRISTONE	200 MG	ORAL	S0190
MILRINONE LACTATE	5 MG	IV	J2260
MINOCIN	1 MG	IV	J2265
MINOCYCLINE HCL	1 MG	IV	J2265
MINOXIDIL	10 MG	ORAL	S0139
MIRCERA	1 MCG	IV	J0887
MIRCERA	1 MCG	SC	J0888
MIRENA	52 MG	OTH	J7298
MIRODERM	SQ CM	OTH	Q4175
MISOPROSTOL	200 MG	ORAL	S0191
MITHRACIN	2.5 MG	IV	J9270
MITOMYCIN	0.2 MG	OTH	J7315
MITOMYCIN	5 MG	IV	J9280
MITOSOL	0.2 MG	OTH	J7315
MITOXANA	1 G	IV	J9208
MITOXANTRONE HCL	5 MG	IV	J9293
~~MOGAMULIZUMAB-KPKC~~	~~1 MG~~	~~IV~~	~~C9038~~
MOGAMULIZUMAB-KPKC	1 MG	IV	J9204

© 2019 Optum360, LLC

Drug Name	Unit Per	Route	Code
MOMETASONE FUROATE SINUS IMPLANT	10 MCG	OTH	J7401
MONARC-M	1 IU	IV	J7190
MONOCLATE-P	1 IU	IV	J7190
MONONINE	1 IU	IV	J7193
MONOPUR	75 IU	SC, IM	S0122
MONOVISC	DOSE	OTH	J7327
MORPHINE SULFATE	10 MG	IM, IV, SC	J2270
MORPHINE SULFATE	500 MG	OTH	S0093
MORPHINE SULFATE, PRESERVATIVE-FREE FOR EPIDURAL OR INTRATHECAL USE	10 MG	OTH	J2274
~~MOXETUMOMAB PASUDOTOX-TDFK~~	~~0.01 MG~~	~~IV~~	~~C9045~~
MOXETUMOMAB PASUDOTOX-TDFK	0.01 MG	IV	J9313
MOXIFLOXACIN	100 MG	IV	J2280
MOZOBIL	1 MG	SC	J2562
MPI INDIUM DTPA	0.5 MCI	IV	A9548
MS CONTIN	500 MG	OTH	S0093
MUCOMYST	1 G	INH	J7608
MUCOSIL	1 G	INH	J7608
MULTIHANCE	1 ML	IV	A9577
MULTIHANCE MULTIPACK	1 ML	IV	A9578
MUROMONAB-CD3	5 MG	OTH	J7505
MUSE	EA	OTH	J0275
MUSTARGEN	10 MG	IV	J9230
MUTAMYCIN	5 MG	IV	J9280
MVASI	10 MG	IV	Q5107
MYCAMINE	1 MG	IV	J2248
MYCOPHENOLATE MOFETIL	250 MG	ORAL	J7517
MYCOPHENOLIC ACID	180 MG	ORAL	J7518
MYFORTIC DELAYED RELEASE	180 MG	ORAL	J7518
MYLERAN	2 MG	ORAL	J8510
MYLOCEL	500 MG	ORAL	S0176
MYLOTARG	0.1 MG	INF	J9203
MYOBLOC	100 U	IM	J0587
MYOCHRYSINE	50 MG	IM	J1600
MYOWN SKIN	SQ CM	OTH	Q4226
MYOZYME	10 MG	IV	J0220
NABILONE	1 MG	ORAL	J8650
NAFCILLIN SODIUM	2 GM	IM, IV	S0032
NAGLAZYME	1 MG	IV	J1458
NALBUPHINE HCL	10 MG	IM, IV, SC	J2300
NALLPEN	2 GM	IM, IV	S0032
NALOXONE HCL	1 MG	IM, IV, SC	J2310
NALTREXONE, DEPOT FORM	1 MG	IM	J2315
NANDROLONE DECANOATE	50 MG	IM	J2320
NARCAN	1 MG	IM, IV, SC	J2310
NAROPIN	1 MG	VAR	J2795
NASALCROM	10 MG	INH	J7631
NATALIZUMAB	1 MG	IV	J2323
NATRECOR	0.1 MG	IV	J2325
NATURAL ESTROGENIC SUBSTANCE	1 MG	IM, IV	J1410
NAVELBINE	10 MG	IV	J9390
ND-STAT	10 MG	IM, SC, IV	J0945

Drug Name	Unit Per	Route	Code
NEBCIN	80 MG	IM, IV	J3260
NEBUPENT	300 MG	IM, IV	S0080
NEBUPENT	300 MG	INH	J2545
NECITUMUMAB	1 MG	IV	J9295
NELARABINE	50 MG	IV	J9261
NEMBUTAL SODIUM	50 MG	IM, IV, OTH	J2515
NEOPATCH	SQ CM	OTH	Q4176
NEORAL	25 MG	ORAL	J7515
NEORAL	250 MG	ORAL	J7516
NEOSAR	100 MG	IV	J9070
NEOSCAN	1 MCI	IV	A9556
NEOSTIGMINE METHYLSULFATE	0.5 MG	IM, IV	J2710
NEOTECT	STUDY DOSE UP TO 35 MCI	IV	A9536
NEOX 100	SQ CM	OTH	Q4156
NEOX CORD 1K	SQ CM	OTH	Q4148
NEOX CORD RT	SQ EM	OTH	Q4148
NEOXFLO	1 MG	OTH	Q4155
NESACAINE	30 ML	VAR	J2400
NESACAINE-MPF	30 ML	VAR	J2400
NESIRITIDE	0.1 MG	IV	J2325
NETSPOT	0.1 MCI	IV	A9587
NETUPITANT AND PALONOSETRON	300 MG/0.5 MG	ORAL	J8655
NEULASTA	6 MG	SC, SQ	J2505
NEUMEGA	5 MG	SC	J2355
NEUPOGEN	1 MCG	SC, IV	J1442
NEURAGEN NERVE GUIDE	1 CM LENGTH	OTH	C9352
NEUROLITE	STUDY DOSE UP TO 25 MCI	IV	A9557
NEUROMATRIX	0.5 CM LENGTH	OTH	C9355
NEUROMEND NERVE WRAP	0.5 CM	OTH	C9361
NEUROWRAP NERVE PROTECTOR	1 CM LENGTH	OTH	C9353
NEUTREXIN	25 MG	IV	J3305
NEUTROSPEC	STUDY DOSE UP TO 25 MCI	IV	A9566
NEXPLANON	IMPLANT	OTH	J7307
NIPENT	10 MG	IV	J9268
NITROGEN MUSTARD	10 MG	IV	J9230
NITROGEN N-13 AMMONIA, DIAGNOSTIC	STUDY DOSE UP TO 40 MCI	INJ	A9526
NIVESTYM	1 MCG	INJ	Q5110
NIVOLUMAB	1 MG	IV	J9299
NOLVADEX	10 MG	ORAL	S0187
NORDITROPIN	1 MG	SC	J2941
NORDYL	50 MG	IV, IM	J1200
NORFLEX	60 MG	IV, IM	J2360
NORMAL SALINE SOLUTION	1000 CC	IV	J7030
NORMAL SALINE SOLUTION	250 CC	IV	J7050
NORMAL SALINE SOLUTION	500 ML	IV	J7040
NOVACHOR	SQ CM	OTH	Q4194
NOVAFIX	SQ CM	OTH	Q4208
NOVANTRONE	5 MG	IV	J9293
NOVAREL	1,000 USP U	IM	J0725
NOVOEIGHT	IU	IV	J7182
NOVOLIN	50 U	SC	J1817

© 2019 Optum360, LLC

Drug Name	Unit Per	Route	Code
NOVOLIN R	5 U	SC	J1815
NOVOLOG	50 U	SC	J1817
NOVOSEVEN	1 MCG	IV	J7189
NPH	5 UNITS	SC	J1815
NPLATE	10 MCG	SC	J2796
NUBAIN	10 MG	IM, IV, SC	J2300
NUCALA	100 MG	SQ	J2182
NULOJIX	1 MG	IV	J0485
NUMORPHAN	1 MG	IV, SC, IM	J2410
NUSHIELD	SQ CM	OTH	Q4160
NUSINERSEN	0.1 MG	INJ	J2326
NUTRI-TWELVE	1,000 MCG	IM, SC	J3420
NUTROPIN	1 MG	SC	J2941
NUTROPIN A.Q.	1 MG	SC	J2941
NUVARING VAGINAL RING	EACH	OTH	J7303
NUWIQ	1 IU	IV	J7209
~~NUZYRA~~	~~1 MG~~	~~IV~~	~~C9051~~
NUZYRA	1 MG	IV	J0121
OASIS BURN MATRIX	SQ CM	OTH	Q4103
OASIS ULTRA TRI-LAYER WOUND MATRIX	SQ CM	OTH	Q4124
OASIS WOUND MATRIX	SQ CM	OTH	Q4102
OBINUTUZUMAB	10 MG	IV	J9301
OBIZUR	IU	IV	J7188
OCRELIZUMAB	1 MG	INJ	J2350
OCREVUS	1 MG	INJ	J2350
OCRIPLASMIN	0.125 MG	OTH	J7316
OCTAFLUOROPROPANE UCISPHERES	1 ML	IV	Q9956
OCTAGAM	500 MG	IV	J1568
OCTREOSCAN	STUDY DOSE UP TO 6 MCI	IV	A9572
OCTREOTIDE ACETATE DEPOT	1 MG	IM	J2353
OCTREOTIDE, NON-DEPOT FORM	25 MCG	SC, IV	J2354
OFATUMUMAB	10 MG	IV	J9302
OFIRMEV	10 MG	IV	J0131
OFLOXACIN	400 MG	IV	S0034
OFORTA	10 MG	ORAL	J8562
OGIVRI	10 MG	IV	Q5114
OLANZAPINE	2.5 MG	IM	S0166
OLANZAPINE LONG ACTING	1 MG	IM	J2358
OLARATUMAB	10 MG	INF	J9285
OMACETAXINE MEPESUCCINATE	0.01 MG	SC	J9262
~~OMADACYCLINE~~	~~1 MG~~	~~IV~~	~~C9051~~
OMADACYCLINE	1 MG	IV	J0121
OMALIZUMAB	5 MG	SC	J2357
OMEGAVEN	10 G	IV	B4187
OMIDRIA	1 ML	OTH	J1097
~~OMIDRIA~~	~~4 ML~~	~~IRR~~	~~C9447~~
OMNIPAQUE 140	PER ML	IV	Q9965
OMNIPAQUE 180	PER ML	IV	Q9965
OMNIPAQUE 240	PER ML	IV	Q9966
~~OMNIPAQUE 300~~	~~PER ML~~	~~IV~~	~~Q9966~~
OMNIPAQUE 300	PER ML	IV	Q9967
OMNIPAQUE 350	PER ML	IV	Q9967
OMNISCAN	1 ML	IV	A9579

Drug Name	Unit Per	Route	Code
OMONTYS (FOR ESRD ON DIALYSIS)	0.1 MG	SC, IV	J0890
ONABOTULINUMTOXINA	1 UNIT	IM, OTH	J0585
ONCASPAR	VIAL	IM, IV	J9266
ONCOSCINT	STUDY DOSE, UP TO 6 MCI	IV	A4642
ONDANSETRON	1 MG	ORAL	Q0162
ONDANSETRON	4 MG	ORAL	S0119
ONDANSETRON HYDROCHLORIDE	1 MG	IV	J2405
ONIVYDE	1 MG	IV	J9205
~~ONPATTRO~~	~~0.1 MG~~	~~IV~~	~~C9036~~
ONPATTRO	0.1 MG	IV	J0222
ONTAK	300 MCG	IV	J9160
ONTRUZANT	10 MG	IV	Q5112
OPDIVO	1 MG	IV	J9299
OPRELVEKIN	5 MG	SC	J2355
OPTIRAY	PER ML	IV	Q9967
OPTIRAY 160	PER ML	IV	Q9965
OPTIRAY 240	PER ML	IV	Q9966
OPTIRAY 300	PER ML	IV	Q9967
OPTIRAY 320	PER ML	IV	Q9967
OPTISON	1 ML	IV	Q9956
ORAL MAGNETIC RESONANCE CONTRAST AGENT, PER 100 ML	100 ML	ORAL	Q9954
ORBACTIV	10 MG	IV	J2407
ORENCIA	10 MG	IV	J0129
ORITAVANCIN	10 MG	IV	J2407
ORPHENADRINE CITRATE	60 MG	IV, IM	J2360
ORTHADAPT BIOIMPLANT	SQ CM	OTH	C1781
ORTHOCLONE OKT3	5 MG	OTH	J7505
ORTHOVISC	DOSE	OTH	J7324
OSELTAMIVIR PHOSPHATE (BRAND NAME) (DEMONSTRATION PROJECT)	75 MG	ORAL	G9035
OSELTAMIVIR PHOSPHATE (GENERIC) (DEMONSTRATION PROJECT)	75 MG	ORAL	G9019
OSMITROL	25% IN 50 ML	IV	J2150
OTIPRIO	6 MG	OTIC	J7342
OXACILLIN SODIUM	250 MG	IM, IV	J2700
OXALIPLATIN	0.5 MG	IV	J9263
OXILAN 300	PER ML	IV	Q9967
OXILAN 350	PER ML	IV	Q9967
OXYMORPHONE HCL	1 MG	IV, SC, IM	J2410
OXYTETRACYCLINE HCL	50 MG	IM	J2460
OXYTOCIN	10 U	IV, IM	J2590
OZURDEX	0.1 MG	OTH	J7312
PACIS BCG	1 MG	OTH	J9030
~~PACIS BCG~~	~~VIAL~~	~~OTH~~	~~J9031~~
PACLITAXEL	1 MG	IV	J9267
PACLITAXEL PROTEIN-BOUND PARTICLES	1 MG	IV	J9264
PALIFERMIN	50 MCG	IV	J2425
PALINGEN OR PALINGEN XPLU	SQ CM	OTH	Q4173
PALINGEN OR PROMATRX	0.36 MG/0.25 CC	OTH	Q4174

© 2019 Optum360, LLC

Drug Name	Unit Per	Route	Code
PALIPERIDONE PALMITATE EXTENDED RELEASED	1 MG	IM	J2426
PALONOSETRON HCL	25 MCG	IV	J2469
PAMIDRONATE DISODIUM	30 MG	IV	J2430
PANHEMATIN	1 MG	IV	J1640
PANITUMUMAB	10 MG	IV	J9303
PANTOPRAZOLE SODIUM	40 MG	IV	S0164
PANTOPRAZOLE SODIUM	VIAL	IV	C9113
PAPAVERINE HCL	60 MG	IV, IM	J2440
PARAGARD T380A	EA	OTH	J7300
PARAPLANTIN	50 MG	IV	J9045
PARICALCITOL	1 MCG	IV, IM	J2501
PARSABIV	0.1 MG	IV	J0606
PASIREOTIDE LONG ACTING	1 MG	IV	J2502
~~PATISIRAN~~	~~0.1 MG~~	~~IV~~	~~C9036~~
PATISIRAN	0.1 MG	IV	J0222
PEDIAPRED	5 MG	ORAL	J7510
PEG-INTRON	180 MCG	SC	S0145
PEGADEMASE BOVINE	25 IU	IM	J2504
PEGAPTANIB SODIUM	0.3 MG	OTH	J2503
PEGASPARGASE	VIAL	IM, IV	J9266
PEGFILGRASTIM	6 MG	SC	J2505
PEGFILGRASTIM-CBQV, BIOSIMILAR	0.5 MG	SC	Q5111
PEGFILGRASTIM-JMDB, BIOSIMILAR	0.5 MG	SC	Q5108
PEGINESATIDE (FOR ESRD ON DIALYSIS)	0.1 MG	SC, IV	J0890
PEGINTERFERON ALFA-2A	180 MCG	SC	S0145
PEGLOTICASE	1 MG	IV	J2507
PEGYLATED INTERFERON ALFA-2A	180 MCG	SC	S0145
PEGYLATED INTERFERON ALFA-2B	10 MCG	SC	S0148
PEMBROLIZUMAB	1 MG	IV	J9271
PEMETREXED	10 MG	IV	J9305
PENICILLIN G BENZATHINE	100,000 U	IM	J0561
PENICILLIN G BENZATHINE AND PENICILLIN G PROCAINE	100,000 UNITS	IM	J0558
PENICILLIN G POTASSIUM	600,000 U	IM, IV	J2540
PENICILLIN G PROCAINE	600,000 U	IM, IV	J2510
PENTACARINAT	300 MG	INH	S0080
PENTAM	300 MG	IM, IV	J2545
PENTAM 300	300 MG	IM, IV	S0080
PENTAMIDINE ISETHIONATE	300 MG	IM, IV	S0080
PENTAMIDINE ISETHIONATE COMPOUNDED	PER 300 MG	INH	J7676
PENTAMIDINE ISETHIONATE NONCOMPOUNDED	300 MG	INH	J2545
PENTASPAN	100 ML	IV	J2513
PENTASTARCH 10% SOLUTION	100 ML	IV	J2513
PENTATE CALCIUM TRISODIUM	STUDY DOSE UP TO 25 MCI	IV	A9539
PENTATE CALCIUM TRISODIUM	STUDY DOSE UP TO 75 MCI	INH	A9567
PENTATE ZINC TRISODIUM	STUDY DOSE UP TO 25 MCI	IV	A9539
PENTATE ZINC TRISODIUM	STUDY DOSE UP TO 75 MCI	INH	A9567
PENTAZOCINE	30 MG	IM, SC, IV	J3070
PENTOBARBITAL SODIUM	50 MG	IM, IV, OTH	J2515
PENTOSTATIN	10 MG	IV	J9268
PEPCID	20 MG	IV	S0028
PERAMIVIR	1 MG	IV	J2547
PERFLEXANE LIPID MICROSPHERE	1 ML	IV	Q9955
PERFLUTREN LIPID MICROSPHERE	1 ML	IV	Q9957
PERFOROMIST	20 MCG	INH	J7606
PERJETA	1 MG	IV	J9306
PERMACOL	SQ CM	OTH	C9364
PERPHENAZINE	4 MG	ORAL	Q0175
PERPHENAZINE	5 MG	IM, IV	J3310
PERSANTINE	10 MG	IV	J1245
~~PERSERIS~~	~~0.5 MG~~	~~SC~~	~~C9037~~
PERSERIS	0.5 MG	SC	J2798
PERTUZUMAB	1 MG	IV	J9306
PFIZERPEN A.S.	600,000 U	IM, IV	J2510
PHENERGAN	12.5 MG	ORAL	Q0169
PHENERGAN	50 MG	IM, IV	J2550
PHENOBARBITAL SODIUM	120 MG	IM, IV	J2560
PHENTOLAMINE MESYLATE	5 MG	IM, IV	J2760
PHENYLEPHRINE 10.16 MG/ML AND KETOROLAC 2.88 MG/ML OPHTHALMIC IRRIGATION SOLUTION	1 ML	OTH	J1097
PHENYLEPHRINE HCL	1 ML	SC, IM, IV	J2370
~~PHENYLEPHRINE KETOROLAC~~	~~4 ML~~	~~IRR~~	~~C9447~~
PHENYTOIN SODIUM	50 MG	IM, IV	J1165
PHOSPHOCOL	1 MCI	IV	A9563
PHOSPHOTEC	STUDY DOSE UP TO 25 MCI	IV	A9538
PHOTOFRIN	75 MG	IV	J9600
PHOTREXA VISCOUS	UP TO 3 ML	OTH	J2787
PHYTONADIONE	1 MG	IM, SC, IV	J3430
PIPERACILLIN SODIUM	500 MG	IM, IV	S0081
PIPERACILLIN SODIUM/TAZOBACTAM SODIUM	1 G/1.125 GM	IV	J2543
PITOCIN	10 U	IV, IM	J2590
PLATINOL AQ	10 MG	IV	J9060
~~PLAZOMICIN~~	~~5 MG~~	~~IV~~	~~C9039~~
PLAZOMICIN	5 MG	IV	J0291
PLERIXAFOR	1 MG	SC	J2562
PLICAMYCIN	2.5 MG	IV	J9270
PNEUMOCOCCAL CONJUGATE	EA	IM	S0195
PNEUMOVAX II	EA	IM	S0195
POLATUZUMAB VEDOTIN-PIIQ	1 MG	IV	J9309
POLIVY	1 MG	IV	J9309
POLOCAINE	10 ML	VAR	J0670
POLYGAM	500 MG	IV	J1566
POLYGAM S/D	500 MG	IV	J1566
PORCINE IMPLANT, PERMACOL	SQ CM	OTH	C9364
PORFIMER SODIUM	75 MG	IV	J9600
PORK INSULIN	5 U	SC	J1815

© 2019 Optum360, LLC

Drug Name	Unit Per	Route	Code
POROUS PURIFIED COLLAGEN MATRIX BONE VOID FILLER	0.5 CC	OTH	C9362
POROUS PURIFIED COLLAGEN MATRIX BONE VOID FILLER, PUTTY	0.5 CC	OTH	C9359
PORTRAZZA.	1 MG	IV	J9295
POTASSIUM CHLORIDE	2 MEQ	IV	J3480
~~POTELIGEO~~	~~1 MG~~	~~IV~~	~~C9038~~
POTELIGEO	1 MG	IV	J9204
PRALATREXATE	1 MG	IV	J9307
PRALIDOXIME CHLORIDE	1 MG	IV, IM, SC	J2730
PREDNISOLONE	5 MG	ORAL	J7510
PREDNISOLONE ACETATE	1 ML	IM	J2650
PREDNISONE, IMMEDIATE RELEASE OR DELAYED RELEASE	1 MG	ORAL	J7512
PREDNORAL	5 MG	ORAL	J7510
PREGNYL	1,000 USP U	IM	J0725
PRELONE	5 MG	ORAL	J7510
PREMARIN	25 MG	IV, IM	J1410
PRENATAL VITAMINS	30 TABS	ORAL	S0197
PRI-METHYLATE	80 MG	IM	J1040
PRIALT	1 MCG	OTH	J2278
PRIMACOR	5 MG	IV	J2260
PRIMATRIX	SQ CM	OTH	Q4110
PRIMAXIN	250 MG	IV, IM	J0743
PRIMESTRIN AQUEOUS	1 MG	IM, IV	J1410
PRIMETHASONE	1 MG	IM, IV, OTH	J1100
PRIVIGEN	500 MG	IV	J1459
PROBUPHINE IMPLANT	74.2 MG	OTH	J0570
PROCAINAMIDE HCL	1 G	IM, IV	J2690
PROCARBAZINE HCL	50 MG	ORAL	S0182
PROCHLOPERAZINE MALEATE	5 MG	ORAL	S0183
PROCHLORPERAZINE	10 MG	IM, IV	J0780
PROCHLORPERAZINE MALEATE	5 MG	ORAL	Q0164
PROCRIT, NON-ESRD USE	1,000 U	SC, IV	J0885
PROFILNINE HEAT-TREATED	1 IU	IV	J7194
PROFILNINE SD	1 IU	IV	J7194
PROFONIX	VIAL	INJ	C9113
PROGENAMATRIX	SQ CM	OTH	Q4222
PROGESTERONE	50 MG	IM	J2675
PROGRAF	1 MG	ORAL	J7507
PROGRAF	5 MG	OTH	J7525
PROLASTIN	10 MG	IV	J0256
PROLEUKIN	1 VIAL	VAR	J9015
PROLIA	1 MG	SC	J0897
PROLIXIN DECANOATE	25 MG	SC, IM	J2680
PROMAZINE HCL	25 MG	IM	J2950
PROMETHAZINE HCL	12.5 MG	ORAL	Q0169
PROMETHAZINE HCL	50 MG	IM, IV	J2550
PRONESTYL	1 G	IM, IV	J2690
PROPECIA	5 MG	ORAL	S0138
PROPLEX SX-T	1 IU	IV	J7194
PROPLEX T	1 IU	IV	J7194
PROPOFOL	10 MG	IV	J2704
PROPRANOLOL HCL	1 MG	IV	J1800
PROREX	50 MG	IM, IV	J2550
PROSCAR	5 MG	ORAL	S0138
PROSTASCINT	STUDY DOSE UP TO 10 MCI	IV	A9507
PROSTIGMIN	0.5 MG	IM, IV	J2710
PROSTIN VR	1.25 MCG	INJ	J0270
PROTAMINE SULFATE	10 MG	IV	J2720
PROTEIN C CONCENTRATE	10 IU	IV	J2724
PROTEINASE INHIBITOR (HUMAN)	10 MG	IV	J0256
PROTIRELIN	250 MCG	IV	J2725
PROTONIX IV	40 MG	IV	S0164
PROTONIX IV	VIAL	IV	C9113
PROTOPAM CHLORIDE	1 G	SC, IM, IV	J2730
PROTROPIN	1 MG	SC, IM	J2940
PROVENGE	INFUSION	IV	Q2043
PROVENTIL NONCOMPOUNDED, CONCENTRATED	1 MG	INH	J7611
PROVENTIL NONCOMPOUNDED, UNIT DOSE	1 MG	INH	J7613
PROVOCHOLINE POWDER	1 MG	INH	J7674
PROZINE-50	25 MG	IM	J2950
PULMICORT	0.25 MG	INH	J7633
PULMICORT RESPULES	0.5 MG	INH	J7627
PULMICORT RESPULES NONCOMPOUNDED, CONCETRATED	0.25 MG	INH	J7626
PULMOZYME	1 MG	INH	J7639
PURAPLY	SQ CM	OTH	Q4195
PURAPLY AM	SQ CM	OTH	Q4196
PURAPLY XT	SQ CM	OTH	Q4197
PURINETHOL	50 MG	ORAL	S0108
PYRIDOXINE HCL	100 MG	IM, IV	J3415
QUADRAMET	PER DOSE UP TO 150 MCI	IV	A9604
QUELICIN	20 MG	IM, IV	J0330
QUINUPRISTIN/DALFOPRISTIN	500 MG	IV	J2770
QUTENZA	1 SQ CM	OTH	J7336
RADICAVA	1 MG	IV	J1301
RADIESSE	0.1 ML	OTH	Q2026
RADIUM (RA) 223 DICHLORIDE THERAPEUTIC	PER MICROCURIE	IV	A9606
RAMUCIRUMAB	5 MG	IV	J9308
RANIBIZUMAB	0.1 MG	OTH	J2778
RANITIDINE HCL	25 MG	INJ	J2780
RAPAMUNE	1 MG	ORAL	J7520
RAPIVAB	1 MG	IV	J2547
RASBURICASE	0.5 MG	IM	J2783
~~RAVULIZUMAB-CWVZ~~	~~10 MG~~	~~IV~~	~~C9052~~
RAVULIZUMAB-CWVZ	10 MG	IV	J1303
REBETRON KIT	1,000,000 U	SC, IM	J9214
REBIF	1 MCG	SC	Q3028
REBIF	30 MCG	SC	J1826
REBINYN	1 IU	IV	J7203
RECLAST	1 MG	IV	J3489
RECOMBINATE	1 IU	IV	J7192
REDISOL	1,000 MCG	SC. IM	J3420
REFACTO	1 IU	IV	J7192
REFLUDAN	50 MG	IM, IV	J1945

© 2019 Optum360, LLC

Drug Name	Unit Per	Route	Code
REGADENOSON	0.1 MG	IV	J2785
REGITINE	5 MG	IM, IV	J2760
REGLAN	10 MG	IV	J2765
REGRANEX GEL	0.5 G	OTH	S0157
REGULAR INSULIN	5 UNITS	SC	J1815
RELAXIN	10 ML	IV, IM	J2800
RELENZA (DEMONSTRATION PROJECT)	10 MG	INH	G9034
RELION	5 U	SC	J1815
RELION NOVOLIN	50 U	SC	J1817
RELISTOR	0.1 MG	SC	J2212
REMICADE	10 MG	IV	J1745
REMODULIN	1 MG	SC	J3285
RENFLEXIS	10 MG	IV	Q5104
REODULIN	1 MG	SC	J3285
REOPRO	10 MG	IV	J0130
REPRIZA	SQ CM	OTH	Q4143
REPRONEX	75 IU	SC, IM, IV	S0122
RESLIZUMAB	1 MG	IV	J2786
RESPIROL NONCOMPOUNDED, CONCENTRATED	1 MG	INH	J7611
RESPIROL NONCOMPOUNDED, UNIT DOSE	1 MG	INH	J7613
RESTORIGIN	1 CC	INJ	Q4192
RESTORIGIN	SQ CM	OTH	Q4191
RETACRIT	100 UNITS	INJ, IV	Q5105
RETACRIT	1000 UNITS	INJ, IV	Q5106
RETAVASE	18.1 MG	IV	J2993
RETEPLASE	18.1 MG	IV	J2993
RETISERT	IMPLANT	OTH	J7311
RETROVIR	10 MG	IV	J3485
RETROVIR	100 MG	ORAL	S0104
REVEFENACIN INHALATION	1 MCG	INH	J7677
REVITA	SQ CM	OTH	Q4180
REVITALON	SQ CM	OTH	Q4157
RHEOMACRODEX	500 ML	IV	J7100
RHEUMATREX	2.5 MG	ORAL	J8610
RHEUMATREX DOSE PACK	2.5 MG	ORAL	J8610
RHO D IMMUNE GLOBULIN	300 MCG	IV	J2790
RHO D IMMUNE GLOBULIN (RHOPHYLAC)	100 IU	IM, IV	J2791
RHO D IMMUNE GLOBULIN MINIDOSE	50 MCG	IM	J2788
RHO D IMMUNE GLOBULIN SOLVENT DETERGENT	100 IU	IV	J2792
RHOGAM	300 MCG	IM	J2790
RHOGAM	50 MCG	IM	J2788
RHOPHYLAC	100 IU	IM, IV	J2791
RIBOFLAVIN 5'-PHOSPHATE, OPHTHALMIC SOLUTION	UP TO 3 ML	OTH	J2787
RILONACEPT	1 MG	SC	J2793
RIMANTADINE HCL (DEMONSTRATION PROJECT)	100 MG	ORAL	G9020
RIMANTADINE HCL (DEMONSTRATION PROJECT)	100 MG	ORAL	G9036
RIMSO 50	50 ML	IV	J1212
RINGERS LACTATE INFUSION	UP TO 1000 CC	IV	J7120
RISPERDAL CONSTA	0.5 MG	IM	J2794
RISPERIDONE	0.5 MG	IM	J2794
~~RISPERIDONE~~	~~0.5 MG~~	~~SC~~	~~C9037~~
RISPERIDONE	0.5 MG	SC	J2798
RITUXAN	10 MG	IV	J9312
RITUXAN HYCELA	10 MG	SC	J9311
RITUXIMAB	10 MG	IV	J9312
RITUXIMAB 10 MG AND HYALURONIDASE	10 MG	SC	J9311
RITUXIMAB-ABBS, BIOSIMILAR	10 MG	IV	Q5115
RIXUBIS	IU	IV	J7200
ROBAXIN	10 ML	IV, IM	J2800
ROCEPHIN	250 MG	IV, IM	J0696
ROFERON-A	3,000,000 U	SC, IM	J9213
ROLAPITANT	0.5 MG	ORAL, IV	J2797
ROLAPITANT	1 MG	ORAL	J8670
ROMIDEPSIN	1 MG	IV	J9315
ROMIPLOSTIM	10 MCG	SC	J2796
ROMOSOZUMAB-AQQG	1 MG	SC	J3111
ROPIVACAINE HYDROCHLORIDE	1 MG	VAR	J2795
RUBEX	10 MG	IV	J9000
RUBIDIUM RB-82	STUDY DOSE UP TO 60 MCI	IV	A9555
RUBRAMIN PC	1,000 MCG	SC, IM	J3420
RUBRATOPE 57	STUDY DOSE UP TO 1 UCI	ORAL	A9559
RUCONEST	10 UNITS	IV	J0596
SAIZEN	1 MG	SC	J2941
SAIZEN SOMATROPIN RDNA ORIGIN	1 MG	SC	J2941
SALINE OR STERILE WATER, METERED DOSE DISPENSER	10 ML	INH	A4218
SALINE, STERILE WATER, AND/OR DEXTROSE DILUENT/FLUSH	10 ML	VAR	A4216
SALINE/STERILE WATER	500 ML	VAR	A4217
SAMARIUM LEXIDRONAM	PER DOSE UP TO 150 MCI	IV	A9604
SANDIMMUNE	100 MG	ORAL	J7502
SANDIMMUNE	25 MG	ORAL	J7515
SANDIMMUNE	250 MG	IV	J7516
SANDOSTATIN	25 MCG	SC, IV	J2354
SANDOSTATIN LAR	1 MG	IM	J2353
SANGCYA	100 MG	ORAL	J7502
SANO-DROL	40 MG	IM	J1030
SANO-DROL	80 MG	IM	J1040
SAQUINAVIR	200 MG	ORAL	S0140
SARGRAMOSTIM (GM-CSF)	50 MCG	IV	J2820
SCANDONEST	PER 10 ML	IV	J0670
SCULPTRA	0.5 ML	OTH	Q2028
SEBELIPASE ALFA	1 MG	IV	J2840
SECREFLO	1 MCG	IV	J2850
SECRETIN, SYNTHETIC, HUMAN	1 MCG	IV	J2850
SENSIPAR	1 MG	ORAL	J0604
SENSORCAINE	30 ML	VAR	S0020
SEPTRA IV	10 ML	IV	S0039

© 2019 Optum360, LLC

Drug Name	Unit Per	Route	Code
SERMORELIN ACETATE	1 MCG	IV	Q0515
SEROSTIM	1 MG	SC	J2941
SEROSTIM RDNA ORIGIN	1 MG	SC	J2941
SIGNIFOR LAR	1 MG	IV	J2502
SILDENAFIL CITRATE	25 MG	ORAL	S0090
SILTUXIMAB	10 MG	IV	J2860
SIMPONI	1 MG	IV	J1602
SIMULECT	20 MG	IV	J0480
SINCALIDE	5 MCG	IV	J2805
SINUVA	10 MCG	OTH	J7401
SIPULEUCEL-T	INFUSION	IV	Q2043
SIROLIMUS	1 MG	ORAL	J7520
SIVEXTRO	1 MG	IV	J3090
SKINTE	SQ CM	OTH	Q4200
SKYLA	13.5 MG	OTH	J7301
SMZ-TMP	10 ML	IV	S0039
SODIUM FERRIC GLUCONATE COMPLEX IN SUCROSE	12.5 MG	IV	J2916
SODIUM FLUORIDE F-18, DIAGNOSTIC	STUDY DOSE UP TO 30 MCI	IV	A9580
SODIUM IODIDE I-131 CAPSULE DIAGNOSTIC	1 MCI	ORAL	A9528
SODIUM IODIDE I-131 CAPSULE THERAPEUTIC	1 MCI	ORAL	A9517
SODIUM IODIDE I-131 SOLUTION THERAPEUTIC	1 MCI	ORAL	A9530
SODIUM PHOSPHATE P32	1 MCI	IV	A9563
SOLGANAL	50 MG	IM	J2910
SOLIRIS	10 MG	IV	J1300
SOLTAMOX	10 MG	ORAL	S0187
SOLU-CORTEF	100 MG	IV, IM, SC	J1720
SOLU-MEDROL	125 MG	IM, IV	J2930
SOLU-MEDROL	40 MG	IM, IV	J2920
SOLUREX	1 MG	IM, IV, OTH	J1100
SOMATREM	1 MG	SC, IM	J2940
SOMATROPIN	1 MG	SC	J2941
SOMATULINE	1 MG	SC	J1930
SOTALOL HYDROCHLORIDE	1 MG	IV	C9482
SPECTINOMYCIN DIHYDROCHLORIDE	2 G	IM	J3320
SPECTRO-DEX	1 MG	IM, IV, OTH	J1100
SPINRAZA	0.1 MG	INJ	J2326
SPORANOX	50 MG	IV	J1835
STADOL	1 MG	IM, IV	J0595
STADOL NS	25 MG	OTH	S0012
~~STELARA~~	~~1 MG~~	~~IV~~	~~C9487~~
STELARA	1 MG	SC	J3357
STELARA	1 MG	SC, IV	J3358
STERILE WATER OR SALINE, METERED DOSE DISPENSER	10 ML	INH	A4218
STERILE WATER, SALINE, AND/OR DEXTROSE DILUENT/FLUSH	10 ML	VAR	A4216
STERILE WATER/SALINE	500 ML	VAR	A4217
STRATTICE TM	SQ CM	OTH	Q4130
STRAVIX	SQ CM	OTH	Q4133
STRAVIXPL	SQ CM	OTH	Q4133
STREPTASE	250,000 IU	IV	J2995
STREPTOKINASE	250,000 IU	IV	J2995
STREPTOMYCIN	1 G	IM	J3000
STREPTOZOCIN	1 G	IV	J9320
STRONTIUM 89 CHLORIDE	1 MCI	IV	A9600
SUBLIMAZE	0.1 MG	IM, IV	J3010
SUBLOCADE	> 100 MG	SC	Q9992
SUBLOCADE	≤ 100 MG	SC	Q9991
SUBOXONE	12 MG	ORAL	J0575
SUBOXONE	2 MG	ORAL	J0572
SUBOXONE	4 MG	ORAL	J0573
SUBOXONE	8 MG	ORAL	J0574
SUBUTEX	1 MG	ORAL	J0571
SUCCINYLCHOLINE CHLORIDE	20 MG	IM, IV	J0330
SULFAMETHOXAZOLE AND TRIMETHOPRIM	10 ML	IV	S0039
SULFUR HEXAFLUORIDE LIPID MICROSPHERES	1 ML	IV	Q9950
SULFUTRIM	10 ML	IV	S0039
SUMATRIPTAN SUCCINATE	6 MG	SC	J3030
SUPARTZ	DOSE	OTH	J7321
SUPPRELIN LA	10 MCG	OTH	J1675
SUREDERM	SQ CM	OTH	Q4220
SURGICORD	SQ CM	OTH	Q4218
SURGIGRAFT	SQ CM	OTH	Q4183
SURGIGRAFT-DUAL	SQ CM	OTH	Q4219
SURGIMEND COLLAGEN MATRIX, FETAL	0.5 SQ CM	OTH	C9358
SURGIMEND COLLAGEN MATRIX, NEONATAL	0.5 SQ CM	OTH	C9360
SURGRAFT	SQ CM	OTH	Q4209
SUSTOL	0.1 MG	SC	J1627
SYLVANT	10 MG	IV	J2860
SYMMETREL (DEMONSTRATION PROJECT)	100 MG	ORAL	G9033
SYNERA	70 MG/70 MG	OTH	C9285
SYNERCID	500 MG	IV	J2770
SYNOJOYNT	1 MG	INJ	J7331
SYNRIBO	0.01 MG	SC	J9262
SYNTOCINON	10 UNITS	IV	J2590
SYNVISC/SYNVISC-ONE	1 MG	OTH	J7325
SYTOBEX	1,000 MCG	SC, IM	J3420
T-GEN	250 MG	ORAL	Q0173
TACRINE HCL	10 MG	ORAL	S0014
TACROLIMUS	1 MG	ORAL	J7507
TACROLIMUS	5 MG	OTH	J7525
TACROLIMUS, EXTENDED RELEASE	0.1 MG	ORAL	J7508
TACROLIMUS, EXTENDED RELEASE	0.25 MG	ORAL	J7503
TAGAMET HCL	300 MG	IM, IV	S0023
~~TAGRAXOFUSP-ERZS~~	~~10 MCG~~	~~IV~~	~~C9049~~
TAGRAXOFUSP-ERZS	10 MCG	IV	J9269
TAKHZYRO	1 MG	SC	J0593
TALIGLUCERASE ALFA	10 U	IV	J3060
TALIMOGENE LAHERPAREPVEC	1 MILLION	INTRALESIONAL	J9325
TALWIN	30 MG	IM, SC, IV	J3070

© 2019 Optum360, LLC

Drug Name	Unit Per	Route	Code
TALYMED	SQ CM	OTH	Q4127
TAMIFLU (DEMONSTRATION PROJECT)	75 MG	ORAL	G9019
TAMIFLU (DEMONSTRATION PROJECT)	75 MG	ORAL	G9035
TAMOXIFEN CITRATE	10 MG	ORAL	S0187
TAXOL	1 MG	IV	J9267
TAXOTERE	1 MG	IV	J9171
TAZICEF	500 MG	IM, IV	J0713
TBO-FILGRASTIM	1 MCG	IV	J1447
TC 99M TILOMANOCEPT	0.5 MCI	SC, OTH	A9520
TEBAMIDE	250 MG	ORAL	Q0173
TEBOROXIME TECHNETIUM TC 99M	STUDY DOSE	IV	A9501
TEBOROXIME, TECHNETIUM	STUDY DOSE	IV	A9501
TECENTRIQ	10 MG	INF	J9022
TECHNEPLEX	STUDY DOSE UP TO 25 MCI	IV	A9539
TECHNESCAN	STUDY DOSE UP TO 30 MCI	IV	A9561
TECHNESCAN FANOLESOMAB	STUDY DOSE UP TO 25 MCI	IV	A9566
TECHNESCAN MAA	STUDY DOSE UP TO 10 MCI	IV	A9540
TECHNESCAN MAG3	STUDY DOSE UP TO 15 MCI	IV	A9562
TECHNESCAN PYP	STUDY DOSE UP TO 25 MCI	IV	A9538
TECHNESCAN PYP KIT	STUDY DOSE UP TO 25 MCI	IV	A9538
TECHNETIUM SESTAMBI	STUDY DOSE	IV	A9500
TECHNETIUM TC 99M APCITIDE	STUDY DOSE UP TO 20 MCI	IV	A9504
TECHNETIUM TC 99M ARCITUMOMAB, DIAGNOSTIC	STUDY DOSE UP TO 45 MCI	IV	A9568
TECHNETIUM TC 99M BICISATE	STUDY DOSE UP TO 25 MCI	IV	A9557
TECHNETIUM TC 99M DEPREOTIDE	STUDY DOSE UP TO 35 MCI	IV	A9536
TECHNETIUM TC 99M EXAMETAZIME	STUDY DOSE UP TO 25 MCI	IV	A9521
TECHNETIUM TC 99M FANOLESOMAB	STUDY DOSE UP TO 25 MCI	IV	A9566
TECHNETIUM TC 99M LABELED RED BLOOD CELLS	STUDY DOSE UP TO 30 MCI	IV	A9560
TECHNETIUM TC 99M MACROAGGREGATED ALBUMIN	STUDY DOSE UP TO 10 MCI	IV	A9540
TECHNETIUM TC 99M MDI-MDP	STUDY DOSE UP TO 30 MCI	IV	A9503
TECHNETIUM TC 99M MEBROFENIN	STUDY DOSE UP TO 15 MCI	IV	A9537
TECHNETIUM TC 99M MEDRONATE	STUDY DOSE UP TO 30 MCI	IV	A9503
TECHNETIUM TC 99M MERTIATIDE	STUDY DOSE UP TO 15 MCI	IV	A9562
TECHNETIUM TC 99M OXIDRONATE	STUDY DOSE UP TO 30 MCI	IV	A9561
TECHNETIUM TC 99M PENTETATE	STUDY DOSE UP TO 25 MCI	IV	A9539
TECHNETIUM TC 99M PYROPHOSPHATE	STUDY DOSE UP TO 25 MCI	IV	A9538
TECHNETIUM TC 99M SODIUM GLUCEPATATE	STUDY DOSE UP TO 25 MCI	IV	A9550
TECHNETIUM TC 99M SUCCIMER	STUDY DOSE UP TO 10 MCI	IV	A9551
TECHNETIUM TC 99M SULFUR COLLOID	STUDY DOSE UP TO 20 MCI	IV	A9541
TECHNETIUM TC 99M TETROFOSMIN, DIAGNOSTIC	STUDY DOSE	IV	A9502
TECHNETIUM TC-99M EXAMETAZIME LABELED AUTOLOGOUS WHITE BLOOD CELLS	STUDY DOSE	IV	A9569
TECHNETIUM TC-99M TEBOROXIME	STUDY DOSE	IV	A9501
TECHNILITE	1 MCI	IV	A9512
TEDIZOLID PHOSPHATE	1 MG	IV	J3090
TEFLARO	10 MG	IV	J0712
TELAVANCIN	10 MG	IV	J3095
TEMODAR	1 MG	IV	J9328
TEMODAR	5 MG	ORAL	J8700
TEMOZOLOMIDE	1 MG	IV	J9328
TEMOZOLOMIDE	5 MG	ORAL	J8700
TEMSIROLIMUS	1 MG	IV	J9330
TENDON, POROUS MATRIX	SQ CM	OTH	C9356
TENDON, POROUS MATRIX CROSS-LINKED AND GLYCOSAMINOGLYCAN MATRIX	SQ CM	OTH	C9356
TENECTEPLASE	1 MG	IV	J3101
TENIPOSIDE	50 MG	IV	Q2017
TENOGLIDE TENDON PROTECTOR	SQ CM	OTH	C9356
TENOGLIDE TENDON PROTECTOR SHEET	SQ CM	OTH	C9356
TENSIX	SQ CM	OTH	Q4146
TEQUIN	10 MG	IV	J1590
TERBUTALINE SULFATE	1 MG	SC, IV	J3105
TERBUTALINE SULFATE, COMPOUNDED, CONCENTRATED	1 MG	INH	J7680
TERBUTALINE SULFATE, COMPOUNDED, UNIT DOSE	1 MG	INH	J7681
TERIPARATIDE	10 MCG	SC	J3110
TERRAMYCIN	50 MG	IM	J2460
TESTOSTERONE CYPIONATE	1 MG	IM	J1071
TESTOSTERONE ENANTHATE	1 MG	IM	J3121
TESTOSTERONE PELLET	75 MG	OTH	S0189
TESTOSTERONE UNDECANOATE	1 MG	IM	J3145
TETANUS IMMUNE GLOBULIN	250 U	IM	J1670
TETRACYCLINE HCL	250 MG	IV	J0120
THALLOUS CHLORIDE	1 MCI	IV	A9505
THALLOUS CHLORIDE TL-201	1 MCI	IV	A9505
THALLOUS CHLORIDE USP	1 MCI	IV	A9505
THEELIN AQUEOUS	1 MG	IM, IV	J1435
THEOPHYLLINE	40 MG	IV	J2810
THERACYS	1 MG	OTH	J9030
~~THERACYS~~	~~VIAL~~	~~OTH~~	~~J9031~~
THERASKIN	SQ CM	OTH	Q4121
THIAMINE HCL	100 MG	INJ	J3411

© 2019 Optum360, LLC

Drug Name	Unit Per	Route	Code
THIETHYLPERAZINE MALEATE	10 MG	IM	J3280
THIETHYLPERAZINE MALEATE	10 MG	ORAL	Q0174
THIMAZIDE	250 MG	ORAL	Q0173
THIOTEPA	15 MG	IV	J9340
THORAZINE	50 MG	IM, IV	J3230
THROMBATE III	1 IU	IV	J7197
THYMOGLOBULIN	25 MG	OTH	J7511
THYROGEN	0.9 MG	IM, SC	J3240
THYROTROPIN ALPHA	0.9 MG	IM, SC	J3240
TICARCILLIN DISODIUM AND CLAVULANATE	3.1 G	IV	S0040
TICE BCG	1 MG	OTH	J9030
~~TICE BCG~~	~~VIAL~~	~~OTH~~	~~J9031~~
TICON	250 MG	IM	Q0173
TIGAN	200 MG	IM	J3250
TIGECYCLINE	1 MG	IV	J3243
TIJECT-20	200 MG	IM	J3250
TILDRAKIZUMAB	1 MG	SC	J3245
TIMENTIN	3.1 G	IV	S0040
TINZAPARIN	1,000 IU	SC	J1655
TIROFIBAN HCL	0.25 MG	IM, IV	J3246
TISAGENLECLEUCEL	UP TO 600 MILLION CELLS	IV	Q2042
TNKASE	1 MG	IV	J3101
TOBI	300 MG	INH	J7682
TOBRAMYCIN COMPOUNDED, UNIT DOSE	300 MG	INH	J7685
TOBRAMYCIN SULFATE	80 MG	IM, IV	J3260
TOBRAMYCIN, NONCOMPOUNDED, UNIT DOSE	300 MG	INH	J7682
TOCILIZUMAB	1 MG	IV	J3262
TOLAZOLINE HCL	25 MG	IV	J2670
TOPOSAR	10 MG	IV	J9181
TOPOTECAN	0.1 MG	IV	J9351
TOPOTECAN	0.25 MG	ORAL	J8705
TORADOL	15 MG	IV	J1885
TORISEL	1 MG	IV	J9330
TORNALATE	PER MG	INH	J7629
TORNALATE CONCENTRATE	PER MG	INH	J7628
TORSEMIDE	10 MG	IV	J3265
TOSITUMOMAB	450 MG	IV	G3001
TOTECT	PER 250 MG	IV	J1190
TRABECTEDIN	0.1 MG	IV	J9352
TRANSCYTE	SQ CM	OTH	Q4182
TRASTUZUMAB AND HYALURONIDASE-OYSK	10 MG	SC	J9356
TRASTUZUMAB, EXCLUDES BIOSIMILAR	10 MG	IV	J9355
TRASTUZUMAB-ANNS, BIOSIMILAR	10 MG	IV	Q5117
TRASTUZUMAB-DKST, BIOSIMILAR	10 MG	IV	Q5114
TRASTUZUMAB-DTTB, BIOSIMILAR	10 MG	IV	Q5112
TRASTUZUMAB-PKRB, BIOSIMILAR	10 MG	IV	Q5113
TRASTUZUMAB-QYYP, BIOSIMILAR	10 MG	IV	Q5116
TRASYLOL	10,000 KIU	IV	J0365
TRAZIMERA	10 MG	IV	Q5116
TREANDA	1 MG	IV	J9033
TRELSTAR DEPOT	3.75 MG	IM	J3315
TRELSTAR DEPOT PLUS DEBIOCLIP KIT	3.75 MG	IM	J3315
TRELSTAR LA	3.75 MG	IM	J3315
TREMFYA	1 MG	SC	J1628
TREPROSTINIL	1 MG	SC	J3285
TREPROSTINIL, INHALATION SOLUTION	1.74 MG	INH	J7686
TRETINOIN	5 G	OTH	S0117
TRETTEN	10 IU	IV	J7181
TRI-KORT	10 MG	IM	J3301
TRIAM-A	10 MG	IM	J3301
TRIAMCINOLONE ACETONIDE	10 MG	IM	J3301
TRIAMCINOLONE ACETONIDE, PRESERVATIVE FREE	1 MG	INJ	J3300
~~TRIAMCINOLONE ACETONIDE, PRESERVATIVE-FREE, EXTENDED-RELEASE, MICROSPHERE FORMULATION~~	~~1 MG~~	~~INJ~~	~~C9469~~
TRIAMCINOLONE ACETONIDE, PRESERVATIVE-FREE, EXTENDED-RELEASE, MICROSPHERE FORMULATION	1 MG	OTH	J3304
TRIAMCINOLONE DIACETATE	5 MG	IM	J3302
TRIAMCINOLONE HEXACETONIDE	5 MG	VAR	J3303
TRIAMCINOLONE, COMPOUNDED, CONCENTRATED	1 MG	INH	J7683
TRIAMCINOLONE, COMPOUNDED, UNIT DOSE	1 MG	INH	J7684
TRIBAN	250 MG	ORAL	Q0173
TRIESENCE	1 MG	OTH	J3300
TRIFERIC POWDER	0.1 MG	IV	J1444
TRIFERIC SOLUTION	0.1 MG	IV	J1443
TRIFLUPROMAZINE HCL	UP TO 20 MG	INJ	J3400
TRILIFON	4 MG	ORAL	Q0175
TRILOG	10 MG	IM	J3301
TRILONE	5 MG	IM	J3302
TRILURON	1 MG	INJ	J7332
TRIMETHOBENZAMIDE HCL	200 MG	IM	J3250
TRIMETHOBENZAMIDE HCL	250 MG	ORAL	Q0173
TRIMETREXATE GLUCURONATE	25 MG	IV	J3305
TRIPTODUR	3.75 MG	IM	J3316
TRIPTORELIN PAMOATE	3.75 MG	IM	J3315
TRIPTORELIN, EXTENDED-RELEASE	3.75 MG	IM	J3316
TRISENOX	1 MG	IV	J9017
TRIVARIS	1 MG	VAR	J3300
TRIVISC	1 MG	INJ	J7329
TROBICIN	2 G	IM	J3320
TROGARZO	10 MG	IV	J1746
TRUSKIN	SQ CM	OTH	Q4167
TRUXADRYL	50 MG	IV, IM	J1200
TRUXIMA	10 MG	IV	Q5115

© 2019 Optum360, LLC

Drug Name	Unit Per	Route	Code
TYGACIL	1 MG	IV	J3243
TYPE A BOTOX	1 UNIT	IM, OTH	J0585
TYSABRI	1 MG	IV	J2323
TYVASO	1.74 MG	INH	J7686
UDENYCA	0.5 MG	SC	Q5111
~~ULTOMIRIS~~	~~10 MG~~	~~IV~~	~~C9052~~
ULTOMIRIS	10 MG	IV	J1303
ULTRA-TECHNEKOW	1 MCI	IV	A9512
ULTRALENTE	5 U	SC	J1815
ULTRATAG	STUDY DOSE UP TO 30 MCI	IV	A9560
ULTRAVIST 150	1 ML	IV	Q9965
ULTRAVIST 240	1 ML	IV	Q9966
ULTRAVIST 300	1 ML	IV	Q9967
ULTRAVIST 370	1 ML	IV	Q9967
UNASYN	1.5 G	IM, IV	J0295
UREA	40 G	IV	J3350
URECHOLINE	UP TO 5 MG	SC	J0520
UROFOLLITROPIN	75 IU	SC, IM	J3355
UROKINASE	250,000 IU	IV	J3365
UROKINASE	5,000 IU	IV	J3364
~~USTEKINUMAB~~	~~1 MG~~	~~IV~~	~~C9487~~
USTEKINUMAB	1 MG	SC	J3357
USTEKINUMAB	1 MG	SC, IV	J3358
VABOMERE	10 MG/10 MG	IV	J2186
VALERGEN	10 MG	IM	J1380
VALIUM	5 MG	IV, IM	J3360
VALRUBICIN INTRAVESICAL	200 MG	OTH	J9357
VALSTAR	200 MG	OTH	J9357
VANCOCIN	500 MG	IM, IV	J3370
VANCOMYCIN HCL	500 MG	IV, IM	J3370
VANTAS	50 MG	OTH	J9225
VAPRISOL	1 MG	INJ	C9488
VARUBI	0.5 MG	ORAL, IV	J2797
VARUBI	1 MG	ORAL	J8670
VECTIBIX	10 MG	IV	J9303
VEDOLIZUMAB	1 MG	IV	J3380
VELAGLUCERASE ALFA	100 U	IV	J3385
VELBAN	I MG	IV	J9360
VELCADE	0.1 MG	IV, SC	J9041
VELETRI	0.5 MG	IV	J1325
VELOSULIN	5 U	SC	J1815
VELOSULIN BR	5 U	SC	J1815
VENOFER	1 MG	IV	J1756
VENTOLIN NONCOMPOUNDED, CONCENTRATED	1 MG	INH	J7611
VENTOLIN NONCOMPOUNDED, UNIT DOSE	1 MG	INH	J7613
VEPESID	10 MG	IV	J9181
VEPESID	50 MG	ORAL	J8560
VERITAS	SQ CM	OTH	C9354
VERSED	1 MG	IM, IV	J2250
VERTEPORFIN	0.1 MG	IV	J3396
VESTRONIDASE ALFA-VJBK	1 MG	IV	J3397
VFEND	200 MG	IV	J3465
VIAGRA	25 MG	ORAL	S0090
VIBATIV	10 MG	IV	J3095
VIDAZA	1 MG	SC	J9025
VIDEX	25 MG	ORAL	S0137
VIMIZIM	1 MG	IV	J1322
VIMPAT	1 MG	IV, ORAL	C9254
VINBLASTINE SULFATE	1 MG	IV	J9360
VINCASCAR	1 MG	IV	J9370
VINCRISTINE SULFATE	1 MG	IV	J9370
VINCRISTINE SULFATE LIPOSOME	5 MG	IV	J9371
VINORELBINE TARTRATE	10 MG	IV	J9390
VIRILON	1 CC, 200 MG	IM	J1080
VISCO-3	DOSE	OTH	J7321
VISTAJECT-25	25 MG	IM	J3410
VISTARIL	25 MG	IM	J3410
VISTARIL	25 MG	ORAL	Q0177
VISTIDE	375 MG	IV	J0740
VISUDYNE	0.1 MG	IV	J3396
VITAMIN B-12 CYANOCOBALAMIN	1,000 MCG	IM, SC	J3420
VITAMIN B-17	VAR	INJ	J3570
VITRASE	1 USP	OTH	J3471
VITRASE	1,000 USP	OTH	J3472
VITRASERT	4.5 MG	OTH	J7310
VITRAVENE	1.65 MG	OTH	J1452
VIVITROL	1 MG	IM	J2315
VON WILLEBRAND FACTOR (RECOMBINANT)	1 IU	IV	J7179
VON WILLEBRAND FACTOR COMPLEX (HUMAN) (WILATE)	1 IU	IV	J7183
VON WILLEBRAND FACTOR COMPLEX, HUMATE-P	1 IU	IV	J7187
VON WILLEBRAND FACTOR VIII COMPLEX, HUMAN	PER FACTOR VIII IU	IV	J7186
VONVENDI	1 IU	IV	J7179
VORAXAZE	10 UNITS	IV	C9293
VORETIGENE NEPARVOVEC-RZYL	1 BILLION VECTOR GENOMES	OTH	J3398
VORICONAZOLE	200 MG	IV	J3465
VPRIV	100 U	IV	J3385
VUMON	50 MG	IV	Q2017
VYXEOS	1 MG/2.27 MG	IV	J9153
WEHAMINE	50 MG	IM, IV	J1240
WEHDRYL	50 MG	IM, IV	J1200
WELBUTRIN SR	150 MG	ORAL	S0106
WILATE	1 IU	IV	J7183
WINRHO SDF	100 IU	IV	J2792
WOUNDEX	SQ CM	OTH	Q4163
WOUNDEX FLOW	0.5 CC	OTH	Q4162
WOUNDFIX, WOUNDFIX PLUS, WOUNDFIX XPLUS	SQ CM	OTH	Q4217
WYCILLIN	600,000 U	IM, IV	J2510
XCM BIOLOGIC TISSUE MATRIX	SQ CM	OTH	Q4142
XELODA	150 MG	ORAL	J8520
XELODA	500 MG	ORAL	J8521
XENLETA	1 MG	IV	C9054

© 2019 Optum360, LLC

Drug Name	Unit Per	Route	Code
XENON XE-133	10 MCI	INH	A9558
XEOMIN	1 UNIT	IM	J0588
XERAVA	1 MG	IV	J0122
XGEVA	1 MG	SC	J0897
XIAFLEX	0.01 MG	OTH	J0775
XOFIGO	PER MICROCURIE	IV	A9606
XOLAIR	5 MG	SC	J2357
XWRAP	SQ CM	OTH	Q4204
XYLOCAINE	10 MG	IV	J2001
XYNTHA	1 IU	IV	J7185
YERVOY	1 MG	IV	J9228
YESCARTA	UP TO 200 MILLION CELLS	IV	Q2041
YONDELIS	0.1 MG	IV	J9352
YTTRIUM 90 IBRITUMOMAB TIUXETAN	TX DOSE UP TO 40 MCI	IV	A9543
YUPELRI	1 MCG	INH	J7677
YUTIQ	0.01 MG	OTH	J7314
ZALTRAP	1 MG	IV	J9400
ZANAMIVIR (BRAND) (DEMONSTRATION PROJECT)	10 MG	INH	G9034
ZANAMIVIR (GENERIC) (DEMONSTRATION PROJECT)	10 MG	INH	G9018
ZANOSAR	1 GM	IV	J9320
ZANTAC	25 MG	INJ	J2780
ZARXIO	1 MCG	IV, SC	Q5101
ZEMAIRA	10 MG	IV	J0256
~~ZEMDRI~~	~~5 MG~~	~~IV~~	~~C9039~~
ZEMDRI	5 MG	IV	J0291
ZEMPLAR	1 MCG	IV, IM	J2501
ZENAPAX	25 MG	OTH	J7513
ZERBAXA	50 MG/25 MG	IV	J0695
ZEVALIN	STUDY DOSE UP TO 5 MCI	IV	A9542
ZEVALIN DIAGNOSTIC	STUDY DOSE UP TO 5 MCI	IV	A9542
ZEVALIN THERAPEUTIC	TX DOSE UP TO 40 MCI	IV	A9543
ZICONOTIDE	1 MCG	IT	J2278
ZIDOVUDINE	10 MG	IV	J3485
ZIDOVUDINE	100 MG	ORAL	S0104
~~ZILRETTA~~	~~1 MG~~	~~INJ~~	~~C9469~~
ZILRETTA	1 MG	OTH	J3304
ZINACEFT	PER 750 MG	IM, IV	J0697
ZINECARD	250 MG	IV	J1190
ZINPLAVA	10 MG	INF	J0565
ZIPRASIDONE MESYLATE	10 MG	IM	J3486
ZIRABEV	10 MG	IV	Q5118
ZITHROMAX	1 G	ORAL	Q0144
ZITHROMAX	500 MG	IV	J0456
ZIV-AFLIBERCEPT	1 MG	IV	J9400
ZOFRAN	1 MG	IV	J2405
ZOFRAN	1 MG	ORAL	Q0162
ZOFRAN	4 MG	ORAL	S0119
ZOLADEX	3.6 MG	SC	J9202
ZOLEDRONIC ACID	1 MG	IV	J3489
ZOMETA	1 MG	IV	J3489
ZORBTIVE	1 MG	SC	J2941
ZORTRESS	0.25 MG	ORAL	J7527
ZOSYN	1 G/1.125 GM	IV	J2543
ZOVIRAX	5 MG	IV	J0133
ZUBSOLV	1.4 MG	ORAL	J0572
ZUBSOLV	5.7 MG	ORAL	J0573
ZULRESSO	1 MG	IV	C9055
ZUPLENZ	1 MG	ORAL	Q0162
ZUPLENZ	4 MG	ORAL	S0119
ZYPREXA	2.5 MG	IM	S0166
ZYPREXA RELPREVV	1 MG	IM	J2358
ZYVOX	200 MG	IV	J2020

NOT OTHERWISE CLASSIFIED DRUGS

Drug Name	Unit Per	Route	Code
ALFENTANIL	500 MCG	IV	J3490
ALLOPURINOL SODIUM	500 MG	IV	J3490
AMINOCAPROIC ACID	250 MG	IV	J3490
AZTREONAM	500 MG	IM, IV	J3490
BORTEZOMIB, NOT OTHERWISE SPECIFIED	0.1 MG	IV, SC	J9044
BUMETANIDE	0.25 MG	IM, IV	J3490
BUPIVACAINE, 0.25%	1 ML	OTH	J3490
BUPIVACAINE, 0.50%	1 ML	OTH	J3490
BUPIVACAINE, 0.75%	1 ML	OTH	J3490
CALCIUM CHLORIDE	100 MG	IV	J3490
CLAVULANTE POTASSIUM/TICARCILLIN DISODIUM	0.1-3 GM	IV	J3490
CLEVIDIPINE BUTYRATE	1 MG	IV	J3490
CLINDAMYCIN PHOSPHATE	150 MG	IV	J3490
COMPOUNDED DRUG, NOT OTHERWISE CLASSIFIED	VAR	VAR	J7999
COPPER SULFATE	0.4 MG	INJ	J3490
DIAGNOSTIC RADIOPHARMACEUTICAL FOR BETA-AMYLOID PET	STUDY DOSE	IV	A9599
DILTIAZEM HCL	5 MG	IV	J3490
DOXAPRAM HCL	20 MG	IV	J3490
DOXYCYCLINE HYCLATE	100 MG	INJ	J3490
DRUG OR BIOLOGICAL, PART B DRUG COMPETITIVE ACQUISITION PROGRAM (CAP)	VAR	VAR	Q4082
ENALAPRILAT	1.25 MG	IV	J3490
ESMOLOL HYDROCHLORIDE	10 MG	IV	J3490
ESOMEPRAZOLE SODIUM	20 MG	IV	J3490
ETOMIDATE	2 MG	IV	J3490
FAMOTIDINE	10 MG	IV	J3490
FLUMAZENIL	0.1 MG	IV	J3490
FOLIC ACID	5 MG	SC, IM, IV	J3490
FOSPROPOFOL DISODIUM	35 MG	IV	J3490
GLUCARPIDASE	10 U	IV	J3490
GLYCOPYRROLATE	0.2 MG	IM, IV	J3490
HEMOPHILIA CLOTTING FACTOR, NOC	VAR	INJ	J7199

© 2019 Optum360, LLC

Drug Name	Unit Per	Route	Code
HEXAMINOLEVULINATE HCL	100 MG PER STUDY DOSE	IV	J3490
INTEGRA MESHED BILAYER WOUND MATRIX	SQ CM	OTH	C9363
LABETALOL HCL	5 MG	INJ	J3490
METOPROLOL TARTRATE	1 MG	IV	J3490
METRONIDAZOLE INJ	500 MG	IV	J3490
MORRHUATE SODIUM	50 MG	OTH	J3490
NITROGLYCERIN	5 MG	IV	J3490
NOC DRUGS, INHALATION SOLUTION ADMINISTERED THROUGH DME	1 EA	OTH	J7699
NONRADIOACTIVE CONTRACT IMAGING MATERIAL	STUDY DOSE	IV	A9698
NOT OTHERWISE CLASSIFIED, ANTINEOPLASTIC DRUGS	VAR	VAR	J9999
OLANZAPINE SHORT ACTING INTRAMUSCULAR INJECTION	0.5 MG	IM	J3490
PHENYLEPHRINE KETOROLAC	4 ML	IRR	J3490
POSITRON EMISSION TOMOGRAPHY RADIOPHARMACEUTICAL, DIAGNOSTIC, FOR NON-TUMOR IDENTIFICATION	STUDY DOSE	IV	A9598
POSITRON EMISSION TOMOGRAPHY RADIOPHARMACEUTICAL, DIAGNOSTIC, FOR TUMOR IDENTIFICATION	STUDY DOSE	IV	A9597
RADIOPHARMACEUTICAL, THERAPEUTIC	STUDY DOSE	IV	A9699
RIFAMPIN	600 MG	IV	J3490
SODIUM ACETATE	2 MEQ	IV	J3490
SODIUM CHLORIDE, HYPERTONIC (3%-5% INFUSION)	250 CC	IV	J3490
SULFAMETHOXAZOLE-TRIMETHOPRIM	80 MG/16 MG	IV	J3490
SURGIMEND	0.5 SQ CM	OTH	J3490
UNCLASSIFIED BIOLOGICS	VAR	VAR	J3590
UNCLASSIFIED DRUG OR BIOLOGICAL USED FOR ESRD ON DIALYSIS	VAR	VAR	J3591
UNCLASSIFIED DRUGS OR BIOLOGICALS	VAR	VAR	C9399
VASOPRESSIN	20 UNITS	SC, IM	J3490
VECURONIUM BROMIDE	1 MG	IV	J3490

© 2019 Optum360, LLC

Appendix 2 — Modifiers

A modifier is a two-position code that is added to the end of a code to clarify the services being billed. Modifiers provide a means by which a service can be altered without changing the procedure code. They add more information, such as the anatomical site, to the code. In addition, they help to eliminate the appearance of duplicate billing and unbundling. Modifiers are used to increase accuracy in reimbursement, coding consistency, editing, and to capture payment data.

A1 Dressing for one wound

A2 Dressing for two wounds

A3 Dressing for three wounds

A4 Dressing for four wounds

A5 Dressing for five wounds

A6 Dressing for six wounds

A7 Dressing for seven wounds

A8 Dressing for eight wounds

A9 Dressing for nine or more wounds

AA Anesthesia services performed personally by anesthesiologist

AD Medical supervision by a physician: more than four concurrent anesthesia procedures

AE Registered dietician

AF Specialty physician

AG Primary physician

AH Clinical psychologist

AI Principal physician of record

AJ Clinical social worker

AK Nonparticipating physician

AM Physician, team member service

AO Alternate payment method declined by provider of service

AP Determination of refractive state was not performed in the course of diagnostic ophthalmological examination

AQ Physician providing a service in an unlisted health professional shortage area (HPSA)

AR Physician provider services in a physician scarcity area

AS Physician assistant, nurse practitioner, or clinical nurse specialist services for assistant at surgery

AT Acute treatment (this modifier should be used when reporting service 98940, 98941, 98942)

AU Item furnished in conjunction with a urological, ostomy, or tracheostomy supply

AV Item furnished in conjunction with a prosthetic device, prosthetic or orthotic

AW Item furnished in conjunction with a surgical dressing

AX Item furnished in conjunction with dialysis services

AY Item or service furnished to an ESRD patient that is not for the treatment of ESRD

AZ Physician providing a service in a dental health professional shortage area for the purpose of an electronic health record incentive payment

BA Item furnished in conjunction with parenteral enteral nutrition (PEN) services

BL Special acquisition of blood and blood products

BO Orally administered nutrition, not by feeding tube

BP The beneficiary has been informed of the purchase and rental options and has elected to purchase the item

BR The beneficiary has been informed of the purchase and rental options and has elected to rent the item

BU The beneficiary has been informed of the purchase and rental options and after 30 days has not informed the supplier of his/her decision

CA Procedure payable only in the inpatient setting when performed emergently on an outpatient who expires prior to admission

~~**CB** Service ordered by a renal dialysis facility (RDF) physician as part of the ESRD beneficiary's dialysis benefit, is not part of the composite rate, and is separately reimbursable~~

CC Procedure code change (use CC when the procedure code submitted was changed either for administrative reasons or because an incorrect code was filed)

CD AMCC test has been ordered by an ESRD facility or MCP physician that is part of the composite rate and is not separately billable

CE AMCC test has been ordered by an ESRD facility or MCP physician that is a composite rate test but is beyond the normal frequency covered under the rate and is separately reimbursable based on medical necessity

CF AMCC test has been ordered by an ESRD facility or MCP physician that is not part of the composite rate and is separately billable

CG Policy criteria applied

CH Zero percent impaired, limited or restricted

CI At least 1 percent but less than 20 percent impaired, limited or restricted

CJ At least 20 percent but less than 40 percent impaired, limited or restricted

CK At least 40 percent but less than 60 percent impaired, limited or restricted

CL At least 60 percent but less than 80 percent impaired, limited or restricted

CM At least 80 percent but less than 100 percent impaired, limited or restricted

CN 100 percent impaired, limited or restricted

CO Outpatient occupational therapy services furnished in whole or in part by an occupational therapy assistant

CQ Outpatient physical therapy services furnished in whole or in part by a physical therapist assistant

CR Catastrophe/disaster related

CS Item or service related, in whole or in part, to an illness, injury, or condition that was caused by or exacerbated by the effects, direct or indirect, of the 2010 oil spill in the Gulf of Mexico, including but not limited to subsequent clean-up activities

CT Computed tomography services furnished using equipment that does not meet each of the attributes of the national electrical manufacturers association (NEMA) XR-29-2013 standard

DA Oral health assessment by a licensed health professional other than a dentist

E1 Upper left, eyelid

E2 Lower left, eyelid

© 2019 Optum360, LLC

E3	Upper right, eyelid
E4	Lower right, eyelid
EA	Erythropoetic stimulating agent (ESA) administered to treat anemia due to anticancer chemotherapy
EB	Erythropoetic stimulating agent (ESA) administered to treat anemia due to anticancer radiotherapy
EC	Erythropoetic stimulating agent (ESA) administered to treat anemia not due to anticancer radiotherapy or anticancer chemotherapy
ED	Hematocrit level has exceeded 39 percent (or hemoglobin level has exceeded 13.0 G/dl) for three or more consecutive billing cycles immediately prior to and including the current cycle
EE	Hematocrit level has not exceeded 39 percent (or hemoglobin level has not exceeded 13.0 G/dl) for three or more consecutive billing cycles immediately prior to and including the current cycle
EJ	Subsequent claims for a defined course of therapy, e.g., EPO, sodium hyaluronate, infliximab
EM	Emergency reserve supply (for ESRD benefit only)
EP	Service provided as part of Medicaid early periodic screening diagnosis and treatment (EPSDT) program
ER	Items and services furnished by a provider-based, off-campus emergency department
ET	Emergency services
EX	Expatriate beneficiary
EY	No physician or other licensed health care provider order for this item or service
F1	Left hand, second digit
F2	Left hand, third digit
F3	Left hand, fourth digit
F4	Left hand, fifth digit
F5	Right hand, thumb
F6	Right hand, second digit
F7	Right hand, third digit
F8	Right hand, fourth digit
F9	Right hand, fifth digit
FA	Left hand, thumb
FB	Item provided without cost to provider, supplier or practitioner, or full credit received for replaced device (examples, but not limited to, covered under warranty, replaced due to defect, free samples)
FC	Partial credit received for replaced device
FP	Service provided as part of family planning program
FX	X-ray taken using film
FY	X-ray taken using computed radiography technology/cassette-based imaging
G0	Telehealth services for diagnosis, evaluation, or treatment, of symptoms of an acute stroke
G1	Most recent URR reading of less than 60
G2	Most recent URR reading of 60 to 64.9
G3	Most recent URR reading of 65 to 69.9
G4	Most recent URR reading of 70 to 74.9
G5	Most recent URR reading of 75 or greater
G6	ESRD patient for whom less than six dialysis sessions have been provided in a month
G7	Pregnancy resulted from rape or incest or pregnancy certified by physician as life threatening
G8	Monitored anesthesia care (MAC) for deep complex, complicated, or markedly invasive surgical procedure
G9	Monitored anesthesia care for patient who has history of severe cardiopulmonary condition
GA	Waiver of liability statement issued as required by payer policy, individual case
GB	Claim being resubmitted for payment because it is no longer covered under a global payment demonstration
GC	This service has been performed in part by a resident under the direction of a teaching physician
~~GD~~	~~Units of service exceeds medically unlikely edit value and represents reasonable and necessary services~~
GE	This service has been performed by a resident without the presence of a teaching physician under the primary care exception
GF	Nonphysician (e.g., nurse practitioner (NP), certified registered nurse anesthetist (CRNA), certified registered nurse (CRN), clinical nurse specialist (CNS), physician assistant (PA)) services in a critical access hospital
GG	Performance and payment of a screening mammogram and diagnostic mammogram on the same patient, same day
GH	Diagnostic mammogram converted from screening mammogram on same day
GJ	"Opt out" physician or practitioner emergency or urgent service
GK	Reasonable and necessary item/service associated with a GA or GZ modifier
GL	Medically unnecessary upgrade provided instead of nonupgraded item, no charge, no advance beneficiary notice (ABN)
GM	Multiple patients on one ambulance trip
GN	Services delivered under an outpatient speech language pathology plan of care
GO	Services delivered under an outpatient occupational therapy plan of care
GP	Services delivered under an outpatient physical therapy plan of care
GQ	Via asynchronous telecommunications system
GR	This service was performed in whole or in part by a resident in a Department of Veterans Affairs medical center or clinic, supervised in accordance with VA policy
GS	Dosage of erythropoietin stimulating agent has been reduced and maintained in response to hematocrit or hemoglobin level
GT	Via interactive audio and video telecommunication systems
GU	Waiver of liability statement issued as required by payer policy, routine notice
GV	Attending physician not employed or paid under arrangement by the patient's hospice provider
GW	Service not related to the hospice patient's terminal condition
GX	Notice of liability issued, voluntary under payer policy
GY	Item or service statutorily excluded, does not meet the definition of any Medicare benefit or, for non-Medicare insurers, is not a contract benefit
GZ	Item or service expected to be denied as not reasonable and necessary
H9	Court-ordered
HA	Child/adolescent program
HB	Adult program, nongeriatric
HC	Adult program, geriatric

© 2019 Optum360, LLC

HD	Pregnant/parenting women's program
HE	Mental health program
HF	Substance abuse program
HG	Opioid addiction treatment program
HH	Integrated mental health/substance abuse program
HI	Integrated mental health and intellectual disability/developmental disabilities program
HJ	Employee assistance program
HK	Specialized mental health programs for high-risk populations
HL	Intern
HM	Less than bachelor degree level
HN	Bachelors degree level
HO	Masters degree level
HP	Doctoral level
HQ	Group setting
HR	Family/couple with client present
HS	Family/couple without client present
HT	Multidisciplinary team
HU	Funded by child welfare agency
HV	Funded state addictions agency
HW	Funded by state mental health agency
HX	Funded by county/local agency
HY	Funded by juvenile justice agency
HZ	Funded by criminal justice agency
J1	Competitive acquisition program no-pay submission for a prescription number
J2	Competitive acquisition program, restocking of emergency drugs after emergency administration
J3	Competitive acquisition program (CAP), drug not available through CAP as written, reimbursed under average sales price methodology
J4	DMEPOS item subject to DMEPOS competitive bidding program that is furnished by a hospital upon discharge
JA	Administered intravenously
JB	Administered subcutaneously
JC	Skin substitute used as a graft
JD	Skin substitute not used as a graft
JE	Administered via dialysate
JF	Compounded drug
JG	Drug or biological acquired with 340B drug pricing program discount
JW	Drug amount discarded/not administered to any patient
K0	Lower extremity prosthesis functional level 0 - does not have the ability or potential to ambulate or transfer safely with or without assistance and a prosthesis does not enhance their quality of life or mobility.
K1	Lower extremity prosthesis functional level 1 - has the ability or potential to use a prosthesis for transfers or ambulation on level surfaces at fixed cadence, typical of the limited and unlimited household ambulator
K2	Lower extremity prosthesis functional level 2 - has the ability or potential for ambulation with the ability to traverse low level environmental barriers such as curbs, stairs or uneven surfaces, typical of the limited community ambulator
K3	Lower extremity prosthesis functional level 3 - has the ability or potential for ambulation with variable cadence, typical of the community ambulator who has the ability to transverse most environmental barriers and may have vocational, therapeutic, or exercise activity that demands prosthetic utilization beyond simple locomotion
K4	Lower extremity prosthesis functional level 4 - has the ability or potential for prosthetic ambulation that exceeds the basic ambulation skills, exhibiting high impact, stress, or energy levels, typical of the prosthetic demands of the child, active adult, or athlete
KA	Add on option/accessory for wheelchair
KB	Beneficiary requested upgrade for ABN, more than four modifiers identified on claim
KC	Replacement of special power wheelchair interface
KD	Drug or biological infused through DME
KE	Bid under round one of the DMEPOS competitive bidding program for use with noncompetitive bid base equipment
KF	Item designated by FDA as Class III device
KG	DMEPOS item subject to DMEPOS competitive bidding program number 1
KH	DMEPOS item, initial claim, purchase or first month rental
KI	DMEPOS item, second or third month rental
KJ	DMEPOS item, parenteral enteral nutrition (PEN) pump or capped rental, months four to fifteen
KK	DMEPOS item subject to DMEPOS competitive bidding program number 2
KL	DMEPOS item delivered via mail
KM	Replacement of facial prosthesis including new impression/moulage
KN	Replacement of facial prosthesis using previous master model
KO	Single drug unit dose formulation
KP	First drug of a multiple drug unit dose formulation
KQ	Second or subsequent drug of a multiple drug unit dose formulation
KR	Rental item, billing for partial month
KS	Glucose monitor supply for diabetic beneficiary not treated with insulin
KT	Beneficiary resides in a competitive bidding area and travels outside that competitive bidding area and receives a competitive bid item
KU	DMEPOS item subject to DMEPOS competitive bidding program number 3
KV	DMEPOS item subject to DMEPOS competitive bidding program that is furnished as part of a professional service
KW	DMEPOS item subject to DMEPOS competitive bidding program number 4
KX	Requirements specified in the medical policy have been met
KY	DMEPOS item subject to DMEPOS competitive bidding program number 5
KZ	New coverage not implemented by managed care
LC	Left circumflex coronary artery
LD	Left anterior descending coronary artery
LL	Lease/rental (use the LL modifier when DME equipment rental is to be applied against the purchase price)
LM	Left main coronary artery

© 2019 Optum360, LLC

	LR	Laboratory round trip
	LS	FDA-monitored intraocular lens implant
	LT	Left side (used to identify procedures performed on the left side of the body)
	M2	Medicare secondary payer (MSP)
●	**MA**	Ordering professional is not required to consult a Clinical Decision Support Mechanism due to service being rendered to a patient with a suspected or confirmed emergency medical condition
●	**MB**	Ordering professional is not required to consult a Clinical Decision Support Mechanism due to the significant hardship exception of insufficient internet access
●	**MC**	Ordering professional is not required to consult a Clinical Decision Support Mechanism due to the significant hardship exception of electronic health record or Clinical Decision Support Mechanism vendor issues
●	**MD**	Ordering professional is not required to consult a Clinical Decision Support Mechanism due to the significant hardship exception of extreme and uncontrollable circumstances
●	**ME**	The order for this service adheres to Appropriate Use Criteria in the Clinical Decision Support Mechanism consulted by the ordering professional
●	**MF**	The order for this service does not adhere to the Appropriate Use Criteria in the Clinical Decision Support Mechanism consulted by the ordering professional
●	**MG**	The order for this service does not have applicable Appropriate Use Criteria in the qualified Clinical Decision Support Mechanism consulted by the ordering professional
●	**MH**	Unknown if ordering professional consulted a Clinical Decision Support Mechanism for this service, related information was not provided to the furnishing professional or provider
	MS	Six month maintenance and servicing fee for reasonable and necessary parts and labor which are not covered under any manufacturer or supplier warranty
	NB	Nebulizer system, any type, FDA-cleared for use with specific drug
	NR	New when rented (use the NR modifier when DME which was new at the time of rental is subsequently purchased)
	NU	New equipment
	P1	A normal healthy patient
	P2	A patient with mild systemic disease
	P3	A patient with severe systemic disease
	P4	A patient with severe systemic disease that is a constant threat to life
	P5	A moribund patient who is not expected to survive without the operation
	P6	A declared brain-dead patient whose organs are being removed for donor purposes
	PA	Surgical or other invasive procedure on wrong body part
	PB	Surgical or other invasive procedure on wrong patient
	PC	Wrong surgery or other invasive procedure on patient
	PD	Diagnostic or related nondiagnostic item or service provided in a wholly owned or operated entity to a patient who is admitted as an inpatient within three days
	PI	Positron emission tomography (PET) or pet/computed tomography (CT) to inform the initial treatment strategy of tumors that are biopsy proven or strongly suspected of being cancerous based on other diagnostic testing
	PL	Progressive addition lenses
	PM	Post mortem
	PN	Nonexcepted service provided at an off-campus, outpatient, provider-based department of a hospital
	PO	Excepted service provided at an off-campus, outpatient, provider-based department of a hospital
	PS	Positron emission tomography (PET) or pet/computed tomography (CT) to inform the subsequent treatment strategy of cancerous tumors when the beneficiary's treating physician determines that the PET study is needed to inform subsequent antitumor strategy
	PT	Colorectal cancer screening test; converted to diagnostic test or other procedure
	Q0	Investigational clinical service provided in a clinical research study that is in an approved clinical research study
	Q1	Routine clinical service provided in a clinical research study that is in an approved clinical research study
	Q2	Demonstration procedure/service
	Q3	Live kidney donor surgery and related services
	Q4	Service for ordering/referring physician qualifies as a service exemption
	Q5	Service furnished under a reciprocal billing arrangement by a substitute physician or by a substitute physical therapist furnishing outpatient physical therapy services in a health professional shortage area, a medically underserved area, or a rural area
	Q6	Service furnished under a fee-for-time compensation arrangement by a substitute physician or by a substitute physical therapist furnishing outpatient physical therapy services in a health professional shortage area, a medically underserved area, or a rural area
	Q7	One Class A finding
	Q8	Two Class B findings
	Q9	One Class B and two Class C findings
	QA	Prescribed amounts of stationary oxygen for daytime use while at rest and nighttime use differ and the average of the two amounts is less than 1 liter per minute (LPM)
	QB	Prescribed amounts of stationary oxygen for daytime use while at rest and nighttime use differ and the average of the two amounts exceeds 4 liters per minute (LPM) and portable oxygen is prescribed
	QC	Single channel monitoring
	QD	Recording and storage in solid state memory by a digital recorder
	QE	Prescribed amount of stationary oxygen while at rest is less than 1 liter per minute (LPM)
	QF	Prescribed amount of stationary oxygen while at rest exceeds 4 liters per minute (LPM) and portable oxygen is prescribed
	QG	Prescribed amount of stationary oxygen while at rest is greater than 4 liters per minute (LPM)
	QH	Oxygen conserving device is being used with an oxygen delivery system
	QJ	Services/items provided to a prisoner or patient in state or local custody; however, the state or local government, as applicable, meets the requirements in 42 CFR 411.4 (B)

© 2019 Optum360, LLC

QK	Medical direction of two, three, or four concurrent anesthesia procedures involving qualified individuals
QL	Patient pronounced dead after ambulance called
QM	Ambulance service provided under arrangement by a provider of services
QN	Ambulance service furnished directly by a provider of services
QP	Documentation is on file showing that the laboratory test(s) was ordered individually or ordered as a CPT-recognized panel other than automated profile codes 80002-80019, G0058, G0059, and G0060.
○ **QQ**	Ordering professional consulted a qualified clinical decision support mechanism for this service and the related data was provided to the furnishing professional
QR	Prescribed amounts of stationary oxygen for daytime use while at rest and nighttime use differ and the average of the two amounts is greater than 4 liters per minute (LPM)
QS	Monitored anesthesiology care service
QT	Recording and storage on tape by an analog tape recorder
QW	CLIA waived test
QX	CRNA service: with medical direction by a physician
QY	Medical direction of one certified registered nurse anesthetist (CRNA) by an anesthesiologist
QZ	CRNA service: without medical direction by a physician
RA	Replacement of a DME, orthotic or prosthetic item
RB	Replacement of a part of a DME, orthotic or prosthetic item furnished as part of a repair
RC	Right coronary artery
RD	Drug provided to beneficiary, but not administered "incident-to"
RE	Furnished in full compliance with FDA-mandated risk evaluation and mitigation strategy (REMS)
RI	Ramus intermedius coronary artery
RR	Rental (use the RR modifier when DME is to be rented)
RT	Right side (used to identify procedures performed on the right side of the body)
SA	Nurse practitioner rendering service in collaboration with a physician
SB	Nurse midwife
SC	Medically necessary service or supply
SD	Services provided by registered nurse with specialized, highly technical home infusion training
SE	State and/or federally-funded programs/services
SF	Second opinion ordered by a professional review organization (PRO) per section 9401, p.l. 99-272 (100 percent reimbursement - no Medicare deductible or coinsurance)
SG	Ambulatory surgical center (ASC) facility service
SH	Second concurrently administered infusion therapy
SJ	Third or more concurrently administered infusion therapy
SK	Member of high risk population (use only with codes for immunization)
SL	State supplied vaccine
SM	Second surgical opinion
SN	Third surgical opinion
SQ	Item ordered by home health
SS	Home infusion services provided in the infusion suite of the IV therapy provider
ST	Related to trauma or injury
SU	Procedure performed in physician's office (to denote use of facility and equipment)
SV	Pharmaceuticals delivered to patient's home but not utilized
SW	Services provided by a certified diabetic educator
SY	Persons who are in close contact with member of high-risk population (use only with codes for immunization)
SZ	Habilitative services
T1	Left foot, second digit
T2	Left foot, third digit
T3	Left foot, fourth digit
T4	Left foot, fifth digit
T5	Right foot, great toe
T6	Right foot, second digit
T7	Right foot, third digit
T8	Right foot, fourth digit
T9	Right foot, fifth digit
TA	Left foot, great toe
TB	Drug or biological acquired with 340B drug pricing program discount, reported for informational purposes
TC	Technical component; under certain circumstances, a charge may be made for the technical component alone; under those circumstances the technical component charge is identified by adding modifier TC to the usual procedure number; technical component charges are institutional charges and not billed separately by physicians; however, portable x-ray suppliers only bill for technical component and should utilize modifier TC; the charge data from portable x-ray suppliers will then be used to build customary and prevailing profiles
TD	RN
TE	LPN/LVN
TF	Intermediate level of care
TG	Complex/high tech level of care
TH	Obstetrical treatment/services, prenatal or postpartum
TJ	Program group, child and/or adolescent
TK	Extra patient or passenger, nonambulance
TL	Early intervention/individualized family service plan (IFSP)
TM	Individualized education program (IEP)
TN	Rural/outside providers' customary service area
TP	Medical transport, unloaded vehicle
TQ	Basic life support transport by a volunteer ambulance provider
TR	School-based individualized education program (IEP) services provided outside the public school district responsible for the student
TS	Follow-up service
TT	Individualized service provided to more than one patient in same setting
TU	Special payment rate, overtime
TV	Special payment rates, holidays/weekends
TW	Back-up equipment
U1	Medicaid level of care 1, as defined by each state
U2	Medicaid level of care 2, as defined by each state

© 2019 Optum360, LLC

U3	Medicaid level of care 3, as defined by each state
U4	Medicaid level of care 4, as defined by each state
U5	Medicaid level of care 5, as defined by each state
U6	Medicaid level of care 6, as defined by each state
U7	Medicaid level of care 7, as defined by each state
U8	Medicaid level of care 8, as defined by each state
U9	Medicaid level of care 9, as defined by each state
UA	Medicaid level of care 10, as defined by each state
UB	Medicaid level of care 11, as defined by each state
UC	Medicaid level of care 12, as defined by each state
UD	Medicaid level of care 13, as defined by each state
UE	Used durable medical equipment
UF	Services provided in the morning
UG	Services provided in the afternoon
UH	Services provided in the evening
UJ	Services provided at night
UK	Services provided on behalf of the client to someone other than the client (collateral relationship)
UN	Two patients served
UP	Three patients served
UQ	Four patients served
UR	Five patients served
US	Six or more patients served
V1	Demonstration modifier 1
V2	Demonstration modifier 2
V3	Demonstration modifier 3
V5	Vascular catheter (alone or with any other vascular access)
V6	Arteriovenous graft (or other vascular access not including a vascular catheter)
V7	Arteriovenous fistula only (in use with two needles)
V8	Infection present
V9	No infection present
VM	Medicare Diabetes Prevention Program (MDPP) virtual make-up session
VP	Aphakic patient
X1	Continuous/broad services: for reporting services by clinicians, who provide the principal care for a patient, with no planned endpoint of the relationship; services in this category represent comprehensive care, dealing with the entire scope of patient problems, either directly or in a care coordination role; reporting clinician service examples include, but are not limited to, primary care, and clinicians providing comprehensive care to patients in addition to specialty care
X2	Continuous/focused services: for reporting services by clinicians whose expertise is needed for the ongoing management of a chronic disease or a condition that needs to be managed and followed with no planned endpoint to the relationship; reporting clinician service examples include, but are not limited to, a rheumatologist taking care of the patient's rheumatoid arthritis longitudinally but not providing general primary care services
X3	Episodic/broad servies: for reporting services by clinicians who have broad responsibility for the comprehensive needs of the patient that is limited to a defined period and circumstance such as a hospitalization; reporting clinician service examples include, but are not limited to, the hospitalist's services rendered providing comprehensive and general care to a patient while admitted to the hospital
X4	Episodic/focused services: for reporting services by clinicians who provide focused care on particular types of treatment limited to a defined period and circumstance; the patient has a problem, acute or chronic, that will be treated with surgery, radiation, or some other type of generally time-limited intervention; reporting clinician service examples include, but are not limited to, the orthopedic surgeon performing a knee replacement and seeing the patient through the postoperative period
X5	Diagnostic services requested by another clinician: for reporting services by a clinician who furnishes care to the patient only as requested by another clinician or subsequent and related services requested by another clinician; this modifier is reported for patient relationships that may not be adequately captured by the above alternative categories; reporting clinician service examples include, but are not limited to, the radiologist's interpretation of an imaging study requested by another clinician
XE	Separate encounter, a service that is distinct because it occurred during a separate encounter
XP	Separate practitioner, a service that is distinct because it was performed by a different practitioner
XS	Separate structure, a service that is distinct because it was performed on a separate organ/structure
XU	Unusual nonoverlapping service, the use of a service that is distinct because it does not overlap usual components of the main service

© 2019 Optum360, LLC

Appendix 3 — Abbreviations and Acronyms

HCPCS Abbreviations and Acronyms

The following abbreviations and acronyms are used in the HCPCS descriptions:

/	or
<	less than
<=	less than equal to
>	greater than
>=	greater than equal to
AC	alternating current
AFO	ankle-foot orthosis
AICC	anti-inhibitor coagulant complex
AK	above the knee
AKA	above knee amputation
ALS	advanced life support
AMP	ampule
ART	artery
ART	Arterial
ASC	ambulatory surgery center
ATT	attached
A-V	Arteriovenous
AVF	arteriovenous fistula
BICROS	bilateral routing of signals
BK	below the knee
BLS	basic life support
BMI	body mass index
BP	blood pressure
BTE	behind the ear (hearing aid)
CAPD	continuous ambulatory peritoneal dialysis
Carb	carbohydrate
CBC	complete blood count
cc	cubic centimeter
CCPD	continuous cycling peritoneal analysis
CHF	congestive heart failure
CIC	completely in the canal (hearing aid)
CIM	Coverage Issue Manual
Clsd	closed
cm	centimeter
CMN	certificate of medical necessity
CMS	Centers for Medicare and Medicaid Services
CMV	Cytomegalovirus
Conc	concentrate
Conc	concentrated
Cont	continuous
CP	clinical psychologist
CPAP	continuous positive airway pressure
CPT	Current Procedural Terminology
CRF	chronic renal failure
CRNA	certified registered nurse anesthetist
CROS	contralateral routing of signals
CSW	clinical social worker
CT	computed tomography
CTLSO	cervical-thoracic-lumbar-sacral orthosis
cu	cubic
DC	direct current
DI	diurnal rhythm
Dx	diagnosis
DLI	donor leukocyte infusion
DME	durable medical equipment
DME MAC	durable medical equipment Medicare administrative contractor
DMEPOS	Durable Medical Equipment, Prosthestics, Orthotics and Other Supplies
DMERC	durable medical equipment regional carrier
DR	diagnostic radiology
DX	diagnostic
e.g.	for example
Ea	each
ECF	extended care facility
EEG	electroencephalogram
EKG	electrocardiogram
EMG	electromyography
EO	elbow orthosis
EP	electrophysiologic
EPO	epoetin alfa
EPSDT	early periodic screening, diagnosis and treatment
ESRD	end-stage renal disease
Ex	extended
Exper	experimental
Ext	external
F	french
FDA	Food and Drug Administration
FDG-PET	Positron emission with tomography with 18 fluorodeoxyglucose
Fem	female
FO	finger orthosis
FPD	fixed partial denture
Fr	french
ft	foot
G-CSF	filgrastim (granulocyte colony-stimulating factor)
gm	gram (g)
H2O	water
HCl	hydrochloric acid, hydrochloride
HCPCS	Healthcare Common Procedural Coding System
HCT	hematocrit
HFO	hand-finger orthosis
HHA	home health agency
HI	high
HI-LO	high-low
HIT	home infusion therapy
HKAFO	hip-knee-ankle foot orthosis
HLA	human leukocyte antigen
HMES	heat and moisture exchange system
HNPCC	hereditary non-polyposis colorectal cancer
HO	hip orthosis
HPSA	health professional shortage area
HST	home sleep test
IA	intra-arterial administration
ip	interphalangeal
I-131	Iodine 131
ICF	intermediate care facility
ICU	intensive care unit
IM	intramuscular

© 2019 Optum360, LLC

in	inch
INF	infusion
INH	inhalation solution
INJ	injection
IOL	intraocular lens
IPD	intermittent peritoneal dialysis
IPPB	intermittent positive pressure breathing
IT	intrathecal administration
ITC	in the canal (hearing aid)
ITE	in the ear (hearing aid)
IU	international units
IV	intravenous
IVF	in vitro fertilization
KAFO	knee-ankle-foot orthosis
KO	knee orthosis
KOH	potassium hydroxide
L	left
LASIK	laser in situ keratomileusis
LAUP	laser assisted uvulopalatoplasty
lbs	pounds
LDL	low density lipoprotein
LDS	lipodystrophy syndrome
Lo	low
LPM	liters per minute
LPN/LVN	Licensed Practical Nurse/Licensed Vocational Nurse
LSO	lumbar-sacral orthosis
MAC	Medicare administrative contractor
mp	metacarpophalangeal
mcg	microgram
mCi	millicurie
MCM	Medicare Carriers Manual
MCP	metacarparpophalangeal joint
MCP	monthly capitation payment
mEq	milliequivalent
MESA	microsurgical epididymal sperm aspiration
mg	milligram
mgs	milligrams
MHT	megahertz
ml	milliliter
mm	millimeter
mmHg	millimeters of Mercury
MRA	magnetic resonance angiography
MRI	magnetic resonance imaging
NA	sodium
NCI	National Cancer Institute
NEC	not elsewhere classified
NG	nasogastric
NH	nursing home
NMES	neuromuscular electrical stimulation
NOC	not otherwise classified
NOS	not otherwise specified
O2	oxygen
OBRA	Omnibus Budget Reconciliation Act
OMT	osteopathic manipulation therapy
OPPS	outpatient prospective payment system
ORAL	oral administration
OSA	obstructive sleep apnea
Ost	ostomy
OTH	other routes of administration
oz	ounce
PA	physician's assistant
PAR	parenteral
PCA	patient controlled analgesia
PCH	pouch
PEN	parenteral and enteral nutrition
PENS	percutaneous electrical nerve stimulation
PET	positron emission tomography
PHP	pre-paid health plan
PHP	physician hospital plan
PI	paramedic intercept
PICC	peripherally inserted central venous catheter
PKR	photorefractive keratotomy
Pow	powder
PQRS	Physician Quality Reporting System
PRK	photoreactive keratectomy
PRO	peer review organization
PSA	prostate specific antigen
PTB	patellar tendon bearing
PTK	phototherapeutic keratectomy
PVC	polyvinyl chloride
R	right
Repl	replace
RN	registered nurse
RP	retrograde pyelogram
Rx	prescription
SACH	solid ankle, cushion heel
SC	subcutaneous
SCT	specialty care transport
SEO	shoulder-elbow orthosis
SEWHO	shoulder-elbow-wrist-hand orthosis
SEXA	single energy x-ray absorptiometry
SGD	speech generating device
SGD	sinus rhythm
SM	samarium
SNCT	sensory nerve conduction test
SNF	skilled nursing facility
SO	sacroilliac othrosis
SO	shoulder orthosis
Sol	solution
SQ	square
SR	screen
ST	standard
ST	sustained release
Syr	syrup
TABS	tablets
Tc	Technetium
Tc 99m	technetium isotope
TENS	transcutaneous electrical nerve stimulator
THKAO	thoracic-hip-knee-ankle orthosis
TLSO	thoracic-lumbar-sacral-orthosis
TM	temporomandibular
TMJ	temporomandibular joint
TPN	total parenteral nutrition
U	unit
uCi	microcurie
VAR	various routes of administration
w	with
w/	with
w/o	without
WAK	wearable artificial kidney
wc	wheelchair
WHFO	wrist-hand-finger orthotic
Wk	week
w/o	without
Xe	xenon (isotope mass of xenon 133)

© 2019 Optum360, LLC

Appendix 4 — Internet-only Manuals (IOMs)

The Centers for Medicare and Medicaid Services restructured its paper-based manual system as a web-based system on October 1, 2003. Called the online CMS manual system, it combines all of the various program instructions into Internet-only Manuals (IOMs), which are used by all CMS programs and contractors. In many instances, the references from the online manuals in appendix 4 contain a mention of the old paper manuals from which the current information was obtained when the manuals were converted. This information is shown in the header of the text, in the following format, when applicable, as A3-3101, HO-210, and B3-2049. Complete versions of all of the manuals can be found at http://www.cms.gov/manuals.

Effective with implementation of the IOMs, the former method of publishing program memoranda (PMs) to communicate program instructions was replaced by the following four templates:

- One-time notification
- Manual revisions
- Business requirements
- Confidential requirements

The web-based system has been organized by functional area (e.g., eligibility, entitlement, claims processing, benefit policy, program integrity) in an effort to eliminate redundancy within the manuals, simplify updating, and make CMS program instructions available more quickly. The web-based system contains the functional areas included below:

Pub. 100	**Introduction**
Pub. 100-01	Medicare General Information, Eligibility, and Entitlement Manual
Pub. 100-02	Medicare Benefit Policy Manual
Pub. 100-03	Medicare National Coverage Determinations (NCD) Manual
Pub. 100-04	Medicare Claims Processing Manual
Pub. 100-05	Medicare Secondary Payer Manual
Pub. 100-06	Medicare Financial Management Manual
Pub. 100-07	State Operations Manual
Pub. 100-08	Medicare Program Integrity Manual
Pub. 100-09	Medicare Contractor Beneficiary and Provider Communications Manual
Pub. 100-10	Quality Improvement Organization Manual
Pub. 100-11	Programs of All-Inclusive Care for the Elderly (PACE) Manual
Pub. 100-12	State Medicaid Manual (under development)
Pub. 100-13	Medicaid State Children's Health Insurance Program (under development)
Pub. 100-14	Medicare ESRD Network Organizations Manual
Pub. 100-15	Medicaid Integrity Program (MIP)
Pub. 100-16	Medicare Managed Care Manual
Pub. 100-17	CMS/Business Partners Systems Security Manual
Pub. 100-18	Medicare Prescription Drug Benefit Manual
Pub. 100-19	Demonstrations
Pub. 100-20	One-Time Notification
Pub. 100-21	Recurring Update Notification
Pub. 100-22	Medicare Quality Reporting Incentive Programs Manual
Pub. 100-24	State Buy-In Manual
Pub. 100-25	Information Security Acceptable Risk Safeguards Manual

A brief description of the Medicare manuals primarily used for *CPC Expert* follows:

The ***National Coverage Determinations Manual*** (NCD), is organized according to categories such as diagnostic services, supplies, and medical procedures. The table of contents lists each category and subject within that category. Revision transmittals identify any new or background material, recap the changes, and provide an effective date for the change.

When complete, the manual will contain two chapters. Chapter 1 currently includes a description of CMS's national coverage determinations. When available, chapter 2 will contain a list of HCPCS codes related to each coverage determination. The manual is organized in accordance with CPT category sequences.

The ***Medicare Benefit Policy Manual*** contains Medicare general coverage instructions that are not national coverage determinations. As a general rule, in the past these instructions have been found in chapter II of the ***Medicare Carriers Manual***, the ***Medicare Intermediary Manual***, other provider manuals, and program memoranda.

The ***Medicare Claims Processing Manual*** contains instructions for processing claims for contractors and providers.

The ***Medicare Program Integrity Manual*** communicates the priorities and standards for the Medicare integrity programs.

100-01, 3, 20.5

Blood Deductibles (Part A and Part B)

(Rev.1, 09-11-02)

Program payment may not be made for the first 3 pints of whole blood or equivalent units of packed red cells received under Part A and Part B combined in a calendar year. However, blood processing (e.g., administration, storage) is not subject to the deductible.

The blood deductibles are in addition to any other applicable deductible and coinsurance amounts for which the patient is responsible.

The deductible applies only to the first 3 pints of blood furnished in a calendar year, even if more than one provider furnished blood.

100-01, 3, 20.5.2

Part B Blood Deductible

(Rev.1, 09-11-02)

Blood is furnished on an outpatient basis or is subject to the Part B blood deductible and is counted toward the combined limit. It should be noted that payment for blood may be made to the hospital under Part B only for blood furnished in an outpatient setting. Blood is not covered for inpatient Part B services.

100-01, 3, 20.5.3

Items Subject to Blood Deductibles

(Rev.18, Issued: 03-04-05, Effective: 07-01-05, Implementation: 07-05-05)

The blood deductibles apply only to whole blood and packed red cells. The term whole blood means human blood from which none of the liquid or cellular components have been removed. Where packed red cells are furnished, a unit of packed red cells is considered equivalent to a pint of whole blood. Other components of blood such as platelets, fibrinogen, plasma, gamma globulin, and serum albumin are not subject to the blood deductible. However, these components of blood are covered as biologicals.

Refer to Pub. 100-04, Medicare Claims Processing Manual, chapter 4, Sec.231 regarding billing for blood and blood products under the Hospital Outpatient Prospective Payment System (OPPS).

100-02, 1, 10

Covered Inpatient Hospital Services Covered Under Part A

(Rev.1, 10-01-03) A3-3101, HO-210

Patients covered under hospital insurance are entitled to have payment made on their behalf for inpatient hospital services. (Inpatient hospital services do not include extended care services provided by hospitals pursuant to swing bed approvals. See Pub. 100-01, Chapter 8, Sec.10.1, "Hospital Providers of Extended Care Services."). However, both inpatient hospital and inpatient SNF benefits are provided under Part A - Hospital Insurance Benefits for the Aged and Disabled, of Title XVIII).

Additional information concerning the following topics can be found in the following manual chapters:

- Benefit periods is found in Chapter 3, "Duration of Covered Inpatient Services";
- Copayment days is found in Chapter 2, "Duration of Covered Inpatient Services";
- Lifetime reserve days is found in Chapter 5, "Lifetime Reserve Days";

© 2019 Optum360, LLC

- Related payment information is housed in the Provider Reimbursement Manual.

Blood must be furnished on a day which counts as a day of inpatient hospital services to be covered as a Part A service and to count toward the blood deductible. Thus, blood is not covered under Part A and does not count toward the Part A blood deductible when furnished to an inpatient after the inpatient has exhausted all benefit days in a benefit period, or where the individual has elected not to use lifetime reserve days. However, where the patient is discharged on their first day of entitlement or on the hospital's first day of participation, the hospital is permitted to submit a billing form with no accommodation charge, but with ancillary charges including blood.

The records for all Medicare hospital inpatient discharges are maintained in CMS for statistical analysis and use in determining future PPS DRG classifications and rates.

Non-PPS hospitals do not pay for noncovered services generally excluded from coverage in the Medicare Program. This may result in denial of a part of the billed charges or in denial of the entire admission, depending upon circumstance. In PPS hospitals, the following are also possible:

1. In appropriately admitted cases where a noncovered procedure was performed, denied services may result in payment of a different DRG (i.e., one which excludes payment for the noncovered procedure); or
2. In appropriately admitted cases that become cost outlier cases, denied services may lead to denial of some or all of an outlier payment.

The following examples illustrate this principle. If care is noncovered because a patient does not need to be hospitalized, the intermediary denies the admission and makes no Part A (i.e., PPS) payment unless paid under limitation on liability. Under limitation on liability, Medicare payment may be made when the provider and the beneficiary were not aware the services were not necessary and could not reasonably be expected to know that he services were not necessary. For detailed instructions, see the Medicare Claims Processing Manual, Chapter 30, "Limitation on Liability." If a patient is appropriately hospitalized but receives (beyond routine services) only noncovered care, the admission is denied.

NOTE: The intermediary does not deny an admission that includes covered care, even if noncovered care was also rendered. Under PPS, Medicare assumes that it is paying for only the covered care rendered whenever covered services needed to treat and/or diagnose the illness were in fact provided.

If a noncovered procedure is provided along with covered nonroutine care, a DRG change rather than an admission denial might occur. If noncovered procedures are elevating costs into the cost outlier category, outlier payment is denied in whole or in part.

When the hospital is included in PPS, most of the subsequent discussion regarding coverage of inpatient hospital services is relevant only in the context of determining the appropriateness of admissions, which DRG, if any, to pay, and the appropriateness of payment for any outlier cases.

If a patient receives items or services in excess of, or more expensive than, those for which payment can be made, payment is made only for the covered items or services or for only the appropriate prospective payment amount. This provision applies not only to inpatient services, but also to all hospital services under Parts A and B of the program. If the items or services were requested by the patient, the hospital may charge him the difference between the amount customarily charged for the services requested and the amount customarily charged for covered services.

An inpatient is a person who has been admitted to a hospital for bed occupancy for purposes of receiving inpatient hospital services. Generally, a patient is considered an inpatient if formally admitted as inpatient with the expectation that he or she will remain at least overnight and occupy a bed even though it later develops that the patient can be discharged or transferred to another hospital and not actually use a hospital bed overnight.

The physician or other practitioner responsible for a patient's care at the hospital is also responsible for deciding whether the patient should be admitted as an inpatient. Physicians should use a 24-hour period as a benchmark, i.e., they should order admission for patients who are expected to need hospital care for 24 hours or more, and treat other patients on an outpatient basis. However, the decision to admit a patient is a complex medical judgment which can be made only after the physician has considered a number of factors, including the patient's medical history and current medical needs, the types of facilities available to inpatients and to outpatients, the hospital's by-laws and admissions policies, and the relative appropriateness of treatment in each setting. Factors to be considered when making the decision to admit include such things as:

The severity of the signs and symptoms exhibited by the patient;

The medical predictability of something adverse happening to the patient;

The need for diagnostic studies that appropriately are outpatient services (i.e., their performance does not ordinarily require the patient to remain at the hospital for 24 hours or more) to assist in assessing whether the patient should be admitted; and

The availability of diagnostic procedures at the time when and at the location where the patient presents.

Admissions of particular patients are not covered or noncovered solely on the basis of the length of time the patient actually spends in the hospital. In certain specific situations coverage of services on an inpatient or outpatient basis is determined by the following rules:

Minor Surgery or Other Treatment - When patients with known diagnoses enter a hospital for a specific minor surgical procedure or other treatment that is expected to keep them in the hospital for only a few hours (less than 24), they are considered outpatients for coverage purposes regardless of: the hour they came to the hospital, whether they used a bed, and whether they remained in the hospital past midnight.

Renal Dialysis - Renal dialysis treatments are usually covered only as outpatient services but may under certain circumstances be covered as inpatient services depending on the patient's condition. Patients staying at home, who are ambulatory, whose conditions are stable and who come to the hospital for routine chronic dialysis treatments, and not for a diagnostic workup or a change in therapy, are considered outpatients. On the other hand, patients undergoing short-term dialysis until their kidneys recover from an acute illness (acute dialysis), or persons with borderline renal failure who develop acute renal failure every time they have an illness and require dialysis (episodic dialysis) are usually inpatients. A patient may begin dialysis as an inpatient and then progress to an outpatient status.

Under original Medicare, the Quality Improvement Organization (QIO), for each hospital is responsible for deciding, during review of inpatient admissions on a case-by-case basis, whether the admission was medically necessary. Medicare law authorizes the QIO to make these judgments, and the judgments are binding for purposes of Medicare coverage. In making these judgments, however, QIOs consider only the medical evidence which was available to the physician at the time an admission decision had to be made. They do not take into account other information (e.g., test results) which became available only after admission, except in cases where considering the post-admission information would support a finding that an admission was medically necessary.

Refer to Parts 4 and 7 of the QIO Manual with regard to initial determinations for these services. The QIO will review the swing bed services in these PPS hospitals as well.

NOTE: When patients requiring extended care services are admitted to beds in a hospital, they are considered inpatients of the hospital. In such cases, the services furnished in the hospital will not be considered extended care services, and payment may not be made under the program for such services unless the services are extended care services furnished pursuant to a swing bed agreement granted to the hospital by the Secretary of Health and Human Services.

100-02, 6, 20.6

Outpatient Observation Services

(Rev.215, Issued, 12-18-15, Effective, 01-01-16, Implementation: 01-04-16)

A. Outpatient Observation Services Defined

Observation care is a well-defined set of specific, clinically appropriate services, which include ongoing short term treatment, assessment, and reassessment before a decision can be made regarding whether patients will require further treatment as hospital inpatients or if they are able to be discharged from the hospital. Observation services are commonly ordered for patients who present to the emergency department and who then require a significant period of treatment or monitoring in order to make a decision concerning their admission or discharge.

Observation services are covered only when provided by the order of a physician or another individual authorized by State licensure law and hospital staff bylaws to admit patients to the hospital or to order outpatient tests. In the majority of cases, the decision whether to discharge a patient from the hospital following resolution of the reason for the observation care or to admit the patient as an inpatient can be made in less than 48 hours, usually in less than 24 hours. In only rare and exceptional cases do reasonable and necessary outpatient observation services span more than 48 hours.

Hospitals may bill for patients who are directly referred to the hospital for outpatient observation services. A direct referral occurs when a physician in the community refers a patient to the hospital for outpatient observation, bypassing the clinic or emergency department (ED) visit. Effective for services furnished on or after January 1, 2003, hospitals may bill for patients directly referred for observation services.

See Pub. 100-04,*Medicare Claims Processing Manual*, chapter 4, section 290, at http://www.cms.hhs.gov/manuals/downloads/clm104c04.pdf for billing and payment instructions for outpatient observation services.

© 2019 Optum360, LLC

Future updates will be issued in a Recurring Update Notification.

B. Coverage of Outpatient Observation Services

When a physician orders that a patient receive observation care, the patient's status is that of an outpatient. The purpose of observation is to determine the need for further treatment or for inpatient admission. Thus, a patient receiving observation services may improve and be released, or be admitted as an inpatient (see Pub. 100-02,*Medicare Benefit Policy Manual*, Chapter 1, Section 10 "Covered Inpatient Hospital Services Covered Under Part A" at http://www.cms.hhs.gov/manuals/Downloads/bp102c01.pdf). For more information on correct reporting of observation services, see Pub. 100-04,*Medicare Claims Processing Manual*, chapter 4, section 290.2.2.)

All hospital observation services, regardless of the duration of the observation care, that are medically reasonable and necessary are covered by Medicare.

Observation services are reported using HCPCS code G0378 (Hospital observation service, per hour). Beginning January 1, 2008, HCPCS code G0378 for hourly observation services is assigned status indicator N, signifying that its payment is always packaged. No separate payment is made for observation services reported with HCPCS code G0378. In most circumstances, observation services are supportive and ancillary to the other separately payable services provided to a patient. In certain circumstances when observation care is billed in conjunction with a high level clinic visit (Level 5), high level Type A emergency department visit (Level 4 or 5), high level Type B emergency department visit (Level 5), critical care services, or direct referral for observation services as an integral part of a patient's extended encounter of care, payment may be made for the entire extended care encounter through one of two composite APCs when certain criteria are met. For information about billing and payment methodology for observation services in years prior to CY 2008, see Pub. 100-04,*Medicare Claims Processing Manual*, Chapter 4, Sec.Sec.290.3-290.4. For information about payment for extended assessment and management under composite APCs, see Sec.290.5.

Payment for all reasonable and necessary observation services is packaged into the payments for other separately payable services provided to the patient in the same encounter. Observation services packaged through assignment of status indicator N are covered OPPS services. Since the payment for these services is included in the APC payment for other separately payable services on the claim, hospitals must not bill Medicare beneficiaries directly for the packaged services.

C. Services Not Covered by Medicare and Notification to the Beneficiary

In making the determination whether an ABN can be used to shift liability to a beneficiary for the cost of non-covered items or services related to an encounter that includes observation care, the provider should follow a two step process. First, the provider must decide whether the item or service meets either the definition of observation care or would be otherwise covered. If the item or service does not meet the definitional requirements of any Medicare-covered benefit under Part B, then the item or service is not covered by Medicare and an ABN is not required to shift the liability to the beneficiary. However, the provider may choose to provide voluntary notification for these items or services.

Second, if the item or service meets the definition of observation services or would be otherwise covered, then the provider must decide whether the item or service is "reasonable and necessary" for the beneficiary on the occasion in question, or if the item or service exceeds any frequency limitation for the particular benefit or falls outside of a timeframe for receipt of a particular benefit. In these cases, the ABN would be used to shift the liability to the beneficiary (see Pub. 100-04,*Medicare Claims Processing Manual*; Chapter 30, "Financial Liability Protections," Section 20, at http://www.cms.hhs.gov/manuals/downloads/clm104c30.pdf for information regarding Limitation On Liability (LOL) Under Sec.1879 Where Medicare Claims Are Disallowed).

If an ABN is not issued to the beneficiary, the provider may be held liable for the cost of the item or service unless the provider/supplier is able to demonstrate that they did not know and could not have reasonably been expected to know that Medicare would not pay for the item or service.

100-02, 7, 40.1.2.8

Wound Care

(Rev.233, Issued: 02-24-17, Effective: 01-01-17, Implementation: 03-27-17)

Care of wounds, (including, but not limited to, ulcers, burns, pressure sores, open surgical sites, fistulas, tube sites, and tumor erosion sites) when the skills of a licensed nurse are needed to provide safely and effectively the services necessary to treat the illness or injury, is considered to be a skilled nursing service. For skilled nursing care to be reasonable and necessary to treat a wound, the size, depth, nature of drainage (color, odor, consistency, and quantity), and condition and appearance of the skin surrounding the wound must be documented in the clinical findings so that an assessment of the need for skilled nursing care can be made. This includes whether wound care is performed via dressing changes, NPWT using conventional DME systems or NPWT using a disposable device. Coverage or denial of skilled nursing visits for wound care may not be based solely on the stage classification of the wound, but rather must be based on all of the documented clinical findings. Moreover, the plan of care must contain the specific instructions for the treatment of the wound. Where the physician has ordered appropriate active treatment (e.g., sterile or complex dressings, NPWT, administration of prescription medications, etc.) of wounds with the following characteristics, the skills of a licensed nurse are usually reasonable and necessary:

- Open wounds which are draining purulent or colored exudate or have a foul odor present or for which the patient is receiving antibiotic therapy;
- Wounds with a drain or T-tube that require shortening or movement of such drains;
- Wounds which require irrigation or instillation of a sterile cleansing or medicated solution into several layers of tissue and skin and/or packing with sterile gauze;
- Recently debrided ulcers;
- Pressure sores (decubitus ulcers) with the following characteristics:
  - There is partial tissue loss with signs of infection such as foul odor or purulent drainage; or
  - There is full thickness tissue loss that involves exposure of fat or invasion of other tissue such as muscle or bone.

NOTE: Wounds or ulcers that show redness, edema, and induration, at times with epidermal blistering or desquamation do not ordinarily require skilled nursing care.

- Wounds with exposed internal vessels or a mass that may have a proclivity for hemorrhage when a dressing is changed (e.g., post radical neck surgery, cancer of the vulva);
- Open wounds or widespread skin complications following radiation therapy, or which result from immune deficiencies or vascular insufficiencies;
- Post-operative wounds where there are complications such as infection or allergic reaction or where there is an underlying disease that has a reasonable potential to adversely affect healing (e.g., diabetes);
- Third degree burns, and second degree burns where the size of the burn or presence of complications causes skilled nursing care to be needed;
- Skin conditions that require application of nitrogen mustard or other chemotherapeutic medication that present a significant risk to the patient;
- Other open or complex wounds that require treatment that can only be provided safely and effectively by a licensed nurse.

EXAMPLE 1:

A patient has a second-degree burn with full thickness skin damage on the back. The wound is cleansed, followed by an application of Sulfamylon. While the wound requires skilled monitoring for signs and symptoms of infection or complications, the dressing change requires skilled nursing services. The home health record at each visit must document the need for the skilled nursing services.

EXAMPLE 2:

A patient experiences a decubitus ulcer where the full thickness tissue loss extends through the dermis to involve subcutaneous tissue. The wound involves necrotic tissue with a physician's order to apply a covering of a debriding ointment following vigorous irrigation. The wound is then packed loosely with wet to dry dressings or continuous moist dressing and covered with dry sterile gauze. Skilled nursing care is necessary for proper treatment. The home health record at each visit must document the need for the skilled nursing services.

NOTE: This section relates to the direct, hands on skilled nursing care provided to patients with wounds, including any necessary dressing changes on those wounds. While a wound might not require this skilled nursing care, the wound may still require skilled monitoring for signs and symptoms of infection or complication (see §40.1.2.1) or for skilled teaching of wound care to the patient or the patient's family (see §40.1.2.3). For an example of when wound care is provided separately from the furnishing of NPWT using a disposable device, see §50.4.4.

100-02, 7, 50.4.4

Negative Pressure Wound Therapy Using a Disposable Device

(Rev.233, Issued: 02-24-17, Effective: 01-01-17, Implementation: 03-27-17)

Sections 1834 and 1861(m)(5) of the Act require a separate payment to an HHA for an applicable disposable device when furnished on or after January 1, 2017, to an individual who receives home health services for which payment is made under the Medicare home health benefit. Section 1834 of the Act defines an applicable device as a disposable NPWT device that is an integrated system comprised of a non-manual vacuum pump, a receptacle for collecting exudate, and dressings for the purposes of

© 2019 Optum360, LLC

wound therapy used in lieu of a conventional NPWT DME system. As required by §1834 of the Act, the separate payment amount for a disposable NPWT device is to be set equal to the amount of the payment that would be made under the Medicare Hospital Outpatient Prospective Payment System (OPPS) using the Level I HCPCS code, otherwise referred to as Current Procedural Terminology (CPT) codes, for which the description for a professional service includes the furnishing of such a device.

Payment for HH visits related to wound care, but not requiring the furnishing of an entirely new disposable NPWT device, will be covered by the HH PPS episode payment and must be billed using the HH claim. Where a home health visit is exclusively for the purpose of furnishing NPWT using a disposable device, the HHA will submit only a type of claim that will be paid for separately outside the HH PPS (TOB 34x). Where, however, the home health visit includes the provision of other home health services in addition to, and separate from, furnishing NPWT using a disposable device, the HHA will submit both a home health claim and a TOB 34x—the home health claim for other home health services and the TOB 34x for furnishing NPWT using a disposable device.

EXAMPLE:

A patient requires NPWT for the treatment of a wound. On Monday, a nurse assesses a patient's wound, applies a new disposable NPWT device, and provides wound care education to the patient and family. The nurse returns on Thursday for wound assessment and replaces the fluid management system (or dressing) for the existing disposable NPWT, but does not replace the entire device. The nurse returns the following Monday, assesses the patient's condition and the wound, and replaces the device that had been applied on the previous Monday with a new disposable NPWT device. In this scenario, the billing procedures are as follows:

For both Monday visits, all the services provided by the nurse were associated with furnishing NPWT using a disposable device. The nurse did not provide any services that were not associated with furnishing NPWT using a disposable device. Therefore, all the nursing services for both Monday visits should be reported on TOB 34x with CPT code 97607 or 97608. None of the services should be reported on the HH claim.

For the Thursday visit, the nurse checked the wound, but did not apply a new disposable NPWT device, so even though the nurse provided care related to the wound, those services would not be considered furnishing NPWT using a disposable device. Therefore, the services should be reported on bill type 32x and no services should be reported on bill type 34x.

For instructions on billing for NPWT using a disposable device, see Pub. 100-04, Medicare Claims Processing Manual, chapter 10, Section 90.3 – Billing Instructions for Disposable Negative Pressure Wound Therapy Services.

100-02, 10, 10.1.1

The Vehicle

(Rev.1, 10-01-03)
B3-2120.1.A, A3-3114.A, HO-236.1.A

Any vehicle used as an ambulance must be designed and equipped to respond to medical emergencies and, in nonemergency situations, be capable of transporting beneficiaries with acute medical conditions. The vehicle must comply with State or local laws governing the licensing and certification of an emergency medical transportation vehicle. At a minimum, the ambulance must contain a stretcher, linens, emergency medical supplies, oxygen equipment, and other lifesaving emergency medical equipment and be equipped with emergency warning lights, sirens, and telecommunications equipment as required by State or local law. This should include, at a minimum, one 2-way voice radio or wireless telephone.

100-02, 10, 10.2.1

Necessity for the Service

(Rev.1, 10-01-03)

Medical necessity is established when the patient's condition is such that use of any other method of transportation is contraindicated. In any case in which some means of transportation other than an ambulance could be used without endangering the individual's health, whether or not such other transportation is actually available, no payment may be made for ambulance services. In all cases, the appropriate documentation must be kept on file and, upon request, presented to the A/B MAC (A) or (B). It is important to note that the presence (or absence) of a physician's order for a transport by ambulance does not necessarily prove (or disprove) whether the transport was medically necessary. The ambulance service must meet all program coverage criteria in order for payment to be made.

In addition, the reason for the ambulance transport must be medically necessary. That is, the transport must be to obtain a Medicare covered service, or to return from such a service.

100-02, 10, 10.2.2

Reasonableness of the Ambulance Trip

(Rev.103; Issued: 02-20-09; Effective Date: 01-05-09; Implementation Date: 03-20-09)

Under the FS payment is made according to the level of medically necessary services actually furnished. That is, payment is based on the level of service furnished (provided they were medically necessary), not simply on the vehicle used. Even if a local government requires an ALS response for all calls, payment under the FS is made only for the level of service furnished, and then only when the service is medically necessary.

100-02, 10, 10.3.3

Separately Payable Ambulance Transport Under Part B versus Patient Transportation that is Covered Under a Packaged Hospital Service

(Rev.103; Issued: 02-20-09; Effective Date: 01-05-09; Implementation Date: 03-20-09)

Transportation of a beneficiary from his or her home, an accident scene, or any other point of origin is covered under Part B as an ambulance service only to the nearest hospital, critical access hospital (CAH), or skilled nursing facility (SNF) that is capable of furnishing the required level and type of care for the beneficiary's illness or injury and only if medical necessity and other program coverage criteria are met.

Medicare-covered ambulance services are paid either as separately billed services, in which case the entity furnishing the ambulance service bills Part B of the program, or as a packaged service, in which case the entity furnishing the ambulance service must seek payment from the provider who is responsible for the beneficiary's care. If either the origin or the destination of the ambulance transport is the beneficiary's home, then the ambulance transport is paid separately by Medicare Part B, and the entity that furnishes the ambulance transport may bill its Medicare carrier or intermediary directly. If both the origin and destination of the ambulance transport are providers, e.g., a hospital, critical access hospital (CAH), skilled nursing facility (SNF), then responsibility for payment for the ambulance transport is determined in accordance with the following sequential criteria.

NOTE: These criteria must be applied in sequence as a flow chart and not independently of one another.

1. Provider Numbers:

   If the Medicare-assigned provider numbers of the two providers are different, then the ambulance service is separately billable to the program. If the provider number of both providers is the same, then consider criterion 2, "campus".

2. Campus:

   Following criterion 1, if the campuses of the two providers (sharing the same provider numbers) are the same, then the transport is not separately billable to the program. In this case the provider is responsible for payment. If the campuses of the two providers are different, then consider criterion 3, "patient status." "Campus" means the physical area immediately adjacent to the provider's main buildings, other areas and structures that are not strictly contiguous to the main buildings, but are located within 250 yards of the main buildings, and any of the other areas determined on an individual case basis by the CMS regional office to be part of the provider's campus.

3. Patient Status: Inpatient vs. Outpatient

   Following criteria 1 and 2, if the patient is an inpatient at both providers (i.e., inpatient status both at the origin and at the destination, providers sharing the same provider number but located on different campuses), then the transport is not separately billable. In this case the provider is responsible for payment. All other combinations (i.e., outpatient-to-inpatient, inpatient-to-outpatient, outpatient-to-outpatient) are separately billable to the program.

In the case where the point of origin is not a provider, Part A coverage is not available because, at the time the beneficiary is being transported, the beneficiary is not an inpatient of any provider paid under Part A of the program and ambulance services are excluded from the 3-day preadmission payment window.

The transfer, i.e., the discharge of a beneficiary from one provider with a subsequent admission to another provider, is also payable as a Part B ambulance transport, provided all program coverage criteria are met, because, at the time that the beneficiary is in transit, the beneficiary is not a patient of either provider and not subject to either the inpatient preadmission payment window or outpatient payment packaging requirements. This includes an outpatient transfer from a remote, off-campus emergency department (ER) to becoming an inpatient or outpatient at the main campus hospital, even if the ER is owned and operated by the hospital.

Once a beneficiary is admitted to a hospital, CAH, or SNF, it may be necessary to transport the beneficiary to another hospital or other site temporarily for specialized care while the beneficiary maintains inpatient status with the original provider. This movement of the patient is considered "patient transportation" and is covered as an

 © 2019 Optum360, LLC

inpatient hospital or CAH service and as a SNF service when the SNF is furnishing it as a covered SNF service and payment is made under Part A for that service. (If the beneficiary is a resident of a SNF and must be transported by ambulance to receive dialysis or certain other high-end outpatient hospital services, the ambulance transport may be separately payable under Part B.) Because the service is covered and payable as a beneficiary transportation service under Part A, the service cannot be classified and paid for as an ambulance service under Part B. This includes intra-campus transfers between different departments of the same hospital, even where the departments are located in separate buildings. Such intra-campus transfers are not separately payable under the Part B ambulance benefit. Such costs are accounted for in the same manner as the costs of such a transfer within a single building.

100-02, 10, 20

Coverage Guidelines for Ambulance Service Claims.

(Rev.103; Issued: 02-20-09; Effective Date: 01-05-09; Implementation Date: 03-20-09)

Payment may be made for expenses incurred by a patient for ambulance service provided conditions I, 2, and 3 in the left-hand column have been met. The right-hand column indicates the documentation needed to establish that the condition has been met

Conditions	Review Action
1. Patient was transported by an approved supplier of ambulance services.	1. Ambulance suppliers are explained in greater detail in §10.1.3
2. The patient was suffering from an illness or injury, which contraindicated transportation by other means. (§10.2)	2. (a) The contractor presumes the requirement was met if the submitted documentation indicates that the patient: • Was transported in an emergency situation, e.g., as a result of an accident, injury or acute illness, or • Needed to be restrained to prevent injury to the beneficiary or others; or • Was unconscious or in shock; or • Required oxygen or other emergency treatment during transport to the nearest appropriate facility; or • Exhibits signs and symptoms of acute respiratory distress or cardiac distress such as shortness of breath or chest pain; or • Exhibits signs and symptoms that indicate the possibility of acute stroke; or • Had to remain immobile because of a fracture that had not been set or the possibility of a fracture; or • Was experiencing severe hemorrhage; or • Could be moved only by stretcher; or • Was bed-confined before and after the ambulance trip.
2. The patient was suffering from an illness or injury, which contraindicated transportation by other means. (§10.2) (Continued)	(b) In the absence of any of the conditions listed in (a) above additional documentation should be obtained to establish medical need where the evidence indicates the existence of the circumstances listed below: (i) Patient's condition would not ordinarily require movement by stretcher, or (ii) The individual was not admitted as a hospital inpatient (except in accident cases), or (iii) The ambulance was used solely because other means of transportation were unavailable, or (iv) The individual merely needed assistance in getting from his room or home to a vehicle. (c) Where the information indicates a situation not listed in 2(a) or 2(b) above, refer the case to your supervisor.
3. The patient was transported from and to points listed below. (a) From patient's residence (or other place where need arose) to hospital or skilled nursing facility.	3. Claims should show the ZIP Code of the point of pickup. (a) i. Condition met if trip began within the institution's service area as shown in the carrier's locality guide. ii. Condition met where the trip began outside the institution's service area if the institution was the nearest one with appropriate facilities.

NOTE: A Patient'sresidence is the place where he or she makes his/her home and dwells permanently, or for an extended period of time. A skilled nursing facility is one, which is listed in the Directory of Medical Facilities as a participating SNF or as an institution which meets §1861(j)(1) of the Act.

NOTE: A claim for ambulance service to a participating hospital or skilled nursing facility should not be denied on the grounds that there is a nearer nonparticipating institution having appropriate facilities.

(b) Skilled nursing facility to a hospital or hospital to a skilled nursing facility.	(b) (i) Condition met if the ZIP Code of the pickup point is within the service area of the destination as shown in the carrier's locality guide. (ii) Condition met where the ZIP Code of the pickup point is outside the service area of the destination if the destination institution was the nearest appropriate facility.
(c) Hospital to hospital or skilled nursing facility to skilled nursing facility.	(c) Condition met if the discharging institution was not an appropriate facility and the admitting institution was the nearest appropriate facility.
(d) From a hospital or skilled nursing facility to patient's residence.	(d) (i) Condition met if patient's residence is within the institution's service area as shown in the carrier's locality guide. (ii) Condition met where the patient's residence is outside the institution's service area if the institution was the nearest appropriate facility.
(e) Round trip for hospital or participating skilled nursing facility inpatients to the nearest hospital or nonhospital treatment facility.	(e) Condition met if the reasonable and necessary diagnostic or therapeutic service required by patient's condition is not available at the institution where the beneficiary is an inpatient.

NOTE: Ambulance service to a physician's office or a physician-directed clinic is not covered. See §10.3.8 above, where a stop is made at a physician's office en route to a hospital and §10.3.3 for additional exceptions.)

4. Ambulance services involving hospital admissions in Canada or Mexico are covered (Medicare Claims Processing Manual, Chapter 1, "General Billing Requirements, "§10.1.3.) if the following conditions are met:	4. (a) The foreign hospitalization has been determined to be covered; and (b) The ambulance service meets the coverage requirements set forth in §§10-10.3. If the foreign hospitalization has been determined to be covered on the basis of emergency services (See the Medicare Claims Processing Manual, Chapter 1, "General Billing Requirements," §10.1.3), the necessity requirement (§10.2) and the destination requirement (§10.3) are considered met.
5. The carrier will make partial payment for otherwise covered ambulance service, which exceeded limits defined in item 6. The carrier will base the payment on the amount payable had the patient been transported:	5 & 6 (a) From the pickup point to the nearest appropriate facility, or 5 & 6 (b) From the nearest appropriate facility to the beneficiary's residence where he or she is being returned home from a distant institution.

© 2019 Optum360, LLC

100-02, 10, 30.1

Definition of Ambulance Services

(Rev.226, Issued: 09-12-16, Effective: 01-01-16, Implementation: 12-12-16)

There are several categories of ground ambulance services and two categories of air ambulance services under the fee schedule. (Note that "ground" refers to both land and water transportation.) All ground and air ambulance transportation services must meet all requirements regarding medical reasonableness and necessity as outlined in the applicable statute, regulations and manual provisions.

100-02, 10, 30.1.1

Ground Ambulance Services

(Rev.236, Issued: 06-16-17, Effective: 09-18-17, Implementation: 09-18-17)

Basic Life Support (BLS)
Definition: BLS is transportation by ground ambulance vehicle (as defined in section 10.1, above) and the provision of medically necessary supplies and services (as defined in section 10.2, above), including BLS ambulance services as defined by the state.

The ambulance vehicle must be staffed by at least two people who meet the requirements of the state and local laws where the services are being furnished, and at least one of the staff members must be certified at a minimum as an emergency medical technician-basic (EMT-Basic) by the state or local authority where the services are being furnished and be legally authorized to operate all lifesaving and life-sustaining equipment on board the vehicle. These laws may vary from state to state or within a state.

Basic Life Support (BLS) - Emergency
Definition: When medically necessary, the provision of BLS services, as specified above, in the context of an emergency response (as defined below).

Advanced Life Support, Level 1 (ALS1)
Definition: Advanced life support, level 1 (ALS1) is the transportation by ground ambulance vehicle (as defined in section 10.1, above) and the provision of medically necessary supplies and services (as defined in section 10.2, above) including the provision of an ALS assessment by ALS personnel or at least one ALS intervention.

Advanced Life Support Assessment
Definition: An ALS assessment is an assessment performed by an ALS crew as part of an emergency response (as defined below) that was necessary because the patient's reported condition at the time of dispatch was such that only an ALS crew was qualified to perform the assessment. An ALS assessment does not necessarily result in a determination that the patient requires an ALS level of service. In the case of an appropriately dispatched ALS Emergency service, as defined below, if the ALS crew completes an ALS Assessment, the services provided by the ambulance transportation service provider or supplier shall be covered at the ALS emergency level, regardless of whether the patient required ALS intervention services during the transport, provided that ambulance transportation itself was medically reasonable and necessary, as defined in section 10.2, above and all other coverage requirements are met.

Advanced Life Support Intervention
Definition: An ALS intervention is a procedure that is in accordance with state and local laws, required to be done by an emergency medical technician-intermediate (EMT-Intermediate) or EMT-Paramedic.

Application: An ALS intervention must be medically necessary to qualify as an intervention for payment for an ALS level of service. An ALS intervention applies only to ground transports.

Advanced Life Support, Level 1 (ALS1) - Emergency
Definition: When medically necessary, the provision of ALS1 services, as specified above, in the context of an emergency response, as defined below.

Advanced Life Support, Level 2 (ALS2)
Definition: Advanced life support, level 2 (ALS2) is the transportation by ground ambulance vehicle and the provision of medically necessary supplies and services including (1) at least three separate administrations of one or more medications by intravenous (IV) push/bolus or by continuous infusion (excluding crystalloid fluids) or (2) ground ambulance transport, medically necessary supplies and services, and the provision of at least one of the ALS2 procedures listed below:

a. Manual defibrillation/cardioversion;

b. Endotracheal intubation;

c. Central venous line;

d. Cardiac pacing;

e. Chest decompression;

f. Surgical airway; or

g. Intraosseous line.

Application: Crystalloid fluids include but are not necessarily limited to 5 percent Dextrose in water (often referred to as D5W), Saline and Lactated Ringer's. To qualify for the ALS2 level of payment, medications must be administered intravenously. Medications that are administered by other means, for example: intramuscularly, subcutaneously, orally, sublingually, or nebulized do not support payment at the ALS2 level rate.

The IV medications are administered in standard doses as directed by local protocol or online medical direction. It is not appropriate to administer a medication in divided doses in order to meet the ALS2 level of payment. For example, if the local protocol for the treatment of supraventricular tachycardia (SVT) calls for a 6 mg dose of adenosine, the administration of three 2 mg doses in order to qualify for the ALS 2 level is not acceptable.

The administration of an intravenous drug by infusion qualifies as one intravenous dose. For example, if a patient is being treated for atrial fibrillation in order to slow the ventricular rate with diltiazem and the patient requires two boluses of the drug followed by an infusion of diltiazem, then the infusion would be counted as the third intravenous administration and the transport would be billed as an ALS 2 level of service.

The fractional administration of a single dose (for this purpose, meaning a "standard" or "protocol" dose) of a medication on three separate occasions does not qualify for ALS2 payment. In other words, the administering 1/3 of a qualifying dose 3 times does not equate to three qualifying doses to support claiming ALS2-level care. For example, administering one-third of a dose of X medication 3 times might = Y (where Y is a standard/protocol drug amount), but the same sequence does not equal 3 times Y. Thus, if 3 administrations of the same drug are required to claim ALS2 level care, each administration must be in accordance with local protocols; the run will not qualify at the ALS2 level on the basis of drug administration if that administration was not according to local protocol. The criterion of multiple administrations of the same drug requires that a suitable quantity of the drug be administered and that there be a suitable amount of time between administrations, and that both are in accordance with standard medical practice guidelines.

An example of a single dose of medication administered fractionally on three separate occasions that would not qualify for the ALS2 payment rate is the administration of a single 1 mg dose of IV Epinephrine in partial increments to treat an adult pulseless Ventricular Tachycardia/Ventricular Fibrillation (VF/VT) patient. The American Heart Association (AHA), Advanced Cardiac Life Support (ACLS) protocol calls for Epinephrine to be administered in 1 mg increments every 3 to 5 minutes. Therefore, administering IV Epinephrine in separate increments of 0.25 mg, 0.25 mg, and 0.50 mg (for a total of 1 mg) over the course of a single 3 to 5 minute episode would not qualify for the ALS2 level of payment. Conversely, administering three separate 1 mg doses of IV Epinephrine over the requisite protocol-based time period to a patient with unresolved VF/VT would qualify for an ALS2 level of service. NOTE: refer to and abide by your authorized protocols; AHA's ACLS protocols are referenced here only by way of widely recognized example.

Another example that would not qualify for the ALS2 payment level is administering Adenosine in three 2 mg increments (for a total of 6 mg) in treating an adult patient with Paroxysmal Supraventricular Tachycardia (PSVT). ACLS guidelines dictate treating PSVT with 6 mg of Adenosine by rapid intravenous push (IVP) over 1 to 2 seconds. Should the initial 6 mg dose not eliminate the PSVT within 1 to 2 minutes, guidelines dictate that another 12 mg of Adenosine IVP should be administered where the PSVT persists, followed by another 12 mg dose 1 to 2 minutes later; for a total of 30 mg of Adenosine. Administering a total of 30 mg of Adenosine, involving three episodes of administration in a complete cycle of treatment as outlined above, would qualify for ALS2 payment.

Endotracheal (ET) intubation (which includes intubating and/or monitoring/maintaining an ET tube inserted prior to transport) is a service that qualifies for the ALS2 level of payment. Therefore, it is not necessary to consider medications administered by ET tube to determine whether the ALS2 rate is payable.

Advanced Life Support (ALS) Personnel
Definition: ALS personnel are individuals trained to the level of the emergency medical technician-intermediate (EMT-Intermediate) or paramedic.

Specialty Care Transport (SCT)
Definition: SCT is the interfacility transportation (as defined below) of a critically injured or ill beneficiary by a ground ambulance vehicle, including the provision of medically necessary supplies and services, at a level of service beyond the scope of the EMT-Paramedic. SCT is necessary when a beneficiary's condition requires ongoing care that must be furnished by one or more health professionals in an appropriate specialty area, for example, emergency or critical care nursing, emergency medicine, respiratory care, cardiovascular care, or an EMT-Paramedic with additional training.

© 2019 Optum360, LLC

Application: SCT is necessary when a beneficiary's condition requires ongoing care that must be furnished by one or more health professionals in an appropriate specialty area. The EMT-Paramedic level of care is set by each state. Medically necessary care that is furnished at a level above the EMT-Paramedic level of care may qualify as SCT. To be clear, if EMT-Paramedics - without specialty care certification or qualification - are permitted to furnish a given service in a state, then that service does not qualify for SCT. The phrase "EMT-Paramedic with additional training" recognizes that a state may permit a person who is not only certified as an EMT-Paramedic, but who also has successfully completed additional education as determined by the state in furnishing higher level medical services required by critically ill or injured patients, to furnish a level of service that otherwise would require a health professional in an appropriate specialty care area (for example, a nurse) to provide. "Additional training" means the specific additional training that a state requires a paramedic to complete in order to qualify to furnish specialty care to a critically ill or injured patient during an SCT.

Paramedic Intercept (PI)
Definition: Paramedic Intercept services are ALS services provided by an entity that does not provide the ambulance transport. This type of service is most often provided for an emergency ambulance transport in which a local volunteer ambulance that can provide only BLS level of service is dispatched to transport a patient. If the patient needs ALS services such as EKG monitoring, chest decompression, or IV therapy, another entity dispatches a paramedic to meet the BLS ambulance at the scene or once the ambulance is on the way to the hospital. The ALS paramedics then provide services to the patient.

This tiered approach to life saving is cost effective in many areas because most volunteer ambulances do not charge for their services and one paramedic service can cover many communities. Prior to March 1, 1999, Medicare payment could be made for these services, but could not be made directly to the intercept service provider; rather, Medicare payment could be made only when the claim was submitted by the entity that actually furnished the ambulance transport. In those areas where state laws prohibited volunteer ambulances from billing Medicare and other health insurance, the intercept service could not receive payment for treating a Medicare beneficiary and was forced to bill the beneficiary for the entire service.

Paramedic intercept services furnished on or after March 1, 1999, are payable separate from the ambulance transport when all of the requirements in the following three conditions are met:

I. The intercept service(s) is:
- Furnished in a rural area (as defined below);
- Furnished under a contract with one or more volunteer ambulance services; and,
- Medically necessary based on the condition of the beneficiary receiving the ambulance service.

II. The volunteer ambulance service involved must:
- Meet Medicare's certification requirements for furnishing ambulance services;
- Furnish services only at the BLS level at the time of the intercept; and,
- Be prohibited by state law from billing anyone for any service.

III. The entity furnishing the ALS paramedic intercept service must:
- Meet Medicare's certification requirements for furnishing ALS services, and,
- Bill all recipients who receive ALS paramedic intercept services from the entity, regardless of whether or not those recipients are Medicare beneficiaries.

For purposes of the paramedic intercept benefit, a rural area is an area that is designated as rural by a state law or regulation or that is located in a rural census tract of a metropolitan statistical area (as determined under the most recent version of the Goldsmith Modification). (The Goldsmith Modification is a methodology to identify small towns and rural areas within large metropolitan counties that are isolated from central areas by distance or other features). The current list of these areas is periodically published in the Federal Register.

See Pub. 100-04, Medicare Claims Processing Manual, Chapter 15, "Ambulance," §20.1.4 for payment of paramedic intercept services.

Services in a Rural Area
Definition: For purposes other than the paramedic intercept benefit (as defined above), services in a rural area are services that are furnished (1) in an area outside a Metropolitan Statistical Area (MSA); or, (2) an area identified as rural using the most recent version of the Goldsmith Modification even though the area is within an MSA.

Emergency Response
Definition: Emergency response is a BLS or ALS1 level of service that has been provided in immediate response to a 911 call or the equivalent. An immediate response is one in which the ambulance provider/supplier begins as quickly as possible to take the steps necessary to respond to the call.

The nature of an ambulance's response (whether emergency or not) does not independently establish or support medical necessity for an ambulance transport. Rather, Medicare coverage always depends on, among other things, whether the service(s) furnished is actually medically reasonable and necessary based on the patient's condition at the time of transport.

Application: The phrase "911 call or the equivalent" is intended to establish the standard that the nature of the call at the time of dispatch is the determining factor. Regardless of the medium by which the call is made (e.g., a radio call could be appropriate) the call is of an emergent nature when, based on the information available to the dispatcher at the time of the call, it is reasonable for the dispatcher to issue an emergency dispatch in light of accepted, standard dispatch protocol. An emergency call need not come through 911 even in areas where a 911 call system exists. However, the determination to respond emergently with a BLS or ALS ambulance must be in accord with the local 911 or equivalent service dispatch protocol. If the call came in directly to the ambulance provider/supplier, then the provider's/supplier's dispatch protocol and the dispatcher's actions must meet, at a minimum, the standards of the dispatch protocol of the local 911 or equivalent service. In areas that do not have a local 911 or equivalent service, the protocol and the dispatcher's actions must meet, at a minimum, the standards of the dispatch protocol in another similar jurisdiction within the state, or if there is no similar jurisdiction, then the standards of any other dispatch protocol within the state. Where the dispatch was inconsistent with this standard of protocol, including where no protocol was used, the beneficiary's condition (for example, symptoms) at the scene determines the appropriate level of payment.

EMT-Intermediate
Definition: EMT-Intermediate is an individual who is qualified, in accordance with state and local laws, as an EMT-Basic and who is also certified in accordance with state and local laws to perform essential advanced techniques and to administer a limited number of medications.

EMT-Paramedic
Definition: EMT-Paramedic possesses the qualifications of the EMT-Intermediate and, in accordance with state and local laws, has enhanced skills that include being able to administer additional interventions and medications.

Interfacility Transportation
Definition: For purposes of SCT payment, an interfacility transportation is one in which the origin and destination are one of the following: a hospital or skilled nursing facility that participates in the Medicare program or a hospital-based facility that meets Medicare's requirements for provider-based status.

100-02, 11, 20.2

Laboratory Services

(Rev.224, Issued: 06-03-16, Effective: 01-01-16, Implementation: 09-06-16)

All laboratory services furnished to individuals for the treatment of ESRD are included in the ESRD PPS as Part B services and are not paid separately as of January 1, 2011. The laboratory services include but are not limited to:

- Laboratory tests included under the composite rate as of December 31, 2010 (discussed below); and
- Former separately billable Part B laboratory tests that were billed by ESRD facilities and independent laboratories for ESRD patients.

Composite rate laboratory tests are listed in §20.2.E of this chapter. More information regarding composite rate laboratory tests can be found in Pub. 100-04, Medicare Claims Processing Manual, chapter 8, §50.1, §60.1, and §80. As discussed below, composite rate laboratory services should not be reported on claims.

To the extent a laboratory test is performed to monitor the levels or effects of any of the drugs that were specifically excluded from the ESRD PPS, these tests would be separately billable. The following table lists the drug categories that were excluded from the ESRD PPS and the rationale for their exclusion. Laboratory services furnished to monitor the medication levels or effects of drugs and biologicals that fall in those categories would not be considered to be furnished for the treatment of ESRD.

DRUG CATEGORIES EXCLUDED FROM THE ESRD PPS BASE RATE FOR THE PURPOSE OF REPORTING LABS

Drug Category	Rationale for Exclusion
Anticoagulant	Drugs labeled for non-renal dialysis conditions and not for vascular access.
Antidiuretic	Used to prevent fluid loss.
Antiepileptic	Used to prevent seizures.
Anti-inflammatory	May be used to treat kidney disease (glomerulonephritis) and other inflammatory conditions.

© 2019 Optum360, LLC

Drug Category	Rationale for Exclusion
Antipsychotic	Used to treat psychosis.
Antiviral	Used to treat viral conditions such as shingles.
Cancer management	Includes oral, parenteral and infusions. Cancer drugs are covered under a separate benefit category.
Cardiac management	Drugs that manage blood pressure and cardiac conditions.
Cartilage	Used to replace synovial fluid in a joint space.
Coagulants	Drugs that cause blood to clot after anti-coagulant overdose or factor VII deficiency.
Cytoprotective agents	Used after chemotherapy treatment.
Endocrine/metabolic management	Used for endocrine/metabolic disorders such as thyroid or endocrine deficiency, hypoglycemia, and hyperglycemia.
Erectile dysfunction management	Androgens were used prior to the development of ESAs for anemia management and currently are not recommended practice. Also used for hypogonadism and erectile dysfunction.
Gastrointestinal management	Used to treat gastrointestinal conditions such as ulcers and gallbladder disease.
Immune system management	Anti-rejection drugs covered under a separate benefit category.
Migraine management	Used to treat migraine headaches and symptoms.
Musculoskeletal management	Used to treat muscular disorders such as prevent muscle spasms, relax muscles, improve muscle tone as in myasthenia gravis, relax muscles for intubation and induce uterine contractions.
Pharmacy handling for oral anti-cancer, anti-emetics and immunosuppressant drugs	Not a function performed by an ESRD facility.
Pulmonary system management	Used for respiratory/lung conditions such as opening airways and newborn apnea.
Radiopharmaceutical procedures	Includes contrasts and procedure preparation.
Unclassified drugs	Should only be used for drugs that do not have a HCPCS code and therefore cannot be identified.
Vaccines	Covered under a separate benefit category.

The distinction of what is considered to be a renal dialysis laboratory test is a clinical decision determined by the ESRD patient's ordering practitioner. If a laboratory test is ordered for the treatment of ESRD, then the laboratory test is not paid separately.

Payment for all renal dialysis laboratory tests furnished under the ESRD PPS is made directly to the ESRD facility responsible for the patient's care. The ESRD facility must furnish the laboratory tests directly or under arrangement and report renal dialysis laboratory tests on the ESRD facility claim (with the exception of composite rate laboratory services).

An ESRD facility must report renal dialysis laboratory services on its claims in order for the laboratory tests to be included in the outlier payment calculation. Renal dialysis laboratory services that were or would have been paid separately under Medicare Part B prior to January 1, 2011, are priced for the outlier payment calculation using the Clinical Laboratory Fee Schedule. Further information regarding the outlier policy can be found in §60.D of this chapter.

Certain laboratory services will be subject to Part B consolidated billing requirements and will no longer be separately payable when provided to ESRD beneficiaries by providers other than the ESRD facility. The list below includes the renal dialysis laboratory tests that are routinely performed for the treatment of ESRD. Payment for the laboratory tests identified on this list is included in the ESRD PPS. The laboratory tests listed in the table are used to enforce consolidated billing edits to ensure that payment is not made for renal dialysis laboratory tests outside of the ESRD PPS. The list of renal dialysis laboratory tests is not an all-inclusive list. If any laboratory test is ordered for the treatment of ESRD, then the laboratory test is considered to be included in the ESRD PPS and is the responsibility of the ESRD facility. Additional renal dialysis laboratory tests may be added through administrative issuances in the future.

LABS SUBJECT TO ESRD CONSOLIDATED BILLING

CPT/ HCPCS	Short Description
80047	Basic Metabolic Panel (Calcium, ionized)
80048	Basic Metabolic Panel (Calcium, total)
80051	Electrolyte Panel
80053	Comprehensive Metabolic Panel
80061*	Lipid Panel*
80069	Renal Function Panel
80076	Hepatic Function Panel
82040	Assay of serum albumin
82108	Assay of aluminum
82306	Vitamin d, 25 hydroxy
82310	Assay of calcium
82330	Assay of calcium, Ionized
82374	Assay, blood carbon dioxide
82379	Assay of carnitine
82435	Assay of blood chloride
82565	Assay of creatinine
82570	Assay of urine creatinine
82575	Creatinine clearance test
82607	Vitamin B-12
82652	Vit d 1, 25-dihydroxy
82668	Assay of erythropoietin
82728	Assay of ferritin
82746	Blood folic acid serum
83540	Assay of iron
83550	Iron binding test
83735	Assay of magnesium
83970	Assay of parathormone
84075	Assay alkaline phosphatase
84100	Assay of phosphorus
84132	Assay of serum potassium
84134	Assay of prealbumin
84155	Assay of protein, serum
84157	Assay of protein by other source
84295	Assay of serum sodium
84466	Assay of transferrin
84520	Assay of urea nitrogen
84540	Assay of urine/urea-n
84545	Urea-N clearance test
85014	Hematocrit
85018	Hemoglobin
85025	Complete (cbc), automated (HgB, Hct, RBC, WBC, and Platelet count) and automated differential WBC count.
85027	Complete (cbc), automated (HgB, Hct, RBC, WBC, and Platelet count)
85041	Automated rbc count
85044	Manual reticulocyte count
85045	Automated reticulocyte count
85046	Reticyte/hgb concentrate
85048	Automated leukocyte count
86704	Hep b core antibody, total
86705	Hep b core antibody, igm
86706	Hep b surface antibody
87040	Blood culture for bacteria
87070	Culture, bacteria, other
87071	Culture bacteri aerobic othr

© 2019 Optum360, LLC

CPT/ HCPCS	Short Description
87073	Culture bacteria anaerobic
87075	Cultr bacteria, except blood
87076	Culture anaerobe ident, each
87077	Culture aerobic identify
87081	Culture screen only
87340	Hepatitis b surface ag, eia
G0306	CBC/diff wbc w/o platelet
G0307	CBC without platelet

* Effective January 1, 2016, the lipid panel is no longer considered to be a renal dialysis service. However, if the panel is furnished for the treatment of ESRD it is the responsibility of the ESRD facility and should be reported on the facility's claim.

A. Automated Multi-Channel Chemistry (AMCC) Tests

During the ESRD PPS transition period (see §70 of this chapter) ESRD facilities are required to report the renal dialysis AMCC tests with the appropriate modifiers (CD, CE, or CF) on their claims for purposes of applying the 50/50 rule under the composite rate portion of the blended payment. Refer to §70.B of this chapter for additional information regarding the composite rate portion of the blended payment during the transition.

The 50/50 rule is necessary for those ESRD facilities that chose to go through the transition period. If the 50/50 rule allows for separate payment, then the laboratory tests are priced using the clinical laboratory fee schedule. Information regarding the 50/50 rule can be found in §20.2.E of this chapter and in Pub. 100-04, Medicare Claims Processing Manual, chapter 16, §40.6.

NOTE: An ESRD facility billing a renal dialysis AMCC test must use the CF modifier when the AMCC is not in the composite rate but is a renal dialysis service. AMCC tests that are furnished to individuals for reasons other than for the treatment of ESRD should be billed with the AY modifier to Medicare directly by the entity furnishing the service with the AY modifier.

B. Laboratory Services Furnished for Reasons Other Than for the Treatment of ESRD

1. Independent Laboratory

   A patient's physician or practitioner may order a laboratory test that is included on the list of items and services subject to consolidated billing edits for reasons other than for the treatment of ESRD. When this occurs, the patient's physician or practitioner should notify the independent laboratory or the ESRD facility (with the appropriate clinical laboratory certification in accordance with the Clinical Laboratory Improvement Act) that furnished the laboratory service that the test is not a renal dialysis service and that entity may bill Medicare separately using the AY modifier. The AY modifier serves as an attestation that the item or service is medically necessary for the patient but is not being used for the treatment of ESRD.

2. Hospital-Based Laboratory

   Hospital outpatient clinical laboratories furnishing renal dialysis laboratory tests to ESRD patients for reasons other than for the treatment of ESRD may submit a claim for separate payment using the AY modifier. The AY modifier serves as an attestation that the item or service is medically necessary for the patient but is not being used for the treatment of ESRD.

C. Laboratory Services Performed in Emergency Rooms or Emergency Departments

In an emergency room or emergency department, the ordering physician or practitioner may not know at the time the laboratory test is being ordered, if it is being ordered as a renal dialysis service. Consequently, emergency rooms or emergency departments are not required to append an AY modifier to these laboratory tests when submitting claims with dates of service on or after January 1, 2012.

When a renal dialysis laboratory service is furnished to an ESRD patient in an emergency room or emergency department on a different date of service, hospitals can append an ET modifier to the laboratory tests furnished to ESRD patients to indicate that the laboratory test was furnished in conjunction with the emergency visit. Appending the ET modifier indicates that the laboratory service being furnished on a day other than the emergency visit is related to the emergency visit and at the time the ordering physician was unable to determine if the test was ordered for reasons of treating the patient's ESRD.

Allowing laboratory testing to bypass consolidated billing edits in the emergency room or department does not mean that ESRD facilities should send patients to other settings for routine laboratory testing for the purpose of not assuming financial responsibility of renal dialysis items and services. For additional information regarding laboratory services furnished in a variety of settings, see Pub. 100-04, Medicare Claims Processing Manual, chapter 16, §30.3 and §40.6.

D. Hepatitis B Laboratory Services for Transient Patients

Laboratory testing for hepatitis B is a renal dialysis service. Effective January 1, 2011, hepatitis B testing is included in the ESRD PPS and therefore cannot be billed separately to Medicare.

The Conditions for Coverage for ESRD facilities require routine hepatitis B testing (42 CFR §494.30(a)(1)). The ESRD facility is responsible for the payment of the laboratory test, regardless of frequency. If an ESRD patient wishes to travel, the patient's home ESRD facility should have systems in place for communicating hepatitis B test results to the destination ESRD facility.

E. Laboratory Services Included Under Composite Rate

Prior to the implementation of the ESRD PPS, the costs of certain ESRD laboratory services furnished for outpatient maintenance dialysis by either the ESRD facility's staff or an independent laboratory, were included in the composite rate calculations. Therefore, payment for all of these laboratory tests was included in the ESRD facility's composite rate and the tests could not have been billed separately to the Medicare program.

All laboratory services that were included under the composite rate are included under the ESRD PPS unless otherwise specified. Payments for these laboratory tests are included in the ESRD PPS and are not paid separately under the composite rate portion of the blended payment and are not eligible for outlier payments. Therefore, composite rate laboratory services should not be reported on the claim. Laboratory tests included in the composite payment rate are identified below.

1. Routinely Covered Tests Paid Under Composite Rate

   The tests listed below are usually performed for dialysis patients and were routinely covered at the frequency specified in the absence of indications to the contrary, (i.e., no documentation of medical necessity was required other than knowledge of the patient's status as an ESRD beneficiary). When any of these tests were performed at a frequency greater than that specified, the additional tests were separately billable and were covered only if they were medically justified by accompanying documentation. A diagnosis of ESRD alone was not sufficient medical evidence to warrant coverage of the additional tests. The nature of the illness or injury (diagnosis, complaint, or symptom) requiring the performance of the test(s) must have been present, along with ICD diagnosis coding, on the claim for payment.

   a. Hemodialysis, IPD, CCPD, and Hemofiltration

      - Per Treatment - All hematocrit, hemoglobin, and clotting time tests furnished incident to dialysis treatments;
      - Weekly - Prothrombin time for patients on anticoagulant therapy and Serum Creatinine;
      - Weekly or Thirteen Per Quarter - BUN;
      - Monthly - Serum Calcium, Serum Potassium, Serum Chloride, CBC, Serum Bicarbonate, Serum Phosphorous, Total Protein, Serum Albumin, Alkaline Phosphatase, aspartate amino transferase (AST) (SGOT) and LDH; and
      - Automated Multi-Channel Chemistry (AMCC) - If an automated battery of tests, such as the SMA-12, is performed and contains most of the tests listed in one of the weekly or monthly categories, it is not necessary to separately identify any tests in the battery that are not listed. Further information concerning automated tests and the "50 percent rule" can be found below and in Pub. 100-04, Medicare Claims Processing Manual, chapter 16, §40.6.1.

   b. CAPD

      - Monthly – BUN, Creatinine, Sodium, Potassium, CO2, Calcium, Magnesium, Phosphate, Total Protein, Albumin, Alkaline Phosphatase, LDH, AST, SGOT, HCT, Hbg, and Dialysate Protein.

Under the ESRD PPS, frequency requirements do not apply for the purpose of payment. However, laboratory tests should be ordered as necessary and should not be restricted because of financial reasons.

2. Separately Billable Tests Under the Composite Rate

   The following list identifies certain separately billable laboratory tests that were covered routinely and without documentation of medical necessity other than knowledge of the patient's status as an ESRD beneficiary, when furnished at specified frequencies. If they were performed at a frequency greater than that specified, they were covered only if accompanied by medical documentation. A diagnosis of ESRD alone was not sufficient documentation. The medical necessity of the test(s), the nature of the illness or injury (diagnosis, complaint or symptom)

© 2019 Optum360, LLC

requiring the performance of the test(s) must have been furnished on claims using the ICD diagnosis coding system.

- Separately Billable Tests for Hemodialysis, IPD, CCPD, and Hemofiltration

  Serum Aluminum - one every 3 months

  Serum Ferritin - one every 3 months

- Separately Billable Tests for CAPD

  WBC, RBC, and Platelet count – One every 3 months

  Residual renal function and 24 hour urine volume – One every 6 months

Under the ESRD PPS frequency requirements do not apply for the purpose of payment. However, laboratory tests should be ordered as necessary and should not be restricted because of financial reasons.

3. Automated Multi-Channel Chemistry (AMCC) Tests Under the Composite Rate

   Clinical diagnostic laboratory tests that comprise the AMCC (listed in Appendix A and B) could be considered to be composite rate and non-composite rate laboratory services. Composite rate payment was paid by the A/B MAC (A). To determine if separate payment was allowed for non-composite rate tests for a particular date of service, 50 percent or more of the covered tests must be non-composite rate tests. This policy also applies to the composite rate portion of the blended payment during the transition. Beginning January 1, 2014, the 50 percent rule will no longer apply and no separate payment will be made under the composite rate portion of the blended payment.

   Medicare applied the following to AMCC tests for ESRD beneficiaries:

   - Payment was the lowest rate for services performed by the same provider, for the same beneficiary, for the same date of service.
   - The A/B MAC identified, for a particular date of service, the AMCC tests ordered that were included in the composite rate and those that were not included. The composite rate tests were defined for Hemodialysis, IPD, CCPD, and Hemofiltration (see Appendix A) and for CAPD (see Appendix B).
   - If 50 percent or more of the covered tests were included under the composite rate payment, then all submitted tests were included within the composite payment. In this case, no separate payment in addition to the composite rate was made for any of the separately billable tests.
   - If less than 50 percent of the covered tests were composite rate tests, all AMCC tests submitted for that Date of Service (DOS) were separately payable.
   - A non-composite rate test was defined as any test separately payable outside of the composite rate or beyond the normal frequency covered under the composite rate that was reasonable and necessary.

   Three pricing modifiers identify the different payment situations for ESRD AMCC tests. The physician who ordered the tests was responsible for identifying the appropriate modifier when ordering the tests.

   - CD - AMCC test had been ordered by an ESRD facility or Medicare capitation payment (MCP) physician that was part of the composite rate and was not separately billable
   - CE - AMCC test had been ordered by an ESRD facility or MCP physician that was a composite rate test but was beyond the normal frequency covered under the rate and was separately reimbursable based on medical necessity
   - CF - AMCC test had been ordered by an ESRD facility or MCP physician that was not part of the composite rate and was separately billable

The ESRD clinical diagnostic laboratory tests identified with modifiers "CD", "CE" or "CF" may not have been billed as organ or disease panels. Effective October 1, 2003, all ESRD clinical diagnostic laboratory tests must be billed individually. See Pub. 100-04, Medicare Claims Processing Manual, chapter 16, §40.6.1, for additional billing and payment instructions as well as examples of the 50/50 rule.

For ESRD dialysis patients, CPT code 82330 Calcium; ionized shall be included in the calculation for the 50/50 rule (Pub. 100-04, Medicare Claims Processing Manual, chapter 16, §40.6.1). When CPT code 82330 is billed as a substitute for CPT code 82310, Calcium; total, it shall be billed with modifier CD or CE. When CPT code 82330 is billed in addition to CPT 82310, it shall be billed with CF modifier.

100-02, 12, 30.1

Rules for Payment of CORF Services

(Rev.255, Issued: 01-25-19, Effective: 01- 01- 19, Implementation: 02-26-19)

The payment basis for CORF services is 80 percent of the lesser of: (1) the actual charge for the service or (2) the physician fee schedule amount for the service when the physician fee schedule establishes a payment amount for such service. Payment for CORF services under the physician fee schedule is made for physical therapy, occupational therapy, speech-language pathology and respiratory therapy services, as well as the nursing and social and/or psychological services, which are a part of, or directly relate to, the rehabilitation plan of treatment.

Payment for covered durable medical equipment, orthotic and prosthetic (DMEPOS) devices and supplies provided by a CORF is based upon: the lesser of 80 percent of actual charges or the payment amount established under the DMEPOS fee schedule; or, the single payment amount established under the DMEPOS competitive bidding program, provided that payment for such an item is not included in the payment amount for other CORF services.

If there is no fee schedule amount for a covered CORF item or service, payment should be based on the lesser of 80 percent of the actual charge for the service provided or an amount determined by the local Medicare contractor.

The following conditions apply to CORF physical therapy, occupational therapy, and speech-language pathology services;

- *Claims must contain the required functional reporting. (Reference: Sections 42 CFR 410.105.) Refer to Pub. 100-04, Medicare Claims Processing Manual, chapter 5, section 10.6. NOTE: Functional reporting and documentation requirements are no longer applicable for claims for dates of service on and after January 1, 2019. For more information, refer to subsection F in section 30 above.*
- *The functional reporting on claims must be consistent with the functional limitations identified as part of the patient's therapy plan of care and expressed as part of the patient's therapy goals; effective for claims with dates of service on and after January, 1, 2013. (Reference: 42 CFR 410.105.) See Pub. 100-04, Medicare Claims Processing Manual, chapter 5, section 10.6. NOTE: Functional reporting and documentation requirements are no longer applicable for claims for dates of service on and after January 1, 2019. For more information, refer to subsection F in section 30 above.*
- *The National Provider Identifier (NPI) of the certifying physician identified for a CORF physical therapy, occupational therapy, and speech-language pathology plan of treatment must be included on the therapy claim. This requirement is effective for claims with dates of service on or after October 1, 2012. (See Pub. 100-04, Medicare Claims Processing Manual, chapter 5, section 10.3.)*

Payment for CORF social and/or psychological services is made under the physician fee schedule only for HCPCS code G0409, as appropriate, and only when billed using revenue codes 0560, 0569, 0910, 0911, 0914 and 0919.

Payment for CORF respiratory therapy services is made under the physician fee schedule when provided by a respiratory therapist as defined at 42CFR485.70(j) and, only to the extent that these services support or are an adjunct to the rehabilitation plan of treatment, when billed using revenue codes 0410, 0412 and 0419. Separate payment is not made for diagnostic tests or for services related to physiologic monitoring services which are bundled into other respiratory therapy services appropriately performed by a respiratory therapist, such as HCPCS codes G0237, G0238 and G0239.

Payment for CORF nursing services is made under the physician fee schedule only when provided by a registered nurse as defined at 42CFR485.70(h) for nursing services only to the extent that these services support or are an adjunct to the rehabilitation plan of treatment. In addition, payment for CORF nursing services is made only when provided by a registered nurse. HCPCS code G0128 is used to bill for these services and only with revenue codes 0550 and 0559.

For specific payment requirements for CORF items and services see Pub. 100-04, Medicare Claims Processing Manual, Chapter 5, Part B Outpatient Rehabilitation and CORF/OPT Services.

100-02, 12, 40.5

Respiratory Therapy Services

(Rev.111, Issued: 09-25-09; Effective Date: 07-07-08; Implementation Date: 10-26-09)

A respiratory therapy plan of treatment is wholly established and signed by the referring physician before the respiratory therapist initiates the actual treatment.

A. Definition

Respiratory therapy services include only those services that can be appropriately provided to CORF patients by a qualified respiratory therapist, as defined at 42CFR485.70(j), under a physician-established respiratory therapy plan of treatment. The facility physician must be present in the facility for a sufficient time to provide, in accordance with accepted principles of medical practice, medical direction, medical care services and consultation. Respiratory therapy services include the physiological monitoring necessary to furnish these services. Payment for these services is bundled into the payment for respiratory therapy services and is not payable separately. Diagnostic and other medical services provided in the CORF setting are not considered CORF services, and therefore may not be included in a respiratory therapy plan of treatment because these are covered under separate benefit categories.

 © 2019 Optum360, LLC

The respiratory therapist assesses the patient to determine the appropriateness of pursed lip breathing activity and may check the patient's oxygen saturation level (via pulse oximetry). If appropriate, the respiratory therapist then provides the initial training in order to ensure that the patient can accurately perform the activity. The respiratory therapist may again check the patient's oxygen saturation level, or perform peak respiratory flow, or check other respiratory parameters. These types of services are considered "physiological monitoring" and are bundled into the payment for HCPCS codes G0237, G0238 and G0239. Physiological monitoring also includes the provision of a 6-minute walk test that is typically conducted before the start of the patient's respiratory therapy activities. The time to provide this walk "test" assessment is included as part of the HCPCS code G0238. When provided as part of a CORF respiratory therapy plan of treatment, payment for these monitoring activities is bundled into the payment for other services provided by the respiratory therapist, such as the three respiratory therapy specific G-codes.

B. Guidelines for Applying Coverage Criteria

There are some conditions for which respiratory therapy services may be indicated. However, respiratory therapy performed as part of a standard protocol without regard to the individual patient's actual condition, capacity for improving, and the need for such services as established, is not reasonable and medically necessary. All respiratory therapy services must meet the test of being "reasonable and medically necessary" pursuant to Sec.1862(a)(1)(A) of the Act. Determinations of medical necessity are made based on local contractor decisions on a claim-by-claim basis.

The three HCPCS codes G0237, G0238, and G0239 are specific to services provided under the respiratory therapy plan of treatment and, as such, are not designated as subject to the therapy caps.

C. Patient Education Programs

Instructing a patient in the use of equipment, breathing exercises, etc. may be considered reasonable and necessary to the patient's respiratory therapy plan of treatment and can usually be given to a patient during the course of treatment by the respiratory therapist. These educational instructions are bundled into the covered service and separate payment is not made.

100-02, 12, 40.8

Nursing Services

(Rev.111, Issued: 09-25-09; Effective Date: 07-07-08; Implementation Date: 10-26-09)

CORF nursing services may only be provided by an individual meeting the qualifications of a registered nurse, as defined at 42CFR485.70(h). They must relate to, or be a part of, the rehabilitation plan of treatment.

CORF nursing services must be reasonable and medically necessary and are provided as an adjunct to the rehabilitation plan of treatment. For example, a registered nurse may perform or instruct a patient, as appropriate, in the proper procedure of "in and out" urethral catheterization, tracheostomy tube suctioning, or the cleaning for ileostomy or colostomy bags.

Nursing services may not substitute for or supplant the services of physical therapists, occupational therapists, speech-language pathologists and respiratory therapists, but instead must support or further the services and goals provided in the rehabilitation plan of treatment.

CORF nursing services must be provided by a registered nurse and may only be coded as HCPCS code G0128 indicating that CORF "nursing services" were provided.

100-02, 12, 40.11

Vaccines

(Rev.111, Issued: 09-25-09; Effective Date: 07-07-08; Implementation Date: 10-26-09)

A CORF may provide pneumococcal pneumonia, influenza virus, and hepatitis B vaccines to its patients. While not included as a service under the CORF benefit, Medicare will make payment to the CORF for certain vaccines and their administration provided to CORF patients (CY 2008 PFS Rule 72 FR 66293).

The following three vaccinations are covered in a CORF if a physician who is a doctor of medicine or osteopathy orders it for a CORF patient:

- Pneumococcal pneumonia vaccine and its administration;
- Hepatitis B vaccine and its administration furnished to a beneficiary who is at high or intermediate risk of contracting hepatitis B; and
- Influenza virus vaccine and its administration

Payment for covered pneumococcal pneumonia, influenza virus, and hepatitis B vaccines provided in the CORF setting is based on 95 percent of the average wholesale price. The CORF registered nurse provides administration of any of these vaccines using HCPCS codes G0008, G0009 or G0010 with payment based on CPT code 90471.

100-02, 13, 220

Preventive Health Services

(Rev.230, Issued: 12-09-16, Effective: 03-09-17, Implementation: 03-09-17)

RHCs and FQHCs are paid for the professional component of allowable preventive services when all of the program requirements are met and frequency limits (where applicable) have not been exceeded. The beneficiary copayment and deductible (where applicable) is waived by the Affordable Care Act for the IPPE and AWV, and for Medicare-covered preventive services recommended by the USPSTF with a grade or A or B.

100-02, 13, 220.1

Preventive Health Services in RHCs

(Rev.239, Issued: 01-09-18, Effective: 1-22-18, Implementation: 1-22-18)

Influenza (G0008) and Pneumococcal Vaccines (G0009)

Influenza and pneumococcal vaccines and their administration are paid at 100 percent of reasonable cost through the cost report. No visit is billed, and these costs should not be included on the claim. The beneficiary coinsurance and deductible are waived.

Hepatitis B Vaccine (G0010)

Hepatitis B vaccine and its administration is included in the RHC visit and is not separately billable. The cost of the vaccine and its administration can be included in the line item for the otherwise qualifying visit. A visit cannot be billed if vaccine administration is the only service the RHC provides. The beneficiary coinsurance and deductible are waived.

Initial Preventive Physical Exam (G0402)

The IPPE is a face-to-face one-time exam that must occur within the first 12 months following the beneficiary's enrollment. The IPPE can be billed as a stand-alone visit if it is the only medical service provided on that day with an RHC practitioner. If an IPPE visit is furnished on the same day as another billable visit, two visits may be billed. The beneficiary coinsurance and deductible are waived.

Annual Wellness Visit (G0438 and G0439)

The AWV is a personalized face-to-face prevention visit for beneficiaries who are not within the first 12 months of their first Part B coverage period and have not received an IPPE or AWV within the past12 months. The AWV can be billed as a stand-alone visit if it is the only medical service provided on that day with an RHC practitioner. If the AWV is furnished on the same day as another medical visit, it is not a separately billable visit. The beneficiary coinsurance and deductible are waived.

Diabetes Self-Management Training (G0108) and Medical Nutrition Therapy (97802 and 97803)

Diabetes self-management training or medical nutrition therapy provided by a registered dietician or nutritional professional at an RHC may be considered incident to a visit with an RHC practitioner provided all applicable conditions are met. DSMT and MNT are not billable visits in an RHC, although the cost may be allowable on the cost report. RHCs cannot bill a visit for services furnished by registered dieticians or nutritional professionals. However, RHCs are permitted to become certified providers of DSMT services and report the cost of such services on their cost report for inclusion in the computation of their AIR. The beneficiary coinsurance and deductible apply.

Screening Pelvic and Clinical Breast Examination (G0101)

Screening pelvic and clinical breast examination can be billed as a stand-alone visit if it is the only medical service provided on that day with an RHC practitioner. If it is furnished on the same day as another medical visit, it is not a separately billable visit. The beneficiary coinsurance and deductible are waived.

Screening Papanicolaou Smear (Q0091)

Screening Papanicolaou smear can be billed as a stand-alone visit if it is the only medical service provided on that day with an RHC practitioner. If it is furnished on the same day as another medical visit, it is not a separately billable visit. The beneficiary coinsurance and deductible are waived.

Prostate Cancer Screening (G0102)

Prostate cancer screening can be billed as a stand-alone visit if it is the only medical service provided on that day with an RHC practitioner. If it is furnished on the same day as another medical visit, it is not a separately billable visit. The beneficiary coinsurance and deductible apply.

Glaucoma Screening (G0117 and G0118)

Glaucoma screening for high risk patients can be billed as a stand-alone visit if it is the only medical service provided on that day with an RHC practitioner. If it is furnished on the same day as another medical visit, it is not a separately billable visit. The beneficiary coinsurance and deductible apply.

© 2019 Optum360, LLC

Lung Cancer Screening Using Low Dose Computed Tomography (LDCT) (G0296)

LDCT can be billed as a stand-alone visit if it is the only medical service provided on that day with an RHC practitioner. If it is furnished on the same day as another medical visit, it is not a separately billable visit. The beneficiary coinsurance and deductible are waived.

NOTE: Hepatitis C Screening (GO472) is a technical service only and therefore it is not paid as part of the RHC visit.

100-02, 13, 220.3

Preventive Health Services in FQHCs

(Rev.238 Issued: 11-17-17, Effective: 2-15-18, Implementation: 2-15-18)

FQHCs must provide preventive health services on site or by arrangement with another provider. These services must be furnished by or under the direct supervision of a physician, NP, PA, CNM, CP, or CSW. Section 330(b)(1)(A)(i)(III) of the Public Health Service (PHS) Act required preventive health services can be found at http://bphc.hrsa.gov/policiesregulations/legislation/index.html, and include:

- prenatal and perinatal services;
- appropriate cancer screening;
- well-child services;
- immunizations against vaccine-preventable diseases;
- screenings for elevated blood lead levels, communicable diseases, and cholesterol;
- pediatric eye, ear, and dental screenings to determine the need for vision and hearing correction and dental care;
- voluntary family planning services; and
- preventive dental services.

NOTE: The cost of providing these services may be included in the FQHC cost report but they do not necessarily qualify as FQHC billable visits or for the waiver of the beneficiary coinsurance.

Influenza (G0008) and Pneumococcal Vaccines (G0009)

Influenza and pneumococcal vaccines and their administration are paid at 100 percent of reasonable cost through the cost report. The cost is included in the cost report and no visit is billed. FQHCs must include these charges on the claim if furnished as part of an encounter. The beneficiary coinsurance is waived.

Hepatitis B Vaccine (G0010)

Hepatitis B vaccine and its administration is included in the FQHC visit and is not separately billable. The cost of the vaccine and its administration can be included in the line item for the otherwise qualifying visit. A visit cannot be billed if vaccine administration is the only service the FQHC provides. The beneficiary coinsurance is waived.

Initial Preventive Physical Exam (G0402)

The IPPE is a one-time exam that must occur within the first 12 months following the beneficiary's enrollment. The IPPE can be billed as a stand-alone visit if it is the only medical service provided on that day with a FQHC practitioner. If an IPPE visit is furnished on the same day as another billable visit, FQHCs may not bill for a separate visit. These FQHCs will have an adjustment of 1.3416 to their PPS rate. The beneficiary coinsurance is waived.

Annual Wellness Visit (G0438 and G0439)

The AWV is a personalized prevention plan for beneficiaries who are not within the first 12 months of their first Part B coverage period and have not received an IPPE or AWV within the past12 months. The AWV can be billed as a stand-alone visit if it is the only medical service provided on that day with a FQHC practitioner. If the AWV is furnished on the same day as another medical visit, it is not a separately billable visit. FQHCs that are authorized to bill under the FQHC PPS will have an adjustment of 1.3416 to their PPS rate. The beneficiary coinsurance is waived.

Diabetes Self-Management Training (G0108) and Medical Nutrition Therapy (97802 and 97803)

DSMT and MNT furnished by certified DSMT and MNT providers are billable visits in FQHCs when they are provided in a one-on-one, face-to-face encounter and all program requirements are met. Other diabetes counseling or medical nutrition services provided by a registered dietician at the FQHC may be considered incident to a visit with a FQHC provider. The beneficiary coinsurance is waived for MNT services and is applicable for DSMT.

DSMT must be furnished by a certified DSMT practitioner, and MNT must be furnished by a registered dietitian or nutrition professional. Program requirements for DSMT services are set forth in 42 CFR 410 Subpart H for DSMT and in Part 410, Subpart G for MNT services, and additional guidance can be found at Pub. 100-02, chapter 15, section 300.

Screening Pelvic and Clinical Breast Examination (G0101)

Screening pelvic and clinical breast examination can be billed as a stand-alone visit if it is the only medical service provided on that day with a FQHC practitioner. If it is furnished on the same day as another medical visit, it is not a separately billable visit. The beneficiary coinsurance is waived.

Screening Papanicolaou Smear (Q0091)

Screening Papanicolaou smear can be billed as a stand-alone visit if it is the only medical service provided on that day with a FQHC practitioner. If it is furnished on the same day as another medical visit, it is not a separately billable visit. The beneficiary coinsurance is waived.

Prostate Cancer Screening (G0102)

Prostate cancer screening can be billed as a stand-alone visit if it is the only medical service provided on that day with a FQHC practitioner. If it is furnished on the same day as another medical visit, it is not a separately billable visit. The beneficiary coinsurance applies.

Glaucoma Screening (G0117 and G0118)

Glaucoma screening for high risk patients can be billed as a stand-alone visit if it is the only medical service provided on that day with a FQHC practitioner. If it is furnished on the same day as another medical visit, it is not a separately billable visit. The beneficiary coinsurance applies.

Lung Cancer Screening Using Low Dose Computed Tomography (LDCT) (G0296)

LDCT can be billed as a stand-alone visit if it is the only medical service provided on that day with a FQHC practitioner. If it is furnished on the same day as another medical visit, it is not a separately billable visit. The beneficiary coinsurance is waived.

NOTE: Hepatitis C Screening (GO472) is a technical service only and therefore not paid as part of the FQHC visit.

100-02, 13, 230.2

General Care Management Services – Chronic Care Management and General Behavioral Health Integration Services

(Rev.239, Issued: 01-09-18, Effective: 1-22-18, Implementation: 1-22-18)

Chronic Care Management (CCM)

Effective January 1, 2016, RHCs and FQHCs are paid for CCM services when a minimum of 20 minutes of qualifying CCM services during a calendar month is furnished to patients with multiple chronic conditions that are expected to last at least 12 months or until the death of the patient, and that place the patient at significant risk of death, acute exacerbation/decompensation, or functional decline. For CCM services furnished between January 1, 2016, and December 31, 2017, payment is based on the PFS national average non-facility payment rate when CPT code 99490 is billed alone or with other payable services on an RHC or FQHC claim.

CCM Service Requirements

- Structured recording of patient health information using Certified EHR Technology including demographics, problems, medications, and medication allergies that inform the care plan, care coordination, and ongoing clinical care;
- 24/7 access to physicians or other qualified health care professionals or clinical staff including providing patients/caregivers with a means to make contact with health care professionals in the practice to address urgent needs regardless of the time of day or day of week, and continuity of care with a designated member of the care team with whom the patient is able to schedule successive routine appointments;
- Comprehensive care management including systematic assessment of the patient's medical, functional, and psychosocial needs; system-based approaches to ensure timely receipt of all recommended preventive care services; medication reconciliation with review of adherence and potential interactions; and oversight of patient self-management of medications;
- Comprehensive care plan including the creation, revision, and/or monitoring of an electronic care plan based on a physical, mental, cognitive, psychosocial, functional, and environmental (re)assessment and an inventory of resources and supports; a comprehensive care plan for all health issues with particular focus on the chronic conditions being managed;
- Care plan information made available electronically (including fax) in a timely manner within and outside the RHC or FQHC as appropriate and a copy of the plan of care given to the patient and/or caregiver;
- Management of care transitions between and among health care providers and settings, including referrals to other clinicians; follow-up after an emergency department visit; and follow-up after discharges from hospitals, skilled nursing facilities, or other health care facilities; timely creation and exchange/transmit continuity of care document(s) with other practitioners and providers;

© 2019 Optum360, LLC

- Coordination with home- and community-based clinical service providers, and documentation of communication to and from home- and community-based providers regarding the patient's psychosocial needs and functional deficits in the patient's medical record; and
- Enhanced opportunities for the patient and any caregiver to communicate with the practitioner regarding the patient's care through not only telephone access, but also through the use of secure messaging, Internet, or other asynchronous non-face-to-face consultation methods.

General Behavioral Health Integration (BHI)
General BHI is a team-based, collaborative approach to care that focuses on integrative treatment of patients with primary care and mental or behavioral health conditions. Patients are eligible to receive BHI services if they have one or more new or pre-existing behavioral health or psychiatric conditions being treated by the RHC or FQHC primary care practitioner, including substance use disorders, that, in the clinical judgment of the RHC or FQHC primary care practitioner, warrants BHI services.

General BHI Service Requirements
- An initial assessment and ongoing monitoring using validated clinical rating scales;
- Behavioral health care planning in relation to behavioral/psychiatric health problems, including revision for patients who are not progressing or whose status changes;
- Facilitating and coordinating treatment such as psychotherapy, pharmacotherapy, counseling and/or psychiatric consultation; and
- Continuity of care with a designated member of the care team.

Care Management Payment
Effective January 1, 2018, RHCs and FQHCs are paid for CCM or general BHI services when general care management G code, G0511, is on an RHC or FQHC claim, either alone or with other payable services, for CCM or BHI services furnished on or after January 1, 2018.

A separately billable initiating visit with an RHC or FQHC primary care practitioner (physician, NP, PA, or CNM) is required before care management services can be furnished. This visit can be an E/M, AWV, or IPPE visit, and must occur no more than one-year prior to commencing care management services.

Documentation that the beneficiary has consented to receive CCM or BHI services must be in the beneficiary's medical record before CCM or BHI services are furnished. This should include that the beneficiary has

- Given permission to consult with relevant specialists as needed;
- Been informed that there may be cost-sharing (e.g. deductible and coinsurance in RHCs, and coinsurance in FQHCs) for both in-person and non-face-to-face services that are provided
- Been informed that only one practitioner/facility can furnish and be paid for these services during a calendar month; and
- Been informed that they can stop care management services at any time, effective at the end of the calendar month.

Payment for G0511 is set at the average of the national non-facility PFS payment rate for CPT codes 99490 (30 minutes or more of CCM services), 99487 (60 minutes or more of complex CCM services), and 99484 (20 minutes or more of general behavioral health integration services). This rate is updated annually based on the PFS amounts.

RHCs and FQHCs can bill G0511 when the requirements for either CPT codes 99490, 99487, or 99484 are met. G0511 can be billed alone or in addition to other services furnished during an RHC or FQHC visit. Coinsurance and deductibles are applied as applicable to RHC claims, and coinsurance is applied as applicable to FQHC claims. General Care Management services furnished by auxiliary personnel may be provided under general supervision and the face-to-face requirements are waived.

RHCs and FQHCs may not bill for care management services for a patient if another practitioner or facility has already billed for care management services for the same beneficiary during the same time period. RHCs and FQHCs may not bill for care management and TCM services, or another program that provides additional payment for care management services (outside of the RHC AIR or FQHC PPS payment), for the same beneficiary during the same time period.

100-02, 13, 230.3

Psychiatric Collaborative Care Model (CoCM) Services

(Rev.239, Issued: 01-09-18, Effective: 1-22-18, Implementation: 1-22-18)

Effective January 1, 2018, RHCs and FQHCs are paid for psychiatric CoCM services when psychiatric CoCM G code, G0512, is on an RHC or FQHC claim, either alone or with other payable services. At least 70 minutes in the first calendar month, and at least 60 minutes in subsequent calendar months, of psychiatric CoCM services must have been furnished in order to bill for this service.

Psychiatric CoCM is a specific model of care provided by a primary care team consisting of a primary care provider and a health care manager who work in collaboration with a psychiatric consultant to integrate primary health care services with care management support for patients receiving behavioral health treatment. It includes regular psychiatric inter-specialty consultation with the primary care team, particularly regarding patients whose conditions are not improving. Patients with mental health, behavioral health, or psychiatric conditions, including substance use disorders, who are being treated by an RHC or FQHC practitioner may be eligible for psychiatric CoCM services, as determined by the RHC or FQHC practitioner.

The psychiatric CoCM team must include the RHC or FQHC practitioner, a behavioral health care manager, and a psychiatric consultant. The primary care team regularly reviews the beneficiary's treatment plan and status with the psychiatric consultant and maintains or adjusts treatment, including referral to behavioral health specialty care, as needed.

RHC or FQHC Practitioner Requirements

The RHC or FQHC practitioner is a primary care physician, NP, PA, or CNM who:

- Directs the behavioral health care manager and any other clinical staff;
- Oversees the beneficiary's care, including prescribing medications, providing treatments for medical conditions, and making referrals to specialty care when needed; and
- Remains involved through ongoing oversight, management, collaboration and reassessment.

Behavioral Health Care Manager Requirements
The behavioral health care manager is a designated individual with formal education or specialized training in behavioral health, including social work, nursing, or psychology, and has a minimum of a bachelor's degree in a behavioral health field (such as in clinical social work or psychology), or is a clinician with behavioral health training, including RNs and LPNs. The behavioral health care manager furnishes both face-to-face and non-face-to-face services under the general supervision of the RHC or FQHC practitioner and may be employed by or working under contract to the RHC or FQHC. The behavioral health care manager:

- Provides assessment and care management services, including the administration of validated rating scales;
- Provides behavioral health care planning in relation to behavioral/psychiatric health problems, including revision for patients who are not progressing or whose status changes;
- Provides brief psychosocial interventions;
- Maintains ongoing collaboration with the RHC or FQHC practitioner;
- Maintains a registry that tracks patient follow-up and progress;
- Acts in consultation with the psychiatric consultant;
- Is available to provide services face-to-face with the beneficiary; and
- Has a continuous relationship with the patient and a collaborative, integrated relationship with the rest of the care team.

Psychiatric Consultant Requirements
The psychiatric consultant is a medical professional trained in psychiatry and qualified to prescribe the full range of medications. The psychiatric consultant is not required to be on site or to have direct contact with the patient and does not prescribe medications or furnish treatment to the beneficiary directly. The psychiatric consultant:

- Participates in regular reviews of the clinical status of patients receiving psychiatric CoCM services;
- Advises the RHC or FQHC practitioner regarding diagnosis and options for resolving issues with beneficiary adherence and tolerance of behavioral health treatment; making adjustments to behavioral health treatment for beneficiaries who are not progressing; managing any negative interactions between beneficiaries' behavioral health and medical treatments; and
- Facilitates referral for direct provision of psychiatric care when clinically indicated.

A separately billable initiating visit with an RHC or FQHC primary care practitioner (physician, NP, PA, or CNM) is required before psychiatric CoCM services can be furnished. This visit can be an E/M, AWV, or IPPE visit, and must occur no more than one-year prior to commencing psychiatric CoCM services.

Documentation that the beneficiary has consented to receive psychiatric CoCM services must be in the beneficiary's medical record before CCM or BHI services are furnished. This should include that the beneficiary has

- Given permission to consult with relevant specialists as needed;

© 2019 Optum360, LLC

- Been informed that there may be cost-sharing (e.g. deductible and coinsurance in RHCs, and coinsurance in FQHCs) for both in-person and non-face-to-face services that are provided;
- Been informed that only one practitioner/facility can furnish and be paid for these services during a calendar month; and
- Been informed that they can stop care management services at any time, effective at the end of the calendar month.

RHCs and FQHCs can bill G0512 when the requirements for either initial or subsequent psychiatric CoCM services are met. G0512 can be billed alone or in addition to other services furnished during an RHC or FQHC visit. To prevent duplication of payment, this code can only be billed once per month per beneficiary, and cannot be billed if other care management services are billed for the same time period.

Payment for G0512 is set at the average of the national non-facility PFS payment rate for CPT code 99492 (70 minutes or more of initial psychiatric CoCM services) and CPT code 99493 (60 minutes or more of subsequent psychiatric CoCM services). This rate is updated annually based on the PFS amounts. Coinsurance is applied as applicable to FQHC claims, and coinsurance and deductibles are applied as applicable to RHC claims. Psychiatric CoCM services furnished by auxiliary personnel may be provided under general supervision and the face-to-face requirements are waived.

100-02, 15, 50.4.4.2

Immunizations

(Rev.202, Iss: 12-31-14, Eff: 09-19-14, Imp: 02-02-15)

Vaccinations or inoculations are excluded as immunizations unless they are directly related to the treatment of an injury or direct exposure to a disease or condition, such as anti-rabies treatment, tetanus antitoxin or booster vaccine, botulin antitoxin, antivenin sera, or immune globulin. In the absence of injury or direct exposure, preventive immunization (vaccination or inoculation) against such diseases as smallpox, polio, diphtheria, etc., is not covered. However, pneumococcal, hepatitis B, and influenza virus vaccines are exceptions to this rule. (See items A, B, and C below.) In cases where a vaccination or inoculation is excluded from coverage, related charges are also not covered.

A. Pneumococcal Pneumonia Vaccinations

Effective for services furnished on or after May 1, 1981, the Medicare Part B program covers pneumococcal pneumonia vaccine and its administration when furnished in compliance with any applicable State law by any provider of services or any entity or individual with a supplier number. This includes revaccination of patients at highest risk of pneumococcal infection. Typically, these vaccines are administered once in a lifetime except for persons at highest risk. Effective July 1, 2000, Medicare does not require for coverage purposes that a doctor of medicine or osteopathy order the vaccine. Therefore, the beneficiary may receive the vaccine upon request without a physician's order and without physician supervision.

An initial vaccine may be administered only to persons at high risk (see below) of pneumococcal disease. Revaccination may be administered only to persons at highest risk of serious pneumococcal infection and those likely to have a rapid decline in pneumococcal antibody levels, provided that at least 5 years have [passed since the previous dose of pneumococcal vaccine.

Persons at high risk for whom an initial vaccine may be administered include all people age 65 and older; immunocompetent adults who are at increased risk of pneumococcal disease or its complications because of chronic illness (e.g., cardiovascular disease, pulmonary disease, diabetes mellitus, alcoholism, cirrhosis, or cerebrospinal fluid leaks); and individuals with compromised immune

(e.g., splenic dysfunction or anatomic asplenia, Hodgkin's disease, lymphoma, multiple myeloma, chronic renal failure, HIV infection, nephrotic syndrome, sickle cell disease, or organ transplantation).

Persons at highest risk and those most likely to have rapid declines in antibody levels are those for whom revaccination may be appropriate. This group includes persons with functional or anatomic asplenia (e.g., sickle cell disease, splenectomy), HIV infection, leukemia, lymphoma, Hodgkin's disease, multiple myeloma, generalized malignancy, chronic renal failure, nephrotic syndrome, or other conditions associated with immunosuppression such as organ or bone marrow transplantation, and those receiving immunosuppressive chemotherapy. It is not appropriate for routine revaccination of people age 65 or older that are not at highest risk.

Those administering the vaccine should not require the patient to present an immunization record prior to administering the pneumococcal vaccine, nor should they feel compelled to review the patient's complete medical record if it is not available. Instead, provided that the patient is competent, it is acceptable to rely on the patient's verbal history to determine prior vaccination status. If the patient is uncertain about his or her vaccination history in the past 5 years, the vaccine should be given. However, if the patient is certain he/she was were vaccinated in the last 5 years, the vaccine should not be given. If the patient is certain that the vaccine was given more than 5 years ago, revaccination is covered only if the patient is at high risk.

B. Hepatitis B Vaccine

Effective for services furnished on or after September 1, 1984, P.L. 98-369 provides coverage under Part B for hepatitis B vaccine and its administration, furnished to a Medicare beneficiary who is at high or intermediate risk of contracting hepatitis B. This coverage is effective for services furnished on or after September 1, 1984. High-risk groups currently identified include (see exception below):

- ESRD patients;
- Hemophiliacs who receive Factor VIII or IX concentrates;
- Clients of institutions for the mentally retarded;
- Persons who live in the same household as a Hepatitis B Virus (HBV) carrier;
- Homosexual men; and
- Illicit injectable drug abusers; and
- Persons diagnosed with diabetes mellitus.

Intermediate risk groups currently identified include:

- Staff in institutions for the mentally retarded; and
- Workers in health care professions who have frequent contact with blood or blood-derived body fluids during routine work.

EXCEPTION: Persons in both of the above-listed groups in paragraph B, would not be considered at high or intermediate risk of contracting hepatitis B, however, if there were laboratory evidence positive for antibodies to hepatitis B. (ESRD patients are routinely tested for hepatitis B antibodies as part of their continuing monitoring and therapy.)

For Medicare program purposes, the vaccine may be administered upon the order of a doctor of medicine or osteopathy, by a doctor of medicine or osteopathy, or by home health agencies, skilled nursing facilities, ESRD facilities, hospital outpatient departments, and persons recognized under the incident to physicians' services provision of law.

A charge separate from the ESRD composite rate will be recognized and paid for administration of the vaccine to ESRD patients.

C. Influenza Virus Vaccine

Effective for services furnished on or after May 1, 1993, the Medicare Part B program covers influenza virus vaccine and its administration when furnished in compliance with any applicable State law by any provider of services or any entity or individual with a supplier number. Typically, these vaccines are administered once a flu season. Medicare does not require, for coverage purposes, that a doctor of medicine or osteopathy order the vaccine. Therefore, the beneficiary may receive the vaccine upon request without a physician's order and without physician supervision

100-02, 15, 50.5

Self-Administered Drugs and Biologicals

(Rev.1, 10-01-03)

B3-2049.5 Medicare Part B does not cover drugs that are usually self-administered by the patient unless the statute provides for such coverage. The statute explicitly provides coverage, for blood clotting factors, drugs used in immunosuppressive therapy, erythropoietin for dialysis patients, certain oral anti-cancer drugs and anti-emetics used in certain situations.

100-02, 15, 50.5.4

Oral Anti-Nausea (Anti-Emetic) Drugs

(Rev.185, Issued: 04-15-14, Effective: 05-29-13, Implementation: 07-07-14)

Effective January 1, 1998, Medicare also covers self-administered anti-emetics, which are necessary for the administration and absorption of the anti-neoplastic chemotherapeutic agents when a high likelihood of vomiting exists. The anti-emetic drug is covered as a necessary means for administration of the anti-neoplastic chemotherapeutic agents. Oral drugs prescribed for use with the primary drug, which enhance the anti-neoplastic effect of the primary drug or permit the patient to tolerate the primary anti-neoplastic drug in higher doses for longer periods, are not covered. Self-administered anti-emetics to reduce the side effects of nausea and vomiting brought on by the primary drug are not included beyond the administration necessary to achieve drug absorption.

Section 1861(s)(2) of the Social Security Act extends coverage to oral anti-emetic drugs that are used as full replacement for intravenous dosage forms of a cancer regimen under the following conditions:

- Coverage is provided only for oral drugs approved by the Food and Drug Administration (FDA) for use as anti-emetics;

© 2019 Optum360, LLC

- The oral anti-emetic must either be administered by the treating physician or in accordance with a written order from the physician as part of a cancer chemotherapy regimen;
- Oral anti-emetic drugs administered with a particular chemotherapy treatment must be initiated within two hours of the administration of the chemotherapeutic agent and may be continued for a period not to exceed 48 hours from that time;
- The oral anti-emetic drugs provided must be used as a full therapeutic replacement for the intravenous anti-emetic drugs that would have otherwise been administered at the time of the chemotherapy treatment.

Only drugs pursuant to a physician's order at the time of the chemotherapy treatment qualify for this benefit. The dispensed number of dosage units may not exceed a loading dose administered within two hours of the treatment, plus a supply of additional dosage units not to exceed 48 hours of therapy.

Oral drugs that are not approved by the FDA for use as anti-emetics and which are used by treating physicians adjunctively in a manner incidental to cancer chemotherapy are not covered by this benefit and are not reimbursable within the scope of this benefit.

It is recognized that a limited number of patients will fail on oral anti-emetic drugs. Intravenous anti-emetics may be covered (subject to the rules of medical necessity) when furnished to patients who fail on oral anti-emetic therapy.

More than one oral anti emetic drug may be prescribed and may be covered for concurrent use if needed to fully replace the intravenous drugs that otherwise would be given. See the Medicare National Coverage Determinations Manual, Publication 100-04, Chapter 1, Section 110.18, for detailed coverage criteria.

100-02, 15, 50.6

Coverage of Intravenous Immune Globulin for Treatment of Primary Immune Deficiency Diseases in the Home

(Rev.194, Issued: 09-03-14, Effective: Upon Implementation of ICD-10)

Beginning for dates of service on or after January 1, 2004, The Medicare Prescription Drug, Improvement, and Modernization Act of 2003 provides coverage of intravenous immune globulin (IVIG) for the treatment of primary immune deficiency diseases in the home (ICD-9 diagnosis codes 279.04, 279.05, 279.06, 279.12, and 279.2 or ICD-10-CM codes D80.0, D80.5, D81.0, D81.1, D81.2, D81.6, D81.7, D81.89, D81.9, D82.0, D83.0, D83.2, D83.8, or D83.9 if only an unspecified diagnosis is necessary). The Act defines "intravenous immune globulin" as an approved pooled plasma derivative for the treatment of primary immune deficiency disease. It is covered under this benefit when the patient has a diagnosed primary immune deficiency disease, it is administered in the home of a patient with a diagnosed primary immune deficiency disease, and the physician determines that administration of the derivative in the patient's home is medically appropriate. The benefit does not include coverage for items or services related to the administration of the derivative. For coverage of IVIG under this benefit, it is not necessary for the derivative to be administered through a piece of durable medical equipment.

100-02, 15, 110

Durable Medical Equipment - General

(Rev.1, 10-01-03)
B3-2100, A3-3113, HO-235, HHA-220

Expenses incurred by a beneficiary for the rental or purchases of durable medical equipment (DME) are reimbursable if the following three requirements are met:

- The equipment meets the definition of DME (Sec.110.1);
- The equipment is necessary and reasonable for the treatment of the patient's illness or injury or to improve the functioning of his or her malformed body member (Sec.110.1); and
- The equipment is used in the patient's home. The decision whether to rent or purchase an item of equipment generally resides with the beneficiary, but the decision on how to pay rests with CMS. For some DME, program payment policy calls for lump sum payments and in others for periodic payment. Where covered DME is furnished to a beneficiary by a supplier of services other than a provider of services, the DMERC makes the reimbursement. If a provider of services furnishes the equipment, the intermediary makes the reimbursement. The payment method is identified in the annual fee schedule update furnished by CMS. The CMS issues quarterly updates to a fee schedule file that contains rates by HCPCS code and also identifies the classification of the HCPCS code within the following categories. Category Code Definition IN Inexpensive and Other Routinely Purchased Items FS Frequently Serviced Items CR Capped Rental Items OX Oxygen and Oxygen Equipment OS Ostomy, Tracheostomy & Urological Items SD Surgical Dressings PO Prosthetics & Orthotics SU Supplies TE Transcutaneous Electrical Nerve Stimulators The DMERCs, carriers, and intermediaries, where appropriate, use the CMS files to determine payment rules. See the Medicare Claims Processing Manual, Chapter 20, "Durable Medical Equipment, Surgical Dressings and Casts, Orthotics and Artificial Limbs, and Prosthetic Devices," for a detailed description of payment rules for each classification. Payment may also be made for repairs, maintenance, and delivery of equipment and for expendable and nonreusable items essential to the effective use of the equipment subject to the conditions in Sec.110.2. See the Medicare Benefit Policy Manual, Chapter 11, "End Stage Renal Disease," for hemodialysis equipment and supplies.

100-02, 15, 140

Therapeutic Shoes for Individuals with Diabetes

(Rev.241, Issued: 02-02-18, Effective: 04-01-18, Implementation: 04-02-18)

B3-2134 Coverage of therapeutic shoes (depth or custom-molded) along with inserts for individuals with diabetes is available as of May 1, 1993. These diabetic shoes are covered if the requirements as specified in this section concerning certification and prescription are fulfilled. In addition, this benefit provides for a pair of diabetic shoes even if only one foot suffers from diabetic foot disease. Each shoe is equally equipped so that the affected limb, as well as the remaining limb, is protected. Claims for therapeutic shoes for diabetics are processed by the Durable Medical Equipment Regional Carriers (DMERCs). Therapeutic shoes for diabetics are not DME and are not considered DME nor orthotics, but a separate category of coverage under Medicare Part B. (See Sec.1861(s)(12) and Sec.1833(o) of the Act.)

A. Definitions

The following items may be covered under the diabetic shoe benefit:

1. Custom-Molded Shoes

Custom-molded shoes are shoes that:

- Are constructed over a positive model of the patient's foot;
- Are made from leather or other suitable material of equal quality;
- Have removable inserts that can be altered or replaced as the patient's condition warrants; and
- Have some form of shoe closure.

2. Depth Shoes

Depth shoes are shoes that:

- Have a full length, heel-to-toe filler that, when removed, provides a minimum of 3/16 inch of additional depth used to accommodate custom-molded or customized inserts;
- Are made from leather or other suitable material of equal quality;
- Have some form of shoe closure; and
- Are available in full and half sizes with a minimum of three widths so that the sole is graded to the size and width of the upper portions of the shoes according to the American standard last sizing schedule or its equivalent. (The American standard last sizing schedule is the numerical shoe sizing system used for shoes sold in the United States.)

3. Inserts

Inserts are total contact, multiple density, removable inlays that are directly molded to the patient's foot or a model of the patient's foot or directly carved from a patientspecific, rectified electronic model and that are made of a suitable material with regard to the patient's condition.

B. Coverage

1. Limitations For each individual, coverage of the footwear and inserts is limited to one of the following within one calendar year:
   - No more than one pair of custom-molded shoes (including inserts provided with such shoes) and two additional pairs of inserts; or
   - No more than one pair of depth shoes and three pairs of inserts (not including the noncustomized removable inserts provided with such shoes).
2. Coverage of Diabetic Shoes and Brace
   Orthopedic shoes, as stated in the Medicare Claims Processing Manual, Chapter 20, "Durable Medical Equipment, Surgical Dressings and Casts, Orthotics and Artificial Limbs, and Prosthetic Devices," generally are not covered. This exclusion does not apply to orthopedic shoes that are an integral part of a leg brace. In situations in which an individual qualifies for both diabetic shoes and a leg brace, these items are covered separately. Thus, the diabetic shoes may be covered if the requirements for this section are met, while the brace may be covered if the requirements of Sec.130 are met.
3. Substitution of Modifications for Inserts
   An individual may substitute modification(s) of custom-molded or depth shoes instead of obtaining a pair(s) of inserts in any combination. Payment for the

© 2019 Optum360, LLC

modification(s) may not exceed the limit set for the inserts for which the individual is entitled. The following is a list of the most common shoe modifications available, but it is not meant as an exhaustive list of the modifications available for diabetic shoes:

- Rigid Rocker Bottoms - These are exterior elevations with apex positions for 51 percent to 75 percent distance measured from the back end of the heel. The apex is a narrowed or pointed end of an anatomical structure. The apex must be positioned behind the metatarsal heads and tapered off sharply to the front tip of the sole. Apex height helps to eliminate pressure at the metatarsal heads. Rigidity is ensured by the steel in the shoe. The heel of the shoe tapers off in the back in order to cause the heel to strike in the middle of the heel;
- Roller Bottoms (Sole or Bar) - These are the same as rocker bottoms, but the heel is tapered from the apex to the front tip of the sole;
- Metatarsal Bars- An exterior bar is placed behind the metatarsal heads in order to remove pressure from the metatarsal heads. The bars are of various shapes, heights, and construction depending on the exact purpose;
- Wedges (Posting) - Wedges are either of hind foot, fore foot, or both and may be in the middle or to the side. The function is to shift or transfer weight bearing upon standing or during ambulation to the opposite side for added support, stabilization, equalized weight distribution, or balance; and
- Offset Heels- This is a heel flanged at its base either in the middle, to the side, or a combination, that is then extended upward to the shoe in order to stabilize extreme positions of the hind foot. Other modifications to diabetic shoes include, but are not limited to flared heels, Velcro closures, and inserts for missing toes.

4. Separate Inserts
Inserts may be covered and dispensed independently of diabetic shoes if the supplier of the shoes verifies in writing that the patient has appropriate footwear into which the insert can be placed. This footwear must meet the definitions found above for depth shoes and custom-molded shoes.

C. Certification

The need for diabetic shoes must be certified by a physician who is a doctor of medicine or a doctor of osteopathy and who is responsible for diagnosing and treating the patient's diabetic systemic condition through a comprehensive plan of care. This managing physician must:

- Document in the patient's medical record that the patient has diabetes;
- Certify that the patient is being treated under a comprehensive plan of care for diabetes, and that the patient needs diabetic shoes; and
- Document in the patient's record that the patient has one or more of the following conditions:
  - Peripheral neuropathy with evidence of callus formation;
  - History of pre-ulcerative calluses;
  - History of previous ulceration;
  - Foot deformity;
  - Previous amputation of the foot or part of the foot; or
  - Poor circulation.

D. Prescription

Following certification by the physician managing the patient's systemic diabetic condition, a podiatrist or other qualified physician who is knowledgeable in the fitting of diabetic shoes and inserts may prescribe the particular type of footwear necessary.

E. Furnishing Footwear

The footwear must be fitted and furnished by a podiatrist or other qualified individual such as a pedorthist, an orthotist, or a prosthetist. The certifying physician may not furnish the diabetic shoes unless the certifying physician is the only qualified individual in the area. It is left to the discretion of each carrier to determine the meaning of "in the area."

100-02, 15, 200

Nurse Practitioner (NP) Services

(Rev.75, Issued: 08-17-07, Effective: 11-19-07, Implementation: 11-19-07)

Effective for services rendered after January 1, 1998, any individual who is participating under the Medicare program as a nurse practitioner (NP) for the first time ever, may have his or her professional services covered if he or she meets the qualifications listed below, and he or she is legally authorized to furnish NP services in the State where the services are performed. NPs who were issued billing provider numbers prior to January 1, 1998, may continue to furnish services under the NP benefit.

Payment for NP services is effective on the date of service, that is, on or after January 1, 1998, and payment is made on an assignment-related basis only.

A. Qualifications for NPs

In order to furnish covered NP services, an NP must meet the conditions as follows:

- Be a registered professional nurse who is authorized by the State in which the services are furnished to practice as a nurse practitioner in accordance with State law; and be certified as a nurse practitioner by a recognized national certifying body that has established standards for nurse practitioners; or
- Be a registered professional nurse who is authorized by the State in which the services are furnished to practice as a nurse practitioner by December 31, 2000.

The following organizations are recognized national certifying bodies for NPs at the advanced practice level:

- American Academy of Nurse Practitioners;
- American Nurses Credentialing Center;
- National Certification Corporation for Obstetric, Gynecologic and Neonatal Nursing Specialties;
- Pediatric Nursing Certification Board (previously named the National Certification Board of Pediatric Nurse Practitioners and Nurses);
- Oncology Nurses Certification Corporation;
- AACN Certification Corporation; and
- National Board on Certification of Hospice and Palliative Nurses.

The NPs applying for a Medicare billing number for the first time on or after January 1, 2001, must meet the requirements as follows:

- Be a registered professional nurse who is authorized by the State in which the services are furnished to practice as a nurse practitioner in accordance with State law; and
- Be certified as a nurse practitioner by a recognized national certifying body that has established standards for nurse practitioners.

The NPs applying for a Medicare billing number for the first time on or after January 1, 2003, must meet the requirements as follows:

- Be a registered professional nurse who is authorized by the State in which the services are furnished to practice as a nurse practitioner in accordance with State law;
- Be certified as a nurse practitioner by a recognized national certifying body that has established standards for nurse practitioners; and
- Possess a master's degree in nursing.

B. Covered Services

Coverage is limited to the services an NP is legally authorized to perform in accordance with State law (or State regulatory mechanism established by State law).

1. General

The services of an NP may be covered under Part B if all of the following conditions are met:

- They are the type that are considered physician's services if furnished by a doctor of medicine or osteopathy (MD/DO);
- They are performed by a person who meets the definition of an NP (see subsection A);
- The NP is legally authorized to perform the services in the State in which they are performed;
- They are performed in collaboration with an MD/DO (see subsection D); and
- They are not otherwise precluded from coverage because of one of the statutory exclusions. (See subsection C.2.)

2. Incident To

If covered NP services are furnished, services and supplies furnished incident to the services of the NP may also be covered if they would have been covered when furnished incident to the services of an MD/DO as described in §60.

C. Application of Coverage Rules

1. Types of NP Services That May Be Covered

State law or regulation governing an NP's scope of practice in the State in which the services are performed applies. Consider developing a list of covered services based on the State scope of practice. Examples of the types of services that NP's may furnish include services that traditionally have been reserved to physicians, such as physical examinations, minor surgery, setting casts for simple fractures, interpreting x-rays, and other activities that involve an independent evaluation or treatment of the patient's condition. Also, if authorized under the scope of their State license, NPs may furnish services billed under all levels of evaluation and

 © 2019 Optum360, LLC

management codes and diagnostic tests if furnished in collaboration with a physician.

See §60.2 for coverage of services performed by NPs incident to the services of physicians.

2. Services Otherwise Excluded From Coverage

The NP services may not be covered if they are otherwise excluded from coverage even though an NP may be authorized by State law to perform them. For example, the Medicare law excludes from coverage routine foot care, routine physical checkups, and services that are not reasonable and necessary for the diagnosis or treatment of an illness or injury or to improve the functioning of a malformed body member. Therefore, these services are precluded from coverage even though they may be within an NP's scope of practice under State law.

D. Collaboration

Collaboration is a process in which an NP works with one or more physicians (MD/DO) to deliver health care services, with medical direction and appropriate supervision as required by the law of the State in which the services are furnished. In the absence of State law governing collaboration, collaboration is to be evidenced by NPs documenting their scope of practice and indicating the relationships that they have with physicians to deal with issues outside their scope of practice.

The collaborating physician does not need to be present with the NP when the services are furnished or to make an independent evaluation of each patient who is seen by the NP.

E. Direct Billing and Payment

Direct billing and payment for NP services may be made to the NP.

F. Assignment

Assignment is mandatory.

100-02,15,220.4

(Rev.255, Issued: 01-25-19, Effective: 01- 01- 19, Implementation: 02-26-19)

Functional Reporting

NOTE: In the calendar year (CY) 2019 Physician Fee Schedule (PFS) final rule, CMS-1693-F, after consideration of stakeholder comments for burden reduction, a review of all of the requirements under section 3005(g) of Middle Class Tax Relief and Jobs Creation Act of 2012 (MCTRJCA), and in light of the statutory amendments to section 1833(g) of the Act, via section 50202 of Bipartisan Budget Act of 2018 to repeal the therapy caps, CMS concluded that continued collection of functional reporting data through the same or reduced format would not yield additional information to inform future analyses or to serve as a basis for reforms to the payment system for therapy services. To reduce the burden of reporting for providers of therapy services, the CY 2019 PFS final rule ended the requirements of reporting the functional limitation nonpayable HCPCS G-codes and severity modifiers on claims for therapy services and the associated documentation requirements in medical records, effective for dates of service on and after January 1, 2019. The rule also revised regulation text at 42 CFR 410.59, 410.60, 410.61, 410.62, 410.105, accordingly.

The instructions below apply only to dates of service when the functional reporting requirements were effective, January 1, 2013 through December 31, 2018.

A. Selecting the G-codes to Use in Functional Reporting.

There are 42 functional G-codes, 14 sets of three codes each, for that can be used in identifying the functional limitation being reported. Six of the G-code sets are generally for PT and OT functional limitations and eight sets of G-codes are for SLP functional limitations. (For a list of these codes and descriptors, see Pub. 100-04, Medicare Claims Processing Manual, chapter 5, section 10.6 F.)

Only one functional limitation shall be reported at a time. Consequently, the clinician must select the G-code set for the functional limitation that most closely relates to the primary functional limitation being treated or the one that is the primary reason for treatment. When the beneficiary has more than one functional limitation, the clinician may need to make a determination as to which functional limitation is primary. In these cases, the clinician may choose the functional limitation that is:

- Most clinically relevant to a successful outcome for the beneficiary;
- The one that would yield the quickest and/or greatest functional progress; or
- The one that is the greatest priority for the beneficiary.

In all cases, this primary functional limitation should reflect the predominant limitation that the furnished therapy services are intended to address.

For services typically reported as PT or OT, the clinician reports one of the "Other PT/OT" functional G-codes sets to report when one of the four PT/OT categorical code sets does not describe the beneficiary's functional limitation, as follows:

- beneficiary's functional limitation that is not defined by one of the four categories;
- beneficiary whose therapy services are not intended to treat a functional limitation; or
- beneficiary's functional limitation where an overall, composite, or other score from a functional assessment tool is used and does not clearly represent a functional limitation defined by one of the above four categorical PT/OT code sets.

In addition, the subsequent "Other PT/OT" G-code set is only reported after the primary "Other PT/OT" G-code set has been reported for the beneficiary during the same episode of care.

For services typically reported as SLP services, the clinician uses the "Other SLP" functional G-code to report when the functional limitation being treated is not represented by one of the seven categorical SLP functional measures. In addition, the "Other SLP" G-code set is used to report where an overall, composite, or other score from an assessment tool that does not clearly represent a functional limitation defined by one of the seven categorical SLP measures.

B. Selecting the severity modifiers to use in functional reporting/documenting.

Each G-code requires one of the following severity modifiers. When the clinician reports any of the following a modifier is used to convey the severity of the functional limitation: current status, the goal status and the discharge status.

Modifier	Impairment Limitation Restriction
CH	0 percent impaired, limited or restricted
CI	At least 1 percent but less than 20 percent impaired, limited or restricted
CJ	At least 20 percent but less than 40 percent impaired, limited or restricted
CK	At least 40 percent but less than 60 percent impaired, limited or restricted
CL	At least 60 percent but less than 80 percent impaired, limited or restricted
CM	At least 80 percent but less than 100 percent impaired, limited or restricted
CN	100 percent impaired, limited or restricted

The severity modifier reflects the beneficiary's percentage of functional impairment as determined by the clinician furnishing the therapy services for each functional status: current, goal, or discharge. In selecting the severity modifier, the clinician:

- Uses the severity modifier that reflects the score from a functional assessment tool or other performance measurement instrument, as appropriate.
- Uses his/her clinical judgment to combine the results of multiple measurement tools used during the evaluative process to inform clinical decision making to determine a functional limitation percentage.
- Uses his/her clinical judgment in the assignment of the appropriate modifier.
- Uses the CH modifier to reflect a zero percent impairment when the therapy services being furnished are not intended to treat (or address) a functional limitation.

In some cases the modifier will be the same for current status and goal status. For example: where improvement is expected but it is not expected to be enough to move to another modifier, such as from 10 percent to 15 percent, the same severity modifier would be used in reporting the current and goal status. Also, when the clinician does not expect improvement, such as for individuals receiving maintenance therapy, the modifier used for projected goal status will be the same as the one for current status. In these cases, the discharge status may also include the same modifier.

Therapists must document in the medical record how they made the modifier selection so that the same process can be followed at succeeding assessment intervals.

C. Documentation of G-code and Severity Modifier Selection.

Documentation of the nonpayable G-codes and severity modifiers regarding functional limitations reported on claims must be included in the patient's medical record of therapy services for each required reporting. (See Pub. 100-04, Medicare Claims Processing Manual, chapter 5, section 10.6 for details about the functional reporting requirements on claims for therapy services, including PT, OT, and SLP services furnished in CORFs.)

Documentation of functional reporting in the medical record of therapy services must be completed by the clinician furnishing the therapy services:

- The qualified therapist furnishing the therapy services
- The physician/NPP personally furnishing the therapy services

- The qualified therapist furnishing services incident to the physician/NPP
- The physician/NPP for incident to services furnished by qualified personnel, who are not qualified therapists.

The qualified therapist furnishing the PT, OT, or SLP services in a CORF

100-02, 15, 232

Cardiac Rehabilitation (CR) and Intensive Cardiac Rehabilitation (ICR) Services Furnished On or After January 1, 2010

(Rev.75, Issued: 08-17-07, Effective: 11-19-07, Implementation: 11-19-07)

Cardiac rehabilitation (CR) services mean a physician-supervised program that furnishes physician prescribed exercise, cardiac risk factor modification, including education, counseling, and behavioral intervention; psychosocial assessment, outcomes assessment, and other items/services as determined by the Secretary under certain conditions. Intensive cardiac rehabilitation (ICR) services mean a physician-supervised program that furnishes the same items/services under the same conditions as a CR program but must also demonstrate, as shown in peer-reviewed published research, that it improves patients' cardiovascular disease through specific outcome measurements described in 42 CFR 410.49(c). Effective January 1, 2010, Medicare Part B pays for CR/ICR programs and related items/services if specific criteria is met by the Medicare beneficiary, the CR/ICR program itself, the setting in which is it administered, and the physician administering the program, as outlined below:

Effective February 9, 2018, section 51004 of the Bipartisan Budget Act (BBA) of 2018, Pub. L. No. 115-123 (2018), amended section 1861(eee)(4)(B) of the Social Security Act to expand coverage in an intensive cardiac rehabilitation program to additional conditions:

- *Stable, chronic heart failure defined as patients with left ventricular ejection fraction of 35% or less and New York Heart Association (NYHA) class II to IV symptoms despite being on optimal heart failure therapy for at least 6 weeks; or*
- *Any additional condition for which the Secretary has determined that a cardiac rehabilitation program shall be covered, unless the Secretary determines, using the same process used to determine that the condition is covered for a cardiac rehabilitation program, that such coverage is not supported by the clinical evidence.*

***NOTE**: CMS plans to amend our intensive cardiac rehabilitation regulations specified at 42 CFR 410.49 to reflect this expanded coverage. CMS anticipates that the changes will be included in the 2020 Medicare Physician Fee Schedule notice of proposed rulemaking. However, because the expanded coverage under the statutory change was effective on enactment, expanded coverage for these conditions will be made effective for services furnished on or after February 9, 2018.*

CR/ICR Program Beneficiary Requirements:

- Medicare covers CR/ICR program services for beneficiaries who have experienced one or more of the following:
- Acute myocardial infarction within the preceding 12 months;
- Coronary artery bypass surgery;
- Current stable angina pectoris;
- Heart valve repair or replacement;
- Percutaneous transluminal coronary angioplasty (PTCA) or coronary stenting;
- Heart or heart-lung transplant.

For cardiac rehabilitation only: Stable, chronic heart failure defined as patients with left ventricular ejection fraction of 35% or less and New York Heart Association (NYHA) class II to IV symptoms despite being on optimal heart failure therapy for at least 6 weeks. (Effective February 18, 2014.)

CR/ICR Program Component Requirements:

Physician-prescribed exercise. This physical activity includes aerobic exercise combined with other types of exercise (i.e., strengthening, stretching) as determined to be appropriate for individual patients by a physician each day CR/ICR items/services are furnished.

Cardiac risk factor modification. This includes education, counseling, and behavioral intervention, tailored to the patients' individual needs.

Psychosocial assessment. This assessment means an evaluation of an individual's mental and emotional functioning as it relates to the individual's rehabilitation. It should include: (1) an assessment of those aspects of the individual's family and home situation that affects the individual's rehabilitation treatment, and, (2) a psychosocial evaluation of the individual's response to, and rate of progress under, the treatment plan.

Outcomes assessment. These should include: (i) minimally, assessments from the commencement and conclusion of CR/ICR, based on patient-centered outcomes which must be measured by the physician immediately at the beginning and end of the program, and, (ii) objective clinical measures of the effectiveness of the CR/ICR program for the individual patient, including exercise performance and self-reported measures of exertion and behavior.

Individualized treatment plan. This plan should be written and tailored to each individual patient and include (i) a description of the individual's diagnosis; (ii) the type, amount, frequency, and duration of the CR/ICR items/services furnished; and (iii) the goals set for the individual under the plan. The individualized treatment plan must be established, reviewed, and signed by a physician every 30 days.

As specified at 42 CFR 410.49(f)(1), CR sessions are limited to a maximum of 2 1-hour sessions per day for up to 36 sessions over up to 36 weeks with the option for an additional 36 sessions over an extended period of time if approved by the contractor under section 1862(a)(1)(A) of the Act. ICR sessions are limited to 72 1-hour sessions (as defined in section 1848(b)(5) of the Act), up to 6 sessions per day, over a period of up to 18 weeks.

CR/ICR Program Setting Requirements:

CR/ICR services must be furnished in a physician's office or a hospital outpatient setting (for ICR, the hospital outpatient setting must provide ICR using an approved ICR program). All settings must have a physician immediately available and accessible for medical consultations and emergencies at all times when items/services are being furnished under the program. This provision is satisfied if the physician meets the requirements for direct supervision of physician office services as specified at 42 CFR 410.26, and for hospital outpatient services as specified at 42 CFR 410.27.

ICR Program Approval Requirements:

All prospective ICR programs must be approved through the national coverage determination (NCD) process. To be approved as an ICR program, it must demonstrate through peer-reviewed, published research that it has accomplished one or more of the following for its patients: (i) positively affected the progression of coronary heart disease, (ii) reduced the need for coronary bypass surgery, or, (iii) reduced the need for percutaneous coronary interventions.

An ICR program must also demonstrate through peer-reviewed, published research that it accomplished a statistically significant reduction in five or more of the following measures for patients from their levels before CR services to after CR services: (i) low density lipoprotein, (ii) triglycerides, (iii) body mass index, (iv) systolic blood pressure, (v) diastolic blood pressure, and (vi) the need for cholesterol, blood pressure, and diabetes medications.

A list of approved ICR programs, identified through the NCD process, will be posted to the CMS Web site and listed in the Federal Register.

Once an ICR program is approved through the NCD process, all prospective ICR sites wishing to furnish ICR items/services via an approved ICR program may enroll with their local contractor to become an ICR program supplier using the designated forms as specified at 42 CFR 424.510, and report specialty code 31 to be identified as an enrolled ICR supplier. For purposes of appealing an adverse determination concerning site approval, an ICR site is considered a supplier (or prospective supplier) as defined in 42 CFR 498.2.

CR/ICR Program Physician Requirements:

Physicians responsible for CR/ICR programs are identified as medical directors who oversee or supervise the CR/ICR program at a particular site. The medical director, in consultation with staff, is involved in directing the progress of individuals in the program. The medical director, as well as physicians acting as the supervising physician, must possess all of the following: (1) expertise in the management of individuals with cardiac pathophysiology, (2) cardiopulmonary training in basic life support or advanced cardiac life support, and (3) licensed to practice medicine in the state in which the CR/ICR program is offered. Direct physician supervision may be provided by a supervising physician or the medical director.

(See Pub. 100-03, Medicare National Coverage Determinations Manual, Chapter 1, Part 1, section 20.10.1, Pub. 100-04, Medicare Claims Processing Manual, Chapter 32, section 140, Pub. 100-08, Medicare Program Integrity Manual, Chapter 15, section 15.4.2.8, for specific claims processing, coding, and billing requirements for CR/ICR program services.)

100-02, 15, 280.1

Glaucoma Screening

(Rev.194, Issued: 09-03-14, Effective: Upon Implementation of ICD-10)

A. Conditions of Coverage

The regulations implementing the Benefits Improvements and Protection Act of 2000, Sec.102, provide for annual coverage for glaucoma screening for beneficiaries in the following high risk categories:

- Individuals with diabetes mellitus;
- Individuals with a family history of glaucoma; or
- African-Americans age 50 and over.

© 2019 Optum360, LLC

In addition, beginning with dates of service on or after January 1, 2006, 42 CFR 410.23(a)(2), revised, the definition of an eligible beneficiary in a high-risk category is expanded to include:

- Hispanic-Americans age 65 and over.

Medicare will pay for glaucoma screening examinations where they are furnished by or under the direct supervision in the office setting of an ophthalmologist or optometrist, who is legally authorized to perform the services under State law. Screening for glaucoma is defined to include:

- A dilated eye examination with an intraocular pressure measurement; and
- A direct ophthalmoscopy examination, or a slit-lamp biomicroscopic examination.

Payment may be made for a glaucoma screening examination that is performed on an eligible beneficiary after at least 11 months have passed following the month in which the last covered glaucoma screening examination was performed.

The following HCPCS codes apply for glaucoma screening:

G0117 Glaucoma screening for high-risk patients furnished by an optometrist or ophthalmologist; and

G0118 Glaucoma screening for high-risk patients furnished under the direct supervision of an optometrist or ophthalmologist.

The type of service for the above G codes is: TOS Q.

For providers who bill intermediaries, applicable types of bill for screening glaucoma services are 13X, 22X, 23X, 71X, 73X, 75X, and 85X. The following revenue codes should be reported when billing for screening glaucoma services:

- Comprehensive outpatient rehabilitation facilities (CORFs), critical access hospitals (CAHs), skilled nursing facilities (SNFs), independent and provider-based RHCs and free standing and provider-based FQHCs bill for this service under revenue code 770. CAHs electing the optional method of payment for outpatient services report this service under revenue codes 96X, 97X, or 98X.
- Hospital outpatient departments bill for this service under any valid/appropriate revenue code. They are not required to report revenue code 770.

B. Calculating the Frequency

Once a beneficiary has received a covered glaucoma screening procedure, the beneficiary may receive another procedure after 11 full months have passed. To determine the 11-month period, start the count beginning with the month after the month in which the previous covered screening procedure was performed.

C. Diagnosis Coding Requirements

Providers bill glaucoma screening using screening ("V") code V80.1 (Special Screening for Neurological, Eye, and Ear Diseases, Glaucoma). Claims submitted without a screening diagnosis code may be returned to the provider as unprocessable.

D. Payment Methodology

1. Carriers
   Contractors pay for glaucoma screening based on the Medicare physician fee schedule. Deductible and coinsurance apply. Claims from physicians or other providers where assignment was not taken are subject to the Medicare limiting charge (refer to the Medicare Claims Processing Manual, Chapter 12, "Physician/Non-physician Practitioners," for more information about the Medicare limiting charge).
2. Intermediaries
   Payment is made for the facility expense as follows:
   - Independent and provider-based RHC/free standing and provider-based FQHC - payment is made under the all inclusive rate for the screening glaucoma service based on the visit furnished to the RHC/FQHC patient;
   - CAH - payment is made on a reasonable cost basis unless the CAH has elected the optional method of payment for outpatient services in which case, procedures outlined in the Medicare Claims Processing Manual, Chapter 3, Sec.30.1.1, should be followed;
   - CORF - payment is made under the Medicare physician fee schedule;
   - Hospital outpatient department - payment is made under outpatient prospective payment system (OPPS);
   - Hospital inpatient Part B - payment is made under OPPS;
   - SNF outpatient - payment is made under the Medicare physician fee schedule (MPFS); and
   - SNF inpatient Part B - payment is made under MPFS.

   Deductible and coinsurance apply.

E. Special Billing Instructions for RHCs and FQHCs

Screening glaucoma services are considered RHC/FQHC services. RHCs and FQHCs bill the contractor under bill type 71X or 73X along with revenue code 770 and HCPCS codes G0117 or G0118 and RHC/FQHC revenue code 520 or 521 to report the related visit. Reporting of revenue code 770 and HCPCS codes G0117 and G0118 in addition to revenue code 520 or 521 is required for this service in order for CWF to perform frequency editing.

Payment should not be made for a screening glaucoma service unless the claim also contains a visit code for the service. Therefore, the contractor installs an edit in its system to assure payment is not made for revenue code 770 unless the claim also contains a visit revenue code (520 or 521).

100-02, 15, 280.2.2

Coverage Criteria

(Rev.196, Issued: 10-17-14, Effective: 01-27-14, Implementation: 11-18-14)

The following are the coverage criteria for these screenings:

A. Screening Fecal-Occult Blood Tests (FOBT) (Codes G0107 & G0328)

Effective for services furnished on or after January 1, 2004, one screening FOBT (code G0107 or G0328) is covered for beneficiaries who have attained age 50, at a frequency of once every 12 months (i.e., at least 11 months have passed following the month in which the last covered screening FOBT was done). Screening FOBT means: (1) a guaiac-based test for peroxidase activity in which the beneficiary completes it by taking samples from two different sites of three consecutive stools or, (2) an immunoassay (or immunochemical) test for antibody activity in which the beneficiary completes the test by taking the appropriate number of samples according to the specific manufacturer's

instructions. This expanded coverage is in accordance with revised regulations at 42 CFR 410.37(a)(2) that includes " other tests determined by the Secretary through a national coverage determination." This screening requires a written order from the beneficiary's attending physician or for claims with dates of service on or after January 27, 2014, from the beneficiary's attending physician assistant, nurse practitioner, or clinical nurse specialist. (The term "attending physician" is defined to mean a doctor of medicine or osteopathy (as defined in §1861(r)(1) of the Act) who is fully knowledgeable about the beneficiary's medical condition, and who would be responsible for using the results of any examination performed in the overall management of the beneficiary's specific medical problem.)

NOTE: For claims with dates of service prior to January 1, 2007, physicians, suppliers, and providers report HCPCS code G0107. Effective January 1, 2007, code G0107, is discontinued and replaced with CPT code 82270. For complete claims processing information refer to Pub. 100-04, Medicare Claims Processing Manual, chapter 18, section 60.

B. Screening Flexible Sigmoidoscopies (code G0104)

For claims with dates of service on or after January 1, 2002, A/B MACs (B) pay for screening flexible sigmoidoscopies (Code G0104) for beneficiaries who have attained age 50 when these services were performed by a doctor of medicine or osteopathy, or by a physician assistant, nurse practitioner, or clinical nurse specialist (as defined in §1861(aa)(5) of the Act and at 42 CFR 410.74, 410.75, and 410.76) at the frequencies noted below. For claims with dates of service prior to January 1, 2002, pay for these services under the conditions noted only when they are performed by a doctor of medicine or osteopathy.

For services furnished from January 1, 1998, through June 30, 2001, inclusive

Once every 48 months (i.e., at least 47 months have passed following the month in which the last covered screening flexible sigmoidoscopy was done).

For services furnished on or after July 1, 2001

Once every 48 months as calculated above unless the beneficiary does not meet the criteria for high risk of developing colorectal cancer (refer to §280.2.3) and the beneficiary has had a screening colonoscopy (code G0121) within the preceding 10 years. If such a beneficiary has had a screening colonoscopy within the preceding 10 years, then he or she can have covered a screening flexible sigmoidoscopy only after at least 119 months have passed following the month that he/she received the screening colonoscopy (code G0121).

NOTE: If during the course of a screening flexible sigmoidoscopy a lesion or growth is detected which results in a biopsy or removal of the growth, the appropriate diagnostic

procedure classified as a flexible sigmoidoscopy with biopsy or removal should be billed and paid rather than code G0104.

© 2019 Optum360, LLC

C. Screening Colonoscopies for Beneficiaries at High Risk of Developing Colorectal Cancer (Code G0105)

The A/B MAC (B) must pay for screening colonoscopies (code G0105) when performed by a doctor of medicine or osteopathy at a frequency of once every 24 months for beneficiaries at high risk for developing colorectal cancer (i.e., at least 23 months have passed following the month in which the last covered G0105 screening colonoscopy was performed). Refer to §280.2.3 for the criteria to use in determining whether or not an individual is at high risk for developing colorectal cancer.

NOTE: If during the course of the screening colonoscopy, a lesion or growth is detected which results in a biopsy or removal of the growth, the appropriate diagnostic procedure classified as a colonoscopy with biopsy or removal should be billed and paid rather than code G0105.

D. Screening Colonoscopies Performed on Individuals Not Meeting the Criteria for Being at High-Risk for Developing Colorectal Cancer (Code G0121)

Effective for services furnished on or after July 1, 2001, screening colonoscopies (code G0121) are covered when performed under the following conditions:

1. On individuals not meeting the criteria for being at high risk for developing colorectal cancer (refer to §280.2.3);
2. At a frequency of once every 10 years (i.e., at least 119 months have passed following the month in which the last covered G0121 screening colonoscopy was performed); and
3. If the individual would otherwise qualify to have covered a G0121 screening colonoscopy based on the above (see §§280.2.2.D.1 and 2) but has had a covered screening flexible sigmoidoscopy (code G0104), then the individual may have a covered G0121 screening colonoscopy only after at least 47 months have passed following the month in which the last covered G0104 flexible sigmoidoscopy was performed.

NOTE: I f during the course of the screening colonoscopy, a lesion or growth is detected which results in a biopsy or removal of the growth, the appropriate diagnostic procedure classified as a colonoscopy with biopsy or removal should be billed and paid rather than code G0121.

E. Screening Barium Enema Examinations (codes G0106 and G0120)

Screening barium enema examinations are covered as an alternative to either a screening sigmoidoscopy (code G0104) or a screening colonoscopy (code G0105) examination. The same frequency parameters for screening sigmoidoscopies and screening colonoscopies above apply.

In the case of an individual aged 50 or over, payment may be made for a screening barium enema examination (code G0106) performed after at least 47 months have passed following the month in which the last screening barium enema or screening flexible sigmoidoscopy was performed. For example, the beneficiary received a screening barium enema examination as an alternative to a screening flexible sigmoidoscopy in January 1999. The count starts beginning February 1999. The beneficiary is eligible for another screening barium enema in January 2003.

In the case of an individual who is at high risk for colorectal cancer, payment may be made for a screening barium enema examination (code G0120) performed after at least 23 months have passed following the month in which the last screening barium enema or the last screening colonoscopy was performed. For example, a beneficiary at high risk for developing colorectal cancer received a screening barium enema examination (code G0120) as an alternative to a screening colonoscopy (code G0105) in January 2000. The count starts beginning February 2000. The beneficiary is eligible for another screening barium enema examination (code G0120) in January 2002.

The screening barium enema must be ordered in writing after a determination that the test is the appropriate screening test. Generally, it is expected that this will be a screening double contrast enema unless the individual is unable to withstand such an exam. This means that in the case of a particular individual, the attending physician must determine that the estimated screening potential for the barium enema is equal to or greater than the screening potential that has been estimated for a screening flexible sigmoidoscopy, or for a screening colonoscopy, as appropriate, for the same individual. The screening single contrast barium enema also requires a written order from the beneficiary's attending physician in the same manner as described above for the screening double contrast barium enema examination.

100-02, 15, 280.4

Screening Pap Smears

(Rev.194, Issued: 09-03-14, Effective: Upon Implementation of ICD-10)

Effective, January 1, 1998, §4102 of the Balanced Budget Act (BBA) of 1997 (P.L. 105-33) amended §1861(nn) of the Act (42 USC 1395X(nn)) to include coverage every 3 years for a screening Pap smear or more frequent coverage for women:

1. At high risk for cervical or vaginal cancer; or

2. Of childbearing age who have had a Pap smear during any of the preceding 3 years indicating the presence of cervical or vaginal cancer or other abnormality.

Effective July 1, 2001, the Consolidated Appropriations Act of 2001 (P.L. 106-554) modifies §1861(nn) to provide Medicare coverage for biennial screening Pap smears. Specifications for frequency limitations are defined below.

For claims with dates of service from January 1, 1998, through June 30, 2001, screening Pap smears are covered when ordered and collected by a doctor of medicine or osteopathy (as defined in §1861(r)(1) of the Act), or other authorized practitioner (e.g., a certified nurse midwife, physician assistant, nurse practitioner, or clinical nurse specialist, who is authorized under State law to perform the examination) under one of the following conditions.

The beneficiary has not had a screening Pap smear test during the preceding 3 years (i.e., 35 months have passed following the month that the woman had the last covered Pap smear – ICD-9-CM code V76.2 or ICD-10 code Z112.4 is used to indicate special screening for malignant neoplasm, cervix); or

There is evidence (on the basis of her medical history or other findings) that she is of childbearing age and has had an examination that indicated the presence of cervical or vaginal cancer or other abnormalities during any of the preceding 3 years; and at least 11 months have passed following the month that the last covered Pap smear was performed; or

She is at high risk of developing cervical or vaginal cancer – ICD-9-CM code V15.89, other specified personal history presenting hazards to health) or as applicable, ICD-10 code Z77.21, Z77.22, Z77.9, Z91.89, OR Z92.89 and at least 11 months have passed following the month that the last covered screening Pap smear was performed. The high risk factors for cervical and vaginal cancer are:

Cervical Cancer High Risk Factors

- Early onset of sexual activity (under 16 years of age);
- Multiple sexual partners (five or more in a lifetime);
- History of a sexually transmitted disease (including HIV infection); and
- Fewer than three negative or any Pap smears within the previous 7 years.

Vaginal Cancer High Risk Factors

- The DES (diethylstilbestrol) - exposed daughters of women who took DES during pregnancy.

The term "woman of childbearing age" means a woman who is premenopausal, and has been determined by a physician, or qualified practitioner, to be of childbearing age, based on her medical history or other findings. Payment is not made for a screening Pap smear for women at high risk or who qualify for coverage under the childbearing provision more frequently than once every 11 months after the month that the last screening Pap smear covered by Medicare was performed.

B. For Claims with Dates of Service on or After July 1, 2001

When the beneficiary does not qualify for a more frequently performed screening Pap smear as noted in items 1 and 2 above, contractors pay for the screening Pap smear only after at least 23 months have passed following the month during which the beneficiary received her last covered screening Pap smear. All other coverage and payment requirements remain the same.

See the Medicare Claims Processing Manual, Chapter 18, "Preventive and Screening Services," for billing procedures.

100-02, 15, 280.5

Annual Wellness Visit (AWV) Providing Personalized Prevention Plan Services (PPPS)

(Rev.170, Issued: 05-10-13, Effective: 01-01-12, Medicare Coverage of the Annual Wellness Visit (AWV))

A. General

Pursuant to section 4103 of the Affordable Care Act of 2010 (the ACA), the Centers for Medicare & Medicaid Services (CMS) amended section 411.15(a)(1) and 411.15(k)(15) of the Code of Federal Regulations (CFR)(list of examples of routine physical examinations excluded from coverage), effective for services furnished on or after January 1, 2011. This expanded coverage, as established at 42 CFR 410.15, is subject to certain eligibility and other limitations that allow payment for an annual wellness visit (AWV), providing personalized prevention plan services (PPPS), when performed by a qualified health professional (as defined in this section), for an individual who is no longer within 12 months after the effective date of his/her first Medicare Part B coverage period, and has not received either an initial preventive physical examination (IPPE) or an AWV within the past 12 months. Medicare coinsurance and Part B deductibles do not apply.

The AWV will include the establishment of, or update to, the individual's medical/family history, measurement of his/her height, weight, body-mass index (BMI) or waist circumference, and blood pressure (BP), with the goal of health

 © 2019 Optum360, LLC

promotion and disease detection and encouraging patients to obtain the screening and preventive services that may already be covered and paid for under Medicare Part B. Definitions relative to the AWV are included below.

Coverage is available for an AWV that meets the following requirements:

1. It is performed by a health professional; and,
2. It is furnished to an eligible beneficiary who is no longer within 12 months after the effective date of his/her first Medicare Part B coverage period, and he/she has not received either an IPPE or an AWV providing PPPS within the past 12 months.

Sections 4103 and 4104 of the ACA also provide for a waiver of the Medicare coinsurance and Part B deductible requirements for an AWV effective for services furnished on or after January 1, 2011.

B. Definitions Relative to the AWV:

Detection of any cognitive impairment: The assessment of an individual's cognitive function by direct observation, with due consideration of information obtained by way of patient reports, concerns raised by family members, friends, caretakers, or others.

Eligible beneficiary: An individual who is no longer within 12 months after the effective date of his/her first Medicare Part B coverage period and who has not received either an IPPE or an AWV providing PPPS within the past 12 months.

Establishment of, or an update to, the individual's medical/family history: At a minimum, the collection and documentation of the following:

a. Past medical and surgical history, including experiences with illnesses, hospital stays, operations, allergies, injuries, and treatments.

b. Use or exposure to medications and supplements, including calcium and vitamins.

c. Medical events in the beneficiary's parents and any siblings and children, including diseases that may be hereditary or place the individual at increased risk.

First AWV providing PPPS: The provision of the following services to an eligible beneficiary by a health professional that include, and take into account the results of, a health risk assessment as those terms are defined in this section:

a. Review (and administration if needed) of a health risk assessment (as defined in this section).

b. Establishment of an individual's medical/family history.

c. Establishment of a list of current providers and suppliers that are regularly involved in providing medical care to the individual.

d. Measurement of an individual's height, weight, BMI (or waist circumference, if appropriate), BP, and other routine measurements as deemed appropriate, based on the beneficiary's medical/family history.

e. Detection of any cognitive impairment that the individual may have as defined in this section.

f. Review of the individual's potential (risk factors) for depression, including current or past experiences with depression or other mood disorders, based on the use of an appropriate screening instrument for persons without a current diagnosis of depression, which the health professional may select from various available standardized screening tests designed for this purpose and recognized by national medical professional organizations.

g. Review of the individual's functional ability and level of safety based on direct observation, or the use of appropriate screening questions or a screening questionnaire, which the health professional may select from various available screening questions or standardized questionnaires designed for this purpose and recognized by national professional medical organizations.

h. Establishment of the following:

(1) A written screening schedule for the individual, such as a checklist for the next 5 to 10 years, as appropriate, based on recommendations of the United States Preventive Services Task Force (USPSTF) and the Advisory Committee on Immunization Practices (ACIP), and the individual's health risk assessment (as that term is defined in this section), the individual's health status, screening history, and age-appropriate preventive services covered by Medicare.

(2) A list of risk factors and conditions for which primary, secondary, or tertiary interventions are recommended or are underway for the individual, including any mental health conditions or any such risk factors or conditions that have been identified through an IPPE, and a list of treatment options and their associated risks and benefits.

i. Furnishing of personalized health advice to the individual and a referral, as appropriate, to health education or preventive counseling services or programs aimed at reducing identified risk factors and improving self-management, or community-based lifestyle interventions to reduce health risks and promote self-management and wellness, including weight loss, physical activity, smoking cessation, fall prevention, and nutrition.

j. Any other element determined appropriate through the National Coverage Determination (NCD) process.

Health professional:

a. A physician who is a doctor of medicine or osteopathy (as defined in section 1861(r)(1) of the Social Security Act (the Act); or,

b. A physician assistant, nurse practitioner, or clinical nurse specialist (as defined in section 1861(aa)(5) of the Act); or,

c. A medical professional (including a health educator, registered dietitian, or nutrition professional or other licensed practitioner) or a team of such medical professionals, working under the direct supervision (as defined in 42CFR 410.32(b)(3)(ii)) of a physician as defined in this section.

Health Risk Assessment means, for the purposes of the annual wellness visit, an evaluation tool that meets the following criteria:

a. collects self-reported information about the beneficiary.

b. can be administered independently by the beneficiary or administered by a health professional prior to or as part of the AWV encounter.

c. is appropriately tailored to and takes into account the communication needs of underserved populations, persons with limited English proficiency, and persons with health literacy needs.

d. takes no more than 20 minutes to complete.

e. addresses, at a minimum, the following topics:

1. demographic data, including but not limited to age, gender, race, and ethnicity.
2. self assessment of health status, frailty, and physical functioning.
3. psychosocial risks, including but not limited to, depression/life satisfaction, stress, anger, loneliness/social isolation, pain, and fatigue.
4. Behavioral risks, including but not limited to, tobacco use, physical activity, nutrition and oral health, alcohol consumption, sexual health, motor vehicle safety (seat belt use), and home safety.
5. Activities of daily living (ADLs), including but not limited to, dressing, feeding, toileting, grooming, physical ambulation (including balance/risk of falls), and bathing.
6. Instrumental activities of daily living (IADLs), including but not limited to, shopping, food preparation, using the telephone, housekeeping, laundry, mode of transportation, responsibility for own medications, and ability to handle finances.

Review of the individual's functional ability and level of safety: At a minimum, includes assessment of the following topics:

a. Hearing impairment,

b. Ability to successfully perform activities of daily living,

c. Fall risk, and, d. Home safety.

Subsequent AWV providing PPPS: The provision of the following services to an eligible beneficiary by a health professional that include, and take into account the results of an updated health risk assessment, as those terms are defined in this section:

a. Review (and administration if needed) of an updated health risk assessment (as defined in this section).

b. An update of the individual's medical/family history.

c. An update of the list of current providers and suppliers that are regularly involved in providing medical care to the individual, as that list was developed for the first AWV providing PPPS or the previous subsequent AWV providing PPPS.

d. Measurement of an individual's weight (or waist circumference), BP, and other routine measurements as deemed appropriate, based on the individual's medical/family history.

e. Detection of any cognitive impairment that the individual may have as defined in this section.

f. An update to the following:

© 2019 Optum360, LLC

(1) The written screening schedule for the individual as that schedule is defined in this section, that was developed at the first AWV providing PPPS, and,

(2) The list of risk factors and conditions for which primary, secondary, or tertiary interventions are recommended or are under way for the individual, as that list was developed at the first AWV providing PPPS or the previous subsequent AWV providing PPPS.

g. Furnishing of personalized health advice to the individual and a referral, as appropriate, to health education or preventive counseling services or programs as that advice and related services are defined for the first AWV providing PPPS.

h. Any other element determined appropriate by the Secretary through the NCD process.

See Pub. 100-04, Medicare Claims Processing Manual, chapter 18, section 140, for detailed claims processing and billing instructions.

100-02, 15, 290

Foot Care

(Rev.1, 10-01-03)

A. Treatment of Subluxation of Foot

Subluxations of the foot are defined as partial dislocations or displacements of joint surfaces, tendons ligaments, or muscles of the foot. Surgical or nonsurgical treatments undertaken for the sole purpose of correcting a subluxated structure in the foot as an isolated entity are not covered.

However, medical or surgical treatment of subluxation of the ankle joint (talo-crural joint) is covered. In addition, reasonable and necessary medical or surgical services, diagnosis, or treatment for medical conditions that have resulted from or are associated with partial displacement of structures is covered. For example, if a patient has osteoarthritis that has resulted in a partial displacement of joints in the foot, and the primary treatment is for the osteoarthritis, coverage is provided.

B. Exclusions from Coverage

The following foot care services are generally excluded from coverage under both Part A and Part B. (See Sec.290.F and Sec.290.G for instructions on applying foot care exclusions.)

1. Treatment of Flat Foot
   The term "flat foot" is defined as a condition in which one or more arches of the foot have flattened out. Services or devices directed toward the care or correction of such conditions, including the prescription of supportive devices, are not covered.
2. Routine Foot Care
   Except as provided above, routine foot care is excluded from coverage. Services that normally are considered routine and not covered by Medicare include the following:
   - The cutting or removal of corns and calluses;
   - The trimming, cutting, clipping, or debriding of nails; and
   - Other hygienic and preventive maintenance care, such as cleaning and soaking the feet, the use of skin creams to maintain skin tone of either ambulatory or bedfast patients, and any other service performed in the absence of localized illness, injury, or symptoms involving the foot.
3. Supportive Devices for Feet
   Orthopedic shoes and other supportive devices for the feet generally are not covered. However, this exclusion does not apply to such a shoe if it is an integral part of a leg brace, and its expense is included as part of the cost of the brace. Also, this exclusion does not apply to therapeutic shoes furnished to diabetics.

C. Exceptions to Routine Foot Care Exclusion

1. Necessary and Integral Part of Otherwise Covered Services
   In certain circumstances, services ordinarily considered to be routine may be covered if they are performed as a necessary and integral part of otherwise covered services, such as diagnosis and treatment of ulcers, wounds, or infections.
2. Treatment of Warts on Foot
   The treatment of warts (including plantar warts) on the foot is covered to the same extent as services provided for the treatment of warts located elsewhere on the body.
3. Presence of Systemic Condition
   The presence of a systemic condition such as metabolic, neurologic, or peripheral vascular disease may require scrupulous foot care by a professional that in the absence of such condition(s) would be considered routine (and, therefore, excluded from coverage). Accordingly, foot care that would otherwise be considered routine may be covered when systemic condition(s) result in severe circulatory embarrassment or areas of diminished sensation in the individual's legs or feet. (See subsection A.)

   In these instances, certain foot care procedures that otherwise are considered routine (e.g., cutting or removing corns and calluses, or trimming, cutting, clipping, or debriding nails) may pose a hazard when performed by a nonprofessional person on patients with such systemic conditions. (See Sec.290.G for procedural instructions.)
4. Mycotic Nails
   In the absence of a systemic condition, treatment of mycotic nails may be covered.
   The treatment of mycotic nails for an ambulatory patient is covered only when the physician attending the patient's mycotic condition documents that (1) there is clinical evidence of mycosis of the toenail, and (2) the patient has marked limitation of ambulation, pain, or secondary infection resulting from the thickening and dystrophy of the infected toenail plate.

   The treatment of mycotic nails for a nonambulatory patient is covered only when the physician attending the patient's mycotic condition documents that (1) there is clinical evidence of mycosis of the toenail, and (2) the patient suffers from pain or secondary infection resulting from the thickening and dystrophy of the infected toenail plate.

   For the purpose of these requirements, documentation means any written information that is required by the carrier in order for services to be covered. Thus, the information submitted with claims must be substantiated by information found in the patient's medical record. Any information, including that contained in a form letter, used for documentation purposes is subject to carrier verification in order to ensure that the information adequately justifies coverage of the treatment of mycotic nails.

D. Systemic Conditions That Might Justify Coverage

Although not intended as a comprehensive list, the following metabolic, neurologic, and peripheral vascular diseases (with synonyms in parentheses) most commonly represent the underlying conditions that might justify coverage for routine foot care.

- Diabetes mellitus *
- Arteriosclerosis obliterans (A.S.O., arteriosclerosis of the extremities, occlusive peripheral arteriosclerosis)
- Buerger's disease (thromboangiitis obliterans)
- Chronic thrombophlebitis *
- Peripheral neuropathies involving the feet -
- Associated with malnutrition and vitamin deficiency *
  - Malnutrition (general, pellagra)
  - Alcoholism
  - Malabsorption (celiac disease, tropical sprue)
  - Pernicious anemia
- Associated with carcinoma *
- Associated with diabetes mellitus *
- Associated with drugs and toxins *
- Associated with multiple sclerosis *
- Associated with uremia (chronic renal disease) *
- Associated with traumatic injury
- Associated with leprosy or neurosyphilis
- Associated with hereditary disorders
- Hereditary sensory radicular neuropathy
- Angiokeratoma corporis diffusum (Fabry's)
- Amyloid neuropathy

When the patient's condition is one of those designated by an asterisk (*), routine procedures are covered only if the patient is under the active care of a doctor of medicine or osteopathy who documents the condition.

E. Supportive Devices for Feet

Orthopedic shoes and other supportive devices for the feet generally are not covered. However, this exclusion does not apply to such a shoe if it is an integral part of a leg brace, and its expense is included as part of the cost of the brace. Also, this exclusion does not apply to therapeutic shoes furnished to diabetics.

F. Presumption of Coverage

In evaluating whether the routine services can be reimbursed, a presumption of coverage may be made where the evidence available discloses certain physical and/or clinical findings consistent with the diagnosis and indicative of severe

© 2019 Optum360, LLC

peripheral involvement. For purposes of applying this presumption the following findings are pertinent:

Class A Findings
Nontraumatic amputation of foot or integral skeletal portion thereof.

Class B Findings
Absent posterior tibial pulse;

Advanced trophic changes as: hair growth (decrease or absence) nail changes (thickening) pigmentary changes (discoloration) skin texture (thin, shiny) skin color (rubor or redness) (Three required); and

Absent dorsalis pedis pulse.

Class C Findings
Claudication;

Temperature changes (e.g., cold feet);

Edema;

Paresthesias (abnormal spontaneous sensations in the feet); and

Burning.

The presumption of coverage may be applied when the physician rendering the routine foot care has identified:

1. A Class A finding;
2. Two of the Class B findings; or
3. One Class B and two Class C findings.

Cases evidencing findings falling short of these alternatives may involve podiatric treatment that may constitute covered care and should be reviewed by the intermediary's medical staff and developed as necessary.

For purposes of applying the coverage presumption where the routine services have been rendered by a podiatrist, the contractor may deem the active care requirement met if the claim or other evidence available discloses that the patient has seen an M.D. or D.O. for treatment and/or evaluation of the complicating disease process during the 6-month period prior to the rendition of the routine-type services. The intermediary may also accept the podiatrist's statement that the diagnosing and treating M.D. or D.O. also concurs with the podiatrist's findings as to the severity of the peripheral involvement indicated.

Services ordinarily considered routine might also be covered if they are performed as a necessary and integral part of otherwise covered services, such as diagnosis and treatment of diabetic ulcers, wounds, and infections.

G. Application of Foot Care Exclusions to Physician's Services

The exclusion of foot care is determined by the nature of the service. Thus, payment for an excluded service should be denied whether performed by a podiatrist, osteopath, or a doctor of medicine, and without regard to the difficulty or complexity of the procedure.

When an itemized bill shows both covered services and noncovered services not integrally related to the covered service, the portion of charges attributable to the noncovered services should be denied. (For example, if an itemized bill shows surgery for an ingrown toenail and also removal of calluses not necessary for the performance of toe surgery, any additional charge attributable to removal of the calluses should be denied.)

In reviewing claims involving foot care, the carrier should be alert to the following exceptional situations:

1. Payment may be made for incidental noncovered services performed as a necessary and integral part of, and secondary to, a covered procedure. For example, if trimming of toenails is required for application of a cast to a fractured foot, the carrier need not allocate and deny a portion of the charge for the trimming of the nails. However, a separately itemized charge for such excluded service should be disallowed. When the primary procedure is covered the administration of anesthesia necessary for the performance of such procedure is also covered.
2. Payment may be made for initial diagnostic services performed in connection with a specific symptom or complaint if it seems likely that its treatment would be covered even though the resulting diagnosis may be one requiring only noncovered care.

The name of the M.D. or D.O. who diagnosed the complicating condition must be submitted with the claim. In those cases, where active care is required, the approximate date the beneficiary was last seen by such physician must also be indicated.

NOTE: Section 939 of P.L. 96-499 removed "warts" from the routine foot care exclusion effective July 1, 1981.

Relatively few claims for routine-type care are anticipated considering the severity of conditions contemplated as the basis for this exception. Claims for this type of foot care should not be paid in the absence of convincing evidence that nonprofessional performance of the service would have been hazardous for the beneficiary because of an underlying systemic disease. The mere statement of a diagnosis such as those mentioned in Sec.D above does not of itself indicate the severity of the condition. Where development is indicated to verify diagnosis and/or severity the carrier should follow existing claims processing practices which may include review of carrier's history and medical consultation as well as physician contacts.

The rules in Sec.290.F concerning presumption of coverage also apply.

Codes and policies for routine foot care and supportive devices for the feet are not exclusively for the use of podiatrists. These codes must be used to report foot care services regardless of the specialty of the physician who furnishes the services. Carriers must instruct physicians to use the most appropriate code available when billing for routine foot care.

100-02, 15, 300

Diabetes Self-Management Training Services

(Rev.72, Issued: 05-25-07; Effective: 07-01-07; Implementation: 07-02-07)

Section 4105 of the Balanced Budget Act of 1997 permits Medicare coverage of diabetes self-management training (DSMT) services when these services are furnished by a certified provider who meets certain quality standards. This program is intended to educate beneficiaries in the successful self-management of diabetes. The program includes instructions in self-monitoring of blood glucose; education about diet and exercise; an insulin treatment plan developed specifically for the patient who is insulin-dependent; and motivation for patients to use the skills for self-management.

Diabetes self-management training services may be covered by Medicare only if the treating physician or treating qualified non-physician practitioner who is managing the beneficiary's diabetic condition certifies that such services are needed. The referring physician or qualified non-physician practitioner must maintain the plan of care in the beneficiary's medical record and documentation substantiating the need for training on an individual basis when group training is typically covered, if so ordered. The order must also include a statement signed by the physician that the service is needed as well as the following:

- The number of initial or follow-up hours ordered (the physician can order less than 10 hours of training);
- The topics to be covered in training (initial training hours can be used for the full initial training program or specific areas such as nutrition or insulin training); and
- A determination that the beneficiary should receive individual or group training.

The provider of the service must maintain documentation in a file that includes the original order from the physician and any special conditions noted by the physician.

When the training under the order is changed, the training order/referral must be signed by the physician or qualified non-physician practitioner treating the beneficiary and maintained in the beneficiary's file in the DSMT's program records.

NOTE: All entities billing for DSMT under the fee-for-service payment system or other payment systems must meet all national coverage requirements.

100-02, 15, 300.2

Certified Providers

(Rev.109; Issued: 08-07-09; Effective Date: 03-30-09; Implementation Date: 09-08-09)

A designated certified provider bills for DSMT provided by an accredited DSMT program. Certified providers must submit a copy of their accreditation certificate to the contractor. The statute states that a "certified provider" is a physician or other individual or entity designated by the Secretary that, in addition to providing outpatient self-management training services, provides other items and services for which payment may be made under title XVIII, and meets certain quality standards. The CMS is designating all providers and suppliers that bill Medicare for other individual services such as hospital outpatient departments, renal dialysis facilities, physicians and durable medical equipment suppliers as certified. All suppliers/providers who may bill for other Medicare services or items and who represent a DSMT program that is accredited as meeting quality standards can bill and receive payment for the entire DSMT program. Registered dietitians are eligible to bill on behalf of an entire DSMT program on or after January 1, 2002, as long as the provider has obtained a Medicare provider number. A dietitian may not be the sole provider of the DSMT service. There is an exception for rural areas. In a rural area, an individual who is qualified as a registered dietitian and as a certified diabetic educator who is currently certified by an organization approved by CMS may furnish training and is deemed to meet the multidisciplinary team requirement.

© 2019 Optum360, LLC

The CMS will not reimburse services on a fee-for-service basis rendered to a beneficiary under Part A.

NOTE: While separate payment is not made for this service to Rural Health Clinics (RHCs), the service is covered but is considered included in the all-inclusive encounter rate. Effective January 1, 2006, payment for DSMT provided in a Federally Qualified Health Clinic (FQHC) that meets all of the requirements identified in Pub. 100-04, chapter 18, section 120 may be made in addition to one other visit the beneficiary had during the same day.

All DSMT programs must be accredited as meeting quality standards by a CMS approved national accreditation organization. Currently, CMS recognizes the American Diabetes Association, American Association of Diabetes Educators and the Indian Health Service as approved national accreditation organizations. Programs without accreditation by a CMS-approved national accreditation organization are not covered. Certified providers may be asked to submit updated accreditation documents at any time or to submit outcome data to an organization designated by CMS.

Enrollment of DMEPOS Suppliers

The DMEPOS suppliers are reimbursed for diabetes training through local carriers. In order to file claims for DSMT, a DMEPOS supplier must be enrolled in the Medicare program with the National Supplier Clearinghouse (NSC). The supplier must also meet the quality standards of a CMS-approved national accreditation organization as stated above. DMEPOS suppliers must obtain a provider number from the local carrier in order to bill for DSMT.

The carrier requires a completed Form CMS-855, along with an accreditation certificate as part of the provider application process. After it has been determined that the quality standards are met, a billing number is assigned to the supplier. Once a supplier has received a provider identification (PIN) number, the supplier can begin receiving reimbursement for this service.

Carriers should contact the National Supplier Clearinghouse (NSC) according to the instruction in Pub 100-08, the Medicare Program Integrity Manual, Chapter 10, "Healthcare Provider/Supplier Enrollment," to verify an applicant is currently enrolled and eligible to receive direct payment from the Medicare program.

The applicant is assigned specialty 87.

Any DMEPOS supplier that has its billing privileges deactivated or revoked by the NSC will also have the billing number deactivated by the carrier.

100-02, 15, 300.3

Frequency of Training

(Rev.72, Issued: 05-25-07; Effective: 07-01-07; Implementation: 07-02-07)

A - Initial Training

The initial year for DSMT is the 12 month period following the initial date.

Medicare will cover initial training that meets the following conditions:

- Is furnished to a beneficiary who has not previously received initial or follow-up training under HCPCS codes G0108 or G0109;
- Is furnished within a continuous 12-month period;
- Does not exceed a total of 10 hours* (the 10 hours of training can be done in any combination of 1/2 hour increments);
- With the exception of 1 hour of individual training, training is usually furnished in a group setting, which can contain other patients besides Medicare beneficiaries, and;
- One hour of individual training may be used for any part of the training including insulin training.

* When a claim contains a DSMT HCPCS code and the associated units cause the total time for the DSMT initial year to exceed '10' hours, a CWF error will set.

B - Follow-Up Training

Medicare covers follow-up training under the following conditions:

- No more than 2 hours individual or group training per beneficiary per year;
- Group training consists of 2 to 20 individuals who need not all be Medicare beneficiaries;
- Follow-up training for subsequent years is based on a 12 month calendar after completion of the full 10 hours of initial training;
- Follow-up training is furnished in increments of no less than one-half hour*; and
- The physician (or qualified non-physician practitioner) treating the beneficiary must document in the beneficiary's medical record that the beneficiary is a diabetic.

*When a claim contains a DSMT HCPCS code and the associated units cause the total time for any follow-up year to exceed 2 hours, a CWF error will set.

100-02, 15, 300.4

Coverage Requirements for Individual Training

(Rev. 72, Issued: 05-25-07; Effective: 07-01-07; Implementation: 07-02-07)

Medicare covers training on an individual basis for a Medicare beneficiary under any of the following conditions:

- No group session is available within 2 months of the date the training is ordered;
- The beneficiary's physician (or qualified non-physician practitioner) documents in the beneficiary's medical record that the beneficiary has special needs resulting from conditions, such as severe vision, hearing or language limitations or other such special conditions as identified by the treating physician or non-physician practitioner, that will hinder effective participation in a group training session; or
- The physician orders additional insulin training.

The need for individual training must be identified by the physician or non-physician practitioner in the referral.

NOTE: If individual training has been provided to a Medicare beneficiary and subsequently the carrier or intermediary determines that training should have been provided in a group, carriers and intermediaries down-code the reimbursement from individual to the group level and provider education would be the appropriate actions instead of denying the service as billed.

100-02, 15, 310

Kidney Disease Patient Education Services

(Rev.117; Issued: 12-18-09; Effective Date: 01-01-10; Implementation Date: 04-05-10)

By definition, chronic kidney disease (CKD) is kidney damage for 3 months or longer, regardless of the cause of kidney damage. CKD typically evolves over a long period of time and patients may not have symptoms until significant, possibly irreversible, damage has been done. Complications can develop from kidneys that do not function properly, such as high blood pressure, anemia, and weak bones. When CKD progresses, it may lead to kidney failure, which requires artificial means to perform kidney functions (dialysis) or a kidney transplant to maintain life.

Patients can be classified into 5 stages based on their glomerular filtration rate (GFR, how quickly blood is filtered through the kidneys), with stage I having kidney damage with normal or increased GFR to stage V with kidney failure, also called end-stage renal disease (ESRD). Once patients with CKD are identified, treatment is available to help prevent complications of decreased kidney function, slow the progression of kidney disease, and reduce the risk of other diseases such as heart disease.

Beneficiaries with CKD may benefit from kidney disease education (KDE) interventions due to the large amount of medical information that could affect patient outcomes, including the increasing emphasis on self-care and patients' desire for informed, autonomous decision-making. Pre-dialysis education can help patients achieve better understanding of their illness, dialysis modality options, and may help delay the need for dialysis. Education interventions should be patient-centered, encourage collaboration, offer support to the patient, and be delivered consistently.

Effective for claims with dates of service on and after January 1, 2010, Section 152(b) of the Medicare Improvements for Patients and Providers Act of 2008 (MIPPA) covers KDE services under Medicare Part B. KDE services are designed to provide beneficiaries with Stage IV CKD comprehensive information regarding: the management of comorbidities, including delaying the need for dialysis; prevention of uremic complications; all therapeutic options (each option for renal replacement therapy, dialysis access options, and transplantation); ensuring that the beneficiary has opportunities to actively participate in his/her choice of therapy; and that the services be tailored to meet the beneficiary's needs.

Regulations for KDE services were established at 42 CFR 410.48. Claims processing instructions and billing requirements can be found in Pub. 100-04, Medicare Claims Processing Manual, Chapter 32 - Billing Requirements for Special Services, Section 20.

100-02, 15, 310.1

Beneficiaries Eligible for Coverage

(Rev.117; Issued: 12-18-09; Effective Date: 01-01-10; Implementation Date: 04-05-10)

Medicare Part B covers outpatient, face-to-face KDE services for a beneficiary that:

- is diagnosed with Stage IV CKD, using the Modification of Diet in Renal Disease (MDRD) Study formula (severe decrease in GFR, GFR value of 15-29 mL/min/1.73 m2), and
- obtains a referral from the physician managing the beneficiary's kidney condition. The referral should be documented in the beneficiary's medical records.

© 2019 Optum360, LLC

100-02, 15, 310.2

Qualified Person

(Rev.117; Issued: 12-18-09; Effective Date: 01-01-10; Implementation Date: 04-05-10)

Medicare Part B covers KDE services provided by a ‚Äòqualified person,' meaning a: physician (as defined in section 30 of this chapter), physician assistant, nurse practitioner, or clinical nurse specialist (as defined in sections 190, 200, and 210 of this chapter), hospital, critical access hospital (CAH), skilled nursing facility (SNF), comprehensive outpatient rehabilitation facility (CORF), home health agency (HHA), or hospice, if the KDE services are provided in a rural area (using the actual geographic location core based statistical area (CBSA) to identify facilities located in rural areas), or hospital or CAH that is treated as being rural (was reclassified from urban to rural status per 42 CFR 412.103).

NOTE: The "incident to" requirements at section 1861(s)(2)(A) of the Social Security Act (the Act) do not apply to KDE services.

The following providers are not ‚Äòqualified persons' and are excluded from furnishing KDE services:

- A hospital, CAH, SNF, CORF, HHA, or hospice located outside of a rural area (using the actual geographic location CBSA to identify facilities located outside of a rural area), unless the services are furnished by a hospital or CAH that is treated as being in a rural area; and
- Renal dialysis facilities.

100-02, 15, 310.4

Standards for Content

(Rev.117; Issued: 12-18-09; Effective Date: 01-01-10; Implementation Date: 04-05-10)

Medicare Part B covers KDE services, provided by a qualified person, which provide comprehensive information regarding:

A. The management of comorbidities, including delaying the need for dialysis, which includes, but is not limited to, the following topics:

- Prevention and treatment of cardiovascular disease,
- Prevention and treatment of diabetes,
- Hypertension management,
- Anemia management,
- Bone disease and disorders of calcium and phosphorus metabolism management,
- Symptomatic neuropathy management, and
- Impairments in functioning and well-being.

B. Prevention of uremic complications, which includes, but is not limited to, the following topics:

- Information on how the kidneys work and what happens when the kidneys fail,
- Understanding if remaining kidney function can be protected, preventing disease
  progression, and realistic chances of survival,
- Diet and fluid restrictions, and
- Medication review, including how each medication works, possible side effects and minimization of side effects, the importance of compliance, and informed decision making if the patient decides not to take a specific drug.

C. Therapeutic options, treatment modalities and settings, advantages and disadvantages of each treatment option, and how the treatments replace the kidney, including, but not limited to, the following topics: Hemodialysis, both at home and in-facility;

- Peritoneal dialysis (PD), including intermittent PD, continuous ambulatory PD, and continuous cycling PD, both at home and in-facility;
- All dialysis access options for hemodialysis and peritoneal dialysis; and
- Transplantation.

D. Opportunities for beneficiaries to actively participate in the choice of therapy and be tailored to meet the needs of the individual beneficiary involved, which includes, but is not limited to, the following topics: Physical symptoms,

- Impact on family and social life,
- Exercise,
- The right to refuse treatment,
- Impact on work and finances,
- The meaning of test results, and
- Psychological impact.

100-02, 15, 310.5

Outcomes Assessment

(Rev.117; Issued: 12-18-09; Effective Date: 01-01-10; Implementation Date: 04-05-10)

Qualified persons that provide KDE services must develop outcomes assessments that are designed to measure beneficiary knowledge about CKD and its treatment. The assessment must be administered to the beneficiary during a KDE session, and be made available to the Centers for Medicare & Medicaid Services (CMS) upon request. The outcomes assessments serve to assist KDE educators and CMS in improving subsequent KDE programs, patient understanding, and assess program effectiveness of:

Preparing the beneficiary to make informed decisions about their healthcare options related to CKD, and

Meeting the communication needs of underserved populations, including persons with disabilities, persons with limited English proficiency, and persons with health literacy needs.

100-03, 10.2

NCD for Transcutaneous Electrical Nerve Stimulation (TENS) for Acute Post-Operative Pain

(Rev.173, Issued: 9-4-14, Effective: With Implementation I-10)

Indications and Limitations of Coverage

The use of Transcutaneous Electrical Nerve Stimulation (TENS) for the relief of acute post-operative pain is covered under Medicare. TENS may be covered whether used as an adjunct to the use of drugs, or as an alternative to drugs, in the treatment of acute pain resulting from surgery.

TENS devices, whether durable or disposable, may be used in furnishing this service. When used for the purpose of treating acute post-operative pain, TENS devices are considered supplies. As such they may be hospital supplies furnished inpatients covered under Part A, or supplies incident to a physician's service when furnished in connection with surgery done on an outpatient basis, and covered under Part B.

It is expected that TENS, when used for acute post-operative pain, will be necessary for relatively short periods of time, usually 30 days or less. In cases when TENS is used for longer periods, Medicare Administrative Contractors should attempt to ascertain whether TENS is no longer being used for acute pain but rather for chronic pain, in which case the TENS device may be covered as durable medical equipment as described in §160.27.

Cross-references:

Medicare Benefit Policy Manual, Chapter 1, "Inpatient Hospital Services," §40;

Medicare Benefit Policy Manual, Chapter 2, "Hospital Services Covered Under Part B," §§20, 20.4, and 80; Medicare Benefit Policy Manual, Chapter 15, "Covered Medical and other Health Services, §110."

100-03, 40.7

NCD for Outpatient Intravenous Insulin Treatment (40.7)

(Rev. 117, Issued: 03-09-10, Effective Date: 12-23-09; Implementation Date: 04-05-10)

A. General

The term outpatient intravenous (IV) insulin therapy (OIVIT) refers to an outpatient regimen that integrates pulsatile or continuous intravenous infusion of insulin via any means, guided by the results of measurement of:

- respiratory quotient; and/or
- urine urea nitrogen (UUN); and/or
- arterial, venous, or capillary glucose; and/or
- potassium concentration; and
- performed in scheduled recurring periodic intermittent episodes.

This regimen is also sometimes termed Cellular Activation Therapy (CAT), Chronic Intermittent Intravenous Insulin Therapy (CIIT), Hepatic Activation Therapy (HAT), Intercellular Activation Therapy (iCAT), Metabolic Activation Therapy (MAT), Pulsatile Intravenous Insulin Treatment (PIVIT), Pulse Insulin Therapy (PIT), and Pulsatile Therapy (PT).

In OIVIT, insulin is intravenously administered in the outpatient setting for a variety of indications. Most commonly, it is delivered in pulses, but it may be delivered as a more conventional drip solution. The insulin administration is adjunctive to the patient's routine diabetic management regimen (oral agent or insulin-based) or other disease management regimen, typically performed on an intermittent basis (often weekly), and frequently performed chronically without duration limits. Glucose or other carbohydrate is available ad libitum (in accordance with patient desire).

B. Nationally Covered Indications

N/A

© 2019 Optum360, LLC

C. Nationally Non-Covered Indications

Effective for claims with dates of service on and after December 23, 2009, the Centers for Medicare and Medicaid Services (CMS) determines that the evidence does not support a conclusion that OIVIT improves health outcomes in Medicare beneficiaries. Therefore, CMS has determined that OIVIT is not reasonable and necessary for any indication under section 1862(a)(1)(A) of the Social Security Act. Services comprising an OIVIT regimen are nationally non-covered under Medicare when furnished pursuant to an OIVIT regimen (see subsection A. above).

D. Other

Individual components of OIVIT may have medical uses in conventional treatment regimens for diabetes and other conditions. Coverage for such other uses may be determined by other local or national Medicare determinations, and do not pertain to OIVIT. For example, see Pub. 100-03, NCD Manual, Section 40.2, Home Blood Glucose Monitors, Section 40.3, Closed-loop Blood Glucose Control Devices (CBGCD), Section 190.20, Blood Glucose Testing, and Section 280.14, Infusion Pumps, as well as Pub. 100-04, Claims Processing Manual, Chapter 18, Section 90, Diabetics Screening.

(This NCD last reviewed December 2009.)

100-03, 70.2.1

Services Provided for the Diagnosis and Treatment of Diabetic Sensory Neuropathy with Loss of Protective Sensation (aka Diabetic Peripheral Neuropathy)

(Rev.1, 10-03-03)

CIM 50-8.1

Presently, peripheral neuropathy, or diabetic sensory neuropathy, is the most common factor leading to amputation in people with diabetes. In diabetes, sensory neuropathy is an anatomically diffuse process primarily affecting sensory and autonomic fibers; however, distal motor findings may be present in advanced cases. Long nerves are affected first, with symptoms typically beginning insidiously in the toes and then advancing proximally. This leads to loss of protective sensation (LOPS), whereby a person is unable to feel minor trauma from mechanical, thermal, or chemical sources. When foot lesions are present, the reduction in autonomic nerve functions may also inhibit wound healing.

Diabetic sensory neuropathy with LOPS is a localized illness of the feet and falls within the regulation's exception to the general exclusionary rule (see 42 CFR 411.15(l)(1)(i)). Foot exams for people with diabetic sensory neuropathy with LOPS are reasonable and necessary to allow for early intervention in serious complications that typically afflict diabetics with the disease.

Effective for services furnished on or after July 1, 2002, Medicare covers, as a physician service, an evaluation (examination and treatment) of the feet no more often than every six months for individuals with a documented diagnosis of diabetic sensory neuropathy and LOPS, as long as the beneficiary has not seen a foot care specialist for some other reason in the interim. LOPS shall be diagnosed through sensory testing with the 5.07 monofilament using established guidelines, such as those developed by the National Institute of Diabetes and Digestive and Kidney Diseases guidelines. Five sites should be tested on the plantar surface of each foot, according to the National Institute of Diabetes and Digestive and Kidney Diseases guidelines. The areas must be tested randomly since the loss of protective sensation may be patchy in distribution, and the patient may get clues if the test is done rhythmically. Heavily callused areas should be avoided. As suggested by the American Podiatric Medicine Association, an absence of sensation at two or more sites out of 5 tested on either foot when tested with the 5.07 Semmes-Weinstein monofilament must be present and documented to diagnose peripheral neuropathy with loss of protective sensation.

The examination includes:

1. A patient history, and
2. A physical examination that must consist of at least the following elements:
   - Visual inspection of forefoot and hindfoot (including toe web spaces);
   - Evaluation of protective sensation;
   - Evaluation of foot structure and biomechanics;
   - Evaluation of vascular status and skin integrity;
   - Evaluation of the need for special footwear; and
3. Patient education.

A. Treatment includes, but is not limited to:

- Local care of superficial wounds;
- Debridement of corns and calluses; and
- Trimming and debridement of nails.

The diagnosis of diabetic sensory neuropathy with LOPS should be established and documented prior to coverage of foot care. Other causes of peripheral neuropathy should be considered and investigated by the primary care physician prior to initiating or referring for foot care for persons with LOPS.

100-03, 80.2

Photodynamic Therapy

(Rev.173, Issued: 09-04-14, Effective: Upon Implementation: of ICD–10)

Photodynamic therapy is a medical procedure which involves the infusion of a photosensitive (light-activated) drug with a very specific absorption peak. This drug is chemically designed to have a unique affinity for the diseased tissue intended for treatment. Once introduced to the body, the drug accumulates and is retained in diseased tissue to a greater degree than in normal tissue. Infusion is followed by the targeted irradiation of this tissue with a non-thermal laser, calibrated to emit light at a wavelength that corresponds to the drug? absorption peak. The drug then becomes active and locally treats the diseased tissue.

Ocular Photodynamic Therapy (OPT)

Ocular Photodynamic Therapy (OPT) is used in the treatment of ophthalmologic diseases. OPT is only covered when used in conjunction with verteporfin (see section 80.3, "Photosensitive Drugs").

- Classic Subfoveal Choroidal Neovascular (CNV) Lesions - OPT is covered with a diagnosis of neovascular age-related macular degeneration (AMD) with predominately classic subfoveal choroidal neovascular (CNV) lesions (where the area of classic CNV occupies = 50 percent of the area of the entire lesion) at the initial visit as determined by a fluorescein angiogram. Subsequent follow-up visits will require either an optical coherence tomography (OCT) or a fluorescein angiogram (FA) to access treatment response. There are no requirements regarding visual acuity, lesion size, and number of re-treatments.
- Occult Subfoveal Choroidal Neovascular (CNV) Lesions - OPT is noncovered for patients with a diagnosis of age-related macular degeneration (AMD) with occult and no classic CNV lesions.
- Other Conditions - Use of OPT with verteporfin for other types of AMD (e.g., patients with minimally classic CNV lesions, atrophic, or dry AMD) is noncovered. OPT with verteporfin for other ocular indications such as pathologic myopia or presumed ocular histoplasmosis syndrome, is eligible for coverage through individual contractor discretion.

100-03, 80.2.1

Ocular Photodynamic Therapy (OPT)- Effective April 3, 2013

(Rev.173, Issued: 09-04-14, Effective: Upon Implementation: of ICD–10)

A. General

Ocular Photodynamic Therapy (OPT) is used in the treatment of ophthalmologic diseases; specifically, for age-related macular degeneration (AMD), a common eye disease among the elderly. OPT involves the infusion of an intravenous photosensitizing drug called verteporfin followed by exposure to a laser. OPT is only covered when used in conjunction with verteporfin.

Effective July 1, 2001, OPT with verteporfin was approved for a diagnosis of neovascular AMD with predominately classic subfoveal choroidal neovascularization (CNV) lesions (where the area of classic CNV occupies = 50% of the area of the entire lesion) at the initial visit as determined by a fluorescein angiogram (FA).

On October 17, 2001, the Centers for Medicare & Medicaid Services (CMS) announced its "intent to cover" OPT with verteporfin for AMD patients with occult and no classic subfoveal CNV as determined by an FA. The October 17, 2001, decision was never implemented.

On March 28, 2002, after thorough review and reconsideration of the October 17, 2001, intent to cover policy, CMS determined that the current non-coverage policy for OPT for verteporfin for AMD patients with occult and no classic subfoveal CNV as determined by an FA should remain in effect.

Effective August 20, 2002, CMS issued a non-covered instruction for OPT with verteporfin for AMD patients with occult and no classic subfoveal CNV as determined by an FA.

B. Nationally Covered Indications

Effective April 1, 2004, OPT with verteporfin continues to be approved for a diagnosis of neovascular AMD with predominately classic subfoveal CNV lesions (where the area of classic CNV occupies = 50% of the area of the entire lesion) at the initial visit as determined by an FA. (CNV lesions are comprised of classic and/or occult components.) Subsequent follow-up visits require either an optical coherence tomography (OCT) (effective April 3. 2013) or an FA (effective April 1, 2004) to access treatment response. There are no requirements regarding visual acuity, lesion size, and number of re-treatments when treating predominantly classic lesions.

© 2019 Optum360, LLC

In addition, after thorough review and reconsideration of the August 20, 2002, non-coverage policy, CMS determines that the evidence is adequate to conclude that OPT with verteporfin is reasonable and necessary for treating:

1. Subfoveal occult with no classic CNV associated with AMD; and,
2. Subfoveal minimally classic CNV (where the area of classic CNV occupies <50% of the area of the entire lesion) associated with AMD.

The above 2 indications are considered reasonable and necessary only when:

1. The lesions are small (4 disk areas or less in size) at the time of initial treatment or within the 3 months prior to initial treatment; and,
2. The lesions have shown evidence of progression within the 3 months prior to initial treatment. Evidence of progression must be documented by deterioration of visual acuity (at least 5 letters on a standard eye examination chart), lesion growth (an increase in at least 1 disk area), or the appearance of blood associated with the lesion.

C. Nationally Non-Covered Indications

Other uses of OPT with verteporfin to treat AMD not already addressed by CMS will continue to be non-covered. These include, but are not limited to, the following AMD indications:

- Juxtafoveal or extrafoveal CNV lesions (lesions outside the fovea),
- Inability to obtain a fluorescein angiogram,
- Atrophic or "dry" AMD.

D. Other

The OPT with verteporfin for other ocular indications, such as pathologic myopia or presumed ocular histoplasmosis syndrome, continue to be eligible for local coverage determinations through individual contractor discretion.

100-03, 80.3

NCD for Photosensitive Drugs (80.3)

(Rev.173, Issued: 09-04-14, Effective: Upon Implementation: of ICD–10)

Photosensitive drugs are the light-sensitive agents used in photodynamic therapy. Once introduced into the body, these drugs selectively identify and adhere to diseased tissue. The drugs remain inactive until they are exposed to a specific wavelength of light, by means of a laser, that corresponds to their absorption peak. The activation of a photosensitive drug results in a photochemical reaction which treats the diseased tissue without affecting surrounding normal tissue.

Verteporfin

Verteporfin, a benzoporphyrin derivative, is an intravenous lipophilic photosensitive drug with an absorption peak of 690 nm. This drug was first approved by the Food and Drug Administration (FDA) on April 12, 2000, and subsequently, approved for inclusion in the United States Pharmacopoeia on July 18, 2000, meeting Medicare's definition of a drug when used in conjunction with ocular photodynamic therapy (OPT) (see section 80.2, "Photodynamic Therapy") when furnished intravenously incident to a physician? service. For patients with age-related macular degeneration (AMD), Verteporfin is only covered with a diagnosis of neovascular age-related macular degeneration with predominately classic subfoveal choroidal neovascular (CNV) lesions (where the area of classic CNV occupies = 50 percent of the area of the entire lesion) at the initial visit as determined by a fluorescein angiogram (FA). Subsequent follow-up visits will require either an optical coherence tomography (OCT) or an FA to access treatment response. OPT with verteporfin is covered for the above indication and will remain non-covered for all other indications related to AMD (see section 80.2). OPT with Verteporfin for use in non-AMD conditions is eligible for coverage through individual contractor discretion.

100-03, 80.3.1

Verteporfin-Effective April 3, 2013

(Rev.173, Issued: 09-04-14, Effective: Upon Implementation: of ICD–10)

A. General

Verteporfin, a benzoporphyrin derivative, is an intravenous lipophilic photosensitive drug with an absorption peak of 690 nm. Verteporfin was first approved by the Food and Drug Administration on April 12, 2000, and subsequently approved for inclusion in the United States Pharmacopoeia on July 18, 2000, meeting Medicare's definition of a drug as defined under Sec. 1861(t)(1) of the Social Security Act. Verteporfin is only covered when used in conjunction with ocular photodynamic therapy OPT) when furnished intravenously incident to a physician's service.

B. Nationally Covered Indications

Effective April 1, 2004, OPT with verteporfin is covered for patients with a diagnosis of neovascular age-related macular degeneration (AMD) with:

- Predominately classic subfoveal choroidal neovascularization (CNV) lesions (where the area of classic CNV occupies = 50% of the area of the entire lesion) at the initial visit as determined by a fluorescein angiogram. (CNV lesions are comprised of classic and/or occult components.) Subsequent follow-up visits require either an optical coherence tomography (OCT) (effective April 3, 2013) or a fluorescein angiogram (FA) (effective April 1, 2004) to access treatment response.

There are no requirements regarding visual acuity, lesion size, and number of retreatments when treating predominantly classic lesions.

- Subfoveal occult with no classic associated with AMD.
- Subfoveal minimally classic CNV CNV (where the area of classic CNV occupies <50% of the area of the entire lesion) associated with AMD.

The above 2 indications are considered reasonable and necessary only when:

1. The lesions are small (4 disk areas or less in size) at the time of initial treatment or within the 3 months prior to initial treatment; and,
2. The lesions have shown evidence of progression within the 3 months prior to initial treatment. Evidence of progression must be documented by deterioration of visual acuity (at least 5 letters on a standard eye examination chart), lesion growth (an increase in at least 1 disk area), or the appearance of blood associated with the lesion.

C. Nationally Non-Covered Indications

Other uses of OPT with verteporfin to treat AMD not already addressed by the Centers for Medicare & Medicaid Services will continue to be non-covered. These include, but are not limited to, the following AMD indications: juxtafoveal or extrafoveal CNV lesions (lesions outside the fovea), inability to obtain an FA, or atrophic or "dry" AMD.

D. Other

The OPT with verteporfin for other ocular indications, such as pathologic myopia or presumed ocular histoplasmosis syndrome, continue to be eligible for local coverage determinations through individual contractor discretion.

100-03, 90.1

Pharmacogenomic Testing to Predict Warfarin Responsiveness (Effective August 3, 2009)

(Rev.111, Issued: 12-18-09, Effective: 08-03-09, Implementation: 04-05-10)

A. General

Warfarin sodium is an orally administered anticoagulant drug that is marketed most commonly as Coumadin(R). (The Food and Drug Administration (FDA) approved labeling for Coumadin(R) includes a Black Box Warning dating back to 2007.) Anticoagulant drugs are sometimes referred to as blood thinners by the lay public. Warfarin affects the vitamin K-dependent clotting factors II, VII, IX, and X. Warfarin is thought to interfere with clotting factor synthesis by inhibition of the C1 subunit of the vitamin K epoxide reductase (VKORC1) enzyme complex, thereby reducing the regeneration of vitamin K1 epoxide. The elimination of warfarin is almost entirely by metabolic conversion to inactive metabolites by cytochrome P450 (CYP) enzymes in liver cells. CYP2C9 is the principal cytochrome P450 enzyme that modulates the anticoagulant activity of warfarin. From results of clinical studies, genetic variation in the CYP2C9 and/or VKORC1 genes can, in concert with clinical factors, predict how each individual responds to warfarin

Pharmacogenomics denotes the study of how an individual's genetic makeup, or genotype, affects the body's response to drugs. Pharmacogenomics as a science examines associations among variations in genes with individual responses to a drug or medication. In application, pharmacogenomic results (i.e., information on the patient's genetic variations) can contribute to predicting a patient's response to a given drug: good, bad, or none at all. Pharmacogenomic testing of CYP2C9 or VKORC1 alleles to predict a patient's response to warfarin occurs ideally prior to initiation of the drug. This would be an once-in-a-lifetime test, absent any reason to believe that the patient's personal genetic characteristics would change over time. Although such pharmacogenomic testing would be used to attempt to better approximate the best starting dose of warfarin, it would not eliminate the need for periodic PT/INR testing, a standard diagnostic test for coagulation activity and for assessing how a patient is reacting to a warfarin dose.

Nationally Covered Indications

Effective August 3, 2009, the Centers for Medicare & Medicaid Services (CMS) believes that the available evidence supports that coverage with evidence development (CED) under Sec.1862(a)(1)(E) of the Social Security Act (the Act) is appropriate for pharmacogenomic testing of CYP2C9 or VKORC1 alleles to predict warfarin responsiveness by any method, and is therefore covered only when provided to Medicare beneficiaries who are candidates for anticoagulation therapy with warfarin who:

1. Have not been previously tested for CYP2C9 or VKORC1 alleles; and
2. Have received fewer than five days of warfarin in the anticoagulation regimen for which the testing is ordered; and

© 2019 Optum360, LLC

3. Are enrolled in a prospective, randomized, controlled clinical study when that study meets the following standards. A clinical study seeking Medicare payment for pharmacogenomic testing of CYP2C9 or VKORC1 alleles to predict warfarin responsiveness provided to the Medicare beneficiary who is a candidate for anticoagulation therapy with warfarin pursuant to CED must address one or more aspects of the following question:

   Prospectively, in Medicare-aged subjects whose warfarin therapy management includes pharmacogenomic testing of CYP2C9 or VKORC1 alleles to predict warfarin response, what is the frequency and severity of the following outcomes, compared to subjects whose warfarin therapy management does not include pharmacogenomic testing?

   Major hemorrhage

   Minor hemorrhage

   Thromboembolism related to the primary indication for anticoagulation

   Other thromboembolic event

   Mortality

   The study must adhere to the following standards of scientific integrity and relevance to the Medicare population:

   a. The principal purpose of the research study is to test whether a particular intervention potentially improves the participants' health outcomes.

   b. The research study is well-supported by available scientific and medical information or it is intended to clarify or establish the health outcomes of interventions already in common clinical use.

   c. The research study does not unjustifiably duplicate existing studies.

   d. The research study design is appropriate to answer the research question being asked in the study.

   e. The research study is sponsored by an organization or individual capable of executing the proposed study successfully.

   f. The research study is in compliance with all applicable Federal regulations concerning the protection of human subjects found in the Code of Federal Regulations (CFR) at 45 CFR Part 46. If a study is regulated by the FDA, it also must be in compliance with 21 CFR Parts 50 and 56.

   g. All aspects of the research study are conducted according to the appropriate standards of scientific integrity.

   h. The research study has a written protocol that clearly addresses, or incorporates by reference, the Medicare standards.

   i. The clinical research study is not designed to exclusively test toxicity or disease pathophysiology in healthy individuals. Trials of all medical technologies measuring therapeutic outcomes as one of the objectives meet this standard only if the disease or condition being studied is life-threatening as defined in 21 CFR Sec. 312.81(a) and the patient has no other viable treatment options.

   j. The clinical research study is registered on the www.ClinicalTrials.gov website by the principal sponsor/investigator prior to the enrollment of the first study subject.

   k. The research study protocol specifies the method and timing of public release of all pre-specified outcomes to be measured including release of outcomes if outcomes are negative or study is terminated early. The results must be made public within 24 months of the end of data collection. If a report is planned to be published in a peer-reviewed journal, then that initial release may be an abstract that meets the requirements of the International Committee of Medical Journal Editors. However, a full report of the outcomes must be made public no later than 3 years after the end of data collection.

   l. The research study protocol must explicitly discuss subpopulations affected by the treatment under investigation, particularly traditionally underrepresented groups in clinical studies, how the inclusion and exclusion criteria affect enrollment of these populations, and a plan for the retention and reporting of said populations on the trial. If the inclusion and exclusion criteria are expected to have a negative effect on the recruitment or retention of underrepresented populations, the protocol must discuss why these criteria are necessary.

   m. The research study protocol explicitly discusses how the results are or are not expected to be generalizable to the Medicare population to infer whether Medicare patients may benefit from the intervention. Separate discussions in the protocol may be necessary for populations eligible for Medicare due to age, disability or Medicaid eligibility. Consistent with section 1142 of the Act, the Agency for Healthcare Research and Quality (AHRQ) supports clinical research studies that CMS determines meet the above-listed standards and address the above-listed research questions.

B. Nationally Non-Covered Indications

The CMS believes that the available evidence does not demonstrate that pharmacogenomic testing of CYP2C9 or VKORC1 alleles to predict warfarin responsiveness improves health outcomes in Medicare beneficiaries outside the context of CED, and is therefore not reasonable and necessary under Sec.1862(a)(1)(A) of the Act.

C. Other

This NCD does not determine coverage to identify CYP2C9 or VKORC1 alleles for other purposes, nor does it determine national coverage to identify other alleles to predict warfarin responsiveness.

(This NCD last reviewed August 2009.)

100-03, 110.3

Anti-Inhibitor Coagulant Complex (AICC)

(Rev.1, 10-03-03)
CIM 45-24

Anti-inhibitor coagulant complex, AICC, is a drug used to treat hemophilia in patients with factor VIII inhibitor antibodies. AICC has been shown to be safe and effective and has Medicare coverage when furnished to patients with hemophilia A and inhibitor antibodies to factor VIII who have major bleeding episodes and who fail to respond to other, less expensive therapies.

100-03, 110.5

Granulocyte Transfusions

(Rev.1, 10-03-03)
CIM 45-18

Granulocyte transfusions to patients suffering from severe infection and granulocytopenia are a covered service under Medicare. Granulocytopenia is usually identified as fewer than 500 granulocytes/mm3 whole blood. Accepted indications for granulocyte transfusions include:

- Granulocytopenia with evidence of gram negative sepsis; and
- Granulocytopenia in febrile patients with local progressive infections unresponsive to appropriate antibiotic therapy, thought to be due to gram negative organisms.

100-03, 110.10

Intravenous Iron Therapy

(Rev.1, 10-03-03)
CIM 45-29

Iron deficiency is a common condition in end stage renal disease (ESRD) patients undergoing hemodialysis. Iron is a critical structural component of hemoglobin, a key protein found in normal red blood cells (RBCs) that transports oxygen. Without this important building block, anemic patients experience difficulty in restoring adequate, healthy RBCs that improve hematocrit levels. Clinical management of iron deficiency involves treating patients with iron replacement products while they undergo hemodialysis. Body iron stores can be supplemented with either oral or intravenous (IV) iron products. The available evidence suggests that the mode of intravenous administration is perhaps the most effective treatment for iron deficiency in hemodialysis patients. Unlike oral iron products which must be absorbed through the GI tract, IV iron products are infused directly into the bloodstream in a form that is readily available to the bone marrow for RBC synthesis, resulting in an earlier correction of iron deficiency and anemia.

Effective December 1, 2000, Medicare covers sodium ferric gluconate complex in sucrose injection as a first line treatment of iron deficiency anemia when furnished intravenously to patients undergoing chronic hemodialysis who are receiving supplemental erythropoeitin therapy.

Effective October 1, 2001, Medicare also covers iron sucrose injection as a first line treatment of iron deficiency anemia when furnished intravenously to patients undergoing chronic hemodialysis who are receiving supplemental erythropoeitin therapy.

100-03, 110.17

Anti-Cancer Chemotherapy for Colorectal Cancer (Effective January 28, 2005)

(Rev.173, Issued: 09-04-14, Effective: Upon Implementation: of ICD–10)

A. General

Oxaliplatin (Eloxatin™), irinotecan (Camptosar®), cetuximab (Erbitux™), and bevacizumab (Avastin™) are anti-cancer chemotherapeutic agents approved by the Food and Drug Administration (FDA) for the treatment of colorectal cancer. Anti-cancer chemotherapeutic agents are eligible for coverage when used in accordance with FDA-approved labeling (see section 1861(t)(2)(B) of the Social Security Act (the Act)), when the off-label use is supported in one of the authoritative drug compendia

 © 2019 Optum360, LLC

listed in section 1861(t)(2)(B)(ii)(I) of the Act, or when the Medicare Administrative Contractor (MAC) determines an off-label use is medically accepted based on guidance provided by the Secretary (section 1861(t)(2)(B)(ii)(II).

B. Nationally Covered Indications

Pursuant to this national coverage determination (NCD), the off-label use of clinical items and services, including the use of the studied drugs oxaliplatin, irinotecan, cetuximab, or bevacizumab, are covered in specific clinical trials identified by the Centers for Medicare & Medicaid Services (CMS). The clinical trials identified by CMS for coverage of clinical items and services are sponsored by the National Cancer Institute (NCI) and study the use of one or more off-label uses of these four drugs in colorectal cancer and in other cancer types. The list of identified trials is on the CMS Web site at: http://www.cms.hhs.gov/coverage/download/id90b.pdf.

C. Other

This policy does not alter Medicare coverage for items and services that may be covered or non-covered according to the existing national coverage policy for Routine Costs in a Clinical Trial (NCD Manual section 310.1). Routine costs will continue to be covered as well as other items and services provided as a result of coverage of these specific trials in this policy. The basic requirements for enrollment in a trial remain unchanged.

The existing requirements for coverage of oxaliplatin, irinotecan, cetuximab, bevacizumab, or other anticancer chemotherapeutic agents for FDA-approved indications or for indications listed in an approved compendium are not modified.

MACs shall continue to make reasonable and necessary coverage determinations under section 1861(t)(2)(B)(ii)(II) of the Act based on guidance provided by the Secretary for medically accepted uses of off-label indications of oxaliplatin, irinotecan, cetuximab, bevacizumab, or other anticancer chemotherapeutic agents provided outside of the identified clinical trials appearing on the CMS website noted above.

100-03, 110.18

NCD for Aprepitant for Chemotherapy-Induced Emesis

(Rev.165, Issued: 04-15-14, Effective: 05-29-13, Implementation: 07-07-14)

A. General

Chemotherapy-induced nausea and vomiting (CINV) can range from mild to severe, with the most severe cases resulting in dehydration, malnutrition, metabolic imbalances, and potential withdrawal from future chemotherapy treatments. The incidence and severity of CINV are influenced by the specific chemotherapeutic agent(s) used; dosage, schedule and route of administration; and drug combinations. Patient specific risk factors such as gender, age, history of motion sickness, and prior `exposure to chemotherapeutic agents can also have an effect on CINV incidence and severity. Progress has been made in reducing CINV, although it can still be hard to control symptoms that occur more than a day after chemotherapy, during repeat cycles of chemotherapy, and when chemotherapy is given on more than one day or in very high doses. No single antiemetic agent is completely effective in all patients. As noted above, many factors influence the incidence and severity of CINV, with the specific chemotherapeutic agent as the primary factor to consider when deciding which antiemetic to administer. Aprepitant (Emend®) is the first Food and Drug Administration-approved drug of its type. Aprepitant has been proposed to function in combination with other oral antiemetics for a specified population of Medicare patients receiving highly emetogenic chemotherapy and/or moderately emetogenic chemotherapy.

CMS is defining highly emetogenic chemotherapy and moderately emetogenic chemotherapy as those anticancer agents so designated in at least two of three guidelines published by the National Comprehensive Cancer Network (NCCN), American Society of Clinical Oncology (ASCO), and European Society of Medical Oncology (ESMO)/Multinational Association of Supportive Care in Cancer (MASCC). The inclusive examples are: NCCN plus ASCO, NCCN plus ESMO/MASCC, or ASCO plus ESMO/MASCC.

B. Nationally Covered Indications

Effective for services performed between April 4, 2005, and May 29, 2013, the Centers for Medicare & Medicaid Services makes the following determinations regarding the use of aprepitant in the treatment of reducing chemotherapy-induced emesis:

The evidence is adequate to conclude that the use of the oral antiemetic three-drug combination of oral aprepitant (Emend®), an oral 5HT3 antagonist, and oral dexamethasone is reasonable and necessary for a specified patient population. We have defined the patient population for which the use of the oral antiemetic three-drug combination of oral aprepitant (Emend®), an oral 5HT3 antagonist, and oral dexamethasone is reasonable and necessary as only those patients who are receiving one or more of the following anti-cancer chemotherapeutic agents:

- Carmustine
- Cisplatin
- Cyclophosphamide
- Dacarbazine
- Mechlorethamine
- Streptozocin
- Doxorubicin
- Epirubicin
- Lomustine

Effective for services performed on or after May 29, 2013, the oral three-drug regimen of oral aprepitant, an oral 5HT3 antagonist and oral dexamethasone is reasonable and necessary for beneficiaries receiving, either singularly or in combination with other drugs the following anticancer chemotherapeutic agents:

- Alemtuzumab
- Azacitidine
- Bendamustine
- Carboplatin
- Carmustine
- Cisplatin
- Clofarabine
- Cyclophosphamide
- Cytarabine
- Dacarbazine
- Daunorubicin
- Doxorubicin
- Epirubicin
- Idarubicin
- Ifosfamide
- Irinotecan
- Lomustine
- Mechlorethamine
- Oxaliplatin
- Streptozocin

The oral three drug regimen must be administered immediately before and within 48 hours after the administration of these chemotherapeutic agents.

C. Nationally Noncovered Indications

The evidence is adequate to conclude that aprepitant cannot function alone as a full replacement for intravenously administered antiemetic agents for patients who are receiving highly emetogenic chemotherapy and/or moderately emetogenic chemotherapy. Medicare does not cover under Part B for oral antiemetic drugs in antiemetic drug combination regimens that are administered in part, via an oral route and in part, via an intravenous route. Medicare does not cover under Part B aprepitant when it is used alone for anticancer chemotherapy related nausea and vomiting.

D. Other

Medicare Administrative Contractors may determine coverage for other all-oral three-drug antiemesis regimens of aprepitant or any other FDA approved oral NK-1 antagonist in combination with an oral 5HT3 antagonist and oral dexamethasone with the chemotherapeutic agents listed above, or any other anticancer chemotherapeutic agents that are FDA approved and are defined as highly or moderately emetogenic.

(Last revised May 2013)

100-03, 110.21

Erythropoiesis Stimulating Agents (ESAs) in Cancer and Related Neoplastic Conditions

(Rev.173, Issued: 09-04-14, Effective: Upon Implementation: of ICD–10)

A. General

Erythropoiesis stimulating agents (ESAs) stimulate the bone marrow to make more red blood cells and are United States Food and Drug Administration (FDA) approved for use in reducing the need for blood transfusion in patients with specific clinical indications. The FDA has issued alerts and warnings for ESAs administered for a number of clinical conditions, including cancer. Published studies report a higher risk of serious and life-threatening events associated with oncologic uses of ESAs.

B. Nationally Covered Indications

ESA treatment for the anemia secondary to myelosuppressive anticancer chemotherapy in solid tumors, multiple myeloma, lymphoma, and lymphocytic leukemia is only reasonable and necessary under the following specified conditions:

© 2019 Optum360, LLC

- The hemoglobin level immediately prior to initiation or maintenance of ESA treatment is <10 g/dL (or the hematocrit is <30%).
- The starting dose for ESA treatment is the recommended FDA label starting dose, no more than 150 U/kg/3 times weekly for epoetin and 2.25 mcg/kg/1 time weekly for darbepoetin alpha. Equivalent doses may be given over other approved time periods.
- Maintenance of ESA therapy is the starting dose if the hemoglobin level remains below 10g/dL (or hematocrit is <30%) 4 weeks after initiation of therapy and the rise in hemoglobin is >1g/dL (hematocrit >3%);
- For patients whose hemoglobin rises <1g/dl (hematocrit rise <3%) compared to pretreatment baseline over 4 weeks of treatment and whose hemoglobin level remains <10g/dL after the 4 weeks of treatment (or the hematocrit is <30%), the recommended FDA label starting dose may be increased once by 25%. Continued use of the drug is not reasonable and necessary if the hemoglobin rises <1g/dl (hematocrit rise <3%) compared to pretreatment baseline by 8 weeks of treatment.
- Continued administration of the drug is not reasonable and necessary if there is a rapid rise in hemoglobin >1g/dl (hematocrit >3%) over 2 weeks of treatment unless the hemoglobin remains below or subsequently falls to <10g/dL (or the hematocrit is <30%). Continuation and reinstitution of ESA therapy must include a dose reduction of 25% from the previously administered dose.
- ESA treatment duration for each course of chemotherapy includes the 8 weeks following the final dose of myelosuppressive chemotherapy in a chemotherapy regimen.

C. Nationally Non-Covered Indications

ESA treatment is not reasonable and necessary for beneficiaries with certain clinical conditions, either because of a deleterious effect of the ESA on their underlying disease or because the underlying disease increases their risk of adverse effects related to ESA use. These conditions include:

- Any anemia in cancer or cancer treatment patients due to folate deficiency, B-12 deficiency, iron deficiency, hemolysis, bleeding, or bone marrow fibrosis;
- The anemia associated with the treatment of acute and chronic myelogenous leukemias (CML, AML), or erythroid cancers;
- The anemia of cancer not related to cancer treatment;
- Any anemia associated only with radiotherapy;
- Prophylactic use to prevent chemotherapy-induced anemia;
- Prophylactic use to reduce tumor hypoxia;
- Patients with erythropoietin-type resistance due to neutralizing antibodies; and
- Anemia due to cancer treatment if patients have uncontrolled hypertension.

D. Other

Local Medicare Administrative Contractors may continue to make reasonable and necessary determinations on all other uses of ESAs not specified in this National Coverage Determination.

See the Medicare Benefit Policy Manual, chapter 11, section 90 and chapter 15, section 50.5.2 for coverage of ESAs for end-stage renal disease-related anemia. 100-03,1121

100-03, 110.22

Autologous Cellular Immunotherapy Treatment (Effective June 30, 2011)

(Rev.140, Issued: 01-06-12, Effective: 06-30-11, Implementation: 08-08-11)

A. General

Prostate cancer is the most common non-cutaneous cancer in men in the United States. In 2009, an estimated 192,280 new cases of prostate cancer were diagnosed and an estimated 27,360 deaths were reported. The National Cancer Institute states that prostate cancer is predominantly a cancer of older men; the median age at diagnosis is 72 years. Once the patient has castration-resistant, metastatic prostate cancer the median survival is generally less than two years.

In 2010 the Food and Drug Administration (FDA) approved sipuleucel-T (PROVENGE®; APC8015), for patients with castration-resistant, metastatic prostate cancer. The posited mechanism of action, immunotherapy, is different from that of anti-cancer chemotherapy such as docetaxel. This is the first immunotherapy for prostate cancer to receive FDA approval.

The goal of immunotherapy is to stimulate the body's natural defenses (such as the white blood cells called dendritic cells, T-lymphocytes and mononuclear cells) in a specific manner so that they attack and destroy, or at least prevent, the proliferation of cancer cells. Specificity is attained by intentionally exposing a patient's white blood cells to a particular protein (called an antigen) associated with the prostate cancer. This exposure "trains" the white blood cells to target and attack the prostate cancer cells. Clinically, this is expected to result in a decrease in the size and/or number of cancer sites, an increase in the time to cancer progression, and/or an increase in survival of the patient.

Sipuleucel-T differs from other infused anti-cancer therapies. Most such anti-cancer therapies are manufactured and sold by a biopharmaceutical company and then purchased by and dispensed from a pharmacy. In contrast, once the decision is made to treat with sipuleucel-T, a multi-step process is used to produce sipuleucel-T. Sipuleucel-T is made individually for each patient with his own white blood cells. The patient's white blood cells are removed via a procedure called leukapheresis. In a laboratory the white blood cells are exposed to PA2024, which is a molecule created by linking prostatic acid phosphatase (PAP) with granulocyte/macrophage-colony stimulating factor (GM-CSF). PAP is an antigen specifically associated with prostate cancer cells; GM-CSF is a protein that targets a receptor on the surface of white blood cells. Hence, PAP serves to externally manipulate the immunological functioning of the patient's white blood cells while GM-CSF serves to stimulate the white blood cells into action. As noted in the FDA's clinical review, each dose of sipuleucel-T contains a minimum of 40 million treated white blood cells, however there is "high inherent variability" in the yield of sipuleucel-T from leukapheresis to leukapheresis in the same patient as well as from patient to patient. The treated white blood cells are then infused back into the same patient. The FDA-approved dosing regimen is three doses with each dose administered two weeks apart.

Indications and Limitations of Coverage

B. Nationally Covered Indications

Effective for services performed on or after June 30, 2011, The Centers for Medicare and Medicaid Services (CMS) proposes that the evidence is adequate to conclude that the use of autologous cellular immunotherapy treatment - sipuleucel-T; PROVENGE® improves health outcomes for Medicare beneficiaries with asymptomatic or minimally symptomatic metastatic castrate-resistant (hormone refractory) prostate cancer, and thus is reasonable and necessary for this on-label indication under 1862(a)(1)(A) of the Social Security Act.

C. Nationally Non-Covered Indications

N/A

D. Other

Effective for services performed on or after June 30, 2011, coverage of all off-label uses of autologous cellular immunotherapy treatment —sipuleucel-T; PROVENGE® for the treatment of prostate cancer is left to the discretion of the local Medicare Administrative Contractors.

(NCD last reviewed June 2011.)

100-03, 150.12

Collagen Meniscus Implant (Effective May 25, 2010)

(Rev.121, Issued: 05-28-10, Effective: 05-25-10, Implementation: 07-06-10)

A. General

The knee menisci are wedge-shaped, semi-lunar discs of fibrous tissue located in the knee joint between the ends of the femur and the tibia and fibula. There is a lateral and medial meniscus in each knee. It is known now that the menisci provide mechanical support, localized pressure distribution, and lubrication of the knee joint. Initially, meniscal tears were treated with total meniscectomy; however, as knowledge of the function of the menisci and the potential long term effects of total meniscectomy on the knee joint evolved, treatment of symptomatic meniscal tears gravitated to repair of the tear, when possible, or partial meniscectomy.

The collagen meniscus implant (also referred to as collagen scaffold (CS), CMI or MenaflexTM meniscus implant throughout the published literature) is used to fill meniscal defects that result from partial meniscectomy. The collagen meniscus implant is not intended to replace the entire meniscus at it requires a meniscal rim for attachment. The literature describes the placement of the collagen meniscus implant through an arthroscopic procedure with an additional incision for capture of the repair needles and tying of the sutures. After debridement of the damaged meniscus, the implant is trimmed to the size of meniscal defect and sutured into place. The collagen meniscus implant is described as a tissue engineered scaffold to support the generation of new meniscus-like tissue. The collagen meniscus implant is manufactured from bovine collagen and should not be confused with the meniscus transplant which involves the replacement of the meniscus with a transplant meniscus from a cadaver donor. The meniscus transplant is not addressed under this national coverage determination.

B. Nationally Covered Indications

N/A

© 2019 Optum360, LLC

C. Nationally Non-Covered Indications

Effective for claims with dates of service performed on or after May 25, 2010, the Centers for Medicare & Medicaid Services has determined that the evidence is adequate to conclude that the collagen meniscus implant does not improve health outcomes and, therefore, is not reasonable and necessary for the treatment of meniscal injury/tear under section 1862(a)(1)(A) of the Social Security Act. Thus, the collagen meniscus implant is non-covered by Medicare.

D. Other

N/A

(This NCD last reviewed May 2010.)

100-03, 150.13

NCD for Percutaneous image-guided lumbar decompression for lumbar spinal stenosis (150.13)

(Rev.200, Issued: 07-25-17, Effective: 12- 07-16, Implementation: 06-27-17)

A. General

PILD is a posterior decompression of the lumbar spine performed under indirect image guidance without any direct visualization of the surgical area. This is a procedure proposed as a treatment for symptomatic LSS unresponsive to conservative therapy. This procedure is generally described as a non-invasive procedure using specially designed instruments to percutaneously remove a portion of the lamina and debulk the ligamentum flavum. The procedure is performed under x-ray guidance (e.g., fluoroscopic, CT) with the assistance of contrast media to identify and monitor the compressed area via epiduragram.

B. Nationally Covered Indications

Effective for dates of service specified below, the Centers for Medicare & Medicaid Services (CMS) has determined that PILD will be covered by Medicare when provided in a clinical study under section 1862(a)(1)(E) of the Social Security Act (the Act) through Coverage with Evidence Development (CED) for beneficiaries with LSS who are enrolled in an approved clinical study that meets the criteria in section I or II below:

I. Effective for services performed on or after January 9, 2014, PILD will be covered by Medicare through CED for beneficiaries with LSS who are enrolled in an approved clinical study that meets the following criteria. CMS has a particular interest in improved beneficiary function and quality of life, specific characteristics that identify patients who may benefit from the procedure, and the duration of benefit. A clinical study seeking Medicare payment for PILD for LSS must address one or more aspects of the following questions in a prospective, randomized, controlled design using current validated and reliable measurement instruments and clinically appropriate comparator treatments, including appropriate medical or surgical interventions or a sham controlled arm, for patients randomized to the non-PILD group.

The study protocol must specify a statistical analysis and a minimum length of patient follow up time that evaluates the effect of beneficiary characteristics on patient health outcomes as well as the duration of benefit.

i. Does PILD provide a clinically meaningful improvement of function and/or quality of life in Medicare beneficiaries with LSS compared to other treatments?

ii. Does PILD provide clinically meaningful reduction in pain in Medicare beneficiaries with LSS compared to other treatments?

iii. Does PILD affect the overall clinical management of LSS and decision making, including use of other medical treatments or services, compared to other treatments?

These studies must be designed so that the contribution of treatments in addition to the procedure under study are either controlled for or analyzed in such a way as to determine their impact.

a. The principal purpose of the research study is to test whether a particular intervention potentially improves the participants' health outcomes.

b. The research study is well supported by available scientific and medical information or it is intended to clarify or establish the health outcomes of interventions already in common clinical use.

c. The research study does not unjustifiably duplicate existing studies.

d. The research study design is appropriate to answer the research question being asked in the study.

e. The research study is sponsored by an organization or individual capable of executing the proposed study successfully.

f. The research study is in compliance with all applicable Federal regulations concerning the protection of human subjects found at 45 Code of Federal Regulations (CFR) Part 46. If a study is regulated by the Food and Drug Administration (FDA), it must be in compliance with 21 CFR parts 50 and 56.

g. All aspects of the research study are conducted according to appropriate standards of scientific integrity (see http://www.icmje.org).

h. The research study has a written protocol that clearly addresses, or incorporates by reference, the standards listed here as Medicare requirements for CED coverage.

i. The clinical research study is not designed to exclusively test toxicity or disease pathophysiology in healthy individuals. Trials of all medical technologies measuring therapeutic outcomes as one of the objectives meet this standard only if the disease or condition being studied is life threatening as defined in 21 CFR§312.81(a) and the patient has no other viable treatment options.

j. The clinical research study is registered on the ClinicalTrials.gov website by the principal sponsor/investigator prior to the enrollment of the first study subject.

k. The research study protocol specifies the method and timing of public release of all prespecified outcomes to be measured including release of outcomes if outcomes are negative or study is terminated early. The results must be made public within 24 months of the end of data collection. If a report is planned to be published in a peer reviewed journal, then that initial release may be an abstract that meets the requirements of the International Committee of Medical Journal Editors (http://www.icmje.org).

l. The research study protocol must explicitly discuss subpopulations affected by the treatment under investigation, particularly traditionally underrepresented groups in clinical studies, how the inclusion and exclusion criteria effect enrollment of these populations, and a plan for the retention and reporting of said populations on the trial. If the inclusion and exclusion criteria are expected to have a negative effect on the recruitment or retention of underrepresented populations, the protocol must discuss why these criteria are necessary.

m. The research study protocol explicitly discusses how the results are or are not expected to be generalizable to the Medicare population to infer whether Medicare patients may benefit from the intervention. Separate discussions in the protocol may be necessary for populations eligible for Medicare due to age, disability or Medicaid eligibility.

Consistent with section 1142 of the Act, the Agency for Healthcare Research and Quality (AHRQ) supports clinical research studies that CMS determines meet the above-listed standards and address the above-listed research questions.

II. Effective for services performed on or after December 7, 2016, CMS will cover through a prospective, longitudinal study for PILD procedures using a FDA-approved/cleared device that completed a CMS-approved randomized control trial (RCT) that met the criteria listed in section I above. ?The CMS-approved prospective, longitudinal study must answer at least one of the following questions:

i. Does PILD provide a clinically meaningful improvement of function (e.g., reduced acute and post-acute hospitalizations, nursing home care or inpatient rehabilitation services) and/or quality of life in Medicare beneficiaries with LSS compared to other treatments?

ii. Does PILD provide a clinically meaningful reduction in pain (e.g., as measured by class, dose, duration of prescription pain medication use) in Medicare beneficiaries with LSS compared to other treatments?

iii. Does PILD affect the overall clinical management of LSS and decision making, including use of other medical treatments or services (e.g., repeat PILD procedures, other interventions and surgical treatments), compared to other treatments?

The prospective, longitudinal study must also meet the following criteria:

1. The protocol must specify a statistical analysis and a minimum length of patient follow-up time that evaluates the effect of beneficiary characteristics on patient health outcomes as well as the duration of the benefit. 2. The eligibility requirements, both inclusion and exclusion criteria that were specified in the CMS-approved RCT protocol, must be maintained in the new prospective, longitudinal study. 3. All study sites and study results must be listed in the ClinicalTrials.gov database.

All CMS-approved clinical research studies must adhere to the following standards of scientific integrity and relevance to the Medicare population:

a. The principal purpose of the study is to test whether the item or service meaningfully improves health outcomes of affected beneficiaries who are represented by the enrolled subjects.

© 2019 Optum360, LLC

b. The rationale for the study is well supported by available scientific and medical evidence.

c. The study results are not anticipated to unjustifiably duplicate existing knowledge.

d. The study design is methodologically appropriate and the anticipated number of enrolled subjects is sufficient to answer the research question(s) being asked in the National Coverage Determination.

e. The study is sponsored by an organization or individual capable of completing it successfully.

f. The research study is in compliance with all applicable Federal regulations concerning the protection of human subjects found in the CFR at 45 CFR Part 46. If a study is regulated by the FDA, it is also in compliance with 21 CFR Parts 50 and 56. In addition, to further enhance the ?protection of human subjects in studies conducted under CED, the study must provide and obtain meaningful informed consent from patients regarding the risks associated with the study items and/or services, and the use and eventual disposition of the collected data.

g. All aspects of the study are conducted according to appropriate standards of scientific integrity.

h. The study has a written protocol that clearly demonstrates adherence to the standards listed here as Medicare requirements.

i. The study is not designed to exclusively test toxicity or disease pathophysiology in healthy individuals. Such studies may meet this requirement only if the disease or condition being studied is life threatening as defined in 21 CFR §312.81(a) and the patient has no other viable treatment options.

j. The clinical research studies and registries are registered on the www.ClinicalTrials.gov website by the principal sponsor/investigator prior to the enrollment of the first study subject. Registries are also registered in the AHRQ Registry of Patient Registries (RoPR).

k. The research study protocol specifies the method and timing of public release of all prespecified outcomes to be measured including release of outcomes if outcomes are negative or study is terminated early. The results must be made public within 12 months of the study's primary completion date, which is the date the final subject had final data collection for the primary endpoint, even if the trial does not achieve its primary aim. The results must include number started/completed, summary results for primary and secondary outcome measures, statistical analyses, and adverse events. Final results must be reported in a publicly accessibly manner; either in a peer-reviewed scientific journal (in print or on-line), in an on-line publicly accessible registry dedicated to the dissemination of clinical trial information such as ClinicalTrials.gov, or in journals willing to publish in abbreviated format (e.g., for studies with negative or incomplete results).

l. The study protocol must explicitly discuss beneficiary subpopulations affected by the item or service under investigation, particularly traditionally underrepresented groups in clinical studies, how the inclusion and exclusion criteria effect enrollment of these populations, and a plan for the retention and reporting of said populations in the trial. If the inclusion and exclusion criteria are expected to have a negative effect on the recruitment or retention of underrepresented populations, the protocol must discuss why these criteria are necessary.

m. The study protocol explicitly discusses how the results are or are not expected to be generalizable to affected beneficiary subpopulations. Separate discussions in the protocol may be necessary for populations eligible for Medicare due to age, disability or Medicaid eligibility. Consistent with section 1142 of the Act, tAHRQ supports clinical research studies that CMS determines meet the above-listed standards and address the above-listed research questions.

All clinical research study protocols must be reviewed and approved by CMS. The principal investigator must submit the complete study protocol, identify the relevant CMS research question(s) that will be addressed and cite the location of the detailed analysis plan for those questions in the protocol, plus provide a statement addressing how the study satisfies each of the standards of scientific integrity (a. through m. listed above), as well as the investigator's contact information, to the address below:

Director, Coverage and Analysis Group
Re: PILD CED
Centers for Medicare & Medicaid Services (CMS)
7500 Security Blvd., Mail Stop S3-02-01
Baltimore MD 21244-1850

Email address for protocol submissions: clinicalstudynotification@cms.hhs.gov

Email subject line: "CED [NCD topic (i.e. PILD)] [name of sponsor/primary investigator]"

The information will be reviewed, and approved studies will be identified on the CMS website -https://www.cms.gov/Medicare/Coverage/Coverage-with-Evidence-Development/index.html.

C. Nationally Non-Covered Indications

Effective for services performed on or after January 9, 2014, PILD for LSS may only be covered under the context of a clinical trial as described in section B above according to section 1862(a)(1)(E) of the Social Security Act. CMS has determined that PILD for LSS is not reasonable and necessary under section 1862(a)(1)(A) of the Act.

D. Other

Endoscopically assisted laminotomy/laminectomy, which requires open and direct visualization, as well as other open lumbar decompression procedures for LSS are not within the scope of this NCD and coverage is at contractor discretion.

(This NCD last reviewed December 2016.)

100-03, 160.13

NCD for Supplies Used in the Delivery of Transcutaneous Electrical Nerve Stimulation (TENS) and Neuromuscular Electrical Stimulation (NMES)

(Rev.173, Issued: 09-04-14, Effective: Upon Implementation: of ICD-10, Implementation: Upon Implemen)

Transcutaneous Electrical Nerve Stimulation (TENS) and/or Neuromuscular Electrical Stimulation (NMES) can ordinarily be delivered to patients through the use of conventional electrodes, adhesive tapes and lead wires. There may be times, however, where it might be medically necessary for certain patients receiving TENS or NMES treatment to use, as an alternative to conventional electrodes, adhesive tapes and lead wires, a form-fitting conductive garment (i.e., a garment with conductive fibers which are separated from the patients' skin by layers of fabric).

A form-fitting conductive garment (and medically necessary related supplies) may be covered under the program only when:

1. It has received permission or approval for marketing by the Food and Drug Administration;
2. It has been prescribed by a physician for use in delivering covered TENS or NMES treatment; and
3. One of the medical indications outlined below is met:
   - The patient cannot manage without the conductive garment because there is such a large area or so many sites to be stimulated and the stimulation would have to be delivered so frequently that it is not feasible to use conventional electrodes, adhesive tapes and lead wires;
   - The patient cannot manage without the conductive garment for the treatment of chronic intractable pain because the areas or sites to be stimulated are inaccessible with the use of conventional electrodes, adhesive tapes and lead wires;
   - The patient has a documented medical condition such as skin problems that preclude the application of conventional electrodes, adhesive tapes and lead wires;
   - The patient requires electrical stimulation beneath a cast either to treat disuse atrophy, where the nerve supply to the muscle is intact, or to treat chronic intractable pain; or
   - The patient has a medical need for rehabilitation strengthening (pursuant to a written plan of rehabilitation) following an injury where the nerve supply to the muscle is intact.

A conductive garment is not covered for use with a TENS device during the trial period specified in §160.3 unless:

4. The patient has a documented skin problem prior to the start of the trial period; and
5. The carrier's medical consultants are satisfied that use of such an item is medically necessary for the patient.

(See conditions for coverage of the use of TENS in the diagnosis and treatment of chronic intractable pain in §§160.3,160.13 and 160.27 and the use of NMES in the treatment of disuse atrophy in §150.4.)

 © 2019 Optum360, LLC

100-03, 160.27

NCD for Transcutaneous Electrical Nerve Stimulation (TENS) for Chronic Low Back Pain (CLBP)

(Rev.149, Issued: 11-30-12, Effective: 06-08-12, Implementation: 01-07-13)

The TENS is a type of electrical nerve stimulator that is employed to treat chronic intractable pain. This stimulator is attached to the surface of the patient's skin over the peripheral nerve to be stimulated. It may be applied in a variety of settings (in the patient's home, a physician's office, or in an outpatient clinic). Payment for TENS may be made under the durable medical equipment benefit.

A. General

For the purposes of this decision chronic low back pain (CLBP) is defined as:

1. an episode of low back pain that has persisted for three months or longer; and
2. is not a manifestation of a clearly defined and generally recognizable primary disease entity. For example, there are cancers that, through metastatic spread to the spine or pelvis, may elicit pain in the lower back as a symptom; and certain systemic diseases such as rheumatoid arthritis and multiple sclerosis manifest many debilitating symptoms of which low back pain is not the primary focus. B. Nationally Covered Indications Effective June 8, 2012, the Centers for Medicare & Medicaid Services (CMS) will allow coverage for Transcutaneous Electrical Nerve Stimulation (TENS) for CLBP only when all of the following conditions are met.

In order to support additional research on the use of TENS for CLBP, we will cover this item under section 1862(a)(1)(E) of the Social Security Act (the Act) subject to all of the following conditions:

1. Coverage under this section expires three years after the publication of this decision on the CMS website.
2. The beneficiary is enrolled in an approved clinical study meeting all of the requirements below. The study must address one or more aspects of the following questions in a randomized, controlled design using validated and reliable instruments. This can include randomized crossover designs when the impact of prior TENS use is appropriately accounted for in the study protocol.
   i. Does the use of TENS provide clinically meaningful reduction in pain in Medicare beneficiaries with CLBP?
   ii. Does the use of TENS provide a clinically meaningful improvement of function in Medicare beneficiaries with CLBP?
   iii. Does the use of TENS impact the utilization of other medical treatments or services used in the medical management of CLBP?

These studies must be designed so that the patients in the control and comparison groups receive the same concurrent treatments and either sham (placebo) TENS or active TENS intervention.

The study must adhere to the following standards of scientific integrity and relevance to the Medicare population:

a. The principal purpose of the research study is to test whether a particular intervention potentially improves the participants' health outcomes.
b. The research study is well supported by available scientific and medical information or it is intended to clarify or establish the health outcomes of interventions already in common clinical use.
c. The research study does not unjustifiably duplicate existing studies.
d. The research study design is appropriate to answer the research question being asked in the study.
e. The research study is sponsored by an organization or individual capable of executing the proposed study successfully. f. The research study is in compliance with all applicable Federal regulations concerning the protection of human subjects found at 45 CFR Part 46. If a study is regulated by the Food and Drug Administration (FDA), it must be in compliance with 21 CFR parts 50 and 56.
g. All aspects of the research study are conducted according to appropriate standards of scientific integrity (see http://www.icmje.org).
h. The research study has a written protocol that clearly addresses, or incorporates by reference, the standards listed here as Medicare requirements for CED coverage.
i. The clinical research study is not designed to exclusively test toxicity or disease pathophysiology in healthy individuals. Trials of all medical technologies measuring therapeutic outcomes as one of the objectives meet this standard only if the disease or condition being studied is life threatening as defined in 21 CFR § 312.81(a) and the patient has no other viable treatment options.
j. The clinical research study is registered on the ClinicalTrials.gov website by the principal sponsor/investigator prior to the enrollment of the first study subject.
k. The research study protocol specifies the method and timing of public release of all prespecified outcomes to be measured including release of outcomes if outcomes are negative or study is terminated early. The results must be made public within 24 months of the end of data collection. If a report is planned to be published in a peer reviewed journal, then that initial release may be an abstract that meets the requirements of the International Committee of Medical Journal Editors (http://www.icmje.org).
l. The research study protocol must explicitly discuss subpopulations affected by the treatment under investigation, particularly traditionally underrepresented groups in clinical studies, how the inclusion and exclusion criteria effect enrollment of these populations, and a plan for the retention and reporting of said populations on the trial. If the inclusion and exclusion criteria are expected to have a negative effect on the recruitment or retention of underrepresented populations, the protocol must discuss why these criteria are necessary
m. The research study protocol explicitly discusses how the results are or are not expected to be generalizable to the Medicare population to infer whether Medicare patients may benefit from the intervention. Separate discussions in the protocol may be necessary for populations eligible for Medicare due to age, disability or Medicaid eligibility. .

C. Nationally Non-Covered Indications

TENS is not reasonable and necessary for the treatment of CLBP under section 1862(a)(1)(A) of the Act.

D. Other

See §160.13 for an explanation of coverage of medically necessary supplies for the effective use of TENS. See §160.7.1 for an explanation of coverage for assessing patients suitability for electrical nerve stimulation therapy. See §10.2 for an explanation of coverage of transcutaneous electrical nerve stimulation (TENS) for acute post-operative pain. Please note, §280.13Transcutaneous Electrical Nerve Stimulators (TENS) NCD has been removed from the NCD manual and incorporated into NCD 160.27.

(This NCD last reviewed June 2012

100-03, 180.2

Enteral and Parenteral Nutritional Therapy

(Rev.173, Issued: 09-04-14, Effective: Upon Implementation: of ICD–10)

Covered As Prosthetic Device

There are patients who, because of chronic illness or trauma, cannot be sustained through oral feeding. These people must rely on either enteral or parenteral nutritional therapy, depending upon the particular nature of their medical condition.

Coverage of nutritional therapy as a Part B benefit is provided under the prosthetic device benefit provision which requires that the patient must have a permanently inoperative internal body organ or function thereof. Therefore, enteral and parenteral nutritional therapy are normally not covered under Part B in situations involving temporary impairments.

Coverage of such therapy, however, does not require a medical judgment that the impairment giving rise to the therapy will persist throughout the patient's remaining years. If the medical record, including the judgment of the attending physician, indicates that the impairment will be of long and indefinite duration, the test of permanence is considered met.

If the coverage requirements for enteral or parenteral nutritional therapy are met under the prosthetic device benefit provision, related supplies, equipment and nutrients are also covered under the conditions in the following paragraphs and the Medicare Benefit Policy Manual, Chapter 15, "Covered Medical and Other Health Services," §120.

Parenteral Nutrition Therapy Daily parenteral nutrition is considered reasonable and necessary for a patient with severe pathology of the alimentary tract which does not allow absorption of sufficient nutrients to maintain weight and strength commensurate with the patient's general condition.

Since the alimentary tract of such a patient does not function adequately, an indwelling catheter is placed percutaneously in the subclavian vein and then advanced into the superior vena cava where intravenous infusion of nutrients is given for part of the day. The catheter is then plugged by the patient until the next infusion. Following a period of hospitalization, which is required to initiate parenteral nutrition and to train the patient in catheter care, solution preparation, and infusion technique, the parenteral nutrition can be provided safely and effectively in the patient's home

© 2019 Optum360, LLC

by nonprofessional persons who have undergone special training. However, such persons cannot be paid for their services, nor is payment available for any services furnished by non-physician professionals except as services furnished incident to a physician's service.

For parenteral nutrition therapy to be covered under Part B, the claim must contain a physician's written order or prescription and sufficient medical documentation to permit an independent conclusion that the requirements of the prosthetic device benefit are met and that parenteral nutrition therapy is medically necessary. An example of a condition that typically qualifies for coverage is a massive small bowel resection resulting in severe nutritional deficiency in spite of adequate oral intake. However, coverage of parenteral nutrition therapy for this and any other condition must be approved on an individual, case-by-case basis initially and at periodic intervals of no more than three months by the Medicare Administrative Contractor (A/B MAC (B)) medical consultant or specially trained staff, relying on such medical and other documentation as the A/B MAC (B) may require. If the claim involves an infusion pump, sufficient evidence must be provided to support a determination of medical necessity for the pump. Program payment for the pump is based on the reasonable charge for the simplest model that meets the medical needs of the patient as established by medical documentation.

Nutrient solutions for parenteral therapy are routinely covered. However, Medicare pays for no more than one month's supply of nutrients at any one time. Payment for the nutrients is based on the reasonable charge for the solution components unless the medical record, including a signed statement from the attending physician, establishes that the beneficiary, due to his/her physical or mental state, is unable to safely or effectively mix the solution and there is no family member or other person who can do so. Payment will be on the basis of the reasonable charge for more expensive premixed solutions only under the latter circumstances.

Enteral Nutrition Therapy

Enteral nutrition is considered reasonable and necessary for a patient with a functioning gastrointestinal tract who, due to pathology to, or non-function of, the structures that normally permit food to reach the digestive tract, cannot maintain weight and strength commensurate with his or her general condition. Enteral therapy may be given by nasogastric, jejunostomy, or gastrostomy tubes and can be provided safely and effectively in the home by nonprofessional persons who have undergone special training. However, such persons cannot be paid for their services, nor is payment available for any services furnished by non-physician professionals except as services furnished incident to a physician's service.

Typical examples of conditions that qualify for coverage are head and neck cancer with reconstructive surgery and central nervous system disease leading to interference with the neuromuscular mechanisms of ingestion of such severity that the beneficiary cannot be maintained with oral feeding. However, claims for Part B coverage of enteral nutrition therapy for these and any other conditions must be approved on an individual, case-by-case basis. Each claim must contain a physician's written order or prescription and sufficient medical documentation (e.g., hospital records, clinical findings from the attending physician) to permit an independent conclusion that the patient's condition meets the requirements of the prosthetic device benefit and that enteral nutrition therapy is medically necessary. Allowed claims are to be reviewed at periodic intervals of no more than 3 months by the A/B MAC (B) medical consultant or specially trained staff, and additional medical documentation considered necessary is to be obtained as part of this review.

Medicare pays for no more than one month's supply of enteral nutrients at any one time.

If the claim involves a pump, it must be supported by sufficient medical documentation to establish that the pump is medically necessary, i.e., gravity feeding is not satisfactory due to aspiration, diarrhea, dumping syndrome. Program payment for the pump is based on the reasonable charge for the simplest model that meets the medical needs of the patient as established by medical documentation.

Nutritional Supplementation

Some patients require supplementation of their daily protein and caloric intake. Nutritional supplements are often given as a medicine between meals to boost protein-caloric intake or the mainstay of a daily nutritional plan. Nutritional supplementation is not covered under Medicare Part B.

100-03, 190.9

NCD for Serologic Testing for Acquired Immunodeficiency Syndrome (AIDS) (190.9)

(Rev.1, 10-03-03)

These tests may be covered when performed to help determine a diagnosis for symptomatic patients. They are not covered when furnished as part of a screening program for asymptomatic persons.

Note: Two enzyme-linked immunosorbent assay (ELISA) tests that were conducted on the same specimen must both be positive before Medicare will cover the Western blot test.

100-03, 190.11

NCD for Home Prothrombin Time International Normalized Ratio (INR) Monitoring for Anticoagulation Management (190.11)

(Rev.90, Issued: 07-25-08, Effective: 03-19-08, Implementation: 08-25-08)

A. General

Use of the International Normalized Ratio (INR) or prothrombin time (PT) - standard measurement for reporting the blood's clotting time) - allows physicians to determine the level of anticoagulation in a patient independent of the laboratory reagents used. The INR is the ratio of the patient's PT (extrinsic or tissue-factor dependent coagulation pathway) compared to the mean PT for a group of normal individuals. Maintaining patients within his/her prescribed therapeutic range minimizes adverse events associated with inadequate or excessive anticoagulation such as serious bleeding or thromboembolic events. Patient self-testing and self-management through the use of a home INR monitor may be used to improve the time in therapeutic rate (TTR) for select groups of patients. Increased TTR leads to improved clinical outcomes and reductions in thromboembolic and hemorrhagic events.

Warfarin (also prescribed under other trade names, e.g., Coumadin(R)) is a self-administered, oral anticoagulant (blood thinner) medication that affects the vitamin K- dependent clotting factors II, VII, IX and X. It is widely used for various medical conditions, and has a narrow therapeutic index, meaning it is a drug with less than a 2-fold difference between median lethal dose and median effective dose. For this reason, since October 4, 2006, it falls under the category of a Food and Drug administration (FDA) "black-box" drug whose dosage must be closely monitored to avoid serious complications. A PT/INR monitoring system is a portable testing device that includes a finger-stick and an FDA-cleared meter that measures the time it takes for a person's blood plasma to clot.

B. Nationally Covered Indications

For services furnished on or after March 19, 2008, Medicare will cover the use of home PT/INR monitoring for chronic, oral anticoagulation management for patients with mechanical heart valves, chronic atrial fibrillation, or venous thromboembolism (inclusive of deep venous thrombosis and pulmonary embolism) on warfarin. The monitor and the home testing must be prescribed by a treating physician as provided at 42 CFR 410.32(a), and all of the following requirements must be met:

1. The patient must have been anticoagulated for at least 3 months prior to use of the home INR device; and,
2. The patient must undergo a face-to-face educational program on anticoagulation management and must have demonstrated the correct use of the device prior to its use in the home; and,
3. The patient continues to correctly use the device in the context of the management of the anticoagulation therapy following the initiation of home monitoring; and,
4. Self-testing with the device should not occur more frequently than once a week.

C. Nationally Non-Covered Indications

N/A

D. Other

1. All other indications for home PT/INR monitoring not indicated as nationally covered above remain at local Medicare contractor discretion.
2. This national coverage determination (NCD) is distinct from, and makes no changes to, the PT clinical laboratory NCD at section 190.17 of Publication 100-03 of the NCD Manual.

100-03, 190.14

NCD for Human Immunodeficiency Virus (HIV) Testing (Diagnosis) (190.14)

(Rev.113, Issued: 02-19-10, Effective: 12-08-09, Implementation; 07-06-10)

Indications and Limitations of Coverage

Indications

Diagnostic testing to establish HIV infection may be indicated when there is a strong clinical suspicion supported by one or more of the following clinical findings:

The patient has a documented, otherwise unexplained, AIDS-defining or AIDS-associated opportunistic infection.

The patient has another documented sexually transmitted disease which identifies significant risk of exposure to HIV and the potential for an early or subclinical infection.

 © 2019 Optum360, LLC

The patient has documented acute or chronic hepatitis B or C infection that identifies a significant risk of exposure to HIV and the potential for an early or subclinical infection.

The patient has a documented AIDS-defining or AIDS-associated neoplasm.

The patient has a documented AIDS-associated neurologic disorder or otherwise unexplained dementia.

The patient has another documented AIDS-defining clinical condition, or a history of other severe, recurrent, or persistent conditions which suggest an underlying immune deficiency (for example, cutaneous or mucosal disorders).

The patient has otherwise unexplained generalized signs and symptoms suggestive of a chronic process with an underlying immune deficiency (for example, fever, weight loss, malaise, fatigue, chronic diarrhea, failure to thrive, chronic cough, hemoptysis, shortness of breath, or lymphadenopathy).

The patient has otherwise unexplained laboratory evidence of a chronic disease process with an underlying immune deficiency (for example, anemia, leukopenia, pancytopenia, lymphopenia, or low CD4+ lymphocyte count).

The patient has signs and symptoms of acute retroviral syndrome with fever, malaise, lymphadenopathy, and skin rash.

The patient has documented exposure to blood or body fluids known to be capable of transmitting HIV (for example, needlesticks and other significant blood exposures) and antiviral therapy is initiated or anticipated to be initiated.

The patient is undergoing treatment for rape. (HIV testing is a part of the rape treatment protocol.)

Limitations

HIV antibody testing in the United States is usually performed using HIV-1 or HIV-¬¾ combination tests. HIV-2 testing is indicated if clinical circumstances suggest HIV-2 is likely (that is, compatible clinical findings and HIV-1 test negative). HIV-2 testing may also be indicated in areas of the country where there is greater prevalence of HIV-2 infections.

The Western Blot test should be performed only after documentation that the initial EIA tests are repeatedly positive or equivocal on a single sample.

The HIV antigen tests currently have no defined diagnostic usage.

Direct viral RNA detection may be performed in those situations where serologic testing does not establish a diagnosis but strong clinical suspicion persists (for example, acute retroviral syndrome, nonspecific serologic evidence of HIV, or perinatal HIV infection).

If initial serologic tests confirm an HIV infection, repeat testing is not indicated.

If initial serologic tests are HIV EIA negative and there is no indication for confirmation of infection by viral RNA detection, the interval prior to retesting is 3-6 months.

Testing for evidence of HIV infection using serologic methods may be medically appropriate in situations where there is a risk of exposure to HIV. However, in the absence of a documented AIDS defining or HIV- associated disease, an HIV associated sign or symptom, or documented exposure to a known HIV-infected source, the testing is considered by Medicare to be screening and thus is not covered by Medicare (for example, history of multiple blood component transfusions, exposure to blood or body fluids not resulting in consideration of therapy, history of transplant, history of illicit drug use, multiple sexual partners, same-sex encounters, prostitution, or contact with prostitutes).

The CPT Editorial Panel has issued a number of codes for infectious agent detection by direct antigen or nucleic acid probe techniques that have not yet been developed or are only being used on an investigational basis. Laboratory providers are advised to remain current on FDA-approval status for these tests.

100-03, 200.1

Nesiritide for Treatment of Heart Failure Patients (Effective March 2, 2006)

(Rev.173, Issued: 09-04-14, Effective: Upon Implementation: of ICD–10)

A. General

Nesiritide (Natrecor®) is Food and Drug Administration (FDA)-approved for the intravenous treatment of patients with acutely decompensated congestive heart failure (CHF) who have dyspnea (shortness of breath) at rest or with minimal activity. Nesiritide is not self-administered.

B. Nationally Covered Indications

N/A

C. Nationally Non-Covered Indications

Effective for dates of service on or after March 2, 2006, the Centers for Medicare & Medicaid Services has determined that there is sufficient evidence to conclude that the use of Nesiritide for the treatment of CHF is not reasonable and necessary for Medicare beneficiaries in any setting.

D. Other

Effective for dates of service on or after March 2, 2006, this determination applies only to the treatment of CHF and does not change Medicare Administrative Contractor discretion to cover other off-label uses of Nesiritide or use consistent with the current FDA indication for intravenous treatment of patients with acutely decompensated CHF who have dyspnea at rest or with minimal activity.

100-03, 200.2

Nebulized Beta Adrenergic Agonist Therapy for Lung Diseases – (Effective September 10, 2007)

(Rev.173, Issued: 09-04-14, Effective: Upon Implementation: of ICD–10)

A. General

Lung diseases such as chronic obstructive pulmonary disease (COPD) and asthma are characterized by airflow limitation that may be partially or completely reversible. Pharmacologic treatment with bronchodilators is used to prevent and/or control daily symptoms that may cause disability for persons with these diseases. These medications are intended to improve the movement of air into and from the lungs by relaxing and dilating the bronchial passageways. Beta adrenergic agonists are a commonly prescribed class of bronchodilator drug. They can be administered via nebulizer, metered dose inhaler, orally, or dry powdered inhaler.

Nebulized beta adrenergic agonist with racemic albuterol has been used for many years. More recently, levalbuterol, the (R) enantiomer of racemic albuterol, has been used in some patient populations. There are concerns regarding the appropriate use of nebulized beta adrenergic agonist therapy for lung disease.

B. Nationally Covered Indications

N/A

C. Nationally Non-Covered Indications

N/A

D. Other

After examining the available medical evidence, the Centers for Medicare & Medicaid Services determines that no national coverage determination is appropriate at this time. Section 1862(a)(1)(A) of the Social Security Act decisions should be made by local Medicare Administrative Contractors through a local coverage determination process or case-by-case adjudication. See Heckler v. Ringer, 466 U.S. 602, 617 (1984) (Recognizing that the Secretary has discretion to either establish a generally applicable rule or to allow individual adjudication.). See also, 68 Fed. Reg. 63692, 63693 (November 7, 2003).

100-03, 210.2

Screening Pap Smears and Pelvic Examinations for Early Detection of Cervical or Vaginal Cancer (210.2)

(Rev.173, Issued: 09-04-14, Effective: Upon Implementation: of ICD–10)

Screening Pap Smear

A screening pap smear and related medically necessary services provided to a woman for the early detection of cervical cancer (including collection of the sample of cells and a physicianâ€™s interpretation of the test results) and pelvic examination (including clinical breast examination) are covered under Medicare Part B when ordered by a physician (or authorized practitioner) under one of the following conditions:

She has not had such a test during the preceding two years or is a woman of childbearing age (§1861(nn) of the Social Security Act (the Act).

There is evidence (on the basis of her medical history or other findings) that she is at high risk of developing cervical cancer and her physician (or authorized practitioner) recommends that she have the test performed more frequently than every two years.

High risk factors for cervical and vaginal cancer are:

- Early onset of sexual activity (under 16 years of age)
- Multiple sexual partners (five or more in a lifetime)
- History of sexually transmitted disease (including HIV infection)
- Fewer than three negative or any pap smears within the previous seven years; and
- DES (diethylstilbestrol) - exposed daughters of women who took DES during pregnancy.

NOTE: Claims for pap smears must indicate the beneficiary's low or high risk status by including the appropriate diagnosis code on the line item (Item 24E of the Form CMS-1500).

© 2019 Optum360, LLC

Definitions

A woman as described in §1861(nn) of the Act is a woman who is of childbearing age and has had a pap smear test during any of the preceding 3 years that indicated the presence of cervical or vaginal cancer or other abnormality, or is at high risk of developing cervical or vaginal cancer.

A woman of childbearing age is one who is premenopausal and has been determined by a physician or other qualified practitioner to be of childbearing age, based upon the medical history or other findings.

Other qualified practitioner, as defined in 42 CFR 410.56(a) includes a certified nurse midwife (as defined in §1861(gg) of the Act), or a physician assistant, nurse practitioner, or clinical nurse specialist (as defined in §1861(aa) of the Act) who is authorized under State law to perform the examination.

Screening Pelvic Examination

Section 4102 of the Balanced Budget Act of 1997 provides for coverage of screening pelvic examinations (including a clinical breast examination) for all female beneficiaries, subject to certain frequency and other limitations. A screening pelvic examination (including a clinical breast examination) should include at least seven of the following eleven elements:

Inspection and palpation of breasts for masses or lumps, tenderness, symmetry, or nipple discharge.

Digital rectal examination including sphincter tone, presence of hemorrhoids, and rectal masses. Pelvic examination (with or without specimen collection for smears and cultures) including:

- External genitalia (for example, general appearance, hair distribution, or lesions).
- Urethral meatus (for example, size, location, lesions, or prolapse).
- Urethra (for example, masses, tenderness, or scarring).
- Bladder (for example, fullness, masses, or tenderness).
- Vagina (for example, general appearance, estrogen effect, discharge lesions, pelvic support, cystocele, or rectocele).
- Cervix (for example, general appearance, lesions, or discharge).
- Uterus (for example, size, contour, position, mobility, tenderness, consistency, descent, or support).
- Adnexa/parametria (for example, masses, tenderness, organomegaly, or nodularity).
- Anus and perineum.

This description is from Documentation Guidelines for Evaluation and Management Services, published in May 1997 and was developed by the Centers for Medicare & Medicaid Services and the American Medical Association.

100-03, 210.2.1

Screening for Cervical Cancer with Human Papillomavirus (HPV) Testing

(Rev.189, Iss: 2-5-16, Eff: 7-5-16; Imp: 3-7-16 - non-shared MAC edits 7-5-16 - CWF analysis)

A. General

Medicare covers a screening pelvic examination and Pap test for all female beneficiaries at 12 or 24 month intervals, based on specific risk factors. See 42 C.F.R. §410.56; Medicare National Coverage Determinations Manual, §210.2.1 Current Medicare coverage does not include the HPV testing. Pursuant to §1861(ddd) of the Social Security Act, the Secretary may add coverage of "additional preventive services" if certain statutory requirements are met.

B. Nationally Covered Indications

Effective for services performed on or after July 9, 2015, CMS has determined that the evidence is sufficient to add Human Papillomavirus (HPV) testing once every five years as an additional preventive service benefit under the Medicare program for asymptomatic beneficiaries aged 30 to 65 years in conjunction with the Pap smear test. CMS will cover screening for cervical cancer with the appropriate U.S. Food and Drug Administration (FDA) approved/cleared laboratory tests, used consistent with FDA approved labeling and in compliance with the Clinical Laboratory Improvement Act (CLIA) regulations.

C. Nationally Non-Covered Indications

Unless specifically covered in this NCD, any other NCD, by statute or regulation, preventive services are non-covered by Medicare.

D. Other

(This NCD last reviewed July 2015.)

100-03, 210.4.1

Counseling to Prevent Tobacco Use (Effective August 25, 2010)

(Rev.202, Issued: 08-25-17, Effective: 09-26-17, Implementation: 09- 26-17)

A. General

Tobacco use remains the leading cause of preventable morbidity and mortality in the U.S. and is a major contributor to the nation's increasing medical costs. Despite the growing list of adverse health effects associated with smoking, more than 45 million U.S. adults continue to smoke and approximately 1,200 die prematurely each day from tobacco-related diseases. Annual smoking-attributable expenditures can be measured both in direct medical costs ($96 billion) and in lost productivity ($97 billion), but the results of national surveys have raised concerns that recent declines in smoking prevalence among U.S. adults may have come to an end. According to the U.S. Department of Health and Human Services (DHHS) Public Health Service (PHS) Clinical Practice Guideline on Treating Tobacco Use and Dependence (2008), 4.5 million adults over 65 years of age smoke cigarettes. Even smokers over age 65, however, can benefit greatly from abstinence, and older smokers who quit can reduce their risk of death from coronary heart disease, chronic obstructive lung disease and lung cancer, as well as decrease their risk of osteoporosis.

B. Nationally Covered Indications

Effective for claims with dates of service on or after August 25, 2010, CMS will cover tobacco cessation counseling for outpatient and hospitalized Medicare beneficiaries

1. Who use tobacco, regardless of whether they have signs or symptoms of tobacco-related disease;
2. Who are competent and alert at the time that counseling is provided; and,
3. Whose counseling is furnished by a qualified physician or other Medicare-recognized practitioner.

Intermediate and intensive smoking cessation counseling services will be covered under Medicare Part B when the above conditions of coverage are met, subject to frequency and other limitations. That is, similar to existing tobacco cessation counseling for symptomatic individuals, CMS will allow 2 individual tobacco cessation counseling attempts per 12-month period. Each attempt may include a maximum of 4 intermediate OR intensive sessions, with a total benefit covering up to 8 sessions per 12-month period per Medicare beneficiary who uses tobacco. The practitioner and patient have the flexibility to choose between intermediate (more than 3 minutes but less than 10 minutes), or intensive (more than 10 minutes) cessation counseling sessions for each attempt.

C. Nationally Non-Covered Indications

Inpatient hospital stays with the principal diagnosis of tobacco use disorder are not reasonable and necessary for the effective delivery of tobacco cessation counseling services. Therefore, we will not cover tobacco cessation services if tobacco cessation is the primary reason for the patient's hospital stay.

D. Other

Section 4104 of the Affordable Care Act provided for a waiver of the Medicare coinsurance and Part B deductible requirements for this service effective on or after January 1, 2011. Until that time, this service will continue to be subject to the standard Medicare coinsurance and Part B deductible requirements.

100-03, 210.6

Screening for Hepatitis B Virus (HBV) Infection

(Rev.198, Issued: 06-29-17, Effective: 09-28-16, Implementation: 10- 02- 17, October 2, 2017 - analysis and design; January 2, 2018 - testing and implementation)

A. General

Hepatitis B Virus (HBV) is transmitted by exposure to blood or bloodcontaining body fluids such as serum, semen or saliva. HBV infection attacks the liver and leads to inflammation. An infected person may initially develop symptoms such as nausea, anorexia, fatigue, fever and abdominal pain, or may be asymptomatic. An acute HBV infection may become a chronic infection and progress to serious and potentially lifethreatening complications including cirrhosis, liver failure, hepatocellular carcinoma and death.

Pursuant to §1861(ddd) of the Social Security Act, the Secretary may add coverage of "additional preventive services" if certain statutory requirements are met.

B. Nationally Covered Indications

Effective for services performed on or after September 28, 2016, CMS has determined that the evidence is sufficient to cover screening for HBV infection with the appropriate U.S. Food and Drug Administration (FDA) approved/cleared laboratory tests, used consistent with FDA approved labeling and in compliance with the Clinical Laboratory Improvement Act (CLIA) regulations, when ordered by the beneficiary's primary care physician or practitioner within the context of a primary care setting, and performed by an eligible Medicare provider for these services, for beneficiaries who meet either of the following conditions.

1. A screening test is covered for asymptomatic, nonpregnant adolescents and adults at high risk for HBV infection. "High risk" is defined as persons born in countries and regions with a high prevalence of HBV infection (i.e., ≥ 2%), USborn persons not

© 2019 Optum360, LLC

vaccinated as infants whose parents were born in regions with a very high prevalence of HBV infection (i.e., ≥ 8%), HIVpositive persons, men who have sex with men, injection drug users, household contacts or sexual partners of persons with HBV infection. In addition, CMS has determined that repeated screening would be appropriate annually only for beneficiaries with continued high risk (i.e., men who have sex with men, injection drug users, household contacts or sexual partners of persons with HBV infection) who do not receive hepatitis B vaccination.

2. A screening test at the first prenatal visit is covered for pregnant women and then rescreening at time of delivery for those with new or continuing risk

factors. In addition, CMS has determined that screening during the first prenatal visit would be appropriate for each pregnancy, regardless of previous hepatitis B vaccination or previous negative HBsAg test results.

The determination of "high risk for HBV" is identified by the primary care physician or practitioner whoassesses the patient's history, which is part of any complete medical history, typically part of an annual wellness visit and considered in the development of a comprehensive prevention plan. The medical record should be a reflection of the service provided.

For the purposes of this decision memorandum, a primary care setting is defined by the provision of integrated, accessible health care services by clinicians who are accountable for addressing a large majority of personal health care needs, developing a sustained partnership with patients, and practicing in the context of family and community. Emergency departments, inpatient hospital settings, ambulatory surgical centers, skilled nursing facilities, inpatient rehabilitation facilities, clinics providing a limited focus of health care services, and hospice are examples of settings not considered primary care settings under this definition.

For the purposes of this decision memorandum, a "primary care physician" and "primary carepractitioner" will be defined consistent with existing sections of the Social Security Act (§1833(u)(6), §1833(x) (2)(A)(i)(I) and §1833(x)(2)(A)(i)(II)).

§1833(u)

(6) Physician Defined.—For purposes of this paragraph, the term "physician" means a physician described in section 1861(r)(1) and the term "primary care physician" means a physician who is identified in the available data as a general practitioner, family practice practitioner, general internist, or obstetrician or gynecologist.

§1833(x)(2)(A)(i)

(I) is a physician (as described in section 1861(r)(1)) who has a primary specialty designation of family medicine, internal medicine, geriatric medicine, or pediatric medicine; or

(II) is a nurse practitioner, clinical nurse specialist, or physician assistant (as those terms are defined in section 1861(aa)(5)).

C. Nationally NonCovered Indications

Effective for claims with dates of service on and after September 28, 2016:

- Medicare beneficiaries who are symptomatic, or who have already been diagnosed with HBV infection, or who are nonpregnant and have already received a hepatitis B vaccination are noncovered.

D. Other

Medicare coinsurance and the Part B deductible are waived for this "additional preventive service."

(NCD updated September 2016)

100-03, 210.7

Screening for the Human Immunodeficiency Virus (HIV) Infection

(Rev.190, Iss: 2-5-16; Eff: 4-13-15; Imp: 3-7-16 - non-shared A/B MAC edits, 7-5-16 - CWF)

A. General

Infection with the human immunodeficiency virus (HIV) is a continuing, worldwide pandemic described by the World Health Organization as "the most serious infectious disease challenge to global public health". Acquired immunodeficiency syndrome (AIDS) is diagnosed when a HIV-infected person's immune system becomes severely compromised and/or a person becomes ill with a HIV-related opportunistic infection. Without treatment, AIDS usually develops within 8-10 years after a person's initial HIV infection. While there is presently no cure for HIV, an infected individual can be recognized by screening, and subsequent access to skilled care plus vigilant monitoring and adherence to continuous antiretroviral therapy may delay the onset of AIDS and increase quality of life for many years.

Significantly, more than half of new HIV infections are estimated to be sexually transmitted from infected individuals who are unaware of their HIV status. Consequently, improved secondary disease prevention and wider availability of screening linked to HIV care and treatment would not only delay disease progression and complications in untested or unaware older individuals, but could also decrease the spread of disease to those living with or partnered with HIV-infected individuals.

HIV antibody testing first became available in 1985. These commonly used, Food and Drug Administration (FDA)-approved HIV antibody screening tests – using serum or plasma from a venipuncture or blood draw – are known as EIA (enzyme immunoassay) or ELISA (enzyme-linked immunosorbent assay) tests.

Developed for point-of-care testing using alternative samples, six rapid HIV-1 and/or HIV-2 antibody tests – using fluid obtained from the oral cavity or using whole blood, serum, or plasma from a blood draw or fingerstick – were approved by the FDA from 2002-2006.

Effective January 1, 2009, the Centers for Medicare & Medicaid Services (CMS) is allowed to add coverage of "additional preventive services" through the national coverage determination (NCD) process if certain statutory requirements are met, as provided under section 101(a) of the Medicare Improvements for Patients and Providers Act. One of those requirements is that the service(s) be categorized as a grade A (strongly recommends) or grade B (recommends) rating by the US Preventive Services Task Force (USPSTF). The USPSTF strongly recommends screening for all adolescents and adults at risk for HIV infection, as well as all pregnant women.

B. Nationally Covered Indications

Effective for claims with dates of service on and after December 8, 2009, CMS determines that the evidence is adequate to conclude that screening for HIV infection is reasonable and necessary for early detection of HIV and is appropriate for individuals entitled to benefits under

Part A or enrolled under Part B. Therefore, CMS proposes to cover both standard and FDA-approved HIV rapid screening tests for:

1. A maximum of one, annual voluntary HIV screening of Medicare beneficiaries at increased risk for HIV infection per USPSTF guidelines as follows:
   - Men who have had sex with men after 1975
   - Men and women having unprotected sex with multiple [more than one] partners
   - Past or present injection drug users
   - Men and women who exchange sex for money or drugs, or have sex partners who do
   - Individuals whose past or present sex partners were HIV-infected, bisexual or injection drug users
   - Persons being treated for sexually transmitted diseases
   - Persons with a history of blood transfusion between 1978 and 1985
   - Persons who request an HIV test despite reporting no individual risk factors, since this group is likely to include individuals not willing to disclose high-risk behaviors; and,
2. A maximum of three, voluntary HIV screenings of pregnant Medicare beneficiaries: (1) when the diagnosis of pregnancy is known, (2) during the third trimester, and (3) at labor, if ordered by the woman's clinician.

C. Nationally Non-Covered Indications

Effective for claims with dates of service on and after December 8, 2009, Medicare beneficiaries with any known diagnosis of a HIV-related illness are not eligible for this screening test.

Medicare beneficiaries (other than those who are pregnant) who have had a prior HIV screening test within one year are not eligible (11 full months must have elapsed following the month in which the previous test was performed in order for the subsequent test to be covered).

Pregnant Medicare beneficiaries who have had three screening tests within their respective term of pregnancy are not eligible (beginning with the date of the first test).

D. Other

N/A

(This NCD last reviewed November 2009.)

100-03, 210.8

Screening and Behavioral Counseling Interventions in Primary Care to Reduce Alcohol Misuse (Effective October 14, 2011)

(Rev.138, Issued: 11-23-11, Effective: 10-14-11, Implementation: 12-27-11 non-system changes, 04-02-1)

A. General

Based upon authority to cover "additional preventive services" for Medicare beneficiaries if certain statutory requirements are met, the Centers for Medicare & Medicaid Services (CMS) initiated a new national coverage analysis on annual screening and brief behavioral counseling in primary care to reduce alcohol misuse in

© 2019 Optum360, LLC

adults, including pregnant women. Annual screening and behavioral counseling for alcohol misuse in adults is recommended with a grade of B by the U.S. Preventive Services Task Force (USPSTF) and is appropriate for individuals entitled to benefits under Part A and Part B.

CMS will cover annual alcohol screening and up to four, brief face-to-face behavioral counseling in primary care settings to reduce alcohol misuse. CMS does not identify specific alcohol misuse screening tools. Rather, the decision to use a specific tool is at the discretion of the clinician in the primary care setting. Various screening tools are available for screening for alcohol misuse.

B. Nationally Covered Indications

Effective for claims with dates of service on or after October 14, 2011, CMS will cover annual alcohol screening, and for those that screen positive, up to four brief, face-to-face, behavioral counseling interventions per year for Medicare beneficiaries, including pregnant women:

- Who misuse alcohol, but whose levels or patterns of alcohol consumption do not meet criteria for alcohol dependence (defined as at least three of the following: tolerance, withdrawal symptoms, impaired control, preoccupation with acquisition and/or use, persistent desire or unsuccessful efforts to quit, sustains social, occupational, or recreational disability, use continues despite adverse consequences); and
- Who are competent and alert at the time that counseling is provided; and,
- Whose counseling is furnished by qualified primary care physicians or other primary care practitioners in a primary care setting.

Each of the behavioral counseling interventions should be consistent with the 5A' approach that has been adopted by the USPSTF to describe such services. They are:

1. Assess: Ask about/assess behavioral health risk(s) and factors affecting choice of behavior change goals/methods.
2. Advise: Give clear, specific, and personalized behavior change advice, including information about personal health harms and benefits.
3. Agree: Collaboratively select appropriate treatment goals and methods based on the patient's interest in and willingness to change the behavior.
4. Assist: Using behavior change techniques (self-help and/or counseling), aid the patient in achieving agreed upon goals by acquiring the skills, confidence, and social/environmental supports for behavior change, supplemented with adjunctive medical treatments when appropriate.
5. Arrange: Schedule follow-up contacts (in person or by telephone) to provide ongoing assistance/support and to adjust the treatment plan as needed, including referral to more intensive or specialized treatment. For the purposes of this policy, a primary care setting is defined as one in which there is provision of integrated, accessible health care services by clinicians who are accountable for addressing a large majority of personal health care needs, developing a sustained partnership with patients, and practicing in the context of family and community. Emergency departments, inpatient hospital settings, ambulatory surgical centers, independent diagnostic testing facilities, skilled nursing facilities, inpatient rehabilitation facilities and hospices are not considered primary care settings under this definition.

For the purposes of this policy a "primary care physician" and "primary care practitioner" are to be defined based on two existing sections of the Social Security Act, §1833(u)(6), §1833(x)(2)(A)(i)(I) and §1833(x)(2)(A)(i)(II):

§1833(u)

(6)Physician Defined.—For purposes of this paragraph, the term "physician" means a physician described in section 1861(r)(1) and the term "primary care physician" means a physician who is identified in the available data as a general practitioner, family practice practitioner, general internist, or obstetrician or gynecologist.

§1833(x)(2)(A)(i)

(I) is a physician (as described in section 1861(r)(1)) who has a primary specialty designation of family medicine, internal medicine, geriatric medicine, or pediatric medicine; or

(II) is a nurse practitioner, clinical nurse specialist, or physician assistant (as those terms are defined in section 1861(aa)(5)).

C. Nationally Non-Covered Indications

1. Alcohol screening is non-covered when performed more than one time in a 12-month period.
2. Brief face-to-face behavioral counseling interventions are non-covered when performed more than once a day; that is, two counseling interventions on the same day are non-covered.
3. Brief face-to-face behavioral counseling interventions are non-covered when performed more than four times in a 12-month period

D. Other

Medicare coinsurance and Part B deductible are waived for this preventive service

(This NCD last reviewed October 2011.)

100-03, 210.10

Screening for Sexually Transmitted Infections (STIs) and High Intensity Behavioral Counseling (HIBC) to Prevent STIs

(Rev.141, Issued: 01-26-12, Effective: 11-08-2011, Implementation: 02-27-12)

A. General

Sexually transmitted infections (STIs) are infections that are passed from one person to another through sexual contact. STIs remain an important cause of morbidity in the United States and have both health and economic consequences. Many of the complications of STIs are borne by women and children Often, STIs do not present any symptoms so can go untreated for long periods of time The presence of an STI during pregnancy may result in significant health complications for the woman and infant. In fact, any person who has an STI may develop health complications. Screening tests for the STIs in this national coverage determination (NCD) are laboratory tests.

Under §1861(ddd) of the Social Security Act (the Act), the Centers for Medicare & Medicaid Services (CMS) has the authority to add coverage of additional preventive services if certain statutory requirements are met. The regulations provide:

§410.64 Additional preventive services

(a) Medicare Part B pays for additional preventive services not described in paragraph (1) or (3) of the definition of "preventive services" under §410.2, that identify medical conditions or risk factors for individuals if the Secretary determines through the national coverage determination process (as defined in section 1869(f)(1)(B) of the Act) that these services are all of the following: (1) reasonable and necessary for the prevention or early detection of illness or disability.(2) recommended with a grade of A or B by the United States Preventive Services Task Force, (3) appropriate for individuals entitled to benefits under Part A or enrolled under Part B.

(b) In making determinations under paragraph (a) of this section regarding the coverage of a new preventive service, the Secretary may conduct an assessment of the relation between predicted outcomes and the expenditures for such services and may take into account the results of such an assessment in making such national coverage determinations.

The scope of the national coverage analysis for this NCD evaluated the evidence for the following STIs and high intensity behavioral counseling (HIBC) to prevent STIs for which the United States Preventive Services Task Force (USPSTF) has issued either an A or B recommendation:

- Screening for chlamydial infection for all sexually active non-pregnant young women aged 24 and younger and for older non-pregnant women who are at increased risk,
- Screening for chlamydial infection for all pregnant women aged 24 and younger and for older pregnant women who are at increased risk,
- Screening for gonorrhea infection in all sexually active women, including those who are pregnant, if they are at increased risk,
- Screening for syphilis infection for all pregnant women and for all persons at increased risk,
- Screening for hepatitis B virus (HBV) infection in pregnant women at their first prenatal visit,
- HIBC for the prevention of STIs for all sexually active adolescents, and for adults at increased risk for STIs.

B. Nationally Covered Indications

CMS has determined that the evidence is adequate to conclude that screening for chlamydia, gonorrhea, syphilis, and hepatitis B, as well as HIBC to prevent STIs, consistent with the grade A and B recommendations by the USPSTF, is reasonable and necessary for the early detection or prevention of an illness or disability and is appropriate for individuals entitled to benefits under Part A or enrolled under Part B.

Therefore, effective for claims with dates of services on or after November 8, 2011, CMS will cover screening for these USPSTF-indicated STIs with the appropriate Food and Drug Administration (FDA)-approved/cleared laboratory tests, used consistent with FDA-approved labeling, and in compliance with the Clinical Laboratory Improvement Act (CLIA) regulations, when ordered by the primary care physician or practitioner, and performed by an eligible Medicare provider for these services.

 © 2019 Optum360, LLC

Screening for chlamydia and gonorrhea:

- Pregnant women who are 24 years old or younger when the diagnosis of pregnancy is known, and then repeat screening during the third trimester if high-risk sexual behavior has occurred since the initial screening test.
- Pregnant women who are at increased risk for STIs when the diagnosis of pregnancy is known, and then repeat screening during the third trimester if high-risk sexual behavior has occurred since the initial screening test.
- Women at increased risk for STIs annually.

Screening for syphilis:

- Pregnant women when the diagnosis of pregnancy is known, and then repeat screening during the third trimester and at delivery if high-risk sexual behavior has occurred since the previous screening test.
- Men and women at increased risk for STIs annually.

Screening for hepatitis B:

- Pregnant women at the first prenatal visit when the diagnosis of pregnancy is known, and then rescreening at time of delivery for those with new or continuing risk factors. In addition, effective for claims with dates of service on or after November 8, 2011, CMS will cover up to two individual 20- to 30-minute, face-to-face counseling sessions annually for Medicare beneficiaries for HIBC to prevent STIs, for all sexually active adolescents, and for adults at increased risk for STIs, if referred for this service by a primary care physician or practitioner, and provided by a Medicare eligible primary care provider in a primary care setting. Coverage of HIBC to prevent STIs is consistent with the USPSTF recommendation.

HIBC is defined as a program intended to promote sexual risk reduction or risk avoidance, which includes each of these broad topics, allowing flexibility for appropriate patient-focused elements:

- education,
- skills training,
- guidance on how to change sexual behavior.

The high/increased risk individual sexual behaviors, based on the USPSTF guidelines, include any of the following:

- Multiple sex partners
- Using barrier protection inconsistently
- Having sex under the influence of alcohol or drugs
- Having sex in exchange for money or drugs
- Age (24 years of age or younger and sexually active for women for chlamydia and gonorrhea)
- Having an STI within the past year
- IV drug use (for hepatitis B only)

In addition for men

- men having sex with men (MSM) and engaged in high risk sexual behavior, but no regard to age

In addition to individual risk factors, in concurrence with the USPSTF recommendations, community social factors such as high prevalence of STIs in the community populations should be considered in determining high/increased risk for chlamydia, gonorrhea, syphilis, and for recommending HIBC.

High/increased risk sexual behavior for STIs is determined by the primary care provider by assessing the patient's sexual history which is part of any complete medical history, typically part of an annual wellness visit or prenatal visit and considered in the development of a comprehensive prevention plan. The medical record should be a reflection of the service provided.

For the purposes of this NCD, a primary care setting is defined as the provision of integrated, accessible health care services by clinicians who are accountable for addressing a large majority of personal health care needs, developing a sustained partnership with patients, and practicing in the context of family and community. Emergency departments, inpatient hospital settings, ambulatory surgical centers, independent diagnostic testing facilities, skilled nursing facilities, inpatient rehabilitation facilities, clinics providing a limited focus of health care services, and hospice are examples of settings not considered primary care settings under this definition.

For the purposes of this NCD, a "primary care physician" and "primary care practitioner" will be defined based on existing sections of the Social Security Act (§1833(u)(6), §1833(x)(2)(A)(i)(I) and §1833(x)(2)(A)(i)(II)).

§1833(u)

(6) Physician Defined.?or purposes of this paragraph, the term "physician" means a physician described in section 1861(r)(1) and the term "primary care physician" means a physician who is identified in the available data as a general practitioner, family practice practitioner, general internist, or obstetrician or gynecologist.

§1833(x)(2)(A)(i)

(I) is a physician (as described in section 1861(r)(1)) who has a primary specialty designation of family medicine, internal medicine, geriatric medicine, or pediatric medicine; or

(II) is a nurse practitioner, clinical nurse specialist, or physician assistant (as those terms are defined in section 1861(aa)(5));

C. Nationally Non-Covered Indications

Unless specifically covered in this NCD, any other NCD, or in statute, preventive services are non-covered by Medicare.

D. Other

Medicare coinsurance and Part B deductible are waived for these preventive services.

HIBC to prevent STIs may be provided on the same date of services as an annual wellness visit, evaluation and management (E&M) service, or during the global billing period for obstetrical car, but only one HIBC may be provided on any one date of service. See the claims processing manual for further instructions on claims processing.

For services provided on an annual basis, this is defined as a 12-month period.

(This NCD last reviewed November 2011.)

100-03, 210.11

Intensive Behavioral Therapy for Cardiovascular Disease (CVD) (Effective November 8, 2011

(Rev.137, Issued: 11-23-11, Effective: 11-08-11, Implementation: 12-27-11 non-shared system edits, 0)

A. General

Cardiovascular disease (CVD) is the leading cause of mortality in the United States. CVD, which is comprised of hypertension, coronary heart disease (such as myocardial infarction and angina pectoris), heart failure and stroke, is also the leading cause of hospitalizations. Although the overall adjusted mortality rate from heart disease has declined over the past decade, opportunities for improvement still exist. Risk factors for CVD include being overweight, obesity, physical inactivity, diabetes, cigarette smoking, high blood pressure, high blood cholesterol, family history of myocardial infarction, and older age.

Under §1861(ddd) of the Social Security Act (the Act), the Centers for Medicare & Medicaid Services (CMS) has the authority to add coverage of additional preventive services through the National Coverage Determination (NCD) process if certain statutory requirements are met. Following its review, CMS has determined that the evidence is adequate to conclude that intensive behavioral therapy for CVD is reasonable and necessary for the prevention or early detection of illness or disability, is appropriate for individuals entitled to benefits under Part A or enrolled under Part B, and is comprised of components that are recommended with a grade of A or B by the U.S. Preventive Services Task Force (USPSTF).

B. Nationally Covered Indications

Effective for claims with dates of service on or after November 8, 2011, CMS covers intensive behavioral therapy for CVD (referred to below as a CVD risk reduction visit), which consists of the following three components:

- encouraging aspirin use for the primary prevention of CVD when the benefits outweigh the risks for men age 45-79 years and women 55-79 years;
- screening for high blood pressure in adults age 18 years and older; and
- intensive behavioral counseling to promote a healthy diet for adults with hyperlipidemia, hypertension, advancing age, and other known risk factors for cardiovascular- and diet-related chronic disease.

We note that only a small proportion (about 4%) of the Medicare population is under 45 years (men) or 55 years (women), therefore the vast majority of beneficiaries should receive all three components. Intensive behavioral counseling to promote a healthy diet is broadly recommended to cover close to 100% of the population due to the prevalence of known risk factors.

Therefore, CMS covers one, face-to-face CVD risk reduction visit per year for Medicare beneficiaries who are competent and alert at the time that counseling is provided, and whose counseling is furnished by a qualified primary care physician or other primary care practitioner in a primary care setting.

The behavioral counseling intervention for aspirin use and healthy diet should be consistent with the Five As approach that has been adopted by the USPSTF to describe such services:

© 2019 Optum360, LLC

- Assess: Ask about/assess behavioral health risk(s) and factors affecting choice of behavior change goals/methods.
- Advise: Give clear, specific, and personalized behavior change advice, including information about personal health harms and benefits.
- Agree: Collaboratively select appropriate treatment goals and methods based on the patient's interest in and willingness to change the behavior.
- Assist: Using behavior change techniques (self-help and/or counseling), aid the patient in achieving agreed-upon goals by acquiring the skills, confidence, and social/environmental supports for behavior change, supplemented with adjunctive medical treatments when appropriate.
- Arrange: Schedule follow-up contacts (in person or by telephone) to provide ongoing assistance/support and to adjust the treatment plan as needed, including referral to more intensive or specialized treatment. For the purpose of this NCD, a primary care setting is defined as the provision of integrated, accessible health care services by clinicians who are accountable for addressing a large majority of personal health care needs, developing a sustained partnership with patients, and practicing in the context of family and community. Emergency departments, inpatient hospital settings, ambulatory surgical centers, independent diagnostic testing facilities, skilled nursing facilities, inpatient rehabilitation facilities, and hospices are not considered primary care settings under this definition.

For the purpose of this NCD, a "primary care physician" and "primary care practitioner" are defined consistent with existing sections of the Act (§1833(u)(6), §1833(x)(2)(A)(i)(I) and §1833(x)(2)(A)(i)(II)).

§1833(u)

(6) Physician Defined.?or purposes of this paragraph, the term "physician" means a physician described in section 1861(r)(1) and the term "primary care physician" means a physician who is identified in the available data as a general practitioner, family practice practitioner, general internist, or obstetrician or gynecologist.

§1833(x)(2)

(A) Primary care practitioner. he term "primary care practitioner" means an individual—

(i) who—

(I) is a physician (as described in section 1861(r)(1)) who has a primary specialty designation of family medicine, internal medicine, geriatric medicine, or pediatric medicine; or

(II) is a nurse practitioner, clinical nurse specialist, or physician assistant (as those terms are defined in section 1861(aa)(5)).

C. Nationally Non-Covered Indications

Unless specifically covered in this NCD, any other NCD, or in statute, preventive services are non-covered by Medicare.

D. Other

Medicare coinsurance and Part B deductible are waived for this preventive service.

(This NCD last reviewed November 2011.)

100-03, 210.12

Intensive Behavioral Therapy for Obesity (Effective November 29, 2011)

(Rev.142, issued: 02-03-12, Effective: 11-29-11, Implementation: 03-06-12)

A. General

Based upon authority to cover "additional preventive services" for Medicare beneficiaries if certain statutory requirements are met, the Centers for Medicare & Medicaid Services (CMS) initiated a new national coverage analysis on intensive behavioral therapy for obesity. Screening for obesity in adults is recommended with a grade of B by the U.S. Preventive Services Task Force (USPSTF) and is appropriate for individuals entitled to benefits under Part A and Part B.

The Centers for Disease Control (CDC) reported that "obesity rates in the U.S. have increased dramatically over the last 30 years, and obesity is now epidemic in the United States." In the Medicare population over 30% of men and women are obese. Obesity is directly or indirectly associated with many chronic diseases including cardiovascular disease, musculoskeletal conditions and diabetes.

B. Nationally Covered Indications

Effective for claims with dates of service on or after November 29, 2011, CMS covers intensive behavioral therapy for obesity, defined as a body mass index (BMI) >= 30 kg/m2, for the prevention or early detection of illness or disability.

Intensive behavioral therapy for obesity consists of the following:

1. Screening for obesity in adults using measurement of BMI calculated by dividing weight in kilograms by the square of height in meters (expressed kg/m2);
2. Dietary (nutritional) assessment; and
3. Intensive behavioral counseling and behavioral therapy to promote sustained weight loss through high intensity interventions on diet and exercise.

The intensive behavioral intervention for obesity should be consistent with the 5-A framework that has been highlighted by the USPSTF:

1. Assess: Ask about/assess behavioral health risk(s) and factors affecting choice of behavior change goals/methods.
2. Advise: Give clear, specific, and personalized behavior change advice, including information about personal health harms and benefits.
3. Agree: Collaboratively select appropriate treatment goals and methods based on the patient's interest in and willingness to change the behavior.
4. Assist: Using behavior change techniques (self-help and/or counseling), aid the patient in achieving agreed-upon goals by acquiring the skills, confidence, and social/environmental supports for behavior change, supplemented with adjunctive medical treatments when appropriate. 5. Arrange: Schedule follow-up contacts (in person or by telephone) to provide ongoing assistance/support and to adjust the treatment plan as needed, including referral to more intensive or specialized treatment. For Medicare beneficiaries with obesity, who are competent and alert at the time that counseling is provided and whose counseling is furnished by a qualified primary care physician or other primary care practitioner and in a primary care setting, CMS covers:
   - One face-to-face visit every week for the first month;
   - One face-to-face visit every other week for months 2-6;
   - One face-to-face visit every month for months 7-12, if the beneficiary meets the 3kg weight loss requirement during the first six months as discussed below.

At the six month visit, a reassessment of obesity and a determination of the amount of weight loss must be performed. To be eligible for additional face-to-face visits occurring once a month for an additional six months, beneficiaries must have achieved a reduction in weight of at least 3kg over the course of the first six months of intensive therapy. This determination must be documented in the physician office records for applicable beneficiaries consistent with usual practice. For beneficiaries who do not achieve a weight loss of at least 3kg during the first six months of intensive therapy, a reassessment of their readiness to change and BMI is appropriate after an additional six month period.

For the purposes of this decision memorandum, a primary care setting is defined as one in which there is provision of integrated, accessible health care services by clinicians who are accountable for addressing a large majority of personal health care needs, developing a sustained partnership with patients, and practicing in the context of family and community. Emergency departments, inpatient hospital settings, ambulatory surgical centers, independent diagnostic testing facilities, skilled nursing facilities, inpatient rehabilitation facilities and hospices are not considered primary care settings under this definition.

For the purposes of this decision memorandum a "primary care physician" and "primary care practitioner" will be defined consistent with existing sections of the Social Security Act (§1833(u)(6), §1833(x)(2)(A)(i)(I) and §1833(x)(2)(A)(i)(II)).

§1833(u)

(6) Physician Defined.—For purposes of this paragraph, the term "physician" means a physician described in section 1861(r)(1) and the term "primary care physician" means a physician who is identified in the available data as a general practitioner, family practice practitioner, general internist, or obstetrician or gynecologist.

§1833(x)(2)(A)

Primary care practitioner—The term "primary care practitioner" means an individual—

(i) who—

(I) is a physician (as described in section 1861(r)(1)) who has a primary specialty designation of family medicine, internal medicine, geriatric medicine, or pediatric medicine; or

(II) is a nurse practitioner, clinical nurse specialist, or physician assistant (as those terms are defined in section 1861(aa)(5))

C. Nationally Non-Covered Indications

All other indications remain non-covered.

D. Other

Medicare coinsurance and Part B deductible are waived for this service

(This NCD last reviewed November 2011)

© 2019 Optum360, LLC

100-03, 210.13

Screening for Hepatitis C Virus (HCV) in Adults

(Rev. 177, Issued: 11-19-14, Effective: 06-02-14, Mult. dates for edits)

A. General

Hepatitis C Virus (HCV) is an infection that attacks the liver and leads to inflammation. The infection is often asymptomatic and can go undiagnosed for decades. It is difficult for the human immune system to eliminate the HCV and it is a major cause of chronic liver disease. The presence of HCV in the liver initiates a response from the immune system which in turn causes inflammation. Inflammation over long periods of time (usually decades) can cause scarring, called cirrhosis. A cirrhotic liver fails to perform the normal functions of the liver which leads to liver failure. Cirrhotic livers are more prone to become cancerous and liver failure leads to serious complications, even death. HCV is reported to be the leading cause of chronic hepatitis, cirrhosis and liver cancer and a primary indication for liver transplant in the Western World.

Under §1861(ddd) of the Social Security Act (the Act), the Centers for Medicare & Medicaid Services (CMS) has the authority to add coverage of additional preventive services if certain statutory requirements are met. The regulations provide:

42 CFR §410.64 Additional preventive services

(a) Medicare Part B pays for additional preventive services not described in paragraph (1) or (3) of the definition of "preventive services" under 42 CFR §410.2, that identify medical conditions or risk factors for individuals if the Secretary determines through the national coverage determination process (as defined in section 1869(f)(1)(B) of the Act) that these services are all of the following: (1) reasonable and necessary for the prevention or early detection of illness or disability,(2) recommended with a grade of A or B by the United States Preventive Services Task Force (USPSTF), (3) appropriate for individuals entitled to benefits under Part A or enrolled under Part B.

(b) In making determinations under paragraph (a) of this section regarding the coverage of a new preventive service, the Secretary may conduct an assessment of the relation between predicted outcomes and the expenditures for such services and may take into account the results of such an assessment in making such national coverage determinations.

The scope of the review for this national coverage determination (NCD) evaluated and determined if the existing body of evidence was sufficient for Medicare coverage for screening for HCV in adults at high risk for HCV infection and one-time screening for HCV infection for adults born between 1945 and 1965, which is recommended with a grade B by the USPSTF.

B. Nationally Covered Indications

Effective for services performed on or after June 2, 2014, CMS has determined the following:

The evidence is adequate to conclude that screening for HCV, consistent with the grade B recommendations by the USPSTF, is reasonable and necessary for the prevention or early detection of an illness or disability and is appropriate for individuals entitled to benefits under Part A or enrolled under Part B, as described below.

Therefore, CMS will cover screening for HCV with the appropriate U.S. Food and Drug Administration (FDA)-approved/cleared laboratory tests, used consistent with FDA-approved labeling and in compliance with the Clinical Laboratory Improvement Act regulations, when ordered by the beneficiary's primary care physician or practitioner within the context of a primary care setting, and performed by an eligible Medicare provider for these services, for beneficiaries who meet either of the following conditions:

1. A screening test is covered for adults at high risk for HCV infection. "High risk" is defined as persons with a current or past history of illicit injection drug use; and persons who have a history of receiving a blood transfusion prior to 1992. Repeat screening for high risk persons is covered annually only for persons who have had continued illicit injection drug use since the prior negative screening test.
2. A single screening test is covered for adults who do not meet the high risk definition above, but who were born from 1945 through 1965.

The determination of "high risk for HCV" is identified by the primary care physician or practitioner who assesses the patient's history, which is part of any complete medical history, typically part of an annual wellness visit and considered in the development of a comprehensive prevention plan. The medical record should be a reflection of the service provided.

A primary care setting is defined by the provision of integrated, accessible health care services by clinicians who are accountable for addressing a large majority of personal health care needs, developing a sustained partnership with patients, and practicing in the context of family and community. Emergency departments, inpatient hospital settings, ambulatory surgical centers, independent diagnostic testing facilities, skilled nursing facilities, inpatient rehabilitation facilities, clinics providing a limited focus of health care services, and hospice are examples of settings not considered primary care settings under this definition.

A "primary care physician" and "primary care practitioner" will be defined consistent with existing sections of the Act (§1833(u)(6), §1833(x)(2)(A)(i)(I) and §1833(x)(2)(A)(i)(II)).

§1833(u)

(6) Physician Defined.—For purposes of this paragraph, the term "physician" means a physician described in section 1861(r)(1) and the term "primary care physician" means a physician who is identified in the available data as a general practitioner, family practice practitioner, general internist, or obstetrician or gynecologist.

§1833(x)(2)(A)(i)

(I) is a physician (as described in section 1861(r)(1)) who has a primary specialty designation of family medicine, internal medicine, geriatric medicine, or pediatric medicine; or

(II) is a nurse practitioner, clinical nurse specialist, or physician assistant (as those terms are defined in section 1861(aa)(5)).

C. Nationally Non-Covered Indications

Unless specifically covered in this NCD, any other NCD, or in statute, preventive services are non-covered by Medicare.

D. Other

N/A

(This NCD last reviewed June 2014.)

100-03, 220.2

NCD for Magnetic Resonance Imaging (MRI)

(Rev.208, Issued: 10-19-18, Effective: 04-10-18, Implementation: 12-10 – 18)

A. General

1. Method of Operation

Magnetic Resonance Imaging (MRI), formerly called nuclear magnetic resonance (NMR), is a non-invasive method of graphically representing the distribution of water and other hydrogen-rich molecules in the human body. In contrast to conventional radiographs or computed tomography (CT) scans, in which the image is produced by x-ray beam attenuation by an object, MRI is capable of producing images by several techniques. In fact, various combinations of MRI image production methods may be employed to emphasize particular characteristics of the tissue or body part being examined. The basic elements by which MRI produces an image are the density of hydrogen nuclei in the object being examined, their motion, and the relaxation times, and the period of time required for the nuclei to return to their original states in the main, static magnetic field after being subjected to a brief additional magnetic field. These relaxation times reflect the physical-chemical properties of tissue and the molecular environment of its hydrogen nuclei. Only hydrogen atoms are present in human tissues in sufficient concentration for current use in clinical MRI.

Magnetic Resonance Angiography (MRA) is a non-invasive diagnostic test that is an application of MRI. By analyzing the amount of energy released from tissues exposed to a strong magnetic field, MRA provides images of normal and diseased blood vessels, as well as visualization and quantification of blood flow through these vessels.

2. General Clinical Utility

Overall, MRI is a useful diagnostic imaging modality that is capable of demonstrating a wide variety of soft-tissue lesions with contrast resolution equal or superior to CT scanning in various parts of the body.

Among the advantages of MRI are the absence of ionizing radiation and the ability to achieve high levels of tissue contrast resolution without injected iodinated radiological contrast agents. Recent advances in technology have resulted in development and Food and Drug Administration (FDA) approval of new paramagnetic contrast agents for MRI which allow even better visualization in some instances. Multi-slice imaging and the ability to image in multiple planes, especially sagittal and coronal, have provided flexibility not easily available with other modalities. Because cortical (outer layer) bone and metallic prostheses do not cause distortion of MR images, it has been possible to visualize certain lesions and body regions with greater certainty than has been possible with CT. The use of MRI on certain soft tissue structures for the purpose of detecting disruptive, neoplastic, degenerative, or inflammatory lesions has now become established in medical practice.

Phase contrast (PC) and time-of-flight (TOF) are some of the available MRA techniques at the time these instructions are being issued. PC measures the difference between the phases of proton spins in tissue and blood and measures

© 2019 Optum360, LLC

both the venous and arterial blood flow at any point in the cardiac cycle. TOF measures the difference between the amount of magnetization of tissue and blood and provides information on the structure of blood vessels, thus indirectly indicating blood flow. Two-dimensional (2D) and three dimensional (3D) images can be obtained using each method.

Contrast-enhanced MRA (CE-MRA) involves blood flow imaging after the patient receives an intravenous injection of a contrast agent. Gadolinium, a non-ionic element, is the foundation of all contrast agents currently in use. Gadolinium affects the way in which tissues respond to magnetization, resulting in better visualization of structures when compared to un-enhanced studies. Unlike ionic (i.e., iodine-based) contrast agents used in conventional contrast angiography (CA), allergic reactions to gadolinium are extremely rare. Additionally, gadolinium does not cause the kidney failure occasionally seen with ionic contrast agents. Digital subtraction angiography (DSA) is a computer-augmented form of CA that obtains digital blood flow images as contrast agent courses through a blood vessel. The computer "subtracts" bone and other tissue from the image, thereby improving visualization of blood vessels. Physicians elect to use a specific MRA or CA technique based upon clinical information from each patient.

B. Nationally Covered MRI and MRA Indications

1. MRI

Although several uses of MRI are still considered investigational and some uses are clearly contraindicated (see subsection C), MRI is considered medically efficacious for a number of uses. Use the following descriptions as general guidelines or examples of what may be considered covered rather than as a restrictive list of specific covered indications. Coverage is limited to MRI units that have received FDA premarket approval, and such units must be operated within the parameters specified by the approval. In addition, the services must be reasonable and necessary for the diagnosis or treatment of the specific patient involved.

a. MRI is useful in examining the head, central nervous system, and spine. Multiple sclerosis can be diagnosed with MRI and the contents of the posterior fossa are visible. The inherent tissue contrast resolution of MRI makes it an appropriate standard diagnostic modality for general neuroradiology.

b. MRI can assist in the differential diagnosis of mediastinal and retroperitoneal masses, including abnormalities of the large vessels such as aneurysms and dissection. When a clinical need exists to visualize the parenchyma of solid organs to detect anatomic disruption or neoplasia, this can be accomplished in the liver, urogenital system, adrenals, and pelvic organs without the use of radiological contrast materials. When MRI is considered reasonable and necessary, the use of paramagnetic contrast materials may be covered as part of the study. MRI may also be used to detect and stage pelvic and retroperitoneal neoplasms and to evaluate disorders of cancellous bone and soft tissues. It may also be used in the detection of pericardial thickening. Primary and secondary bone neoplasm and aseptic necrosis can be detected at an early stage and monitored with MRI. Patients with metallic prostheses, especially of the hip, can be imaged in order to detect the early stages of infection of the bone to which the prosthesis is attached.

c. MRI may also be covered to diagnose disc disease without regard to whether radiological imaging has been tried first to diagnose the problem.

d. MRI with gating devices and surface coils, and gating devices that eliminate distorted images caused by cardiac and respiratory movement cycles are now considered state of the art techniques and may be covered. Surface and other specialty coils may also be covered, as they are used routinely for high resolution imaging where small limited regions of the body are studied. They produce high signal-to-noise ratios resulting in images of enhanced anatomic detail.

2. MRA (MRI for Blood Flow)

Currently covered indications include using MRA for specific conditions to evaluate flow in internal carotid vessels of the head and neck, peripheral arteries of lower extremities, abdomen and pelvis, and the chest. Coverage is limited to MRA units that have received FDA premarket approval, and such units must be operated within the parameters specified by the approval. In addition, the services must be reasonable and necessary for the diagnosis or treatment of the specific patient involved.

a. Head and Neck

Studies have proven that MRA is effective for evaluating flow in internal carotid vessels of the head and neck. However, not all potential applications of MRA have been shown to be reasonable and necessary. All of the following criteria must apply in order for Medicare to provide coverage for MRA of the head and neck:

- MRA is used to evaluate the carotid arteries, the circle of Willis, the anterior, middle or posterior cerebral arteries, the vertebral or basilar arteries or the venous sinuses;
- MRA is performed on patients with conditions of the head and neck for which surgery is anticipated and may be found to be appropriate based on the MRA. These conditions include, but are not limited to, tumor, aneurysms, vascular malformations, vascular occlusion or thrombosis. Within this broad category of disorders, medical necessity is the underlying determinant of the need for an MRA in specific diseases. The medical records should clearly justify and demonstrate the existence of medical necessity; and
- MRA and CA are not expected to be performed on the same patient for diagnostic purposes prior to the application of anticipated therapy. Only one of these tests will be covered routinely unless the physician can demonstrate the medical need to perform both tests.

b. Peripheral Arteries of Lower Extremities

Studies have proven that MRA of peripheral arteries is useful in determining the presence and extent of peripheral vascular disease in lower extremities. This procedure is non-invasive and has been shown to find occult vessels in some patients for which those vessels were not apparent when CA was performed. Medicare will cover either MRA or CA to evaluate peripheral arteries of the lower extremities. However, both MRA and CA may be useful in some cases, such as:

- A patient has had CA and this test was unable to identify a viable run-off vessel for bypass. When exploratory surgery is not believed to be a reasonable medical course of action for this patient, MRA may be performed to identify the viable runoff vessel; or
- A patient has had MRA, but the results are inconclusive.

c. Abdomen and Pelvis

i. Pre-operative Evaluation of Patients Undergoing Elective Abdominal Aortic Aneurysm (AAA) Repair

MRA is covered for pre-operative evaluation of patients undergoing elective AAA repair if the scientific evidence reveals MRA is considered comparable to CA in determining the extent of AAA, as well as in evaluating aortoiliac occlusion disease and renal artery pathology that may be necessary in the surgical planning of AAA repair. These studies also reveal that MRA could provide a net benefit to the patient. If preoperative CA is avoided, then patients are not exposed to the risks associated with invasive procedures, contrast media, end-organ damage, or arterial injury.

ii. Imaging the Renal Arteries and the Aortoiliac Arteries in the Absence of AAA or Aortic Dissection

MRA coverage is expanded to include imaging the renal arteries and the aortoiliac arteries in the absence of AAA or aortic dissection. MRA should be obtained in those circumstances in which using MRA is expected to avoid obtaining CA, when physician history, physical examination, and standard assessment tools provide insufficient information for patient management, and obtaining an MRA has a high probability of positively affecting patient management. However, CA may be ordered after obtaining the results of an MRA in those rare instances where medical necessity is demonstrated.

d. Chest

i. Diagnosis of Pulmonary Embolism

Current scientific data has shown that diagnostic pulmonary MRAs are improving due to recent developments such as faster imaging capabilities and gadolinium-enhancement. However, these advances in MRA are not significant enough to warrant replacement of pulmonary angiography in the diagnosis of pulmonary embolism for patients who have no contraindication to receiving intravenous iodinated contrast material. Patients who are allergic to iodinated contrast material face a high risk of developing complications if they undergo pulmonary angiography or computed tomography angiography. Therefore, Medicare will cover MRA of the chest for diagnosing a suspected pulmonary embolism when it is contraindicated for the patient to receive intravascular iodinated contrast material.

ii. Evaluation of Thoracic Aortic Dissection and Aneurysm

Studies have shown that MRA of the chest has a high level of diagnostic accuracy for pre-operative and post-operative evaluation of aortic dissection of aneurysm. Depending on the clinical presentation, MRA may be used as an alternative to other non-invasive imaging technologies, such as transesophageal echocardiography and CT. Generally, Medicare will provide coverage only for MRA or for CA when used as a diagnostic test. However, if both MRA and CA of the chest are used, the physician must demonstrate the medical need for performing these tests.

While the intent of this policy is to provide reimbursement for either RA or CA, the Centers for Medicare & Medicaid Services (CMS) is also allowing flexibility

© 2019 Optum360, LLC

for physicians to make appropriate decisions concerning the use of these tests based on the needs of individual patients. CMS anticipates, however, low utilization of the combined use of MRA and CA. As a result, CMS encourages the Medicare Administrative Contractors (MACs) to monitor the use of these tests and, where indicated, require evidence of the need to perform both MRA and CA.

3. MRI for Patients with an Implanted Pacemaker, Implantable Cardioverter Defibrillator (ICD), Cardiac Resynchronization Therapy Pacemaker (CRT-P), or Cardiac Resynchronization Therapy Defibrillators (CRT-D)

i. An MRI is covered when used according to the FDA labeling in an MRI environment for patients with an implanted pacemaker, implantable cardioverter defibrillator (ICD) cardiac resynchronization therapy pacemaker (CRT-P), or cardiac resynchronization therapy defibrillator (CRT-D). ii. Any MRI for patients with an implanted pacemaker, ICD, CRT-P, or CRT-D that does not have FDA labeling specific to use in an MRI environment is only covered under the following conditions:

a. MRI field strength is 1.5 Tesla using Normal Operating Mode;

b. The implanted pacemaker, ICD, CRT-P, or CRT-D system has no fractured, epicardial, or abandoned leads;

c. The facility has implemented a checklist which includes the following: • patient assessment is performed to identify the presence of an implanted pacemaker, ICD, CRT-P, or CRT-D;

- before the scan benefits and harms of the MRI scan are communicated with the patient or the patient's delegated decision-maker;
- prior to the MRI scan, the implanted pacemaker, ICD, CRT-P, or CRT-D is interrogated and programmed into the appropriate MRI scanning mode;
- a qualified physician, nurse practitioner, or physician assistant with expertise with implanted pacemakers, ICDs, CRT-Ps, or CRT-Ds must directly supervise the MRI scan as defined in 42 CFR § §410.28 and 410.32;
- patients are observed throughout the MRI scan via visual and voice contact and monitored with equipment to assess vital signs and cardiac rhythm;
- an advanced cardiac life support provider must be present for the duration of the MRI scan;
- a discharge plan that includes before being discharged from the hospital/facility, the patient is evaluated and the implanted pacemaker, ICD, CRT-P, or CRT-D is reinterrogated immediately after the MRI scan to detect and correct any abnormalities that might have developed.

C. Contraindications and Nationally Non-Covered Indications

1. Contraindications

The MRI is not covered when the following patient-specific contraindications are present

- • MRI during a viable pregnancy.
- The danger inherent in bringing ferromagnetic materials within range of MRI units generally constrains the use of MRI on acutely ill patients requiring life support systems and monitoring devices that employ ferromagnetic materials.
- The long imaging time and the enclosed position of the patient may result in claustrophobia, making patients who have a history of claustrophobia unsuitable candidates for MRI procedures.

2. Nationally Non-Covered Indications

CMS has determined that MRI of cortical bone and calcifications, and procedures involving spatial resolution of bone and calcifications, are not considered reasonable and necessary indications within the meaning of section 1862(a)(1)(A) of the Act, and are therefore non-covered.

MRI is not covered for patients with metallic clips on vascular aneurysms.

D. Other

All other uses of MRI or MRA for which CMS has not specifically indicated coverage or non-coverage continue to be eligible for coverage through individual MAC discretion.

(This NCD last reviewed April 2018.)

100-03, 220.6.1

PET for Perfusion of the Heart (Various Effective Dates)

(Rev.177, Issued: 11-19-14, Effective: 06-02-14, Mult. dates for edits)

Indications and Limitations of Coverage

1. Rubidium 82 (Effective March 14, 1995)

Effective for services performed on or after March 14, 1995, PET scans performed at rest or with pharmacological stress used for noninvasive imaging of the perfusion of the heart for the diagnosis and management of patients with known or suspected coronary artery disease using the FDA-approved radiopharmaceutical Rubidium 82 (Rb 82) are covered, provided the requirements below are met:

The PET scan, whether at rest alone, or rest with stress, is performed in place of, but not in addition to, a single photon emission computed tomography (SPECT); or

The PET scan, whether at rest alone or rest with stress, is used following a SPECT that was found to be inconclusive. In these cases, the PET scan must have been considered necessary in order to determine what medical or surgical intervention is required to treat the patient. (For purposes of this requirement, an inconclusive test is a test(s) whose results are equivocal, technically uninterpretable, or discordant with a patient's other clinical data and must be documented in the beneficiary's file.)

For any PET scan for which Medicare payment is claimed for dates of services prior to July 1, 2001, the claimant must submit additional specified information on the claim form (including proper codes and/or modifiers), to indicate the results of the PET scan. The claimant must also include information on whether the PET scan was performed after an inconclusive noninvasive cardiac test. The information submitted with respect to the previous noninvasive cardiac test must specify the type of test performed prior to the PET scan and whether it was inconclusive or unsatisfactory. These explanations are in the form of special G codes used for billing PET scans using Rb 82. Beginning July 1, 2001, claims should be submitted with the appropriate codes.

2. Ammonia N-13 (Effective October 1, 2003)

Effective for services performed on or after October 1, 2003, PET scans performed at rest or with pharmacological stress used for noninvasive imaging of the perfusion of the heart for the diagnosis and management of patients with known or suspected coronary artery disease using the FDA-approved radiopharmaceutical ammonia N-13 are covered, provided the requirements below are met:

The PET scan, whether at rest alone, or rest with stress, is performed in place of, but not in addition to, a SPECT; or

The PET scan, whether at rest alone or rest with stress, is used following a SPECT that was found to be inconclusive. In these cases, the PET scan must have been considered necessary in order to determine what medical or surgical intervention is required to treat the patient. (For purposes of this requirement, an inconclusive test is a test whose results are equivocal, technically uninterpretable, or discordant with a patient's other clinical data and must be documented in the beneficiary's file.)

(This NCD last reviewed March 2005.)

100-03, 220.6.9

FDG PET for Refractory Seizures (Effective July 1, 2001)

(Rev.120; Issued: 05-06-10; Effective Date: 04-03-09; Implementation Date: 10-30-09)

Beginning July 1, 2001, Medicare covers FDG PET for pre-surgical evaluation for the purpose of localization of a focus of refractory seizure activity.

Limitations: Covered only for pre-surgical evaluation.

Documentation that these conditions are met should be maintained by the referring physician in the beneficiary's medical record, as is normal business practice.

(This NCD last reviewed June 2001.)

100-03, 220.6.13

FDG Positron Emission Tomography (PET) for Dementia and Neurodegenerative Diseases

(Rev.173, Issued: 09-04-14, Effective: Upon Implementation: of ICD–10)

A. General

Medicare covers FDG Positron Emission Tomography (PET) scans for either the differential diagnosis of fronto-temporal dementia (FTD) and Alzheimer's disease (AD) under specific requirements; OR, its use in a Centers for Medicare & Medicaid Services (CMS)-approved practical clinical trial focused on the utility of FDG PET in the diagnosis or treatment of dementing neurodegenerative diseases. Specific requirements for each indication are clarified below:

B. Nationally Covered Indications

1. FDG PET Requirements for Coverage in the Differential Diagnosis of AD and FTD

An FDG PET scan is considered reasonable and necessary in patients with a recent diagnosis of dementia and documented cognitive decline of at least 6 months, who meet diagnostic criteria for both AD and FTD. These patients have been evaluated for specific alternate neurodegenerative diseases or other causative factors, but the cause of the clinical symptoms remains uncertain.

The following additional conditions must be met before an FDG PET scan will be covered:

a. The patient's onset, clinical presentation, or course of cognitive impairment is such that FTD is suspected as an alternative neurodegenerative cause of the cognitive decline. Specifically, symptoms such as social disinhibition, awkwardness, difficulties with language, or loss of executive function are more prominent early in the course of FTD than the memory loss typical of AD;

b. The patient has had a comprehensive clinical evaluation (as defined by the American Academy of Neurology encompassing a medical history from the patient and a well-acquainted informant (including assessment of activities of daily living), physical and mental status examination (including formal documentation of cognitive decline occurring over at least 6 months) aided by cognitive scales or neuropsychological testing, laboratory tests, and structural imaging such as magnetic resonance imaging (MRI) or computed tomography (CT);

c. The evaluation of the patient has been conducted by a physician experienced in the diagnosis and assessment of dementia;

d. The evaluation of the patient did not clearly determine a specific neurodegenerative disease or other cause for the clinical symptoms, and information available through FDG PET is reasonably expected to help clarify the diagnosis between FTD and AD and help guide future treatment;

e. The FDG PET scan is performed in a facility that has all the accreditation necessary to operate nuclear medicine equipment. The reading of the scan should be done by an expert in nuclear medicine, radiology, neurology, or psychiatry, with experience interpreting such scans in the presence of dementia;

f. A brain single photon emission computed tomography (SPECT) or FDG PET scan has not been obtained for the same indication. (The indication can be considered to be different in patients who exhibit important changes in scope or severity of cognitive decline, and meet all other qualifying criteria listed above and below (including the judgment that the likely diagnosis remains uncertain.) The results of a prior SPECT or FDG PET scan must have been inconclusive or, in the case of SPECT, difficult to interpret due to immature or inadequate technology. In these instances, an FDG PET scan may be covered after one year has passed from the time the first SPECT or FDG PET scan was performed.)

g. The referring and billing provider(s) have documented the appropriate evaluation of the Medicare beneficiary. Providers should establish the medical necessity of an FDG PET scan by ensuring that the following information has been collected and is maintained in the beneficiary medical record:

- Date of onset of symptoms;
- Diagnosis of clinical syndrome (normal aging; mild cognitive impairment (MCI); mild, moderate or severe dementia);
- Mini mental status exam (MMSE) or similar test score;
- Presumptive cause (possible, probable, uncertain AD);
- Any neuropsychological testing performed;
- Results of any structural imaging (MRI or CT) performed;
- Relevant laboratory tests (B12, thyroid hormone); and,
- Number and name of prescribed medications.

The billing provider must furnish a copy of the FDG PET scan result for use by CMS and its Medicare Administrative Contractors upon request. These verification requirements are consistent with Federal requirements set forth in 42 Code of Federal Regulations section 410.32 generally for diagnostic x-ray tests, diagnostic laboratory tests, and other tests. In summary, section 410.32 requires the billing physician and the referring physician to maintain information in the medical record of each patient to demonstrate medical necessity [410.32(d) (2)] and submit the information demonstrating medical necessity to CMS and/or its agents upon request [410.32(d)(3)(I)] (OMB number 0938-0685).

2. FDG PET Requirements for Coverage in the Context of a CMS-approved Practical Clinical Trial Utilizing a Specific Protocol to Demonstrate the Utility of FDG PET in the Diagnosis, and Treatment of Neurodegenerative Dementing Diseases

An FDG PET scan is considered reasonable and necessary in patients with MCI or early dementia (in clinical circumstances other than those specified in subparagraph 1) only in the context of an approved clinical trial that contains patient safeguards and protections to ensure proper administration, use and evaluation of the FDG PET scan.

The clinical trial must compare patients who do and do not receive an FDG PET scan and have as its goal to monitor, evaluate, and improve clinical outcomes. In addition, it must meet the following basic criteria:

- Written protocol on file;
- Institutional Review Board review and approval;
- Scientific review and approval by two or more qualified individuals who are not part of the research team; and,

Certification that investigators have not been disqualified.

C. Nationally Non- Covered Indications

All other uses of FDG PET for patients with a presumptive diagnosis of dementia-causing neurodegenerative disease (e.g., possible or probable AD, clinically typical FTD, dementia of Lewy bodies, or Creutzfeld-Jacob disease) for which CMS has not specifically indicated coverage continue to be noncovered.

D. Other

Not applicable.

(This NCD last reviewed September 2004.)

100-03, 220.6.17

Positron Emission Tomography (FDG PET) for Oncologic Conditions

(Effective June 11, 2013)

(Rev.173, Issued: 09-04-14, Effective: Upon Implementation: of ICD-10, Implementation: Upon Implementation of ICD-10)

A. General

FDG (2-[F18] fluoro-2-deoxy-D-glucose) Positron Emission Tomography (PET) is a minimally-invasive diagnostic imaging procedure used to evaluate glucose metabolism in normal tissue as well as in diseased tissues in conditions such as cancer, ischemic

heart disease, and some neurologic disorders. FDG is an injected radionuclide (or radiopharmaceutical) that emits sub-atomic particles, known as positrons, as it decays. FDG PET uses a positron camera (tomograph) to measure the decay of FDG. The rate of FDG decay provides biochemical information on glucose metabolism in the tissue being studied. As malignancies can cause abnormalities of metabolism and blood flow, FDG PET evaluation may indicate the probable presence or absence of a malignancy based upon observed differences in biologic activity compared to adjacent tissues.

The Centers for Medicare and Medicaid Services (CMS) was asked by the National Oncologic PET Registry (NOPR) to reconsider section 220.6 of the National Coverage Determinations (NCD) Manual to end the prospective data collection requirements under Coverage with Evidence Development (CED) across all oncologic indications of FDG PET imaging. The CMS received public input indicating that the current coverage framework of prospective data collection under CED be ended for all oncologic uses of FDG PET imaging.

1. Framework

Effective for claims with dates of service on and after June 11, 2013, CMS is adopting a coverage framework that ends the prospective data collection requirements by NOPR under CED for all oncologic uses of FDG PET imaging. CMS is making this change for all NCDs that address coverage of FDG PET for oncologic uses addressed in this decision. This decision does not change coverage for any use of PET imaging using radiopharmaceuticals NaF-18 (fluorine-18 labeled sodium fluoride), ammonia N-13, or rubidium-82 (Rb-82).

2. Initial Anti-Tumor Treatment Strategy

CMS continues to believe that the evidence is adequate to determine that the results of FDG PET imaging are useful in determining the appropriate initial anti-tumor treatment strategy for beneficiaries with suspected cancer and improve health outcomes and thus are reasonable and necessary under §1862(a)(1)(A) of the Social Security Act (the Act).

Therefore, CMS continues to nationally cover one FDG PET study for beneficiaries who have cancers that are biopsy proven or strongly suspected based on other diagnostic testing when the beneficiary's treating physician determines that the FDG PET study is needed to determine the location and/or extent of the tumor for the following therapeutic purposes related to the initial anti-tumor treatment strategy:

- To determine whether or not the beneficiary is an appropriate candidate for an invasive diagnostic or therapeutic procedure; or
- To determine the optimal anatomic location for an invasive procedure; or

© 2019 Optum360, LLC

– To determine the anatomic extent of tumor when the recommended anti-tumor treatment reasonably depends on the extent of the tumor.

See the table at the end of this section for a synopsis of all nationally covered and non-covered oncologic uses of FDG PET imaging.

B.1. Initial Anti-Tumor Treatment Strategy Nationally Covered Indications

a. CMS continues to nationally cover FDG PET imaging for the initial anti-tumor treatment strategy for male and female breast cancer only when used in staging distant metastasis.

b CMS continues to nationally cover FDG PET to determine initial anti-tumor treatment strategy for melanoma other than for the evaluation of regional lymph nodes.

c. CMS continues to nationally cover FDG PET imaging for the detection of pre-treatment metastasis (i.e., staging) in newly diagnosed cervical cancers.

d. C.1 Initial Anti-Tumor Treatment Strategy Nationally Non-Covered Indications

a. CMS continues to nationally non-cover initial anti-tumor treatment strategy in Medicare beneficiaries who have adenocarcinoma of the prostate.

b. CMS continues to nationally non-cover FDG PET imaging for diagnosis of breast cancer and initial staging of axillary nodes.

c. CMS continues to nationally non-cover FDG PET imaging for initial anti-tumor treatment strategy for the evaluation of regional lymph nodes in melanoma.

d. CMS continues to nationally non-cover FDG PET imaging for the diagnosis of cervical cancer related to initial anti-tumor treatment strategy.

3. Subsequent Anti-Tumor Treatment Strategy

B.2. Subsequent Anti-Tumor Treatment Strategy Nationally Covered Indications

Three FDG PET scans are nationally covered when used to guide subsequent management of anti-tumor treatment strategy after completion of initial anti-cancer therapy. Coverage of more than three FDG PET scans to guide subsequent management of anti-tumor treatment strategy after completion of initial anti-cancer therapy shall be determined by the local Medicare Administrative Contractors.

4. Synopsis of Coverage of FDG PET for Oncologic Conditions

Effective for claims with dates of service on and after June 11, 2013, the chart below summarizes national FDG PET coverage for oncologic conditions:

FDG PET for Cancers Tumor Type	Initial Treatment Strategy (formerly "diagnosis" & "staging"	Subsequent Treatment Strategy (formerly "restaging" & "monitoring response to treatment"
Colorectal	Cover	Cover
Esophagus	Cover	Cover
Head and Neck (not thyroid, CNS)	Cover	Cover
Lymphoma	Cover	Cover
Non-small cell lung	Cover	Cover
Ovary	Cover	Cover
Brain	Cover	Cover
Cervix	Cover with exceptions *	Cover
Small cell lung	Cover	Cover
Soft tissue sarcoma	Cover	Cover
Pancreas	Cover	Cover
Testes	Cover	Cover
Prostate	Non-cover	Cover
Thyroid	Cover	Cover
Breast (male and female)	Cover with exceptions *	Cover
Melanoma	Cover with exceptions *	Cover
All other solid tumors	Cover	Cover
Myeloma	Cover	Cover
All other cancers not listed	Cover	Cover

* Cervix: Nationally non-covered for the initial diagnosis of cervical cancer related to initial anti-tumor treatment strategy. All other indications for initial anti-tumor treatment strategy for cervical cancer are nationally covered.
* Breast: Nationally non-covered for initial diagnosis and/or staging of axillary lymph nodes. Nationally covered for initial staging of metastatic disease. All other indications for initial anti-tumor treatment strategy for breast cancer are nationally covered.
* Melanoma: Nationally non-covered for initial staging of regional lymph nodes. All other indications for initial anti-tumor treatment strategy for melanoma are nationally covered.

D. Other

N/A

100-03, 220.6.19

Positron Emission Tomography NaF-18 (NaF-18 PET) to Identify Bone Metastasis of Cancer (Effective February 26, 2010)

(Rev.119, Issued: 03-26-10, Effective: 02-26-10, Implementation: 07-06-10)

A. General

Positron Emission Tomography (PET) is a non-invasive, diagnostic imaging procedure that assesses the level of metabolic activity and perfusion in various organ systems of the body. A positron camera (tomograph) is used to produce cross-sectional tomographic images, which are obtained from positron-emitting radioactive tracer substances (radiopharmaceuticals) such as

F-18 sodium fluoride. NaF-18 PET has been recognized as an excellent technique for imaging areas of altered osteogenic activity in bone. The clinical value of detecting and assessing the initial extent of metastatic cancer in bone is attested by a number of professional guidelines for oncology. Imaging to detect bone metastases is also recommended when a patient, following completion of initial treatment, is symptomatic with bone pain suspicious for metastases from a known primary tumor.

B. Nationally Covered Indications

Effective February 26, 2010, the Centers for Medicare & Medicaid Services (CMS) will cover NaF-18 PET imaging when the beneficiary's treating physician determines that the NaF-18 PET study is needed to inform to inform the initial antitumor treatment strategy or to guide subsequent antitumor treatment strategy after the completion of initial treatment, and when the beneficiary is enrolled in, and the NaF-18 PET provider is participating in, the following type of prospective clinical study:

A NaF-18 PET clinical study that is designed to collect additional information at the time of the scan to assist in initial antitumor treatment planning or to guide subsequent treatment strategy by the identification, location and quantification of bone metastases in beneficiaries in whom bone metastases are strongly suspected based on clinical symptoms or the results of other diagnostic studies. Qualifying clinical studies must ensure that specific hypotheses are addressed; appropriate data elements are collected; hospitals and providers are qualified to provide the PET scan and interpret the results; participating hospitals and providers accurately report data on all enrolled patients not included in other qualifying trials through adequate auditing mechanisms; and all patient confidentiality, privacy, and other Federal laws must be followed.

The clinical studies for which Medicare will provide coverage must answer one or more of the following questions:

Prospectively, in Medicare beneficiaries whose treating physician determines that the NaF-18 PET study results are needed to inform the initial antitumor treatment strategy or to guide subsequent antitumor treatment strategy after the completion of initial treatment, does the addition of NaF-18 PET imaging lead to:

A change in patient management to more appropriate palliative care; or A change in patient management to more appropriate curative care; or Improved quality of life; or Improved survival?

The study must adhere to the following standards of scientific integrity and relevance to the Medicare population:

a. The principal purpose of the research study is to test whether a particular intervention potentially improves the participants' health outcomes.

b. The research study is well-supported by available scientific and medical information or it is intended to clarify or establish the health outcomes of interventions already in common clinical use.

c. The research study does not unjustifiably duplicate existing studies.

d. The research study design is appropriate to answer the research question being asked in the study.

e. The research study is sponsored by an organization or individual capable of executing the proposed study successfully.

f. The research study is in compliance with all applicable Federal regulations concerning the protection of human subjects found in the Code of Federal

© 2019 Optum360, LLC

Regulations (CFR) at 45 CFR Part 46. If a study is regulated by the Food and Drug Administration (FDA), it also must be in compliance with 21 CFR Parts 50 and 56.

g. All aspects of the research study are conducted according to the appropriate standards of scientific integrity.

h. The research study has a written protocol that clearly addresses, or incorporates by reference, the Medicare standards.

i. The clinical research study is not designed to exclusively test toxicity or disease pathophysiology in healthy individuals. Trials of all medical technologies measuring therapeutic outcomes as one of the objectives meet this standard only if the disease or condition being studied is life-threatening as defined in 21 CFR Sec.312.81(a) and the patient has no other viable treatment options.

j. The clinical research study is registered on the www.ClinicalTrials.gov Web site by the principal sponsor/investigator prior to the enrollment of the first study subject.

k. The research study protocol specifies the method and timing of public release of all pre-specified outcomes to be measured including release of outcomes if outcomes are negative or study is terminated early. The results must be made public within 24 months of the end of data collection. If a report is planned to be published in a peer-reviewed journal, then that initial release may be an abstract that meets the requirements of the International Committee of Medical Journal Editors. However, a full report of the outcomes must be made public no later than three (3) years after the end of data collection.

l. The research study protocol must explicitly discuss subpopulations affected by the treatment under investigation, particularly traditionally underrepresented groups in clinical studies, how the inclusion and exclusion criteria affect enrollment of these populations, and a plan for the retention and reporting of said populations on the trial. If the inclusion and exclusion criteria are expected to have a negative effect on the recruitment or retention of underrepresented populations, the protocol must discuss why these criteria are necessary.

m. The research study protocol explicitly discusses how the results are or are not expected to be generalizable to the Medicare population to infer whether Medicare patients may benefit from the intervention. Separate discussions in the protocol may be necessary for populations eligible for Medicare due to age, disability or Medicaid eligibility.

Consistent with section 1142 of the Social Security Act (the Act), the Agency for Healthcare Research and Quality (AHRQ) supports clinical research studies that the Centers for Medicare and Medicaid Services (CMS) determines meet the above-listed standards and address the above-listed research questions.

C. Nationally Non-Covered Indications

Effective February 26, 2010, CMS determines that the evidence is not sufficient to determine that the results of NaF-18 PET imaging to identify bone metastases improve health outcomes of beneficiaries with cancer and is not reasonable and necessary under Sec.1862(a)(1)(A) of the Act unless it is to inform initial antitumor treatment strategy or to guide subsequent antitumor treatment strategy after completion of initial treatment, and then only under CED. All other uses and clinical indications of NaF-18 PET are nationally non-covered.

D. Other

The only radiopharmaceutical diagnostic imaging agents covered by Medicare for PET cancer imaging are 2-[F-18] Fluoro-D-Glucose (FDG) and NaF-18 (sodium fluoride-18). All other PET radiopharmaceutical diagnostic imaging agents are non-covered for this indication.

(This NCD was last reviewed in February 2010.)

100-03, 230.6

Vabra Aspirator

(Rev.1, 10-03-03)

The VABRA aspirator is a sterile, disposable, vacuum aspirator which is used to collect uterine tissue for study to detect endometrial carcinoma. The use of this device is indicated where the patient exhibits clinical symptoms or signs suggestive of endometrial disease, such as irregular or heavy vaginal bleeding.

Program payment cannot be made for the aspirator or the related diagnostic services when furnished in connection with the examination of an asymptomatic patient. Payment for routine physical checkups is precluded under the statute (§1862(a)(7) of the Act).

Cross-reference:

See the Medicare Benefit Policy Manual, Chapter 16, "General Exclusions From Coverage," §90, and §230.5 of this manual.

100-03, 240.4

Continuous Positive Airway Pressure (CPAP) Therapy For Obstructive Sleep Apnea (OSA) (Effective April 4, 2005) (Effective March 13, 2008)

(Rev.96, Issued: 10-15-08, Effective: 03-13-08, Implementation: 08-04-08)

A. General

Continuous Positive Airway Pressure (CPAP) is a non-invasive technique for providing single levels of air pressure from a flow generator, via a nose mask, through the nares. The purpose is to prevent the collapse of the oropharyngeal walls and the obstruction of airflow during sleep, which occurs in obstructive sleep apnea (OSA).

The apnea hypopnea index (AHI) is equal to the average number of episodes of apnea and hypopnea per hour. The respiratory disturbance index (RDI) is equal to the average number of respiratory disturbances per hour.

Apnea is defined as a cessation of airflow for at least 10 seconds. Hypopnea is defined as an abnormal respiratory event lasting at least 10 seconds with at least a 30% reduction in thoracoabdominal movement or airflow as compared to baseline, and with at least a 4% oxygen desaturation.

The AHI and/or RDI may be measured by polysomnography (PSG) in a facility-based sleep study laboratory, or by a Type II home sleep test (HST) monitor, a Type III HST monitor, or a Type IV HST monitor measuring at least 3 channels.

B. Nationally Covered Indications

Effective for claims with dates of service on and after March 13, 2008, the Centers for Medicare & Medicaid Services (CMS) determines that CPAP therapy when used in adult patients with OSA is considered reasonable and necessary under the following situations:

1 The use of CPAP is covered under Medicare when used in adult patients with OSA. Coverage of CPAP is initially limited to a 12-week period to identify beneficiaries diagnosed with OSA as subsequently described who benefit from CPAP. CPAP is subsequently covered only for those beneficiaries diagnosed with OSA who benefit from CPAP during this 12-week period.

2. The provider of CPAP must conduct education of the beneficiary prior to the use of the CPAP device to ensure that the beneficiary has been educated in the proper use of the device. A caregiver, for example a family member, may be compensatory, if consistently available in the beneficiary's home and willing and able to safely operate the CPAP device.

3. A positive diagnosis of OSA for the coverage of CPAP must include a clinical evaluation and a positive:

   a. attended PSG performed in a sleep laboratory; or

   b. unattended HST with a Type II home sleep monitoring device; or

   c. unattended HST with a Type III home sleep monitoring device; or

   d. unattended HST with a Type IV home sleep monitoring device that measures at least 3 channels.

4. The sleep test must have been previously ordered by the beneficiary?s treating physician and furnished under appropriate physician supervision.

5. An initial 12-week period of CPAP is covered in adult patients with OSA if either of the following criterion using the AHI or RDI are met:

   a. AHI or RDI greater than or equal to 15 events per hour, or

   b. AHI or RDI greater than or equal to 5 events and less than or equal to 14 events per hour with documented symptoms of excessive daytime sleepiness, impaired cognition, mood disorders or insomnia, or documented hypertension, ischemic heart disease, or history of stroke.

6. The AHI or RDI is calculated on the average number of events of per hour. If the AHI or RDI is calculated based on less than 2 hours of continuous recorded sleep, the total number of recorded events to calculate the AHI or RDI during sleep testing must be at a minimum the number of events that would have been required in a 2-hour period.

7. Apnea is defined as a cessation of airflow for at least 10 seconds. Hypopnea is defined as an abnormal respiratory event lasting at least 10 seconds with at least a 30% reduction in thoracoabdominal movement or airflow as compared to baseline, and with at least a 4% oxygen desaturation.

8. Coverage with Evidence Development (CED): Medicare provides the following limited coverage for CPAP in adult beneficiaries who do not qualify for CPAP coverage based on criteria 1-7 above. A clinical study seeking Medicare payment for CPAP provided to a beneficiary who is an enrolled subject in that study must address one or more of the following questions

   a. In Medicare-aged subjects with clinically identified risk factors for OSA, how does the diagnostic accuracy of a clinical trial of CPAP compare with PSG and Type II, III & IV HST in identifying subjects with OSA who will respond to CPAP?

© 2019 Optum360, LLC

b. In Medicare-aged subjects with clinically identified risk factors for OSA who have not undergone confirmatory testing with PSG or Type II, III & IV HST, does CPAP cause clinically meaningful harm?

The study must meet the following additional standards:

c. The principal purpose of the research study is to test whether a particular intervention potentially improves the participants? health outcomes.

d. The research study is well-supported by available scientific and medical information or it is intended to clarify or establish the health outcomes of interventions already in common clinical use.

e. The research study does not unjustifiably duplicate existing studies.

f. The research study design is appropriate to answer the research question being asked in the study.

g. The research study is sponsored by an organization or individual capable of executing the proposed study successfully.

h. The research study is in compliance with all applicable Federal regulations concerning the protection of human subjects found at 45 CFR Part 46. If a study is Food and Drug Administration-regulated, it also must be in compliance with 21 CFR Parts 50 and 56.

i. All aspects of the research study are conducted according to the appropriate standards of scientific integrity.

j. The research study has a written protocol that clearly addresses, or incorporates by reference, the Medicare standards.

k. The clinical research study is not designed to exclusively test toxicity or disease pathophysiology in healthy individuals. Trials of all medical technologies measuring therapeutic outcomes as one of the objectives meet this standard only if the disease or condition being studied is life-threatening as defined in 21 CFR ? 312.81(a) and the patient has no other viable treatment options.

l. The clinical research study is registered on the ClinicalTrials.gov Web site by the principal sponsor/investigator prior to the enrollment of the first study subject.

m. The research study protocol specifies the method and timing of public release of all pre-specified outcomes to be measured, including release of outcomes if outcomes are negative or study is terminated early. The results must be made public within 24 months of the end of data collection. If a report is planned for publication in a peer-reviewed journal, then that initial release may be an abstract that meets the requirements of the International Committee of Medical Journal Editors. However, a full report of the outcomes must be made public no later than 3 years after the end of data collection.

n. The research study protocol must explicitly discuss subpopulations affected by the treatment under investigation, particularly traditionally underrepresented groups in clinical studies, how the inclusion and exclusion criteria affect enrollment of these populations, and a plan for the retention and reporting of said populations in the trial. If the inclusion and exclusion criteria are expected to have a negative effect on the recruitment or retention of underrepresented populations, the protocol must discuss why these criteria are necessary.

o. The research study protocol explicitly discusses how the results are or are not expected to be generalizable to the Medicare population to infer whether Medicare patients may benefit from the intervention. Separate discussions in the protocol may be necessary for populations eligible for Medicare due to age, disability, or Medicaid eligibility.

C. Nationally Non-covered Indications

Effective for claims with dates of services on and after March 13, 2008, other diagnostic tests for the diagnosis of OSA, other than those noted above for prescribing CPAP, are not sufficient for the coverage of CPAP.

D. Other

N/A

(This NCD last reviewed March 2008.)

100-03, 250.5

Dermal Injections for the Treatment of Facial Lipodystrophy Syndrome (LDS) - Effective March 23, 2010

(Rev.122, Issued: 06-04-10, Effective: 03-23-10, Implementation: 07-06-10)

A. General

Treatment of persons infected with the human immunodeficiency virus (HIV) or persons who have Acquired Immune Deficiency Syndrome (AIDS) may include highly active antiretroviral therapy (HAART). Drug reactions commonly associated with long-term use of HAART include metabolic complications such as, lipid abnormalities, e.g., hyperlipidemia, hyperglycemia, diabetes, lipodystrophy, and heart disease. Lipodystrophy is characterized by abnormal fat distribution in the body. The LDS is often characterized by a loss of fat that results in a facial abnormality such as severely sunken cheeks. The patient's physical appearance may contribute to psychological conditions (e.g., depression) or adversely impact a patient's adherence to antiretroviral regimens (therefore jeopardizing their health) and both of these are important health-related outcomes of interest in this population. Therefore, improving a patient's physical appearance through the use of dermal injections could improve these health-related outcomes.

B. Nationally Covered Indications

Effective for claims with dates of service on and after March 23, 2010, dermal injections for LDS are only reasonable and necessary using dermal fillers approved by the Food and Drug Administration (FDA) for this purpose, and then only in HIV-infected beneficiaries when LDS caused by antiretroviral HIV treatment is a significant contributor to their depression.

C. Nationally Non-Covered Indications

1. Dermal fillers that are not approved by the FDA for the treatment of LDS.
2. Dermal fillers that are used for any indication other than LDS in HIV-infected individuals who manifest depression as a result of their antiretroviral HIV treatments.

D. Other

N/A

(This NCD last reviewed March 2010.)

100-03, 270.3

NCD for Blood-Derived Products for Chronic Non-Healing Wounds (Various Effective Dates Below)

(Rev.154, Issued: 06-10-13, Effective: 08-02-12, Implementation: 07-01- 13)

A. General

Wound healing is a dynamic, interactive process that involves multiple cells and proteins. There are three progressive stages of normal wound healing, and the typical wound healing duration is about 4 weeks. While cutaneous wounds are a disruption of the normal, anatomic structure and function of the skin, subcutaneous wounds involve tissue below the skin? surface. Wounds are categorized as either acute, in where the normal wound healing stages are not yet completed but it is presumed they will be, resulting in orderly and timely wound repair, or chronic, in where a wound has failed to progress through the normal wound healing stages and repair itself within a sufficient time period.

Platelet-rich plasma (PRP) is produced in an autologous or homologous manner. Autologous PRP is comprised of blood from the patient who will ultimately receive the PRP. Alternatively, homologous PRP is derived from blood from multiple donors.

Blood is donated by the patient and centrifuged to produce an autologous gel for treatment of chronic, non-healing cutaneous wounds that persists for 30 days or longer and fail to properly complete the healing process. Autologous blood derived products for chronic, non-healing wounds includes both: (1) platelet derived growth factor (PDGF) products (such as Procuren), and (2) PRP (such as AutoloGel).

The PRP is different from previous products in that it contains whole cells including white cells, red cells, plasma, platelets, fibrinogen, stem cells, macrophages, and fibroblasts.

The PRP is used by physicians in clinical settings in treating chronic, non-healing wounds, open, cutaneous wounds, soft tissue, and bone. Alternatively, PDGF does not contain cells and was previously marketed as a product to be used by patients at home.

B. Nationally Covered Indications

Effective August 2, 2012, upon reconsideration, The Centers for Medicare and Medicaid Services (CMS) has determined that platelet-rich plasma (PRP) ?an autologous blood-derived product, will be covered only for the treatment of chronic non-healing diabetic, venous and/or pressure wounds and only when the following conditions are met:

The patient is enrolled in a clinical trial that addresses the following questions using validated and reliable methods of evaluation. Clinical study applications for coverage pursuant to this National coverage Determination (NCD) must be received by August 2, 2014.

The clinical research study must meet the requirements specified below to assess the effect of PRP for the treatment of chronic non-healing diabetic, venous and/or pressure wounds. The clinical study must address:

Prospectively, do Medicare beneficiaries that have chronic non-healing diabetic, venous and/or pressure wounds who receive well-defined optimal usual care along with PRP therapy, experience clinically significant health outcomes compared to patients who receive well-defined optimal usual care for chronic non-healing diabetic, venous and/or pressure wounds as indicated by addressing at least one of the following:

a. Complete wound healing

b. Ability to return to previous function and resumption of normal activities

c. Reduction of wound size or healing trajectory which results in the patient's ability to return to previous function and resumption of normal activities

The required clinical trial of PRP must adhere to the following standards of scientific integrity and relevance to the Medicare population:

a. The principal purpose of the CLINICAL STUDY is to test whether PRP improves the participants?health outcomes.

b. The CLINICAL STUDY is well supported by available scientific and medical information or it is intended to clarify or establish the health outcomes of interventions already in common clinical use.

c. The CLINICAL STUDY does not unjustifiably duplicate existing studies.

d. The CLINICAL STUDY design is appropriate to answer the research question being asked in the study.

e. The CLINICAL STUDY is sponsored by an organization or individual capable of executing the proposed study successfully.

f. The CLINICAL STUDY is in compliance with all applicable Federal regulations concerning the protection of human subjects found at 45 CFR Part 46.

g. All aspects of the CLINICAL STUDY are conducted according to appropriate standards of scientific integrity set by the International Committee of Medical Journal Editors (http://www.icmje.org).

h. The CLINICAL STUDY has a written protocol that clearly addresses, or incorporates by reference, the standards listed here as Medicare requirements for coverage with evidence development (CED).

i. The CLINICAL STUDY is not designed to exclusively test toxicity or disease pathophysiology in healthy individuals. Trials of all medical technologies measuring therapeutic outcomes as one of the objectives meet this standard only if the disease or condition being studied is life threatening as defined in 21 CFR ?312.81(a) and the patient has no other viable treatment options.

j. The CLINICAL STUDY is registered on the ClinicalTrials.gov website by the principal sponsor/investigator prior to the enrollment of the first study subject.

k. The CLINICAL STUDY protocol specifies the method and timing of public release of all pre-specified outcomes to be measured including release of outcomes if outcomes are negative or study is terminated early. The results must be made public within 24 months of the end of data collection. If a report is planned to be published in a peer reviewed journal, then that initial release may be an abstract that meets the requirements of the International Committee of Medical Journal Editors (http://www.icmje.org). However a full report of the outcomes must be made public no later than three (3) years after the end of data collection.

l. The CLINICAL STUDY protocol must explicitly discuss subpopulations affected by the treatment under investigation, particularly traditionally underrepresented groups in clinical studies, how the inclusion and exclusion criteria effect enrollment of these populations, and a plan for the retention and reporting of said populations on the trial. If the inclusion and exclusion criteria are expected to have a negative effect on the recruitment or retention of underrepresented populations, the protocol must discuss why these criteria are necessary.

m. The CLINICAL STUDY protocol explicitly discusses how the results are or are not expected to be generalizable to the Medicare population to infer whether Medicare patients may benefit from the intervention. Separate discussions in the protocol may be necessary for populations eligible for Medicare due to age, disability or Medicaid eligibility. Consistent with ?1142 of the Social Security Act (the Act), the Agency for Healthcare Research and Quality (AHRQ) supports clinical research studies that CMS determines meet the above-listed standards and address the above-listed research questions.

Any clinical study undertaken pursuant to this NCD must be approved no later than August 2, 2014. If there are no approved clinical studies on or before August 2, 2014, this CED will expire. Any clinical study approved will adhere to the timeframe designated in the approved clinical study protocol.

C. Nationally Non-Covered Indications

1. Effective December 28, 1992, the Centers for Medicare & Medicaid Services (CMS) issued a national non-coverage determination for platelet-derived wound-healing formulas intended to treat patients with chronic, non-healing wounds. This decision was based on a lack of sufficient published data to determine safety and efficacy, and a public health service technology assessment.

100-04, 1, 30.3.5

Effect of Assignment Upon Purchase of Cataract Glasses FromParticipating Physician or Supplier on Claims Submitted to Carriers
(Rev.1, 10-01-03)B3-3045.4

A pair of cataract glasses is comprised of two distinct products: a professional product (the prescribed lenses) and a retail commercial product (the frames). The frames serve not only as a holder of lenses but also as an article of personal apparel. As such, they are usually selected on the basis of personal taste and style. Although Medicare will pay only for standard frames, most patients want deluxe frames. Participating physicians and suppliers cannot profitably furnish such deluxe frames unless they can make an extra (noncovered) charge for the frames even though they accept assignment.

Therefore, a participating physician or supplier (whether an ophthalmologist, optometrist, or optician) who accepts assignment on cataract glasses with deluxe frames may charge the Medicare patient the difference between his/her usual charge to private pay patients for glasses with standard frames and his/her usual charge to such patients for glasses with deluxe frames, in addition to the applicable deductible and coinsurance on glasses with standard frames, if all of the following requirements are met:

A. The participating physician or supplier has standard frames available, offers them for saleto the patient, and issues and ABN to the patient that explains the price and other differences between standard and deluxe frames. Refer to Chapter 30.

B. The participating physician or supplier obtains from the patient (or his/her representative) and keeps on file the following signed and dated statement:

Name of Patient Medicare Claim Number

Having been informed that an extra charge is being made by the physician or supplier for deluxe frames, that this extra charge is not covered by Medicare, and that standard frames are available for purchase from the physician or supplier at no extra charge, I have chosen to purchase deluxe frames.

Signature Date

C. The participating physician or supplier itemizes on his/her claim his/her actual charge for the lenses, his/her actual charge for the standard frames, and his/her actual extra charge for the deluxe frames (charge differential). Once the assigned claim for deluxe frames has been processed, the carrier will follow the ABN instructions as described in Sec.60.

100-04, 3, 20.7.3

Payment for Blood Clotting Factor Administered to Hemophilia Inpatients
(Rev.3481, Issued: 03-18-16. Effective: 06-20-16, Implementation: 06-20-16)

Section 6011 of Public Law (P.L.) 101-239 amended §1886(a)(4) of the Social Security Act (the Act) to provide that prospective payment system (PPS) hospitals receive an additional payment for the costs of administering blood clotting factor to Medicare hemophiliacs who are hospital inpatients. Section 6011(b) of P.L. 101.239 specified that the payment be based on a predetermined price per unit of clotting factor multiplied by the number of units provided. This add-on payment originally was effective for blood clotting factors furnished on or after June 19, 1990, and before December 19, 1991. Section 13505 of P. L. 103-66 amended §6011 (d) of P.L. 101-239 to extend the period covered by the add-on payment for blood clotting factors administered to Medicare inpatients with hemophilia through September 30, 1994. Section 4452 of P.L. 105-33 amended §6011(d) of P.L. 101-239 to reinstate the add-on payment for the costs of administering blood-clotting factor to Medicare beneficiaries who have hemophilia and who are hospital inpatients for discharges occurring on or after October 1, 1998.

A/B MACs (B) shall process non-institutional blood clotting factor claims.

The A/B MACs (A) shall process institutional blood clotting factor claims payable under either Part A or Part B.

A. Inpatient Bills

Under the Inpatient Prospective Payment System (IPPS), hospitals receive a special add-on payment for the costs of furnishing blood clotting factors to Medicare beneficiaries with hemophilia, admitted as inpatients of PPS hospitals. The clotting factor add-on payment is calculated using the number of units (as defined in the HCPCS code long descriptor) billed by the provider under special instructions for units of service.

The PPS Pricer software does not calculate the payment amount. The Fiscal Intermediary Shared System (FISS) calculates the payment amount and subtracts the

 © 2019 Optum360, LLC

charges from those submitted to Pricer so that the clotting factor charges are not included in cost outlier computations.

Blood clotting factors not paid on a cost or PPS basis are priced as a drug/biological under the Medicare Part B Drug Pricing File effective for the specific date of service. As of January 1, 2005, the average sales price (ASP) plus 6 percent shall be used.

If a beneficiary is in a covered Part A stay in a PPS hospital, the clotting factors are paid in addition to the DRG/HIPPS payment (For FY 2004, this payment is based on 95 percent of average wholesale price.) For a SNF subject to SNF/PPS, the payment is bundled into the SNF/PPS rate.

For SNF inpatient Part A, there is no add-on payment for blood clotting factors.

The codes for blood-clotting factors are found on the Medicare Part B Drug Pricing File. This file is distributed on a quarterly basis.

For discharges occurring on or after October 1, 2000, and before December 31, 2005, report HCPCS Q0187 based on 1 billing unit per 1.2 mg. Effective January 1, 2006, HCPCS code J7189 replaces Q0187 and is defined as 1 billing unit per 1 microgram (mcg).

The examples below include the HCPCS code and indicate the dosage amount specified in the descriptor of that code. Facilities use the units field as a multiplier to arrive at the dosage amount.

EXAMPLE 1

HCPCS	Drug	Dosage
J7189	Factor VIIa	1 mcg

Actual dosage: 13,365 mcg

On the bill, the facility shows J7189 and 13,365 in the units field (13,365 mcg divided by 1 mcg = 13,365 units).

NOTE: The process for dealing with one international unit (IU) is the same as the process of dealing with one microgram.

EXAMPLE 2

HCPCS	Drug	Dosage
J7189	Trastuzumab	10 mg

Actual dosage: 140 mg

On the bill, the facility shows J9355 and 14 in the units field (140 mg divided by 10mg = 14 units).

When the dosage amount is greater than the amount indicated for the HCPCS code, the facility rounds up to determine units. When the dosage amount is less than the amount indicated for the HCPCS code, use 1 as the unit of measure.

EXAMPLE 3

HCPCS	Drug	Dosage
J3100	Tenecteplase	50 mg

Actual Dosage: 40 mg

The provider would bill for 1 unit, even though less than 1 full unit was furnished.

At times, the facility provides less than the amount provided in a single use vial and there is waste, i.e.; some drugs may be available only in packaged amounts that exceed the needs of an individual patient. Once the drug is reconstituted in the hospital's pharmacy, it may have a limited shelf life. Since an individual patient may receive less than the fully reconstituted amount, we encourage hospitals to schedule patients in such a way that the hospital can use the drug most efficiently. However, if the hospital must discard the remainder of a vial after administering part of it to a Medicare patient, the provider may bill for the amount of drug discarded plus the amount administered.

Example 1:
Drug X is available only in a 100-unit size. A hospital schedules three Medicare patients to receive drug X on the same day within the designated shelf life of the product. An appropriate hospital staff member administers 30 units to each patient. The remaining 10 units are billed to Medicare on the account of the last patient. Therefore, 30 units are billed on behalf of the first patient seen and 30 units are billed on behalf of the second patient seen. Forty units are billed on behalf of the last patient seen because the hospital had to discard 10 units at that point.

Example 2:
An appropriate hospital staff member must administer 30 units of drug X to a Medicare patient, and it is not practical to schedule another patient who requires the same drug. For example, the hospital has only one patient who requires drug X, or the hospital sees the patient for the first time and did not know the patient's condition. The hospital bills for 100 units on behalf of the patient, and Medicare pays for 100 units.

When the number of units of blood clotting factor administered to hemophiliac inpatients exceeds 99,999, the hospital reports the excess as a second line for revenue code 0636 and repeats the HCPCS code. One hundred thousand fifty (100,050) units are reported on one line as 99,999, and another line shows 1,051.

Revenue Code 0636 is used. It requires HCPCS. Some other inpatient drugs continue to be billed without HCPCS codes under pharmacy.

No changes in beneficiary notices are required. Coverage is applicable to hospital Part A claims only. Coverage is also applicable to inpatient Part B services in SNFs and all types of hospitals, including CAHs. Separate payment is not made to SNFs for beneficiaries in an inpatient Part A stay.

B. A/B MAC (A) Action
The contractor is responsible for the following:

- It accepts HCPCS codes for inpatient services;
- It edits to require HCPCS codes with Revenue Code 0636. Multiple iterations of the revenue code are possible with the same or different HCPCS codes. It does not edit units except to ensure a numeric value;
- It reduces charges forwarded to Pricer by the charges for hemophilia clotting factors in revenue code 0636. It retains the charges and revenue and HCPCS codes for CWF; and
- It modifies data entry screens to accept HCPCS codes for hospital (including CAH) swing bed, and SNF inpatient claims (bill types 11X, 12X, 18x, 21x and, 22x).

The September 1, 1993, IPPS final rule (58 FR 46304) states that payment will be made for the blood clotting factor only if diagnosis code for hemophilia is included on the bill.

Inpatient blood-clotting factors are covered only for beneficiaries with hemophilia. One of the following hemophilia diagnosis codes must be reported on the claim for payment to be made for blood clotting factors.

Table 1 - Effective for discharges September 1 1993 through the implementation of ICD-10

ICD-9-CM code	Description
286.0	Congenital factor VIII disorder
286.1	Congenital factor IX disorder
286.2	Congenital factor XI deficiency
286.3	Congenital deficiency of other clotting factors
286.4	von Willebrands' disease

Table 2 - Effective for discharges August 1, 2001 through the implementation of ICD-10, payment may be made if a diagnosis codes from either Table 1 or Table 2 is reported is reported:

ICD-9-CM code	Description
286.5	Hemorrhagic disorder due to intrinsic circulating anticoagulants (terminate effective September 30, 2011)
286.7	Acquired coagulation factor deficiency

Table 3 - Effective for discharges on October 1, 2011, through the implementation of ICD-10 payment may be made if a diagnosis code from any of Table 1, Table 2 or Table 3 is reported:

ICD-9-CM code	Description
286.52	Acquired hemophilia
286.53	Antiphospholipid antibody with hemorrhagic disorder
286.59	Other hemorrhagic disorder due to intrinsic circulating anticoagulants, antibodies, or inhibitors

Effective for discharges on or after the implementation of ICD-10-CM, the following codes are applicable, and payment may be made for blood clotting factors only if a hemophilia code from the range D66 - D68.4 is reported

© 2019 Optum360, LLC

A crosswalk of ICD 9 to ICD10 hemophilia diagnosis codes follows:

ICD-9-CM Code	Description	ICD-10-CM Code	Description
286.0	Congenital factor VIII disorder	D66	Hereditary factor VIII deficiency
286.1	Congenital factor IX disorder	D67	Hereditary factor IX deficiency
286.2	Congenital factor XI deficiency	D68.1	Hereditary factor XI deficiency
286.3	Congenital deficiency of other clotting factors	D68.2	Hereditary deficiency of other clotting factors
286.4	von Willebrands' disease	D68.0	Von Willebrand's disease
286.5	Hemorrhagic disorder due to intrinsic circulating anticoagulants (terminate effective September 30, 2011)	N/A	
286.52	Acquired hemophilia	D68.311	Acquired hemophilia
286.53	Antiphospholipid antibody with hemorrhagic disorder	D68.312	Antiphospholipid antibody with hemorrhagic disorder
286.59	Other hemorrhagic disorder due to intrinsic circulating anticoagulants, antibodies, or inhibitors	D68.318	Other hemorrhagic disorder due to intrinsic circulating anticoagulants, antibodies, or inhibitors
286.7	Acquired coagulation factor deficiency	D68.32	Antiphospholipid antibody with hemorrhagic disorder
286.7	Acquired coagulation factor deficiency	D68.4	Acquired coagulation factor deficiency

C. Part A Remittance Advice

For remittance reporting PIP and/or non-PIP payments, the Hemophilia Add On is included in the overall claim payment (Provider Reimbursement, CLP04).

If an inpatient claim has a Hemophilia Add On payment, the payment to the provider is increased in the PLB segment with a PLB adjustment HM. The Hemophilia Add On amount will always be included in the CLP04 Claim Payment Amount.

For remittance reporting PIP payments, the Hemophilia Add On will also be reported in the provider level adjustment (element identifier PLB) segment with the provider level adjustment reason code HM. For remittances reporting PIP payments, the sum of inpatient claims, CLP04, is backed out at PLB with PI/PA. If an inpatient claim has a Hemophilia Add On payment, the payment to the provider is increased in the PLB segment with a PLB adjustment HM.

D. Standard Hard Copy Remittance Advice

For paper remittances reporting non-PIP payments involving Hemophilia Add On, add a "Hemophilia Add On" category to the end of the "Pass Thru Amounts" listings in the "Summary" section of the paper remittance. Enter the total of the Hemophilia Add On amounts due for the claims covered by this remittance next to the Hemophilia Add On heading.

The following reflects the remittance advice messages and associated codes that will appear when processing claims under this policy. The CARC below is not included in the CAQH CORE Business Scenarios.

Group Code: OA

CARC: 94

RARC: MA103

MSN: N/A

This will be the full extent of Hemophilia Add On reporting on paper remittance notices; providers wishing more detailed information must subscribe to the Medicare Part A specifications for the ASC X12 835 remittance advice, where additional information is available.

See chapter 22, for detailed instructions and definitions.

100-04, 3, 40.2.2

Charges to Beneficiaries for Part A Services

(Rev.1495; Issued: 05-02-08; Effective Date: 10-01-08; Implementation Date: 10-06-08)

The hospital submits a bill even where the patient is responsible for a deductible which covers the entire amount of the charges for non-PPS hospitals, or in PPS hospitals, where the DRG payment amount will be less than the deductible.

A hospital receiving payment for a covered hospital stay (or PPS hospital that includes at least one covered day, or one treated as covered under guarantee of payment or limitation on liability) may charge the beneficiary, or other person, for items and services furnished during the stay only as described in subsections A through H. If limitation of liability applies, a beneficiary's liability for payment is governed by the limitation on liability notification rules in Chapter 30 of this manual. For related notices for inpatient hospitals, see CMS Transmittal 594, Change Request3903, dated June 24, 2005.

A. Deductible and Coinsurance

The hospital may charge the beneficiary or other person for applicable deductible and coinsurance amounts. The deductible is satisfied only by charges for covered services. The FI deducts the deductible and coinsurance first from the PPS payment. Where the deductible exceeds the PPS amount, the excess will be applied to a subsequent payment to the hospital. (See Chapter 3 of the Medicare General Information, Eligibility, and Entitlement Manual for specific policies.)

B. Blood Deductible

The Part A blood deductible provision applies to whole blood and red blood cells, and reporting of the number of pints is applicable to both PPS and non-PPS hospitals. (See Chapter 3 of the Medicare General Information, Eligibility, and Entitlement Manual for specific policies.) Hospitals shall report charges for red blood cells using revenue code 381, and charges for whole blood using revenue code 382.

C. Inpatient Care No Longer Required

The hospital may charge for services that are not reasonable and necessary or that constitute custodial care. Notification may be required under limitation of liability. See CMS Transmittal 594, Change Request3903, dated June 24, 2005, section V. of the attachment, for specific notification requirements. Note this transmittal will be placed in Chapter 30 of this manual at a future point. Chapter 1, section 150 of this manual also contains related billing information in addition to that provided below.

In general, after proper notification has occurred, and assuming an expedited decision is received from a Quality Improvement Organization (QIO), the following entries are required on the bill the hospital prepares:

- Occurrence code 3I (and date) to indicate the date the hospital notified the patient in accordance with the first bullet above;
- Occurrence span code 76 (and dates) to indicate the period of noncovered care for which it is charging the beneficiary;
- Occurrence span code 77 (and dates) to indicate the period of noncovered care for which the provider is liable, when it is aware of this prior to billing; and
- Value code 3I (and amount) to indicate the amount of charges it may bill the beneficiary for days for which inpatient care was no longer required. They are included as noncovered charges on the bill.

D. Change in the Beneficiary's Condition

If the beneficiary remains in the hospital after receiving notice as described in subsection C, and the hospital, the physician who concurred in the hospital's determination, or the QIO, subsequently determines that the beneficiary again requires inpatient hospital care, the hospital may not charge the beneficiary or other person for services furnished after the beneficiary again required inpatient hospital care until proper notification occurs (see subsection C).

If a patient who needs only a SNF level of care remains in the hospital after the SNF bed becomes available, and the bed ceases to be available, the hospital may continue to charge the beneficiary. It need not provide the beneficiary with another notice when the patient chose not to be discharged to the SNF bed.

E. Admission Denied

If the entire hospital admission is determined to be not reasonable or necessary, limitation of liability may apply. See 2005 CMS transmittal 594, section V. of the attachment, for specific notification requirements.

NOTE: This transmittal will be placed in Chapter 30 of this manual at a future point.

In such cases the following entries are required on the bill:

- Occurrence code 3I (and date) to indicate the date the hospital notified the beneficiary.
- Occurrence span code 76 (and dates) to indicate the period of noncovered care for which the hospital is charging the beneficiary.
- Occurrence span code 77 (and dates) to indicate any period of noncovered care for which the provider is liable (e.g., the period between issuing the notice and the time it may charge the beneficiary) when the provider is aware of this prior to billing.
- Value code 3I (and amount) to indicate the amount of charges the hospital may bill the beneficiary for hospitalization that was not necessary or reasonable. They are included as noncovered charges on the bill.

© 2019 Optum360, LLC

F. Procedures, Studies and Courses of Treatment That Are Not Reasonable or Necessary

If diagnostic procedures, studies, therapeutic studies and courses of treatment are excluded from coverage as not reasonable and necessary (even though the beneficiary requires inpatient hospital care) the hospital may charge the beneficiary or other person for the services or care according the procedures given in CMS Transmittal 594, Change Request3903, dated June 24, 2005.

The following bill entries apply to these circumstances:

- Occurrence code 32 (and date) to indicate the date the hospital provided the notice to the beneficiary.
- Value code 3I (and amount) to indicate the amount of such charges to be billed to the beneficiary. They are included as noncovered charges on the bill.

G. Nonentitlement Days and Days after Benefits Exhausted

If a hospital stay exceeds the day outlier threshold, the hospital may charge for some, or all, of the days on which the patient is not entitled to Medicare Part A, or after the Part A benefits are exhausted (i.e., the hospital may charge its customary charges for services furnished on those days). It may charge the beneficiary for the lesser of:

- The number of days on which the patient was not entitled to benefits or after the benefits were exhausted; or
- The number of outlier days. (Day outliers were discontinued at the end of FY 1997.)

If the number of outlier days exceeds the number of days on which the patient was not entitled to benefits, or after benefits were exhausted, the hospital may charge for all days on which the patient was not entitled to benefits or after benefits were exhausted. If the number of days on which the beneficiary was not entitled to benefits, or after benefits were exhausted, exceeds the number of outlier days, the hospital determines the days for which it may charge by starting with the last day of the stay (i.e., the day before the day of discharge) and identifying and counting off in reverse order, days on which the patient was not entitled to benefits or after the benefits were exhausted, until the number of days counted off equals the number of outlier days. The days counted off are the days for which the hospital may charge.

H. Contractual Exclusions

In addition to receiving the basic prospective payment, the hospital may charge the beneficiary for any services that are excluded from coverage for reasons other than, or in addition to, absence of medical necessity, provision of custodial care, non-entitlement to Part A, or exhaustion of benefits. For example, it may charge for most cosmetic and dental surgery.

I. Private Room Care

Payment for medically necessary private room care is included in the prospective payment. Where the beneficiary requests private room accommodations, the hospital must inform the beneficiary of the additional charge. (See the Medicare Benefit Policy Manual, Chapter 1.) When the beneficiary accepts the liability, the hospital will supply the service, and bill the beneficiary directly. If the beneficiary believes the private room was medically necessary, the beneficiary has a right to a determination and may initiate a Part A appeal.

J. Deluxe Item or Service

Where a beneficiary requests a deluxe item or service, i.e., an item or service which is more expensive than is medically required for the beneficiary's condition, the hospital may collect the additional charge if it informs the beneficiary of the additional charge. That charge is the difference between the customary charge for the item or service most commonly furnished by the hospital to private pay patients with the beneficiary's condition, and the charge for the more expensive item or service requested. If the beneficiary believes that the more expensive item or service was medically necessary, the beneficiary has a right to a determination and may initiate a Part A appeal.

K - Inpatient Acute Care Hospital Admission Followed By a Death or Discharge Prior To Room Assignment

A patient of an acute care hospital is considered an inpatient upon issuance of written doctor's orders to that effect. If a patient either dies or is discharged prior to being assigned and/or occupying a room, a hospital may enter an appropriate room and board charge on the claim. If a patient leaves of their own volition prior to being assigned and/or occupying a room, a hospital may enter an appropriate room and board charge on the claim as well as a patient status code 07 which indicates they left against medical advice. A hospital is not required to enter a room and board charge, but failure to do so may have a minimal impact on future DRG weight calculations.

100-04, 4, 20.6.4

Use of Modifiers for Discontinued Services

(Rev. 4204, Issued: 01-17-19, Effective: 01-01-19, Implementation: 01-07-19)

A. General

Modifiers provide a way for hospitals to report and be paid for expenses incurred in preparing a patient for a procedure and scheduling a room for performing the procedure where the service is subsequently discontinued. This instruction is applicable to both outpatient hospital departments and to ambulatory surgical centers.

Modifier -73 is used by the facility to indicate that a procedure requiring anesthesia was terminated due to extenuating circumstances or to circumstances that threatened the well being of the patient after the patient had been prepared for the procedure (including procedural pre-medication when provided), and been taken to the room where the procedure was to be performed, but prior to administration of anesthesia. For purposes of billing for services furnished in the hospital outpatient department, anesthesia is defined to include local, regional block(s), moderate sedation/analgesia ("conscious sedation"), deep sedation/analgesia, or general anesthesia. This modifier code was created so that the costs incurred by the hospital to prepare the patient for the procedure and the resources expended in the procedure room and recovery room (if needed) could be recognized for payment even though the procedure was discontinued.

Modifier -74 is used by the facility to indicate that a procedure requiring anesthesia was terminated after the induction of anesthesia or after the procedure was started (e.g., incision made, intubation started, scope inserted) due to extenuating circumstances or circumstances that threatened the well being of the patient. This modifier may also be used to indicate that a planned surgical or diagnostic procedure was discontinued, partially reduced or cancelled at the physician's discretion after the administration of anesthesia. For purposes of billing for services furnished in the hospital outpatient department, anesthesia is defined to include local, regional block(s), moderate sedation/analgesia ("conscious sedation"), deep sedation/analgesia, and general anesthesia. This modifier code was created so that the costs incurred by the hospital to initiate the procedure (preparation of the patient, procedure room, recovery room) could be recognized for payment even though the procedure was discontinued prior to completion.

Coinciding with the addition of the modifiers -73 and -74, modifiers -52 and -53 were revised. Modifier -52 is used to indicate partial reduction, cancellation, or discontinuation of services for which anesthesia is not planned. The modifier provides a means for reporting reduced services without disturbing the identification of the basic service. Modifier -53 is used to indicate discontinuation of physician services and is not approved for use for outpatient hospital services.

The elective cancellation of a procedure should not be reported.

Modifiers -73 and -74 are only used to indicate discontinued procedures for which anesthesia is planned or provided.

B. Effect on Payment

Procedures that are discontinued after the patient has been prepared for the procedure and taken to the procedure room but before anesthesia is provided will be paid at 50 percent of the full OPPS payment amount. Modifier -73 is used for these procedures. As of January 1, 2016, for device-intensive procedures that append modifier -73, we will reduce the APC payment amount for the discontinued device-intensive procedure, by 100 percent of the device offset amount prior to applying the additional payment adjustments that apply when the procedure is discontinued as modified by means of a final rule with comment period and published in the November 13, 2015 "Federal Register" (80 FR 70424). Beginning January 1, 2017, device-intensive procedures are defined as those procedures requiring the insertion of an implantable device, that also have a HCPCS- level device offset greater than 40 percent. From January 1, 2016 through December 31, 2016 device-intensive procedures were defined as those procedures that involve implantable devices that are assigned to a device-intensive APC (defined as those APCs with a device offset greater than 40 percent). Beginning January 1, 2019, device-intensive procedures are defined as procedures that involve the surgical implantation or insertion of an implantable device that is assigned a CPT or HCPCS code (including single-use devices) and has a device offset amount that exceeds 30 percent of the procedure's mean cost.

Procedures that are discontinued, partially reduced or cancelled after the procedure has been initiated and/or the patient has received anesthesia will be paid at the full OPPS payment amount. Modifier -74 is used for these procedures.

Procedures for which anesthesia is not planned that are discontinued, partially reduced or cancelled after the patient is prepared and taken to the room where the procedure is to be performed will be paid at 50 percent of the full OPPS payment amount. Modifier -52 is used for these procedures.

© 2019 Optum360, LLC

100-04, 4, 160

Clinic and Emergency Visits

(Rev.1445, Issued: 02-08-08; Effective: 01-01-08; Implementation: 03-10-08)

CMS has acknowledged from the beginning of the OPPS that CMS believes that CPT Evaluation and Management (E/M) codes were designed to reflect the activities of physicians and do not describe well the range and mix of services provided by hospitals during visits of clinic and emergency department patients. While awaiting the development of a national set of facility-specific codes and guidelines, providers should continue to apply their current internal guidelines to the existing CPT codes. Each hospital's internal guidelines should follow the intent of the CPT code descriptors, in that the guidelines should be designed to reasonably relate the intensity of hospital resources to the different levels of effort represented by the codes. Hospitals should ensure that their guidelines accurately reflect resource distinctions between the five levels of codes.

Effective January 1, 2007, CMS is distinguishing between two types of emergency departments: Type A emergency departments and Type B emergency departments.

A Type A emergency department is defined as an emergency department that is available 24 hours a day, 7 days a week and is either licensed by the State in which it is located under applicable State law as an emergency room or emergency department or it is held out to the public (by name, posted signs, advertising, or other means) as a place that provides care for emergency medical conditions on an urgent basis without requiring a previously scheduled appointment.

A Type B emergency department is defined as an emergency department that meets the definition of a "dedicated emergency department" as defined in 42 CFR 489.24 under the EMTALA regulations. It must meet at least one of the following requirements: (1) It is licensed by the State in which it is located under applicable State law as an emergency room or emergency department; (2) It is held out to the public (by name, posted signs, advertising, or other means) as a place that provides care for emergency medical conditions on an urgent basis without requiring a previously scheduled appointment; or (3) During the calendar year immediately preceding the calendar year in which a determination under 42 CFR 489.24 is being made, based on a representative sample of patient visits that occurred during that calendar year, it provides at least one-third of all of its outpatient visits for the treatment of emergency medical conditions on an urgent basis without requiring a previously scheduled appointment.

Hospitals must bill for visits provided in Type A emergency departments using CPT emergency department E/M codes. Hospitals must bill for visits provided in Type B emergency departments using the G-codes that describe visits provided in Type B emergency departments.

Hospitals that will be billing the new Type B ED visit codes may need to update their internal guidelines to report these codes.

Emergency department and clinic visits are paid in some cases separately and in other cases as part of a composite APC payment. See section 10.2.1 of this chapter for further details.

100-04, 4, 160.1

Critical Care Services

(Rev.2141, Issued: 01-24-11, Effective: 01-01-11, Implementation: 01-03-11)

Hospitals should separately report all HCPCS codes in accordance with correct coding principles, CPT code descriptions, and any additional CMS guidance, when available. Specifically with respect to CPT code 99291 (Critical care, evaluation and management of the critically ill or critically injured patient; first 30-74 minutes), hospitals must follow the CPT instructions related to reporting that CPT code. Prior to January 1, 2011, any services that CPT indicates are included in the reporting of CPT code 99291 (including those services that would otherwise be reported by and paid to hospitals using any of the CPT codes specified by CPT) should not be billed separately by the hospital. Instead, hospitals should report charges for any services provided as part of the critical care services. In establishing payment rates for critical care services, and other services, CMS packages the costs of certain items and services separately reported by HCPCS codes into payment for critical care services and other services, according to the standard OPPS methodology for packaging costs.

Beginning January 1, 2011, in accordance with revised CPT guidance, hospitals that report in accordance with the CPT guidelines will begin reporting all of the ancillary services and their associated charges separately when they are provided in conjunction with critical care. CMS will continue to recognize the existing CPT codes for critical care services and will establish payment rates based on historical data, into which the cost of the ancillary services is intrinsically packaged. The I/OCE conditionally packages payment for the ancillary services that are reported on the same date of service as critical care services in order to avoid overpayment. The payment status of the ancillary services does not change when they are not provided in conjunction with critical care services. Hospitals may use HCPCS modifier -59 to indicate when an ancillary procedure or service is distinct or independent from critical care when performed on the same day but in a different encounter.

Beginning January 1, 2007, critical care services will be paid at two levels, depending on the presence or absence of trauma activation. Providers will receive one payment rate for critical care without trauma activation and will receive additional payment when critical care is associated with trauma activation.

To determine whether trauma activation occurs, follow the National Uniform Billing Committee (NUBC) guidelines in the Claims Processing Manual, Pub 100-04, Chapter 25, §75.4 related to the reporting of the trauma revenue codes in the 68x series. The revenue code series 68x can be used only by trauma centers/hospitals as licensed or designated by the state or local government authority authorized to do so, or as verified by the American College of Surgeons. Different subcategory revenue codes are reported by designated Level 1-4 hospital trauma centers. Only patients for whom there has been prehospital notification based on triage information from prehospital caregivers, who meet either local, state or American College of Surgeons field triage criteria, or are delivered by inter-hospital transfers, and are given the appropriate team response can be billed a trauma activation charge.

When critical care services are provided without trauma activation, the hospital may bill CPT code 99291, Critical care, evaluation and management of the critically ill or critically injured patient; first 30-74 minutes (and 99292, if appropriate). If trauma activation occurs under the circumstances described by the NUBC guidelines that would permit reporting a charge under 68x, the hospital may also bill one unit of code G0390, which describes trauma activation associated with hospital critical care services. Revenue code 68x must be reported on the same date of service. The OCE will edit to ensure that G0390 appears with revenue code 68x on the same date of service and that only one unit of G0390 is billed. CMS believes that trauma activation is a one-time occurrence in association with critical care services, and therefore, CMS will only pay for one unit of G0390 per day.

The CPT code 99291 is defined by CPT as the first 30-74 minutes of critical care. This 30 minute minimum has always applied under the OPPS. The CPT code 99292, Critical care, evaluation and management of the critically ill or critically injured patient; each additional 30 minutes, remains a packaged service under the OPPS, so that hospitals do not have the ongoing administrative burden of reporting precisely the time for each critical service provided. As the CPT guidelines indicate, hospitals that provide less than 30 minutes of critical care should bill for a visit, typically an emergency department visit, at a level consistent with their own internal guidelines.

Under the OPPS, the time that can be reported as critical care is the time spent by a physician and/or hospital staff engaged in active face-to-face critical care of a critically ill or critically injured patient. If the physician and hospital staff or multiple hospital staff members are simultaneously engaged in this active face-to-face care, the time involved can only be counted once.

- Beginning in CY 2007 hospitals may continue to report a charge with RC 68x without any HCPCS code when trauma team activation occurs. In order to receive additional payment when critical care services are associated with trauma activation, the hospital must report G0390 on the same date of service as RC 68x, in addition to CPT code 99291 (or 99292, if appropriate.)
- Beginning in CY 2007 hospitals should continue to report 99291 (and 99292 as appropriate) for critical care services furnished without trauma team activation. CPT 99291 maps to APC 0617 (Critical Care). (CPT 99292 is packaged and not paid separately, but should be reported if provided.)

Critical care services are paid in some cases separately and in other cases as part of a composite APC payment. See Section 10.2.1 of this chapter for further details.

Future updates will be issued in a Recurring Update Notification.

100-04, 4, 200.1

Billing for Corneal Tissue

(Rev.3425, Iss.: 12-18-15, Eff: 01-01-16, Implementation: 01-04-16)

Corneal tissue will be paid on a cost basis, not under OPPS. To receive cost based reimbursement hospitals must bill charges for corneal tissue using HCPCS code V2785.

100-04, 4, 200.2

Hospital Dialysis Services For Patients with and without End Stage Renal Disease (ESRD)

(Rev.2455, Issued: 04-26-12, Effective: 10-01-12, Implementation; 10-01-12)

Effective with claims with dates of service on or after August 1, 2000, hospital-based End Stage Renal Disease (ESRD) facilities must submit services covered under the ESRD benefit in 42 CFR 413.174 (maintenance dialysis and those items and services

© 2019 Optum360, LLC

directly related to dialysis such as drugs, supplies) on a separate claim from services not covered under the ESRD benefit. Items and services not covered under the ESRD benefit must be billed by the hospital using the hospital bill type and be paid under the Outpatient Prospective Payment System (OPPS) (or to a CAH at reasonable cost). Services covered under the ESRD benefit in 42 CFR 413.174 must be billed on the ESRD bill type and must be paid under the ESRD PPS. This requirement is necessary to properly pay only unrelated ESRD services (those not covered under the ESRD benefit) under OPPS (or to a CAH at reasonable cost).

Medicare does not allow payment for routine or related dialysis treatments, which are covered and paid under the ESRD PPS, when furnished to ESRD patients in the outpatient department of a hospital. However, in certain medical situations in which the ESRD outpatient cannot obtain her or his regularly scheduled dialysis treatment at a certified ESRD facility, the OPPS rule for 2003 allows payment for non-routine dialysis treatments (which are not covered under the ESRD benefit) furnished to ESRD outpatients in the outpatient department of a hospital. Payment for unscheduled dialysis furnished to ESRD outpatients and paid under the OPPS is limited to the following circumstances:

- Dialysis performed following or in connection with a dialysis-related procedure such as vascular access procedure or blood transfusions;
- Dialysis performed following treatment for an unrelated medical emergency; e.g., if a patient goes to the emergency room for chest pains and misses a regularly scheduled dialysis treatment that cannot be rescheduled, CMS allows the hospital to provide and bill Medicare for the dialysis treatment; or
- Emergency dialysis for ESRD patients who would otherwise have to be admitted as inpatients in order for the hospital to receive payment.

In these situations, non-ESRD certified hospital outpatient facilities are to bill Medicare using the Healthcare Common Procedure Coding System (HCPCS) code G0257 (Unscheduled or emergency dialysis treatment for an ESRD patient in a hospital outpatient department that is not certified as an ESRD facility).

HCPCS code G0257 may only be reported on type of bill 13X (hospital outpatient service) or type of bill 85X (critical access hospital) because HCPCS code G0257 only reports services for hospital outpatients with ESRD and only these bill types are used to report services to hospital outpatients. Effective for services on and after October 1, 2012, claims containing HCPCS code G0257 will be returned to the provider for correction if G0257 is reported with a type of bill other than 13X or 85X (such as a 12x inpatient claim).

HCPCS code 90935 (Hemodialysis procedure with single physician evaluation) may be reported and paid only if one of the following two conditions is met:

1) The patient is a hospital inpatient with or without ESRD and has no coverage under Part A, but has Part B coverage. The charge for hemodialysis is a charge for the use of a prosthetic device. See Benefits Policy Manual 100-02 Chapter 15 section 120. A. The service must be reported on a type of bill 12X or type of bill 85X. See the Benefits Policy Manual 100-02 Chapter 6 section 10 (Medical and Other Health Services Furnished to Inpatients of Participating Hospitals) for the criteria that must be met for services to be paid when a hospital inpatient has Part B coverage but does not have coverage under Part A; or 2) A hospital outpatient does not have ESRD and is receiving hemodialysis in the hospital outpatient department. The service is reported on a type of bill 13X or type of bill 85X. CPT code 90945 (Dialysis procedure other than hemodialysis (e.g. peritoneal dialysis, hemofiltration, or other continuous replacement therapies)), with single physician evaluation, may be reported by a hospital paid under the OPPS or CAH method I or method II on type of bill 12X, 13X or 85X.

100-04, 4, 200.4

Billing for Amniotic Membrane

(Rev.1445, Issued: 02-08-08; Effective: 01-01-08; Implementation: 03-10-08)

Hospitals should report HCPCS code V2790 (Amniotic membrane for surgical reconstruction, per procedure) to report amniotic membrane tissue when the tissue is used. A specific procedure code associated with use of amniotic membrane tissue is CPT code 65780 (Ocular surface reconstruction; amniotic membrane transplantation).

Payment for the amniotic membrane tissue is packaged into payment for CPT code 65780 or other procedures with which the amniotic membrane is used.

100-04, 4, 200.6

Billing and Payment for Alcohol and/or Substance Abuse Assessment and Intervention Services

(Rev.1445, Issued: 02-08-08; Effective: 01-01-08; Implementation: 03-10-08)

For CY 2008, the CPT Editorial Panel has created two new Category I CPT codes for reporting alcohol and/or substance abuse screening and intervention services. They are CPT code 99408 (Alcohol and/or substance (other than tobacco) abuse structured screening (e.g., AUDIT, DAST), and brief intervention (SBI) services; 15 to 30 minutes); and CPT code 99409 (Alcohol and/or substance (other than tobacco) abuse structured screening (e.g., AUDIT, DAST), and brief intervention (SBI) services; greater than 30 minutes). However, screening services are not covered by Medicare without specific statutory authority, such as has been provided for mammography, diabetes, and colorectal cancer screening. Therefore, beginning January 1, 2008, the OPPS recognizes two parallel G-codes (HCPCS codes G0396 and G0397) to allow for appropriate reporting and payment of alcohol and substance abuse structured assessment and intervention services that are not provided as screening services, but that are performed in the context of the diagnosis or treatment of illness or injury.

Contractors shall make payment under the OPPS for HCPCS code G0396 (Alcohol and/or substance (other than tobacco) abuse structured assessment (e.g., AUDIT, DAST) and brief intervention, 15 to 30 minutes) and HCPCS code G0397, (Alcohol and/or substance(other than tobacco) abuse structured assessment (e.g., AUDIT, DAST) and intervention greater than 30 minutes), only when reasonable and necessary (i.e., when the service is provided to evaluate patients with signs/symptoms of illness or injury) as per section 1862(a)(1)(A) of the Act.

HCPCS codes G0396 and G0397 are to be used for structured alcohol and/or substance (other than tobacco) abuse assessment and intervention services that are distinct from other clinic and emergency department visit services performed during the same encounter. Hospital resources expended performing services described by HCPCS codes G0396 and G0397 may not be counted as resources for determining the level of a visit service and vice versa (i.e., hospitals may not double count the same facility resources in order to reach a higher level clinic or emergency department visit). However, alcohol and/or substance structured assessment or intervention services lasting less than 15 minutes should not be reported using these HCPCS codes, but the hospital resources expended should be included in determining the level of the visit service reported.

100-04, 4, 200.7.2

Cardiac Echocardiography With Contrast

(Rev.1657, Issued: 12-31-08, Effective: 01-01-09, Implementation: 01-05-09)

Hospitals are instructed to bill for echocardiograms with contrast using the applicable HCPCS code(s) included in Table 200.7.2 below. Hospitals should also report the appropriate units of the HCPCS codes for the contrast agents used in the performance of the echocardiograms.

Table 200.7.2 - HCPCS Codes For Echocardiograms With Contrast

PCS	Long Descriptor
C8921	Transthoracic echocardiography with contrast, or without contrast followed by with contrast, for congenital cardiac anomalies; complete
C8922	Transthoracic echocardiography with contrast, or without contrast followed by with contrast, for congenital cardiac anomalies; follow-up or limited study
C8923	Transthoracic echocardiography with contrast, or without contrast followed by with contrast, real-time with image documentation (2D), includes M-mode recording, when performed, complete, without spectral or color Doppler echocardiography
C8924	Transthoracic echocardiography with contrast, or without contrast followed by with contrast, real-time with image documentation (2D), includes M-mode recording, when performed, follow-up or limited study
C8925	Transesophageal echocardiography (TEE) with contrast, or without contrast followed by with contrast, real time with image documentation (2D) (with or without M-mode recording); including probe placement, image acquisition, interpretation and report
C8926	Transesophageal echocardiography (TEE) with contrast, or without contrast followed by with contrast, for congenital cardiac anomalies; including probe placement, image acquisition, interpretation and report
C8927	Transesophageal echocardiography (TEE) with contrast, or without contrast followed by with contrast, for monitoring purposes, including probe placement, real time 2-dimensional image acquisition and interpretation leading to ongoing (continuous) assessment of (dynamically changing) cardiac pumping function and to therapeutic measures on an immediate time basis
C8928	Transthoracic echocardiography with contrast, or without contrast followed by with contrast, real-time with image documentation (2D), includes M-mode recording, when performed, during rest and cardiovascular stress test using treadmill, bicycle exercise and/or pharmacologically induced stress, with interpretation and report

© 2019 Optum360, LLC

PCS	Long Descriptor
C8929	Transthoracic echocardiography with contrast, or without contrast followed by with contrast, real-time with image documentation (2D), includes M-mode recording, when performed, complete, with spectral Doppler echocardiography, and with color flow Doppler echocardiography
C8930	Transthoracic echocardiography, with contrast, or without contrast followed by with contrast, real-time with image documentation (2D), includes M-mode recording, when performed, during rest and cardiovascular stress test using treadmill, bicycle exercise and/or pharmacologically induced stress, with interpretation and report; including performance of continuous electrocardiographic monitoring, with physician supervision

100-04, 4, 230.2

Coding and Payment for Drug Administration

(Rev.2141, Issued: 01-24-11, Effective: 01-01-11, Implementation: 01-03-11)

A. Overview

Drug administration services furnished under the Hospital Outpatient Prospective Payment System (OPPS) during CY 2005 were reported using CPT codes 90780, 90781, and 96400-96459.

Effective January 1, 2006, some of these CPT codes were replaced with more detailed CPT codes incorporating specific procedural concepts, as defined and described by the CPT manual, such as initial, concurrent, and sequential.

Hospitals are instructed to use the full set of CPT codes, including those codes referencing concepts of initial, concurrent, and sequential, to bill for drug administration services furnished in the hospital outpatient department beginning January 1, 2007. In addition, hospitals are instructed to continue billing the HCPCS codes that most accurately describe the service(s) provided.

Hospitals are reminded to bill a separate Evaluation and Management code (with modifier 25) only if a significant, separately identifiable E/M service is performed in the same encounter with OPPS drug administration services.

B. Billing for Infusions and Injections

Beginning in CY 2007, hospitals were instructed to use the full set of drug administration CPT codes (90760-90779; 96401-96549), (96413-96523 beginning in CY 2008) (96360-96549 beginning in CY 2009) when billing for drug administration services provided in the hospital outpatient department. In addition, hospitals are to continue to bill HCPCS code C8957 (Intravenous infusion for therapy/diagnosis; initiation of prolonged infusion (more than 8 hours), requiring use of portable or implantable pump) when appropriate. Hospitals are expected to report all drug administration CPT codes in a manner consistent with their descriptors, CPT instructions, and correct coding principles. Hospitals should note the conceptual changes between CY 2006 drug administration codes effective under the OPPS and the CPT codes in effect beginning January 1, 2007, in order to ensure accurate billing under the OPPS. Hospitals should report all HCPCS codes that describe the drug administration services provided, regardless of whether or not those services are separately paid or their payment is packaged.

Medicare's general policy regarding physician supervision within hospital outpatient departments meets the physician supervision requirements for use of CPT codes 90760-90779, 96401-96549, (96413-96523 beginning in CY 2008). (Reference: Pub.100-02, Medicare Benefit Policy Manual, Chapter 6, §20.4.)

Drug administration services are to be reported with a line item date of service on the day they are provided. In addition, only one initial drug administration service is to be reported per vascular access site per encounter, including during an encounter where observation services span more than 1 calendar day.

C. Payments For Drug Administration Services

For CY 2007, OPPS drug administration APCs were restructured, resulting in a six-level hierarchy where active HCPCS codes have been assigned according to their clinical coherence and resource use. Contrary to the CY 2006 payment structure that bundled payment for several instances of a type of service (non-chemotherapy, chemotherapy by infusion, non-infusion chemotherapy) into a per-encounter APC payment, structure introduced in CY 2007 provides a separate APC payment for each reported unit of a separately payable HCPCS code.

Hospitals should note that the transition to the full set of CPT drug administration codes provides for conceptual differences when reporting, such as those noted below.

- In CY 2006, hospitals were instructed to bill for the first hour (and any additional hours) by each type of infusion service (non-chemotherapy, chemotherapy by infusion, non-infusion chemotherapy). Beginning in CY 2007, the first hour concept no longer exists. CPT codes in CY 2007 and beyond allow for only one initial service per encounter, for each vascular access site, no matter how many types of infusion services are provided; however, hospitals will receive an APC payment for the initial service and separate APC payment(s) for additional hours of infusion or other drug administration services provided that are separately payable.
- In CY 2006, hospitals providing infusion services of different types (non-chemotherapy, chemotherapy by infusion, non-infusion chemotherapy) received payment for the associated per-encounter infusion APC even if these infusions occurred during the same time period. Beginning in CY 2007, hospitals should report only one initial drug administration service, including infusion services, per encounter for each distinct vascular access site, with other services through the same vascular access site being reported via the sequential, concurrent or additional hour codes. Although new CPT guidance has been issued for reporting initial drug administration services, Medicare contractors shall continue to follow the guidance given in this manual.

(NOTE: This list above provides a brief overview of a limited number of the conceptual changes between CY 2006 OPPS drug administration codes and CY 2007 OPPS drug administration codes - this list is not comprehensive and does not include all items hospitals will need to consider during this transition)

For APC payment rates, refer to the most current quarterly version of Addendum B on the CMS Web site at http://www.cms.hhs.gov/HospitalOutpatientPPS/.

D. Infusions Started Outside the Hospital

Hospitals may receive Medicare beneficiaries for outpatient services who are in the process of receiving an infusion at their time of arrival at the hospital (e.g., a patient who arrives via ambulance with an ongoing intravenous infusion initiated by paramedics during transport). Hospitals are reminded to bill for all services provided using the HCPCS code(s) that most accurately describe the service(s) they provided. This includes hospitals reporting an initial hour of infusion, even if the hospital did not initiate the infusion, and additional HCPCS codes for additional or sequential infusion services if needed.

100-04, 4, 231.4

Billing for Split Unit of Blood

(Rev.1487, Issued: 04-08-08, Effective: 04-01-08, Implementation: 04-07-08)

HCPCS code P9011 was created to identify situations where one unit of blood or a blood product is split and some portion of the unit is transfused to one patient and the other portions are transfused to other patients or to the same patient at other times. When a patient receives a transfusion of a split unit of blood or blood product, OPPS providers should bill P9011 for the blood product transfused, as well as CPT 86985 (Splitting, blood products) for each splitting procedure performed to prepare the blood product for a specific patient.

Providers should bill split units of packed red cells and whole blood using Revenue Code 389 (Other blood), and should not use Revenue Codes 381 (Packed red cells) or 382 (Whole blood). Providers should bill split units of other blood products using the applicable revenue codes for the blood product type, such as 383 (Plasma) or 384 (Platelets), rather than 389. Reporting revenue codes according to these specifications will ensure the Medicare beneficiary's blood deductible is applied correctly.

EXAMPLE: OPPS provider splits off a 100cc aliquot from a 250 cc unit of leukocytereduced red blood cells for a transfusion to Patient X. The hospital then splits off an 80cc aliquot of the remaining unit for a transfusion to Patient Y. At a later time, the remaining 70cc from the unit is transfused to Patient Z.

In billing for the services for Patient X and Patient Y, the OPPS provider should report the charges by billing P9011 and 86985 in addition to the CPT code for the transfusion service, because a specific splitting service was required to prepare a split unit for transfusion to each of those patients. However, the OPPS provider should report only P9011 and the CPT code for the transfusion service for Patient Z because no additional splitting was necessary to prepare the split unit for transfusion to Patient Z. The OPPS provider should bill Revenue Code 0389 for each split unit of the leukocyte-reduced red blood cells that was transfused.

100-04, 4, 250.18

Incomplete Colonoscopies (Codes 44388, 45378, G0105 and G0121)

(Rev.4153, Issued: 10-26-18, Effective: 04-01-19, Implementation: 04-01-19)

An incomplete colonoscopy, e.g., the inability to advance the colonoscope to the cecum or colon-small intestine anastomosis due to unforeseen circumstances, is billed and paid using colonoscopy through stoma code 44388, colonoscopy code 45378, and screening colonoscopy codes G0105 and G0121 with modifier "-53." (Code 44388 is valid with modifier 53 beginning January 1, 2016.) The Medicare physician fee schedule database has specific values for codes 44388-53, 45378-53,

© 2019 Optum360, LLC

G0105-53 and G0121-53. An incomplete colonoscopy performed prior to January 1, 2016, is paid at the same rate as a sigmoidoscopy. Beginning January 1, 2016, Medicare will pay for the interrupted colonoscopy at a rate that is calculated using one-half the value of the inputs for the codes.

As such, instruct CAHs that elect Method II payment to use modifier "-53" to identify an incomplete screening colonoscopy (physician professional service(s) billed in revenue code 096X, 097X, and/or 098X).

CAH Method II shall be consistent with the guidelines outlined in PUB. 100-04, chapter 12, section 30.1 and chapter 18, section 60.2.

100-04, 4, 260.1

Special Partial Hospitalization Billing Requirements forHospitals, Community Mental Health Centers, and Critical Access Hospitals

(Rev.4204, Issued: 01-17-19, Effective: 01-01-19, Implementation: 01-07-19)

Medicare Part B coverage is available for hospital outpatient partial hospitalization services.

A. Billing Requirement

Section 1861 (http://www.socialsecurity.gov/OP_Home/ssact/title18/1800.htm) of the Act defines the services under the partial hospitalization benefit in a hospital.

Section 1866(e)(2) of the Act (http://www.socialsecurity.gov/OP_Home/ssact/title18/1800.htm)recognizes CMHCs as "providers of services" but only for furnishing partial hospitalization services. See §261.1.1 of this chapter for CMHC partial hospitalization bill review directions.

Hospitals and CAHs report condition code 41 in FLs 18-28 (or electronic equivalent) to indicate the claim is for partial hospitalization services. They must also report a revenue code and the charge for each individual covered service furnished. In addition, hospital outpatient departments are required to report HCPCS codes. CAHs are not required to report HCPCS code for this benefit.

Under component billing, hospitals are required to report a revenue code and the charge for each individual covered service furnished under a partial hospitalization program. In addition, hospital outpatient departments are required to report HCPCS codes. Component billing assures that only those partial hospitalization services covered under §1861(ff) of the Act are paid by the Medicare program.

Effective January 1, 2017, non-excepted off-campus provider-based departments of a hospital are required to report a "PN" modifier on each claim line for non-excepted items and services. The use of modifier "PN" will trigger a payment rate under the Medicare Physician Fee Schedule. We expect the PN modifier to be reported with each non-excepted item and service including those for which payment will not be adjusted, such as separately payable drugs, clinical laboratory tests, and therapy services.

Excepted off-campus provider-based departments of a hospital must continue to report existing modifier "PO" (Services, procedures and/or surgeries provided at off-campus provider-based outpatient departments) for all excepted items and services furnished. Use of the off-campus PBD modifier became mandatory beginning January 1, 2016.

All hospitals are required to report condition code 41 in FLs 18-28 to indicate the claim is for partial hospitalization services. Hospitals use bill type 13X and CAHs use bill type 85X. The following special procedures apply.

Bills must contain an acceptable revenue code. They are as follows:

Revenue Code	Description
0250	Drugs and Biologicals

Revenue Code	Description
043X	Occupational Therapy
0900	Behavioral Health Treatment/Services
0904	Activity Therapy
0910	Psychiatric/Psychological Services (Dates of Service prior to October 16, 2003)
0914	Individual Therapy
0915	Group Therapy
0916	Family Therapy
0918	Behavioral Health/Testing
0942	Education/Training

Psychiatric diagnostic evaluation (no medical services) completed by a non-physician.

*****The definition of code 90792 is as follows:

Psychiatric diagnostic evaluation (with medical services) completed by a physician.

Codes G0129 and G0176 are used only for partial hospitalization programs.

Code G0177 may be used in both partial hospitalization program and outpatient mental health settings.

Revenue code 250 does not require HCPCS coding. However, Medicare does not cover drugs that can be self-administered.

Edit to assure that HCPCS are present when the above revenue codes are billed and that they are valid HCPCS codes. Do not edit for the matching of revenue code to HCPCS.

B. Professional Services

The professional services listed below when provided in all hospital outpatient departments are separately covered and paid as the professional services of physicians and other practitioners. These professional services are unbundled and these practitioners (other than physician assistants (PA) bill the Medicare A/B MAC (B) directly for the professional services furnished to hospital outpatient partial hospitalization patients. The hospital can also serve as a billing agent for these professionals by billing the A/B MAC (B) on their behalf under their billing number for their professional services. The professional services of a PA can be billed to the A/B MAC (B) only by the PAs employer. The employer of a PA may be such entities or individuals as a physician, medical group, professional corporation, hospital, SNF, or nursing facility. For example, if a physician is the employer of the PA and the PA renders services in the hospital, the physician and not the hospital would be responsible for billing the A/B MAC (B) on Form CMS-1500 for the services of the PA. The following direct professional services are unbundled and not paid as partial hospitalization services.

- Physician services that meet the criteria of 42 CFR 415.102, for payment on a fee schedule basis; • Physician assistant (PA) services as defined in §1861(s)(2)(K)(i) of the Act;
- Nurse practitioner and clinical nurse specialist services, as defined in §1861(s)(2)(K)(ii) of the Act; and
- Clinical psychologist services as defined in §1861(ii) of the Act.

The services of other practitioners (including clinical social workers and occupational therapists), are bundled when furnished to hospital patients, including partial hospitalization patients. The hospital must bill the contractor for such nonphysician practitioner services as partial hospitalization services. Make payment for the services to the hospital.

C. Outpatient Mental Health Treatment Limitation

The outpatient mental health treatment limitation may apply to services to treat mental, psychoneurotic, and

personality disorders when furnished by physicians, clinical psychologists, NPs, CNSs, and PAs to partial hospitalization patients. However, the outpatient mental health treatment limitation does not apply to such mental health treatment services billed to the A/B MAC (A) by a CMHC or hospital outpatient department as partial hospitalization services.

D. Reporting of Service Units

Hospitals report the number of times the service or procedure, as defined by the HCPCS code, was performed. CAHs report the number of times the revenue code visit was performed.

NOTE: Service units are not required to be reported for drugs and biologicals (Revenue Code 250).

E. Line Item Date of Service Reporting

Hospitals other than CAHs are required to report line item dates of service per revenue code line for partial hospitalization claims. This means each service (revenue code) provided must be repeated on a separate line item along with the specific date the service was provided for every occurrence. Line item dates of service are reported in FL 45 "Service Date" (MMDDYY). See §260.5 for a detailed explanation.

F. Payment

Starting in CY 2017 and subsequent years, the payment structure for partial hospitalization services provided in hospital outpatient departments and CMHCs has been reduced from four APCs (two for CMHCs and two for hospital-based PHPs) to a single APC by provider type. Effective January 2, 2017, we are replacing existing CMHC APCs 5851 (Level 1 Partial Hospitalization (3 services)) and 5852 (Level 2 Partial Hospitalization (4 or more services)) with a new CMHC APC 5853 (Partial Hospitalization (3 or More Services Per Day)), and replacing existing hospital-based PHP APCs 5861 (Level 1 Partial Hospitalization (3 services)) and 5862 (Level 2 Partial Hospitalization (4 or more services)) with a new hospital-based PHP APC 5863 (Partial

© 2019 Optum360, LLC

Hospitalization (3 or More Services Per Day)). The following chart displays the CMHC and hospital-based PHPAPCs:

Hospital-Based and Community Mental Health Center PHP APCs CY 2017

APC	Group Title
5853	Partial Hospitalization (3 or more services per day) for CMHCs
5863	Partial Hospitalization (3 or more services per day) for hospital-based PHPs

Apply Part B deductible, if any, and coinsurance.

G. Data for CWF and PS&R

Include revenue codes, HCPCS/CPT codes, units, and covered charges in the financial data section (fields 65a - 65j), as appropriate. Report the billed charges in field 65h, "Charges," of the CWF record.

Include in the financial data portion of the PS&R UNIBILL, revenue codes, HCPCS/CPT codes, units, and charges, as appropriate.

Future updates will be issued in a Recurring Update Notification.

100-04, 4, 260.1.1

Bill Review for Partial Hospitalization Services Provided in Community Mental Health Centers (CMHC)

(Rev.4204, Issued: 01-17-19, Effective: 01-01-19, Implementation: 01-07-19)

A. General

Medicare Part B coverage for partial hospitalization services provided by CMHCs is available effective for services provided on or after October 1, 1991.

B. Special Requirements

Section 1866(e)(2) (http://www.socialsecurity.gov/OP_Home/ssact/title18/1800.htm) of the Act recognizes CMHCs as "providers of services" but only for furnishing partial hospitalization services. Applicable provider ranges are 1400-1499, 4600-4799, and 4900-4999.

C. Billing Requirements

The CMHCs bill for partial hospitalization services under bill type 76X. The A/B MACs (A) follow bill review instructions in chapter 25 of this manual, except for those listed below.

The acceptable revenue codes are as follows:

Revenue Code	Description
0250	Drugs and Biologicals
043X	Occupational Therapy
0900	Behavioral Health Treatments/Services
0904	Activity Therapy
0910	Psychiatric/Psychological Services (Dates of Service prior to October 16, 2003)
0914	Individual Therapy
0915	Group Therapy
0916	Family Therapy
0918	Behavioral Health/Testing
0942	Education/Training

The A/B MAC(s) (A) edit to assure that HCPCS are present when the above revenue codes are billed and

that they are valid HCPCS codes. They do not edit for the matching of revenue codes to HCPCS.

Definitions each of the asterisked HCPCS codes follows:

* The definition of code G0129 is as follows:

Occupational therapy services requiring the skills of a qualified occupational therapist, furnished as a component of a partial hospitalization treatment program, per session (45 minutes or more).

** The definition of code G0176 is as follows:

Activity therapy, such as music, dance, art or play therapies not for recreation, related to the care and treatment of patient's disabling mental health problems, per session (45 minutes or more).

*** The definition of code G0177 is as follows:

Training and educational services related to the care and treatment of patient's disabling mental health problems, per session (45 minutes or more).

****The definition of code 90791 is as follows:

Psychiatric diagnostic evaluation (no medical services) completed by a non-physician.

*****The definition of code 90792 is as follows:

Psychiatric diagnostic evaluation (with medical services) completed by a physician.

Codes G0129 and G0176 are used only for partial hospitalization programs.

Code G0177 may be used in both partial hospitalization program and outpatient mental health settings.

Revenue code 0250 does not require HCPCS coding. However, drugs that can be self-administered are not covered by Medicare.

HCPCS includes CPT-4 codes. See the ASC X12 837 institutional claim guide for how to report HCPCS electronically. CMHCs report HCPCS codes on Form CMS-1450 in FL44, "HCPCS/Rates." HCPCS code reporting is effective for claims with dates of service on or after April 1, 2000.

The A/B MACs (A) are to advise their CMHCs of these requirements. CMHCs should complete the remaining items on the claim in accordance with the ASC X12 837 Institutional Claim implementation guide and the Form CMS-1450 instructions in Chapter 25 of this manual.

The professional services listed below are separately covered and are paid as the professional services of physicians and other practitioners. These professional services are unbundled and these practitioners (other than physician assistants (PAs)) bill the A/B MAC (B) directly for the professional services furnished to CMHC partial hospitalization patients. The ASC X12 837 professional claim format or the paper form 1500 is used. The CMHC can also serve as a billing agent for these professionals by billing the A/B MAC (B) on their behalf for their professional services. The professional services of a PA can be billed to the A/B MAC (B) only by the PAs employer. The employer of a PA may be such entities or individuals as a physician, medical group, professional corporation, hospital, SNF, or nursing facility. For example, if a physician is the employer of the PA and the PA renders services in the CMHC, the physician and not the CMHC would be responsible for billing the A/B MAC (B) for the services of the PA.

The following professional services are unbundled and not paid as partial hospitalization services:

- Physician services that meet the criteria of 42 CFR 415.102, for payment on a fee schedule basis;
- PA services, as defined in §1861(s)(2)(K)(i) (http://www.socialsecurity.gov/OP_Home/ssact/title18/1800.htm) of the Act;
- Nurse practitioner and clinical nurse specialist services, as defined in §1861(s)(2)(K)(ii) (http://www.socialsecurity.gov/OP_Home/ssact/title18/1800.htm) of the Act; and,
- Clinical psychologist services, as defined in §1861(ii) (http://www.socialsecurity.gov/OP_Home/ssact/title18/1800.htm) of the Act.

The services of other practitioners (including clinical social workers and occupational therapists) are bundled when furnished to CMHC patients. The CMHC must bill the A/B MAC (A) for such nonphysician practitioner services as partial hospitalization services. The A/B MAC (A) makes payment for the services to the CMHC.

D. Outpatient Mental Health Treatment Limitation

The outpatient mental health treatment limitation **may apply** to services to treat mental, psychoneurotic, and personality disorders when furnished by physicians, clinical psychologists, NPs, CNSs, and PAs to partial hospitalization patients. However, the outpatient mental health treatment limitation **does not** apply to such mental health treatment services billed to the A/B MAC (A) as partial hospitalization services.

E. Reporting of Service Units

Visits should no longer be reported as units. Instead, CMHCs report in the field, "Service Units," the number of times the service or procedure, as defined by the HCPCS code, was performed when billing for partial hospitalization services identified by revenue code in subsection C.

EXAMPLE: A beneficiary received psychological testing *performed by a physician for a total of 3 hours during one day* (HCPCS code *96130, first hour; HCPCS code 96131 for 2 additional hours)*. The CMHC reports revenue code 0918, HCPCS code *96130, and 1 unit; and a second line on the claim showing revenue code 918, HCPCS code 96131, and 2 units.*

When reporting service units for HCPCS codes where the definition of the procedure does not include any reference to time (either minutes, hours or days), CMHCs should not bill for sessions of less than 45 minutes.

© 2019 Optum360, LLC

The CMHC need not report service units for drugs and biologicals (Revenue Code 0250)

NOTE: Information regarding the Form CMS-1450 form locators that correspond with these fields is found in Chapter 25 of this manual. See the ASC X12 837 Institutional Claim implementation guide for related guidelines for the electronic claim.

F. Line Item Date of Service Reporting

Dates of service per revenue code line for partial hospitalization claims that span two or more dates. This means each service (revenue code) provided must be repeated on a separate line item along with the specific date the service was provided for every occurrence. Line item dates of service are reported in "Service Date". See examples below of reporting line item dates of service. These examples are for group therapy services provided twice during a billing period.

For claims, report as follows:

Revenue Code	HCPCS	Dates of Service	Units	Total Charges
0915	G0176	20090505	1	$80
0915	G0176	20090529	2	$160

NOTE: Information regarding the Form CMS-1450 form locators that correspond with these fields is found in Chapter 25 of this manual. See the ASC X12 837 Institutional Claim Implementation Guide for related guidelines for the electronic claim.

The A/B MACs (A) return to provider claims that span two or more dates if a line item date of service is not entered for each HCPCS code reported or if the line item dates of service reported are outside of the statement covers period. Line item date of service reporting is effective for claims with dates of service on or after June 5, 2000.

G. Payment

Section 1833(a)(2)(B) (http://www.socialsecurity.gov/OP_Home/ssact/title18/1800.htm) of the Act provides the statutory authority governing payment for partial hospitalization services provided by a CMHC. A/B MAC(s) (A) made payment on a reasonable cost basis until OPPS was implemented. The Part B deductible and coinsurance applied.

Payment principles applicable to partial hospitalization services furnished in CMHCs are contained in §2400 of the Medicare Provider Reimbursement Manual.

The A/B MACs (A) make payment on a per diem basis under the hospital outpatient prospective payment system for partial hospitalization services. CMHCs must continue to maintain documentation to support medical necessity of each service provided, including the beginning and ending time.

Effective January 1, 2011, there were four separate APC payment rates for PHP: two for CMHCs (for Level I and Level II services based on only CMHC data) and two for hospital-based PHPs (for Level I and Level II services based on only hospital-based PHP data).

The two CMHC APCS for providing partial hospitalization services were: APC 5851 (Level 1 Partial Hospitalization (3 services)) and APC 5852 (Level 2 Partial Hospitalization (4 or more services)). Effective January 1, 2017, we are combining APCs 5851 and 5852 into one new APC 5853 (Partial Hospitalization (3 or more services) for CMHCs).

Community Mental Health Center PHP APC

APC	Group Title
5853	Partial Hospitalization (3 or more services per day) for CMHCs

NOTE: Occupational therapy services provided to partial hospitalization patients are not subject to the prospective payment system for outpatient rehabilitation services, and therefore the financial limitation required under §4541 of the Balanced Budget Act (BBA) does not apply.

H. Medical Review

The A/B MACs (A) follow medical review guidelines in Pub. 100-08, Medicare Program Integrity Manual.

I. Coordination with CWF

See chapter 27 of this manual. All edits for bill type 74X apply, except provider number ranges 4600-4799 are acceptable only for services provided on or after October 1, 1991.

100-04, 4, 260.5

Line Item Date of Service Reporting for Partial Hospitalization

(Rev.3019, Issued: 08-07-14, Effective: 01-01-12, ICD-10: Upon Implementation of ICD- 10, Implementation: 09-08-14, ICD-10: Upon Implementation of ICD- 10)

Hospitals other than CAHs are required to report line item dates of service per revenue code line for partial hospitalization claims. Where services are provided on more than one day included in the billing period, the date of service must be identified. Each service (revenue code) provided must be repeated on a separate line item along with the specific date the service was provided for every occurrence. See examples below of reporting line item dates of service. These examples are for group therapy services provided twice during a billing period.

For the claims, report as follows:

Revenue Code	HCPCS	Dates of Service	Units	Total Charges
0915	G0176	20090505	1	$80.00
0915	G0176	20090529	2	$160.00

NOTE: Information regarding the Form CMS-1450 form locators that correspond with these fields is found in Chapter 25 of this manual. See the ASC X12 837 Institutional Claim Implementation Guide for related guidelines for the electronic claim.

The A/B MAC (A) must return to the hospital (RTP) claims where a line item date of service is not entered for each HCPCS code reported, or if the line item dates of service reported are outside of the statement covers period. Line item date of service reporting is effective for claims with dates of service on or after June 5, 2000.

100-04, 4, 290.1

Observation Services Overview

(Rev.1760, Issued: 06-23-09; Effective Date: 07-01-09; Implementation Date: 07-06-09)

Observation care is a well-defined set of specific, clinically appropriate services, which include ongoing short term treatment, assessment, and reassessment, that are furnished while a decision is being made regarding whether patients will require further treatment as hospital inpatients or if they are able to be discharged from the hospital. Observation status is commonly assigned to patients who present to the emergency department and who then require a significant period of treatment or monitoring in order to make a decision concerning their admission or discharge. Observation services are covered only when provided by the order of a physician or another individual authorized by State licensure law and hospital staff bylaws to admit patients to the hospital or to order outpatient services.

Observation services must also be reasonable and necessary to be covered by Medicare. In only rare and exceptional cases do reasonable and necessary outpatient observation services span more than 48 hours. In the majority of cases, the decision whether to discharge a patient from the hospital following resolution of the reason for the observation care or to admit the patient as an inpatient can be made in less than 48 hours, usually in less than 24 hours.

100-04, 4, 290.2.2

Reporting Hours of Observation

(Rev.2234, Issued: 05-27-11, Effective: 07-01-11, Implementation: 07-05-11)

Observation time begins at the clock time documented in the patient's medical record, which coincides with the time the patient is placed in a bed for the purpose of initiating observation care in accordance with a physician's order. Hospitals should round to the nearest hour. For example, a patient who was placed in an observation bed at 3:03 p.m. according to the nurses' notes and discharged to home at 9:45 p.m. should have a "7" placed in the units field of the reported observation HCPCS code.

General standing orders for observation services following all outpatient surgery are not recognized. Hospitals should not report as observation care, services that are part of another Part B service, such as postoperative monitoring during a standard recovery period (e.g., 4-6 hours), which should be billed as recovery room services. Similarly, in the case of patients who undergo diagnostic testing in a hospital outpatient department, routine preparation services furnished prior to the testing and recovery afterwards are included in the payments for those diagnostic services. Observation services should not be billed concurrently with diagnostic or therapeutic services for which active monitoring is a part of the procedure (e.g., colonoscopy, chemotherapy). In situations where such a procedure interrupts observation services, hospitals would record for each period of observation services the beginning and ending times during the hospital outpatient encounter and add the length of time for the periods of observation services together to reach the total number of units reported on the claim for the hourly observation services HCPCS code G0378 (Hospital observation service, per hour).

Observation time ends when all medically necessary services related to observation care are completed. For example, this could be before discharge when the need for observation has ended, but other medically necessary services not meeting the definition of observation care are provided (in which case, the additional medically necessary services would be billed separately or included as part of the emergency department or clinic visit). Alternatively, the end time of observation services may coincide with the time the patient is actually discharged from the hospital or admitted as an inpatient.

© 2019 Optum360, LLC

Observation time may include medically necessary services and follow-up care provided after the time that the physician writes the discharge order, but before the patient is discharged. However, reported observation time would not include the time patients remain in the observation area after treatment is finished for reasons such as waiting for transportation home.

If a period of observation spans more than 1 calendar day, all of the hours for the entire period of observation must be included on a single line and the date of service for that line is the date that observation care begins.

100-04, 4, 290.4.1

Billing and Payment for All Hospital Observation Services Furnished Between January 1, 2006 and December 31, 2007

(Rev.1760, Issued: 06-23-09; Effective Date: 07-01-09; Implementation Date: 07-06-09)

Since January 1, 2006, two G-codes have been used to report observation services and direct referral for observation care. For claims for dates of service January 1, 2006 through December 31, 2007, the Integrated Outpatient Code Editor (I/OCE) determines whether the observation care or direct referral services are packaged or separately payable. Thus, hospitals provide consistent coding and billing under all circumstances in which they deliver observation care.

Beginning January 1, 2006, hospitals should not report CPT codes 99217-99220 or 99234-99236 for observation services. In addition, the following HCPCS codes were discontinued as of January 1, 2006: G0244 (Observation care by facility to patient), G0263 (Direct Admission with congestive heart failure, chest pain or asthma), and G0264 (Assessment other than congestive heart failure, chest pain, or asthma).

The three discontinued G-codes and the CPT codes that were no longer recognized were replaced by two new G-codes to be used by hospitals to report all observation services, whether separately payable or packaged, and direct referral for observation care, whether separately payable or packaged:

G0378- Hospital observation service, per hour; and

G0379- Direct admission of patient for hospital observation care.

The I/OCE determines whether observation services billed as units of G0378 are separately payable under APC 0339 (Observation) or whether payment for observation services will be packaged into the payment for other services provided by the hospital in the same encounter. Therefore, hospitals should bill HCPCS code G0378 when observation services are ordered and provided to any patient regardless of the patient's condition. The units of service should equal the number of hours the patient receives observation services.

Hospitals should report G0379 when observation services are the result of a direct referral for observation care without an associated emergency room visit, hospital outpatient clinic visit, critical care service, or hospital outpatient surgical procedure (status indicator T procedure) on the day of initiation of observation services. Hospitals should only report HCPCS code G0379 when a patient is referred directly for observation care after being seen by a physician in the community (see Sec.290.4.2 below)

Some non-repetitive OPPS services provided on the same day by a hospital may be billed on different claims, provided that all charges associated with each procedure or service being reported are billed on the same claim with the HCPCS code which describes that service. See chapter 1, section 50.2.2 of this manual. It is vitally important that all of the charges that pertain to a non-repetitive, separately paid procedure or service be reported on the same claim with that procedure or service. It should also be emphasized that this relaxation of same day billing requirements for some non-repetitive services does not apply to non-repetitive services provided on the same day as either direct referral to observation care or observation services because the OCE claim-by-claim logic cannot function properly unless all services related to the episode of observation care, including diagnostic tests, lab services, hospital clinic visits, emergency department visits, critical care services, and status indicator T procedures, are reported on the same claim. Additional guidance can be found in chapter 1, section 50.2.2 of this manual.

100-04, 4, 290.4.2

Separate and Packaged Payment for Direct Admission to Observation

(Rev.1760, Issued: 06-23-09; Effective Date: 07-01-09; Implementation Date: 07-06-09)

In order to receive separate payment for a direct referral for observation care (APC 0604), the claim must show:

1. Both HCPCS codes G0378 (Hourly Observation) and G0379 (Direct Admit to Observation) with the same date of service;
2. That no services with a status indicator T or V or Critical care (APC 0617) were provided on the same day of service as HCPCS code G0379; and
3. The observation care does not qualify for separate payment under APC 0339.

Only a direct referral for observation services billed on a 13X bill type may be considered for a separate APC payment.

Separate payment is not allowed for HCPCS code G0379, direct admission to observation care, when billed with the same date of service as a hospital clinic visit, emergency room visit, critical care service, or "T" status procedure.

If a bill for the direct referral for observation services does not meet the three requirements listed above, then payment for the direct referral service will be packaged into payments for other separately payable services provided to the beneficiary in the same encounter.

100-04, 4, 290.4.3

Separate and Packaged Payment for Observation Services Furnished Between January 1, 2006 and December 31, 2007

(Rev.1745, Issued: 05-22-09, Effective: 07-01-09, Implementation: 07-06-09)

Separate payment may be made for observation services provided to a patient with congestive heart failure, chest pain, or asthma. The list of ICD-9-CM diagnosis codes eligible for separate payment is reviewed annually. Any changes in applicable ICD-9-CM diagnosis codes are included in the October quarterly update of the OPPS and also published in the annual OPPS Final Rule. The list of qualifying ICD-9-CM diagnosis codes is also published on the OPPS Web page.

All of the following requirements must be met in order for a hospital to receive a separate APC payment for observation services through APC 0339:

1. Diagnosis Requirements
   a. The beneficiary must have one of three medical conditions: congestive heart failure, chest pain, or asthma.
   b. Qualifying ICD-9-CM diagnosis codes must be reported in Form Locator (FL) 76, Patient Reason for Visit, or FL 67, principal diagnosis, or both in order for the hospital to receive separate payment for APC 0339. If a qualifying ICD-9-CM diagnosis code(s) is reported in the secondary diagnosis field, but is not reported in either the Patient Reason for Visit field (FL 76) or in the principal diagnosis field (FL 67), separate payment for APC 0339 is not allowed.
2. Observation Time
   a. Observation time must be documented in the medical record.
   b. Hospital billing for observation services begins at the clock time documented in the patient's medical record, which coincides with the time that observation services are initiated in accordance with a physician's order for observation services.
   c. A beneficiary's time receiving observation services (and hospital billing) ends when all clinical or medical interventions have been completed, including follow-up care furnished by hospital staff and physicians that may take place after a physician has ordered the patient be released or admitted as an inpatient.
   d. The number of units reported with HCPCS code G0378 must equal or exceed 8 hours.
3. Additional Hospital Services
   a. The claim for observation services must include one of the following services in addition to the reported observation services. The additional services listed below must have a line item date of service on the same day or the day before the date reported for observation:

      An emergency department visit (APC 0609, 0613, 0614, 0615, 0616) or

      A clinic visit (APC 0604, 0605, 0606, 0607, 0608); or

      Critical care (APC 0617); or

      Direct referral for observation care reported with HCPCS code G0379 (APC 0604); must be reported on the same date of service as the date reported for observation services.
   b. No procedure with a T status indicator can be reported on the same day or day before observation care is provided.
4. Physician Evaluation
   a. The beneficiary must be in the care of a physician during the period of observation, as documented in the medical record by outpatient registration, discharge, and other appropriate progress notes that are timed, written, and signed by the physician.
   b. The medical record must include documentation that the physician explicitly assessed patient risk to determine that the beneficiary would benefit from observation care.

© 2019 Optum360, LLC

Only observation services that are billed on a 13X bill type may be considered for a separate APC payment.

Hospitals should bill all of the other services associated with the observation care, including direct referral for observation, hospital clinic visits, emergency room visits, critical care services, and T status procedures, on the same claim so that the claims processing logic may appropriately determine the payment status (either packaged or separately payable) of HCPCS codes G0378 and G0379.

If a bill for observation care does not meet all of the requirements listed above, then payment for the observation care will be packaged into payments for other separately payable services provided to the beneficiary in the same encounter.

100-04, 4, 290.5.1

Billing and Payment for Observation Services Beginning January 1, 2008

(Rev.3425, Iss.: 12-18-15, Eff: 01-01-16, Imp: 01-04-16)

Observation services are reported using HCPCS code G0378 (Hospital observation service, per hour). Beginning January 1, 2008, HCPCS code G0378 for hourly observation services is assigned status indicator N, signifying that its payment is always packaged. No separate payment is made for observation services reported with HCPCS code G0378, and APC 0339 is deleted as of January 1, 2008. In most circumstances, observation services are supportive and ancillary to the other services provided to a patient. Beginning January 1, 2014, in certain circumstances when observation care is billed in conjunction with a clinic visit, high level Type A emergency department visit (Level 4 or 5), high level Type B emergency department visit (Level 5), critical care services, or a direct referral as an integral part of a patient's extended encounter of care, payment may be made for the entire extended care encounter through APC 8009 (Extended Assessment and Management Composite) when certain criteria are met. Prior to January 1, 2014, in certain circumstances when observation care was billed in conjunction with a high level clinic visit (Level 5), high level Type A emergency department visit (Level 4 or 5), high level Type B emergency department visit (Level 5), critical care services, or a direct referral as an integral part of a patient's extended encounter of care, payment could be made for the entire extended care encounter through one of two composite APCs (APCs 8002 and 8003) when certain criteria were met. APCs 8002 and 8003 are deleted as of January 1, 2014. For information about payment for extended assessment and management composite APC, see §10.2.1 (Composite APCs) of this chapter.

There is no limitation on diagnosis for payment of APC 8009; however, composite APC payment will not be made when observation services are reported in association with a surgical procedure (T status procedure) or the hours of observation care reported are less than 8. The I/OCE evaluates every claim received to determine if payment through a composite APC is appropriate. If payment through a composite APC is inappropriate, the I/OCE, in conjunction with the Pricer, determines the appropriate status indicator, APC, and payment for every code on a claim.

All of the following requirements must be met in order for a hospital to receive an APC payment for an extended assessment and management composite APC:

1. Observation Time
   a. Observation time must be documented in the medical record.
   b. Hospital billing for observation services begins at the clock time documented in the patient's medical record, which coincides with the time that observation services are initiated in accordance with a physician's order for observation services.
   c. A beneficiary's time receiving observation services (and hospital billing) ends when all clinical or medical interventions have been completed, including follow-up care furnished by hospital staff and physicians that may take place after a physician has ordered the patient be released or admitted as an inpatient.
   d. The number of units reported with HCPCS code G0378 must equal or exceed 8 hours.
2. Additional Hospital Services
   a. The claim for observation services must include one of the following services in addition to the reported observation services. The additional services listed below must have a line item date of service on the same day or the day before the date reported for observation:

      A Type A or B emergency department visit (CPT codes 99284 or 99285 or HCPCS code G0384); or

      A clinic visit (CPT code 99205 or 99215); or

      Critical care (CPT code 99291); or

      Direct referral for observation care reported with HCPCS code G0379 (APC 0604) must be reported on the same date of service as the date reported for observation services.
   b. No procedure with a T status indicator can be reported on the same day or day before observation care is provided.
3. Physician Evaluation
   a. The beneficiary must be in the care of a physician during the period of observation, as documented in the medical record by outpatient registration, discharge, and other appropriate progress notes that are timed, written, and signed by the physician.
   b. The medical record must include documentation that the physician explicitly assessed patient risk to determine that the beneficiary would benefit from observation care.

Criteria 1 and 3 related to observation care beginning and ending time and physician evaluation apply regardless of whether the hospital believes that the criteria will be met for payment of the extended encounter through extended assessment and management composite payment.

Only visits, critical care and observation services that are billed on a 13X bill type may be considered for a composite APC payment.

Non-repetitive services provided on the same day as either direct referral for observation care or observation services must be reported on the same claim because the OCE claim-by-claim logic cannot function properly unless all services related to the episode of observation care, including hospital clinic visits, emergency department visits, critical care services, and T status procedures, are reported on the same claim. Additional guidance can be found in chapter 1, section 50.2.2 of this manual.

If a claim for services provided during an extended assessment and management encounter including observation care does not meet all of the requirements listed above, then the usual APC logic will apply to separately payable items and services on the claim; the special logic for direct admission will apply, and payment for the observation care will be packaged into payments for other separately payable services provided to the beneficiary in the same encounter.

100-04, 4, 290.5.2

Billing and Payment for Direct Referral for Observation Care Furnished Beginning January 1, 2008

(Rev.3425, Iss.: 12-18-15, Eff: 01-01-16, Imp: 01-04-16)

Direct referral for observation care continues to be reported using HCPCS code G0379 (Direct admission of patient for hospital observation care). Hospitals should report G0379 when observation services are the result of a direct referral for observation care without an associated emergency room visit, hospital outpatient clinic visit, or critical care service on the day of initiation of observation services. Hospitals should only report HCPCS code G0379 when a patient is referred directly to observation care after being seen by a physician in the community.

Payment for direct referral for observation care will be made either separately as a low level hospital clinic visit under APC 0604 or packaged into payment for composite APC 8002 (Level I Prolonged Assessment and Management Composite) or packaged into the payment for other separately payable services provided in the same encounter. For information about payment for extended assessment and management composite APCs, see, Sec.10.2.1 (Composite APCs) of this chapter.

The criteria for payment of HCPCS code G0379 under either APC 0604 or APC 8002 include:

1. Both HCPCS codes G0378 (Hospital observation services, per hr) and G0379 (Direct admission of patient for hospital observation care) are reported with the same date of service.
2. No service with a status indicator of T or V or Critical Care (APC 0617) is provided on the same day of service as HCPCS code G0379.

If either of the above criteria is not met, HCPCS code G0379 will be assigned status indicator N and will be packaged into payment for other separately payable services provided in the same encounter.

Only a direct referral for observation services billed on a 13X bill type may be considered for a composite APC payment.

100-04, 4, 290.5.3

Billing and Payment for Observation Services Furnished Beginning January 1, 2016

(Rev.3425, Issued: 12-18-15, Effective: 01-01-16, Implementation: 01-04-16)

Observation services are reported using HCPCS code G0378 (Hospital observation service, per hour). Beginning January 1, 2008, HCPCS code G0378 for hourly observation services is assigned status indicator N, signifying that its payment is always packaged. No separate payment is made for observation services reported with HCPCS APCs, see §10.2.3 (Comprehensive APCs) of this chapter.

There is no limitation on diagnosis for payment of APC 8011; however, comprehensive APC payment will not be made when observation services are reported in association with a surgical procedure (T status procedure) or the hours of observation care reported are less than 8. The I/OCE evaluates every claim received to determine if payment through a comprehensive APC is appropriate. If payment through a comprehensive APC is inappropriate, the I/OCE, in conjunction with the Pricer, determines the appropriate status indicator, APC, and payment for every code on a claim.

All of the following requirements must be met in order for a hospital to receive a comprehensive APC payment through the Comprehensive Observation Services APC (APC 8011):

1. Observation Time
   a. Observation time must be documented in the medical record.
   b. Hospital billing for observation services begins at the clock time documented in the patient's medical record, which coincides with the time that observation services are initiated in accordance with a physician's order for observation services.
   c. A beneficiary's time receiving observation services (and hospital billing) ends when all clinical or medical interventions have been completed, including follow-up care furnished by hospital staff and physicians that may take place after a physician has ordered the patient be released or admitted as an inpatient.
   d. The number of units reported with HCPCS code G0378 must equal or exceed 8 hours.
2. Additional Hospital Services
   a. The claim for observation services must include one of the following services in addition to the reported observation services. The additional services listed below must have a line item date of service on the same day or the day before the date reported for observation:

- A Type A or B emergency department visit (CPT codes 99281 through 99285 or HCPCS codes G0380 through G0384); or
- A clinic visit (HCPCS code G0463); or
- Critical care (CPT code 99291); or
- Direct referral for observation care reported with HCPCS code G0379 (APC 5013) must be reported on the same date of service as the date reported for observation services.

   b. No procedure with a T status indicator or a J1 status indicator can be reported on the claim.
3. Physician Evaluation
   a. The beneficiary must be in the care of a physician during the period of observation, as documented in the medical record by outpatient registration, discharge, and other appropriate progress notes that are timed, written, and signed by the physician.
   b. The medical record must include documentation that the physician explicitly assessed patient risk to determine that the beneficiary would benefit from observation care.

Criteria 1 and 3 related to observation care beginning and ending time and physician evaluation apply regardless of whether the hospital believes that the criteria will be met for payment of the extended encounter through the Comprehensive Observation Services APC (APC 8011).

Only visits, critical care and observation services that are billed on a 13X bill type may be considered for a comprehensive APC payment through the Comprehensive Observation Services APC (APC 8011).

Non-repetitive services provided on the same day as either direct referral for observation care or observation services must be reported on the same claim because the OCE claim-by-claim logic cannot function properly unless all services related to the episode of observation care, including hospital clinic visits, emergency department visits, critical care services, and T status procedures, are reported on the same claim. Additional guidance can be found in chapter 1, section 50.2.2 of this manual.

If a claim for services provided during an extended assessment and management encounter including observation care does not meet all of the requirements listed above, then the usual APC logic will apply to separately payable items and services on the claim; the special logic for direct admission will apply, and payment for the observation care will be packaged into payments for other separately payable services provided to the beneficiary in the same encounter.

100-04, 4, 300.6

Common Working File (CWF) Edits

(Rev.1846; Issued: 11-06-09; Effective Date: 04-01-10; Implementation Date: 04-05-10)

The CWF edit will allow 3 hours of therapy for MNT in the initial calendar year. The edit will allow more than 3 hours of therapy if there is a change in the beneficiary's medical condition, diagnosis, or treatment regimen and this change must be documented in the beneficiary's medical record. Two new G codes have been created for use when a beneficiary receives a second referral in a calendar year that allows the beneficiary to receive more than 3 hours of therapy. Another edit will allow 2 hours of follow up MNT with another referral in subsequent years.

Advance Beneficiary Notice (ABN)

The beneficiary is liable for services denied over the limited number of hours with referrals for MNT. An ABN should be issued in these situations. In absence of evidence of a valid ABN, the provider will be held liable.

An ABN should not be issued for Medicare-covered services such as those provided by hospital dietitians or nutrition professionals who are qualified to render the service in their state but who have not obtained Medicare provider numbers.

Duplicate Edits

Although beneficiaries are allowed to receive training and therapy during the same time period Diabetes Self-Management and Training (DSMT) and Medical Nutrition Therapy (MNT) services may not be provided on the same day to the same beneficiary. Effective April 1, 2010 CWF shall implement a new duplicate crossover edit to identify and prevent claims for DSMT/MNT services from being billed with the same dates of services for the same beneficiaries submitted from institutional providers and from a professional provider.

100-04, 4, 320.1

HCPCS Coding for OIVIT

(Rev.1930, Issued: 03-09-10, Effective Date: 12-23-09; Implementation Date: 04-05-10)

HCPCS code G9147, effective with the April IOCE and MPFSDB updates, is to be used on claims with dates of service on and after December 23, 2009, billing for non-covered OIVIT and any services comprising an OIVIT regimen.

NOTE: HCPCS codes 99199 or 94681(with or without diabetes related conditions 250.00-250.93) are not to be used on claims billing for non-covered OIVIT and any services comprising an OIVIT regimen when furnished pursuant to an OIVIT regimen. Claims billing for HCPCS codes 99199 and 94681 for non-covered OIVIT are to be returned to provider/returned as unprocessable.

100-04, 4, 320.2

Outpatient Intravenous Insulin Treatment (OIVIT)

(Rev.3475, Issued: 03-04-16, Effective: 06-06-16, Implementation: 06-06-16)

Effective for claims with dates of service on and after December 23, 2009, the Centers for Medicare and Medicaid Services (CMS) determines that the evidence does not support a conclusion that OIVIT improves health outcomes in Medicare beneficiaries. Therefore, CMS has determined that OIVIT is not reasonable and necessary for any indication under section 1862(a)(1)(A) of the Social Security Act. Services comprising an OIVIT regimen are nationally non-covered under Medicare when furnished pursuant to an OIVIT regimen.

See Pub. 100-03, Medicare National Coverage Determinations Manual, Section 40.7, Outpatient Intravenous Insulin Treatment (Effective December 23, 2009), for general information and coverage indications.

100-04, 5, 10.2

The Financial Limitation Legislation

(Rev.2073, Issued:10-22-10, Effective: 01-01-11, Implementation: 01-03-11)

A. Legislation on Limitations

The dollar amount of the limitations (caps) on outpatient therapy services is established by statute. The updated amount of the caps is released annually via Recurring Update Notifications and posted on the CMS Website www.cms.gov/TherapyServices, on contractor Websites, and on each beneficiary's Medicare Summary Notice. Medicare contractors shall publish the financial limitation amount in educational articles. It is also available at 1-800-Medicare.

Section 4541(a)(2) of the Balanced Budget Act (BBA) (P.L. 105-33) of 1997, which added §1834(k)(5) to the Act, required payment under a prospective payment system (PPS) for outpatient rehabilitation services (except those furnished by or under arrangements with a hospital). Outpatient rehabilitation services include the following services:

- Physical therapy

© 2019 Optum360, LLC

- Speech-language pathology; and
- Occupational therapy.

Section 4541(c) of the BBA required application of financial limitations to all outpatient rehabilitation services (except those furnished by or under arrangements with a hospital).

In 1999, an annual per beneficiary limit of $1,500 was applied, including all outpatient physical therapy services and speech-language pathology services. A separate limit applied to all occupational therapy services. The limits were based on incurred expenses and included applicable deductible and coinsurance. The BBA provided that the limits be indexed by the Medicare Economic Index (MEI) each year beginning in 2002.

Since the limitations apply to outpatient services, they do not apply to skilled nursing facility (SNF) residents in a covered Part A stay, including patients occupying swing beds. Rehabilitation services are included within the global Part A per diem payment that the SNF receives under the prospective payment system (PPS) for the covered stay. Also, limitations do not apply to any therapy services covered under prospective payment systems for home health or inpatient hospitals, including critical access hospitals.

The limitation is based on therapy services the Medicare beneficiary receives, not the type of practitioner who provides the service. Physical therapists, speech-language pathologists, and occupational therapists, as well as physicians and certain nonphysician practitioners, could render a therapy service.

B. Moratoria and Exceptions for Therapy Claims

Since the creation of therapy caps, Congress has enacted several moratoria. The Deficit Reduction Act of 2005 directed CMS to develop exceptions to therapy caps for calendar year 2006 and the exceptions have been extended periodically. The cap exception for therapy services billed by outpatient hospitals was part of the original legislation and applies as long as caps are in effect. Exceptions to caps based on the medical necessity of the service are in effect only when Congress legislates the exceptions.

C. Repeal of Original Legislation and Replacement with Thresholds to Ensure Appropriate Therapy.

Section 50202 of the Bipartisan Budget Act of 2018 repeals application of the Medicare outpatient therapy caps but retains the former cap amounts as a threshold of incurred expenses above which claims must include a modifier as a confirmation that services are medically necessary as justified by appropriate documentation in the medical record. This is termed the KX modifier threshold.

Along with this KX modifier threshold, the new law retains the targeted medical review process but at a lower threshold amount of $3,000. For more information about the medical review (MR) threshold see the below section 10.3.4.

100-04, 5, 10.3.2

Exceptions Process

(Rev.3670, Issued: 12-01-16, Effective: 01-01-17, Implementation: 01-03-17)

An exception may be made when the patient's condition is justified by documentation indicating that the beneficiary requires continued skilled therapy, i.e., therapy beyond the amount payable under the therapy cap, to achieve their prior functional status or maximum expected functional status within a reasonable amount of time.

No special documentation is submitted to the contractor for exceptions. The clinician is responsible for consulting guidance in the Medicare manuals and in the professional literature to determine if the beneficiary may qualify for the exception because documentation justifies medically necessary services above the caps. The clinician's opinion is not binding on the Medicare contractor who makes the final determination concerning whether the claim is payable.

Documentation justifying the services shall be submitted in response to any Additional Documentation Request (ADR) for claims that are selected for medical review. Follow the documentation requirements in Pub. 100-02, chapter 15, section 220.3. If medical records are requested for review, clinicians may include, at their discretion, a summary that specifically addresses the justification for therapy cap exception.

In making a decision about whether to utilize the exception, clinicians shall consider, for example, whether services are appropriate to--

The patient's condition, including the diagnosis, complexities, and severity;

The services provided, including their type, frequency, and duration;

The interaction of current active conditions and complexities that directly and significantly influence the treatment such that it causes services to exceed caps. In addition, the following should be considered before using the exception process:

1. Exceptions for Evaluation Services

Evaluation. The CMS will except therapy evaluations from caps after the therapy caps are reached when evaluation is necessary, e.g., to determine if the current status of the beneficiary requires therapy services. For example, the following CPT codes for evaluation procedures may be appropriate:

92521, 92522, 92523, 92524, 92597, 92607, 92608, 92610, 92611, 92612, 92614, 92616, 96105, 96125. 97161, 97162, 97163, 97164, 97165, 97166, 97167, and 97168.

These codes will continue to be reported as outpatient therapy procedures as listed in the Annual Therapy Update for the current year at: http://www.cms.gov/TherapyServices/05_Annual_Therapy_Update.asp#TopOfPage.

They are not diagnostic tests. Definitions of evaluations and documentation are found in Pub. 100-02, chapter 15, sections 220 and 230.

Other Services. There are a number of sources that suggest the amount of certain services that may be typical, either per service, per episode, per condition, or per discipline. For example, see the CSC - Therapy Cap Report, 3/21/2008, and CSC – Therapy Edits Tables 4/14/2008 at www.cms.hhs.gov/TherapyServices (Studies and Reports), or more recent utilization reports. Professional literature and guidelines from professional associations also provide a basis on which to estimate whether the type, frequency, and intensity of services are appropriate to an individual. Clinicians and contractors should utilize available evidence related to the patient's condition to justify provision of medically necessary services to individual beneficiaries, especially when they exceed caps. Contractors shall not limit medically necessary services that are justified by scientific research applicable to the beneficiary. Neither contractors nor clinicians shall utilize professional literature and scientific reports to justify payment for continued services after an individual's goals have been met earlier than is typical. Conversely, professional literature and scientific reports shall not be used as justification to deny payment to patients whose needs are greater than is typical or when the patient's condition is not represented by the literature.

2. Exceptions for Medically Necessary Services

Clinicians may utilize the process for exception for any diagnosis or condition for which they can justify services exceeding the cap. Regardless of the diagnosis or condition, the patient must also meet other requirements for coverage.

Bill the most relevant diagnosis. As always, when billing for therapy services, the diagnosis code that best relates to the reason for the treatment shall be on the claim, unless there is a compelling reason to report another diagnosis code. For example, when a patient with diabetes is being treated with therapy for gait training due to amputation, the preferred diagnosis is abnormality of gait (which characterizes the treatment). Where it is possible in accordance with State and local laws and the contractors' local coverage determinations, avoid using vague or general diagnoses. When a claim includes several types of services, or where the physician/NPP must supply the diagnosis, it may not be possible to use the most relevant therapy diagnosis code in the primary position. In that case, the relevant diagnosis code should, if possible, be on the claim in another position.

Codes representing the medical condition that caused the treatment are used when there is no code representing the treatment. Complicating conditions are preferably used in non-primary positions on the claim and are billed in the primary position only in the rare circumstance that there is no more relevant code.

The condition or complexity that caused treatment to exceed caps must be related to the therapy goals and must either be the condition that is being treated or a complexity that directly and significantly impacts the rate of recovery of the condition being treated such that it is appropriate to exceed the caps. Documentation for an exception should indicate how the complexity (or combination of complexities) directly and significantly affects treatment for a therapy condition.

If the contractor has determined that certain codes do not characterize patients who require medically necessary services, providers/suppliers may not use those codes, but must utilize a billable diagnosis code allowed by their contractor to describe the patient's condition. Contractors shall not apply therapy caps to services based on the patient's condition, but only on the medical necessity of the service for the condition. If a service would be payable before the cap is reached and is still medically necessary after the cap is reached, that service is excepted.

Contact your contractor for interpretation if you are not sure that a service is applicable for exception.

It is very important to recognize that most conditions would not ordinarily result in services exceeding the cap. Use the KX modifier only in cases where the condition of the individual patient is such that services are APPROPRIATELY provided in an episode that exceeds the cap. Routine use of the KX modifier for all patients with these conditions will likely show up on data analysis as aberrant and invite inquiry. Be sure that documentation is sufficiently detailed to support the use of the modifier.

In justifying exceptions for therapy caps, clinicians and contractors should not only consider the medical diagnoses and medical complications that might directly and significantly influence the amount of treatment required. Other variables (such as the availability of a caregiver at home) that affect appropriate treatment shall also be considered. Factors that influence the need for treatment should be supportable by published research, clinical guidelines from professional sources, and/or clinical or common sense. See Pub. 100-02, chapter 15, section 220.3 for information related to documentation of the evaluation, and section 220.2 on medical necessity for some factors that complicate treatment.

NOTE: The patient's lack of access to outpatient hospital therapy services alone, when outpatient hospital therapy services are excluded from the limitation, does not justify excepted services. Residents of skilled nursing facilities prevented by consolidated billing from accessing hospital services, debilitated patients for whom transportation to the hospital is a physical hardship, or lack of therapy services at hospitals in the beneficiary's county may or may not qualify as justification for continued services above the caps. The patient's condition and complexities might justify extended services, but their location does not. For dates of service on or after October 1, 2012, therapy services furnished in an outpatient hospital are not excluded from the limitation.

100-04, 5, 10.3.3

Use of the KX Modifier

(Rev.4214, Issued: 01-25-19, Effective: 01-01-19, Implementation: 02-26-19)

***NOTE**: Effective for dates of service on or after January 1, 2018, the KX modifier continues to be used. It no longer represents an exception request but serves as a confirmation that services are medically necessary after the beneficiary has exceeded the KX modifier threshold of incurred expenses. Medicare claims systems process claims with and without the KX modifier in the same manner described below and in section 10.4.*

When exceptions are in effect and the beneficiary qualifies for a therapy cap exception, the provider shall add a KX modifier to the therapy HCPCS code subject to the cap limits. The KX modifier shall not be added to any line of service that is not a medically necessary service; this applies to services that, according to a local coverage determination by the contractor, are not medically necessary services.

The codes subject to the therapy cap tracking requirements for a given calendar year are listed at:
http://www.cms.hhs.gov/TherapyServices/05_Annual_Therapy_Update.asp#TopOfPage.

The GN, GO, or GP therapy modifiers are currently required to be appended to therapy services. In addition to the KX modifier, the GN, GP and GO modifiers shall continue to be used. Providers may report the modifiers on claims in any order. If there is insufficient room on a claim line for multiple modifiers, additional modifiers may be reported in the remarks field. Follow the routine procedure for placing HCPCS modifiers on a claim as described below.

- • For professional claims, sent to the A/B MAC(B), refer to:
  - Pub.100-04, Medicare Claims Processing Manual, chapter 26, for more detail regarding completing Form CMS 1500, including the placement of HCPCS modifiers. NOTE: The Form CMS 1500 currently has space for providing four modifiers in block 24D, but, if the provider has more than four to report, he/she can do so by placing the -99 modifier (which indicates multiple modifiers) in block 24D and placing the additional modifiers in block 19.
  - The ASC X12N 837 Health Care Claim: Professional Implementation Guide for more detail regarding how to electronically submit a health care claim transaction, including the placement of HCPCS modifiers. The ASC X12N 837 implementation guides are the standards adopted under the Health Insurance Portability and Accountability Act of 1996 (HIPAA) for submitting health care claims electronically. The 837 professional transaction currently permits the placement of up to four modifiers, in the 2400 loop, SV1 segment, and data elements SV101-3, SV101-4, SV101-5, and SV101-6. Copies of the ASC X12N 837 implementation guides may be obtained from the Washington Publishing Company.
  - For claims paid by a carrier or an A/B MAC(B), it is only appropriate to append the KX modifier to a service that reasonably may exceed the cap. Use of the KX modifier when there is no indication that the cap is likely to be exceeded is abusive. For example, use of the KX modifier for low cost services early in an episode when there is no evidence of a previous episode that might have exceeded the cap is inappropriate.
- For institutional claims, sent to the A/B MAC(A):
  - When the cap is exceeded by at least one line on the claim, use the KX modifier on all of the lines on that institutional claim that refer to the same therapy cap (PT/SLP or OT), regardless of whether the other services exceed the cap. For example, if one PT service line exceeds the cap, use the KX modifier on all the PT and SLP service lines (also identified with the GP or GN modifier) for that claim. When the PT/SLP cap is exceeded by PT services, the SLP lines on the claim may meet the requirements for an exception due to the complexity of two episodes of service.
  - Use the KX modifier on either all or none of the SLP lines on the claim, as appropriate. In contrast, if all the OT lines on the claim are below the cap, do not use the KX modifier on any of the OT lines, even when the KX modifier is appropriately used on all of the PT lines. Refer to Pub.100-04, Medicare Claims Processing Manual, chapter 25, for more detail.

By appending the KX modifier, the provider is attesting that the services billed:

- Are reasonable and necessary services that require the skills of a therapist; (See Pub. 100-02, chapter 15, section 220.2); and
- Are justified by appropriate documentation in the medical record, (See Pub. 100-02, chapter 15, section 220.3); and
- Qualify for an exception using the automatic process exception.

If this attestation is determined to be inaccurate, the provider/supplier is subject to sanctions resulting from providing inaccurate information on a claim.

When the KX modifier is appended to a therapy HCPCS code, the contractor will override the CWF system reject for services that exceed the caps and pay the claim if it is otherwise payable.

Providers and suppliers shall continue to append correct coding initiative (CCI) HCPCS modifiers under current instructions.

If a claim is submitted without KX modifiers and the cap is exceeded, those services will be denied. In cases where appending the KX modifier would have been appropriate, contractors may reopen and/or adjust the claim, if it is brought to their attention.

Services billed after the cap has been exceeded which are not eligible for exceptions may be billed for the purpose of obtaining a denial using condition code 21.

100-04, 5, 10.6

Functional Reporting

(Rev.3670, Issued: 12-01-16, Effective: 01-01-17, Implementation: 01-03-17)

A. General

Section 3005(g) of the Middle Class Tax Relief and Jobs Creation Act (MCTRJCA) amended Section 1833(g) of the Act to require a claims-based data collection system for outpatient therapy services, including physical therapy (PT), occupational therapy (OT) and speech-language pathology (SLP) services. 42 CFR 410.59, 410.60, 410.61, 410.62 and 410.105 implement this requirement. The system will collect data on beneficiary function during the course of therapy services in order to better understand beneficiary conditions, outcomes, and expenditures.

Beneficiary unction information is reported using 42 nonpayable functional G-codes and seven severity/complexity modifiers on claims for PT, OT, and SLP services. Functional reporting on one functional limitation at a time is required periodically throughout an entire PT, OT, or SLP therapy episode of care.

The nonpayable G-codes and severity modifiers provide information about the beneficiary's functional status at the outset of the therapy episode of care, including projected goal status, at specified points during treatment, and at the time of discharge. These G-codes, along with the associated modifiers, are required at specified intervals on all claims for outpatient therapy services – not just those over the cap.

In the CY 2019 Physician Fee Schedule final rule, CMS-1693-F, after consideration of stakeholders' requests for burden reduction, a review of all of the MCTRJCA requirements, and in light of the statutory amendments to section 1833(g) of the Act, via section 50202 of Bipartisan Budget Act of 2018 to repeal the therapy caps, CMS concluded that continued collection of functional reporting data through the same format would not yield additional information to inform future analyses or to serve as a basis for reforms to the payment system for therapy services. The rule ended the functional reporting requirements to reduce burden of reporting for providers of therapy services and revised regulation text at 42 CFR 410.59, 410.60, 410.61, 410.62, 410.105, accordingly.

The instructions below apply only to dates of service when the reporting requirement was effective, January 1, 2013 through December 31, 2018.

B. Application of New Coding Requirements

This functional data reporting and collection system is effective for therapy services with dates of service on and after January 1, 2013. A testing period will be in effect from January 1, 2013 and before January 1, 2019.

© 2019 Optum360, LLC

C. Services Affected

These requirements apply to all claims for services furnished under the Medicare Part B outpatient therapy benefit and the PT, OT, and SLP services furnished under the CORF benefit. They also apply to the therapy services furnished personally by and incident to the service of a physician or a nonphysician practitioner (NPP), including a nurse practitioner (NP), a certified nurse specialist (CNS), or a physician assistant (PA), as applicable.

D. Providers and Practitioners Affected.

The functional reporting requirements apply to the therapy services furnished by the following providers: hospitals, CAHs, SNFs, CORFs, rehabilitation agencies, and HHAs (when the beneficiary is not under a home health plan of care). It applies to the following practitioners: physical therapists, occupational therapists, and speech-language pathologists in private practice (TPPs), physicians, and NPPs as noted above. The term "clinician" is applied to these practitioners throughout this manual section. (See definition section of Pub. 100-02, chapter 15, section 220.)

E. Function-related G-codes

There are 42 functional G-codes, 14 sets of three codes each. Six of the G-code sets are generally for PT and OT functional limitations and eight sets of G-codes are for SLP functional limitations.

The following G-codes are for functional limitations typically seen in beneficiaries receiving PT or OT services. The first four of these sets describe categories of functional limitations and the final two sets describe "other" functional limitations, which are to be used for functional limitations not described by one of the four categories.

NONPAYABLE G-CODES FOR FUNCTIONAL LIMITATIONS

	Long Descriptor	Short Descriptor
Mobility G-code Set		
G8978	Mobility: walking & moving around functional limitation, current status, at therapy episode outset and at reporting intervals	Mobility current status
G8979	Mobility: walking & moving around functional limitation, projected goal status, at therapy episode outset, at reporting intervals, and at discharge or to end reporting	Mobility goal status
G8980	Mobility: walking & moving around functional limitation, discharge status, at discharge from therapy or to end reporting	Mobility D/C status
Changing & Maintaining Body Position G-code Set		
G8981	Changing & maintaining body position functional limitation, current status, at therapy episode outset and at reporting intervals	Body pos current status
G8982	Changing & maintaining body position functional limitation, projected goal status, at therapy episode outset, at reporting intervals, and at discharge or to end reporting	Body pos goal status
G8983	Changing & maintaining body position functional limitation, discharge status, at discharge from therapy or to end reporting	Body pos D/C status
Carrying, Moving & Handling Objects G-code Set		
G8984	Carrying, moving & handling objects functional limitation, current status, at therapy episode outset and at reporting intervals	Carry current status
G8985	Carrying, moving & handling objects functional limitation, projected goal status, at therapy episode outset, at reporting intervals, and at discharge or to end reporting	Carry goal status
G8986	Carrying, moving & handling objects functional limitation, discharge status, at discharge from therapy or to end reporting	Carry D/C status
Self Care G-code Set		
G8987	Self care functional limitation, current status, at therapy episode outset and at reporting intervals	Self care current status
G8988	Self care functional limitation, projected goal status, at therapy episode outset, at reporting intervals, and at discharge or to end reporting	Self care goal status
G8989	Self care functional limitation, discharge status, at discharge from therapy or to end reporting	Self care D/C status

- The following "other PT/OT" functional G-codes are used to report:
- a beneficiary's functional limitation that is not defined by one of the above four categories;
- a beneficiary whose therapy services are not intended to treat a functional limitation;
- or a beneficiary's functional limitation when an overall, composite or other score from a functional assessment too is used and it does not clearly represent a functional limitation defined by one of the above four code sets.

	Long Descriptor	Short Descriptor
Other PT/OT Primary G-code Set		
G8990	Other physical or occupational therapy primary functional limitation, current status, at therapy episode outset and at reporting intervals	Other PT/OT current status
G8991	Other physical or occupational therapy primary functional limitation, projected goal status, at therapy episode outset, at reporting intervals, and at discharge or to end reporting	Other PT/OT goal status
G8992	Other physical or occupational therapy primary functional limitation, discharge status, at discharge from therapy or to end reporting	Other PT/OT D/C status
Other PT/OT Subsequent G-code Set		
G8993	Other physical or occupational therapy subsequent functional limitation, current status, at therapy episode outset and at reporting intervals	Sub PT/OT current status
G8994	Other physical or occupational therapy subsequent functional limitation, projected goal status, at therapy episode outset, at reporting intervals, and at discharge or to end reporting	Sub PT/OT goal status
G8995	Other physical or occupational subsequent functional limitation, discharge from therapy or end reporting.	Sub PT/OT D/C status

The following G-codes are for functional limitations typically seen in beneficiaries receiving SLP services. Seven are for specific functional communication measures, which are modeled after the National Outcomes Measurement System (NOMS), and one is for any "other" measure not described by one of the other seven.

	Long Descriptor	Short Descriptor
Swallowing G-code Set		
G8996	Swallowing functional limitation, current status, at therapy episode outset and at reporting intervals	Swallow current status
G8997	Swallowing functional limitation, projected goal status, at therapy episode outset, at reporting intervals, and at discharge or to end reporting	Swallow goal status
G8998	Swallowing functional limitation, discharge status, at discharge from therapy or to end reporting	Swallow D/C status
Motor Speech G-code Set (Note: These codes are not sequentially numbered)		
G8999	Motor speech functional limitation, current status, at therapy episode outset and at reporting intervals	Motor speech current status
G9186	Motor speech functional limitation, projected goal status at therapy episode outset, at reporting intervals, and at discharge or to end reporting	Motor speech goal status
G9158	Motor speech functional limitation, discharge status, at discharge from therapy or to end reporting	Motor speech D/C status
Spoken Language Comprehension G-code Set		
G9159	Spoken language comprehension functional limitation, current status, at therapy episode outset and at reporting intervals	Lang comp current status

© 2019 Optum360, LLC

	Long Descriptor	Short Descriptor
G9160	Spoken language comprehension functional limitation, projected goal status, at therapy episode outset, at reporting intervals, and at discharge or to end reporting	Lang comp goal status
G9161	Spoken language comprehension functional limitation, discharge status, at discharge from therapy or to end reporting	Lang comp D/C status
Spoken Language Expressive G-code Set		
G9162	Spoken language expression functional limitation, current status, at therapy episode outset and at reporting intervals	Lang express current status
G9163	Spoken language expression functional limitation, projected goal status, at therapy episode outset, at reporting intervals, and at discharge or to end reporting	Lang press goal status
G9164	Spoken language expression functional limitation, discharge status, at discharge from therapy or to end reporting	Lang express D/C status
Attention G-code Set		
G9165	Attention functional limitation, current status, at therapy episode outset and at reporting intervals	Atten current status
G9166	Attention functional limitation, projected goal status, at therapy episode outset, at reporting intervals, and at discharge or to end reporting	Atten goal status
G9167	Attention functional limitation, discharge status, at discharge from therapy or to end reporting	Atten D/C status
Memory G-code Set		
G9168	Memory functional limitation, current status, at therapy episode outset and at reporting intervals	Memory current status
G9169	Memory functional limitation, projected goal status, at therapy episode outset, at reporting intervals, and at discharge or to end reporting	Memory goal status
G9170	Memory functional limitation, discharge status, at discharge from therapy or to end reporting	Memory D/C status
Voice G-code Set		
G9171	Voice functional limitation, current status, at therapy episode outset and at reporting intervals	Voice current status
G9172	Voice functional limitation, projected goal status, at therapy episode outset, at reporting intervals, and at discharge or to end reporting	Voice goal status
G9173	Voice functional limitation, discharge status, at discharge from therapy or to end reporting	Voice D/C status

The following "other SLP" G-code set is used to report:

- on one of the other eight NOMS-defined functional measures not described by the above code sets; or
- to report an overall, composite or other score from assessment tool that does not clearly represent one of the above seven categorical SLP functional measures.

	Long Descriptor	Short Descriptor
Other Speech Language Pathology G-code Set		
G9174	Other speech language pathology functional limitation, current status, at therapy episode outset and at reporting intervals	Speech lang current status
G9175	Other speech language pathology functional limitation, projected goal status, at therapy episode outset, at reporting intervals, and at discharge or to end reporting	Speech lang goal status
G9176	Other speech language pathology functional limitation, discharge status, at discharge from therapy or to end reporting	Speech lang D/C status

F. Severity/Complexity Modifiers

For each nonpayable functional G-code, one of the modifiers listed below must be used to report the severity/complexity for that functional limitation.

Modifier	Impairment Limitation Restriction
CH	0 percent impaired, limited or restricted
CI	At least 1 percent but less than 20 percent impaired, limited or restricted
CJ	At least 20 percent but less than 40 percent impaired, limited or restricted
CK	At least 40 percent but less than 60 percent impaired, limited or restricted
CL	At least 60 percent but less than 80 percent impaired, limited or restricted
CM	At least 80 percent but less than 100 percent impaired, limited or restricted
CN	100 percent impaired, limited or restricted

The severity modifiers reflect the beneficiary's percentage of functional impairment as determined by the clinician furnishing the therapy services.

G. Required Reporting of Functional G-codes and Severity Modifiers

The functional G-codes and severity modifiers listed above are used in the required reporting on therapy claims at certain specified points during therapy episodes of care. Claims containing these functional G-codes must also contain another billable and separately payable (non-bundled) service. Only one functional limitation shall be reported at a given time for each related therapy plan of care (POC).

Functional reporting using the G-codes and corresponding severity modifiers is required reporting on specified therapy claims. Specifically, they are required on claims:

- At the outset of a therapy episode of care (i.e., on the claim for the date of service (DOS) of the initial therapy service);
- At least once every 10 treatment days, which corresponds with the progress reporting period;
- When an evaluative procedure, including a re-evaluative one, (HCPCS/CPT codes 92521, 92522, 92523, 92524, 92597, 92607, 92608, 92610, 92611, 92612, 92614, 92616, 96105, 96125, 97161, 97162, 97163, 97164, 97165, 97166, 97167, 97168) is furnished and billed;
- At the time of discharge from the therapy episode of care–(i.e., on the date services related to the discharge [progress] report are furnished); and
- At the time reporting of a particular functional limitation is ended in cases where the need for further therapy is necessary.
- At the time reporting is begun for a new or different functional limitation within the same episode of care (i.e., after the reporting of the prior functional limitation is ended)

Functional reporting is required on claims throughout the entire episode of care. When the beneficiary has reached his or her goal or progress has been maximized on the initially selected functional limitation, but the need for treatment continues, reporting is required for a second functional limitation using another set of G-codes. In these situations two or more functional limitations will be reported for a beneficiary during the therapy episode of care. Thus, reporting on more than one functional limitation may be required for some beneficiaries but not simultaneously.

When the beneficiary stops coming to therapy prior to discharge, the clinician should report the functional information on the last claim. If the clinician is unaware that the beneficiary is not returning for therapy until after the last claim is submitted, the clinician cannot report the discharge status.

When functional reporting is required on a claim for therapy services, two G-codes will generally be required.

Two exceptions exist:

1. Therapy services under more than one therapy POC. Claims may contain more than two nonpayable functional G-codes when in cases where a beneficiary receives therapy services under multiple POCs (PT, OT, and/or SLP) from the same therapy provider.
2. One-Time Therapy Visit. When a beneficiary is seen and future therapy services are either not medically indicated or are going to be furnished by another provider, the clinician reports on the claim for the DOS of the visit, all three G-codes in the appropriate code set (current status, goal status and discharge status), along with corresponding severity modifiers. Each reported functional G-code must also contain the following line of service information:
   - Functional severity modifier

© 2019 Optum360, LLC

- Therapy modifier indicating the related discipline/POC -- GP, GO or GN -- for PT, OT, and SLP services, respectively
- Date of the related therapy service
- Nominal charge, e.g., a penny, for institutional claims submitted to the FIs and A/MACs. For professional claims, a zero charge is acceptable for the service line. If provider billing software requires an amount for professional claims, a nominal charge, e.g., a penny, may be included. Note: The KX modifier is not required on the claim line for nonpayable G-codes, but would be required with the procedure code for medically necessary therapy services furnished once the beneficiary's annual cap has been reached.

The following example demonstrates how the G-codes and modifiers are used. In this example, the clinician determines that the beneficiary's mobility restriction is the most clinically relevant functional limitation and selects the Mobility G-code set (G8978 – G8980) to represent the beneficiary's functional limitation. The clinician also determines the severity/complexity of the beneficiary's functional limitation and selects the appropriate modifier. In this example, the clinician determines that the beneficiary has a 75 percent mobility restriction for which the CL modifier is applicable. The clinician expects that at the end of therapy the beneficiaries will have only a 15 percent mobility restriction for which the CI modifier is applicable. When the beneficiary attains the mobility goal, therapy continues to be medically necessary to addresss a functional limitation for which there is no categorical G-code. The clinician reports this using (G8990 – G8992).

At the outset of therapy. On the DOS for which the initial evaluative procedure is furnished or the initial treatment day of a therapy POC, the claim for the service will also include two G-codes as shown below.

- G8978-CL to report the functional limitation (Mobility with current mobility limitation of "at least 60 percent but less than 80 percent impaired, limited or restricted")
- G8979-CI to report the projected goal for a mobility restriction of "at least 1 percent but less than 20 percent impaired, limited or restricted."

At the end of each progress reporting period. On the claim for the DOS when the services related to the progress report (which must be done at least once each 10 treatment days) are furnished, the clinician will report the same two G-codes but the modifier for the current status may be different.

- G8978 with the appropriate modifier are reported to show the beneficiary's current status as of this DOS. So if thebeneficiary has made no progress, this claim will include G8978-CL. If the beneficiary made progress and now has a mobility restriction of 65 percent CL would still be the appropriate modifier for 65 percent, and G8978-CL would be reported in this case. If the beneficiary now has a mobility restriction of 45 percent, G8978-CK would be reported.
- G8979-CI would be reported to show the projected goal. This severity modifier would not change unless the clinician adjusts the beneficiary's goal. This step is repeated as necessary and clinically appropriate, adjusting the current status modifier used as the beneficiary progresses through therapy.
- At the time the beneficiary is discharged from the therapy episode. The final claim for therapy episode will include two G-codes.
- G8979-CI would be reported to show the projected goal. G8980-CI would be reported if the beneficiary attained the 15 percent mobility goal. Alternatively, if the beneficiary's mobility restriction only reached 25 percent; G8980-CJ would be reported. To end reporting of one functional limitation. As noted above, functional reporting is required to continue throughout the entire episode of care. Accordingly, when further therapy is medically necessary after the beneficiary attains the goal for the first reported functional limitation, the clinician would end reporting of the first functional limitation by using the same G-codes and modifiers that would be used at the time of discharge. Using the mobility example, to end reporting of the mobility functional limitation, G8979-CI and G8980-CI would be reported on the same DOS that coincides with end of that progress reporting period.

To begin reporting of a second functional limitation. At the time reporting is begun for a new and different functional limitation, within the same episode of care (i.e., after the reporting of the prior functional limitation is ended). Reporting on the second functional limitation, however, is not begun until the DOS of the next treatment day -- which is day one of the new progress reporting period. When the next functional limitation to be reported is NOT defined by one of the other three PT/OT categorical codes, the G-code set (G8990 - G8992) for the "other PT/OT primary" functional limitation is used, rather than the G-code set for the "other PT/OT subsequent" because it is the first reported "other PT/OT" functional limitation. This reporting begins on the DOS of the first treatment day following the mobility "discharge" reporting, which is counted as the initial service for the "other PT/OT primary" functional limitation and the first treatment day of the new progress reporting period. In this case, G8990 and G8991, along with the corresponding modifiers, are reported on the claim for therapy services.

The table below illustrates when reporting is required using this example and what G-codes would be used.

Example of Required Reporting

Key: Reporting Period (RP)	Begin RP #1 for Mobility at Episode Outset	End RP#1for Mobility at Progress Report	Mobility RP #2 Begins Next Treatment Day	End RP#2 for Mobility at Progress Report	Mobility RP #3 Begins Next Treatment Day	D/C or End Reporting for \Mobility	Begin RP #1 for Other PT/OT Primary
Mobility: Walking & Moving Around							
G8978 – Current Status	X	X		X			
G 8979– Goal Status	X	X		X		X	
G8980 – Discharge Status						X	
Other PT/OT Primary							
G8990 – Current Status							X
G8991 – Goal Status							X
G8992 – Discharge Status							
No Functional Reporting Req'd			X		X		

H. Required Tracking and Documentation of Functional G-codes and Severity Modifiers

The clinician who furnishes the services must not only report the functional information on the therapy claim, but, he/she must track and document the G-codes and severity modifiers used for this reporting in the beneficiary's medical record of therapy services.

For details related to the documentation requirements, refer to Pub. 100-02, Medicare Benefit Policy Manual, chapter 15, section 220.4, - MCTRJCA-required Functional Reporting. For coverage rules related to MCTRJCA and therapy goals, refer to Pub. 100-02: a) for outpatient therapy services, see chapter 15, section 220.1.2 B and b) for instructions specific to PT, OT, and SLP services in the CORF, see chapter 12, section 10.

100-04, 5, 20.4

Coding Guidance for Certain CPT Codes - All Claims

(Rev.3475, Issued: 03-04-16, Effective: 06-06-16, Implementation: 06-06-16)

The following provides guidance about the use of codes 96105, 97026, 97150, 97545, 97546, and G0128.

CPT Codes 96105, 97545, and 97546.

Providers report code 96105, assessment of aphasia with interpretation and report in 1-hour units. This code represents formal evaluation of aphasia with an instrument such as the Boston Diagnostic Aphasia Examination. If this formal assessment is performed during treatment, it is typically performed only once during treatment and its medical necessity should be documented. If the test is repeated during treatment, the medical necessity of the repeat administration of the test must also be documented. It is common practice for regular assessment of a patient's progress in therapy to be documented in the chart, and this may be done using test items taken from the formal examinations. This is considered to be part of the treatment and should not be billed as 96105 unless a full, formal assessment is completed.

Other timed physical medicine codes are 97545 and 97546. The interval for code 97545 is 2 hours and for code 97546, 1 hour. These are specialized codes to be used in the context of rehabilitating a worker to return to a job. The expectation is that the entire time period specified in the codes 97545 or 97546 would be the treatment period, since a shorter period of treatment could be coded with another code such as codes 97110, 97112, or 97537. (Codes 97545 and 97546 were developed for reporting services to persons in the worker's compensation program, thus we do not expect to see them reported for Medicare patients except under very unusual circumstances. Further, we would not expect to see code 97546 without also seeing code 97545 on the same claim. Code 97546, when used, is used in conjunction with 97545.)

CPT Code 97026

Effective for services performed on or after October 24, 2006, the Centers for Medicare & Medicaid Services announce a NCD stating the use of infrared and/or near-infrared light and/or heat, including monochromatic infrared energy (MIRE), is non-covered for the treatment, including symptoms such as pain arising from these conditions, of diabetic and/or non-diabetic peripheral sensory neuropathy, wounds and/or ulcers of the skin and/or subcutaneous tissues in Medicare beneficiaries. Further coverage guidelines can be found in the National Coverage Determination Manual (Publication 100-03), section 270.6.

Contractors shall deny claims with CPT 97026 (infrared therapy incident to or as a PT/OT benefit) and HCPCS E0221 or A4639, if the claim contains any of the following ICD-9 codes: 250.60-250.63, 354.4, 354.5, 354.9, 355.1-355.4, 355.6-355.9, 356.0, 356.2-356.4, 356.8-356.9, 357.0-357.7, 674.10, 674.12, 674.14, 674.20, 674.22, 674.24, 707.00-707.07, 707.09-707.15, 707.19, 870.0-879.9, 880.00-887.7, 890.0-897.7, 998.31-998.32. Contractors can use the following messages when denying the service:

- Medicare Summary Notice # 21.11 "This service was not covered by Medicare at the time you received it."
- Reason Claim Adjustment Code #50 "These are noncovered services because this is not deemed a medical necessity by the payer."

Advanced Beneficiary Notice (ABN): Physicians, physical therapists, occupational therapists, outpatient rehabilitation facilities (ORFs), comprehensive outpatient rehabilitation facilities (CORFs), home health agencies (HHA), and hospital outpatient departments are liable if the service is performed, unless the beneficiary signs an ABN.

Similarly, DME suppliers and HHA are liable for the devices when they are supplied, unless the beneficiary signs an ABN.

100-04, 5, 100.3

Proper Reporting of Nursing Services by CORFs - A/B MAC (A)

(Rev.1459; Issued: 02-22-08; Effective: 07-01-08; Implementation: 07-07-08)

Nursing services performed in the CORF shall be billed utilizing the following HCPCS code:

G0128 – Direct (Face to Face w/ patient) skilled nursing services of a registered nurse provided in a CORF, each 10 minutes beyond the first 5 minutes.

In addition, HCPCS G0128 is billable with revenue codes 0550 and 0559 only.

100-04, 5, 100.4

Outpatient Mental Health TreatmentLimitation

(Rev.2736, Issued: 06-28-13, Effective: 10-01-12, Implementation10-07-13)

The Outpatient Mental Health Treatment Limitation (the limitation) is not applicable to CORF services because CORFs do not provide services to treat mental, psychoneurotic and personality disorders that are subject to the limitation in section 1833(c) of the Act. For dates of service on or after October 1, 2012, HCPCS code G0409 is the only code allowed for social work and psychological services furnished in a CORF. This service is not subject to the limitation because it is not a psychiatric mental health treatment service.

For additional information on the limitation, see Publication 100-01, Chapter 3, section 30 and Publication 100-02, Chapter 12, sections 50-50.5.

100-04, 5, 100.11

Billing for Social Work and Psychological Services in a CORF

(Rev 2736, Issued: 06-28-13, Effective: 10-01-12, Implementation10-07-13)

The CORF providers shall only bill social work and psychological services with the following HCPCS code:

G0409 Social work and psychological services, directly relating to and/or the patient's rehabilitation goals, each 15 minutes, face-to-face; individual (services provided by a CORF-qualified social worker or psychologist in a CORF).

In addition, HCPCS code G0409 shall only be billed with revenue code 0569 or 0911.

100-04, 6, 20.1.1.2

Hospital's "Facility Charge" in Connection with Clinic Services of a Physician

(Rev.3230, Issued: 04-03-15, Effective: 06-15-15, Implementation: 06-15-15)

As noted above in section 20.1.1, physician services are excluded from Part A PPS payment and the requirement for consolidated billing. When a beneficiary receives clinic services from a hospital-based physician, the physician in this situation would bill his or her own professional services directly to the A/B MAC (B) and would be reimbursed at the facility rate of the Medicare physician fee schedule--which does not include overhead expenses. The hospital historically has submitted a separate Part B "facility charge" for the associated overhead expenses to its A/B MAC (A). The hospital's facility charge does not involve a separate service (such as a diagnostic test) furnished in addition to the physician's professional service; rather, it represents solely the overhead expenses associated with furnishing the professional service itself. Accordingly, hospitals bill for "facility charges" under the physician evaluation and management (E&M) codes in the range of 99201-99245 and G0463 (for hospitals paid under the Outpatient Prospective Payment System).

E&M codes, representing the hospital's "facility charge" for the overhead expenses associated with furnishing the professional service itself, are excluded from SNF CB. Effective for claims with dates of service on or after January 1, 2006, the CWF will bypass CB edits when billed with revenue code 0510 (clinic visit) with an E&M HCPCS code in the range of 99201-99245 and, effective January 1, 2014 with HCPCS code G0463.

NOTE: Unless otherwise excluded in one of the Five Major Categories for billing services to FIs, physician services codes are to be billed to the carrier by the physician. Facility charges associated with the physician's clinic visit must be reported as explained above.

100-04, 7, 80.2

Mammography Screening

(Rev.3053, Iss. 08-28-14, Eff. ICD -10: Upon Imp. ICD - 10 ASC-X 12: 1-1-12, ASC X12: 9-30 -14)

Section 4163 of the Omnibus Budget Reconciliation Act of 1990 added §1834(c) of the Act to provide for Part B coverage of mammography screening for certain women entitled to Medicare for screenings performed on or after January 1, 1991. The term "screening mammography" means a radiologic procedure provided to an asymptomatic woman for the purpose of early detection of breast cancer and includes a physician's interpretation of the results of the procedure. Unlike diagnostic mammographies, there do not need to be signs, symptoms, or history of breast disease in order for the exam to be covered.

The technical component portion of the screening mammography should be billed on the ASC X12 837 institutional claim format or if permissible Form CMS-1450 under bill type 22X for SNF Part A and Part B inpatients or 23X for SNF outpatients. Claims for mammography screening should include only the charges for the screening mammography.

100-04, 8, 60.2.1.1

Separately Billable ESRD Drugs

(Rev.3053, Iss. 08-28-14, Eff. ICD -10: Upon Imp. ICD - 10 ASC-X 12: 1-1-12, ASC X12: 9-30 -14)

The following categories of drugs (including but not limited to) are separately billable when used to treat the patient's renal condition:

- Antibiotics;
- Analgesics;
- Anabolics;
- Hematinics;
- Muscle relaxants;
- Sedatives;
- Tranquilizers; and
- Thrombolytics: used to declot central venous catheters. **Note:** Thrombolytics were removed from the separately billable drugs for claims with dates of service on or after January 1, 2013.

For claims with dates of service on or after July 1, 2013, when these drugs are administered through the dialysate the provider must append the modifier JE (Administered via Dialysate).

These separately billable drugs may only be billed by an ESRD facility if they are actually administered in the facility by the facility staff. Staff time used to administer separately billable drugs is covered under the composite rate and may not be billed separately. However, the supplies used to administer these drugs may be billed in addition to the composite rate.

Effective January 1, 2011, section 153b of the MIPPA requires that all ESRD-related drugs and biologicals be billed by the renal dialysis facility. When a drug or biological is billed by providers other than the ESRD facility and the drug or biological furnished is designated as a drug or biological that is included in the ESRD PPS (ESRD-related), the claim will be rejected or denied. In the event that an ESRD-related drug or biological was furnished to an ESRD beneficiary for reasons other than for the treatment of ESRD, the provider may submit a claim for separate payment using modifier AY.

All drugs reported on the renal dialysis facility claim are considered included in the ESRD PPS. The list of drugs and biologicals for consolidated billing are designated as always ESRD-related and therefore not allowing separate payment to be made to ESRD facilities. However, CMS has determined that some of these drugs may warrant separate payment.

© 2019 Optum360, LLC

Exceptions to "Always ESRD Related" Drugs:
The following drugs have been approved for separate payment consideration when billed with the AY modifier attesting to the drug not being used for the treatment of ESRD. The ESRD facility is required to indicate (in accordance with ICD-9 guidelines) the diagnosis code for which the drug is indicated.

- Vancomycin, effective January 1, 2012
- Daptomycin, effective January 1, 2013

Items and services subject to the consolidated billing requirements for the ESRD PPS can be found on the CMS website at:
http://www.cms.gov/ESRDPayment/50_Consolidated_Billing.asp#TopOfPage.

Other drugs and biologicals may be considered separately payable to the dialysis facility if the drug was not for the treatment of ESRD. The facility must include the modifier AY to indicate it was not for the treatment of ESRD.

Drugs are assigned HCPCS codes. If no HCPCS code is listed for a drug (e.g., a new drug) the facility bills using HCPCS code J3490, "Unclassified Drugs," and submits documentation identifying the drug. To establish a code for the drug, the FI checks HCPCS to verify that there is no acceptable HCPCS code for billing and if a code is not found checks with the local carrier, which may have a code and price that is appropriate. If no code is found the drug is processed under HCPCS code J3490. See Chapter 17 for a complete description of drug pricing.

100-04, 8, 60.2.4.2

Physician Billing Requirements to the A/B MAC (B)

(Rev.3650, Issued: 11-10-16, Effective: 02-10-17, Implementation: 02-10-17)

A. Sodium Ferric Gluconate Complex in Sucrose Injection
Sodium Ferric Gluconate Complex in sucrose injection may be payable for claims with dates of service on or after December 1, 2000 when furnished intravenously, for first line treatment of iron deficiency anemia in patients undergoing chronic hemodialysis who are receiving supplemental erythropoeitin therapy. Physicians bill and A/B MACs (B) pay for HCPCS code J1756 when submitted with a primary diagnosis for chronic renal failure and a secondary diagnosis for iron deficiency anemia.

These diagnoses are listed below. Use ICD-9-CM or ICD-10-CM as applicable for the service date.

Chronic Renal Failure (Primary Diagnosis)

- ICD-9-CM – 585
- ICD-10-CM – N18.3, N18.4, N18.5, N18.6,

Iron Deficiency Anemia (Secondary Diagnosis)

- ICD-9-CM – 280.0, 280.1, 280.8, or 280.9
- ICD-10-CM – D50.0, D50.1, D50.8, D50.9,D63.1

This benefit is subject to the Part B deductible and coinsurance and should be paid per current Medicare drug payment reimbursement rules. A/B MACs (B) may cover other uses of this drug at their discretion.

B. Iron Sucrose Injection
Iron Sucrose injections are payable for claims with dates of service on or after October 1, 2001, when furnished intravenously, for first line treatment of iron deficiency anemia in patients undergoing chronic hemodialysis who are receiving supplemental erythropoeitin therapy. Until a specific code for iron sucrose injection is developed, providers must submit HCPCS code J1756, with the appropriate explanation of drug name and dosage

entered on the claim. The primary diagnosis code for chronic renal failure and one of the following secondary diagnosis codes for iron deficiency must be entered.

These diagnoses are listed below. Use ICD-9-CM or ICD-10-CM as applicable for the service date.

Chronic Renal Failure (Primary Diagnosis)

- ICD-9-CM - 585
- ICD-10-CM - N18.3, N18.4, N18.5, N18.6,

Iron Deficiency Anemia (Secondary Diagnosis)

- ICD-9-CM – 280.0, 280.1, 280.8, or 280.9
- ICD-10-CM – D50.0, D50.1, D50.8, D50.9,D63.1

Iron sucrose injection is subject to the Part B deductible and coinsurance and should be paid per current Medicare drug payment reimbursement rules. A/B MACs (B) may cover other uses of this drug at their discretion.

C. Messages for Use with Denials
The contractor shall deny claims for sodium ferric gluconate complex in sucrose injection or iron sucrose injection due to a missing diagnosis code.

The contractor shall use the following remittance advice messages and associated codes when rejecting/denying claims under this policy. This CARC/RARC combination is compliant with CAQH CORE Business Scenario Two.

Group Code: CO
CARC: 16
RARC: M76
MSN: 9.2

100-04, 8, 60.4

Erythropoietin Stimulating Agents (ESAs)

(Rev.2582, Issued: 11-02-12, Effective: 04-01-13, Implementation: 04-01-13)

Coverage rules for ESAs are explained in the Medicare Benefit Policy Manual, Publication 100-02, chapter 11.

Fiscal intermediaries (FIs) pay for ESAs, to end-stage renal disease (ESRD) facilities as separately billable drugs to the composite rate. No additional payment is made to administer an ESA, whether in a facility or a home. Effective January 1, 2005, the cost of supplies to administer EPO may be billed to the FI. HCPCS A4657 and Revenue Code 270 should be used to capture the charges for syringes used in the administration of EPO.

ESAs and their administration supplies are included in the payment for the ESRD Prospective Payment System effective January 1, 2011. Providers must continue to report ESAs on the claim as ESAs are subject to a national claims monitoring program and are entitled to outlier payment consideration. The Medicare allowed payment (MAP) amount for outlier includes the ESA rate provided on the Average Sale Price (ASP) list, subject to reduction based on the ESA monitoring policy.

Medicare has an established national claims monitoring policy for erythropoietin stimulating agents for the in-facility dialysis population as outlined in the sections below.

100-04, 8, 60.4.1

ESA Claims Monitoring Policy

(Rev.2582, Issued: 11-02-12, Effective: 04-01-13, Implementation: 04-01-13)

Effective for services provided on or after April 1, 2006, Medicare has implemented a national claims monitoring policy for ESAs administered in Medicare renal dialysis facilities. This policy does not apply to claims for ESAs for patients who receive their dialysis at home and self-administer their ESA.

While Medicare is not changing its coverage policy on erythropoietin use to maintain a target hematocrit level between 30% and 36%, we believe the variability in response to ESAs warrants postponing requiring monitoring until the hematocrit reaches higher levels. For dates of services April 1, 2006, and later, the Centers for Medicare & Medicaid Services (CMS) claims monitoring policy applies when the hematocrit level exceeds 39.0% or the hemoglobin level exceeds 13.0g/dL. This does not preclude the contractors from performing medical review at lower levels.

Effective for services provided on or after April 1, 2006, for claims reporting hematocrit or hemoglobin levels exceeding the monitoring threshold, the dose shall be reduced by 25% over the preceding month. Providers may report that a dose reduction did occur in response to the reported elevated hematocrit or hemoglobin level by adding a GS modifier on the claim. The definition of the GS modifier is defined as: "Dosage of ESA has been reduced and maintained in response to hematocrit or hemoglobin level." Thus, for claims reporting a hematocrit level or hemoglobin level exceeding the monitoring threshold without the GS modifier, CMS will reduce the covered dosage reported on the claim by 25%. The excess dosage is considered to be not reasonable and necessary. Providers are reminded that the patient's medical records should reflect hematocrit/hemoglobin levels and any dosage reduction reported on the claim during the same time period for which the claim is submitted.

Effective for dates of service provided on and after January 1, 2008, requests for payments or claims for ESAs for ESRD patients receiving dialysis in renal dialysis facilities reporting a hematocrit level exceeding 39.0% (or hemoglobin exceeding 13.0g/dL) shall also include modifier ED or EE. Claims reporting neither modifier or both modifiers will be returned to the provider for correction.

The definition of modifier ED is "The hematocrit level has exceeded 39.0% (or hemoglobin 1evel has exceeded 13.0g/dL) 3 or more consecutive billing cycles immediately prior to and including the current billing cycle." The definition of modifier EE is "The hematocrit level has exceeded 39.0% (or hemoglobin level has exceeded 13.0g/dL) less than 3 consecutive billing cycles immediately prior to and including the current billing cycle." The GS modifier continues to be defined as stated above.

Providers may continue to report the GS modifier when the reported hematocrit or hemoglobin levels exceed the monitoring threshold for less than 3 months and a

© 2019 Optum360, LLC

dose reduction has occurred. When both modifiers GS and EE are included, no reduction in the covered dose will occur. Claims reporting a hematocrit or hemoglobin level exceeding the monitoring threshold and the ED modifier shall have an automatic 50% reduction in the covered dose applied, even if the claim also reports the GS modifier.

Below is a chart illustrating the resultant claim actions under all possible reporting scenarios:

Hct Exceeds 39.0% or Hgb Exceeds 13.0g/dL	ED Modifier? (Hct >39% or Hgb >13g/dL =3 cycles)	EE Modifier? Hct >39% or Hgb >13g/dL <3 cycles)	GS Modifier? (Dosage reduced and maintained)	Claim Action
No	N/A	N/A	N/A	Do not reduce reported dose.
Yes	No	No	No	Return to provider for correction. Claim must report either modifier ED or EE.
Yes	No	No	Yes	Return to provider for correction. Claim must report either modifier ED or EE.
Yes	No	Yes	Yes	Do not reduce reported dose.
Yes	No	Yes	No	Reduce reported dose 25%.
Yes	Yes	No	Yes	Reduce reported dose 50%.
Yes	Yes	No	No	Reduce reported dose 50%.

In some cases, physicians may believe there is medical justification to maintain a hematocrit above 39.0% or hemoglobin above 13.0g/dL. Beneficiaries, physicians, and/or renal facilities may submit additional medical documentation to justify this belief under the routine appeal process. You may reinstate any covered dosage reduction amounts under this first level appeal process when you believe the documentation supports a higher hematocrit/hemoglobin level.

Providers are reminded that, in accordance with FDA labeling, CMS expects that as the hematocrit approaches 36.0% (hemoglobin 12.0g/dL), a dosage reduction occurs. Providers are expected to maintain hematocrit levels between 30.0 to 36.0% (hemoglobin 10.0-12.0g/dL). Hematocrit levels that remain below 30.0% (hemoglobin levels below 10.0g/dL)) despite dosage increases, should have causative factors evaluated. The patient's medical record should reflect the clinical reason for dose changes and hematocrit levels outside the range of 30.0-36.0% (hemoglobin levels 10.0-12.0g/dL). Medicare contractors may review medical records to assure appropriate dose reductions are applied and maintained and hematological target ranges are maintained.

These hematocrit requirements apply only to ESAs furnished as an ESRD benefit under §1881(b) of the Social Security Act.

Medically Unlikely Edits (MUE)

For dates of service on and after January 1, 2008, the MUE for claims billing for Epogen® is reduced to 400,000 units from 500,000. The MUE for claims for Aranesp® is reduced to 1200 mcg from 1500 mcg.

For dates of service on and after April 1, 2013, the MUE for claims billing for peginesatide is applicable when units billed are equal to or greater than 26 mg.

It is likely that claims reporting doses exceeding the threshold reflect typographical errors and will be returned to providers for correction.

100-04, 8, 60.4.2

60.4.2 - Facility Billing Requirements for ESAs

(Rev.4105, Issued: 08- 03-18, Effective: 01-01-19, Implementation: 01-07-19)

Hematocrit and Hemoglobin Levels

Renal dialysis facilities are required to report hematocrit or hemoglobin levels for their Medicare patients receiving erythropoietin products. Hematocrit levels are reported in value code 49 and reflect the most recent reading taken before the start of the billing period. Hemoglobin readings before the start of the billing period are reported in value code 48.

To report a hemoglobin or hematocrit reading for a new patient on or after January 1, 2006, the provider should report the reading that prompted the treatment of epoetin alfa. The provider may use results documented on form CMS 2728 or the patient's medical records from a transferring facility.

Effective January 1, 2012, ESRD facilities are required to report hematocrit or hemoglobin levels on all ESRD claims. Reporting the value 99.99 is not permitted when billing for an ESA.

The revenue codes for reporting Epoetin Alfa are 0634 and 0635. All other ESAs are reported using revenue code 0636. The HCPCS code for the ESA must be included:

HCPCS	HCPCS Description	Dates of Service
Q4055	Injection, Epoetin Alfa, 1,000 units (for ESRD on Dialysis)	1/1/2004 - 12/31/2005
J0886	Injection, Epoetin Alfa, 1,000 units (for ESRD on Dialysis)	1/1/2006 - 12/31/2006
Q4081	Injection, Epoetin alfa, 100 units (for ESRD on Dialysis)	1/1/2007 to through 7/1/2015
Q5105	Injection, epoetin alfa, biosimilar, (Retacrit) (For ESRD on Dialysis), 100 units	7/1/2018 to present

Each administration of an ESA is reported on a separate line item with the units reported used as a multiplier by the dosage description in the HCPCS to arrive at the dosage per administration.

Route of Administration Modifiers

Patients with end stage renal disease (ESRD) receiving administrations of erythropoiesis stimulating agents (ESA) for the treatment of anemia may receive intravenous administration or subcutaneous administrations of the ESA. Effective for claims with dates of services on or after January 1, 2012, all facilities billing for injections of ESA for ESRD beneficiaries must include the modifier JA on the claim to indicate an intravenous administration or modifier JB to indicate a subcutaneous administration. ESRD claims containing ESA administrations that are submitted without the route of administration modifiers will be returned to the provider for correction. Renal dialysis facilities claim including charges for administrations of the ESA by both methods must report separate lines to identify the number of administration provided using each method.

Effective July 1, 2013, providers must identify when a drug is administered via the dialysate by appending the modifier JE (administered via dialysate).

ESA Monitoring Policy Modifiers

Append modifiers ED, EE and GS as applicable, see instructions in section 60.4.1.

Maximum Allowable Administrations

The maximum number of administrations of EPO for a billing cycle is 13 times in 30 days and 14 times in 31 days.

The maximum number of administrations of Aranesp for a billing cycle is 5 times in 30/ 31days.

The maximum number of administrations of Peginesatide is 1 time in 30/ 31days.

100-04, 8, 60.4.4

Payment Amount for Epoetin Alfa (EPO)

(Rev.2582, Issued: 11-02-12, Effective: 04-01-13, Implementation: 04-01-13)

Dates of service prior to January 1, 2005, the Medicare contractor pays the facility $10 per 1,000 units of EPO administered, rounded to the nearest 100 units (i.e., $1.00 per 100 units). Effective January 1, 2005, EPO will be paid based on the ASP Pricing File. Also effective January 1, 2005, the cost of supplies to administer EPO may be billed to the Medicare contractor. HCPCS A4657 and Revenue Code 270 should be used to capture the charges for syringes used in the administration of EPO. Where EPO is furnished by a supplier that is not a facility, the DMERC pays at the same rate.

Physician payment is calculated through the drug payment methodology described in Chapter 17 of the Claims Processing Manual.

EXAMPLE: The billing period is 2/1/94 - 2/28/94.

The facility provides the following:

Date	Units	Date	Units
2/1	3000	2/15	2500
2/4	3000	2/18	2500
2/6	3000	2/20	2560
2/8	3000	2/22	2500
2/11	2500	2/25	2000
2/13	2500	2/27	2000

Total 31,060 units

For value code 68, the facility enters 31,060. The 31,100 are used to determine the rate payable. This is 31,060 rounded to the nearest 100 units. The amount payable is 31.1 x $10 =$311.00. In their systems, FIs have the option of setting up payment of $1.00 per 100 units. Effective January 1, 2005, EPO will be paid based on the ASP Pricing File.

© 2019 Optum360, LLC

Effective January 1, 2008, payment is calculated on a renal dialysis facility claim at the line level by multiplying the rate from the ASP pricing file by the number of units reported on the line billing for EPO.

EXAMPLE: 311 x $1.00 = $311.00

If an ESRD beneficiary requires 10,000 units or more of EPO per administration, special documentation must be made in the medical records. It must consist of a narrative report that addresses the following:

- Iron deficiency. Most patients need supplemental iron therapy while being treated, even if they do not start out iron deficient;
- Concomitant conditions such as infection, inflammation, or malignancy. These conditions must be addressed to assure that EPO has maximum effect;
- Unrecognized blood loss. Patients with kidney disease and anemia may easily have chronic blood loss (usually gastrointestinal) as a major cause of anemia. In those circumstances, EPO is limited in effectiveness;
- Concomitant hemolysis, bone morrow dysplasia, or refractory anemia for a reason other than renal disease, e.g., aluminum toxicity;
- Folic acid or vitamin B12 deficiencies;
- Circumstances in which the bone morrow is replaced with other tissue, e.g., malignancy or osteitis fibrosa cystica; and

Patient's weight, the current dose required, a historical record of the amount that has been given, and the hematocrit response to date.

Payment for ESRD-related EPO is included in the ESRD PPS for claims with dates of service on or after January 1, 2011.

100-04, 8, 60.4.4.1

Payment for Epoetin Alfa (EPO) in Other Settings

(Rev.2582, Issued: 11-02-12, Effective: 04-01-13, Implementation: 04-01-13)

With the implementation of the ESRD PPS, ESRD-related EPO is included in ESRD PPS payment amount and is not separately payable on Part B claims with dates of service on or after January 1, 2011 for other providers with the exception of a hospital billing for an emergency or unscheduled dialysis session.

In the hospital inpatient setting, payment under Part A is included in the DRG.

In the hospital inpatient setting, payment under Part B is made on bill type 12x. Hospitals report the drug units based on the units defined in the HCPCS description. Hospitals do not report value code 68 for units of EPO. For dates of service prior to April 1, 2006, report EPO under revenue code 0636. For dates of service from April 1, 2006 report EPO under the respective revenue code 0634 for EPO less than 10,000 units and revenue code 0635 for EPO over 10,000 units. Payment will be based on the ASP Pricing File.

In a skilled nursing facility (SNF), payment for EPO covered under the Part B EPO benefit is not included in the prospective payment rate for the resident's Medicare-covered SNF stay.

In a hospice, payment is included in the hospice per diem rate.

For a service furnished by a physician or incident to a physician's service, payment is made to the physician by the carrier in accordance with the rules for 'incident to" services. When EPO is administered in the renal facility, the service is not an "incident to" service and not under the "incident to" provision.

100-04, 8, 60.4.4.2

Epoetin Alfa (EPO) Provided in the Hospital Outpatient Departments

(Rev.2582, Issued: 11-02-12, Effective: 04-01-13, Implementation: 04-01-13)

When ESRD patients come to the hospital for an unscheduled or emergency dialysis treatment they may also require the administration of EPO. Effective January 1, 2005, EPO will be paid based on the ASP Pricing File.

Hospitals use type of bill 13X (or 85X for Critical Access Hospitals) and report charges under the respective revenue code 0634 for EPO less than 10,000 units and revenue code 0635 for EPO over 10,000 units. Hospitals report the drug units based on the units defined in the HCPCS description. Hospitals do not report value code 68 for units of EPO. Value code 49 must be reported with the hematocrit value for the hospital outpatient visits prior to January 1, 2006, and for all claims with dates of service on or after January 1, 2008.

100-04, 8, 60.4.5.1

Self Administered ESA Supply

(Rev.2582, Issued: 11-02-12, Effective: 04-01-13, Implementation: 04-01-13)

Initially, facilities may bill for up to a 2-month supply of an ESA for Method I beneficiaries who meet the criteria for selection for self-administration. After the initial two months' supply, the facility will bill for one month's supply at a time. Condition code 70 is used to indicate payment requested for a supply of an ESA furnished a beneficiary. Usually, revenue code 0635 would apply to EPO since the supply would be over 10,000 units. Facilities leave FL 46, Units of Service, blank since they are not administering the drug.

For claims with dates of service on or after January 1, 2008, supplies of an ESA for self administration should be billed according to the pre-determined plan of care schedule provided to the beneficiary. Submit a separate line item for each date an administration is expected to be performed with the expected dosage. In the event that the schedule was changed, the provider should note the changes in the medical record and bill according to the revised schedule. For patients beginning to self administer an ESA at home receiving an extra month supply of the drug, bill the one month reserve supply on one claim line and include modifier EM defined as "Emergency Reserve Supply (for ESRD benefit only)".

When billing for drug wastage in accordance with the policy in chapter 17 of this manual, section 40.1 the provider must show the wastage on a separate line item with the modifier JW. The line item date of service should be the date of the last covered administration according to the plan of care or if the patient dies use the date of death.

Condition code 70 should be reported on claims billing for home dialysis patients that self administer anemia management drugs including ESAs.

100-04, 8, 60.4.6.3

Payment Amount for Darbepoetin Alfa (Aranesp)

(Rev.2582, Issued: 11-02-12, Effective: 04-01-13, Implementation: 04-01-13)

For Method I patients, the FI pays the facility per one mcg of Aranesp administered, in accordance with the MMA Drug Payment Limits Pricing File rounded up to the next highest whole mcg. Effective January 1, 2005, Aranesp will be paid based on the ASP Pricing File. Effective January 1, 2005, the cost of supplies to administer Aranesp may be billed to the FI. HCPCS A4657 and Revenue Code 270 should be used to capture the charges for syringes used in the administration of Aranesp.

Physician payment is calculated through the drug payment methodology described in Chapter 17, of the Claims Processing Manual.

The coinsurance and deductible are based on the Medicare allowance payable, not on the provider's charges. The provider may not charge the beneficiary more than 20 percent of the Medicare Aranesp allowance. This rule applies to independent and hospital based renal facilities.

Payment for ESRD-related Aranesp is included in the ESRD PPS for claims with dates of service on or after January 1, 2011.

100-04, 8, 60.4.6.4

Payment for Darbepoetin Alfa (Aranesp) in Other Settings

(Rev.2582, Issued: 11-02-12, Effective: 04-01-13, Implementation: 04-01-13)

In the hospital inpatient setting, payment under Part A for Aranesp is included in the DRG.

In the hospital inpatient setting, payment under Part B is made on bill type 12x when billed with revenue code 0636. The total number of units as a multiple of 1mcg is placed in the unit field. Reimbursement is based on the payment allowance limit for Medicare Part B drugs as found in the ASP pricing file.

In a skilled nursing facility (SNF), payment for Aranesp covered under the Part B EPO benefit is not included in the prospective payment rate for the resident's Medicare-covered SNF stay.

In a hospice, payment is included in the hospice per diem rate.

For a service furnished by a physician or incident to a physician's service, payment is made to the physician by the carrier in accordance with the rules for 'incident to" services. When Aranesp is administered in the renal facility, the service is not an "incident to" service and not under the "incident to" provision.

With the implementation of the ESRD PPS, ESRD-related Aranesp is included in the ESRD PPS payment amount and is not separately payable on Part B claims with dates of service on or after January 1,2011 for other providers, with the exception of a hospital billing for an emergency or unscheduled dialysis session.

100-04, 8, 60.4.6.5

Payment for Darbepoetin Alfa (Aranesp) in the Hospital Outpatient Department

(Rev.2582, Issued: 11-02-12, Effective: 04-01-13, Implementation: 04-01-13)

When ESRD patients come to the hospital for an unscheduled or emergency dialysis treatment they may also require the administration of Aranesp. For patients with ESRD who are on a regular course of dialysis, Aranesp administered in a hospital outpatient department is paid the MMA Drug Pricing File rate. Effective January 1, 2005, Aranesp will be paid based on the ASP Pricing File.

© 2019 Optum360, LLC

Hospitals use bill type 13X (or 85X for Critical Access Hospitals) and report charges under revenue code 0636. The total number of units as a multiple of 1mcg is placed in the unit field. Value code 49 must be reported with the hematocrit value for the hospital outpatient visits prior to January 1, 2006, and for all claims with dates of service on or after January 1, 2008.

100-04, 8, 60.4.7

Payment for Peginesatide in the Hospital Outpatient Department

(Rev.2582, Issued: 11-02-12, Effective: 04-01-13, Implementation: 04-01-13)

When ESRD patients come to the hospital for an unscheduled or emergency dialysis treatment they may also require the administration of an ESA, such as peginesatide. When hospitals bill for an unscheduled or emergency outpatient dialysis session (G0257) they may include the administration of an ESA.

100-04, 10, 20.1.2

Responsibilities of Providers/Suppliers of Services Subject to Consolidated Billing

(Rev.4312, Issued: 05-23-19, Effective: 01-01-20, Implementation: 08-16-19)

Since Medicare payment for services subject to home health consolidated billing is made to the primary HHA, providers or suppliers of these services must be aware that separate Medicare payment will not be made to them. Therefore, before they provide services to a Medicare beneficiary, these providers or suppliers need to determine whether or not a home health episode/*period* of care exists for that beneficiary. This information may be available to providers or suppliers from a number of sources.

The first avenue a therapy provider or a supplier may pursue is to ask the beneficiary (or his/her authorized representative) if he/she is presently receiving home health services under a home health plan of care. Beneficiaries and their representatives should have the most complete information as to whether or not they are receiving home health care. Therapy providers or suppliers may, but are not required to, document information from the beneficiary that states the beneficiary is not receiving home health care, but such documentation in itself does not shift liability to either the beneficiary or Medicare.

Additionally, information about current home health episodes/*periods of care* may be available from MACs. Institutional providers (providers who bill using the institutional claim format) may access this information electronically through the home health CWF inquiry process (See §30.1). Independent therapists or suppliers who bill using the professional claim format also have access to a similar electronic inquiry via the

HIPAA standard eligibility transaction - the 270/271 transaction. They may also, as a last resort, call their A/B MAC's (B)'s provider toll free line to request home health eligibility information available on the Common Working File. The A/B MAC's (B)'s information is based only on claims Medicare has received from home health agencies at the day of the contact.

Beginning October 2010, another source of information is available via the CWF. Medicare systems will maintain a data file that captures and displays the dates when Medicare paid physicians for the certification or recertification of the beneficiary's HH plan of care. Physicians submit claims for these services to A/B MACs (B) on the professional claim format separate from the HHA's billing their Request for Anticipated Payment (RAP) and claim on the institutional claim format for the HH services themselves. HHAs have a strong payment incentive to submit their RAP for an HH episode/*period of care* promptly in order to receive their initial 60% or 50% payment.

But there may be instances in which the physician claim for the certification service is received before any HHA billing and this claim is the earliest indication Medicare systems have that HH *services* will be provided. As an aid to suppliers and providers subject to HH consolidated billing, Medicare systems display, for each Medicare beneficiary, the code for certification (G0180) or recertification (G0179) and the date of service for either of the two codes.

Suppliers and providers should note that this information is supplementary to the previously existing sources of information about HH episodes. Like HH episode/*period of care* information maintained on CWF, certification information is only as complete and timely as billing by providers allows it to be. For many episodes, a physician certification claim may never be billed. As a result, the beneficiary and their caregivers remain the first and best source of information about the beneficiary's home health status.

If a therapy provider or a supplier learns of a home health episode/*period of care* from any of these sources, or if they believe they don't have reliable information, they should advise the beneficiary that if the beneficiary decides not to have the services provided by the primary HHA and the beneficiary is in an HH episode/period, the beneficiary will be liable for payment for the services. Beneficiaries should be notified of their potential liability before the services are provided.

If a therapy provider or a supplier learns of a home health episode and has sufficient information to contact the primary HHA, they may inquire about the possibility of making a payment arrangement for the service with the primary HHA. Such contacts may foster relationships between therapy providers, suppliers and HHAs that are beneficial both to providers involved and to Medicare beneficiaries.

100-04, 10, 40.2

HH PPS Claims

(Rev.4312, Issued: 05-23-19, Effective: 01-01-20, Implementation: 08-16-19)

The following data elements are required to submit a claim under home health PPS. For billing of home health claims not under an HH plan of care (not under HH PPS), see §90. Home health services under a plan of care are paid based on a 60-day episode of care (before January 1, 2020) or a 30-day period of care (on or after January 1, 2020). Payment for this episode or period will usually be made in two parts. After a RAP has been paid and an episode or period has been completed, or the patient has been discharged, the HHA submits a claim to receive the balance of payment due.

HH PPS claims will be processed in Medicare claims processing systems as debit/credit adjustments against the record created by the RAP, except in the case of "No-RAP" LUPA claims (see §40.3). As the claim is processed the payment on the RAP will be reversed in full and the full payment due for the episode will be made on the claim. Both the debit and credit actions will be reflected on the RA so the net payment on the claim can be easily understood. Detailed RA information is contained in chapter 22 of this manual.

Billing Provider Name, Address, and Telephone Number

Required – The HHA's minimum entry is the agency's name, city, state, and ZIP Code. The post office box number or street name and number may be included. The state may be abbreviated using standard post office abbreviations. Five or nine-digit ZIP Codes are acceptable. A/B MACs (HHH) use this information in connection with the provider identifier to verify provider identity.

Patient Control Number and Medical/Health Record Number

Required - The patient's control number may be shown if the patient is assigned one and the number is needed for association and reference purposes.

The HHA may enter the number assigned to the patient's medical/health record. If this number is entered, the A/B MAC (HHH) must carry it through their system and return it on the remittance record.

Type of Bill

Required - This 4-digit alphanumeric code gives two pieces of information. The first three digits indicate the base type of bill. The fourth digit indicates the sequence of this bill in this particular episode of care. The types of bill accepted for HH PPS claims are:

032x - Home Health Services under a Plan of Treatment

4th Digit - Definition

7 - Replacement of Prior Claim - HHAs use to correct a previously submitted bill. Apply this code for the corrected or "new" bill. These adjustment claims must be accepted at any point within the timely filing period after the payment of the original claim.

8 - Void/Cancel of a Prior Claim - HHAs use this code to indicate this bill is an exact duplicate of an incorrect bill previously submitted. A replacement RAP or claim must be submitted for the episode to be paid.

9 - Final Claim for an HH PPS Episode - This code indicates the HH bill should be processed as a debit/credit adjustment to the RAP. This code is specific to home health and does not replace codes 7, or 8.

HHAs must submit HH PPS claims with the 4th digit of "9." These claims may be adjusted with code "7" or cancelled with code "8." A/B MACs (HHH) do not accept late charge bills, submitted with code "5," on HH PPS claims. To add services within the period of a paid HH claim, the HHA must submit an adjustment.

NOTE: Type of bill 033x is no longer valid, effective October 1, 2013.

Statement Covers Period

The Patient-Driven Groupings Model is effective for periods of care beginning January 1, 2020. The HHA should follow all prior claims submission instructions for claims with "From" dates before January 1, 2020, including episodes that span into 2020. The HHA should follow PDGM instructions for claims with "From" dates on or after January 1, 2020.

Required - The beginning and ending dates of the period covered by this claim. The "from" date must match the date submitted on the RAP for the episode. For continuous care episodes, the "through" date must be 59 days after the "from" date for a 60-day episode or 29 days after the "From" date for a 30-day period of care

© 2019 Optum360, LLC

In cases where the beneficiary has been discharged or transferred within the episode or period, HHAs will report the date of discharge in accordance with internal discharge procedures as the "through" date. If the beneficiary has died, the HHA reports the date of death in the "through date."

The HHA may submit claims for payment immediately after the claim "through" date. It is not required to hold claims until the end of the episode or period unless the beneficiary continues under care.

Patient Name/Identifier
Required - The HHA enters the patient's last name, first name, and middle initial.

Patient Address
Required - The HHA enters the patient's full mailing address, including street number and name, post office box number or RFD, City, State, and ZIP Code.

Patient Birth Date
Required -The HHA enters the month, day, and year of birth of patient. If the full correct date is not known, leave blank.

Patient Sex
Required - "M" for male or "F" for female must be present. This item is used in conjunction with diagnoses and surgical procedures to identify inconsistencies.

Admission/Start of Care Date
Required - The HHA enters the same date of admission that was submitted on the RAP for the episode.

Point of Origin for Admission or Visit
Required - The HHA enters the same point of origin code that was submitted on the RAP for the episode.

Patient Discharge Status
Required - The HHA enters the code that most accurately describes the patient's status as of the "Through" date of the billing period. Any applicable NUBC approved code may be used.

Patient status code 06 should be reported in all cases where the HHA is aware that the episode will be paid as a PEP adjustment. These are cases in which the agency is aware that the beneficiary has transferred to another HHA within the 60-day episode or 30-day period, or the agency is aware that the beneficiary was discharged with the goals of the original plan of care met and has been readmitted within the episode or period. Situations may occur in which the HHA is unaware at the time of billing the discharge that these circumstances exist. In these situations, Medicare claims processing systems will adjust the discharge claim automatically to reflect the PEP adjustment, changing the patient status code on the paid claims record to 06.

In cases where an HHA is changing the A/B MAC (HHH) to which they submit claims, the service dates on the claims must fall within the provider's effective dates at each A/B MAC (HHH). To ensure this, RAPs for all episodes with "from" dates before the provider's termination date must be submitted to the A/B MAC (HHH) the provider is leaving. The resulting episode must be resolved by the provider submitting claims for shortened periods, with "through" dates on or before the termination date. The provider must indicate that these claims will be PEP adjustments by using patient status code 06. Billing for the beneficiary is being "transferred" to the new A/B MAC (HHH).

In cases where the ownership of an HHA is changing and the CMS certification number (CCN) also changes, the service dates on the claims must fall within the effective dates of the terminating CCN. To ensure this, RAPs for all episodes with "from" dates before the termination date of the CCN must be resolved by the provider submitting claims for shortened periods, with "through" dates on or before the termination date. The provider must indicate that these claims will be PEP adjustments by using patient status 06. Billing for the beneficiary is being "transferred" to the new agency ownership. In changes of ownership which do not affect the CCN, billing for episodes is also unaffected.

In cases where an HHA is aware in advance that a beneficiary will become enrolled in a Medicare Advantage (MA) Organization as of a certain date, the provider should submit a claim for the shortened period prior to the MA Organization enrollment date. The claim should be coded with patient status 06. Payment responsibility for the beneficiary is being "transferred" from Medicare fee-for-service to MA Organization, since HH PPS applies only to Medicare fee-for-service.

If HHAs require guidance on OASIS assessment procedures in these cases, they should contact the appropriate state OASIS education coordinator.

Condition Codes
Conditional – The HHA enters any NUBC approved code to describe conditions that apply to the claim.

If the RAP is for an episode in which the patient has transferred from another HHA, the HHA enters condition code 47.

If the claim is for an episode in which there are no skilled HH visits in billing period, but a policy exception that allows billing for covered services is documented at the HHA, the HHA enters condition code 54.

HHAs that are adjusting previously paid claims enter one of the condition codes representing Claim Change Reasons (code values D0 through E0). If adjusting the claim to correct a HIPPS code, HHAs use condition code D2 and enter "Remarks" indicating the reason for the HIPPS code change. HHAs use D9 if multiple changes are necessary.

When submitting an HH PPS claim as a demand bill, HHAs use condition code 20. See §50 for more detailed instructions regarding demand billing.

When submitting an HH PPS claim for a denial notice, HHAs use condition code 21. See §60 for more detailed instructions regarding no-payment billing.

Required - If canceling the claim (TOB 0328), HHAs report the condition codes D5 or D6 and enter "Remarks" indicating the reason for cancellation of the claim.

Occurrence Codes and Dates
Required – On claims with "From" dates on or after January 1, 2020, the HHA enters occurrence code 50 and the date the OASIS assessment corresponding to the period of care was completed (OASIS item M0090). If occurrence code 50 is not reported on a claim or adjustment, the claim will be returned to the provider for correction.

On claims for initial periods of care (i.e. when the From and Admission dates match), the HHA reports an inpatient admission that ended within 14 days of the "From" date by using one of the following codes.

Code	Short Descriptor	Long Descriptor
61	Hospital Discharge Date	The Through date of a hospital stay that ended within 14 days prior to the From date this HHA claim.
62	Other Institutional Discharge Date	The Through date of skilled nursing facility (SNF), inpatient rehabilitation facility (IRF), long term care hospital (LTCH) or inpatient psychiatric facility (IPF) stay that ended within 14 days prior to this HHA admission.

On claims for continuing periods of care, the HHA reports an inpatient hospital admission that ended within 14 days of the "From" date by using occurrence code 61.

If more than one inpatient discharge occurs during the 14 day period, the HHA reports only the most recent discharge date. Claims reporting more than one of any combination of occurrence codes 61 and 62 will be returned to the provider for correction.

Conditional - The HHA enters any other NUBC approved code to describe occurrences that apply to the claim.

Occurrence Span Code and Dates

Conditional - The HHA enters any NUBC approved Occurrence Span code to describe occurrences that apply to the claim. Reporting of occurrence span code 74 is not required to show the dates of an inpatient admission during an episode.

Value Codes and Amounts

Required - Home health episode payments must be based upon the site at which the beneficiary is served. For certain dates of service when required by law, payments may be further adjusted if the site is in a rural CBSA or rural county. For episodes in which the beneficiary's site of service changes from one CBSA or county to another within the episode period, HHAs should submit the CBSA code or State and County code corresponding to the site of service at the end of the episode on the claim.

Provider-submitted codes:

Code	Title	Definition
61	Location Where Service is Furnished (HHA and Hospice)	HHAs report the MSA number or Core Based Statistical Area (CBSA) number (or rural state code) of the location where the home health or hospice service is delivered. The HHA reports the number in dollar portion of the form locator right justified to the left of the dollar/cents delimiter, add two zeros to the cents field if no cents.
85	County Where Service is Rendered	Where required by law or regulation, report the Federal Information Processing Standards (FIPS) State and County Code of the place of residence where the home health service is delivered.

© 2019 Optum360, LLC

Medicare-applied codes: The following codes are added during processing and may be visible in the A/B MAC (HHH)'s online claim history. They are never submitted by the HHA.

Code	Title	Definition
17	Outlier Amount	The amount of any outlier payment returned by the Pricer with this code. A/B MACs (HHH) always place condition code 61 on the claim along with this value code.)
61	Location Where Service is Furnished (HHA and Hospice)	HHAs report the MSA number or Core Based Statistical Area (CBSA) number (or rural state code) of the location where the home health or hospice service is delivered. The HHA reports the number in dollar portion of the form locator right justified to the left of the dollar/cents delimiter, add two zeros to the cents field if no cents.
62	HH Visits - Part A	The number of visits determined by Medicare to be payable from the Part A trust fund to reflect the shift of payments from the Part A to the Part B trust fund as mandated by §1812 (a)(3) of the Social Security Act.
63	HH Visits - Part B	The number of visits determined by Medicare to be payable from the Part B trust fund to reflect the shift of payments from the Part A to the Part B trust fund as mandated by §1812 (a)(3) of the Social Security Act.
64	HH Reimbursement - Part A	The dollar amounts determined to be associated with the HH visits identified in a value code 62 amount. This Part A payment reflects the shift of payments from the Part A to the Part B trust fund as mandated by §1812 (a)(3) of the Social Security Act.
65	HH Reimbursement - Part B	The dollar amounts determined to be associated with the HH visits identified in a value code 63 amount. This Part B payment reflects the shift of payments from the Part A to the Part B trust fund as mandated by §1812 (a)(3) of the Social Security Act.

If information returned from the CWF indicates all visits on the claim are Part A, the shared system must place value codes 62 and 64 on the claim record, showing the total visits and total PPS payment amount as the values, and send the claim to CWF with RIC code V.

If information returned from CWF indicates all visits on the claim are Part B, the shared system must place value codes 63 and 65 on the claim record, showing the total visits and total PPS payment amount as the values, and send the claim to CWF with RIC code W.

If information returned from CWF indicates certain visits on the claim are payable from both Part A and Part B, the shared system must place value codes 62, 63, 64, and 65 on the claim record. The shared system also must populate the values for code 62 and 63 based on the numbers of visits returned from CWF and prorate the total PPS reimbursement amount based on the numbers of visits to determine the dollars amounts to be associated with value codes 64 and 65. The shared system will return the claim to CWF with RIC code U.

Revenue Code and Revenue Description

Required

HH PPS claims must report a 0023 revenue code line on which the first four positions of the HIPPS code match the code submitted on the RAP. *This HIPPS code is used to match the claim to the corresponding RAP that was previously paid. After this match is completed, grouping to determine the HIPPS code used for final payment of the period of care will occur in Medicare systems. At that time, the submitted HIPPS code on the claim will be replaced with the system-calculated code.*

For claims with "From" dates before January 1, 2020, the fifth position of the code represents the NRS severity level. This fifth position may differ to allow the HHA to change a code that represents that supplies were provided to a code that represents that supplies were not provided, or vice versa. However, the fifth position may only change between the two values that represent the same NRS severity level. Section 10.1.9 of this chapter contains the pairs of corresponding values. If these criteria are not met, Medicare claims processing systems will return the claim.

HHAs enter only one 0023 revenue code per claim in all cases.

Unlike RAPs, claims must also report all services provided to the beneficiary within the episode/*period. All services must be billed on one claim for the entire episode/period. The A/B MAC (HHH) will return to the provider TOB 0329 when submitted without any visit charges.*

Each service must be reported in line item detail. Each service visit (revenue codes 042x, 043x, 044x, 055x, 056x and 057x) must be reported as a separate line. Any of the following revenue codes may be used:

027x	Medical/Surgical Supplies (Also see 062x, an extension of 027x) Required detail: With the exception of revenue code 0274 (prosthetic and orthotic devices), only service units and a charge must be reported with this revenue code. If also reporting revenue code 0623 to separately identify specific wound care supplies, not just supplies for wound care patients, ensure that the charge amounts for revenue code 0623 lines are mutually exclusive from other lines for supply revenue codes reported on the claim. Report only nonroutine supply items in this revenue code or in 0623. Revenue code 0274 requires an HCPCS code, the date of service units and a charge amount. NOTE: Revenue Codes 0275 through 0278 are not used for Medicare billing on HH PPS types of bills
042x	Physical Therapy Required detail: One of the physical therapy HCPCS codes defined below in the instructions for the HCPCS code field, the date of service, service units which represent the number of 15 minute increments that comprised the visit, and a charge amount.
043x	Occupational Therapy Required detail: One of the occupational therapy HCPCS codes defined below in the instructions for the HCPCS code field, the date of service, service units which represent the number of 15 minute increments that comprised the visit, and a charge amount.
044x	Speech-Language Pathology Required detail: One of the speech-language pathology HCPCS codes defined below in the instructions for the HCPCS code field, the date of service, service units which represent the number of 15 minute increments that comprised the visit, and a charge amount.
055x	Skilled Nursing Required detail: One of the skilled nursing HCPCS codes defined below in the instructions for the HCPCS code field, the date of service, service units which represent the number of 15 minute increments that comprised the visit, and a charge amount.
056x	Medical Social Services Required detail: The medical social services HCPCS code defined below in the instructions for the HCPCS code field, the date of service, service units which represent the number of 15 minute increments that comprised the visit, and a charge amount.
057x	Home Health Aide (Home Health) Required detail: The home health aide HCPCS code defined below in the instructions for the HCPCS code field, the date of service, service units which represent the number of 15 minute increments that comprised the visit, and a charge amount.

NOTE: A/B MACs (HHH) do not accept revenue codes 058x or 059x when submitted with covered charges on Medicare home health claims under HH PPS. They also do not accept revenue code 0624, investigational devices, on HH claims under HH PPS.

Revenue Codes for Optional Billing of DME

Billing of DME provided in the episode is not required on the HH PPS claim. Home health agencies retain the option to bill these services to their A/B MAC (HHH) processing home health claims or to have the services provided under arrangement with a supplier that bills these services to the DME MAC. Agencies that choose to bill DME services on their HH PPS claims must use the revenue codes below. These services will be paid separately in addition to the HH PPS amount, based on the

 © 2019 Optum360, LLC

applicable Medicare fee schedule. For additional instructions for billing DME services see chapter 20 of this manual.

0274	Prosthetic/Orthotic Devices Required detail: The applicable HCPCS code for the item, a date of service, a number of service units, and a charge amount.
029x	Durable Medical Equipment (DME) (Other Than Renal) Required detail: The applicable HCPCS code for the item, a date of service indicating the purchase date or the beginning date of a monthly rental, a number of service units, and a charge amount. Monthly rental items should be reported with a separate line for each month's rental and service units of one. Revenue code 0294 is used to bill drugs/supplies for the effective use of DME.
060x	Oxygen (Home Health) Required detail: The applicable HCPCS code for the item, a date of service, a number of service units, and a charge amount.

Revenue Code for Optional Reporting of Wound Care Supplies

0623	Medical/Surgical Supplies - Extension of 027x Required detail: Only service units and a charge must be reported with this revenue code. If also reporting revenue code 027x to identify nonroutine supplies other than those used for wound care, the HHA must ensure that the charge amounts for the two revenue code lines are mutually exclusive.

HHAs may voluntarily report a separate revenue code line for charges for nonroutine wound care supplies, using revenue code 0623. Notwithstanding the standard abbreviation "surg dressings," HHAs use this code to report charges for ALL nonroutine wound care supplies, including but not limited to surgical dressings.

Pub. 100-02, Medicare Benefit Policy Manual, chapter 7, defines routine vs. nonroutine supplies. HHAs use that definition to determine whether any wound care supply item should be reported in this line because it is nonroutine.

HHAs can assist Medicare's future refinement of payment rates if they consistently and accurately report their charges for nonroutine wound care supplies under revenue center code 0623. HHAs should ensure that charges reported under revenue code 027x for nonroutine supplies are also complete and accurate.

Validating Required Reporting of Supply Revenue Code

For claims with "From" dates before January 1, 2020, the HH PPS includes a separate case-mix adjustment for non-routine supplies. Non-routine supply severity levels are indicated on HH PPS claims through a code value in the fifth position of the HIPPS code. The fifth position of the HIPPS code can contain two sets of values. One set of codes (the letters S through X) indicate that supplies were provided. The second set of codes (the numbers 1 through 6) indicate the HHA is intentionally reporting that they did not provide supplies during the episode. See section 10.1.9 for the complete composition of HIPPS under the HH PPS.

HHAs must ensure that if they are submitting a HIPPS code with a fifth position containing the letters S through X, the claim must also report a non-routine supply revenue code with covered charges. This revenue code may be either revenue code 27x, excluding 274, or revenue code 623, consistent with the instructions for optional separate reporting of wound care supplies.

Medicare systems will return the claim to the HHA if the HIPPS code indicates non-routine supplies were provided and supply charges are not reported on the claim. When the HHA receives a claim returned for this reason, the HHA must review their records regarding the supplies provided to the beneficiary. The HHA may take one of the following actions, based on the review of their records:

- If non-routine supplies were provided, the supply charges must be added to the claim using the appropriate supply revenue code.
- If non-routine supplies were not provided, the HHA must indicate that on the claim by changing the fifth position of the HIPPS code to the appropriate numeric value in the range 1 through 6.

After completing one of these actions, the HHA may return the claim to the A/B MAC (HHH) for continued adjudication.

HCPCS/Accommodation Rates/HIPPS Rate Codes

Required - On the 0023 revenue code line, the HHA must report the HIPPS code that was reported on the RAP. The first four positions of the code must be identical to the value reported on the RAP. For claims with "From" dates before January 1, 2020, the fifth position may vary from the letter value reported on the RAP to the corresponding number which represents the same non-routine supply severity level but which reports that non-routine supplies were not provided.

HHAs enter only one HIPPS code per claim in all cases. Claims submitted with additional HIPPS codes will be returned to the provider.

For episodes with "From" dates before January 1, 2020, Medicare may change the HIPPS used for payment of the claim in the course of claims processing, but the HIPPS code submitted by the provider in this field is never changed or replaced. If the HIPPS code is changed, the code used for payment is recorded in the APC-HIPPS field of the electronic claim record.

For episodes with "From" dates on or after January 1, 2020, Medicare will determine the appropriate HIPPS code for payment based on claims and OASIS data and will replace the provider-submitted HIPPS code as necessary. If the HIPPS code further changed based on medical review or other processes, the code used for payment is recorded in the APC-HIPPS field of the electronic claim record.

For revenue code lines other than 0023, the HHA reports HCPCS codes as appropriate to that revenue code.

To report HH visits, the HHA reports one of the following HCPCS codes to represent a visit by each HH care discipline:

Physical Therapy (revenue code 042x)

G0151 Services performed by a qualified physical therapist in the home health or hospice setting, each 15 minutes.

G0157 Services performed by a qualified physical therapist assistant in the home health or hospice setting, each 15 minutes.

G0159 Services performed by a qualified physical therapist, in the home health setting, in the establishment or delivery of a safe and effective physical therapy maintenance program, each 15 minutes.

Occupational Therapy (revenue code 043x)

G0152 Services performed by a qualified occupational therapist in the home health or hospice setting, each 15 minutes.

G0158 Services performed by a qualified occupational therapist assistant in the home health or hospice setting, each 15 minutes.

G0160 Services performed by a qualified occupational therapist, in the home health setting, in the establishment or delivery of a safe and effective occupational therapy maintenance program, each 15 minutes.

Speech-Language Pathology (revenue code 044x)

G0153 Services performed by a qualified speech-language pathologist in the home health or hospice setting, each 15 minutes.

G0161 Services performed by a qualified speech-language pathologist, in the home health setting, in the establishment or delivery of a safe and effective speech-language pathology maintenance program, each 15 minutes.

Note that modifiers indicating services delivered under a therapy plan of care (modifiers GN, GO or GP) are not required on HH PPS claims.

Skilled Nursing (revenue code 055x)

General skilled nursing:

For dates of service before January 1, 2016: G0154 Direct skilled services of a licensed nurse (LPN or RN) in the home health or hospice setting, each 15 minutes.

For dates of service on or after January 1, 2016: Visits previously reported with G0154 are reported with one of the following codes:

G0299 Direct skilled nursing services of a registered nurse (RN) in the home health or hospice setting

G0300 Direct skilled nursing of a licensed practical nurse (LPN) in the home health or hospice setting.

Care plan oversight:

For dates of service before January 1, 2017:

G0162 Skilled services by a licensed nurse (RN only) for management and evaluation of the plan of care, each 15 minutes (the patient's underlying condition or complication requires an RN to ensure that essential non-skilled care achieves its purpose in the home health or hospice setting).

G0163 Skilled services of a licensed nurse (LPN or RN) for the observation and assessment of the patient's condition, each 15 minutes (the change in the patient's condition requires skilled nursing personnel to identify and evaluate the patient's need for possible modification of treatment in the home health or hospice setting).

© 2019 Optum360, LLC

For dates of service on or after January 1, 2017, HHAs report visits previously reported with G0163 with one of the following codes:

G0493 Skilled services of a registered nurse (RN) for the observation and assessment of the patient's condition, each 15 minutes (the change in the patient's condition requires skilled nursing personnel to identify and evaluate the patient's need for possible modification of treatment in the home health or hospice setting).

G0494 Skilled services of a licensed practical nurse (LPN) for the observation and assessment of the patient's condition, each 15 minutes (the change in the patient's condition requires skilled nursing personnel to identify and evaluate the patient's need for possible modification of treatment in the home health or hospice setting).

Training:

For dates of service before January 1, 2017: G0164 Skilled services of a licensed nurse (LPN or RN), in the training and/or education of a patient or family member, in the home health or hospice setting, each 15 minutes.

For dates of service on or after January 1, 2017, HHAs report visits previously reported with G0164 with one of the following codes:

G0495 Skilled services of a registered nurse (RN), in the training and/or education of a patient or family member, in the home health or hospice setting, each 15 minutes.

G0496 Skilled services of a licensed practical nurse (LPN), in the training and/or education of a patient or family member, in the home health or hospice setting, each 15 minutes.

Medical Social Services (revenue code 056x)

G0155 Services of a clinical social worker under a home health plan of care, each 15 minutes.

Home Health Aide (revenue code 057x)

G0156 Services of a home health aide under a home health plan of care, each 15 minutes.

Regarding all skilled nursing and skilled therapy visits

In the course of a single visit, a nurse or qualified therapist may provide more than one of the nursing or therapy services reflected in the codes above. HHAs must not report more than one G-code for each visit regardless of the variety of services provided during the visit. In cases where more than one nursing or therapy service is provided in a visit, the HHA must report the G-code which reflects the service for which the clinician spent most of his/her time.

For instance, if direct skilled nursing services are provided, and the nurse also provides training/education of a patient or family member during that same visit, Medicare would expect the HHA to report the G-code which reflects the service for which most of the time was spent during that visit. Similarly, if a qualified therapist is performing a therapy service and also establishes a maintenance program during the same visit, the HHA should report the G-code that reflects the service for which most of the time was spent during that visit. In all cases, however, the number of 15-minute increments reported for the visit should reflect the total time of the visit.

For episodes beginning on or after July 1, 2013, HHAs must report where home health services were provided. The following codes are used for this reporting:

Q5001: Hospice or home health care provided in patient's home/residence

Q5002: Hospice or home health care provided in assisted living facility

Q5009: Hospice or home health care provided in place not otherwise specified

The location where services were provided must always be reported along with the first visit reported on the claim. In addition to reporting a visit line using the G codes as described above, HHAs must report an additional line item with the same revenue code and date of service, reporting one of the three Q codes (Q5001, Q5002, and Q5009), one unit and a nominal covered charge (e.g., a penny). If the location where services were provided changes during the episode, the new location should be reported with an additional line corresponding to the first visit provided in the new location.

Service Date

Required - For initial episodes, the HHA reports on the 0023 revenue code line the date of the first covered visit provided during the episode. For subsequent episodes, the HHA reports on the 0023 revenue code the date of the first visit provided during the episode line, regardless of whether the visit was covered or non-covered.

For other line items detailing all services within the episode period, it reports service dates as appropriate to that revenue code. For service visits that begin in 1 calendar day and span into the next calendar day, report one visit using the date the visit ended as the service date.

When the claim Admission Date matches the Statement Covers "From" Date, Medicare systems ensure that the Service Date on the 0023 revenue code line also matches these dates.

Service Units

Required - Transaction standards require the reporting of a number greater than zero as the units on the 0023 revenue code line. However, Medicare systems will disregard the submitted units in processing the claim. For line items detailing all services within the episode period, the HHA reports units of service as appropriate to that revenue code. Coding detail for each revenue code under HH PPS is defined above under Revenue Codes.

For the revenue codes that represent home health visits (042x, 043x, 044x, 055x, 056x, and 057x), the HHA reports as service units a number of 15 minute increments that comprise the time spent treating the beneficiary. Time spent completing the OASIS assessment in the home as part of an otherwise covered and billable visit and time spent updating medical records in the home as part of such a visit may also be reported.

Visits of any length are to be reported, rounding the time to the nearest 15-minute increment. If any visits report over 96 units (over 24 hours) on a single line item, Medicare systems return the claim returned to the provider.

Effective January 1, 2017, covered and noncovered increments of the same visit must be reported on separate lines. This is to ensure that only covered increments are included in the per-unit based calculation of outlier payments.

Total Charges

Required - The HHA must report zero charges on the 0023 revenue code line (the field must contain zero).

For line items detailing all services within the episode period, the HHA reports charges as appropriate to that revenue code. Coding detail for each revenue code under HH PPS is defined above under Revenue Codes. Charges may be reported in dollars and cents (i.e., charges are not required to be rounded to dollars and zero cents). Medicare claims processing systems will not make any payments based upon submitted charge amounts.

Non-covered Charges

Required – The HHA reports the total non-covered charges pertaining to the related revenue code here. Examples of non-covered charges on HH PPS claims may include:

- Visits provided exclusively to perform OASIS assessments
- Visits provided exclusively for supervisory or administrative purposes
- Therapy visits provided prior to the required re-assessments

Payer Name

Required - See chapter 25.

Release of Information Certification Indicator

Required - See chapter 25.

National Provider Identifier – Billing Provider

Required - The HHA enters their provider identifier.

Insured's Name

Required only if MSP involved. See Pub. 100-05, Medicare Secondary Payer Manual.

Patient's Relationship To Insured

Required only if MSP involved. See Pub. 100-05, Medicare Secondary Payer Manual.

Insured's Unique Identifier

Required only if MSP involved. See Pub. 100-05, Medicare Secondary Payer Manual.

Insured's Group Name

Required only if MSP involved. See Pub. 100-05, Medicare Secondary Payer Manual.

Insured's Group Number

Required only if MSP involved. See Pub. 100-05, Medicare Secondary Payer Manual.

Treatment Authorization Code

Required - On claims with "From" dates before January 1, 2020, the code on the claim will match that submitted on the RAP.

In cases of billing for denial notice, using condition code 21, this code may be filled with a placeholder value as defined in section 60.

The investigational device (IDE) revenue code, 0624, is not allowed on HH PPS claims. Therefore, treatment authorization codes associated with IDE items must never be submitted in this field.

 © 2019 Optum360, LLC

Medicare systems validate the length of the treatment authorization code and ensure that each position is in the correct format. If the format is incorrect, the contractor returns the claim to the provider.

On claims with "From" dates on of after January 1, 2020, treatment authorization codes are no longer required on all claims. The HHA submits a code in this field only if the period is subject to Pre-Claim Review. In that case, the required tracking number is submitted in the first position of the field in all submission formats.

Document Control Number (DCN)

Required - If submitting an adjustment (TOB 0327) to a previously paid HH PPS claim, the HHA enters the control number assigned to the original HH PPS claim here.

Since HH PPS claims are processed as adjustments to the RAP, Medicare claims processing systems will match all HH PPS claims to their corresponding RAP and populate this field on the electronic claim record automatically. Providers do not need to submit a DCN on all HH PPS claims, only on adjustments to paid claims.

Employer Name

Required only if MSP involved. See Pub. 100-05, Medicare Secondary Payer Manual.

Principal Diagnosis Code

Required - The HHA enters the ICD code for the principal diagnosis. The code must be reported according to Official ICD Guidelines for Coding and Reporting, as required by the HIPAA. The code must be the full diagnosis code, including all five digits for ICD-9-CM or all seven digits for ICD-10 CM where applicable. Where the proper code has fewer than the maximum number of digits, the HHA does not fill it with zeros.

Medicare systems may return claims to the provider when the principal diagnosis code is not sufficient to determine the HHRG assignment under the PDGM.

For claim "From" dates before January 1, 2020, the ICD code and principle diagnosis reported must match the primary diagnosis code reported on the OASIS form item M1020 (Primary Diagnosis).

For claim "From" dates on or after January 1, 2020, the ICD code and principle diagnosis used for payment grouping will be claim coding rather than the OASIS item. As a result, the claim and OASIS diagnosis codes will no longer be expected to match in all cases.

Typically, the codes will match between the first claim in an admission and the start of care (Reason for Assessment –RFA 01) assessment and claims corresponding to recertification (RFA 04) assessments. Second 30-day claims in any 60-day period will not necessarily match the OASIS assessment. When diagnosis codes change between one 30-day claim and the next, there is no absolute requirement for the HHA to complete an 'other follow-up' (RFA 05) assessment to ensure that diagnosis coding on the claim matches to the assessment. However, the HHA would be required to complete an 'other follow-up' (RFA 05) assessment when such a change would be considered a major decline or improvement in the patient's health status.

Other Diagnosis Codes

Required - The HHA enters the full diagnosis codes for additional conditions if they coexisted at the time of the establishment of the plan of care. These codes may not duplicate the principal diagnosis as an additional or secondary diagnosis.

In listing the diagnoses, the HHA places them in order to best reflect the seriousness of the patient's condition and to justify the disciplines and services provided in accordance with the Official ICD Guidelines for Coding and Reporting. The sequence of codes should follow ICD guidelines for reporting manifestation codes. Medicare does not have any additional requirements regarding the reporting or sequence of the codes beyond those contained in ICD guidelines.

For claim "From" dates before January 1, 2020, the other diagnoses and ICD codes reported on the claim must match the additional diagnoses reported on the OASIS, form item M1022 (Other Diagnoses).

For claim "From" dates on or after January 1, 2020, claim and OASIS diagnosis codes may vary as described under Principal Diagnosis.

Attending Provider Name and Identifiers

Required - The HHA enters the name and national provider identifier (NPI) of the attending physician who signed the plan of care.

Other Provider (Individual) Names and Identifiers

Required - The HHA enters the name and NPI of the physician who certified/re-certified the patient's eligibility for home health services.

NOTE: Both the attending physician and other provider fields should be completed unless the patient's designated attending physician is the same as the physician who certified/re-certified the patient's eligibility. When the attending physician is also the certifying/re-certifying physician, only the attending physician is required to be reported.

Remarks

Conditional - Remarks are required only in cases where the claim is cancelled or adjusted.

100-04, 10, 40.3

HH PPS Claims When No RAP is Submitted - "No-RAP" LUPAs

(Rev.4312, Issued: 05-23-19, Effective: 01-01-20, Implementation: 08-16-19)

A RAP and a claim must be submitted for all episodes*/periods of care* for which Medicare makes payment based on HIPPS codes. However, if the HHA is aware prior to billing Medicare that it will supply fewer visits *than the LUPA threshold* in the episode*/period*, it may submit only a claim. In these cases, the claim is called a "No-RAP LUPA," since the HHA is aware the claim will be paid a LUPA payment adjustment based on national standard visit rates. HHAs may submit both a RAP and a claim in these instances if they choose, but only the claim is required. HHAs should be aware that submission of a RAP in these instances will result in a recoupment of funds since the payment for a RAP will exceed payment for four or fewer visits. HHAs should also be aware that the receipt of the RAP or a "no-RAP LUPA" claim causes the creation of an episode*/period* record in CWF and establishes an agency as the primary HHA. If submission of a "No-RAP LUPA" delays submission of the claim significantly, the agency is at risk of not being established as the primary HHA for that period.

If the agency chooses to submit this "No-RAP LUPA" claim, the claim form should be coded like other claim as described in §40.2.

100-04, 10, 40.5

RESERVED

(Rev.4312, Issued: 05-23-19, Effective: 01-01-20, Implementation: 08-16-19)

100-04, 10, 70.2

Input/Output Record Layout

(Rev.4312, Issued: 05-23-19, Effective: 01-01-20, Implementation: 08-16-19)

The required data and format for the HH Pricer input/output record for episodes beginning before January 1, 2020 are shown below:

File Position	Format	Title	Description
1-10	X(10)	NPI	This field will be used for the National Provider Identifier if it is sent to the HH Pricer in the future.
11-22	X(12)	HIC	Input item: The Health Insurance Claim number of the beneficiary, copied from the claim form.
23-28	X(6)	PROV-NO	Input item: The six-digit CMS certification number, copied from the claim form.
29-31	X(3)	TOB	Input item: The type of bill code, copied from the claim form.
32	X	PEP-INDICATOR	Input item: A single Y/N character to indicate if a claim must be paid a partial episode payment (PEP) adjustment. Medicare claims processing systems must set a Y if the patient discharge status code of the claim is 06. An N is set in all other cases.
33-35	9(3)	PEP-DAYS	Input item: The number of days to be used for PEP payment calculation. Medicare claims processing systems determine this number by the span of days from and including the first line item service date on the claim to and including the last line item service date on the claim.
36	X	INIT-PAY-INDICATOR	Input item: A single character to indicate if normal percentage payments should be made on RAP or whether payment should be based on data drawn by the Medicare claims processing systems from field 19 of the provider specific file. Valid values: 0 = Make normal percentage payment 1 = Pay 0% 2 = Make final payment reduced by 2% 3 = Make final payment reduced by 2%, pay RAPs at 0%
37-46	X(9)	FILLER	Blank.

© 2019 Optum360, LLC

File Position	Format	Title	Description
47-50	X(5)	CBSA	Input item: The core based statistical area (CBSA) code, copied from the value code 61 amount on the claim form.
51-52	X(2)	FILLER	Blank.
53-60	X(8)	SERV-FROM-DATE	Input item: The statement covers period "From" date, copied from the claim form. Date format must be CCYYMMDD.
61-68	X(8)	SERV-THRU DATE	Input item: The statement covers period "through" date, copied from the claim form. Date format must be CCYYMMDD.
69-76	X(8)	ADMIT-DATE	Input item: The admission date, copied from claim form. Date format must be CCYYMMDD.
77	X	HRG-MED - REVIEW - INDICATOR	Input item: A single Y/N character to indicate if a HIPPS code has been changed by medical review. Medicare claims processing systems must set a Y if an ANSI code on the line item indicates a medical review change. An N must be set in all other cases.
78-82	X(5)	HRG-INPUT-CODE	Input item: Medicare claims processing systems must copy the HIPPS code reported by the provider on each 0023 revenue code line. If an ANSI code on the line item indicates a medical review change, Medicare claims processing systems must copy the additional HIPPS code placed on the 0023 revenue code line by the medical reviewer.
83-87	X(5)	HRG - OUTPUT - CODE	Output item: The HIPPS code used by the Pricer to determine the payment amount on the claim. This code will match the input code unless the claim is recoded due to therapy thresholds or changes in episode sequence. If recoded, the Medicare claims processing system stores this output item in the APC-HIPPS field on the claim record.
88-90	9(3)	HRG-NO-OF - DAYS	Input item: A number of days calculated by the shared systems for each HIPPS code. The number is determined by the span of days from and including the first line item service date provided under that HIPPS code to and including the last line item service date provided under that HIPPS code.
91-96	9(2)V9(4)	HRG-WGTS	Output item: The weight used by the Pricer to determine the payment amount on the claim.
97-105	9(7)V9(2)	HRG-PAY	Output item: The payment amount calculated by the Pricer for each HIPPS code on the claim.
106-250	Defined above	Additional HRG data	Fields for five more occurrences of all HRG/HIPPS code related fields defined above. Not used.
251-254	X(4)	REVENUE - CODE	Input item: One of the six home health discipline revenue codes (042x, 043x, 044x, 055x, 056x, 057x). All six revenue codes must be passed by the Medicare claims processing systems even if the revenue codes are not present on the claim.
255-257	9(3)	REVENUE-QTY - COV-VISITS	Input item: A quantity of covered visits corresponding to each of the six revenue codes. Medicare claims processing systems must count the number of covered visits in each discipline on the claim. If the revenue codes are not present on the claim, a zero must be passed with the revenue code.
258-262	9(5)	REVENUE-QTY - OUTLIER-UNITS	Input item: The sum of the units reported on all covered lines corresponding to each of the six revenue codes. Medicare claims processing systems accumulate the number of units in each discipline on the claim, subject to a limit of 32 units per date of service. If any revenue code is not present on the claim, a zero must be passed with that revenue code.
263-270	9(8)	REVENUE-EARLIEST-DATE	Input item: The earliest line item date for the corresponding revenue code. Date format must be CCYYMMDD.
271-279	9(7)V9(2)	REVENUE - DOLL-RATE	Output item: The dollar rates used by the Pricer to calculate the payment for the visits in each discipline if the claim is paid as a LUPA. Otherwise, the dollar rates used by the Pricer to impute the costs of the claim for purposes of calculating an outlier payment, if any.
280-288	9(7)V9(2)	REVENUE - COST	Output item: The dollar amount determined by the Pricer to be the payment for the visits in each discipline if the claim is paid as a LUPA. Otherwise, the dollar amounts used by the Pricer to impute the costs of the claim for purposes of calculating an outlier payment, if any.
289-297	9(7)V9(2)	REVENUE-ADD-ON-VISIT-AMT	Output item: The add-on amount to be applied to the earliest line item date with the corresponding revenue code. If revenue code 055x, then this is the national per-visit amount multiplied by 1.8451. If revenue code 042x, then this is the national per-visit amount multiplied by 1.6700. If revenue code 044x, then this is the national per-visit amount multiplied by 1.6266.
298-532	Defined above	Additional REVENUE data	Five more occurrences of all REVENUE related data defined above.
533-534	9(2)	PAY-RTC	Output item: A return code set by Pricer to define the payment circumstances of the claim or an error in input data.
			Payment return codes:
			00 Final payment where no outlier applies
			01 Final payment where outlier applies
			02 Final payment where outlier applies, but is not payable due to limitation.
			03 Initial percentage payment, 0%
			04 Initial percentage payment, 50%
			05 Initial percentage payment, 60%
			06 LUPA payment only
			07 Not used.
			08 Not used.

© 2019 Optum360, LLC

File Position	Format	Title	Description
			09 Final payment, PEP
			11 Final payment, PEP with outlier
			12 Not used.
			13 Not used.
			14 LUPA payment, 1st episode add-on payment applies
			Error return codes:
			10 Invalid TOB
			15 Invalid PEP days
			16 Invalid HRG days, greater than 60
			20 PEP indicator invalid
			25 Med review indicator invalid
			30 Invalid MSA/CBSA code
			35 Invalid Initial Payment Indicator
			40 Dates before Oct 1, 2000 or invalid
			70 Invalid HRG code
			75 No HRG present in 1st occurrence
			80 Invalid revenue code
			85 No revenue code present on 03x9 or adjustment TOB
535-539	9(5)	REVENUE - SUM 1-3-QTY-THR	Output item: The total therapy visits used by the Pricer to determine if the therapy threshold was met for the claim. This amount will be the total of the covered visit quantities input in association with revenue codes 042x, 043x, and 044x.
540-544	9(5)	REVENUE - SUM 1-6-QTY-ALL	Output item: The total number of visits used by the Pricer to determine if the claim must be paid as a LUPA. This amount will be the total of all the covered visit quantities input with all six HH discipline revenue codes.
545-553	9(7)V9(2)	OUTLIER - PAYMENT	Output item: The outlier payment amount determined by the Pricer to be due on the claim in addition to any HRG payment amounts.
554-562	9(7)V9(2)	TOTAL - PAYMENT	Output item: The total payment determined by the Pricer to be due on the RAP or claim.
563-567	9(3)V9(2)	LUPA-ADD-ON-PAYMENT	Output item: For claim "Through" dates before January 1, 2014, the add-on amount to be paid for LUPA claims that are the first episode in a sequence. This amount is added by the Shared System to the payment for the first visit line on the claim. For claim "Through" dates on or after January 1, 2014, zero filled.
568	X	LUPA-SRC-ADM	Input Item: Medicare systems set this indicator to 'B' when condition code 47 is present on the RAP or claim. The indicator is set to '1' in all other cases.
569	X	RECODE-IND	Input Item: A recoding indicator set by Medicare claims processing systems in response to the Common Working File identifying that the episode sequence reported in the first position of the HIPPS code must be changed. Valid values: 0 = default value 1 = HIPPS code shows later episode, should be early episode 2 = HIPPS code shows early episode, but this is not a first or only episode 3 = HIPPS code shows early episode, should be later episode
570	9	EPISODE-TIMING	Input item: A code indicating whether a claim is an early or late episode. Medicare systems copy this code from the 10th position of the treatment authorization code. Valid values: 1 = early episode 2 = late episode
571	X	CLINICAL-SEV-EQ1	Input item: A hexavigesimal code that converts to a number representing the clinical score for this patient calculated under equation 1 of the case-mix system. Medicare systems copy this code from the 11th position of the treatment authorization code.
572	X	FUNCTION-SEV-EQ1	Input item: A hexavigesimal code that converts to a number representing the functional score for this patient calculated under equation 1 of the case-mix system. Medicare systems copy this code from the 12th position of the treatment authorization code.
573	X	CLINICAL-SEV-EQ2	Input item: A hexavigesimal code that converts to a number representing the clinical score for this patient calculated under equation 2 of the case-mix system. Medicare systems copy this code from the 13th position of the treatment authorization code.
574	X	FUNCTION-SEV-EQ2	Input item: A hexavigesimal code that converts to a number representing the functional score for this patient calculated under equation 2 of the case-mix system. Medicare systems copy this code from the 14th position of the treatment authorization code.
575	X	CLINICAL-SEV-EQ3	Input item: A hexavigesimal code that converts to a number representing the clinical score for this patient calculated under equation 3 of the case-mix system. Medicare systems copy this code from the 15th position of the treatment authorization code.
576	X	FUNCTION-SEV-EQ3	Input item: A hexavigesimal code that converts to a number representing the functional score for this patient calculated under equation 3 of the case-mix system. Medicare systems copy this code from the 16th position of the treatment authorization code.

© 2019 Optum360, LLC

File Position	Format	Title	Description
577	X	CLINICAL-SEV-EQ4	Input item: A hexavigesimal code that converts to a number representing the clinical score for this patient calculated under equation 4 of the case-mix system. Medicare systems copy this code from the 17th position of the treatment authorization code.
578	X	FUNCTION-SEV-EQ4	Input item: A hexavigesimal code that converts to a number representing the functional score for this patient calculated under equation 4 of the case-mix system. Medicare systems copy this code from the 18th position of the treatment authorization code.
579-588	9(8)V99	PROV-OUTLIER-PAY-TOTAL	Input item: The total amount of outlier payments that have been made to this HHA for episodes ending during the current calendar year.
589-599	9(9)V99	PROV-PAYMENT-TOTAL	Input item: The total amount of HH PPS payments that have been made to this HHA for episodes ending during the current calendar year.
600-604	9V9(5)	PROV-VBP-ADJ-FAC	Input item: Medicare systems move this information from field 30 of the provider specific file.
605-613	S9(7)V9(2)	VBP-ADJ-AMT	Output item: The HHVBP adjustment amount, determined by subtracting the HHVBP adjustment total payment from the HH PPS payment that would otherwise apply to the claim. Added to the claim as a value code QV amount.
614-622	9(7)V9(2)	PPS-STD-VALUE	Output item: Standardized payment amount – the HH PPS payment without applying any provider-specific adjustments. Informational only. Subject to additional calculations before entered on the claim in PPS-STNDRD-VALUE field.
623-650		X(28)	FILLER

The required data and format for the HH Pricer input/output record for periods of care beginning on or after January 1, 2020 are shown below:

File Position	Format	Title	Description
1-10	X(10)	NPI	Input item: The National Provider Identifier, copied from the claim form.
11-22	X(12)	HIC	Input item: The Health Insurance Claim number of the beneficiary, copied from the claim form.
23-28	X(6)	PROV-NO	Input item: The six-digit CMS certification number, copied from the claim form.
29	X	INIT-PAY-QRP-INDICATOR	Input item: A single character to indicate if normal percentage payments should be made on RAP and/or whether payment should be reduced under the Quality Reporting Program. Medicare systems move this value from field 19 of the provider specific file. Valid values: 0 = Make normal percentage payment 1 = Pay 0% 2 = Make final payment reduced by 2% 3 = Make final payment reduced by 2%, pay RAPs at 0% NOTE: All new HHAs enrolled after January 1, 2019 must have this value set to 1 or 3 (no RAP payments).
30-35	9V9(5)	PROV-VBP-ADJ-FAC	Input item: Medicare systems move this information from from field 30 of the provider specific file.
36-45	9(8)V99	PROV-OUTL-PAY-TOT	Input item: The total amount of outlier payments that have been made to this HHA for episodes ending during the current calendar year.
46-56	9(9)V99	PROV-PAYMENT-TOTAL	Input item: The total amount of HH PPS payments that have been made to this HHA for episodes ending during the current calendar year.
57-59	X(3)	TOB	Input item: The type of bill code, copied from the claim form.
60-64	X(5)	CBSA	Input item: The core based statistical area (CBSA) code, copied from the value code 61 amount on the claim form.
65-69	X(5)	COUNTY-CODE	Input item: The FIPS State and County Code copied from the value code 85 amount on the claim form.
70-77	X(8)	SERV-FROM-DATE	Input item: The statement covers period "From" date, copied from the claim form. Date format must be CCYYMMDD.
78-85	X(8)	SERV-THRU DATE	Input item: The statement covers period "through" date, copied from the claim form. Date format must be CCYYMMDD.
86-93	X(8)	ADMIT-DATE	Input item: The admission date, copied from claim form. Date format must be CCYYMMDD.
94	X	LUPA-SRC-ADM	Input Item: Medicare systems set this indicator to 'B' when condition code 47 is present on the claim. The indicator is set to '1' in all other cases.
95	X	ADJ-IND	Input Item: Medicare systems set the adjustment indicator to '2' when a LUPA add-on claim is identified as not being the first or only episode in a sequence. The indicator is set to '0' in all other cases.
96	X	PEP-IND	Input item: A single Y/N character to indicate if a claim must be paid a partial episode payment (PEP) adjustment. Medicare claims processing systems must set a Y if the patient discharge status code of the claim is 06. An N is set in all other cases.
97-101	X(5)	HRG-INPUT-CODE	Input item: Medicare claims processing systems must copy the HIPPS code from the 0023 revenue code line.
102-104	9(3)	HRG-NO-OF - DAYS	Input item: A number of days calculated by the shared systems for each HIPPS code. The number is determined by the span of days from and including the first line item service date provided under that HIPPS code to and including the last line item service date provided under that HIPPS code.
105-110	9(2)V9(4)	HRG-WGTS	Output item: The weight used by the Pricer to determine the payment amount on the claim.
111-119	9(7)V9(2)	HRG-PAY	Output item: The payment amount calculated by the Pricer for the HIPPS code.

© 2019 Optum360, LLC

File Position	Format	Title	Description
120-123	X(4)	REVENUE - CODE	Input item: One of the six home health discipline revenue codes (042x, 043x, 044x, 055x, 056x, 057x). All six revenue codes must be passed by the Medicare claims processing systems even if the revenue codes are not present on the claim.
124-126	9(3)	REVENUE-QTY - COV-VISITS	Input item: A quantity of covered visits corresponding to each of the six revenue codes. Medicare claims processing systems must count the number of covered visits in each discipline on the claim. If the revenue codes are not present on the claim, a zero must be passed with the revenue code.
127-131	9(5)	REVENUE-QTY - OUTLIER-UNITS	Input item: The sum of the units reported on all covered lines corresponding to each of the six revenue codes. Medicare claims processing systems accumulate the number of units in each discipline on the claim, subject to a limit of 32 units per date of service. If any revenue code is not present on the claim, a zero must be passed with that revenue code.
132-139	9(8)	REVENUE-EARLIEST-DATE	Input item: The earliest line item date for the corresponding revenue code. Date format must be CCYYMMDD.
140-148	9(7)V9(2)	REVENUE - DOLL-RATE	Output item: The dollar rates used by the Pricer to calculate the payment for the visits in each discipline if the claim is paid as a LUPA. Otherwise, the dollar rates used by the Pricer to impute the costs of the claim for purposes of calculating an outlier payment, if any.
149-157	9(7)V9(2)	REVENUE - COST	Output item: The dollar amount determined by the Pricer to be the payment for the visits in each discipline if the claim is paid as a LUPA. Otherwise, the dollar amounts used by the Pricer to impute the costs of the claim for purposes of calculating an outlier payment, if any.
158-166	9(7)V9(2)	REVENUE-ADD-ON-VISIT-AMT	Output item: The add-on amount to be applied to the earliest line item date with the corresponding revenue code. If revenue code 055x, then this is the national per-visit amount multiplied by 1.8714. If revenue code 042x, then this is the national per-visit amount multiplied by 1.6841. If revenue code 044x, then this is the national per-visit amount multiplied by 1.6293.
167-401	Defined above	Additional REVENUE data	Five more occurrences of all REVENUE related data defined above.
402-403	9(2)	PAY-RTC	Output item: A return code set by Pricer to define the payment circumstances of the claim or an error in input data.
			Payment return codes:
			00 Final payment where no outlier applies
			01 Final payment where outlier applies
			02 Final payment where outlier applies, but is not payable due to limitation.
			03 Initial percentage payment, 0%
			04 Initial percentage payment, 50%
			05 Initial percentage payment, 60%
			06 LUPA payment only
			07 Not used.
			08 Not used.
			09 Final payment, PEP
			11 Final payment, PEP with outlier
			12 Not used.
			13 Not used.
			14 LUPA payment, 1st episode add-on payment applies
			Error return codes:
			10 Invalid TOB
			15 Invalid PEP days
			16 Invalid HRG days, greater than 30
			20 PEP indicator invalid
			25 Med review indicator invalid
			30 Invalid CBSA code
			31 Invalid/missing County Code
			35 Invalid Initial Payment Indicator
			40 Dates before January 2020 or invalid
			70 Invalid HRG code
			75 No HRG present in 1st occurrence
			80 Invalid revenue code
			85 No revenue code present on adjustment TOB
404-408	9(5)	REVENUE - SUM 1-6-QTY-ALL	Output item: The total number of visits used by the Pricer to determine if the claim must be paid as a LUPA. This amount will be the total of all the covered visit quantities input with all six HH discipline revenue codes.
409-417	9(7)V9(2)	OUTLIER - PAYMENT	Output item: The outlier payment amount determined by the Pricer to be due on the claim in addition to any HRG payment amounts. Added to the claim as a value code 17 amount.
418-426	9(7)V9(2)	TOTAL - PAYMENT	Output item: The total payment determined by the Pricer to be due on the claim.
427-435	S9(7)V9(2)	VBP-ADJ-AMT	Output item: The HHVBP adjustment amount, determined by subtracting the HHVBP adjustment total payment from the HH PPS payment that would otherwise apply to the claim. Added to the claim as a value code QV amount.
436-444	9(7)V9(2)	PPS-STD-VALUE	Output item: Standardized payment amount – the HH PPS payment without applying any provider-specific adjustments. Informational only. Subject to additional calculations before entered on the claim in PPS-STNDRD-VALUE field.
445-650	X(206)	FILLER	

Input records on RAPs will include all input items except for "REVENUE" related items. Input records on claims must include all input items. Output records will contain all input and output items. If an output item does not apply to a particular record, Pricer will return zeroes.

The Medicare claims processing system will move the following Pricer output items to the claim record. The return code will be placed in the claim header. The HRG-PAY

© 2019 Optum360, LLC

amount for the HIPPS code will be placed in the total charges and the covered charges field of the revenue code 0023 line. The OUTLIER-PAYMENT amount, if any, will be placed in a value code 17 amount. If the return code is 06 (indicating a low utilization payment adjustment), the Medicare claims processing system will apportion the REVENUE-COST amounts to the appropriate line items in order for the per-visit payments to be accurately reflected on the remittance advice. If the return code is 14, the Medicare claims processing system will apply the H-HHA-REVENUE-ADD-ON-VISIT-AMT to the earliest line item with the corresponding revenue code.

100-04, 10, 40.2

HH PPS Claims

(Rev.4312, Issued: 05-23-19, Effective: 01-01-20, Implementation: 08-16-19)

The following data elements are required to submit a claim under home health PPS. For billing of home health claims not under an HH plan of care (not under HH PPS), see §90. Home health services under a plan of care are paid based on a 60-day episode of care (before January 1, 2020) or a 30-day period of care (on or after January 1, 2020). Payment for this episode or period will usually be made in two parts. After a RAP has been paid and an episode or period has been completed, or the patient has been discharged, the HHA submits a claim to receive the balance of payment due.

HH PPS claims will be processed in Medicare claims processing systems as debit/credit adjustments against the record created by the RAP, except in the case of "No-RAP" LUPA claims (see §40.3). As the claim is processed the payment on the RAP will be reversed in full and the full payment due for the episode will be made on the claim. Both the debit and credit actions will be reflected on the RA so the net payment on the claim can be easily understood. Detailed RA information is contained in chapter 22 of this manual.

Billing Provider Name, Address, and Telephone Number

Required – The HHA's minimum entry is the agency's name, city, state, and ZIP Code. The post office box number or street name and number may be included. The state may be abbreviated using standard post office abbreviations. Five or nine-digit ZIP Codes are acceptable. A/B MACs (HHH) use this information in connection with the provider identifier to verify provider identity.

Patient Control Number and Medical/Health Record Number

Required - The patient's control number may be shown if the patient is assigned one and the number is needed for association and reference purposes.

The HHA may enter the number assigned to the patient's medical/health record. If this number is entered, the A/B MAC (HHH) must carry it through their system and return it on the remittance record.

Type of Bill

Required - This 4-digit alphanumeric code gives two pieces of information. The first three digits indicate the base type of bill. The fourth digit indicates the sequence of this bill in this particular episode of care. The types of bill accepted for HH PPS claims are:

032x - Home Health Services under a Plan of Treatment

4th Digit - Definition

7 - Replacement of Prior Claim - HHAs use to correct a previously submitted bill. Apply this code for the corrected or "new" bill. These adjustment claims must be accepted at any point within the timely filing period after the payment of the original claim.

8 - Void/Cancel of a Prior Claim - HHAs use this code to indicate this bill is an exact duplicate of an incorrect bill previously submitted. A replacement RAP or claim must be submitted for the episode to be paid.

9 - Final Claim for an HH PPS Episode - This code indicates the HH bill should be processed as a debit/credit adjustment to the RAP. This code is specific to home health and does not replace codes 7, or 8.

HHAs must submit HH PPS claims with the 4th digit of "9." These claims may be adjusted with code "7" or cancelled with code "8." A/B MACs (HHH) do not accept late charge bills, submitted with code "5," on HH PPS claims. To add services within the period of a paid HH claim, the HHA must submit an adjustment.

NOTE: Type of bill 033x is no longer valid, effective October 1, 2013.

Statement Covers Period

The Patient-Driven Groupings Model is effective for periods of care beginning January 1, 2020. The HHA should follow all prior claims submission instructions for claims with "From" dates before January 1, 2020, including episodes that span into 2020. The HHA should follow PDGM instructions for claims with "From" dates on or after January 1, 2020.

Required - The beginning and ending dates of the period covered by this claim. The "from" date must match the date submitted on the RAP for the episode. For continuous care episodes, the "through" date must be 59 days after the "from" date for a 60-day episode or 29 days after the "From" date for a 30-day period of care

In cases where the beneficiary has been discharged or transferred within the episode or period, HHAs will report the date of discharge in accordance with internal discharge procedures as the "through" date. If the beneficiary has died, the HHA reports the date of death in the "through date."

The HHA may submit claims for payment immediately after the claim "through" date. It is not required to hold claims until the end of the episode or period unless the beneficiary continues under care.

Patient Name/Identifier

Required - The HHA enters the patient's last name, first name, and middle initial.

Patient Address

Required - The HHA enters the patient's full mailing address, including street number and name, post office box number or RFD, City, State, and ZIP Code.

Patient Birth Date

Required - The HHA enters the month, day, and year of birth of patient. If the full correct date is not known, leave blank.

Patient Sex

Required - "M" for male or "F" for female must be present. This item is used in conjunction with diagnoses and surgical procedures to identify inconsistencies.

Admission/Start of Care Date

Required - The HHA enters the same date of admission that was submitted on the RAP for the episode.

Point of Origin for Admission or Visit

Required - The HHA enters the same point of origin code that was submitted on the RAP for the episode.

Patient Discharge Status

Required - The HHA enters the code that most accurately describes the patient's status as of the "Through" date of the billing period. Any applicable NUBC approved code may be used.

Patient status code 06 should be reported in all cases where the HHA is aware that the episode will be paid as a PEP adjustment. These are cases in which the agency is aware that the beneficiary has transferred to another HHA within the 60-day episode or 30-day period, or the agency is aware that the beneficiary was discharged with the goals of the original plan of care met and has been readmitted within the episode or period. Situations may occur in which the HHA is unaware at the time of billing the discharge that these circumstances exist. In these situations, Medicare claims processing systems will adjust the discharge claim automatically to reflect the PEP adjustment, changing the patient status code on the paid claims record to 06.

In cases where an HHA is changing the A/B MAC (HHH) to which they submit claims, the service dates on the claims must fall within the provider's effective dates at each A/B MAC (HHH). To ensure this, RAPs for all episodes with "from" dates before the provider's termination date must be submitted to the A/B MAC (HHH) the provider is leaving. The resulting episode must be resolved by the provider submitting claims for shortened periods, with "through" dates on or before the termination date. The provider must indicate that these claims will be PEP adjustments by using patient status code 06. Billing for the beneficiary is being "transferred" to the new A/B MAC (HHH).

In cases where the ownership of an HHA is changing and the CMS certification number (CCN) also changes, the service dates on the claims must fall within the effective dates of the terminating CCN. To ensure this, RAPs for all episodes with "from" dates before the termination date of the CCN must be resolved by the provider submitting claims for shortened periods, with "through" dates on or before the termination date. The provider must indicate that these claims will be PEP adjustments by using patient status 06. Billing for the beneficiary is being "transferred" to the new agency ownership. In changes of ownership which do not affect the CCN, billing for episodes is also unaffected.

In cases where an HHA is aware in advance that a beneficiary will become enrolled in a Medicare Advantage (MA) Organization as of a certain date, the provider should submit a claim for the shortened period prior to the MA Organization enrollment date. The claim should be coded with patient status 06. Payment responsibility for the beneficiary is being "transferred" from Medicare fee-for-service to MA Organization, since HH PPS applies only to Medicare fee-for-service.

If HHAs require guidance on OASIS assessment procedures in these cases, they should contact the appropriate state OASIS education coordinator.

Condition Codes

Conditional – The HHA enters any NUBC approved code to describe conditions that apply to the claim.

© 2019 Optum360, LLC

If the RAP is for an episode in which the patient has transferred from another HHA, the HHA enters condition code 47.

If the claim is for an episode in which there are no skilled HH visits in billing period, but a policy exception that allows billing for covered services is documented at the HHA, the HHA enters condition code 54.

HHAs that are adjusting previously paid claims enter one of the condition codes representing Claim Change Reasons (code values D0 through E0). If adjusting the claim to correct a HIPPS code, HHAs use condition code D2 and enter "Remarks" indicating the reason for the HIPPS code change. HHAs use D9 if multiple changes are necessary.

When submitting an HH PPS claim as a demand bill, HHAs use condition code 20. See §50 for more detailed instructions regarding demand billing.

When submitting an HH PPS claim for a denial notice, HHAs use condition code 21. See §60 for more detailed instructions regarding no-payment billing.

Required - If canceling the claim (TOB 0328), HHAs report the condition codes D5 or D6 and enter "Remarks" indicating the reason for cancellation of the claim.

Occurrence Codes and Dates

Required – On claims with "From" dates on or after January 1, 2020, the HHA enters occurrence code 50 and the date the OASIS assessment corresponding to the period of care was completed (OASIS item M0090). If occurrence code 50 is not reported on a claim or adjustment, the claim will be returned to the provider for correction.

On claims for initial periods of care (i.e. when the From and Admission dates match), the HHA reports an inpatient admission that ended within 14 days of the "From" date by using one of the following codes.

Code	Short Descriptor	Long Descriptor
61	Hospital Discharge Date	The Through date of a hospital stay that ended within 14 days prior to the From date this HHA claim.
62	Other Institutional Discharge Date	The Through date of skilled nursing facility (SNF), inpatient rehabilitation facility (IRF), long term care hospital (LTCH) or inpatient psychiatric facility (IPF) stay that ended within 14 days prior to this HHA admission.

On claims for continuing periods of care, the HHA reports an inpatient hospital admission that ended within 14 days of the "From" date by using occurrence code 61.

If more than one inpatient discharge occurs during the 14 day period, the HHA reports only the most recent discharge date. Claims reporting more than one of any combination of occurrence codes 61 and 62 will be returned to the provider for correction.

Conditional - The HHA enters any other NUBC approved code to describe occurrences that apply to the claim.

Occurrence Span Code and Dates

Conditional - The HHA enters any NUBC approved Occurrence Span code to describe occurrences that apply to the claim. Reporting of occurrence span code 74 is not required to show the dates of an inpatient admission during an episode.

Value Codes and Amounts

Required - Home health episode payments must be based upon the site at which the beneficiary is served. For certain dates of service when required by law, payments may be further adjusted if the site is in a rural CBSA or rural county. For episodes in which the beneficiary's site of service changes from one CBSA or county to another within the episode period, HHAs should submit the CBSA code or State and County code corresponding to the site of service at the end of the episode on the claim.

Provider-submitted codes:

Code	Title	Definition
61	Location Where Service is Furnished (HHA and Hospice)	HHAs report the MSA number or Core Based Statistical Area (CBSA) number (or rural state code) of the location where the home health or hospice service is delivered. The HHA reports the number in dollar portion of the form locator right justified to the left of the dollar/cents delimiter, add two zeros to the cents field if no cents.
85	County Where Service is Rendered	Where required by law or regulation, report the Federal Information Processing Standards (FIPS) State and County Code of the place of residence where the home health service is delivered.

Medicare-applied codes: The following codes are added during processing and may be visible in the A/B MAC (HHH)'s online claim history. They are never submitted by the HHA.

Code	Title	Definition
17	Outlier Amount	The amount of any outlier payment returned by the Pricer with this code. A/B MACs (HHH) always place condition code 61 on the claim along with this value code.)
61	Location Where Service is Furnished (HHA and Hospice)	HHAs report the MSA number or Core Based Statistical Area (CBSA) number (or rural state code) of the location where the home health or hospice service is delivered. The HHA reports the number in dollar portion of the form locator right justified to the left of the dollar/cents delimiter, add two zeros to the cents field if no cents.
62	HH Visits - Part A	The number of visits determined by Medicare to be payable from the Part A trust fund to reflect the shift of payments from the Part A to the Part B trust fund as mandated by §1812 (a)(3) of the Social Security Act.
63	HH Visits - Part B	The number of visits determined by Medicare to be payable from the Part B trust fund to reflect the shift of payments from the Part A to the Part B trust fund as mandated by §1812 (a)(3) of the Social Security Act.
64	HH Reimbursement - Part A	The dollar amounts determined to be associated with the HH visits identified in a value code 62 amount. This Part A payment reflects the shift of payments from the Part A to the Part B trust fund as mandated by §1812 (a)(3) of the Social Security Act.
65	HH Reimbursement - Part B	The dollar amounts determined to be associated with the HH visits identified in a value code 63 amount. This Part B payment reflects the shift of payments from the Part A to the Part B trust fund as mandated by §1812 (a)(3) of the Social Security Act.

If information returned from the CWF indicates all visits on the claim are Part A, the shared system must place value codes 62 and 64 on the claim record, showing the total visits and total PPS payment amount as the values, and send the claim to CWF with RIC code V.

If information returned from CWF indicates all visits on the claim are Part B, the shared system must place value codes 63 and 65 on the claim record, showing the total visits and total PPS payment amount as the values, and send the claim to CWF with RIC code W.

If information returned from CWF indicates certain visits on the claim are payable from both Part A and Part B, the shared system must place value codes 62, 63, 64, and 65 on the claim record. The shared system also must populate the values for code 62 and 63 based on the numbers of visits returned from CWF and prorate the total PPS reimbursement amount based on the numbers of visits to determine the dollars amounts to be associated with value codes 64 and 65. The shared system will return the claim to CWF with RIC code U.

Revenue Code and Revenue Description

Required

© 2019 Optum360, LLC

HH PPS claims must report a 0023 revenue code line on which the first four positions of the HIPPS code match the code submitted on the RAP. *This HIPPS code is used to match the claim to the corresponding RAP that was previously paid. After this match is completed, grouping to determine the HIPPS code used for final payment of the period of care will occur in Medicare systems. At that time, the submitted HIPPS code on the claim will be replaced with the system-calculated code.*

For claims with "From" dates before January 1, 2020, the fifth position of the code represents the NRS severity level. This fifth position may differ to allow the HHA to change a code that represents that supplies were provided to a code that represents that supplies were not provided, or vice versa. However, the fifth position may only change between the two values that represent the same NRS severity level. Section 10.1.9 of this chapter contains the pairs of corresponding values. If these criteria are not met, Medicare claims processing systems will return the claim.

HHAs enter only one 0023 revenue code per claim in all cases.

Unlike RAPs, claims must also report all services provided to the beneficiary within the episode/*period. All services must be billed on one claim for the entire episode/period. The A/B MAC (HHH) will return to the provider TOB 0329 when submitted without any visit charges.*

Each service must be reported in line item detail. Each service visit (revenue codes 042x, 043x, 044x, 055x, 056x and 057x) must be reported as a separate line. Any of the following revenue codes may be used:

027x	Medical/Surgical Supplies (Also see 062x, an extension of 027x) Required detail: With the exception of revenue code 0274 (prosthetic and orthotic devices), only service units and a charge must be reported with this revenue code. If also reporting revenue code 0623 to separately identify specific wound care supplies, not just supplies for wound care patients, ensure that the charge amounts for revenue code 0623 lines are mutually exclusive from other lines for supply revenue codes reported on the claim. Report only nonroutine supply items in this revenue code or in 0623. Revenue code 0274 requires an HCPCS code, the date of service units and a charge amount. NOTE: Revenue Codes 0275 through 0278 are not used for Medicare billing on HH PPS types of bills
042x	Physical Therapy Required detail: One of the physical therapy HCPCS codes defined below in the instructions for the HCPCS code field, the date of service, service units which represent the number of 15 minute increments that comprised the visit, and a charge amount.
043x	Occupational Therapy Required detail: One of the occupational therapy HCPCS codes defined below in the instructions for the HCPCS code field, the date of service, service units which represent the number of 15 minute increments that comprised the visit, and a charge amount.
044x	Speech-Language Pathology Required detail: One of the speech-language pathology HCPCS codes defined below in the instructions for the HCPCS code field, the date of service, service units which represent the number of 15 minute increments that comprised the visit, and a charge amount.
055x	Skilled Nursing Required detail: One of the skilled nursing HCPCS codes defined below in the instructions for the HCPCS code field, the date of service, service units which represent the number of 15 minute increments that comprised the visit, and a charge amount.
056x	Medical Social Services Required detail: The medical social services HCPCS code defined below in the instructions for the HCPCS code field, the date of service, service units which represent the number of 15 minute increments that comprised the visit, and a charge amount.
057x	Home Health Aide (Home Health) Required detail: The home health aide HCPCS code defined below in the instructions for the HCPCS code field, the date of service, service units which represent the number of 15 minute increments that comprised the visit, and a charge amount.

NOTE: A/B MACs (HHH) do not accept revenue codes 058x or 059x when submitted with covered charges on Medicare home health claims under HH PPS. They also do not accept revenue code 0624, investigational devices, on HH claims under HH PPS.

Revenue Codes for Optional Billing of DME

Billing of DME provided in the episode is not required on the HH PPS claim. Home health agencies retain the option to bill these services to their A/B MAC (HHH) processing home health claims or to have the services provided under arrangement with a supplier that bills these services to the DME MAC. Agencies that choose to bill DME services on their HH PPS claims must use the revenue codes below. These services will be paid separately in addition to the HH PPS amount, based on the applicable Medicare fee schedule. For additional instructions for billing DME services see chapter 20 of this manual.

0274	Prosthetic/Orthotic Devices Required detail: The applicable HCPCS code for the item, a date of service, a number of service units, and a charge amount.
029x	Durable Medical Equipment (DME) (Other Than Renal) Required detail: The applicable HCPCS code for the item, a date of service indicating the purchase date or the beginning date of a monthly rental, a number of service units, and a charge amount. Monthly rental items should be reported with a separate line for each month's rental and service units of one. Revenue code 0294 is used to bill drugs/supplies for the effective use of DME.
060x	Oxygen (Home Health) Required detail: The applicable HCPCS code for the item, a date of service, a number of service units, and a charge amount.

Revenue Code for Optional Reporting of Wound Care Supplies

0623	Medical/Surgical Supplies - Extension of 027x Required detail: Only service units and a charge must be reported with this revenue code. If also reporting revenue code 027x to identify nonroutine supplies other than those used for wound care, the HHA must ensure that the charge amounts for the two revenue code lines are mutually exclusive.

HHAs may voluntarily report a separate revenue code line for charges for nonroutine wound care supplies, using revenue code 0623. Notwithstanding the standard abbreviation "surg dressings," HHAs use this code to report charges for ALL nonroutine wound care supplies, including but not limited to surgical dressings.

Pub. 100-02, Medicare Benefit Policy Manual, chapter 7, defines routine vs. nonroutine supplies. HHAs use that definition to determine whether any wound care supply item should be reported in this line because it is nonroutine.

HHAs can assist Medicare's future refinement of payment rates if they consistently and accurately report their charges for nonroutine wound care supplies under revenue center code 0623. HHAs should ensure that charges reported under revenue code 027x for nonroutine supplies are also complete and accurate.

Validating Required Reporting of Supply Revenue Code

For claims with "From" dates before January 1, 2020, the HH PPS includes a separate case-mix adjustment for non-routine supplies. Non-routine supply severity levels are indicated on HH PPS claims through a code value in the fifth position of the HIPPS code. The fifth position of the HIPPS code can contain two sets of values. One set of codes (the letters S through X) indicate that supplies were provided. The second set of codes (the numbers 1 through 6) indicate the HHA is intentionally reporting that they did not provide supplies during the episode. See section 10.1.9 for the complete composition of HIPPS under the HH PPS.

HHAs must ensure that if they are submitting a HIPPS code with a fifth position containing the letters S through X, the claim must also report a non-routine supply revenue code with covered charges. This revenue code may be either revenue code 27x, excluding 274, or revenue code 623, consistent with the instructions for optional separate reporting of wound care supplies.

Medicare systems will return the claim to the HHA if the HIPPS code indicates non-routine supplies were provided and supply charges are not reported on the claim. When the HHA receives a claim returned for this reason, the HHA must review their records regarding the supplies provided to the beneficiary. The HHA may take one of the following actions, based on the review of their records:

- If non-routine supplies were provided, the supply charges must be added to the claim using the appropriate supply revenue code.

 © 2019 Optum360, LLC

- If non-routine supplies were not provided, the HHA must indicate that on the claim by changing the fifth position of the HIPPS code to the appropriate numeric value in the range 1 through 6.

After completing one of these actions, the HHA may return the claim to the A/B MAC (HHH) for continued adjudication.

HCPCS/Accommodation Rates/HIPPS Rate Codes

Required - On the 0023 revenue code line, the HHA must report the HIPPS code that was reported on the RAP. The first four positions of the code must be identical to the value reported on the RAP. For claims with "From" dates before January 1, 2020, the fifth position may vary from the letter value reported on the RAP to the corresponding number which represents the same non-routine supply severity level but which reports that non-routine supplies were not provided.

HHAs enter only one HIPPS code per claim in all cases. Claims submitted with additional HIPPS codes will be returned to the provider.

For episodes with "From" dates before January 1, 2020, Medicare may change the HIPPS used for payment of the claim in the course of claims processing, but the HIPPS code submitted by the provider in this field is never changed or replaced. If the HIPPS code is changed, the code used for payment is recorded in the APC-HIPPS field of the electronic claim record.

For episodes with "From" dates on or after January 1, 2020, Medicare will determine the appropriate HIPPS code for payment based on claims and OASIS data and will replace the provider-submitted HIPPS code as necessary. If the HIPPS code further changed based on medical review or other processes, the code used for payment is recorded in the APC-HIPPS field of the electronic claim record.

For revenue code lines other than 0023, the HHA reports HCPCS codes as appropriate to that revenue code.

To report HH visits, the HHA reports one of the following HCPCS codes to represent a visit by each HH care discipline:

Physical Therapy (revenue code 042x)

G0151 Services performed by a qualified physical therapist in the home health or hospice setting, each 15 minutes.

G0157 Services performed by a qualified physical therapist assistant in the home health or hospice setting, each 15 minutes.

G0159 Services performed by a qualified physical therapist, in the home health setting, in the establishment or delivery of a safe and effective physical therapy maintenance program, each 15 minutes.

Occupational Therapy (revenue code 043x)

G0152 Services performed by a qualified occupational therapist in the home health or hospice setting, each 15 minutes.

G0158 Services performed by a qualified occupational therapist assistant in the home health or hospice setting, each 15 minutes.

G0160 Services performed by a qualified occupational therapist, in the home health setting, in the establishment or delivery of a safe and effective occupational therapy maintenance program, each 15 minutes.

Speech-Language Pathology (revenue code 044x)

G0153 Services performed by a qualified speech-language pathologist in the home health or hospice setting, each 15 minutes.

G0161 Services performed by a qualified speech-language pathologist, in the home health setting, in the establishment or delivery of a safe and effective speech-language pathology maintenance program, each 15 minutes.

Note that modifiers indicating services delivered under a therapy plan of care (modifiers GN, GO or GP) are not required on HH PPS claims.

Skilled Nursing (revenue code 055x)

General skilled nursing:

For dates of service before January 1, 2016: G0154 Direct skilled services of a licensed nurse (LPN or RN) in the home health or hospice setting, each 15 minutes.

For dates of service on or after January 1, 2016: Visits previously reported with G0154 are reported with one of the following codes:

G0299 Direct skilled nursing services of a registered nurse (RN) in the home health or hospice setting

G0300 Direct skilled nursing of a licensed practical nurse (LPN) in the home health or hospice setting.

Care plan oversight:

For dates of service before January 1, 2017:

G0162 Skilled services by a licensed nurse (RN only) for management and evaluation of the plan of care, each 15 minutes (the patient's underlying condition or complication requires an RN to ensure that essential non-skilled care achieves its purpose in the home health or hospice setting).

G0163 Skilled services of a licensed nurse (LPN or RN) for the observation and assessment of the patient's condition, each 15 minutes (the change in the patient's condition requires skilled nursing personnel to identify and evaluate the patient's need for possible modification of treatment in the home health or hospice setting).

For dates of service on or after January 1, 2017, HHAs report visits previously reported with G0163 with one of the following codes:

G0493 Skilled services of a registered nurse (RN) for the observation and assessment of the patient's condition, each 15 minutes (the change in the patient's condition requires skilled nursing personnel to identify and evaluate the patient's need for possible modification of treatment in the home health or hospice setting).

G0494 Skilled services of a licensed practical nurse (LPN) for the observation and assessment of the patient's condition, each 15 minutes (the change in the patient's condition requires skilled nursing personnel to identify and evaluate the patient's need for possible modification of treatment in the home health or hospice setting).

Training:

For dates of service before January 1, 2017: G0164 Skilled services of a licensed nurse (LPN or RN), in the training and/or education of a patient or family member, in the home health or hospice setting, each 15 minutes.

For dates of service on or after January 1, 2017, HHAs report visits previously reported with G0164 with one of the following codes:

G0495 Skilled services of a registered nurse (RN), in the training and/or education of a patient or family member, in the home health or hospice setting, each 15 minutes.

G0496 Skilled services of a licensed practical nurse (LPN), in the training and/or education of a patient or family member, in the home health or hospice setting, each 15 minutes.

Medical Social Services (revenue code 056x)

G0155 Services of a clinical social worker under a home health plan of care, each 15 minutes.

Home Health Aide (revenue code 057x)

G0156 Services of a home health aide under a home health plan of care, each 15 minutes.

Regarding all skilled nursing and skilled therapy visits

In the course of a single visit, a nurse or qualified therapist may provide more than one of the nursing or therapy services reflected in the codes above. HHAs must not report more than one G-code for each visit regardless of the variety of services provided during the visit. In cases where more than one nursing or therapy service is provided in a visit, the HHA must report the G-code which reflects the service for which the clinician spent most of his/her time.

For instance, if direct skilled nursing services are provided, and the nurse also provides training/education of a patient or family member during that same visit, Medicare would expect the HHA to report the G-code which reflects the service for which most of the time was spent during that visit. Similarly, if a qualified therapist is performing a therapy service and also establishes a maintenance program during the same visit, the HHA should report the G-code that reflects the service for which most of the time was spent during that visit. In all cases, however, the number of 15-minute increments reported for the visit should reflect the total time of the visit.

For episodes beginning on or after July 1, 2013, HHAs must report where home health services were provided. The following codes are used for this reporting:

Q5001: Hospice or home health care provided in patient's home/residence

Q5002: Hospice or home health care provided in assisted living facility

Q5009: Hospice or home health care provided in place not otherwise specified

The location where services were provided must always be reported along with the first visit reported on the claim. In addition to reporting a visit line using the G codes as described above, HHAs must report an additional line item with the same revenue code and date of service, reporting one of the three Q codes (Q5001, Q5002, and Q5009), one unit and a nominal covered charge (e.g., a penny). If the location where services were provided changes during the episode, the new location should be reported with an additional line corresponding to the first visit provided in the new location.

© 2019 Optum360, LLC

Service Date

Required - For initial episodes, the HHA reports on the 0023 revenue code line the date of the first covered visit provided during the episode. For subsequent episodes, the HHA reports on the 0023 revenue code the date of the first visit provided during the episode line, regardless of whether the visit was covered or non-covered.

For other line items detailing all services within the episode period, it reports service dates as appropriate to that revenue code. For service visits that begin in 1 calendar day and span into the next calendar day, report one visit using the date the visit ended as the service date.

When the claim Admission Date matches the Statement Covers "From" Date, Medicare systems ensure that the Service Date on the 0023 revenue code line also matches these dates.

Service Units

Required - Transaction standards require the reporting of a number greater than zero as the units on the 0023 revenue code line. However, Medicare systems will disregard the submitted units in processing the claim. For line items detailing all services within the episode period, the HHA reports units of service as appropriate to that revenue code. Coding detail for each revenue code under HH PPS is defined above under Revenue Codes.

For the revenue codes that represent home health visits (042x, 043x, 044x, 055x, 056x, and 057x), the HHA reports as service units a number of 15 minute increments that comprise the time spent treating the beneficiary. Time spent completing the OASIS assessment in the home as part of an otherwise covered and billable visit and time spent updating medical records in the home as part of such a visit may also be reported.

Visits of any length are to be reported, rounding the time to the nearest 15-minute increment. If any visits report over 96 units (over 24 hours) on a single line item, Medicare systems return the claim returned to the provider.

Effective January 1, 2017, covered and noncovered increments of the same visit must be reported on separate lines. This is to ensure that only covered increments are included in the per-unit based calculation of outlier payments.

Total Charges

Required - The HHA must report zero charges on the 0023 revenue code line (the field must contain zero).

For line items detailing all services within the episode period, the HHA reports charges as appropriate to that revenue code. Coding detail for each revenue code under HH PPS is defined above under Revenue Codes. Charges may be reported in dollars and cents (i.e., charges are not required to be rounded to dollars and zero cents). Medicare claims processing systems will not make any payments based upon submitted charge amounts.

Non-covered Charges

Required – The HHA reports the total non-covered charges pertaining to the related revenue code here. Examples of non-covered charges on HH PPS claims may include:

- Visits provided exclusively to perform OASIS assessments
- Visits provided exclusively for supervisory or administrative purposes
- Therapy visits provided prior to the required re-assessments

Payer Name

Required - See chapter 25.

Release of Information Certification Indicator

Required - See chapter 25.

National Provider Identifier – Billing Provider

Required - The HHA enters their provider identifier.

Insured's Name

Required only if MSP involved. See Pub. 100-05, Medicare Secondary Payer Manual.

Patient's Relationship To Insured

Required only if MSP involved. See Pub. 100-05, Medicare Secondary Payer Manual.

Insured's Unique Identifier

Required only if MSP involved. See Pub. 100-05, Medicare Secondary Payer Manual.

Insured's Group Name

Required only if MSP involved. See Pub. 100-05, Medicare Secondary Payer Manual.

Insured's Group Number

Required only if MSP involved. See Pub. 100-05, Medicare Secondary Payer Manual.

Treatment Authorization Code

Required - On claims with "From" dates before January 1, 2020, the code on the claim will match that submitted on the RAP.

In cases of billing for denial notice, using condition code 21, this code may be filled with a placeholder value as defined in section 60.

The investigational device (IDE) revenue code, 0624, is not allowed on HH PPS claims. Therefore, treatment authorization codes associated with IDE items must never be submitted in this field.

Medicare systems validate the length of the treatment authorization code and ensure that each position is in the correct format. If the format is incorrect, the contractor returns the claim to the provider.

On claims with "From" dates on of after January 1, 2020, treatment authorization codes are no longer required on all claims. The HHA submits a code in this field only if the period is subject to Pre-Claim Review. In that case, the required tracking number is submitted in the first position of the field in all submission formats.

Document Control Number (DCN)

Required - If submitting an adjustment (TOB 0327) to a previously paid HH PPS claim, the HHA enters the control number assigned to the original HH PPS claim here.

Since HH PPS claims are processed as adjustments to the RAP, Medicare claims processing systems will match all HH PPS claims to their corresponding RAP and populate this field on the electronic claim record automatically. Providers do not need to submit a DCN on all HH PPS claims, only on adjustments to paid claims.

Employer Name

Required only if MSP involved. See Pub. 100-05, Medicare Secondary Payer Manual.

Principal Diagnosis Code

Required - The HHA enters the ICD code for the principal diagnosis. The code must be reported according to Official ICD Guidelines for Coding and Reporting, as required by the HIPAA. The code must be the full diagnosis code, including all five digits for ICD-9-CM or all seven digits for ICD-10 CM where applicable. Where the proper code has fewer than the maximum number of digits, the HHA does not fill it with zeros.

Medicare systems may return claims to the provider when the principal diagnosis code is not sufficient to determine the HHRG assignment under the PDGM.

For claim "From" dates before January 1, 2020, the ICD code and principle diagnosis reported must match the primary diagnosis code reported on the OASIS form item M1020 (Primary Diagnosis).

For claim "From" dates on or after January 1, 2020, the ICD code and principle diagnosis used for payment grouping will be claim coding rather than the OASIS item. As a result, the claim and OASIS diagnosis codes will no longer be expected to match in all cases.

Typically, the codes will match between the first claim in an admission and the start of care (Reason for Assessment –RFA 01) assessment and claims corresponding to recertification (RFA 04) assessments. Second 30-day claims in any 60-day period will not necessarily match the OASIS assessment. When diagnosis codes change between one 30-day claim and the next, there is no absolute requirement for the HHA to complete an 'other follow-up' (RFA 05) assessment to ensure that diagnosis coding on the claim matches to the assessment. However, the HHA would be required to complete an 'other follow-up' (RFA 05) assessment when such a change would be considered a major decline or improvement in the patient's health status.

Other Diagnosis Codes

Required - The HHA enters the full diagnosis codes for additional conditions if they coexisted at the time of the establishment of the plan of care. These codes may not duplicate the principal diagnosis as an additional or secondary diagnosis.

In listing the diagnoses, the HHA places them in order to best reflect the seriousness of the patient's condition and to justify the disciplines and services provided in accordance with the Official ICD Guidelines for Coding and Reporting. The sequence of codes should follow ICD guidelines for reporting manifestation codes. Medicare does not have any additional requirements regarding the reporting or sequence of the codes beyond those contained in ICD guidelines.

For claim "From" dates before January 1, 2020, the other diagnoses and ICD codes reported on the claim must match the additional diagnoses reported on the OASIS, form item M1022 (Other Diagnoses).

For claim "From" dates on or after January 1, 2020, claim and OASIS diagnosis codes may vary as described under Principal Diagnosis.

Attending Provider Name and Identifiers

Required - The HHA enters the name and national provider identifier (NPI) of the attending physician who signed the plan of care.

Other Provider (Individual) Names and Identifiers

 © 2019 Optum360, LLC

Required - The HHA enters the name and NPI of the physician who certified/re-certified the patient's eligibility for home health services.

NOTE: Both the attending physician and other provider fields should be completed unless the patient's designated attending physician is the same as the physician who certified/re-certified the patient's eligibility. When the attending physician is also the certifying/re-certifying physician, only the attending physician is required to be reported.

Remarks

Conditional - Remarks are required only in cases where the claim is cancelled or adjusted.

100-04, 10, 40.3

HH PPS Claims When No RAP is Submitted - "No-RAP" LUPAs

(Rev.4312, Issued: 05-23-19, Effective: 01-01-20, Implementation: 08-16-19)

A RAP and a claim must be submitted for all episodes/*periods of care* for which Medicare makes payment based on HIPPS codes. However, if the HHA is aware prior to billing Medicare that it will supply fewer visits *than the LUPA threshold* in the episode/*period*, it may submit only a claim. In these cases, the claim is called a "No-RAP LUPA," since the HHA is aware the claim will be paid a LUPA payment adjustment based on national standard visit rates. HHAs may submit both a RAP and a claim in these instances if they choose, but only the claim is required. HHAs should be aware that submission of a RAP in these instances will result in a recoupment of funds since the payment for a RAP will exceed payment for four or fewer visits. HHAs should also be aware that the receipt of the RAP or a "no-RAP LUPA" claim causes the creation of an episode/*period* record in CWF and establishes an agency as the primary HHA. If submission of a "No-RAP LUPA" delays submission of the claim significantly, the agency is at risk of not being established as the primary HHA for that period.

If the agency chooses to submit this "No-RAP LUPA" claim, the claim form should be coded like other claim as described in §40.2.

100-04, 10, 40.5

RESERVED

(Rev.4312, Issued: 05-23-19, Effective: 01-01-20, Implementation: 08-16-19)

100-04, 10, 70.2

Input/Output Record Layout

(Rev.4312, Issued: 05-23-19, Effective: 01-01-20, Implementation: 08-16-19)

The required data and format for the HH Pricer input/output record for episodes beginning before January 1, 2020 are shown below:

File Position	Format	Title	Description
1-10	X(10)	NPI	This field will be used for the National Provider Identifier if it is sent to the HH Pricer in the future.
11-22	X(12)	HIC	Input item: The Health Insurance Claim number of the beneficiary, copied from the claim form.
23-28	X(6)	PROV-NO	Input item: The six-digit CMS certification number, copied from the claim form.
29-31	X(3)	TOB	Input item: The type of bill code, copied from the claim form.
32	X	PEP-INDICATOR	Input item: A single Y/N character to indicate if a claim must be paid a partial episode payment (PEP) adjustment. Medicare claims processing systems must set a Y if the patient discharge status code of the claim is 06. An N is set in all other cases.
33-35	9(3)	PEP-DAYS	Input item: The number of days to be used for PEP payment calculation. Medicare claims processing systems determine this number by the span of days from and including the first line item service date on the claim to and including the last line item service date on the claim.
36	X	INIT-PAY-INDICATOR	Input item: A single character to indicate if normal percentage payments should be made on RAP or whether payment should be based on data drawn by the Medicare claims processing systems from field 19 of the provider specific file. Valid values: 0 = Make normal percentage payment 1 = Pay 0% 2 = Make final payment reduced by 2% 3 = Make final payment reduced by 2%, pay RAPs at 0%
37-46	X(9)	FILLER	Blank.
47-50	X(5)	CBSA	Input item: The core based statistical area (CBSA) code, copied from the value code 61 amount on the claim form.
51-52	X(2)	FILLER	Blank.
53-60	X(8)	SERV-FROM-DATE	Input item: The statement covers period "From" date, copied from the claim form. Date format must be CCYYMMDD.
61-68	X(8)	SERV-THRU DATE	Input item: The statement covers period "through" date, copied from the claim form. Date format must be CCYYMMDD.
69-76	X(8)	ADMIT-DATE	Input item: The admission date, copied from claim form. Date format must be CCYYMMDD.
77	X	HRG-MED - REVIEW - INDICATOR	Input item: A single Y/N character to indicate if a HIPPS code has been changed by medical review. Medicare claims processing systems must set a Y if an ANSI code on the line item indicates a medical review change. An N must be set in all other cases.
78-82	X(5)	HRG-INPUT-CODE	Input item: Medicare claims processing systems must copy the HIPPS code reported by the provider on each 0023 revenue code line. If an ANSI code on the line item indicates a medical review change, Medicare claims processing systems must copy the additional HIPPS code placed on the 0023 revenue code line by the medical reviewer.
83-87	X(5)	HRG - OUTPUT - CODE	Output item: The HIPPS code used by the Pricer to determine the payment amount on the claim. This code will match the input code unless the claim is recoded due to therapy thresholds or changes in episode sequence. If recoded, the Medicare claims processing system stores this output item in the APC-HIPPS field on the claim record.
88-90	9(3)	HRG-NO-OF - DAYS	Input item: A number of days calculated by the shared systems for each HIPPS code. The number is determined by the span of days from and including the first line item service date provided under that HIPPS code to and including the last line item service date provided under that HIPPS code.
91-96	9(2)V9(4)	HRG-WGTS	Output item: The weight used by the Pricer to determine the payment amount on the claim.
97-105	9(7)V9(2)	HRG-PAY	Output item: The payment amount calculated by the Pricer for each HIPPS code on the claim.

© 2019 Optum360, LLC

File Position	Format	Title	Description
106-250	Defined above	Additional HRG data	Fields for five more occurrences of all HRG/HIPPS code related fields defined above. Not used.
251-254	X(4)	REVENUE - CODE	Input item: One of the six home health discipline revenue codes (042x, 043x, 044x, 055x, 056x, 057x). All six revenue codes must be passed by the Medicare claims processing systems even if the revenue codes are not present on the claim.
255-257	9(3)	REVENUE-QTY - COV-VISITS	Input item: A quantity of covered visits corresponding to each of the six revenue codes. Medicare claims processing systems must count the number of covered visits in each discipline on the claim. If the revenue codes are not present on the claim, a zero must be passed with the revenue code.
258-262	9(5)	REVENUE-QTY - OUTLIER-UNITS	Input item: The sum of the units reported on all covered lines corresponding to each of the six revenue codes. Medicare claims processing systems accumulate the number of units in each discipline on the claim, subject to a limit of 32 units per date of service. If any revenue code is not present on the claim, a zero must be passed with that revenue code.
263-270	9(8)	REVENUE-EARLIEST-DATE	Input item: The earliest line item date for the corresponding revenue code. Date format must be CCYYMMDD.
271-279	9(7)V9(2)	REVENUE - DOLL-RATE	Output item: The dollar rates used by the Pricer to calculate the payment for the visits in each discipline if the claim is paid as a LUPA. Otherwise, the dollar rates used by the Pricer to impute the costs of the claim for purposes of calculating an outlier payment, if any.
280-288	9(7)V9(2)	REVENUE - COST	Output item: The dollar amount determined by the Pricer to be the payment for the visits in each discipline if the claim is paid as a LUPA. Otherwise, the dollar amounts used by the Pricer to impute the costs of the claim for purposes of calculating an outlier payment, if any.
289-297	9(7)V9(2)	REVENUE-ADD-ON-VISIT-AMT	Output item: The add-on amount to be applied to the earliest line item date with the corresponding revenue code. If revenue code 055x, then this is the national per-visit amount multiplied by 1.8451. If revenue code 042x, then this is the national per-visit amount multiplied by 1.6700. If revenue code 044x, then this is the national per-visit amount multiplied by 1.6266.
298-532	Defined above	Additional REVENUE data	Five more occurrences of all REVENUE related data defined above.
533-534	9(2)	PAY-RTC	Output item: A return code set by Pricer to define the payment circumstances of the claim or an error in input data.
			Payment return codes:
			00 Final payment where no outlier applies
			01 Final payment where outlier applies
			02 Final payment where outlier applies, but is not payable due to limitation.
			03 Initial percentage payment, 0%
			04 Initial percentage payment, 50%
			05 Initial percentage payment, 60%
			06 LUPA payment only
			07 Not used.
			08 Not used.
			09 Final payment, PEP
			11 Final payment, PEP with outlier
			12 Not used.
			13 Not used.
			14 LUPA payment, 1st episode add-on payment applies
			Error return codes:
			10 Invalid TOB
			15 Invalid PEP days
			16 Invalid HRG days, greater than 60
			20 PEP indicator invalid
			25 Med review indicator invalid
			30 Invalid MSA/CBSA code
			35 Invalid Initial Payment Indicator
			40 Dates before Oct 1, 2000 or invalid
			70 Invalid HRG code
			75 No HRG present in 1st occurrence
			80 Invalid revenue code
			85 No revenue code present on 03x9 or adjustment TOB
535-539	9(5)	REVENUE - SUM 1-3-QTY-THR	Output item: The total therapy visits used by the Pricer to determine if the therapy threshold was met for the claim. This amount will be the total of the covered visit quantities input in association with revenue codes 042x, 043x, and 044x.
540-544	9(5)	REVENUE - SUM 1-6-QTY-ALL	Output item: The total number of visits used by the Pricer to determine if the claim must be paid as a LUPA. This amount will be the total of all the covered visit quantities input with all six HH discipline revenue codes.
545-553	9(7)V9(2)	OUTLIER - PAYMENT	Output item: The outlier payment amount determined by the Pricer to be due on the claim in addition to any HRG payment amounts.
554-562	9(7)V9(2)	TOTAL - PAYMENT	Output item: The total payment determined by the Pricer to be due on the RAP or claim.
563-567	9(3)V9(2)	LUPA-ADD-ON-PAYMENT	Output item: For claim "Through" dates before January 1, 2014, the add-on amount to be paid for LUPA claims that are the first episode in a sequence. This amount is added by the Shared System to the payment for the first visit line on the claim. For claim "Through" dates on or after January 1, 2014, zero filled.
568	X	LUPA-SRC-ADM	Input Item: Medicare systems set this indicator to 'B' when condition code 47 is present on the RAP or claim. The indicator is set to '1' in all other cases.

© 2019 Optum360, LLC

File Position	Format	Title	Description
569	X	RECODE-IND	Input Item: A recoding indicator set by Medicare claims processing systems in response to the Common Working File identifying that the episode sequence reported in the first position of the HIPPS code must be changed. Valid values: 0 = default value 1 = HIPPS code shows later episode, should be early episode 2 = HIPPS code shows early episode, but this is not a first or only episode 3 = HIPPS code shows early episode, should be later episode
570	9	EPISODE-TIMING	Input item: A code indicating whether a claim is an early or late episode. Medicare systems copy this code from the 10th position of the treatment authorization code. Valid values: 1 = early episode 2 = late episode
571	X	CLINICAL-SEV-EQ1	Input item: A hexavigesimal code that converts to a number representing the clinical score for this patient calculated under equation 1 of the case-mix system. Medicare systems copy this code from the 11th position of the treatment authorization code.
572	X	FUNCTION-SEV-EQ1	Input item: A hexavigesimal code that converts to a number representing the functional score for this patient calculated under equation 1 of the case-mix system. Medicare systems copy this code from the 12th position of the treatment authorization code.
573	X	CLINICAL-SEV-EQ2	Input item: A hexavigesimal code that converts to a number representing the clinical score for this patient calculated under equation 2 of the case-mix system. Medicare systems copy this code from the 13th position of the treatment authorization code.
574	X	FUNCTION-SEV-EQ2	Input item: A hexavigesimal code that converts to a number representing the functional score for this patient calculated under equation 2 of the case-mix system. Medicare systems copy this code from the 14th position of the treatment authorization code.
575	X	CLINICAL-SEV-EQ3	Input item: A hexavigesimal code that converts to a number representing the clinical score for this patient calculated under equation 3 of the case-mix system. Medicare systems copy this code from the 15th position of the treatment authorization code.
576	X	FUNCTION-SEV-EQ3	Input item: A hexavigesimal code that converts to a number representing the functional score for this patient calculated under equation 3 of the case-mix system. Medicare systems copy this code from the 16th position of the treatment authorization code.
577	X	CLINICAL-SEV-EQ4	Input item: A hexavigesimal code that converts to a number representing the clinical score for this patient calculated under equation 4 of the case-mix system. Medicare systems copy this code from the 17th position of the treatment authorization code.
578	X	FUNCTION-SEV-EQ4	Input item: A hexavigesimal code that converts to a number representing the functional score for this patient calculated under equation 4 of the case-mix system. Medicare systems copy this code from the 18th position of the treatment authorization code.
579-588	9(8)V99	PROV-OUTLIER-PAY-TOTAL	Input item: The total amount of outlier payments that have been made to this HHA for episodes ending during the current calendar year.
589-599	9(9)V99	PROV-PAYMENT-TOTAL	Input item: The total amount of HH PPS payments that have been made to this HHA for episodes ending during the current calendar year.
600-604	9V9(5)	PROV-VBP-ADJ-FAC	Input item: Medicare systems move this information from field 30 of the provider specific file.
605-613	S9(7)V9(2)	VBP-ADJ-AMT	Output item: The HHVBP adjustment amount, determined by subtracting the HHVBP adjustment total payment from the HH PPS payment that would otherwise apply to the claim. Added to the claim as a value code QV amount.
614-622	9(7)V9(2)	PPS-STD-VALUE	Output item: Standardized payment amount – the HH PPS payment without applying any provider-specific adjustments. Informational only. Subject to additional calculations before entered on the claim in PPS-STNDRD-VALUE field.
623-650		X(28)	FILLER

The required data and format for the HH Pricer input/output record for periods of care beginning on or after January 1, 2020 are shown below:

File Position	Format	Title	Description
1-10	X(10)	NPI	Input item: The National Provider Identifier, copied from the claim form.
11-22	X(12)	HIC	Input item: The Health Insurance Claim number of the beneficiary, copied from the claim form.
23-28	X(6)	PROV-NO	Input item: The six-digit CMS certification number, copied from the claim form.
29	X	INIT-PAY-QRP-INDICATOR	Input item: A single character to indicate if normal percentage payments should be made on RAP and/or whether payment should be reduced under the Quality Reporting Program. Medicare systems move this value from field 19 of the provider specific file. Valid values: 0 = Make normal percentage payment 1 = Pay 0% 2 = Make final payment reduced by 2% 3 = Make final payment reduced by 2%, pay RAPs at 0% NOTE: All new HHAs enrolled after January 1, 2019 must have this value set to 1 or 3 (no RAP payments).

© 2019 Optum360, LLC

File Position	Format	Title	Description
30-35	9V9(5)	PROV-VBP-ADJ-FAC	Input item: Medicare systems move this information from from field 30 of the provider specific file.
36-45	9(8)V99	PROV-OUTL-PAY-TOT	Input item: The total amount of outlier payments that have been made to this HHA for episodes ending during the current calendar year.
46-56	9(9)V99	PROV-PAYMENT-TOTAL	Input item: The total amount of HH PPS payments that have been made to this HHA for episodes ending during the current calendar year.
57-59	X(3)	TOB	Input item: The type of bill code, copied from the claim form.
60-64	X(5)	CBSA	Input item: The core based statistical area (CBSA) code, copied from the value code 61 amount on the claim form.
65-69	X(5)	COUNTY-CODE	Input item: The FIPS State and County Code copied from the value code 85 amount on the claim form.
70-77	X(8)	SERV-FROM-DATE	Input item: The statement covers period "From" date, copied from the claim form. Date format must be CCYYMMDD.
78-85	X(8)	SERV-THRU DATE	Input item: The statement covers period "through" date, copied from the claim form. Date format must be CCYYMMDD.
86-93	X(8)	ADMIT-DATE	Input item: The admission date, copied from claim form. Date format must be CCYYMMDD.
94	X	LUPA-SRC-ADM	Input Item: Medicare systems set this indicator to 'B' when condition code 47 is present on the claim. The indicator is set to '1' in all other cases.
95	X	ADJ-IND	Input Item: Medicare systems set the adjustment indicator to '2' when a LUPA add-on claim is identified as not being the first or only episode in a sequence. The indicator is set to '0' in all other cases.
96	X	PEP-IND	Input item: A single Y/N character to indicate if a claim must be paid a partial episode payment (PEP) adjustment. Medicare claims processing systems must set a Y if the patient discharge status code of the claim is 06. An N is set in all other cases.
97-101	X(5)	HRG-INPUT-CODE	Input item: Medicare claims processing systems must copy the HIPPS code from the 0023 revenue code line.
102-104	9(3)	HRG-NO-OF - DAYS	Input item: A number of days calculated by the shared systems for each HIPPS code. The number is determined by the span of days from and including the first line item service date provided under that HIPPS code to and including the last line item service date provided under that HIPPS code.
105-110	9(2)V9(4)	HRG-WGTS	Output item: The weight used by the Pricer to determine the payment amount on the claim.
111-119	9(7)V9(2)	HRG-PAY	Output item: The payment amount calculated by the Pricer for the HIPPS code.
120-123	X(4)	REVENUE - CODE	Input item: One of the six home health discipline revenue codes (042x, 043x, 044x, 055x, 056x, 057x). All six revenue codes must be passed by the Medicare claims processing systems even if the revenue codes are not present on the claim.
124-126	9(3)	REVENUE-QTY - COV-VISITS	Input item: A quantity of covered visits corresponding to each of the six revenue codes. Medicare claims processing systems must count the number of covered visits in each discipline on the claim. If the revenue codes are not present on the claim, a zero must be passed with the revenue code.
127-131	9(5)	REVENUE-QTY - OUTLIER-UNITS	Input item: The sum of the units reported on all covered lines corresponding to each of the six revenue codes. Medicare claims processing systems accumulate the number of units in each discipline on the claim, subject to a limit of 32 units per date of service. If any revenue code is not present on the claim, a zero must be passed with that revenue code.
132-139	9(8)	REVENUE-EARLIEST-DATE	Input item: The earliest line item date for the corresponding revenue code. Date format must be CCYYMMDD.
140-148	9(7)V9(2)	REVENUE - DOLL-RATE	Output item: The dollar rates used by the Pricer to calculate the payment for the visits in each discipline if the claim is paid as a LUPA. Otherwise, the dollar rates used by the Pricer to impute the costs of the claim for purposes of calculating an outlier payment, if any.
149-157	9(7)V9(2)	REVENUE - COST	Output item: The dollar amount determined by the Pricer to be the payment for the visits in each discipline if the claim is paid as a LUPA. Otherwise, the dollar amounts used by the Pricer to impute the costs of the claim for purposes of calculating an outlier payment, if any.
158-166	9(7)V9(2)	REVENUE-ADD-ON-VISIT-AMT	Output item: The add-on amount to be applied to the earliest line item date with the corresponding revenue code. If revenue code 055x, then this is the national per-visit amount multiplied by 1.8714. If revenue code 042x, then this is the national per-visit amount multiplied by 1.6841. If revenue code 044x, then this is the national per-visit amount multiplied by 1.6293.
167-401	Defined above	Additional REVENUE data	Five more occurrences of all REVENUE related data defined above.
402-403	9(2)	PAY-RTC	Output item: A return code set by Pricer to define the payment circumstances of the claim or an error in input data.
			Payment return codes:
			00 Final payment where no outlier applies
			01 Final payment where outlier applies
			02 Final payment where outlier applies, but is not payable due to limitation.

© 2019 Optum360, LLC

File Position	Format	Title	Description
			03 Initial percentage payment, 0%
			04 Initial percentage payment, 50%
			05 Initial percentage payment, 60%
			06 LUPA payment only
			07 Not used.
			08 Not used.
			09 Final payment, PEP
			11 Final payment, PEP with outlier
			12 Not used.
			13 Not used.
			14 LUPA payment, 1st episode add-on payment applies
			Error return codes:
			10 Invalid TOB
			15 Invalid PEP days
			16 Invalid HRG days, greater than 30
			20 PEP indicator invalid
			25 Med review indicator invalid
			30 Invalid CBSA code
			31 Invalid/missing County Code
			35 Invalid Initial Payment Indicator
			40 Dates before January 2020 or invalid
			70 Invalid HRG code
			75 No HRG present in 1st occurrence
			80 Invalid revenue code
			85 No revenue code present on adjustment TOB
404-408	9(5)	REVENUE - SUM 1-6-QTY-ALL	Output item: The total number of visits used by the Pricer to determine if the claim must be paid as a LUPA. This amount will be the total of all the covered visit quantities input with all six HH discipline revenue codes.
409-417	9(7)V9(2)	OUTLIER - PAYMENT	Output item: The outlier payment amount determined by the Pricer to be due on the claim in addition to any HRG payment amounts. Added to the claim as a value code 17 amount.
418-426	9(7)V9(2)	TOTAL - PAYMENT	Output item: The total payment determined by the Pricer to be due on the claim.
427-435	S9(7)V9(2)	VBP-ADJ-AMT	Output item: The HHVBP adjustment amount, determined by subtracting the HHVBP adjustment total payment from the HH PPS payment that would otherwise apply to the claim. Added to the claim as a value code QV amount.
436-444	9(7)V9(2)	PPS-STD-VALUE	Output item: Standardized payment amount – the HH PPS payment without applying any provider-specific adjustments. Informational only. Subject to additional calculations before entered on the claim in PPS-STNDRD-VALUE field.
445-650	X(206)	FILLER	

Input records on RAPs will include all input items except for "REVENUE" related items. Input records on claims must include all input items. Output records will contain all input and output items. If an output item does not apply to a particular record, Pricer will return zeroes.

The Medicare claims processing system will move the following Pricer output items to the claim record. The return code will be placed in the claim header. The HRG-PAY amount for the HIPPS code will be placed in the total charges and the covered charges field of the revenue code 0023 line. The OUTLIER-PAYMENT amount, if any, will be placed in a value code 17 amount. If the return code is 06 (indicating a low utilization payment adjustment), the Medicare claims processing system will apportion the REVENUE-COST amounts to the appropriate line items in order for the per-visit payments to be accurately reflected on the remittance advice. If the return code is 14, the Medicare claims processing system will apply the H-HHA-REVENUE-ADD-ON-VISIT-AMT to the earliest line item with the corresponding revenue code.

100-04, 10, 90.1

Osteoporosis Injections as HHA Benefit

(Rev.2977, Issued; 06-20-14, Effective: 09-23-14; ICD-10: Upon Implementation of ICD-10)

A - Billing Requirements

The administration of the drug is included in the charge for the skilled nursing visit billed using TOB 032x. The cost of the drug is billed using TOB 034x, using revenue code 0636. Drugs that have the ingredient calcitonin are billed using HCPCS code J0630. Drugs that have the ingredient teriparatide may be billed using HCPCS code J3110, if all existing guidelines for coverage under the home health benefit are met. All other osteoporosis drugs that are FDA approved and are awaiting a HCPCS code must use the miscellaneous code of J3490 until a specific HCPCS code is approved for use.

HCPCS code J0630 is defined as up to 400 units. Therefore, the provider must calculate units for the bill as follows:

Units Furnished During Billing Period	Units of Service Entry on Bill
100-400	1
401-800	2
801-1200	3
1201-1600	4
1601-2000	5
2001-2400	6

HCPCS code J3110 is defined as 10 mcg. Providers should report 1 unit for each 10 mcg dose provided during the billing period.

These codes are paid on a reasonable cost basis, using the provider's submitted charges to make initial payments, which are subject to annual cost settlement.

Coverage requirements for osteoporosis drugs are found in Pub. 100-02, Medicare Benefit Policy Manual, chapter 7, section 50.4.3. Coverage requirements for the home health benefit in general are found in Pub. 100-02, Medicare Benefit Policy Manual, chapter 7, section 30.

B - Edits

Medicare system edits require that the date of service on a 034x claim for covered osteoporosis drugs falls within the start and end dates of an existing home health PPS episode. Once the system ensures the service dates on the 034x claim fall within an HH PPS episode that is open for the beneficiary on CWF, CWF edits to assure that the provider number on the 034x claim matches the provider number on the episode file. This is to reflect that although the osteoporosis drug is paid separately from the HH PPS episode rate it is included in consolidated billing requirements (see §10.1.25 regarding consolidated billing).

Claims are also edited to assure that if the claim is an HH claim (TOB 034x), the beneficiary is female and that the diagnosis code for post-menopausal osteoporosis is present.

100-04, 11, 10

Overview

(Rev.304, Issued: 09-24-04, Effective: 12-08-03, Implementation: 06-28-04)

Medicare beneficiaries entitled to hospital insurance (Part A) who have terminal illnesses and a life expectancy of six months or less have the option of electing hospice benefits in lieu of standard Medicare coverage for treatment and management of their terminal condition. Only care provided by a Medicare certified hospice is covered under the hospice benefit provisions.

Hospice care is available for two 90-day periods and an unlimited number of 60-day periods during the remainder of the hospice patient's lifetime. However, a beneficiary may voluntarily terminate his hospice election period. Election/termination dates are retained on CWF.

When hospice coverage is elected, the beneficiary waives all rights to Medicare Part B payments for services that are related to the treatment and management of his/her terminal illness during any period his/her hospice benefit election is in force, except for professional services of an attending physician, which may include a nurse practitioner. If the attending physician, who may be a nurse practitioner, is an

© 2019 Optum360, LLC

employee of the designated hospice, he or she may not receive compensation from the hospice for those services under Part B. These physician professional services are billed to Medicare Part A by the hospice.

To be covered, hospice services must be reasonable and necessary for the palliation or management of the terminal illness and related conditions. The individual must elect hospice care and a certification that the individual is terminally ill must be completed by the patient's attending physician (if there is one), and the Medical Director (or the physician member of the Interdisciplinary Group (IDG)). Nurse practitioners serving as the attending physician may not certify or re-certify the terminal illness. A plan of care must be established before services are provided. To be covered, services must be consistent with the plan of care. Certification of terminal illness is based on the physician's or medical director's clinical judgment regarding the normal course of an individual's illness. It should be noted that predicting life expectancy is not always exact.

See the Medicare Benefit Policy Manual, Chapter 9, for additional general information about the Hospice benefit.

See Chapter 29 of this manual for information on the appeals process that should be followed when an entity is dissatisfied with the determination made on a claim.

See Chapter 9 of the Medicare Benefit Policy Manual for hospice eligibility requirements and election of hospice care.

100-04, 11, 30.3

Data Required on the Institutional Claim to A/B MAC (HHH)

(Rev.4280, Issued: 04-19-2019, Effective: 07-21-19, Implementation: 07-21-19)

See Pub. 100-02, Medicare Benefit Policy Manual, chapter 9, for coverage requirements for Hospice benefits. This section addresses only claims submission. Before submitting claims, the hospice must submit a Notice of Election (NOE) to the A/B MAC (HHH). See section 20, of this chapter for information on NOE transaction types.

The Social Security Act at §1862 (a)(22) requires that all claims for Medicare payment must be submitted in an electronic form specified by the Secretary of Health and Human Services, unless an exception described at §1862 (h) applies. The electronic format required for billing hospice services is the ASC X12 837 institutional claim transaction.

Since the data structure of this transaction is difficult to express in narrative form and to provide assistance to small providers excepted from the electronic claim requirement, the instructions below are given relative to the data element names on the Form CMS-1450 hardcopy form. Each data element name is shown in bold type. Information regarding the form locator numbers that correspond to these data element names is found in Chapter 25.

Because claim formats serve the needs of many payers, some data elements may not be needed by a particular payer. Detailed information is given only for items required for Medicare hospice claims. Items not listed need not be completed although hospices may complete them when billing multiple payers.

Provider Name, Address, and Telephone Number
The hospice enters this information for their agency.

Type of Bill
The hospice enters on of the following Type of Bill codes:

081x – Hospice (non-hospital based)

082x – Hospice (hospital based)

4th Digit – Frequency	Definition
0 - Nonpayment/Zero Claims	Used when no payment from Medicare is anticipated.
I - Admit Through Discharge Claim	This code is used for a bill encompassing an entire course of hospice treatment for which the provider expects payment from the payer, i.e., no further bills will be submitted for this patient.
2 - Interim – First Claim	This code is used for the first of an expected series of payment bills for a hospice course of treatment.
3 - Interim - Continuing Claim	This code is used when a payment bill for a hospice course of treatment has already been submitted and further bills are expected to be submitted.
4 - Interim - Last Claim	This code is used for a payment bill that is the last of a series for a hospice course of treatment. The "Through" date of this bill is the discharge date, transfer date, or date of death.
7 - Replacement of Prior Claim	This code is used by the provider when it wants to correct a previously submitted bill. This is the code used on the corrected or "new" bill.
8 - Void/Cancel of a Prior Claim	This code is used to cancel a previously processed claim.

Statement Covers Period (From-Through)
The hospice shows the beginning and ending dates of the period covered by this bill in numeric fields (MM-DD-YY). The hospice does not show days before the patient's entitlement began.

Statement periods should follow the frequency of billing instructions in section 90.

Patient Name/Identifier
The hospice enters the beneficiary's name exactly as it appears on the Medicare card.

Patient Address

Patient Birth date

Patient Sex
The hospice enters the appropriate address, date of birth and gender information describing the beneficiary.

Admission/Start of Care Date
The hospice enters the admission date, which must be the same date as the effective date of the hospice election or change of election. The date of admission may not precede the physician's certification by more than 2 calendar days.

The admission date stays the same on all continuing claims for the same hospice election.

Patient Discharge Status
This code indicates the patient's status as of the "Through" date of the billing period. The hospice enters the most appropriate National Uniform Billing Committee (NUBC) approved code.

NOTE: that patient discharge status code 20 is not used on hospice claims. If the patient has died during the billing period, use codes 40, 41 or 42 as appropriate.

Medicare regulations at 42 CFR 418.26 define three reasons for discharge from hospice care:

1) The beneficiary moves out of the hospice's service area or transfers to another hospice,

2) The hospice determines that the beneficiary is no longer terminally ill or

3) The hospice determines the beneficiary meets their internal policy regarding discharge for cause.

Each of these discharge situations requires different coding on Medicare claims.

Reason 1: A beneficiary may move out of the hospice's service area either with, or without, a transfer to another hospice. In the case of a discharge when the beneficiary moves out of the hospice's service area without a transfer, the hospice uses the NUBC approved discharge status code that best describes the beneficiary's situation and appends condition code 52. The hospice does not report occurrence code 42 on their claim. This discharge claim will terminate the beneficiary's current hospice benefit period as of the "Through" date on the claim. The beneficiary may re-elect the hospice benefit at any time as long they remain eligible for the benefit.

In the case of a discharge when the beneficiary moves out of the hospice's service area and transfers to another hospice, the hospice uses discharge status code 50 or 51, depending on whether the beneficiary is transferring to home hospice or hospice in a medical facility. The hospice does not report occurrence code 42 on their claim. This discharge claim does not terminate the beneficiary's current hospice benefit period. The admitting hospice submits a transfer Notice of Election (type of bill 8xC) after the transfer has occurred and the beneficiary's hospice benefit is not affected.

Reason 2: In the case of a discharge when the hospice determines the beneficiary is no longer terminally ill, the hospice uses the NUBC approved discharge status code that best describes the beneficiary's situation. The hospice does not report occurrence code 42 on their claim. This discharge claim will terminate the beneficiary's current hospice benefit period as of the "Through" date on the claim.

Reason 3: In the case of a discharge for cause, the hospice uses the NUBC approved discharge status code that best describes the beneficiary's situation. The hospice does not report occurrence code 42 on their claim. Instead, the hospice reports condition code H2 to indicate a discharge for cause. The effect of this discharge claim on the beneficiary's current hospice benefit period depends on the discharge status.

If the beneficiary is transferred to another hospice (discharge status codes 50 or 51) the claim does not terminate the beneficiary's current hospice benefit period. The admitting hospice submits a transfer Notice of Election (type of bill 8xC) after the

© 2019 Optum360, LLC

transfer has occurred and the beneficiary's hospice benefit is not affected. If any other appropriate discharge status code is used, this discharge claim will terminate the beneficiary's current hospice benefit period as of the "Through" date on the claim. The beneficiary may re-elect the hospice benefit if they are certified as terminally ill and eligible for the benefit again in the future and are willing to be compliant with care.

If the beneficiary has chosen to revoke their hospice election, the provider uses the NUBC approved discharge patient status code and the occurrence code 42 indicating the date the beneficiary revoked the benefit. The beneficiary may re-elect the hospice benefit if they are certified as terminally ill and eligible for the benefit again in the future.

Discharge Reason	Coding Required in Addition to Patient Status Code
Beneficiary Moves Out of Service Area	Condition Code 52
Beneficiary Transfers Hospices	Patient Status Code 50 or 51; no other indicator
Beneficiary No Longer Terminally Ill	No other indicator
Beneficiary Discharged for Cause	Condition code H2
Beneficiary Revokes	Occurrence code 42

If a hospice beneficiary is discharged alive or if a hospice beneficiary revokes the election of hospice care, the hospice shall file a timely-filed Notice of Election Termination / Revocation (NOTR) using type of bill 8xB, unless it has already filed a final claim. A timely-filed NOTR is a NOTR that is submitted to the A/B MAC (HHH) and accepted by the A/B MAC (HHH) within 5 calendar days after the effective date of discharge or revocation. While a timely-filed NOTR is one that is submitted to and accepted by the A/B MAC (HHH) within 5 calendar days after the hospice election, posting to the CWF may not occur within that same timeframe. The date of posting to the CWF is not a reflection of whether the NOTR is considered timely-filed. A NOTR (type of bill 8xB) is entered via Direct Data Entry in the same way as an NOE (type of bill 8xA). Hospices continue to have 12 months from the date of service in which to file their claims timely.

A patient can also be admitted and discharged on the same day. They would submit an 8x1 Type of Bill ("Admission through Discharge Claim"), matching "From" and "Through" dates, and whatever the appropriate level of care the revenue code was, with 1 unit. A patient cannot be discharged and re-admitted to the same hospice on the same day.

Untimely Face-to-Face Encounters and Discharge

When a required face-to-face encounter occurs prior to, but no more than 30 calendar days prior to, the third benefit period recertification and every benefit period recertification thereafter, it is considered timely. A timely face-to-face encounter would be evident when examining the face-to-face attestation, which is part of the recertification, as that attestation includes the date of the encounter. While the face-to-face encounter itself must occur no more than 30 calendar days prior to the start of the third benefit period recertification and each subsequent recertification, its accompanying attestation must be completed before the claim is submitted.

If the required face-to-face encounter is not timely, the hospice would be unable to recertify the patient as being terminally ill, and the patient would cease to be eligible for the Medicare hospice benefit. In such instances, the hospice must discharge the patient from the Medicare hospice benefit because he or she is not considered terminally ill for Medicare purposes.

When a discharge from the Medicare hospice benefit occurs due to failure to perform a required face-to-face encounter timely, the claim should include the most appropriate patient discharge status code. Occurrence span code 77 does not apply when the face-to-face encounter has not occurred timely.

The hospice can re-admit the patient to the Medicare hospice benefit once the required encounter occurs, provided the patient continues to meet all of the eligibility requirements and the patient (or representative) files an election statement in accordance with CMS regulations. Where the only reason the patient ceases to be eligible for the Medicare hospice benefit is the hospice's failure to meet the face-to-face requirement, CMS would expect the hospice to continue to care for the patient at its own expense until the required encounter occurs, enabling the hospice to re-establish Medicare eligibility.

Condition Codes

The hospice enters any appropriate NUBC approved code(s) identifying conditions related to this bill that may affect processing.

Codes listed below are only those most frequently applicable to hospice claims. For a complete list of codes, see the NUBC manual.

07	Treatment of Non-terminal Condition for Hospice	Code indicates the patient has elected hospice care but the provider is not treating the terminal condition, and is, therefore, requesting regular Medicare payment.
20	Beneficiary Requested Billing	Code indicates the provider realizes the services on this bill are at a noncovered level of care or otherwise excluded from coverage, but the beneficiary has requested a formal determination.
21	Billing for Denial Notice	Code indicates the provider realizes services are at a noncovered level of care or excluded, but requests a denial notice from Medicare in order to bill Medicaid or other insurers.
H2	Discharge by a Hospice Provider for Cause	Discharge by a Hospice Provider for Cause. NOTE: Used by the provider to indicate the patient meets the hospice's documented policy addressing discharges for cause.
52	Out of Hospice Service Area	Code indicates the patient is discharged for moving out of the hospice service area. This can include patients who relocate or who go on vacation outside of the hospice's service area, or patients who are admitted to a hospital or SNF that does not have contractual arrangements with the hospice.
85	Delayed recertification of hospice terminal illness	Code indicates the hospice received the recertification of terminal illness later than 2 days after the first day of a new benefit period. This code is reported with occurrence span code 77, which reports the provider liable days associated with the untimely recertification.

Occurrence Codes and Dates

The hospice enters any appropriate NUBC approved code(s) and associated date(s) defining specific event(s) relating to this billing period. Event codes are two numeric digits, and dates are six numeric digits (MM-DD-YY). If there are more occurrences than there are spaces on the form, use the occurrence span code fields to record additional occurrences and dates.

Codes listed below are only those most frequently applicable to hospice claims. For a complete list of codes, see the NUBC manual.

Code	Title	Definition
23	Cancellation of Hospice Election Period (A/B MAC (HHH) USE ONLY)	Code indicates date on which a hospice period of election is cancelled by an A/B MAC (HHH) as opposed to revocation by the beneficiary.
24	Date Insurance Denied	Code indicates the date of receipt of a denial of coverage by a higher priority payer.
27	Date of Hospice Certification or Re-Certification	Code indicates the date of certification or re-certification of the hospice benefit period, beginning with the first 2 initial benefit periods of 90 days each and the subsequent 60-day benefit periods. NOTE: regarding transfers from one hospice to another hospice: If a patient is in the first certification period when they transfer to another hospice, the receiving hospice would use the same certification date as the previous hospice until the next certification period. However, if they were in the next certification at the time of transfer, then they would enter that date in the Occurrence Code 27 and date.

© 2019 Optum360, LLC

Code	Title	Definition
42	Date of Termination of Hospice Benefit	Enter code to indicate the date on which beneficiary terminated his/her election to receive hospice benefits. This code can be used only when the beneficiary has revoked the benefit. It is not used in transfer situations.
55	Beneficiary is Deceased	Report the appropriate NUBC discharge status code that best describes the place in which the beneficiary died (40, 41, or 42). Discharge status code 20 is not used on hospice claims.

Occurrence code 27 is required on the claim for the billing period in which the certification or re-certification was obtained. It may be optionally reported on other claims.

When the re-certification is late and not obtained during the month it was due, the occurrence span code 77 should be reported with the through date of the span code equal to the through date of the claim.

Occurrence Span Code and Dates

The hospice enters any appropriate NUBC approved code(s) and associated beginning and ending date(s) defining a specific event relating to this billing period are shown. Event codes are two alphanumeric digits and dates are shown numerically as MM-DD-YY.

Codes listed below are only those most frequently applicable to hospice claims. For a complete list of codes, see the NUBC manual.

Code	Title	Definition
M2	Dates of Inpatient Respite Care	Code indicates From/Through dates of a period of inpatient respite care for hospice patients to differentiate separate respite periods of less than 5 days each. M2 is used when respite care is provided more than once during a benefit period.
77	Provider Liability – Utilization Charged	Code indicates From/Through dates for a period of non-covered hospice care for which the provider accepts payment liability (other than for medical necessity or custodial care).

Respite care is payable only for periods of respite up to 5 consecutive days. Claims reporting respite periods greater than 5 consecutive days will be returned to the provider. Days of respite care beyond 5 days must be billed at the appropriate home care rate for payment consideration.

For example: If the patient enters a respite period on July 1 and is returned to routine home care on July 6, the units of respite reported on the line item would be 5 representing July 1 through July 5, July 6 is reported as a day of routine home care regardless of the time of day entering respite or returning to routine home care.

When there is more than one respite period in the billing period, the provider must include the M2 occurrence span code for all periods of respite. The individual respite periods reported shall not exceed 5 days, including consecutive respite periods.

For example: If the patient enters a respite period on July 1 and is returned to routine home care on July 6 and later returns to respite care from July 15 to July 18, and completes the month on routine home care, the provider must report two separate line items for the respite periods and two occurrence span code M2, as follows:

Revenue Line items:

- Revenue code 0655 with line item date of service 07/01/XX (for respite period July 1 through July 5) and line item units reported as 5
- Revenue code 0651 with line item date of service 07/06/XX (for routine home care July 6 through July 14) and line item units reported as 9
- Revenue code 0655 with line item date of service 07/15/XX (for respite period July 15 through 17th) and line item units reported as 3
- Revenue code 0651 with line item date of service 07/18/XX (for routine home care on date of discharge from respite through July 31 and line item units reported as 14.

Occurrence Span Codes:

- M2 0701XX – 07/05/XX
- M2 0715XX – 07/17/XX

Provider Liability Periods Using Occurrence Span Code 77: Hospices must use occurrence span code 77 to identify days of care that are not covered by Medicare due to:

- Untimely physician recertification. This is particularly important when the non-covered days fall at the beginning of a billing period other than the initial certification period.

Example:

A new benefit period begins on 6/14/20XX

The hospice is required to obtain the recertification (verbal or written) by 6/16/20XX.

The hospice obtains the recertification 6/19/20XX.

The hospice reports 6/14 – 6/18 as non-covered days using occurrence span code 77.

The hospice reports the date the certification was actually obtained, 6/19/20XX, in occurrence code 27.

Condition code 85 is only reported in this case because the certification was untimely.

- Late-filing of a Notice of Election (NOE). A timely-filed NOE is a NOE that is submitted to the A/B MAC (HHH) and accepted by the A/B MAC (HHH) within 5 calendar days after the hospice admission date. When the hospice files a NOE late, Medicare shall not cover and pay for the days of hospice care from the hospice admission date to the date the NOE is submitted to and accepted by the A/B MAC (HHH). The date the NOE is submitted to and accepted by the A/B MAC (HHH) is an allowable day for payment.

Example:

Admission date is 10/10/20XX (Fri).

Day 1 = Sat. 10/11/20XX

Day 2 = Sun. 10/12/20XX

Day 3 = Mon. 10/13/20XX

Day 4 = Tues. 10/14/20XX

Day 5 = Weds. 10/15/20XX 10/15/20XX is the NOE Due Date.

IF NOE Receipt date is 10/16/20XX, the hospice reports 10/10- 10/15 as non-covered days using occurrence span code 77 or Medicare systems return the claim to the provider for correction.

Value Codes and Amounts

The hospice enters any appropriate NUBC approved code(s) and the associated value amounts identifying numeric information related to this bill that may affect processing.

Provider-submitted codes:

The most commonly used value codes on hospice claims are value codes 61 and G8, which are used to report the location of the site of hospice services. Otherwise, value codes are commonly used only to indicate Medicare is secondary to another payer. For detailed information on reporting Medicare secondary payer information, see the Medicare Secondary Payer Manual.

Code	Title	Definition
61	Place of Residence where Service is Furnished (Routine Home Care and Continuous Home Care)	MSA or Core-Based Statistical Area (CBSA) number (or rural State code) of the location where the hospice service is delivered. A residence can be an inpatient facility if an individual uses that facility as a place of residence. It is the level of care that is required and not the location where hospice services are provided that determines payment. In other words, if an individual resides in a freestanding hospice facility and requires routine home care, then claims are submitted for routine home care. Hospices must report value code 61 when billing revenue codes 0651 and 0652.
G8	Facility where Inpatient Hospice Service is Delivered (General Inpatient and Inpatient Respite Care).	MSA or Core Based Statistical Area (CBSA) number (or rural State code) of the facility where inpatient hospice services are delivered. Hospices must report value code G8 when billing revenue codes 0655 and 0656.

© 2019 Optum360, LLC

Medicare-applied codes: The following codes are added during processing and may be visible in the A/B MAC (HHH)'s online claim history. They are never submitted by the hospice. Code

Code	Title	Definition
62	Number of High Routine Home Care Days	Days that fall within the first 60 days of a routine home care hospice claim. The Medicare system puts the high days returned by Pricer on the claim as a value code 62 amount.
63	Number of Low Routine Home Care Days	Days that come after the first 60 days of a routine home care hospice claim. The Medicare system puts the low days returned by Pricer on the claim as a value code 63 amount.

If hospice services are provided to the beneficiary in more than one CBSA area during the billing period, the hospice reports the CBSA that applies at the end of the billing period. For routine home care and continuous home care (e.g., the beneficiary's residence changes between locations in different CBSAs), report the CBSA of the beneficiary's residence at the end of the billing period. For general inpatient and inpatient respite care (e.g., the beneficiary is served in inpatient facilities in different CBSAs), report the CBSA of the latest facility that served the beneficiary. If the beneficiary receives both home and inpatient care during the billing period, the latest home CBSA is reported with value code 61 and the latest facility CBSA is reported with value code G8.

Revenue Codes

The hospice assigns a revenue code for each type of service provided and enters the appropriate four-digit numeric revenue code to explain each charge.

Hospice claims are required to report separate line items for the level of care each time the level of care changes. This includes revenue codes 0651, 0655 and 0656. For example, if a patient begins the month receiving routine home care followed by a period of general inpatient care and then later returns to routine home care all in the same month, in addition to the one line reporting the general inpatient care days, there should be two separate line items for routine home care. Each routine home care line reports a line item date of service to indicate the first date that level of care began for that consecutive period.

Code	Description	Standard Abbreviation
0651	Routine Home Care	RTN Home
0652	Continuous Home Care	CTNS Home A minimum of 8 hours of primarily nursing care within a 24-hour period. The 8-hours of care do not need to be continuous within the 24-hour period, but a need for an aggregate of 8 hours of primarily nursing care is required. Nursing care must be provided by a registered nurse or a licensed practical nurse. If skilled intervention is required for less than 8 aggregate hours (or less than 32 units) within a 24 hour period, then the care rendered would be covered as a routine home care day. Services provided by a nurse practitioner as the attending physician are not included in the CHC computation nor is care that is not directly related to the crisis included in the computation. CHC billing should reflect direct patient care during a period of crisis and should not reflect time related to staff working hours, time taken for meal breaks, time used for educating staff, time used to report etc.
0655**	Inpatient Respite Care	IP Respite
0656**	General Inpatient Care	GNL IP
0657	Physician Services	PHY SER (must be accompanied by a physician procedure code)

** The date of discharge from general inpatient or inpatient respite care is paid at the appropriate home care rate and must be billed with the appropriate home care revenue code unless the patient is deceased at time of discharge in which case, the appropriate inpatient respite or general inpatient care revenue code should be used.

NOTE: Hospices use revenue code 0657 to identify hospice charges for services furnished to patients *by physicians, nurse practitioners, or physician assistants employed by the hospice; or physicians, nurse practitioners or physician assistants* receiving compensation from the hospice. Procedure codes are required in order for the A/B MAC (HHH) to determine the reimbursement rate for the physician services. Appropriate procedure codes are available from the A/B MAC (HHH).

Additional revenue codes are reported describing the visits provided under each level of care.

To constitute a visit, the discipline, (as defined above) must have provided care to the beneficiary. Services provided by a social worker to the beneficiary's family also constitute a visit. For example, documentation in the medical/clinical record, interdisciplinary group meetings, obtaining physician orders, rounds in a facility or any other activity that is not related to the provision of items or services to a beneficiary, do not count towards a visit to be placed on the claim. During an initial or comprehensive assessment, it would not be best practice to wait until later (after the clinician has left the home) to document the findings of an assessment or the interventions provided during a patient visit. It is recommended that this information be documented as close to the time of the assessment or intervention as possible. In addition, the visit must be reasonable and necessary for the palliation and management of the terminal illness and related conditions as described in the patient's plan of care.

If a hospice patient is receiving routine home care while residing in a nursing home, the hospice would record visits for all of its physicians, nurses, social workers, and home health aides who visit the patient to provide care for the palliation and management of the terminal illness and related conditions, as described in the patient's plan of care. In this example the nursing home is acting as the patient's home. Only the patient care provided by the hospice staff constitutes a visit.

When making the determination as to whether or not a particular visit should be reported, a hospice should consider whether the visit would have been reported, and how it would have been reported, if the patient were receiving RHC in his or her private home. If a group of tasks would normally be performed in a single visit to a patient living in his or her private home, then the hospice should count the tasks as a single visit for the patient residing in a facility. Hospices should not record a visit every time a staff member enters the patient's room. Hospices should use clinical judgment in counting visits and summing time.

Hospices report social worker phone calls and all visits performed by hospice staff in 15 minute increments using the following revenue codes and associated HCPCS. This includes visits by hospice nurses, aides, social workers, physical therapists, occupational therapists, and speech-language pathologists

All visits to provide care related to the palliation and management of the terminal illness or related conditions, whether provided by hospice employees or provided under arrangement, must be reported. The two exceptions are related to General Inpatient Care and Respite care. CMS is not requiring hospices to report visit data at this time for visits made by non-hospice staff providing General Inpatient Care or respite care in contract facilities. However, General Inpatient Care or respite care visits related to the palliation and management of the terminal illness or related conditions provided by hospice staff in contract facilities must be reported, and all General Inpatient Care and respite care visits related to the palliation and management of the terminal illness or related conditions provided in hospice-owned facilities must be reported.

Social worker phone calls made to the patient or the patient's family should be reported using revenue code 0569, and HCPCS G-code G0155 for the length of the call, with each call being a separate line item. Only phone calls that are necessary for the palliation and management of the terminal illness and related conditions as described in the patient's plan of care (such as counseling or speaking with a patient's family or arranging for a placement) should be reported. Report only social worker phone calls related to providing and or coordinating care to the patient and family and documented as such in the clinical records.

When recording any visit or social worker phone call time, providers should sum the time for each visit or call, rounding to the nearest 15 minute increment. Providers should not include travel time or documentation time in the time recorded for any visit or call. Additionally, hospices may not include interdisciplinary group time in time and visit reporting.

For dates of service before October 1, 2018, Hospice agencies shall report injectable and non-injectable prescription drugs for the palliation and management of the terminal illness and related conditions on their claims. Both injectable and non-injectable prescription drugs shall be reported on claims on a line-item basis per fill, based on the amount dispensed by the pharmacy.

When a facility (hospital, SNF, NF, or hospice inpatient facility) uses a medication management system where each administration of a hospice medication is

© 2019 Optum360, LLC

considered a fill for hospice patients receiving care, the hospice shall report a monthly total for each drug (i.e., report a total for the period covered by the claim), along with the total dispensed.

Hospices shall report multi-ingredient compound prescription drugs (non-injectable) using revenue code 0250. The hospice shall specify the same prescription number for each ingredient of a compound drug according to the 837i guidelines in loop 2410. In addition, the hospice shall provide the NDC for each ingredient in the compound; the NDC qualifier represents the quantity of the drug filled (meaning the amount dispensed) and shall be reported as the unit measure.

When reporting prescription drugs in a comfort kit/pack, the hospice shall report the NDC of each prescription drug within the package, in accordance with the procedures for non-injectable prescriptions.

Hospice agencies shall report infusion pumps (a type of DME) on a line-item basis for each pump and for each medication fill and refill. The hospice claim shall reflect the total charge for the infusion pump for the period covered by the claim, whether the hospice is billed for it daily, weekly, biweekly, with each

medication refill, or in some other fashion. The hospice shall include on the claim the infusion pump charges on whatever basis is easiest for its billing systems, so long as in total, the claim reflects the charges for the pump for the time period of that claim.

Effective for dates of service on and after 10/1/2018, hospices are no longer required to report drugs using line item detail. Hospices may report summary charges for drugs as shown in the table below.

Hospices must enter the following visit revenue codes, when applicable:

Revenue Code	Required HCPCS	Required Detail
0250 Non-injectable Prescription Drugs	N/A	Required detail: Report on a line-item basis per fill, using revenue code 0250 and the National Drug Code (NDC). The NDC qualifier represents the quantity of the drug filled, and should be reported as the unit measure. For dates of service on and after 10/1/2018: Report a monthly charge total for all drugs (i.e., report a total charge amount for the period covered by the claim) using revenue code 0250.
029X Infusion pumps	Applicable HCPCS N/A	Required detail: Report on the claim on a line-item basis per pump order and per medication refill, using revenue code 029X for the equipment and 0294 for the drugs along with the appropriate HCPCS. For dates of service on and after 10/1/18: Report a monthly charge total for infusion DME (i.e., report a total charge amount for the period covered by the claim), including DME infusion drugs, using revenue center 029X for the infusion pumps and 0294 for DME infusion drugs.
042x Physical Therapy	G0151	Required detail: Each visit is identified on a separate line item with the appropriate line item date of service and a charge amount. The units reported on the claim are the multiplier for the total time of the visit defined in the HCPCS description.
043x Occupational Therapy	G0152	Required detail: Each visit is identified on a separate line item with the appropriate line item date of service and a charge amount. The units reported on the claim are the multiplier for the total time of the visit defined in the HCPCS description.
044x Speech Therapy – Language Pathology	G0153	Required detail: Each visit is identified on a separate line item with the appropriate line item date of service and a charge amount. The units reported on the claim are the multiplier for the total time of the visit defined in the HCPCS description.
055x Skilled Nursing	G0154 (before 01/01/2016) G0299 or G0300 (on or after 01/01/2016)	Required detail: Each visit is identified on a separate line item with the appropriate line item date of service and a charge amount. The units reported on the claim are the multiplier for the total time of the visit defined in the HCPCS description.
056x Medical Social Services	G0155	Required detail: Each visit is identified on a separate line item with the appropriate line item date of service and a charge amount. The units reported on the claim are the multiplier for the total time of the visit defined in the HCPCS description.
0569 Other Medical Social Services	G0155	Required detail: Each social service phone call is identified on a separate line item with the appropriate line item date of service and a charge amount. The units reported on the claim are the multiplier for the total time of the call defined in the HCPCS description.
057x Aide	G0156	Required detail: Each visit is identified on a separate line item with the appropriate line item date of service and a charge amount. The units reported on the claim are the multiplier the total time of the visit defined in the HCPCS description.
0636 Injectable Drugs	Applicable HCPCS	Required detail: Report on a line item basis per fill with units representing the amount filled. (i.e., Q1234 Drug 100mg and the fill was for 200 mg, units reported = 2). For dates of service on and after 10/1/2018: Revenue code 0636 is not required.

Visits by registered nurses, licensed vocational nurses and nurse practitioners (unless the nurse practitioner is acting as the beneficiary's attending physician) are reported under revenue code 055x.

Charges associated with the reported visits are covered under the hospice bundled payment and reflected in the payment for the level of care billed on the claim. No additional payment is made on the visit revenue lines.

The contractor shall use the following remittance advice messages and associated codes when bundling line items under this policy. This CARC/RARC combination is compliant with CAQH CORE Business Scenario Four.

Group Code: CO
CARC: 97
RARC: N/A
MSN: N/A

Effective January 1, 2016, Medicare requires hospices to use G0299 for "direct skilled nursing services of a registered nurse (RN) in the home health or hospice setting" and G0300 "direct skilled nursing of a licensed practical nurse (LPN) in the home health or hospice setting." G0154 is retired as of 12/31/2015.

Hospices should report in the unit field on the line level the units as a multiplier of the visit time defined in the HCPCS description.

HCPCS/Accommodation Rates/HIPPS Rate Codes

Hospices must report a HCPCS code along with each level of care revenue code (651, 652, 655 and 656) to identify the type of service location where that level of care was provided.

The following HCPCS codes will be used to report the type of service location for hospice services:

HCPCS Code	Definition
Q5001	HOSPICE CARE PROVIDED IN PATIENT'S HOME/RESIDENCE
Q5002	HOSPICE CARE PROVIDED IN ASSISTED LIVING FACILITY
Q5003	HOSPICE CARE PROVIDED IN NURSING LONG TERM CARE FACILITY (LTC) OR NON-SKILLED NURSING FACILITY (NF)
Q5004	HOSPICE CARE PROVIDED IN SKILLED NURSING FACILITY (SNF)

© 2019 Optum360, LLC

HCPCS Code	Definition
Q5005	HOSPICE CARE PROVIDED IN INPATIENT HOSPITAL
Q5006	HOSPICE CARE PROVIDED IN INPATIENT HOSPICE FACILITY
Q5007	HOSPICE CARE PROVIDED IN LONG TERM CARE HOSPITAL (LTCH)
Q5008	HOSPICE CARE PROVIDED IN INPATIENT PSYCHIATRIC FACILITY
Q5009	HOSPICE CARE PROVIDED IN PLACE NOT OTHERWISE SPECIFIED (NOS)
Q5010	Hospice home care provided in a hospice facility

If care is rendered at multiple locations, each location is to be identified on the claim with a corresponding HCPCS code. For example, routine home care may be provided for a portion of the billing period in the patient's residence and another portion in an assisted living facility. In this case, report one revenue code 651 line with HCPCS code Q5001 and the number of days of routine home care provided in the residence and another revenue code 651 line with HCPCS code Q5002 and the number of days of routine home care provided in the assisted living facility.

Q5004 shall be used for hospice patients in a skilled nursing facility (SNF), or hospice patients in the SNF portion of a dually-certified nursing facility. There are 4 situations where this would occur:

1) If the beneficiary is receiving hospice care in a solely-certified SNF.
2) If the beneficiary is receiving general inpatient care in the SNF.
3) If the beneficiary is in a SNF receiving SNF care under the Medicare SNF benefit for a condition unrelated to the terminal illness and related conditions, and is receiving hospice routine home care; this is uncommon.
4) If the beneficiary is receiving inpatient respite care in a SNF.

If a beneficiary is in a nursing facility but doesn't meet the criteria above for Q5004, the site shall be coded as Q5003, for a long term care nursing facility.

General inpatient care provided by hospice staff requires line item visit reporting in units of 15 minute increments when provided in the following sites of service: Skilled Nursing Facility (Q5004), Inpatient Hospital (Q5005), Long Term Care Hospital (Q5007), Inpatient Psychiatric Facility (Q5008).

These service location HCPCS codes are not required on revenue code lines describing the visits provided under each level of care. These lines report the HCPCS codes shown in the table under Revenue Codes.

Modifiers

The following modifier is required reporting for claims:

PM – Post-mortem visits. Hospices shall report visits and length of visits (rounded to the nearest 15 minute increment), for nurses, aides, social workers, and therapists who are employed by the hospice, that occur on the date of death, after the patient has passed away. Post mortem visits occurring on a date subsequent to the date of death are not to be reported. The reporting of post-mortem visits, on the date of death, should occur regardless of the patient's level of care or site of service. Date of death is defined as the date of death reported on the death certificate. Hospices shall report hospice visits that occur before death on a separate line from those which occur after death.

For example, assume that a nurse arrives at the home at 9 pm to provide routine home care (RHC) to a dying patient, and that the patient passes away at 11 pm. The nurse stays with the family until 1:30 am. The hospice should report a nursing visit with eight 15-minute time units for the visit from 9 pm to 11 pm. On a separate line, the hospice should report a nursing visit with a PM modifier with four 15-minute time units for the portion of the visit from 11 pm to midnight to account for the 1 hour post mortem visit.

If the patient passes away suddenly, and the hospice nurse does not arrive until after his death at 11:00 pm, and remains with the family until 1:30 am, then the hospice should report a line item nursing visit with a PM modifier and four 15-minute increments of time as the units to account for the 1 hour post mortem visit from 11:00 pm to midnight.

The following modifier may be used to identify requests for an exception to the consequences of not filing the NOE timely:

KX - Even if a hospice believes that exceptional circumstances beyond its control are the cause of its late-filed NOE, the hospice shall file the associated claim with occurrence span code 77 used to identify the non-covered, provider liable days. The hospice shall also report a KX modifier with the Q HCPCS code reported on the earliest dated level of care line on the claim. The KX modifier shall prompt the A/B MAC (HHH) to request the documentation supporting the request for an exception. Based on that documentation, the A/B MAC (HHH) shall determine if a circumstance encountered by a hospice qualifies for an exception.

If the request for an exception is approved by the A/B MAC (HHH), the A/B MAC (HHH) shall process the claim with the CWF override code and remove the submitted provider liable days, which will allow payment for the days associated with the late-filed NOE. If the A/B MAC (HHH) finds that the documentation does not support allowing an exceptional circumstance, the A/B MAC (HHH) shall process the claim as submitted.

The contractor shall use the following remittance advice messages and associated codes under this policy. This CARC/RARC combination is compliant with CAQH CORE Business Scenario Three

Group Code: CO
CARC: 96
RARC: MA54
MSN: N/A

Hospices may appeal the contractor's determination that an exceptional circumstance did not apply.

Modifier GV may be used to identify attending physician services performed by a *doctor of medicine, doctor of osteopathy,* nurse practitioner *or physician assistant.*

Service Date

The HIPAA standard 837 Institutional claim format requires line item dates of service for all outpatient claims. Medicare classifies hospice claims as outpatient claims (see Chapter 1, §60.4).

Service date reporting requirements will vary between continuous home care lines (revenue code 652) and other revenue code lines.

Revenue code 652 – report a separately dated line item for each day that continuous home care is provided, reporting the number of hours, or parts of hours rounded to 15-minute increments, of continuous home care that was provided on that date.

Other level of care revenue codes – report a separate line for each level of care provided at each service location type, as described in the instructions for HCPCS coding reported above. Hospices report the earliest date that each level of care was provided at each service location. Attending physician services should be individually dated, reporting the date that each HCPCS code billed was delivered.

Service reporting revenue codes – report dates as described in the table above under Revenue Codes.

For service visits that begin in one calendar day and span into the next calendar day, report one visit using the date the visit ended as the service date.

Service Units

The hospice enters the number of units for each type of service. Units are measured in days for revenue codes 651, 655, and 656. , Units for revenue code 652 are reported in 15-minute increments.

When days are non-covered due to not filing a timely NOE, the hospice reports two lines for the affected level of care. For example, if a billing period contains 31 days of routine home care and the first 5 days are non-covered due to not filing a timely NOE:

- The hospice reports one revenue code 0651 line containing the earliest non-covered date of service, 5 units and all non-covered charges
- The hospice reports a second revenue code 0651 line containing the first covered date of service, 26 units and all covered charges.
- Report units for service reporting lines as a multiplier of the visit time defined in the HCPCS description.

For dates of service on and after 10/1/2018, units for summary drug charges lines may be reported using '1' to satisfy the required field or using a number of drugs provided during the billing period, at the option of the hospice. Service unit data will not be used by Medicare for payment or data analysis.

Total Charges

The hospice enters the total charge for the service described on each revenue code line. This information is being collected for purposes of research and will not affect the amount of reimbursement.

Non-Covered Charges

The hospice enters a charge amount equal to the Total Charges for any revenue code line with a Service Date within a non-covered period (e.g., an occurrence span code 77 period).

Payer Name

The hospice identifies the appropriate payer(s) for the claim.

National Provider Identifier – Billing Provider

The hospice enters its own National Provider Identifier (NPI).

Principal Diagnosis Code

The hospice enters diagnosis coding as required by ICD-9-CM / ICD-10-CM Coding Guidelines.

© 2019 Optum360, LLC

CMS accepts only HIPAA approved ICD-9-CM or ICD-10-CM/ICD-10-PCS codes, depending on the date of service. The official ICD-9-CM codes, which were updated annually through October 1, 2013, are posted at http://www.cms.gov/Medicare/Coding/ICD9ProviderDiagnosticCodes/codes.html

The official annual updates to ICD-10-CM and ICD-10-PCS codes are posted at http://www.cms.gov/Medicare/Coding/ICD10/index.html.

Use full diagnosis codes including all applicable digits, up to five digits for ICD-9-CM and up to seven digits for ICD-10-CM.

The principal diagnosis listed is the diagnosis most contributory to the terminal prognosis.

Non-reportable Principal Diagnosis Codes to be returned to the provider for correction:

- Hospices may not report ICD-9CM v-codes and ICD-10-CM z-codes as the principal diagnosis on hospice claims.
- Hospices may not report debility, failure to thrive, or dementia codes classified as unspecified as principal hospice diagnoses on the hospice claim.
- Hospices may not report diagnosis codes that cannot be used as the principal diagnosis according to ICD-9-CM or ICD-10-CM Coding Guidelines or require further compliance with various ICD-9-CM or ICD-10-CM coding conventions, such as those that have principal diagnosis code sequencing guidelines.

Other Diagnosis Codes

The hospice enters diagnosis coding as required by ICD-9-CM and ICD-10-CM Coding Guidelines. Hospices will report all diagnoses identified in the initial and comprehensive assessments on hospice claims, whether related or unrelated to the terminal prognosis of the individual effective October 1, 2015. This will also include the reporting of any mental health disorders and conditions that would affect the plan of care.

Attending Provider Name and Identifiers

The hospice enters the National Provider Identifier (NPI) and name of the physician currently responsible for certifying the terminal illness, and signing the individual's plan of care for medical care and treatment.

The hospice shall enter the NPI and name of the attending physician designated by the patient as having the most significant role in the determination and delivery of the patient's medical care. If there is no attending physician listed, then the hospice shall report the certifying MD.

Other Provider Name and Identifiers

If the attending physician is a nurse practitioner *or physician assistant*, the hospice enters the NPI and name of the nurse practitioner *or physician assistant.*

The hospice enters the NPI and name of the hospice physician responsible for certifying that the patient is terminally ill, with a life expectancy of 6 months or less if the disease runs its normal course. Note: Both the attending physician and other physician fields should be completed unless the patient's designated attending physician is the same as the physician certifying the terminal illness. When the attending physician is also the physician certifying the terminal illness, only the attending physician is required to be reported.

NOTE: for electronic claims, this information is reported in Loop ID 2310F – Referring Provider Name.

Hospices shall report the NPI of any nursing facility, hospital, or hospice inpatient facility where the patient is receiving hospice services, regardless of the level of care provided when the site of service is not the billing hospice. The billing hospice shall obtain the NPI for the facility where the patient is receiving care and report the facility's name, address and NPI on the 837 Institutional claim format in loop 2310 E Service Facility Location. When the patient has received care in more than one facility during the billing month, the hospice shall report the NPI of the facility where the patient was last treated. Failure to report this information for claims reporting place of service HCPCS Q5003 (long term care nursing facility), Q5004 (skilled nursing facility), Q5005 (inpatient hospital), Q5007 (long term care hospital) and Q5008 (inpatient psychiatric facility) will result in the claim being returned to the provider.

100-04, 11, 100.1

Billing for Denial of Hospice Room and Board Charges

(Rev.2410, Issued: 02-03-12, Effective: 07-01-12, Implementation: 07-02-12)

Hospice providers wishing to receive a line item denial for room and board charges may submit the charges as non-covered using revenue code 0659 with HCPCS A9270 and modifier GY on an otherwise covered hospice claim.

100-04, 12, 30.6.15.4

Power Mobility Devices (PMDs) (Code G0372)

(Rev.748, Issued: 11-04-05; Effective/Implementation Dates: 10-25-05)

Section 302(a)(2)(E)(iv) of the Medicare Prescription Drug, Improvement, and Modernization Act of 2003 (MMA) sets forth revised conditions for Medicare payment of Power Mobility Devices (PMDs). This section of the MMA states that payment for motorized or power wheelchairs may not be made unless a physician (as defined in §1861(r)(1) of the Act), a physician assistant, nurse practitioner, or a clinical nurse specialist (as those terms are defined in §1861(aa)(5)) has conducted a face-to-face examination of the beneficiary and written a prescription for the PMD.

Payment for the history and physical examination will be made through the appropriate evaluation and management (E&M) code corresponding to the history and physical examination of the patient. Due to the MMA requirement that the physician or treating practitioner create a written prescription and a regulatory requirement that the physician or treating practitioner prepare pertinent parts of the medical record for submission to the durable medical equipment supplier, code G0372 (physician service required to establish and document the need for a power mobility device)has been established to recognize additional physician services and resources required to establish and document the need for the PMD.

The G code indicates that all of the information necessary to document the PMD prescription is included in the medical record, and the prescription and supporting documentation is delivered to the PMD supplier within 30 days after the face-to-face examination.

Effective October 25, 2005, G0372 will be used to recognize additional physician services and resources required to establish and document the need for the PMD and will be added to the Medicare physician fee schedule.

100-04, 12, 100.1.1

Evaluation and Management (E/M) Services

(Rev.4283, Issued: 04- 26-19, Effective: 01-01-19, 07-29-19)

A. General Documentation *Requirements*

Evaluation and Management (E/M) Services -- For a given encounter, the selection of the appropriate level of E/M service should be determined according to the code definitions in the American Medical Association's Current Procedural Terminology (CPT) *book* and any applicable documentation guidelines.

For purposes of payment, E/M services billed by teaching physicians require that *the medical records must demonstrate:*

- That the *teaching physician* performed the service or *was* physically present during the key or critical portions of the service when performed by the resident; and
- The participation of the teaching physician in the management of the patient.

The presence of the teaching physician during E/M services may be demonstrated by the notes in the medical records made by physicians, residents, or nurses.

B. E/M Service Documentation Provided By Students

Any contribution and participation of *students* to the performance of a billable service (other than the review of systems and/or past family/social history which are not separately billable, but are taken as part of an E/M service) must be performed in the physical presence of a teaching physician or physical presence of a resident in a service meeting the requirements set forth in this section for teaching physician billing.

Students may document services in the medical record. However, the teaching physician must verify in the medical record all student documentation or findings, including history, physical exam and/or medical decision making. The teaching physician must personally perform (or re-perform) the physical exam and medical decision making activities of the E/M service being billed, but may verify any student documentation of them in the medical record, rather than re-documenting this work.

C. Exception for E/M Services Furnished in Certain Primary CareCenters

Teaching physicians providing E/M services with a GME program granted a primary care exception may bill Medicare for lower and mid-level E/M services provided by residents. For the E/M codes listed below, teaching physicians may submit claims for services furnished by residents in the absence of a teaching physician:

New Patient	Established Patient
99201	99211
99202	99212
99203	99213

© 2019 Optum360, LLC

Effective January 1, 2005, the following code is included under the primary care exception: HCPCS code G0402 (Initial preventive physical examination; face-to-face visit services limited to new beneficiary during the first 12 months of Medicare enrollment).

Effective January 1, 2011, the following codes are included under the primary care exception: HCPCS codes G0438 (Annual wellness visit, including personal preventive plan service, first visit) and G0439 (Annual wellness visit, including personal preventive plan service, subsequent visit).

If a service other than those listed above needs to be furnished, then the general teaching physician policy set forth in §100.1 applies. For this exception to apply, a center must attest in writing that all the following conditions are met for a particular residency program. Prior approval is not necessary, but centers exercising the primary care exception must maintain records demonstrating that they qualify for the exception.

The services must be furnished in a center located in the outpatient department of a hospital or another ambulatory care entity in which the time spent by residents in patient care activities is included in determining direct GME payments to a teaching hospital by the hospital's A/B MAC (A). This requirement is not met when the resident is assigned to a physician's office away from the center or makes home visits. In the case of a nonhospital entity, verify with the A/B MAC (A) that the entity meets the requirements of a written agreement between the hospital and the entity set forth at 42 CFR 413.78(e)(3)(ii).

Under this exception, residents providing the billable patient care service without the physical presence of a teaching physician must have completed at least 6 months of a GME approved residency program. Centers must maintain information under the provisions at 42 CFR 413.79(a)(6).

Teaching physicians submitting claims under this exception may not supervise more than four residents at any given time and must direct the care from such proximity as to constitute immediate availability. Teaching physicians may include residents with less than 6 months in a GME approved residency program in the mix of four residents under the teaching physician's supervision. However, the teaching physician must be physically present for the critical or key portions of services furnished by the residents with less than 6 months in a GME approved residency program. That is, the primary care exception does not apply in the case of residents with less than 6 months in a GME approved residency program.

Teaching physicians submitting claims under this exception must:

- Not have other responsibilities (including the supervision of other personnel) at the time the service was provided by the *residents*;
- Have the primary medical responsibility for patients cared for by the residents;
- Ensure that the care provided was reasonable and necessary;
- Review the care provided by the *residents* during or immediately after each visit. This must include a review of the patient's medical history, the resident's findings on physical examination, the patient's diagnosis, and treatment plan (i.e., record of tests and therapies); and

Patients under this exception should consider the center to be their primary location for health care services. The residents must be expected to generally provide care to the same group of established patients during their residency training. The types of services furnished by residents under this exception include:

- Acute care for undifferentiated problems or chronic care for ongoing conditions including chronic mental illness;
- Coordination of care furnished by other physicians and providers; and,
- Comprehensive care not limited by organ system or diagnosis.

Residency programs most likely qualifying for this exception include family practice, general internal medicine, geriatric medicine, pediatrics, and obstetrics/gynecology.

Certain GME programs in psychiatry may qualify in special situations such as when the program furnishes comprehensive care for chronically mentally ill patients. These would be centers in which the range of services the residents are trained to furnish, and actually do furnish, include comprehensive medical care as well as psychiatric care. For example, antibiotics are being prescribed as well as psychotropic drugs.

The patient medical record must document the extent of the teaching physician's participation in the review and direction of the services furnished to each beneficiary. The extent of the teaching physician's participation may be demonstrated by the notes in the medical records made by physicians, residents, or nurses.

100-04, 12, 180

Care Plan Oversight Services

(Rev.999, Issued: 07-14-06; Effective: 01-01-05; Implementation: 10-02-06)

The Medicare Benefit Policy Manual, Chapter 15, contains requirements for coverage for medical and other health services including those of physicians and non-physician practitioners.

Care plan oversight (CPO) is the physician supervision of a patient receiving complex and/or multidisciplinary care as part of Medicare-covered services provided by a participating home health agency or Medicare approved hospice.

CPO services require complex or multidisciplinary care modalities involving: Regular physician development and/or revision of care plans; Review of subsequent reports of patient status; Review of related laboratory and other studies; Communication with other health professionals not employed in the same practice who are involved in the patient's care; Integration of new information into the medical treatment plan; and/or Adjustment of medical therapy.

The CPO services require recurrent physician supervision of a patient involving 30 or more minutes of the physician's time per month. Services not countable toward the 30 minutes threshold that must be provided in order to bill for CPO include, but are not limited to: Time associated with discussions with the patient, his or her family or friends to adjust medication or treatment; Time spent by staff getting or filing charts; Travel time; and/or Physician's time spent telephoning prescriptions into the pharmacist unless the telephone conversation involves discussions of pharmaceutical therapies.

Implicit in the concept of CPO is the expectation that the physician has coordinated an aspect of the patient's care with the home health agency or hospice during the month for which CPO services were billed. The physician who bills for CPO must be the same physician who signs the plan of care.

Nurse practitioners, physician assistants, and clinical nurse specialists, practicing within the scope of State law, may bill for care plan oversight. These non-physician practitioners must have been providing ongoing care for the beneficiary through evaluation and management services. These non-physician practitioners may not bill for CPO if they have been involved only with the delivery of the Medicare-covered home health or hospice service.

A. Home Health CPO

Non-physician practitioners can perform CPO only if the physician signing the plan of care provides regular ongoing care under the same plan of care as does the NPP billing for CPO and either: The physician and NPP are part of the same group practice; or If the NPP is a nurse practitioner or clinical nurse specialist, the physician signing the plan of care also has a collaborative agreement with the NPP; or If the NPP is a physician assistant, the physician signing the plan of care is also the physician who provides general supervision of physician assistant services for the practice.

Billing may be made for care plan oversight services furnished by an NPP when: The NPP providing the care plan oversight has seen and examined the patient; The NPP providing care plan oversight is not functioning as a consultant whose participation is limited to a single medical condition rather than multidisciplinary coordination of care; and The NPP providing care plan oversight integrates his or her care with that of the physician who signed the plan of care.

NPPs may not certify the beneficiary for home health care.

B. Hospice CPO

The attending physician or nurse practitioner (who has been designated as the attending physician) may bill for hospice CPO when they are acting as an "attending physician".

An "attending physician" is one who has been identified by the individual, at the time he/she elects hospice coverage, as having the most significant role in the determination and delivery of their medical care. They are not employed nor paid by the hospice. The care plan oversight services are billed using Form CMS-1500 or electronic equivalent.

For additional information on hospice CPO, see Chapter 11, 40.1.3.1 of this manual.

100-04, 12, 180.1

Care Plan Oversight Billing Requirements

(Rev.999, Issued: 07-14-06; Effective: 01-01-05; Implementation: 10-02-06)

A. Codes for Which Separate Payment May Be Made

Effective January 1, 1995, separate payment may be made for CPO oversight services for 30 minutes or more if the requirements specified in the Medicare Benefits Policy Manual, Chapter 15 are met.

Providers billing for CPO must submit the claim with no other services billed on that claim and may bill only after the end of the month in which the CPO services were

© 2019 Optum360, LLC

rendered. CPO services may not be billed across calendar months and should be submitted (and paid) only for one unit of service.

Physicians may bill and be paid separately for CPO services only if all the criteria in the Medicare Benefit Policy Manual, Chapter 15 are met.

B. Physician Certification and Recertification of Home Health Plans of Care
Effective 2001, two new HCPCS codes for the certification and recertification and development of plans of care for Medicare-covered home health services were created.

See the Medicare General Information, Eligibility, and Entitlement Manual, Pub. 100-01, Chapter 4, "Physician Certification and Recertification of Services," 10-60, and the Medicare Benefit Policy Manual, Pub. 100-02, Chapter 7, "Home Health Services", 30.

The home health agency certification code can be billed only when the patient has not received Medicare-covered home health services for at least 60 days. The home health agency recertification code is used after a patient has received services for at least 60 days (or one certification period) when the physician signs the certification after the initial certification period. The home health agency recertification code will be reported only once every 60 days, except in the rare situation when the patient starts a new episode before 60 days elapses and requires a new plan of care to start a new episode.

C. Provider Number of Home Health Agency (HHA) or Hospice
For claims for CPO submitted on or after January 1, 1997, physicians must enter on the Medicare claim form the 6-character Medicare provider number of the HHA or hospice providing Medicare-covered services to the beneficiary for the period during which CPO services was furnished and for which the physician signed the plan of care. Physicians are responsible for obtaining the HHA or hospice Medicare provider numbers.

Additionally, physicians should provide their UPIN to the HHA or hospice furnishing services to their patient.

NOTE: There is currently no place on the HIPAA standard ASC X12N 837 professional format to specifically include the HHA or hospice provider number required for a care plan oversight claim. For this reason, the requirement to include the HHA or hospice provider number on a care plan oversight claim is temporarily waived until a new version of this electronic standard format is adopted under HIPAA and includes a place to provide the HHA and hospice provider numbers for care plan oversight claims.

100-04, 12, 190.3

List of Medicare Telehealth Services

(Rev.3476, Issued: 03-11-16, Effective: 01-01-15, Effective: 04-11-16)

The use of a telecommunications system may substitute for an in-person encounter for professional consultations, office visits, office psychiatry services, and a limited number of other physician fee schedule (PFS) services. The various services and corresponding current procedure terminology (CPT) or Healthcare Common Procedure Coding System (HCPCS) codes are listed below.

- Consultations (CPT codes 99241 - 99275) - Effective October 1, 2001 – December 31, 2005;
- Consultations (CPT codes 99241 - 99255) - Effective January 1, 2006 – December 31, 2009;
- Telehealth consultations, emergency department or initial inpatient (HCPCS codes G0425 – G0427) - Effective January 1, 2010;
- Follow-up inpatient telehealth consultations (HCPCS codes G0406, G0407, and G0408) - Effective January 1, 2009;
- Office or other outpatient visits (CPT codes 99201 - 99215);
- Subsequent hospital care services, with the limitation of one telehealth visit every 3 days (CPT codes 99231, 99232, and 99233) – Effective January 1, 2011;
- Subsequent nursing facility care services, with the limitation of one telehealth visit every 30 days (CPT codes 99307, 99308, 99309, and 99310) – Effective January 1, 2011;
- Pharmacologic management (CPT code 90862) – Effective March 1, 2003 – December 31, 2012;
- Individual psychotherapy (CPT codes 90804 - 90809); Psychiatric diagnostic interview examination (CPT code 90801) – Effective March 1, 2003 – December 31, 2012;
- Individual psychotherapy (CPT codes 90832 – 90834, 90836 – 90838); Psychiatric diagnostic interview examination (CPT codes 90791 -- 90792) – Effective January 1, 2013.
- Neurobehavioral status exam (CPT code 96116) - Effective January 1, 2008;
- End Stage Renal Disease (ESRD) related services (HCPCS codes G0308, G0309, G0311, G0312, G0314, G0315, G0317, and G0318) – Effective January 1, 2005 – December 31, 2008;
- End Stage Renal Disease (ESRD) related services (CPT codes 90951, 90952, 90954, 90955, 90957, 90958, 90960, and 90961) – Effective January 1, 2009;
- Individual and group medical nutrition therapy (HCPCS codes G0270, 97802, 97803, and 97804) – Individual effective January 1, 2006; group effective January 1, 2011;
- Individual and group health and behavior assessment and intervention (CPT codes 96150 – 96154) – Individual effective January 1, 2010; group effective January 1, 2011.
- Individual and group kidney disease education (KDE) services (HCPCS codes G0420 and G0421) – Effective January 1, 2011; and
- Individual and group diabetes self-management training (DSMT) services, with a minimum of 1 hour of in-person instruction to be furnished in the initial year training period to ensure effective injection training (HCPCS codes G0108 and G0109) - Effective January 1, 2011.
- Smoking Cessation Services (CPT codes 99406 and 99407and HCPCS codes G0436 and G0437) – Effective January 1, 2012.
- Alcohol and/or substance (other than tobacco) abuse structured assessment and intervention services (HCPCS codes G0396 and G0397) – Effective January 1, 2013.
- Annual alcohol misuse screening (HCPCS code G0442) – Effective January 1, 2013.
- Brief face-to-face behavioral counseling for alcohol misuse (HCPCS code G0443) – Effective January 1, 2013.
- Annual Depression Screening (HCPCS code G0444) – Effective January 1, 2013.
- High-intensity behavioral counseling to prevent sexually transmitted infections (HCPCS code G0445) – Effective January 1, 2013.
- Annual, face-to-face Intensive behavioral therapy for cardiovascular disease (HCPCS code G0446) – Effective January 1, 2013.
- Face-to-face behavioral counseling for obesity (HCPCS code G0447) – Effective January 1, 2013.
- Transitional Care Management Services (CPT codes 99495 -99496) – Effective January 1, 2014.

NOTE: Beginning January 1, 2010, CMS eliminated the use of all consultation codes, except for inpatient telehealth consultation G-codes. CMS no longer recognizes office/outpatient or inpatient consultation CPT codes for payment of office/outpatient or inpatient visits. Instead, physicians and practitioners are instructed to bill a new or established patient office/outpatient visit CPT code or appropriate hospital or nursing facility care code, as appropriate to the particular patient, for all office/outpatient or inpatient visits.

100-04, 12, 190.3.1

Telehealth Consultation Services, Emergency Department or Initial Inpatient versus Inpatient Evaluation and Management (E/M) Visits

(Rev.2354, Issued:11-18-11 Effective: 01-01-12, Implementation: 01-03-12)

A consultation service is an evaluation and management (E/M) service furnished to evaluate and possibly treat a patient's problem(s). It can involve an opinion, advice, recommendation, suggestion, direction, or counsel from a physician or qualified nonphysician practitioner (NPP) at the request of another physician or appropriate source.

Section 1834(m) of the Social Security Act includes "professional consultations" in the definition of telehealth services. Inpatient or emergency department consultations furnished via telehealth can facilitate the provision of certain services and/or medical expertise that might not otherwise be available to a patient located at an originating site.

The use of a telecommunications system may substitute for an in-person encounter for emergency department or initial and follow-up inpatient consultations.

Medicare contractors pay for reasonable and medically necessary inpatient or emergency department telehealth consultation services furnished to beneficiaries in hospitals or SNFs when all of the following criteria for the use of a consultation code are met:

- An inpatient or emergency department consultation service is distinguished from other inpatient or emergency department evaluation and management (E/M) visits because it is provided by a physician or qualified nonphysician practitioner (NPP) whose opinion or advice regarding evaluation and/or management of a specific problem is requested by another physician or other appropriate source. The qualified NPP may perform consultation services

 © 2019 Optum360, LLC

within the scope of practice and licensure requirements for NPPs in the State in which he/she practices;

- A request for an inpatient or emergency department telehealth consultation from an appropriate source and the need for an inpatient or emergency department telehealth consultation (i.e., the reason for a consultation service) shall be documented by the consultant in the patient's medical record and included in the requesting physician or qualified NPP's plan of care in the patient's medical record; and
- After the inpatient or emergency department telehealth consultation is provided, the consultant shall prepare a written report of his/her findings and recommendations, which shall be provided to the referring physician.

The intent of an inpatient or emergency department telehealth consultation service is that a physician or qualified NPP or other appropriate source is asking another physician or qualified NPP for advice, opinion, a recommendation, suggestion, direction, or counsel, etc. in evaluating or treating a patient because that individual has expertise in a specific medical area beyond the requesting professional's knowledge.

Unlike inpatient or emergency department telehealth consultations, the majority of subsequent inpatient hospital, emergency department and nursing facility care services require in-person visits to facilitate the comprehensive, coordinated, and personal care that medically volatile, acutely ill patients require on an ongoing basis.

Subsequent hospital care services are limited to one telehealth visit every 3 days. Subsequent nursing facility care services are limited to one telehealth visit every 30 days.

100-04, 12, 190.3.2

Telehealth Consultation Services, Emergency Department or Initial Inpatient Defined

(Rev.3929; Issued: 11-29-17; Effective: 01-01-18; Implementation: 01-02-18)

Emergency department or initial inpatient telehealth consultations are furnished to beneficiaries in hospitals or SNFs via telehealth at the request of the physician of record, the attending physician, or another appropriate source. The physician or practitioner who furnishes the emergency department or initial inpatient consultation via telehealth cannot be the physician of record or the attending physician, and the emergency department or initial inpatient telehealth consultation would be distinct from the care provided by the physician of record or the attending physician. Counseling and coordination of care with other providers or agencies is included as well, consistent with the nature of the problem(s) and the patient's needs. Emergency department or initial inpatient telehealth consultations are subject to the criteria for emergency department or initial inpatient telehealth consultation services, as described in section 190.3.1 of this chapter.

Payment for emergency department or initial inpatient telehealth consultations includes all consultation related services furnished before, during, and after communicating with the patient via telehealth. Pre-service activities would include, but would not be limited to, reviewing patient data (for example, diagnostic and imaging studies, interim labwork) and communicating with other professionals or family members. Intra-service activities must include the three key elements described below for each procedure code. Post-service activities would include, but would not be limited to, completing medical records or other documentation and communicating results of the consultation and further care plans to other health care professionals. No additional E/M service could be billed for work related to an emergency department or initial inpatient telehealth consultation.

Emergency department or initial inpatient telehealth consultations could be provided at various levels of complexity:

- Practitioners taking a problem focused history, conducting a problem focused examination, and engaging in medical decision making that is straightforward, would bill HCPCS code G0425 (Telehealth consultation, emergency department or initial inpatient, typically 30 minutes communicating with the patient via telehealth).
- Practitioners taking a detailed history, conducting a detailed examination, and engaging in medical decision making that is of moderate complexity, would bill HCPCS code G0426 (Telehealth consultation, emergency department or initial inpatient, typically 50 minutes communicating with the patient via telehealth).
- Practitioners taking a comprehensive history, conducting a comprehensive examination, and engaging in medical decision making that is of high complexity, would bill HCPCS code G0427 (Telehealth consultation, emergency department or initial inpatient, typically 70 minutes or more communicating with the patient via telehealth).

Although emergency department or initial inpatient telehealth consultations are specific to telehealth, these services must be billed with either the -GT or -GQ modifier to identify the telehealth technology used to provide the service. See section 190.6 of this chapter for instructions on how to use these modifiers.

100-04, 12, 190.3.3

Follow-Up Inpatient Telehealth Consultations Defined

(Rev.3929; Issued: 11-29-17; Effective: 01-01-18; Implementation: 01-02-18)

Follow-up inpatient telehealth consultations are furnished to beneficiaries in hospitals or SNFs via telehealth to follow up on an initial consultation, or subsequent consultative visits requested by the attending physician. The initial inpatient consultation may have been provided in person or via telehealth.

Follow-up inpatient telehealth consultations include monitoring progress, recommending management modifications, or advising on a new plan of care in response to changes in the patient's status or no changes on the consulted health issue. Counseling and coordination of care with other providers or agencies is included as well, consistent with the nature of the problem(s) and the patient's needs.

The physician or practitioner who furnishes the inpatient follow-up consultation via telehealth cannot be the physician of record or the attending physician, and the follow-up inpatient consultation would be distinct from the follow-up care provided by the physician of record or the attending physician. If a physician consultant has initiated treatment at an initial consultation and participates thereafter in the patient's ongoing care management, such care would not be included in the definition of a follow-up inpatient consultation and is not appropriate for delivery via telehealth. Follow-up inpatient telehealth consultations are subject to the criteria for inpatient telehealth consultation services, as described in Sec.190.3.1

Payment for follow-up inpatient telehealth consultations includes all consultation related services furnished before, during, and after communicating with the patient via telehealth. Pre-service activities would include, but would not be limited to, reviewing patient data (for example, diagnostic and imaging studies, interim labwork) and communicating with other professionals or family members. Intra-service activities must include at least two of the three key elements described below for each procedure code. Post-service activities would include, but would not be limited to, completing medical records or other documentation and communicating results of the consultation and further care plans to other health care professionals. No additional evaluation and management service could be billed for work related to a follow-up inpatient telehealth consultation.

Follow-up inpatient telehealth consultations could be provided at various levels of complexity:

Practitioners taking a problem focused interval history, conducting a problem focused examination, and engaging in medical decision making that is straightforward or of low complexity, would bill a limited service, using HCPCS G0406, Follow-up inpatient telehealth consultation, limited. At this level of service, practitioners would typically spend 15 minutes communicating with the patient via telehealth.

Practitioners taking an expanded focused interval history, conducting an expanded problem focused examination, and engaging in medical decision making that is of moderate complexity, would bill an intermediate service using HCPCS G0407, Follow-up inpatient telehealth consultation, intermediate. At this level of service, practitioners would typically spend 25 minutes communicating with the patient via telehealth.

Practitioners taking a detailed interval history, conducting a detailed examination, and engaging in medical decision making that is of high complexity, would bill a complex service, using HCPCS G0408, Follow-up inpatient telehealth consultation, complex. At this level of service, practitioners would typically spend 35 minutes or more communicating with the patient via telehealth.

Although follow-up inpatient telehealth consultations are specific to telehealth, these services must be billed with either the "GT" or "GQ" modifier to identify the telehealth technology used to provide the service. (See Sec.190.6 et. al. for instructions on how to use these modifiers.)

100-04, 12, 190.6

Payment Methodology for Physician/Practitioner at the Distant Site

(Rev.3586, Issued: 08-12-16, Effective: 01-01-17, Implementation: 01-03-17)

1. Distant Site Defined

The term "distant site" means the site where the physician or practitioner, providing the professional service, is located at the time the service is provided via a telecommunications system.

© 2019 Optum360, LLC

2. Payment Amount (professional fee)

The payment amount for the professional service provided via a telecommunications system by the physician or practitioner at the distant site is equal to the current fee schedule amount for the service provided at the facility rate. Payment for an office visit, consultation, individual psychotherapy or pharmacologic management via a telecommunications system should be made at the same facility amount as when these services are furnished without the use of a telecommunications system. For Medicare payment to occur, the service must be within a practitioner's scope of practice under State law. The beneficiary is responsible for any unmet deductible amount and applicable coinsurance.

3. Medicare Practitioners Who May Receive Payment at the Distant Site (i.e., at a site other than where beneficiary is)

As a condition of Medicare Part B payment for telehealth services, the physician or practitioner at the distant site must be licensed to provide the service under state law. When the physician or practitioner at the distant site is licensed under state law to provide a covered telehealth service (i.e., professional consultation, office and other outpatient visits, individual psychotherapy, and pharmacologic management) then he or she may bill for and receive payment for this service when delivered via a telecommunications system.

If the physician or practitioner at the distant site is located in a CAH that has elected Method II, and the physician or practitioner has reassigned his/her benefits to the CAH, the CAH bills its regular A/B/MAC (A) for the professional services provided at the distant site via a telecommunications system, in any of the revenue codes 096x, 097x or 098x. All requirements for billing distant site telehealth services apply.

4. Medicare Practitioners Who May Bill for Covered Telehealth Services are Listed Below (subject to State law)

Physician
Nurse practitioner
Physician assistant
Nurse-midwife
Clinical nurse specialist
Clinical psychologist*
Clinical social worker*
Registered dietitian or nutrition professional
Certified registered nurse anesthetist

*Clinical psychologists and clinical social workers cannot bill for psychotherapy services that include medical evaluation and management services under Medicare. These practitioners may not bill or receive payment for the following CPT codes: 90805, 90807, and 90809.

100-04, 12, 190.6.1

Submission of Telehealth Claims for Distant Site Practitioners

(Rev.3929; Issued: 11-29-17; Effective: 01-01-18; Implementation: 01-02-18)

Claims for telehealth services are submitted to the contractors that process claims for the performing physician/practitioner's service area. Physicians/practitioners submit the appropriate HCPCS procedure code for covered professional telehealth services with place of service code 02 (Telehealth). By billing place of service code 02 with a covered telehealth procedure code, the distant site physician/practitioner certifies that the beneficiary was present at an eligible originating site when the telehealth service was furnished. By billing the place of service code 02 with a covered ESRD-related service telehealth code, the distant site physician/practitioner certifies that 1 visit per month was furnished face-to-face "hands on" to examine the vascular access site. Refer to section 190.3.4 of this chapter for the conditions of telehealth payment for ESRD-related services.

In situations where a CAH has elected payment Method II for CAH outpatients, and the practitioner has reassigned his/her benefits to the CAH, CAHs submit the appropriate HCPCS procedure code for the covered telehealth services with the GT modifier, and A/B/MACs (A) should make payment for telehealth services provided by the physician or practitioner at 80 percent of the MPFS facility amount for the distant site service. In all other cases, except for MNT services as discussed in Section 190.7-A/B MAC (B) Editing of Telehealth Claims, telehealth services provided by the physician or practitioner at the distant site are billed to the A/B/MAC (B).

Physicians and practitioners at the distant site bill their A/B/MAC (B) for covered telehealth services. Physicians' and practitioners' offices serving as a telehealth originating site bill their A/B/MAC (B) for the originating site facility fee.

100-04, 12, 190.7

A/B MAC (B) Editing of Telehealth Claims

(Rev.3929; Issued: 11-29-17; Effective: 01-01-18; Implementation: 01-02-18)

Medicare telehealth services (as listed in section 190.3) are billed with either the "GT" or "GQ" modifier. The contractor shall approve covered telehealth services if the physician or practitioner is licensed under State law to provide the service. Contractors must familiarize themselves with licensure provisions of States for which they process claims and disallow telehealth services furnished by physicians or practitioners who are not authorized to furnish the applicable telehealth service under State law. For example, if a nurse practitioner is not licensed to provide individual psychotherapy under State law, he or she would not be permitted to receive payment for individual psychotherapy under Medicare. The contractor shall install edits to ensure that only properly licensed physicians and practitioners are paid for covered telehealth services.

If a contractor receives claims for professional telehealth services coded with the "GQ" modifier (representing "via asynchronous telecommunications system"), it shall approve/pay for these services only if the physician or practitioner is affiliated with a Federal telemedicine demonstration conducted in Alaska or Hawaii. The contractor may require the physician or practitioner at the distant site to document his or her participation

in a Federal telemedicine demonstration program conducted in Alaska or Hawaii prior to paying for telehealth services provided via asynchronous, store and forward technologies.

Contractors shall deny telehealth services if the physician or practitioner is not eligible to bill for them.

The following reflects the remittance advice messages and associated codes that will appear when rejecting/denying claims under this policy. This CARC/RARC combination is compliant with CAQH CORE Business Scenario 3.

Group Code: CO
CARC: 185
RARC: N/A
MSN: 21.18

If a service is billed with one of the telehealth modifiers and the procedure code is not designated as a covered telehealth service, the contractor denies the service.

The following reflects the remittance advice messages and associated codes that will appear when rejecting/denying claims under this policy. This CARC/RARC combination is compliant with CAQH CORE Business Scenario 3.

Group Code: CO
CARC: 96
RARC: N776
MSN: 9.4

The only claims from institutional facilities that FIs shall pay for telehealth services at the distant site, except for MNT services, are for physician or practitioner services when the distant site is located in a CAH that has elected Method II, and the physician or practitioner has reassigned his/her benefits to the CAH. The CAH bills its regular FI for the professional services provided at the distant site via a telecommunications system, in any of the revenue codes 096x, 097x or 098x. All requirements for billing distant site telehealth services apply.

Claims from hospitals or CAHs for MNT services are submitted to the hospital's or CAH's regular FI. Payment is based on the non-facility amount on the Medicare Physician Fee Schedule for the particular HCPCS codes.

100-04, 13, 30.1.3.1

A/B MAC (A) Payment for Low Osmolar Contrast Material (LOCM) (Radiology)

(Rev.3227, Issued: 04-02-15, Effective--multiple effective dates)

The LOCM is paid on a reasonable cost basis when rendered by a SNF to its Part B patients (in addition to payment for the radiology procedure) when it is used in one of the situations listed below.

The following HCPCS are used when billing for LOCM.

HCPCS Code	Description (January 1. 1994, and later)
A4644	Supply of low osmolar contrast material (100-199 mgs of iodine);
A4645	Supply of low osmolar contrast material (200-299 mgs of iodine); or
A4646	Supply of low osmolar contrast material (300-399 mgs of iodine).

When billing for LOCM, SNFs use revenue code 0636. If the SNF charge for the radiology procedure includes a charge for contrast material, the SNF must adjust the charge for the radiology procedure to exclude any amount for the contrast material.

NOTE: LOCM is never billed with revenue code 0255 or as part of the radiology procedure.

The A/B MAC (A) will edit for the intrathecal procedure codes and the following codes to determine if payment for LOCM is to be made. If an intrathecal procedure code is not present, or one of the ICD codes is not present to indicate that a required medical

© 2019 Optum360, LLC

condition is met, the A/B MAC (A) will deny payment for LOCM. In these instances, LOCM is not covered and should not be billed to Medicare.

When LOCM Is Separately Billable and Related Coding Requirements

- In all intrathecal injections. HCPCS codes that indicate intrathecal injections are:
  - 70010 70015 72240 72255 72265 72270 72285 72295

One of these must be included on the claim; or

- In intravenous and intra-arterial injections only when certain medical conditions are present in an outpatient. The SNF must verify the existence of at least one of the following medical conditions, and report the applicable diagnosis code(s) either as a principal diagnosis code or other diagnosis codes on the claim:
  - A history of previous adverse reaction to contrast material. The applicable ICD-9-CM codes are V14.8 and V14.9. The applicable ICD-10-CM codes are Z88.8 and Z88.9. The conditions which should not be considered adverse reactions are a sensation of heat, flushing, or a single episode of nausea or vomiting. If the adverse reaction occurs on that visit with the induction of contrast material, codes describing hives, urticaria, etc. should also be present, as well as a code describing the external cause of injury and poisoning, ICD-9-CM code E947.8. The applicable ICD-10 CM codes are: T50.8X5A Adverse effect of diagnostic agents, initial encounter, T50.8X5S Adverse effect of diagnostic agents, sequela , T50.995A Adverse effect of other drugs, medicaments and biological substances, initial encounter, or T50.995S Adverse effect of other drugs, medicaments and biological substances, sequela;
  - A history or condition of asthma or allergy. The applicable ICD-9-CM codes are V07.1, V14.0 through V14.9, V15.0, 493.00, 493.01, 493.10, 493.11, 493.20, 493.21, 493.90, 493.91, 495.0, 495.1, 495.2, 495.3, 495.4, 495.5, 495.6, 495.7, 495.8, 495.9, 995.0, 995.1, 995.2, and 995.3. The applicable ICD-10-CM codes are in the table below:

ICD-10-CM Codes				
J44.0	J44.9	J45.20	J45.22	J45.30
J45.32	J45.40	J45.42	J45.50	J45.52
J45.902	J45.909	J45.998	J67.0	J67.1
JJ67.2	J67.3	J67.4	J67.5	J67.6
J67.7	J67.8	J67.9	J96.00	J96.01
J96.02	J96.90	J96.91	J96.92	T36.0X5A
T36.1X5A	T36.2X5A	T36.3X5A	T36.4X5A	T36.5X5A
T36.6X5A	T36.7X5A	T36.8X5A	T36.95XA	T37.0X5A
T37.1X5A	T37.2X5A	T37.3X5A	T37.8X5A	T37.95XA
T38.0X5A	T38.1X5A	T38.2X5A	T38.3X5A	T38.4X5A
T38.6X5A	T38.7X5A	T38.805A	T38.815A	T38.895A
T38.905A	T38.995A	T39.015A	T39.095A	T39.1X5A
T39.2X5A	T39.2X5A	T39.315A	T39.395A	T39.4X5A
T39.8X5A	T39.95XA	T40.0X5A	T40.1X5A	T40.2X5A
T40.3X5A	T40.4X5A	T40.5X5A	T40.605A	T40.695A
T40.7X5A	T40.8X5A	T40.905A	T40.995A	T41.0X5A
T41.1X5A	T41.205A	T41.295A	T41.3X5A	T41.4X5A
T41.X5A	T41.5X5A	T42.0X5A	T42.1X5A	T42.2X5A
T42.3X5A	T42.4X5A	T42.5X5A	T42.6X5A	427.5XA
428.X5A	T43.015A	T43.025A	T43.1X5A	T43.205A
T43.215A	T43.225A	T43.295A	T43.3X5A	T43.4X5A
T43.505A	T43.595A	T43.605A	T43.615A	T43.625A
T43.635A	T43.695A	T43.8X5A	T43.95XA	T44.0X5A
T44.1X5A	T44.2X5A	T44.3X5A	T44.6X5A	T44.7X5A
T44.8X5A	T44.905A	T44.995A	T45.0X5A	T45.1X5A
T45.2X5A	T45.3X5A	T45.4X5A	T45.515A	T45.525A
T45.605A	T45.615A	T45.625A	T45.695A	T45.7X5A
T45.8X5A	T45.95XA	T46.0X5A	T46.1X5A	T46.2X5A
T46.3X5A	T46.4X5A	T46.5X5A	T46.6X5A	T46.7X5A
T46.8X5A	T46.905A	T46.995A	T47.0X5A	T47.1X5A
T47.2X5A	T47.3X5A	T47.4X5A	T47.5X5A	T47.6X5A
T47.7X5A	T47.8X5A	T47.95XA	T48.0X5A	T48.1X5A
T48.205A	T48.295A	T48.3X5A	T48.4X5A	T48.5X5A

ICD-10-CM Codes				
T48.6X5A	T48.905A	T48.995A	T49.0X5A	T49.1X5A
T49.2X5A	T49.3X5A	T49.4X5A	T49.5X5A	T49.6X5A
T49.6X5A	T47.X5A9	T49.8X5A	T49.95XA	T50.0X5A
T50.1X5A	T50.2X5A	T50.3X5A	T50.4X5A	T50.5X5A
T50.6X5A	T50.7X5A	T50.8X5A	T50.905a	T50.995A
T50.A15A	T50.A25A	T50.A95A	T50.B15A	T50.B95A
T50.Z15A	T50.Z95A	T78.2XXA	T78.3XXA	T78.40XA
T78.41XA	T88.52XA	T88.59XA	T88.6XXA	Z51.89
Z88.0	Z88.1	Z88.2	Z88.3	Z88.4
Z88.5	Z88.6	Z88.7	Z88.8	Z88.9
Z91.010				

  - Significant cardiac dysfunction including recent or imminent cardiac decompensation, severe arrhythmia, unstable angina pectoris, recent myocardial infarction, and pulmonary hypertension. The applicable ICD-9-CM codes are:

ICD-9-CM				
402.00	402.01	402.10	402.11	402.90
402.91	404.00	404.01	404.02	404.03
404.10	404.11	404.12	404.13	404.90
404.91	404.92	404.93	410.00	410.01
410.02	410.10	410.11	410.12	410.20
410.21	410.22	410.30	410.31	410.32
410.40	410.41	410.42	410.50	410.51
410.52	410.60	410.61	410.62	410.70
410.71	410.72	410.80	410.81	410.82
410.90	410.91	410.92	411.1	415.0
416.0	416.1	416.8	416.9	420.0
420.90	420.91	420.99	424.90	424.91
424.99	427.0	427.1	427.2	427.31
427.32	427.41	427.42	427.5	427.60
427.61	427.69	427.81	427.89	427.9
428.0	428.1	428.9	429.0	429.1
429.2	429.3	429.4	429.5	429.6
429.71	429.79	429.81	429.82	429.89
429.9	785.50	785.51	785.59	

  - The applicable ICD-10-CM codes are in the table below:

ICD-10-CM Codes				
A18.84	I11.0	I11.9	I13.0	I13.10
I13.11	I13.2	I20.0	I21.01	I21.02
I21.09	I21.11	I21.19	I21.21	I21.29
I21.3	I21.4	I22.1	I22.2	I22.8
I23.0	I23.1	I23.2	I23.3	I23.4
I23.5	I23.6	I23.7	I23.8	I25.10
I25.110	I25.700	I25.710	I25.720	I25.730
I25.750	I25.760	I25.790	I26.01	I26.02
I26.09	I27.0	I27.1	I27.2	I27.81
I27.89	I27.9	I30.0	I30.1	I30.8
I30.9	I32	I38	I39	I46.2
I46.8	I46.9	I47.0	I471	I472
I47.9	I48.0	I48.1	I48.1	I48.2
I48.3	I48.4	I48.91	I48.92	I49.01
I49.02	I49.1	I49.2	I49.3	I49.40
I49.49	I49.5	I49.8	I49.9	I50.1
I50.20	I50.21	I50.22	I50.23	I50.30
I50.31	I50.32	I50.33	I50.40	I50.41
I50.42	I50.43	I50.9	I51	I51.0
I51.1	I51.2	I51.3	I51.4	I51.5
I51.7	I51.89	I51.9	I52	I97.0

© 2019 Optum360, LLC

ICD-10-CM Codes				
I97.110	I97.111	I97.120	I97.121	I97.130
I97.131	I97.190	I97.191	M32.11	M32.12
R00.1	R57.0	R57.8	R57.9	

- Generalized severe debilitation. The applicable ICD-9-CM codes are: 203.00, 203.01, all codes for diabetes mellitus, 518.81, 585, 586, 799.3, 799.4, and V46.1. The applicable ICD-10-CM codes are: J96.850, J96.00 through J96.02, J96.90 through J96.91, N18.1 through N19, R53.81, R64, and Z99.11 through Z99.12. Or
- Sickle Cell disease. The applicable ICD-9-CM codes are 282.4, 282.60, 282.61, 282.62, 282.63, and 282.69. The applicable ICD-10-CM codes are D56.0 through D56.3, D56.5 through D56.9, D57.00 through D57.1, D57.20, D57.411 through D57.419, and D57.811 through D57.819.

100-04, 13, 40

Magnetic Resonance Imaging (MRI) Procedures

(Rev.4147, Issued: 10-19-18, Effective: 04- 10-18, Implementation: 12-10-18)

The Centers for Medicare & Medicaid Services (CMS) finds that the non-coverage of magnetic resonance imaging (MRI) for blood flow determination is no longer supported by the available evidence. CMS is removing the phrase "blood flow measurement" and local Medicare contractors will have the discretion to cover (or not cover).

Consult Publication (Pub.) 100-03, National Coverage Determinations (NCD) Manual, chapter 1, section 220.2, for specific coverage and non-coverage indications associated with MRI and MRA (Magnetic Resonance Angiography).

A/B MACs (B) do not make additional payments for three or more MRI sequences. The relative value units (RVUs) reflect payment levels for two sequences.

The technical component (TC) RVUs for MRI procedures that specify "with contrast" include payment for paramagnetic contrast media. A/B MACs (B) do not make separate payment under code A4647.

A diagnostic technique has been developed under which an MRI of the brain or spine is first performed without contrast material, then another MRI is performed with a standard (0.1mmol/kg) dose of contrast material and, based on the need to achieve a better image, a third MRI is performed with an additional double dosage (0.2mmol/kg) of contrast material. When the high-dose contrast technique is utilized, A/B MACs (B):

- Do not pay separately for the contrast material used in the second MRI procedure;
- Pay for the contrast material given for the third MRI procedure through supply code Q9952, the replacement code for A4643, when billed with Current Procedural Terminology (CPT) codes 70553, 72156, 72157, and 72158;
- Do not pay for the third MRI procedure. For example, in the case of an MRI of the brain, if CPT code 70553 (without contrast material, followed by with contrast material(s) and further sequences) is billed, make no payment for CPT code 70551 (without contrast material(s)), the additional procedure given for the purpose of administering the double dosage, furnished during the same session. Medicare does not pay for the third procedure (as distinguished from the contrast material) because the CPT definition of code 70553 includes all further sequences; and
- Do not apply the payment criteria for low osmolar contrast media in §30.1.2 to billings for code Q9952, the replacement code for A4643. Effective January 1, 2008, Q9952 is replaced with A9579.

With the implementation for calendar year 2007 of a bottom-up methodology, which utilizes the direct inputs to determine the practice expense (PE) relative value units (RVUs), the cost of the contrast media is not included in the PE RVUs. Therefore, a separate payment for the contrast media used in various imaging procedures is paid. In addition to the CPT code representing the imaging procedure, separately bill the appropriate HCPCS "Q" code (Q9945 – Q9954; Q9958-Q9964) for the contrast medium utilized in performing the service. Effective January 1, 2008, HCPCS code ranges changed to Q9950-Q9954, Q9958-Q9967.

For claims with dates of service on or after February 24, 2011, through April 9, 2018, Medicare will allow for coverage of MRI for beneficiaries with implanted pacemakers (PMs) or cardioverter defibrillators

(ICDs) for use in an MRI environment in a Medicare-approved clinical study as described in section 220.C.1 of the NCD Manual.

For claims with dates of service on or after July 7, 2011, through April 9, 2018, Medicare will allow for coverage of MRI for beneficiaries with implanted PMs when the PMs are used according to the Food and Drug Administration (FDA)-approved labeling for use in an MRI environment as described in section 220.2.C.1 of the NCD Manual.

For claims with dates of service on or after April 10, 2018, Medicare will allow for coverage for MRIs for beneficiaries with implanted PMs, ICDs, cardiac resynchronization therapy pacemakers (CRT-Ps), or cardiac resynchronization therapy defibrillators (CRT-Ds), both on and off FDA label, for use in an MRI environment as described in section 220.2.B.3 of the NCD Manual. The data collection requirement under coverage with evidence development ceases April 9, 2018.

100-04, 13, 40.1.1

Magnetic Resonance Angiography (MRA) Coverage Summary

(Rev.2171, Issued: 03-04-11, Effective: 02-24-11, Implementation: 04-04-11)

Section 1861(s)(2)(C) of the Social Security Act provides for coverage of diagnostic testing. Coverage of magnetic resonance angiography (MRA) of the head and neck, and MRA of the peripheral vessels of the lower extremities is limited as described in Publication (Pub.) 100-03, the Medicare National Coverage Determinations (NCD) Manual. This instruction has been revised as of July 1, 2003, based on a determination that coverage is reasonable and necessary in additional circumstances. Under that instruction, MRA is generally covered only to the extent that it is used as a substitute for contrast angiography, except to the extent that there are documented circumstances consistent with that instruction that demonstrates the medical necessity of both tests. Prior to June 3, 2010, there was no coverage of MRA outside of the indications and circumstances described in that instruction.

Effective for claims with dates of service on or after June 3, 2010, contractors have the discretion to cover or not cover all indications of MRA (and magnetic resonance imaging (MRI)) that are not specifically nationally covered or nationally non-covered as stated in section 220.2 of the NCD Manual.

Because the status codes for HCPCS codes 71555, 71555-TC, 71555-26, 74185, 74185-TC, and 74185-26 were changed in the Medicare Physician Fee Schedule Database from 'N' to 'R' on April 1, 1998, any MRA claims with those HCPCS codes with dates of service between April 1, 1998, and June 30, 1999, are to be processed according to the contractor's discretionary authority to determine payment in the absence of national policy.

Effective for claims with dates of service on or after February 24, 201l, Medicare will provide coverage for MRIs for beneficiaries with implanted cardiac pacemakers or implantable cardioverter defibrillators if the beneficiary is enrolled in an approved clinical study under the Coverage with Study Participation form of Coverage with Evidence Development that meets specific criteria per Pub. 100-03, the NCD Manual, chapter 1, section 220.2.C.1

100-04, 13, 40.1.2

HCPCS Coding Requirements

(Rev.1472, Issued: 03-06-08, Effective: 05-23-07, Implementation: 04-07-08)

Providers must report HCPCS codes when submitting claims for MRA of the chest, abdomen, head, neck or peripheral vessels of lower extremities. The following HCPCS codes should be used to report these services:

MRA of head	70544, 70544-26, 70544-TC
MRA of head	70545, 70545-26, 70545-TC
MRA of head	70546, 70546-26, 70546-TC
MRA of neck	70547, 70547-26, 70547-TC
MRA of neck	70548, 70548-26, 70548-TC
MRA of neck	70549, 70549-26, 70549-TC
MRA of chest	71555, 71555-26, 71555-TC
MRA of pelvis	72198, 72198-26, 72198-TC
MRA of abdomen (dates of service on or after July 1, 2003) —see below.	74185, 74185-26, 74185-TC
MRA of peripheral vessels of lower extremities	73725, 73725-26, 73725-TC

100-04, 13, 60

Positron Emission Tomography (PET) Scans - General Information

(Rev.1833; Issued: 10-16-09; Effective Date: 04-03-09; Implementation Date: 10-30-09)

Positron emission tomography (PET) is a noninvasive imaging procedure that assesses perfusion and the level of metabolic activity in various organ systems of the human body. A positron camera (tomograph) is used to produce cross-sectional tomographic images which are obtained by detecting radioactivity from a

© 2019 Optum360, LLC

radioactive tracer substance radiopharmaceutical) that emits a radioactive tracer substance (radiopharmaceutical FDG) such as 2 -[F-18] flouro-D-glucose FDG, that is administered intravenously to the patient.

The Medicare National Coverage Determinations (NCD) Manual, Chapter 1, Sec.220.6, contains additional coverage instructions to indicate the conditions under which a PET scan is performed.

A. Definitions

For all uses of PET, excluding Rubidium 82 for perfusion of the heart, myocardial viability and refractory seizures, the following definitions apply:

Diagnosis: PET is covered only in clinical situations in which the PET results may assist in avoiding an invasive diagnostic procedure, or in which the PET results may assist in determining the optimal anatomical location to perform an invasive diagnostic procedure. In general, for most solid tumors, a tissue diagnosis is made prior to the performance of PET scanning. PET scans following a tissue diagnosis are generally performed for the purpose of staging, rather than diagnosis. Therefore, the use of PET in the diagnosis of lymphoma, esophageal and colorectal cancers, as well as in melanoma, should be rare. PET is not covered for other diagnostic uses, and is not covered for screening (testing of patients without specific signs and symptoms of disease).

Staging: PET is covered in clinical situations in which (1) (a) the stage of the cancer remains in doubt after completion of a standard diagnostic workup, including conventional imaging (computed tomography, magnetic resonance imaging, or ultrasound) or, (b) the use of PET would also be considered reasonable and necessary if it could potentially replace one or more conventional imaging studies when it is expected that conventional study information is insufficient for the clinical management of the patient and, (2) clinical management of the patient would differ depending on the stage of the cancer identified.

NOTE: Effective for services on or after April 3, 2009, the terms "diagnosis" and "staging" will be replaced with "Initial Treatment Strategy." For further information on this new term, refer to Pub. 100-03, NCD Manual, section 220.6.17.

Restaging: PET will be covered for restaging: (1) after the completion of treatment for the purpose of detecting residual disease, (2) for detecting suspected recurrence, or metastasis, (3) to determine the extent of a known recurrence, or (4) if it could potentially replace one or more conventional imaging studies when it is expected that conventional study information is to determine the extent of a known recurrence, or if study information is insufficient for the clinical management of the patient. Restaging applies to testing after a course of treatment is completed and is covered subject to the conditions above.

Monitoring: Use of PET to monitor tumor response to treatment during the planned course of therapy (i.e., when a change in therapy is anticipated).

NOTE: Effective for services on or after April 3, 2009, the terms "restaging" and "monitoring" will be replaced with "Subsequent Treatment Strategy." For further information on this new term, refer to Pub. 100-03, NCD Manual, section 220.6.17.

B. Limitations

For staging and restaging: PET is covered in either/or both of the following circumstances:

The stage of the cancer remains in doubt after completion of a standard diagnostic workup, including conventional imaging (computed tomography, magnetic resonance imaging, or ultrasound); and/or

The clinical management of the patient would differ depending on the stage of the cancer identified. PET will be covered for restaging after the completion of treatment for the purpose of detecting residual disease, for detecting suspected recurrence, or to determine the extent of a known recurrence. Use of PET would also be considered reasonable and necessary if it could potentially replace one or more conventional imaging studies when it is expected that conventional study information is insufficient for the clinical management of the patient.

The PET is not covered for other diagnostic uses, and is not covered for screening (testing of patients without specific symptoms). Use of PET to monitor tumor response during the planned course of therapy (i.e. when no change in therapy is being contemplated) is not covered.

100-04, 13, 60.3

PET Scan Qualifying Conditions and HCPCS Code Chart

(Rev.527, Issued: 04-15-05, Effective: 01-28-05, Implementation: 04-18-05)

Below is a summary of all covered PET scan conditions, with effective dates.

NOTE: The G codes below except those a # can be used to bill for PET Scan services through January 27, 2005. Effective for dates of service on or after January 28, 2005, providers must bill for PET Scan services using the appropriate CPT codes. See section 60.3.1. The G codes with a # can continue to be used for billing after January 28, 2005 and these remain non-covered by Medicare. (NOTE: PET Scanners must be FDA-approved.)

Conditions	Coverage Effective Date	****HCPCS/CPT
*Myocardial perfusion imaging (following previous PET G0030-G0047) single study, rest or stress (exercise and/or pharmacologic)	3/14/95	G0030
*Myocardial perfusion imaging (following previous PET G0030-G0047) multiple studies, rest or stress (exercise and/or pharmacologic)	3/14/95	G0031
*Myocardial perfusion imaging (following rest SPECT, 78464); single study, rest or stress (exercise and/or pharmacologic)	3/14/95	G0032
*Myocardial perfusion imaging (following rest SPECT 78464); multiple studies, rest or stress (exercise and/or pharmacologic)	3/14/95	G0033
*Myocardial perfusion (following stress SPECT 78465); single study, rest or stress (exercise and/or pharmacologic)	3/14/95	G0034
*Myocardial Perfusion Imaging (following stress SPECT 78465); multiple studies, rest or stress (exercise and/or pharmacologic)	3/14/95	G0035
*Myocardial Perfusion Imaging (following coronary angiography 93510-93529); single study, rest or stress (exercise and/or pharmacologic)	3/14/95	G0036
*Myocardial Perfusion Imaging, (following coronary angiography), 93510-93529); multiple studies, rest or stress (exercise and/or pharmacologic)	3/14/95	G0037
*Myocardial Perfusion Imaging (following stress planar myocardial perfusion, 78460); single study, rest or stress (exercise and/or pharmacologic)	3/14/95	G0038
*Myocardial Perfusion Imaging (following stress planar myocardial perfusion, 78460); multiple studies, rest or stress (exercise and/or pharmacologic)	3/14/95	G0039
*Myocardial Perfusion Imaging (following stress echocardiogram 93350); single study, rest or stress (exercise and/or pharmacologic)	3/14/95	G0040
*Myocardial Perfusion Imaging (following stress echocardiogram, 93350); multiple studies, rest or stress (exercise and/or pharmacologic)	3/14/95	G0041
*Myocardial Perfusion Imaging (following stress nuclear ventriculogram 78481 or 78483); single study, rest or stress (exercise and/or pharmacologic)	3/14/95	G0042
*Myocardial Perfusion Imaging (following stress nuclear ventriculogram 78481 or 78483); multiple studies, rest or stress (exercise and/or pharmacologic)	3/14/95	G0043
*Myocardial Perfusion Imaging (following stress ECG, 93000); single study, rest or stress (exercise and/or pharmacologic)	3/14/95	G0044
*Myocardial perfusion (following stress ECG, 93000), multiple studies; rest or stress (exercise and/or pharmacologic)	3/14/95	G0045
*Myocardial perfusion (following stress ECG, 93015), single study; rest or stress (exercise and/or pharmacologic)	3/14/95	G0046
*Myocardial perfusion (following stress ECG, 93015); multiple studies, rest or stress (exercise and/or pharmacologic)	3/14/95	G0047
PET imaging regional or whole body; single pulmonary nodule	1/1/98	G0125

© 2019 Optum360, LLC

Conditions	Coverage Effective Date	****HCPCS/CPT
Lung cancer, non-small cell (PET imaging whole body) Diagnosis, Initial Staging, Restaging	7/1/01	G0210 G0211 G0212
Colorectal cancer (PET imaging whole body) Diagnosis, Initial Staging, Restaging	7/1/01	G0213 G0214 G0215
Melanoma (PET imaging whole body) Diagnosis, Initial Staging, Restaging	7/1/01	G0216 G0217 G0218
Melanoma for non-covered indications Lymphoma (PET imaging whole body)	7/1/01	#G0219
Diagnosis, Initial Staging, Restaging	7/1/01	G0220 G0221 G0222
Head and neck cancer; excluding thyroid and CNS cancers (PET imaging whole body or regional) Diagnosis, Initial Staging, Restaging	7/1/01	G0223 G0224 G0225

100-04, 13, 60.3.1

Appropriate CPT Codes Effective for PET Scans for Services Performed on or After January 28, 2005

(Rev.1301, Issued: 07-20-07, Effective: 01-28-05 CPT Code 78609/01-01-08 HCPCS Code A4641, Implementation: 01-07-08)

NOTE: All PET scan services require the use of a radiopharmaceutical diagnostic imaging agent (tracer). The applicable tracer code should be billed when billing for a PET scan service. See section 60.3.2 below for applicable tracer codes.

CPT Code	Description
78459	Myocardial imaging, positron emission tomography (PET), metabolic evaluation
78491	Myocardial imaging, positron emission tomography (PET), perfusion, single study at rest or stress
78492	Myocardial imaging, positron emission tomography (PET), perfusion, multiple studies at rest and/or stress
78608	Brain imaging, positron emission tomography (PET); metabolic evaluation
78811	Tumor imaging, positron emission tomography (PET); limited area (eg, chest, head/neck)
78812	Tumor imaging, positron emission tomography (PET); skull base to mid-thigh
78813	Tumor imaging, positron emission tomography (PET); whole body
78814	Tumor imaging, positron emission tomography (PET) with concurrently acquired computed tomography (CT) for attenuation correction and anatomical localization; limited area (eg, chest, head/neck)
78815	Tumor imaging, positron emission tomography (PET) with concurrently acquired computed tomography (CT) for attenuation correction and anatomical localization; skull base to mid-thigh
78816	Tumor imaging, positron emission tomography (PET) with concurrently acquired computed tomography (CT) for attenuation correction and anatomical localization; whole body

100-04, 13, 60.3.2

Tracer Codes Required for Positron Emission Tomography (PET) Scans

(Rev.3911, Issued: 11-09-17, Effective: 01-01-18, Implementation: 12-11-17)

An applicable tracer/radiopharmaceutical code, along with an applicable Current Procedural Technology (CPT) code, is necessary for claims processing of any Positron Emission Tomography (PET) scan services. While there are a number of PET tracers already billable for a diverse number of medical indications, there have been, and may be in the future, additional PET indications that might require a new PET tracer. Under those circumstances, the process to request/approve/implement a new code could be time-intensive. To help alleviate inordinate spans of time between when a national coverage determination is made, or when the Food and Drug Administration (FDA) approves a particular radiopharmaceutical for an oncologic indication already approved by the Centers for Medicare & Medicaid Services (CMS), and when it can be fully implemented via valid claims processing, CMS has created two new PET radiopharmaceutical unclassified tracer codes that can be used temporarily. This time period would be pending the creation/approval/implementation of permanent CPT codes that would later specifically define their function by CMS in official instructions.

Effective with dates of service on or after January 1, 2018, the following Healthcare Common Procedure Coding System (HCPCS) codes shall be used ONLY AS NECESSARY FOR AN INTERIM PERIOD OF TIME under the circumstances explained here. Specifically, there are two circumstances that would warrant use of the below codes: (1) After FDA approval of a PET oncologic indication, or, (2) after CMS approves coverage of a new PET indication, and ONLY if either of those situations requires the use of a dedicated PET radiopharmaceutical/tracer that is currently non-existent. Once permanent replacement codes are officially implemented by CMS, use of the temporary code for that particular indication will simultaneously be discontinued.

NOTE: The following two codes were effective as of January 1, 2017, with the January 2017 quarterly HCPCS update.

A9597 - Positron emission tomography radiopharmaceutical, diagnostic, for tumor identification, not otherwise classified

A9598 - Positron emission tomography radiopharmaceutical, diagnostic, for non-tumor identification, not otherwise classified

Effective for claims with dates of service on and after January 1, 2018, when PET tracer code A9597 or A9598 are present on a claim, that claim must also include:

-an appropriate PET HCPCS code, either 78459, 78491, 78492, 78608, 78811, 78812, 78813, 78814, 78815, or 78816,

-if tumor-related, either the -PI or -PS modifier as appropriate,

-if clinical trial, registry, or study-related outside of NCD220.6.17, PET for Solid Tumors, clinical trial modifier –Q0,

-if clinical trial, registry, or study-related, all claims require the 8-digit clinical trial number,

-if Part A OP and clinical trial, registry, or study-related outside of NCD220.6.17, PET for Solid Tumors, also include condition code 30 and ICD-10 diagnosis Z00.6.

Effective for claims with dates of service on and after January 1, 2018, A/Medicare Administrative Contractors (MACs) shall line-item deny, and B/MACs shall line-item reject, PET claims for A9597 or A9598 that don't include the elements noted above as appropriate.

Contractors shall use the following messaging when line-item denying (Part A) or line-item rejecting (Part B) PET claims containing HCPCS A9597 or A9598:

Remittance Advice Remark Codes (RARC) N386

Claim Adjustment Reason Code (CARC) 50, 96, and/or 119.

Group Code CO (Contractual Obligation) assigning financial liability to the provider (if a claim is received with a GZ modifier indicating no signed ABN is on file).

(The above new verbiage will supersede any existing verbiage in chapter 13, section 60.3.2.)

100-04, 13, 60.12

Coverage for PET Scans for Dementia and Neurodegenerative Diseases

(Rev.3942; Issued: 12-22-17; Effective: 01-01-18; Implementation: 01-22-18)

Effective for dates of service on or after September 15, 2004, Medicare will cover FDG PET scans for a differential diagnosis of fronto-temporal dementia (FTD) and Alzheimer's disease OR; its use in a CMS-approved practical clinical trial focused on the utility of FDG-PET in the diagnosis or treatment of dementing neurodegenerative diseases. Refer to Pub. 100-03, NCD Manual, section 220.6.13, for complete coverage conditions and clinical trial requirements and section 60.15 of this manual for claims processing information.

A. A/B MAC (A and B) Billing Requirements for PET Scan Claims for FDG-PET for the Differential Diagnosis of Fronto-temporal Dementia and Alzheimer's Disease:

CPT Code for PET Scans for Dementia and Neurodegenerative Diseases

Contractors shall advise providers to use the appropriate CPT code from section 60.3.1 for dementia and neurodegenerative diseases for services performed on or after January 28, 2005.

Diagnosis Codes for PET Scans for Dementia and Neurodegenerative Diseases

The contractor shall ensure one of the following appropriate diagnosis codes is present on claims for PET Scans for AD:

- If ICD-9-CM is applicable, ICD-9 codes are: 290.0, 290.10 - 290.13, 290.20 - 290, 21, 290.3, 331.0, 331.11, 331.19, 331.2, 331.9, 780.93
- If ICD-10-CM is applicable, ICD-10 codes are: F03.90, F03.90 plus F05, G30.9, G31.01, G31.9, R41.2 or R41.3

© 2019 Optum360, LLC

Medicare contractors shall deny claims when submitted with an appropriate CPT code from section 60.3.1 and with a diagnosis code other than the range of codes listed above.

Medicare contractors shall instruct providers to issue an Advanced Beneficiary Notice to beneficiaries advising them of potential financial liability prior to delivering the service if one of the appropriate diagnosis codes will not be present on the claim.

The contractor shall use the following remittance advice messages and associated codes when rejecting/denying claims under this policy. This CARC/RARC combination is compliant with CAQH CORE Business Scenario Three.

Group Code: PR (if claim is received with a GA modifier) otherwise CO

CARC: 11

RARC: N/A

MSN: 16.48

Provider Documentation Required with the PET Scan Claim

Medicare contractors shall inform providers to ensure the conditions mentioned in the NCD Manual, section 220.6.13, have been met. The information must also be maintained in the beneficiary's medical record:

- Date of onset of symptoms;
- Diagnosis of clinical syndrome (normal aging, mild cognitive impairment or MCI: mild, moderate, or severe dementia);
- Mini mental status exam (MMSE) or similar test score;
- Presumptive cause (possible, probably, uncertain AD);
- Any neuropsychological testing performed;
- Results of any structural imaging (MRI, CT) performed;
- Relevant laboratory tests (B12, thyroid hormone); and,
- Number and name of prescribed medications.

B. Billing Requirements for Beta Amyloid Positron Emission Tomography (PET) in Dementia and Neurodegenerative Disease:

Effective for claims with dates of service on and after September 27, 2013, Medicare will only allow coverage with evidence development (CED) for Positron Emission Tomography (PET) beta amyloid (also referred to as amyloid-beta (Aβ)) imaging (HCPCS A9586)or (HCPCS A9599) (one PET Aβ scan per patient).

NOTE: Please note that effective January 1, 2014 the following code A9599 will be updated in the IOCE and HCPCS update. This code will be contractor priced.

Medicare Summary Notices, Remittance Advice Remark Codes, and Claim Adjustment Reason Codes

Effective for dates of service on or after September 27, 2013, contractors shall return as unprocessable/return to provider claims for PET Aβ imaging, through CED during a clinical trial, not containing the following:

- Condition code 30, (A/B MAC (A) only)
- Modifier Q0 and/or modifier Q1 as appropriate
- ICD-9 dx code V70.7/ICD-10 dx code Z00.6 (on either the primary/secondary position)
- A PET HCPCS code (78811 or 78814)
- At least, one Dx code from the table below,

ICD-9 Codes	Corresponding ICD-10 Codes
290.0 Senile dementia, uncomplicated	F03.90 Unspecified dementia without behavioral disturbance
290.10 Presenile dementia, uncomplicated	F03.90 Unspecified dementia without behavioral disturbance
290.11 Presenile dementia with delirium	F03.90 Unspecified dementia without behavioral disturbance
290.12 Presenile dementia with delusional features	F03.90 Unspecified dementia without behavioral disturbance
290.13 Presenile dementia with depressive features	F03.90 Unspecified dementia without behavioral disturbance
290.20 Senile dementia with delusional features	F03.90 Unspecified dementia without behavioral disturbance
290.21 Senile dementia with depressive features	F03.90 Unspecified dementia without behavioral disturbance
290.3 Senile dementia with delirium	F03.90 Unspecified dementia without behavioral disturbance
290.40 Vascular dementia, uncomplicated	F01.50 Vascular dementia without behavioral disturbance
290.41 Vascular dementia with delirium	F01.51 Vascular dementia with behavioral disturbance
290.42 Vascular dementia with delusions	F01.51 Vascular dementia with behavioral disturbance
290.43 Vascular dementia with depressed mood	F01.51 Vascular dementia with behavioral disturbance
294.10 Dementia in conditions classified elsewhere without behavioral disturbance	F02.80 Dementia in other diseases classified elsewhere without behavioral disturbance
294.11 Dementia in conditions classified elsewhere with behavioral disturbance	F02.81 Dementia in other diseases classified elsewhere with behavioral disturbance
294.20 Dementia, unspecified, without behavioral disturbance	F03.90 Unspecified dementia without behavioral disturbance
294.21 Dementia, unspecified, with behavioral disturbance	F03.91 Unspecified dementia with behavioral disturbance
331.11 Pick's Disease	G31.01 Pick's disease
331.19 Other Frontotemporal dementia	G31.09 Other frontotemporal dementia
331.6 Corticobasal degeneration	G31.85 Corticobasal degeneration
331.82 Dementia with Lewy Bodies	G31.83 Dementia with Lewy bodies
331.83 Mild cognitive impairment, so stated	G31.84 Mild cognitive impairment, so stated
780.93 Memory Loss	R41.1 Anterograde amnesia R41.2 Retrograde amnesia R41.3 Other amnesia (Amnesia NOS, Memory loss NOS)
V70.7 Examination for normal comparison or control in clinical	Z00.6 Encounter for examination for normal comparison and control in clinical research program

and

- Aβ HCPCS code A9586 or A9599

The contractor shall use the following remittance advice messages and associated codes when returning claims under this policy. This CARC/RARC combination is compliant with CAQH CORE Business Scenario Two.

Group Code: CO
CARC: 4
RARC: N517, N519
MSN: N/A

Contractors shall line-item deny claims for PET Aβ, HCPCS code A9586 or A9599, where a previous PET Aβ, HCPCS code A9586 or A9599 is paid in history.

The contractor shall use the following remittance advice messages and associated codes when rejecting/denying claims under this policy. This CARC/RARC combination is compliant with CAQH CORE Business Scenario Three.

Group Code: PR (if claim is received with a GA modifier) otherwise CO
CARC: 149
RARC: N587
MSN: 20.12

100-04, 13, 60.13

Billing Requirements for PET Scans for Specific Indications of Cervical Cancer for Services Performed on or After January 28, 2005

(Rev.1888; Issued: 01-06-10, Effective date: 11-10-09; Implementation Date: 01-04-10)

Contractors shall accept claims for these services with the appropriate CPT code listed in section 60.3.1. Refer to Pub. 100-03, section 220.6.17, for complete coverage guidelines for this new PET oncology indication. The implementation date for these CPT codes will be April 18, 2005. Also see section 60.17, of this chapter for further claims processing instructions for cervical cancer indications.

© 2019 Optum360, LLC

100-04, 13, 60.14

Billing Requirements for PET Scans for Non-Covered Indications

(Rev.527, Issued: 04-15-05, Effective: 01-28-05, Implementation: 04-18-05)

For services performed on or after January 28, 2005, contractors shall accept claims with the following HCPCS code for non-covered PET indications: - G0235: PET imaging, any site not otherwise specified Short Descriptor: PET not otherwise specified Type of Service: 4

NOTE: This code is for a non-covered service.

100-04, 13, 60.15

Billing Requirements for CMS - Approved Clinical Trials and Coverage With Evidence Development Claims for PET Scans for Neurodegenerative Diseases, Previously Specified Cancer Indications, and All Other Cancer Indications Not Previously Specified

Parts A and B Medicare Administrative Contractors (MACs)

(Rev.3227, Issued: 04-02-15, Multiple effective dates)

Effective for services on or after January 28, 2005, contractors shall accept and pay for claims for Positron Emission Tomography (PET) scans for lung cancer, esophageal cancer, colorectal cancer, lymphoma, melanoma, head & neck cancer, breast cancer, thyroid cancer, soft tissue sarcoma, brain cancer, ovarian cancer, pancreatic cancer, small cell lung cancer, and testicular cancer, as well as for neurodegenerative diseases and all other cancer indications not previously mentioned in this chapter, if these scans were performed as part of a Centers for Medicare & Medicaid (CMS)-approved clinical trial. (See Pub. 100-03, National Coverage Determinations (NCD) Manual, sections 220.6.13 and 220.6.17.)

Contractors shall also be aware that PET scans for all cancers not previously specified at Pub. 100-03, NCD Manual, section 220.6.17, remain nationally non-covered unless performed in conjunction with a CMS-approved clinical trial.

Effective for dates of service on or after June 11, 2013, Medicare has ended the coverage with evidence development (CED) requirement for FDG (2-[F18] fluoro-2-deoxy-D-glucose) PET and PET/computed tomography (CT) and PET/magnetic resonance imaging (MRI) for all oncologic indications contained in section 220.6.17 of the NCD Manual. Modifier -Q0 (Investigational clinical service provided in a clinical research study that is in an approved clinical research study) or -Q1 (routine clinical service provided in a clinical research study that is in an approved clinical research study) is no longer mandatory for these services when performed on or after June 11, 2013.

Part B MACs Only

Part B MACs shall pay claims for PET scans for beneficiaries participating in a CMS-approved clinical trial submitted with an appropriate current procedural terminology (CPT) code from section 60.3.1 of this chapter and modifier -Q0/-Q1 for services performed on or after January 1, 2008, through June 10, 2013. (NOTE: Modifier -QR (Item or service provided in a Medicare specified study) and -QA (FDA investigational device exemption) were replaced by modifier -Q0 effective January 1, 2008.) Modifier -QV (item or service provided as routine care in a Medicare qualifying clinical trial) was replaced by modifier -Q1 effective January 1, 2008.) Beginning with services performed on or after June 11, 2013, modifier -Q0/-Q1 is no longer required for PET FDG services.

Part A MACs Only

In order to pay claims for PET scans on behalf of beneficiaries participating in a CMS-approved clinical trial, Part A MACs require providers to submit claims with ICD-9/ICD-10 code V70.7/Z00.6 in the primary/secondary diagnosis position on the CMS-1450 (UB-04), or the electronic equivalent, with the appropriate principal diagnosis code and an appropriate CPT code from section 60.3.1. Effective for PET scan claims for dates of service on or after January 28, 2005, through December 31, 2007, FIs shall accept claims with the –QR, -QV, or -QA modifier on other than inpatient claims. Effective for services on or after January 1, 2008, through June 10, 2013, modifier -Q0 replaced the -QR and –QA modifier, modifier –Q1 replaced the –QV modifier. Modifier -Q0/-Q1 is no longer required for services performed on or after June 11, 2013.

100-04, 13, 60.16

Billing and Coverage Changes for PET Scans Effective for Services on or After April 3, 2009

(Rev.3650, Issued: 11-10-16, Effective: 02-10-17, Implementation: 02-10-17)

A. Summary of Changes

Effective for services on or after April 3, 2009, Medicare will not cover the use of FDG PET imaging to determine initial treatment strategy in patients with adenocarcinoma of the prostate.

Medicare will also not cover FDG PET imaging for subsequent treatment strategy for tumor types other than breast, cervical, colorectal, esophagus, head and neck (non-CNS/thyroid), lymphoma, melanoma, myeloma, non-small cell lung, and ovarian, unless

the FDG PET is provided under the coverage with evidence development (CED) paradigm (billed with modifier -Q0/-Q1, see section 60.15 of this chapter).

Medicare will cover FDG PET imaging for initial treatment strategy for myeloma.

Effective for services performed on or after June 11, 2013, Medicare has ended the CED requirement for FDG PET and PET/CT and PET/MRI for all oncologic indications contained in section 220.6.17 of the NCD Manual. Effective for services on or after June 11, 2013, the Q0/Q1 modifier is no longer required.

Beginning with services performed on or after June 11, 2013, contractors shall pay for up to three (3) FDG PET scans when used to guide subsequent management of anti-tumor treatment strategy (modifier PS) after completion of initial anti-cancer therapy (modifier PI) for the exact same cancer diagnosis.

Coverage of any additional FDG PET scans (that is, beyond 3) used to guide subsequent management of anti-tumor treatment strategy after completion of initial anti-tumor therapy for the same cancer diagnosis will be determined by the A/B MACs (A or B). Claims will include the KX modifier indicating the coverage criteria is met for coverage of four or more FDG PET scans for subsequent treatment strategy for the same cancer diagnosis under this NCD.

A different cancer diagnosis whether submitted with a PI or a PS modifier will begin the count of one initial and three subsequent FDG PET scans not requiring the KX modifier and four or more FDG PET scans for subsequent treatment strategy for the same cancer diagnosis requiring the KX modifier.

NOTE: The presence or absence of an initial treatment strategy claim in a beneficiary's record does not impact the frequency criteria for subsequent treatment strategy claims for the same cancer diagnosis.

NOTE: Providers please refer to the following link for a list of appropriate diagnosis codes, http://cms.gov/medicare/coverage/determinationprocess/downloads/petforsolidtumorsoncologicdxcodesattachment_NCD220_6_17.pdf

For further information regarding the changes in coverage, refer to Pub.100-03, NCD Manual, section 220.6.17.

B. Modifiers for PET Scans

Effective for claims with dates of service on or after April 3, 2009, the following modifiers have been created for use to inform for the initial treatment strategy of biopsy-proven or strongly suspected tumors or subsequent treatment strategy of cancerous tumors:

PI Positron Emission Tomography (PET) or PET/Computed Tomography (CT) to inform the initial treatment strategy of tumors that are biopsy proven or strongly suspected of being cancerous based on other diagnostic testing.

Short descriptor: PET tumor init tx strat

PS Positron Emission Tomography (PET) or PET/Computed Tomography (CT) to inform the subsequent treatment strategy of cancerous tumors when the beneficiary's treatment physician determines that the PET study is needed to inform subsequent anti-tumor strategy.

Short descriptor: PS - PET tumor subsq tx strategy

C. Billing for A/B MACs (A and B)

Effective for claims with dates of service on or after April 3, 2009, contractors shall accept FDG PET claims billed to inform initial treatment strategy with the following CPT codes AND modifier PI: 78608, 78811, 78812, 78813, 78814, 78815, 78816.

Effective for claims with dates of service on or after April 3, 2009, contractors shall accept FDG PET claims with modifier PS for the subsequent treatment strategy for solid tumors using a CPT code above AND a cancer diagnosis code.

Contractors shall also accept FDG PET claims billed to inform initial treatment strategy or subsequent treatment strategy when performed under CED with one of the PET or PET/CT CPT codes above AND modifier PI OR modifier PS AND a cancer diagnosis code AND modifier Q0/Q1. Effective for services performed on or after June 11, 2013, the CED requirement has ended and modifier Q0/Q1, along with condition code 30 (institutional claims only), or ICD-9 code V70.7, (both institutional and practitioner claims) are no longer required.

D. Medicare Summary Notices, Remittance Advice Remark Codes, and Claim Adjustment Reason Codes

Effective for dates of service on or after April 3, 2009, contractors shall return as unprocessable/return to provider claims that do not include the PI modifier with one of the PET/PET/CT CPT codes listed in subsection C. above when billing for the initial treatment strategy for solid tumors in accordance with Pub.100-03, NCD Manual, section 220.6.17.

© 2019 Optum360, LLC

In addition, contractors shall return as unprocessable/return to provider claims that do not include the PS modifier with one of the CPT codes listed in subsection C. above when billing for the subsequent treatment strategy for solid tumors in accordance with Pub.100-03, NCD Manual, section 220.6.17.

The contractor shall use the following remittance advice messages and associated codes when returning claims under this policy. This CARC/RARC combination is compliant with CAQH CORE Business Scenario Two.

Group Code: CO
CARC: 4
RARC: MA130
MSN: N/A

Effective for claims with dates of service on or after April 3, 2009, through June 10, 2013, contractors shall return as unprocessable/return to provider FDG PET claims billed to inform initial treatment strategy or subsequent treatment strategy when performed under CED without one of the PET/PET/CT CPT codes listed in subsection C. above AND modifier PI OR modifier PS AND a cancer diagnosis code AND modifier Q0/Q1.

The contractor shall use the following remittance advice messages and associated codes when returning claims under this policy. This CARC/RARC combination is compliant with CAQH CORE Business Scenario Two.

Group Code: CO
CARC: 4
RARC: MA130
MSN: N/A

Effective April 3, 2009, contractors shall deny claims with ICD-9/ICD-10 diagnosis code 185/C61 for FDG PET imaging for the initial treatment strategy of patients with adenocarcinoma of the prostate.

For dates of service prior to June 11, 2013, contractors shall also deny claims for FDG PET imaging for subsequent treatment strategy for tumor types other than breast, cervical, colorectal, esophagus, head and neck (non-CNS/thyroid), lymphoma, melanoma, myeloma, non-small cell lung, and ovarian, unless the FDG PET is provided under CED (submitted with the Q0/Q1 modifier) and use the following messages:

The contractor shall use the following remittance advice messages and associated codes when rejecting/denying claims under this policy. This CARC/RARC combination is compliant with CAQH CORE Business Scenario Three.

Group Code: PR (if claim is received with a GA modifier) otherwise CO
CARC: 50
RARC: N/A
MSN: 15.4

Effective for dates of service on or after June 11, 2013, contractors shall use the following messages when denying claims in excess of three for PET FDG scans for subsequent treatment strategy when the KX modifier is not included, identified by CPT codes 78608, 78811, 78812, 78813, 78814, 78815, or 78816, modifier PS, HCPCS A9552, and the same cancer diagnosis code.

The contractor shall use the following remittance advice messages and associated codes when rejecting/denying claims under this policy. This CARC/RARC combination is compliant with CAQH CORE Business Scenario Three.

Group Code: PR (if claim is received with a GA modifier) otherwise CO
CARC: 96
RARC: N435
MSN: 23.17

100-04, 13, 60.17

Billing and Coverage Changes for PET Scans for Cervical Cancer Effective for Services on or After November 10, 2009

(Rev.3650, Issued: 11-10-16, Effective: 02-10-17, Implementation: 02-10-17)

A. Billing Changes for A/B MACs (A and B)

Effective for claims with dates of service on or after November 10, 2009, contractors shall accept FDG PET oncologic claims billed to inform initial treatment strategy; specifically for staging in beneficiaries who have biopsy-proven cervical cancer when the beneficiary's treating physician determines the FDG PET study is needed to determine the location and/or extent of the tumor as specified in Pub. 100-03, section 220.6.17.

EXCEPTION: CMS continues to non-cover FDG PET for initial diagnosis of cervical cancer related to initial treatment strategy.

NOTE: Effective for claims with dates of service on and after November 10, 2009, the –Q0 modifier is no longer necessary for FDG PET for cervical cancer.

B. Medicare Summary Notices, Remittance Advice Remark Codes, and Claim Adjustment Reason Codes

Additionally, contractors shall return as unprocessable /return to provider for FDG PET for cervical cancer for initial treatment strategy billed without the following: one of the PET/PET/ CT CPT codes listed in 60.16 C above AND modifier PI AND a cervical cancer diagnosis code.

The contractor shall use the following remittance advice messages and associated codes when returning claims under this policy. This CARC/RARC combination is compliant with CAQH CORE Business Scenario Two.

Group Code: CO
CARC: 4
RARC: MA130
MSN: N/A

100-04, 13, 60.18

Billing and Coverage Changes for PET (NaF-18) Scans to Identify Bone Metastasis of Cancer Effective for Claims With Dates of Services on or After February 26, 2010

(Rev.3650, Issued: 11-10-16, Effective: 02-10-17, Implementation: 02-10-17)

A. Billing Changes for A/B MACs (A and B)

Effective for claims with dates of service on and after February 26, 2010, contractors shall pay for NaF-18 PET oncologic claims to inform of initial treatment strategy (PI) or subsequent treatment strategy (PS) for suspected or biopsy proven bone metastasis ONLY in the context of a clinical study and as specified in Pub. 100-03, section 220.6. All other claims for NaF-18 PET oncology claims remain non-covered.

B. Medicare Summary Notices, Remittance Advice Remark Codes, and Claim Adjustment Reason Codes

Effective for claims with dates of service on or after February 26, 2010, contractors shall return as unprocessable NaF-18 PET oncologic claims billed with modifier TC or globally (for A/B MACs (A) modifier TC or globally does not apply) and HCPCS A9580 to inform the initial treatment strategy or subsequent treatment strategy for bone metastasis that do not include ALL of the following:

- PI or PS modifier AND
- PET or PET/CT CPT code (78811, 78812, 78813, 78814, 78815, 78816) AND
- Cancer diagnosis code AND
- Q0 modifier - Investigational clinical service provided in a clinical research study, are present on the claim.

NOTE: For institutional claims, continue to include ICD-9 diagnosis code V70.7 or ICD-10 diagnosis code Z00.6 and condition code 30 to denote a clinical study.

The contractor shall use the following remittance advice messages and associated codes when returning claims under this policy. This CARC/RARC combination is compliant with CAQH CORE Business Scenario Two

Group Code: CO
CARC: 4
RARC: MA130
MSN: N/A

Effective for claims with dates of service on or after February 26, 2010, contractors shall accept PET oncologic claims billed with modifier 26 and modifier KX to inform the initial treatment strategy or subsequent treatment strategy for bone metastasis that include the following:

- PI or PS modifier AND
- PET or PET/CT CPT code (78811, 78812, 78813, 78814, 78815, 78816) AND
- Cancer diagnosis code AND
- Q0 modifier - Investigational clinical service provided in a clinical research study, are present on the claim.

NOTE: If modifier KX is present on the professional component service, Contractors shall process the service as PET NaF-18 rather than PET with FDG.

Contractors shall also return as unprocessable NaF-18 PET oncologic professional component claims (i.e., claims billed with modifiers 26 and KX) to inform the initial treatment strategy or subsequent treatment strategy for bone metastasis billed with HCPCS A9580.

The contractor shall use the following remittance advice messages and associated codes when returning claims under this policy. This CARC/RARC combination is compliant with CAQH CORE Business Scenario Two.

Group Code: CO
CARC: 4
RARC: MA130
MSN: N/A

© 2019 Optum360, LLC

100-04, 13, 90.3

Transportation Component (HCPCS Codes R0070 - R0076)

(Rev.3387, Issued: 10-30-15, Effective: 01-01-16, Implementation: 01-01-16)

This component represents the transportation of the equipment to the patient. Establish local RVUs for the transportation R codes based on Medicare Administrative Contractor (MAC) knowledge of the nature of the service furnished. The MACs shall allow only a single transportation payment for each trip the portable x-ray supplier makes to a particular location. When more than one patient is x-rayed at the same location, e.g., a nursing home, prorate the single fee schedule transportation payment among all patients (Medicare Parts A and B, and non-Medicare) receiving the portable x-ray services during that trip, regardless of their insurance status. For example, for portable x-ray services furnished at a Skilled Nursing Facility (SNF), the transportation fee should be allocated among all patients receiving portable x-ray services at the same location in a single trip irrespective of whether the patient is in a Part A stay, a Part B patient, or not a Medicare beneficiary at all. If the patient is in a Part A SNF stay, the transportation and set up costs are subject to consolidated billing and not separately billable to Medicare Part B. For a privately insured patient, it would be the responsibility of that patient's insurer. For a Medicare Part B patient, payment would be made under Part B for the share of the transportation fee attributable to that patient.

R0075 must be billed in conjunction with the CPT radiology codes (7000 series) and only when the x-ray equipment used was actually transported to the location where the x-ray was taken. R0075 would not apply to the x-ray equipment stored in the location where the x-ray was done (e.g., a nursing home) for use as needed.

Below are the definitions for each modifier that must be reported with R0075. Only one of these five modifiers shall be reported with R0075. NOTE: If only one patient is served, R0070 should be reported with no modifier since the descriptor for this code reflects only one patient seen.

UN - Two patients served

UP - Three patients served

UQ - Four patients served

UR - Five Patients served

US - Six or more patients served

Payment for the above modifiers must be consistent with the definition of the modifiers. Therefore, for R0075 reported with modifiers, -UN, -UP, -UQ, and –UR, the total payment for the service shall be divided by 2, 3, 4, and 5 respectively. For modifier –US, the total payment for the service shall be divided by 6 regardless of the number of patients served. For example, if 8 patients were served, R0075 would be reported with modifier –US and the total payment for this service would be divided by 6.

The units field for R0075 shall always be reported as "1" except in extremely unusual cases. The number in the units field should be completed in accordance with the provisions of 100-04, chapter 23, section 10.2 item 24 G which defines the units field as the number of times the patient has received the itemized service during the dates listed in the from/to field. The units field must never be used to report the number of patients served during a single trip. Specifically, the units field must reflect the number of services that the specific beneficiary received, not the number of services received by other beneficiaries.

As a contractor priced service, MACs must initially determine a payment rate for portable x-ray transportation services that is associated with the cost of providing the service. In order to determine an appropriate cost, the MAC should, at a minimum, cost out the vehicle, vehicle modifications, gasoline and the staff time involved in only the transportation for a portable x-ray service. A review of the pricing of this service should be done every five years

Direct costs related to the vehicle carrying the x-ray machine are fully allocable to determining the payment rate. This includes the cost of the vehicle using a recognized depreciation method, the salary and fringe benefits associated with the staff who drive the vehicle, the communication equipment used between the vehicle and the home office, the salary and fringe benefits of the staff who determine the vehicles route (this could be proportional of office staff), repairs and maintenance of the vehicle(s), insurance for the vehicle(s), operating expenses for the vehicles and any other reasonable costs associated with this service as determined by the MAC. The MAC will have discretion for allocating indirect costs (those costs that cannot be directly attributed to portable x-ray transportation) between the transportation service and the technical component of the x-ray tests.

Suppliers may send MACs unsolicited cost information. The MACs may use this cost data as a comparison to its contractor priced determination. The data supplied should reflect a year's worth (either calendar or corporate fiscal) of information. Each provider who submits such data is to be informed that the data is subject to verification and will be used to supplement other information that is used to determine Medicare's payment rate.

The MACs are required to update the rate on an annual basis using independently determined measures of the cost of providing the service. A number of readily available measures (e.g., ambulance inflation factor, the Medicare economic index) that are used by the Medicare program to adjust payment rates for other types of services may be appropriate to use to update the rate for years that the MAC does not recalibrate the payment. Each MAC has the flexibility to identify the index it will use to update the rate. In addition, the MAC can consider locally identified factors that are measured independently of CMS as an adjunct to the annual adjustment.

NOTE: No transportation charge is payable unless the portable x-ray equipment used was actually transported to the location where the x-ray was taken. For example, MACs do not allow a transportation charge when the x-ray equipment is stored in a nursing home for use as needed. However, a set-up payment (see §90.4, below) is payable in such situations. Further, for services furnished on or after January 1, 1997, MACs may not make separate payment under HCPCS code R0076 for the transportation of EKG equipment by portable x-ray suppliers or any other entity.

100-04, 13, 90.4

Set-Up Component (HCPCS Code Q0092)

(Rev.1, 10-01-03)

Carriers must pay a set-up component for each radiologic procedure (other than retakes of the same procedure) during both single patient and multiple patient trips under Level II HCPCS code Q0092. Carriers do not make the set-up payment for EKG services furnished by the portable x-ray supplier.

100-04, 13, 140.1

Payment Methodology and HCPCS Coding

(Rev.4150, Issued: 10-26-2018, Effective: 04-01-19, Implementation: 04-01-19)

A/B MACs (B) pay for BMM procedures based on the Medicare physician fee schedule. Claims from physicians, other practitioners, or suppliers where assignment was not taken are subject to the Medicare limiting charge.

The A/B MACs (A) pay for BMM procedures under the current payment methodologies for radiology services according to the type of provider.

Do not pay BMM procedure claims for dual photon absorptiometry, CPT procedure code 78351.

Deductible and coinsurance *do not* apply.

Any of the following CPT procedure codes may be used when billing for BMMs through December 31, 2006. All of these codes are bone densitometry measurements except code 76977, which is bone sonometry measurements. CPT procedure codes are applicable to billing A/B MACs (A and B).

76070 76071 76075 76076 76078 76977 78350 G0130

Effective for dates of services on and after January 1, 2007, the following changes apply to BMM:

New 2007 CPT bone mass procedure codes have been assigned for BMM. The following codes will replace current codes, however the CPT descriptors for the services remain the same:

77078 replaces 76070

77079 replaces 76071

77080 replaces 76075

77081 replaces 76076

77083 replaces 76078

Effective for dates of service on and after January 1, 2015, contractors shall pay for bone mass procedure code 77085 (Dual-energy X-ray absorptiometry (DXA), bone density study, 1 or more sites, axial skeleton, (e.g., hips, pelvis, spine), including vertebral fracture assessment.)

Certain BMM tests are covered when used to screen patients for osteoporosis subject to the frequency standards described in chapter 15, section 80.5.5 of the Medicare Benefit Policy Manual.

Contractors will pay claims for screening tests when coded as follows:

Contains CPT procedure code 77078, 77079, 77080, 77081, 77083, 76977 or G0130, and

Contains a valid diagnosis code indicating the reason for the test is postmenopausal female, vertebral fracture, hyperparathyroidism, or steroid therapy. Contractors are to maintain local lists of valid codes for the benefit's screening categories.

Contractors will deny claims for screening tests when coded as follows:

© 2019 Optum360, LLC

Contains CPT procedure code 77078, 77079, 77081, 77083, 76977 or G0130, but

Does not contain a valid diagnosis code from the local lists of valid diagnosis codes maintained by the contractor for the benefit's screening categories indicating the reason for the test is postmenopausal female, vertebral fracture, hyperparathyroidism, or steroid therapy.

Dual-energy x-ray absorptiometry (axial) tests are covered when used to monitor FDA-approved osteoporosis drug therapy subject to the 2-year frequency standards described in chapter 15, section 80.5.5 of the Medicare Benefit Policy Manual.

Contractors will pay claims for monitoring tests when coded as follows:

Contains CPT procedure code 77080 *or 77085*, and

Contains 733.00, 733.01, 733.02, 733.03, 733.09, 733.90, or 255.0 as the ICD-9-CM diagnosis code or M81.0, M81.8, M81.6 or M94.9 as the ICD-10-CM diagnosis code.

Contractors will deny claims for monitoring tests when coded as follows:

Contains CPT procedure code 77078, 77079, 77081, 77083, 76977 or G0130, and

Contains 733.00, 733.01, 733.02, 733.03, 733.09, 733.90, or 255.0 as the ICD-9-CM diagnosis code, but

Does not contain a valid ICD-9-CM diagnosis code from the local lists of valid ICD-9-CM diagnosis codes maintained by the contractor for the benefit's screening categories indicating the reason for the test is postmenopausal female, vertebral fracture, hyperparathyroidism, or steroid therapy.

Does not contain a valid ICD-10-CM diagnosis code from the local lists of valid ICD-10-CM diagnosis codes maintained by the contractor for the benefit's screening categories indicating the reason for the test is postmenopausal female, vertebral fracture, hyperparathyroidism, or steroid therapy.

Single photon absorptiometry tests are not covered. Contractors will deny CPT procedure code 78350.

The A/B MACs (A) are billed using the ASC X12 837 institutional claim format or hardcopy Form CMS-1450. The appropriate bill types are: 12X, 13X, 22X, 23X, 34X, 71X (Provider-based and independent), 72X, 77X (Provider-based and freestanding), 83X, and 85X. Effective April 1, 2006, type of bill 14X is for non-patient laboratory specimens and is no longer applicable for bone mass measurements. Information regarding the claim form locators that correspond to the HCPCS/CPT code or Type of Bill are found in chapter 25.

Providers must report HCPCS codes for bone mass measurements under revenue code 320 with number of units and line item dates of service per revenue code line for each bone mass measurement reported.

A/B MACs (B) are billed for bone mass measurement procedures using the ASC X12 837 professional claim format or hardcopy Form CMS-1500.

100-04, 14, 40.8

Payment When a Device is Furnished With No Cost or With Full or Partial Credit Beginning January 1, 2008

(Rev.1669, Issued: 01-13-09, Effective: 01-01-09, Implementation: 01-05-09)

Contractors pay ASCs a reduced amount for certain specified procedures when a specified device is furnished without cost or for which either a partial or full credit is received (e.g., device recall). For specified procedure codes that include payment for a device, ASCs are required to include modifier -FB on the procedure code when a specified device is furnished without cost or for which full credit is received. If the ASC receives a partial credit of 50 percent or more of the cost of a specified device, the ASC is required to include modifier -FC on the procedure code if the procedure is on the list of specified procedures to which the -FC reduction applies. A single procedure code should not be submitted with both modifiers -FB and -FC. The pricing determination related to modifiers -FB and -FC is made prior to the application of multiple procedure payment reductions. Contractors adjust beneficiary coinsurance to reflect the reduced payment amount. Tables listing the procedures and devices to which the payment adjustments apply, and the full and partial adjustment amounts, are available on the CMS Web site.

In order to report that the receipt of a partial credit of 50 percent or more of the cost of a device, ASCs have the option of either: 1) Submitting the claim for the procedure to their Medicare contractor after the procedure's performance but prior to manufacturer acknowledgement of credit for a specified device, and subsequently contacting the contractor regarding a claims adjustment once the credit determination is made; or 2) holding the claim for the procedure until a determination is made by the manufacturer on the partial credit and submitting the claim with modifier -FC appended to the implantation procedure HCPCS code if the partial credit is 50 percent or more of the cost of the device. If choosing the first billing option, to request a claims adjustment once the credit determination is made, ASCs should keep in mind that the initial Medicare payment for the procedure involving the device is conditional and subject to adjustment.

100-04, 15, 20.1.4

Components of the Ambulance Fee Schedule

(Rev.3800, Issued: 06 -23 -17, Effective: 07 - 25- 17, Implementation: 07- 25- 17)

The mileage rates provided in this section are the base rates that are adjusted by the yearly ambulance inflation factor (AIF). The payment amount under the fee schedule is determined as follows:

- For ground ambulance services, the fee schedule amount includes:
  1. A money amount that serves as a nationally uniform base rate, called a "conversion factor" (CF), for all ground ambulance services;
  2. A relative value unit (RVU) assigned to each type of ground ambulance service;
  3. A geographic adjustment factor (GAF) for each ambulance fee schedule locality area (geographic practice cost index (GPCI));
  4. A nationally uniform loaded mileage rate;
  5. An additional amount for certain mileage for a rural point-of-pickup; and
  6. For specified temporary periods, certain additional payment amounts as described in section 20.1.4A, below.
- For air ambulance services, the fee schedule amount includes:
  1. A nationally uniform base rate for fixed wing and a nationally uniform base rate for rotary wing;
  2. A geographic adjustment factor (GAF) for each ambulance fee schedule locality area (GPCI);
  3. A nationally uniform loaded mileage rate for each type of air service; and
  4. A rural adjustment to the base rate and mileage for services furnished for a rural point-of-pickup.

A. Ground Ambulance Services

1. Conversion Factor

The conversion factor (CF) is a money amount used to develop a base rate for each category of ground ambulance service. The CF is updated annually by the ambulance inflation factor and for other reasons as necessary.

2. Relative Value Units

Relative value units (RVUs) set a numeric value for ambulance services relative to the value of a base level ambulance service. Since there are marked differences in resources necessary to furnish the various levels of ground ambulance services, different levels of payment are appropriate for the various levels of service. The different payment amounts are based on level of service. An RVU expresses the constant multiplier for a particular type of service (including, where appropriate, an emergency response). An RVU of 1.00 is assigned to the BLS of ground service, e.g., BLS has an RVU of 1; higher RVU values are assigned to the other types of ground ambulance services, which require more service than BLS.

The RVUs are as follows:

Service Level	RVU
BLS	1.00
BLS - Emergency	1.60
ALS1	1.20
ALS1- Emergency	1.90
ALS2	2.75
SCT	3.25
PI	1.75

3. Geographic Adjustment Factor (GAF)

The GAF is one of two factors intended to address regional differences in the cost of furnishing ambulance services. The GAF for the ambulance FS uses the non-facility practice expense (PE) of the geographic practice cost index (GPCI) of the Medicare physician fee schedule to adjust payment to account for regional differences. Thus, the geographic areas applicable to the ambulance FS are the same as those used for the physician fee schedule.

The location where the beneficiary was put into the ambulance (POP) establishes which GPCI applies. For multiple vehicle transports, each leg of the transport is separately evaluated for the applicable GPCI. Thus, for the second (or any subsequent) leg of a transport, the POP establishes the applicable GPCI for that portion of the ambulance transport.

© 2019 Optum360, LLC

For ground ambulance services, the applicable GPCI is multiplied by 70 percent of the base rate. Again, the base rate for each category of ground ambulance services is the CF multiplied by the applicable RVU. The GPCI is not applied to the ground mileage rate.

4. Mileage

In the context of all payment instructions, the term "mileage" refers to loaded mileage. The ambulance FS provides a separate payment amount for mileage. The mileage rate per statute mile applies for all types of ground ambulance services, except Paramedic Intercept, and is provided to all Medicare contractors electronically by CMS as part of the ambulance FS. Providers and suppliers must report all medically necessary mileage, including the mileage subject to a rural adjustment, in a single line item.

5. Adjustment for Certain Ground Mileage for Rural Points of Pickup (POP)

The payment rate is greater for certain mileage where the POP is in a rural area to account for the higher costs per ambulance trip that are typical of rural operations where fewer trips are made in any given period.

If the POP is a rural ZIP Code, the following calculations should be used to determine the rural adjustment portion of the payment allowance. For loaded miles 1-17, the rural adjustment for ground mileage is 1.5 times the rural mileage allowance.

For services furnished during the period July 1, 2004 through December 31, 2008, a 25 percent increase is applied to the appropriate ambulance FS mileage rate to each mile of a transport (both urban and rural POP) that exceeds 50 miles (i.e., mile 51 and greater).

The following chart summarizes the above information:

Service	Dates of Service	Bonus	Calculation
Loaded miles 1-17, Rural POP	Beginning 4/1/02	50%	FS Rural mileage * 1.5
Loaded miles 18-50, Rural POP	4/1/02 – 12/31/03	25%	FS Rural mileage * 1.25
All loaded miles (Urban or Rural POP) 51+	7/1/04 – 12/31/08	25%	FS Urban or Rural mileage * 1.25

The POP, as identified by ZIP Code, establishes whether a rural adjustment applies to a particular service. Each leg of a multi-leg transport is separately evaluated for a rural adjustment application. Thus, for the second (or any subsequent) leg of a transport, the ZIP Code of the POP establishes whether a rural adjustment applies to such second (or subsequent) transport.

For the purpose of all categories of ground ambulance services except paramedic intercept, a rural area is defined as a U.S. Postal Service (USPS) ZIP Code that is located, in whole or in part, outside of either a Metropolitan Statistical Area (MSA) or in New England, a New England County Metropolitan Area (NECMA), or is an area wholly within an MSA or NECMA that has been identified as rural under the "Goldsmith modification." (The Goldsmith modification establishes an operational definition of rural areas within large counties that contain one or more metropolitan areas. The Goldsmith areas are so isolated by distance or physical features that they are more rural than urban in character and lack easy geographic access to health services.)

For Paramedic Intercept, an area is a rural area if:

- It is designated as a rural area by any law or regulation of a State;
- It is located outside of an MSA or NECMA; or
- It is located in a rural census tract of an MSA as determined under the most recent Goldsmith modification.

See IOM Pub. 100-02, Medicare Benefit Policy Manual, chapter 10 – Ambulance Services, section 30.1.1 – Ground Ambulance Services for coverage requirements for the Paramedic Intercept benefit. Presently, only the State of New York meets these requirements.

Although a transport with a POP located in a rural area is subject to a rural adjustment for mileage, Medicare still pays the lesser of the billed charge or the applicable FS amount for mileage. Thus, when rural mileage is involved, the contractor compares the calculated FS rural mileage payment rate to the provider's/supplier's actual charge for mileage and pays the lesser amount.

The CMS furnishes the ambulance FS files to claims processing contractors electronically. A version of the Ambulance Fee Schedule is also posted to the CMS website (http://www.cms.hhs.gov/AmbulanceFeeSchedule/02_afspuf.asp) for public consumption. To clarify whether a particular ZIP Code is rural or urban, please refer to the most recent version of the Medicare supplied ZIP Code file.

6. Regional Ambulance FS Payment Rate Floor for Ground Ambulance Transports

For services furnished during the period July 1, 2004 through December 31, 2009, the base rate portion of the payment under the ambulance FS for ground ambulance transports is subject to a minimum amount. This minimum amount depends upon the area of the country in which the service is furnished. The country is divided into 9 census divisions and each of the census divisions has a regional FS that is constructed using the same methodology as the national FS. Where the regional FS is greater than the national FS, the base rates for ground ambulance transports are determined by a blend of the national rate and the regional rate in accordance with the following schedule:

Year	National FS Percentage	Regional FS Percentage
7/1/04 - 12/31/04	20%	80%
CY 2005	40%	60%
CY 2006	60%	40%
CY 2007 – CY 2009	80%	20%
CY 2010 and thereafter	100%	0%

Where the regional FS is not greater than the national FS, there is no blending and only the national FS applies. Note that this provision affects only the FS portion of the blended transition payment rate. This floor amount is calculated by CMS centrally and is incorporated into the FS amount that appears in the FS file maintained by CMS and downloaded by CMS contractors. There is no calculation to be done by the Medicare B/MAC or A/MAC in order to implement this provision.

7. Adjustments for FS Payment Rate for Certain Rural Ground Ambulance Transports

For services furnished during the period July 1, 2004 through December 31, 2010, the base rate portion of the payment under the FS for ground ambulance transports furnished in certain rural areas is increased by a percentage amount determined by CMS . Section 3105 (c) and 10311 (c) of the Affordable Care Act amended section 1834 (1) (13) (A) of the Act to extend this rural bonus for an additional year through December 31, 2010. This increase applies if the POP is in a rural county (or Goldsmith area) that is comprised by the lowest quartile by population of all such rural areas arrayed by population density. CMS will determine this bonus amount and the designated POP rural ZIP Codes in which the bonus applies. Beginning on July 1, 2004, rural areas qualifying for the additional bonus amount will be identified with a "B" indicator on the national ZIP Code file. Contractors must apply the additional rural bonus amount as a multiplier to the base rate portion of the FS payment for all ground transports originating in the designated POP ZIP Codes.

Subsequently, section of 106 (c) of the MMEA again amended section 1843 (l) (13) (A) of the Act to extend the rural bonus an additional year, through December 31, 2011.

8. Adjustments for FS Payment Rates for Ground Ambulance Transports

The payment rates under the FS for ground ambulance transports (both the fee schedule base rates and the mileage amounts) are increased for services furnished during the period July 1, 2004 through December 31, 2006 as well as July 1, 2008 through December 31, 2010. For ground ambulance transport services furnished where the POP is urban, the rates are increased by 1 percent for claims with dates of service July 1, 2004 through December 31, 2006 in accordance with Section 414 of the Medicare Modernization Act (MMA) of 2004 and by 2 percent for claims with dates of service July 1, 2008 through December 31, 2010 in accordance with Section 146(a) of the Medicare Improvements for Patients and Providers Act of 2008 and Sections 3105(a) and 10311(a) of the Patient Protection and Affordable Care Act (ACA) of

2010. For ground ambulance transport services furnished where the POP is rural, the rates are increased by 2 percent for claims with dates of service July 1, 2004 through December 31, 2006 in accordance with Section 414 of the Medicare Modernization Act (MMA) of 2004 and by 3 percent for claims with dates of service July 1, 2008 through December 31, 2010 in accordance with Section 146(a) of the Medicare Improvements for Patients and Providers Act of 2008 and Sections 3105(a) and 10311(a) of the Patient Protection and Affordable Care Act (ACA) of 2010. Subsequently, section 106 (a) of the Medicare and Medicaid Extenders Act of 2010 (MMEA) again amended section 1834 (1) (12) (A) of the Act to extend the payment increases for an additional year, through December 31, 2011. These amounts are incorporated into the fee schedule amounts that appear in the Ambulance FS file maintained by CMS and downloaded by CMS contractors. There is no calculation to be done by the Medicare carrier or intermediary in order to implement this provision.

The following chart summarizes the Medicare Prescription Drug, Improvement, and Modernization Act (MMA) of 2003 payment changes for ground ambulance services that became effective on July 1, 2004 as well as the Medicare Improvement for Patients and Providers Act (MIPPA) of 2008 changes that became effective July 1, 2008 and were extended by the Patient Protection and Affordable Care Act of 2010 and the Medicare and Medicaid Extenders Act of 2010 (MMEA).

 © 2019 Optum360, LLC

Summary Chart of Additional Payments for Ground Ambulance Services Provided by MMA, MIPPA and MMEA

Service	Effective Dates	Payment Increase*
All rural miles	7/1/04 - 12/31/06	2%
All rural miles	7/1/08 – 12/31/11	3%
Rural miles 51+	7/1/04 - 12/31/08	25% **
All urban miles	7/1/04 - 12/31/06	1%
All urban miles	7/1/08 – 12/31/11	2%
Urban miles 51+	7/1/04 - 12/31/08	25% **
All rural base rates	7/1/04 - 12/31/06	2%
All rural base rates	7/1/08 – 12/31/11	3%
Rural base rates (lowest quartile)	7/1/04 - 12/31/11	22.6%**
All urban base rates	7/1/04 - 12/31/06	1%
All urban base rates	7/1/08 – 12/31/11	2%
All base rates (regional fee schedule blend)	7/1/04 - 12/31/09	Floor

NOTES: * All payments are percentage increases and all are cumulative.

**Contractor systems perform this calculation. All other increases are incorporated into the CMS Medicare Ambulance FS file.

B. Air Ambulance Services

1. Base Rates
   Each type of air ambulance service has a base rate. There is no conversion factor (CF) applicable to air ambulance services.
2. Geographic Adjustment Factor (GAF)
   The GAF, as described above for ground ambulance services, is also used for air ambulance services. However, for air ambulance services, the applicable GPCI is applied to 50 percent of each of the base rates (fixed and rotary wing).
3. Mileage
   The FS for air ambulance services provides a separate payment for mileage.
4. Adjustment for Services Furnished in Rural Areas
   The payment rates for air ambulance services where the POP is in a rural area are greater than in an urban area. For air ambulance services (fixed or rotary wing), the rural adjustment is an increase of 50 percent to the unadjusted FS amount, e.g., the applicable air service base rate multiplied by the GAF plus the mileage amount or, in other words, 1.5 times both the applicable air service base rate and the total mileage amount.

The basis for a rural adjustment for air ambulance services is determined in the same manner as for ground services. That is, whether the POP is within a rural ZIP Code as described above for ground services.

100-04, 15, 20.3

Air Ambulance

(Rev.3380, Iss: 10-23-15, Eff: 01-01-16, Imp: 01-04-16)

PHs AB-01-165, AB-02-036, and AB-02-131; B3-5116.5, B3-5205 partial

Refer to IOM Pub. 100-02, Medicare Benefit Policy Manual, chapter 10 - Ambulance Services, section 10.4 - Air Ambulance Services, for additional information on the coverage of air ambulance services. Under certain circumstances, transportation by airplane or helicopter may qualify as covered ambulance services. If the conditions of coverage are met, payment may be made for the air ambulance services.

Air ambulance services are paid at different rates according to two air ambulance categories:

- AIR ambulance service, conventional air services, transport, one way, fixed wing (FW) (HCPCS code A0430)
- AIR ambulance service, conventional air services, transport, one way, rotary wing (RW) (HCPCS code A0431)

Covered air ambulance mileage services are paid when the appropriate HCPCS code is reported on the claim:

HCPCS code A0435 identifies FIXED WING AIR MILEAGE

HCPCS code A0436 identifies ROTARY WING AIR MILEAGE

Air mileage must be reported in whole numbers of loaded statute miles flown. Contractors must ensure that the appropriate air transport code is used with the appropriate mileage code.

Air ambulance services may be paid only for ambulance services to a hospital. Other destinations e.g., skilled nursing facility, a physician's office, or a patient's home may not be paid air ambulance. The destination is identified by the use of an appropriate modifier as defined in Section 30(A) of this chapter.

Claims for air transports may account for all mileage from the point of pickup, including where applicable: ramp to taxiway, taxiway to runway, takeoff run, air miles, roll out upon landing, and taxiing after landing. Additional air mileage may be allowed by the contractor in situations where additional mileage is incurred, due to circumstances beyond the pilot's control. These circumstances include, but are not limited to, the following:

Military base and other restricted zones, air-defense zones, and similar FAA restrictions and prohibitions;

Hazardous weather; or

Variances in departure patterns and clearance routes required by an air traffic controller.

If the air transport meets the criteria for medical necessity, Medicare pays the actual miles flown for legitimate reasons as determined by the Medicare contractor, once the Medicare beneficiary is loaded onto the air ambulance.

IOM Pub. 100-08, Medicare Program Integrity Manual, chapter 6 - Intermediary MR Guidelines for Specific Services contains instructions for Medical Review of Air Ambulance Services.

100-04, 15, 20.4

Ambulance Inflation Factor (AIF)

(Rev.4172, Issued: 11-30-18, Effective: 01-01-19, Implementation: 01-07-19)

Section 1834(l)(3)(B) of the Social Security Act (the Act) provides the basis for an update to the payment limits for ambulance services that is equal to the percentage increase in the consumer price index for all urban consumers (CPI-U) for the 12-month period ending with June of the previous year. Section 3401 of the Affordable Care Act amended Section 1834(l)(3) of the Act to apply a productivity adjustment to this update equal to the 10-year moving average of changes in economy-wide private nonfarm business multi- factor productivity beginning January 1, 2011. The resulting update percentage is referred to as the Ambulance Inflation Factor (AIF). These updated percentages are issued via Recurring Update Notifications.

Part B coinsurance and deductible requirements apply to payments under the ambulance fee schedule. Following is a chart tracking the history of the AIF:

CY	AIF
2003	1.1
2004	2.1
2005	3.3
2006	2.5
2007	4.3
2008	2.7
2009	5.0
2010	0.0
2011	-0.1
2012	2.4
2013	0.8
2014	1.0
2015	1.5
2016	-0.4
2017	0.7
2018	1.1
2019	2.3

100-04, 15, 20.6

Payment for Non-Emergency Trips to/from ESRD Facilities

(Rev.4017; Issued: 04-06-18; Effective: 10-01-18; Implementation: 10-01-18)

Section 637 of the American Taxpayer Relief Act of 2012 requires that, effective for transports occurring on and after October 1, 2013, fee schedule payments for non-emergency basic life support (BLS) transports of individuals with end-stage renal disease (ESRD) to and from renal dialysis treatment be reduced by 10%. The payment reduction affects transports (base rate and mileage) to and from hospital-based and freestanding renal dialysis treatment facilities for dialysis services provided on a non-emergency basis. Non-emergency BLS ground transports are identified by Healthcare Common Procedure Code System (HCPCS) code A0428. Ambulance transports to and from renal dialysis treatment are identified by modifier codes "G" (hospital-based

© 2019 Optum360, LLC

ESRD) and "J" (freestanding ESRD facility) in either the first position (origin code) or second position (destination code) within the two-digit ambulance modifier. (See Section 30 (A) for information regarding modifiers specific to ambulance.)

Effective for claims with dates of service on and after October 1, 2013 through September 20, 2018, the 10% reduction will be calculated and applied to HCPCS code A0428 when billed with modifier code "G" or "J". The reduction will also be applied to any mileage billed in association with a non-emergency transport of a beneficiary with ESRD to and from renal dialysis treatment. BLS mileage is identified by HCPCS code A0425.

The 10% reduction will be taken after calculation of the normal fee schedule payment amount, including any add-on or bonus payments, and will apply to transports in rural and urban areas as well as areas designated as "super rural".

Payment for emergency transports is not affected by this reduction. Payment for non-emergency BLS transports to other destinations is also not affected. This reduction does not affect or change the Ambulance Fee Schedule.

Note: The 10% reduction applies to beneficiaries with ESRD that are receiving non-emergency BLS transport to and from renal dialysis treatment. While it is possible that a beneficiary who is not diagnosed with ESRD will require routine transport to and from renal dialysis treatment, it is highly unlikely. However, contractors have discretion to override or reverse the reduction on appeal if they deem it appropriate based on supporting documentation.

Section 53108 of the Bipartisan Budget Act of 2018 increased the amount of the reduction described above to 23% for transports occurring on and after October 1, 2018.

100-04, 15, 30

General Billing Guidelines

(Rev.3076, Issued: 09-24-14, Effective: Upon Implementation of ICD-10 ASC X12: 01-01-12, Implementation: ICD-10: Upon Implementation of ICD-10 ASC X12: 09-16-14)

Independent ambulance suppliers may bill on the ASC X12 837 professional claim transaction or the CMS-1500 form. These claims are processed using the Multi-Carrier System (MCS).

Institution based ambulance providers may bill on the ASC X12 837 institutional claim transaction or Form CMS 1450. These claims are processed using the Fiscal Intermediary Shared System (FISS).

A. Modifiers Specific to Ambulance Service Claims

For ambulance service claims, institutional-based providers and suppliers must report an origin and destination modifier for each ambulance trip provided in HCPCS/Rates. Origin and destination modifiers used for ambulance services are created by combining two alpha characters. Each alpha character, with the exception of "X", represents an origin code or a destination code. The pair of alpha codes creates one modifier. The first position alpha code equals origin; the second position alpha code equals destination. Origin and destination codes and their descriptions are listed below:

D= Diagnostic or therapeutic site other than P or H when these are used as origin codes;

E = Residential, domiciliary, custodial facility (other than 1819 facility);

G = Hospital based ESRD facility;

H = Hospital;

I = Site of transfer (e.g. airport or helicopter pad) between modes of ambulance transport;

J = Freestanding ESRD facility;

N = Skilled nursing facility;

P = Physician's office;

R = Residence;

S = Scene of accident or acute event;

X = Intermediate stop at physician's office on way to hospital (destination code only)

In addition, institutional-based providers must report one of the following modifiers with every HCPCS code to describe whether the service was provided under arrangement or directly:

QM - Ambulance service provided under arrangement by a provider of services; or

QN - Ambulance service furnished directly by a provider of services.

While combinations of these items may duplicate other HCPCS modifiers, when billed with an ambulance transportation code, the reported modifiers can only indicate origin/destination.

B. HCPCS Codes

The following codes and definitions are effective for billing ambulance services on or after January 1, 2001.

AMBULANCE HCPCS CODES AND DEFINITIONS

Code	Description
A0425	BLS mileage (per mile)
A0425	ALS mileage (per mile)
A0426	Ambulance service, Advanced Life Support (ALS), non-emergency transport, Level 1
A0427	Ambulance service, ALS, emergency transport, Level 1
A0428	Ambulance service, Basic Life Support (BLS), non-emergency transport
A0429	Ambulance service, basic life support (BLS), emergency transport
A0430	Ambulance service, conventional air services, transport, one way, fixed wing (FW)
A0431	Ambulance service, conventional air services, transport, one way, rotary wing (RW)
A0432	Paramedic ALS intercept (PI), rural area transport furnished by a volunteer ambulance company, which is prohibited by state law from billing third party payers.
A0433	Ambulance service, advanced life support, level 2 (ALS2)
A0434	Ambulance service, specialty care transport (SCT)
A0435	Air mileage; FW, (per statute mile)
A0436	Air mileage; RW, (per statute mile)

NOTE: PI, ALS2, SCT, FW, and RW assume an emergency condition and do not require an emergency designator.

Refer to IOM Pub. 100-02, Medicare Benefit Policy Manual, Chapter 10 – Ambulance Service, section 30.1 – Definitions of Ambulance Services, for the definitions of levels of ambulance services under the fee schedule.

100-04, 15, 30.1.2

Coding Instructions for Paper and Electronic Claim Forms

(Rev.3855, Issued: 09-01-17, Effective: 10-02-17, Implementation:10-02-17)

Except as otherwise noted, beginning with dates of service on or after January 1, 2001, the following coding instructions must be used.

Origin

Electronic billers should refer to the Implementation Guide to determine how to report the origin information (e.g., the ZIP Code of the point of pickup). Beginning with the early implementation of version 5010 of the ASC X12 837 professional claim format on January 1, 2011, electronic billers are required to submit, in addition to the loaded ambulance trip's origin information (e.g., the ZIP Code of the point of pickup), the loaded ambulance trip's destination information (e.g., the ZIP code of the point of drop-off). Refer to the appropriate Implementation Guide to determine how to report the destination information. Only the ZIP Code of the point of pickup will be used to adjudicate and price the ambulance claim, not the point of drop-off. However, the point of drop-off is an additional reporting requirement on version 5010 of the ASC X12 837 professional claim format.

Where the CMS-1500 Form is used the ZIP code is reported in item 23. Since the ZIP Code is used for pricing, more than one ambulance service may be reported on the same paper claim for a beneficiary if all points of pickup have the same ZIP Code. Suppliers must prepare a separate paper claim for each trip if the points of pickup are located in different ZIP Codes.

Claims without a ZIP Code in item 23 on the CMS-1500 Form item 23, or with multiple ZIP Codes in item 23, must be returned as unprocessable.

The contractor shall use the following remittance advice messages and associated codes when rejecting/denying claims under this policy. This CARC/RARC combination is compliant with CAQH CORE Business Scenario Two.

Group Code: CO

CARC: 16

RARC: N53

MSN: N/A

ZIP Codes must be edited for validity.

© 2019 Optum360, LLC

The format for a ZIP Code is five numerics. If a nine-digit ZIP Code is submitted, the last four digits are ignored. If the data submitted in the required field does not match that format, the claim is rejected.

Mileage

Generally, each ambulance trip will require two lines of coding, e.g., one line for the service and one line for the mileage. Suppliers who do not bill mileage would have one line of code for the service.

Beginning with dates of service on or after January 1, 2011, mileage billed must be reported as fractional units in the following situations:

- Where billing is by ASC X12 claims transaction (professional or institutional), and
- Where billing is by CMS-1500 paper form.

Electronic billers should see the appropriate Implementation Guide to determine where to report the fractional units. Item 24G of the Form CMS-1500 paper claim is used.

Fractional units are not required on Form CMS-1450.

For trips totaling up to 100 covered miles suppliers must round the total miles up to the nearest tenth of a mile and report the resulting number with the appropriate HCPCS code for ambulance mileage. The decimal must be used in the appropriate place (e.g., 99.9).

For trips totaling 100 covered miles and greater, suppliers must report mileage rounded up to the next whole number mile without the use of a decimal (e.g., 998.5 miles should be reported as 999).

For trips totaling less than 1 mile, enter a "0" before the decimal (e.g., 0.9).

For mileage HCPCS billed on a the ASC X12 837 professional transaction or the CMS-1500 paper form only, contractors shall automatically default to "0.1" units when the total mileage units are missing.

Multiple Patients on One Trip

Ambulance suppliers submitting a claim using the ASC X12 professional format or the CMS-1500 paper form for an ambulance transport with more than one patient onboard must use the "GM" modifier ("Multiple Patients on One Ambulance Trip") for each service line item. In addition, suppliers are required to submit documentation to A/B MACs (Part B) to specify the particulars of a multiple patient transport. The documentation must include the total number of patients transported in the vehicle at the same time and the Health Insurance Claim Numbers (HICN) for each Medicare beneficiary. A/B/MACs (Part B) shall calculate payment amounts based on policy instructions found in Pub.100-02, Medicare Benefit Policy Manual, Chapter 10 – Ambulance Services, Section 10.3.10 – Multiple Patient Ambulance Transport.

Ambulance claims submitted on or after January 1, 2011, in version 5010 of the ASC X12 837 professional claim format require the presence of a diagnosis code and the absence of diagnosis code will cause the ambulance claim to not be accepted into the claims processing system. The presence of a diagnosis code on an ambulance claim is not required as a condition of ambulance payment policy. The adjudicative process does not take into account the presence (or absence) of a diagnosis code, but a diagnosis code is required on the ASC X12 837 professional claim format.

100-04, 15, 30.2

Intermediary Guidelines

(Rev.3076, Issued: 09-24-14, Effective: Upon Implementation of ICD-10)

For SNF Part A, the cost of transportation to receive most services included in the RUG rate is included in the cost for the service. This includes transportation in an ambulance. Payment for the SNF claim is based on the RUGs, and recalibration for future years takes into account the cost of transportation to receive the ancillary services.

If the services are excluded from the SNF PPS rate, the ambulance service may be billed separately as can the excluded service.

Refer to section 10.5, of chapter 3, of the Medicare Claims Processing Manual, for additional information on hospital inpatient bundling of ambulance services.

In general, the intermediary processes claims for Part B ambulance services provided by an ambulance supplier under arrangements with hospitals or SNFs. These providers bill intermediaries using only Method 2.

The provider must furnish the following data in accordance with intermediary instructions. The intermediary will make arrangements for the method and media for submitting the data: A detailed statement of the condition necessitating the ambulance service; A statement indicating whether the patient was admitted as an inpatient. If yes the name and address of the facility must be shown; Name and address of certifying physician; Name and address of physician ordering service if other than certifying physician; Point of pickup (identify place and completed address); Destination (identify place and complete address); Number of loaded miles (the number of miles traveled when the beneficiary was in the ambulance); Cost per mile; Mileage charge; Minimum or base charge; and Charge for special items or services. Explain.

A. General

The reasonable cost per trip of ambulance services furnished by a provider of services may not exceed the prior year's reasonable cost per trip updated by the ambulance inflation factor. This determination is effective with services furnished during Federal Fiscal Year (FFY) 1998 (between October 1, 1997, and September 30, 1998).

Providers are to bill for Part B ambulance services using the billing method of base rate including supplies, with mileage billed separately as described below.

The following instructions provide billing procedures implementing the above provisions.

B. Applicable Bill Types

The appropriate type of bill (13X, 22X, 23X, 83X, and 85X) must be reported. For SNFs, ambulance cannot be reported on a 21X type of bill.

C. Value Code Reporting

For claims with dates of service on or after January 1, 2001, providers must report on every Part B ambulance claim value code A0 (zero) and the related ZIP code of the geographic location from which the beneficiary was placed on board the ambulance in FLs 39-41 "Value Codes." The value code is defined as "ZIP Code of the location from which the beneficiary is initially placed on board the ambulance." Providers report the number in dollar portion of the form location right justified to the left to the dollar/cents delimiter. Providers utilizing the UB-92 flat file use Record Type 41 fields 16-39. On the X-12 institutional claims transactions, providers show HI*BE:A0:::12345, 2300 Loop, HI segment.

More than one ambulance trip may be reported on the same claim if the ZIP code of all points of pickup are the same. However, since billing requirements do not allow for value codes (ZIP codes) to be line item specific and only one ZIP code may be reported per claim, providers must prepare a separate claim for a beneficiary for each trip if the points of pickup are located in different ZIP codes.

D. Revenue Code/HCPCS Code Reporting

Providers must report revenue code 054X and, for services provided before January 1, 2001, one of the following CMS HCPCS codes in FL 44 "HCPCS/Rates" for each ambulance trip provided during the billing period: A0030 (discontinued 12/31/2000); A0040 (discontinued 12/31/2000); A0050 (discontinued 12/31/2000); A0320 (discontinued 12/31/2000); A0322 (discontinued 12/31/2000); A0324 (discontinued 12/31/2000); A0326 (discontinued 12/31/2000); A0328, (discontinued 12/31/2000); or A0330 (discontinued 12/31/2000).

In addition, providers report one of A0380 or A0390 for mileage HCPCS codes. No other HCPCS codes are acceptable for reporting ambulance services and mileage.

Providers report one of the following revenue codes: 0540; 0542; 0543; 0545; 0546; or 0548.

Do not report revenue codes 0541, 0544, or 0547.

For claims with dates of service on or after January 1, 2001, providers must report revenue code 540 and one of the following HCPCS codes in FL 44 "HCPCS/Rates" for each ambulance trip provided during the billing period: A0426; A0427; A0428; A0429; A0430; A0431; A0432; A0433; or A0434.

Providers using an ALS vehicle to furnish a BLS level of service report HCPCS code, A0426 (ALS1) or A0427 (ALS1 emergency), and are paid accordingly.

In addition, all providers report one of the following mileage HCPCS codes: A0380; A0390; A0435; or A0436.

Since billing requirements do not allow for more than one HCPCS code to be reported for per revenue code line, providers must report revenue code 0540 (ambulance) on two separate and consecutive lines to accommodate both the Part B ambulance service and the mileage HCPCS codes for each ambulance trip provided during the billing period. Each loaded (e.g., a patient is onboard) 1-way ambulance trip must be reported with a unique pair of revenue code lines on the claim. Unloaded trips and mileage are NOT reported.

However, in the case where the beneficiary was pronounced dead after the ambulance is called but before the ambulance arrives at the scene: Payment may be made for a BLS service if a ground vehicle is dispatched or at the fixed wing or rotary wing base rate, as applicable, if an air ambulance is dispatched. Neither mileage nor a rural adjustment would be paid. The blended rate amount will otherwise apply. Providers report the A0428 (BLS) HCPCS code. Providers report modifier QL (Patient pronounced dead after ambulance called) in Form Locator (FL) 44 "HCPCS/Rates" instead of the origin and destination modifier. In addition to the QL modifier, providers report modifier QM or QN.

© 2019 Optum360, LLC

E. Modifier Reporting

Providers must report an origin and destination modifier for each ambulance trip provided in FL 44 "HCPCS/Rates." Origin and destination modifiers used for ambulance services are created by combining two alpha characters. Each alpha character, with the exception of x, represents an origin code or a destination code. The pair of alpha codes creates one modifier. The first position alpha code equals origin; the second position alpha code equals destination. Origin and destination codes and their descriptions are listed below: D - Diagnostic or therapeutic site other than "P" or "H" when these are used as origin codes; E - Residential, Domiciliary, Custodial Facility (other than an 1819 facility); H - Hospital; I - Site of transfer (e.g. airport or helicopter pad) between modes of ambulance transport; J - Nonhospital based dialysis facility; N - Skilled Nursing Facility (SNF) (1819 facility); P - Physician's office (Includes HMO nonhospital facility, clinic, etc.); R - Residence; S - Scene of accident or acute event; or X - (Destination Code Only) intermediate stop at physician's office enroute to the hospital. (Includes HMO nonhospital facility, clinic, etc.) In addition, providers must report one of the following modifiers with every HCPCS code to describe whether the service was provided under arrangement or directly: QM - Ambulance service provided under arrangement by a provider of services; or QN - Ambulance service furnished directly by a provider of services.

F. Line-Item Dates of Service Reporting

Providers are required to report line-item dates of service per revenue code line. This means that they must report two separate revenue code lines for every ambulance trip provided during the billing period along with the date of each trip. This includes situations in which more than one ambulance service is provided to the same beneficiary on the same day. Line-item dates of service are reported on the hard copy UB-92 in FL 45 "Service Date" (MMDDYY), and on RT 61, field 13, "Date of Service" (YYYYMMDD) on the UB-92 flat file.

G. Service Units Reporting

For line items reflecting HCPCS code A0030, A0040, A0050, A0320, A0322, A0324, A0326, A0328, or A0330 (services before January 1, 2001) or code A0426, A0427, A0428, A0429, A0430, A0431, A0432, A0433, or A0434 (services on and after January 1, 2001), providers are required to report in FL 46 "Service Units" each ambulance trip provided during the billing period. Therefore, the service units for each occurrence of these HCPCS codes are always equal to one. In addition, for line items reflecting HCPCS code A0380 or A0390, the number of loaded miles must be reported. (See examples below.) Therefore, the service units for each occurrence of these HCPCS codes are always equal to one.

In addition, for line items reflecting HCPCS code A0380, A0390, A0435, or A0436, the number of loaded miles must be reported.

H. Total Charges Reporting

For line items reflecting HCPCS code: A0030, A0040, A0050, A0320, A0322, A0324, A0326, A0328, or A0330 (services before January 1, 2001); OR HCPCS code A0426, A0427, A0428, A0429, A0430, A0431, A0432, A0433, or A0434 (on or after January 1, 2001); Providers are required to report in FL 47 "Total Charges" the actual charge for the ambulance service including all supplies used for the ambulance trip but excluding the charge for mileage.

For line items reflecting HCPCS code A0380, A0390, A0435, or A0436, report the actual charge for mileage.

NOTE:There are instances where the provider does not incur any cost for mileage, e.g., if the beneficiary is pronounced dead after the ambulance is called but before the ambulance arrives at the scene. In these situations, providers report the base rate ambulance trip and mileage as separate revenue code lines. Providers report the base rate ambulance trip in accordance with current billing requirements. For purposes of reporting mileage, they must report the appropriate HCPCS code, modifiers, and units as a separate line item. For the related charges, providers report $1.00 in FL48 for noncovered charges. Intermediaries should assign ANSI Group Code OA to the $1.00 noncovered mileage line, which in turn informs the beneficiaries and providers that they each have no liability.

Prior to submitting the claim to CWF, the intermediary will remove the entire revenue code line containing the mileage amount reported in FL 48 "Noncovered Charges" to avoid nonacceptance of the claim.

EXAMPLES:The following provides examples of how bills for Part B ambulance services should be completed based on the reporting requirements above. These examples reflect ambulance services furnished directly by providers. Ambulance services provided under arrangement between the provider and an ambulance company are reported in the same manner except providers report a QM modifier instead of a QN modifier. The following examples are for claims submitted with dates of service on or after January 1, 2001.

EXAMPLE 1: Claim containing only one ambulance trip:

For the UB-92 Flat File, providers report as follows:

Modifier Record Type	Revenue Code	HCPCS Modifier	Date of Service	Units	Total Charges
61	0540	A0428RHQN	082701	1 (trip)	100.00
61	0540	A0380RHQN	082701	4 (mileage)	8.00

For the hard copy UB-92 (Form CMS-1450), providers report as follows:

Modifier Record Type	Revenue Code	HCPCS Modifier	Date of Service	Units	Total Charges
FL 42, FL 44	0540	A0428RHQN	082701	1 (trip)	100.00
FL 45, FL 46 FL 47	0540	A0380RHQN	082701	4 (mileage)	8.00

EXAMPLE 2: Claim containing multiple ambulance trips:
For the UB-92 Flat File, providers report as follows:

Modifier Record Type	Revenue Code	HCPCS Code	Modifiers		Date of Service	Units	Total Charges
			#1	#2			
61	0540	A0429	RH	QN	082801	1 (trip)	100.00
61	0540	A0380	RH	QN	082801	2 (mileage)	4.00
61	0540	A0330	RH	QN	082901	1 (trip)	400.00
61	0540	A0390	RH	QN	082901	3 (mileage)	6.00
61	0540	A0426	RH	QN	083001	1 (trip)	500.00
61	0540	A0390	RH	QN	083001	5 (mileage)	10.00
61	0540	A0390	RH	QN	082901	3 (mileage)	6.00
61	0540	A0426	RH	QN	083001	1 (trip)	500.00

For the hard copy UB-92 (Form CMS-1450), providers report as follows:

Modifier	Revenue Code	HCPCS Code	#1	#2	Date of Service	Units	Total Charges
FL42, FL 44, FL 45, FL 46, FL 47	0540	A0429	RH	QN	082801	1 (trip)	100.00
	0540	A0380	RH	QN	082801	2 (mileage)	4.00

EXAMPLE 3: Claim containing more than one ambulance trip provided on the same day: For the UB-92 Flat File, providers report as follows:

Modifier Record Type	Revenue Code	HCPCS Code	#1	#2	Date of Service	Units	Total Charges
61	0540	A0429	RH	QN	090201	1 (trip)	100.00
61	0540	A0380	RH	QN	090201	2 (mileage)	4.00
61	0540	A0429	HR	QN	090201	1 (trip)	100.00
61	0540	A0380	HR	QN	090201	2 (mileage)	4.00

For the hard copy UB-92 (Form CMS-1450), providers report as follows:

Modifier	Revenue Code	HCPCS Code	#1	#2	Date of Service	Units	Total Charges
FL42, FL 44, FL 45, FL 46, FL 47	0540	A0429	RH	QN	090201	1 (trip)	100.00
	0540	A0380	RH	QN	090201	2 (mileage)	4.00
	0540	A0429	HR	QN	090201	1 (trip)	100.00
	0540	A0380	HR	QN	090201	2 (mileage)	4.00

I. Edits Intermediaries edit to assure proper reporting as follows:

For claims with dates of service before January 1, 2001, each pair of revenue codes 0540 must have one of the following ambulance trip HCPCS codes - A0030, A0040, A0050, A0320, A0322, A0324, A0326, A0328 or A0330; and one of the following mileage HCPCS codes - A0380 or A0390; For claims with dates of service on or after January 1, 2001, each pair of revenue codes 0540 must have one of the following ambulance HCPCS codes - A0426, A0427, A0428, A0429, A0430, A0431, A0432, A0433, or A0434; and one of the following mileage HCPCS codes - A0435, A0436 or for claims with dates of service before April 1, 2002, A0380, or A0390, or for claims with dates of service on or after April 1, 2002, A0425; For claims with dates of service on or after January 1, 2001, the presence of an origin and destination modifier and a QM or QN modifier for every line item containing revenue code 0540; The units field is

© 2019 Optum360, LLC

completed for every line item containing revenue code 0540; For claims with dates of service on or after January 1, 2001, the units field is completed for every line item containing revenue code 0540; Service units for line items containing HCPCS codes A0030, A0040, A0050, A0320, A0322, A0324, A0326, A0328, A0330, A0426, A0427, A0428, A0429, A0430, A0431, A0432, A0433, or A0434 always equal "1" For claims with dates of service on or after July 1, 2001, each 1-way ambulance trip, line-item dates of service for the ambulance service, and corresponding mileage are equal.

100-04, 15, 30.2.1

A/MAC Bill Processing Guidelines Effective April 1, 2002, as a Result of Fee Schedule Implementation

(Rev.3076, Iss: 9-24-14, Eff: Upon Imp of I-10 ASC X12: 1-1-12, I-10: Imp of ICD-10 ASC X12: 9-1-14)

For SNF Part A, the cost of medically necessary ambulance transportation to receive most services included in the RUG rate is included in the cost for the service. Payment for the SNF claim is based on the RUGs, which takes into account the cost of such transportation to receive the ancillary services.

Refer to IOM Pub. 100-04, Medicare Claims Processing Manual, chapter 6—SNF Inpatient Part A Billing, Section 20.3.1—Ambulance Services for additional information on SNF consolidated billing and ambulance transportation.

Refer to IOM Pub. 100-04, Medicare Claims Processing Manual, chapter 3—Inpatient Hospital Billing, section 10.5—Hospital Inpatient Bundling, for additional information on hospital inpatient bundling of ambulance services.

In general, the A/MAC processes claims for Part B ambulance services provided by an ambulance supplier under arrangements with hospitals or SNFs. These providers bill A/MACs using only Method 2.

The provider must furnish the following data in accordance with A/MAC instructions. The A/MAC will make arrangements for the method and media for submitting the data:

- A detailed statement of the condition necessitating the ambulance service;
- A statement indicating whether the patient was admitted as an inpatient. If yes the name and address of the facility must be shown;
- Name and address of certifying physician;
- Name and address of physician ordering service if other than certifying physician;
- Point of pickup (identify place and completed address);
- Destination (identify place and complete address);
- Number of loaded miles (the number of miles traveled when the beneficiary was in the ambulance);
- Cost per mile;
- Mileage charge;
- Minimum or base charge; and
- Charge for special items or services. Explain.

A. Revenue Code Reporting

Providers report ambulance services under revenue code 540 in FL 42 "Revenue Code."

B. HCPCS Codes Reporting

Providers report the HCPCS codes established for the ambulance fee schedule. No other HCPCS codes are acceptable for the reporting of ambulance services and mileage. The HCPCS code must be used to reflect the type of service the beneficiary received, not the type of vehicle used.

Providers must report one of the following HCPCS codes in FL 44 "HCPCS/Rates" for each base rate ambulance trip provided during the billing period:

A0426; A0427; A0428; A0429; A0430; A0431; A0432; A0433; or A0434.

These are the same codes required effective for services January 1, 2001.

In addition, providers must report one of HCPCS mileage codes:

A0425; A0435; or A0436.

Since billing requirements do not allow for more than one HCPCS code to be reported per revenue code line, providers must report revenue code 540 (ambulance) on two separate and consecutive line items to accommodate both the ambulance service and the mileage HCPCS codes for each ambulance trip provided during the billing period. Each loaded (e.g., a patient is onboard) 1-way ambulance trip must be reported with a unique pair of revenue code lines on the claim. Unloaded trips and mileage are NOT reported.

For UB-04 hard copy claims submission prior to August 1, 2011, providers code one mile for trips less than a mile. Miles must be entered as whole numbers. If a trip has a fraction of a mile, round up to the nearest whole number.

Beginning with dates of service on or after January 1, 2011, for UB-04 hard copy claims submissions August 1, 2011 and after, mileage must be reported as fractional units. When reporting fractional mileage, providers must round the total miles up to the nearest tenth of a mile and the decimal must be used in the appropriate place (e.g., 99.9).

For trips totaling less than 1 mile, enter a "0" before the decimal (e.g., 0.9).

For electronic claims submissions prior to January 1, 2011, providers code one mile for trips less than a mile. Miles must be entered as whole numbers. If a trip has a fraction of a mile, round up to the nearest whole number.

Beginning with dates of service on or after January 1, 2011, for electronic claim submissions only, mileage must be reported as fractional units in the ANSI X12N 837I element SV205 for trips totaling up to 100 covered miles. When reporting fractional mileage, providers must round the total miles up to the nearest tenth of a mile and the decimal must be used in the appropriate place (e.g., 99.9).

For trips totaling 100 covered miles and greater, providers must report mileage rounded up to the nearest whole number mile (e.g., 999) and not use a decimal when reporting whole number miles over 100 miles.

For trips totaling less than 1 mile, enter a "0" before the decimal (e.g., 0.9).

C. Modifier Reporting

Providers must report an origin and destination modifier for each ambulance trip provided and either a QM (Ambulance service provided under arrangement by a provider of services) or QN (Ambulance service furnished directly by a provider of services) modifier in FL 44 "HCPCS/Rates".

D. Service Units Reporting

For line items reflecting HCPCS codes A0426, A0427, A0428, A0429, A0430, A0431, A0432, A0433, or A0434, providers are required to report in FL 46 "Service Units" for each ambulance trip provided. Therefore, the service units for each occurrence of these HCPCS codes are always equal to one. In addition, for line items reflecting HCPCS code A0425, A0435, or A0436, providers must also report the number of loaded miles.

E. Total Charges Reporting

For line items reflecting HCPCS codes A0426, A0427, A0428, A0429, A0430, A0431, A0432, A0433, or A0434, providers are required to report in FL 47, "Total Charges," the actual charge for the ambulance service including all supplies used for the ambulance trip but excluding the charge for mileage. For line items reflecting HCPCS codes A0425, A0435, or A0436, providers are to report the actual charge for mileage.

NOTE: There are instances where the provider does not incur any cost for mileage, e.g., if the beneficiary is pronounced dead after the ambulance is called but before the ambulance arrives at the scene. In these situations, providers report the base rate ambulance trip and mileage as separate revenue code lines. Providers report the base rate ambulance trip in accordance with current billing requirements. For purposes of reporting mileage, they must report the appropriate HCPCS code, modifiers, and units. For the related charges, providers report $1.00 in non-covered charges. A/MACs should assign ANSI Group Code OA to the $1.00 non-covered mileage line, which in turn informs the beneficiaries and providers that they each have no liability.

F. Edits (A/MAC Claims with Dates of Service On or After 4/1/02)

For claims with dates of service on or after April 1, 2002, A/MACs perform the following edits to assure proper reporting:

Edit to assure each pair of revenue codes 540 have one of the following ambulance HCPCS codes - A0426, A0427, A0428, A0429, A0430, A0431, A0432, A0433, or A0434; and one of the following mileage HCPCS codes - A0425, A0435, or A0436.

Edit to assure the presence of an origin, destination modifier, and a QM or QN modifier for every line item containing revenue code 540;

Edit to assure that the unit's field is completed for every line item containing revenue code 540;

Edit to assure that service units for line items containing HCPCS codes A0426, A0427, A0428, A0429, A0430, A0431, A0432, A0433, or A0434 always equal "1"; and

Edit to assure on every claim that revenue code 540, a value code of A0 (zero), and a corresponding ZIP Code are reported. If the ZIP Code is not a valid ZIP Code in accordance with the USPS assigned ZIP Codes, intermediaries verify the ZIP Code to determine if the ZIP Code is a coding error on the claim or a new ZIP Code from the USPS not on the CMS supplied ZIP Code File.

Beginning with dates of service on or after April 1, 2012, edit to assure that only non-emergency trips (i.e., HCPCS A0426, A0428 [when A0428 is billed without modifier QL]) require an NPI in the Attending Physician field. Emergency trips do not require an NPI in the Attending Physician field (i.e., A0427, A0429, A0430, A0431, A0432, A0433, A0434 and A0428 [when A0428 is billed with modifier QL])

© 2019 Optum360, LLC

G. CWF (A/MACs)

A/MACs report the procedure codes in the financial data section (field 65a-65j). They include revenue code, HCPCS code, units, and covered charges in the record. Where more than one HCPCS code procedure is applicable to a single revenue code, the provider reports each HCPCS code and related charge on a separate line, and the A/MAC reports this to CWF. Report the payment amount before adjustment for beneficiary liability in field 65g "Rate" and the actual charge in field 65h, "Covered Charges."

100-04, 15, 30.2.4

30.2.4 - Non-covered Charges on Institutional Ambulance Claims

(Rev.1921, Issued: 02-19-10, Effective: 04-01-10, Implementation: 04-05-10)

Medicare law contains a restriction that miles beyond the closest available facility cannot be billed to Medicare. Non-covered miles beyond the closest facility are billed with HCPCS procedure code A0888 ("non-covered ambulance mileage per mile, e.g., for miles traveled beyond the closest appropriate facility"). These non-covered line items can be billed on claims also containing covered charges. Ambulance claims may use the -GY modifier on line items for such non-covered mileage, and liability for the service will be assigned correctly to the beneficiary.

The method of billing all miles for the same trip, with covered and non-covered portions, on the same claim is preferable in this scenario. However, billing the non-covered mileage using condition code 21 claims is also permitted, if desired, as long as all line items on the claims are non-covered and the beneficiary is liable. Additionally, unless requested by the beneficiary or required by specific Medicare policy, services excluded by statute do not have to be billed to Medicare.

When the scenario is point of pick up outside the United States, including U.S. territories but excepting some points in Canada and Mexico in some cases, mileage is also statutorily excluded from Medicare coverage. Such billings are more likely to be submitted on entirely non-covered claims using condition code 21. This scenario requires the use of a different message on the Medicare Summary Notice (MSN) sent to beneficiaries.

Another scenario in which billing non-covered mileage to Medicare may occur is when the beneficiary dies after the ambulance has been called but before the ambulance arrives. The -QL modifier should be used on the base rate line in this scenario, in place of origin and destination modifiers, and the line is submitted with covered charges. The -QL modifier should also be used on the accompanying mileage line, if submitted, with non-covered charges. Submitting this non-covered mileage line is optional for providers.

Non-covered charges may also apply is if there is a subsidy of mileage charges that are never charged to Medicare. Because there are no charges for Medicare to share in, the only billing option is to submit non-covered charges, if the provider bills Medicare at all (it is not required in such cases). These non-covered charges are unallowable, and should not be considered in settlement of cost reports. However, there is a difference in billing if such charges are subsidized, but otherwise would normally be charged to Medicare as the primary payer. In this latter case, CMS examination of existing rules relating to grants policy since October 1983, supported by Federal regulations (42CFR 405.423), generally requires providers to reduce their costs by the amount of grants and gifts restricted to pay for such costs. Thereafter, section 405.423 was deleted from the regulations.

Thus, providers were no longer required to reduce their costs for restricted grants and gifts, and charges tied to such grants/gifts/subsidies should be submitted as covered charges. This is in keeping with Congress's intent to encourage hospital philanthropy, allowing the provider receiving the subsidy to use it, and also requiring Medicare to share in the unreduced cost. Treatment of subsidized charges as non-covered Medicare charges serves to reduce Medicare payment on the Medicare cost report contrary to the 1983 change in policy.

Medicare requires the use of the -TQ modifier so that CMS can track the instances of the subsidy scenario for non-covered charges. The -TQ should be used whether the subsidizing entity is governmental or voluntary. The -TQ modifier is not required in the case of covered charges submitted when a subsidy has been made, but charges are still normally made to Medicare as the primary payer.

If providers believe they have been significantly or materially penalized in the past by the failure of their cost reports to consider covered charges occurring in the subsidy case, since Medicare had previous billing instructions that stated all charges in the case of a subsidy, not just charges when the entity providing the subsidy never charges another entity/primary payer, should be submitted as non-covered charges, they may contact their FI about reopening the reports in question for which the time period in 42 CFR 405.1885 has not expired. FIs have the discretion to determine if the amount in question warrants reopening. The CMS does not expect many such cases to occur.

Billing requirements for all these situations, including the use of modifiers, are presented in the chart below:

Mileage Scenario	HCPCS	Modifiers*	Liability	Billing	Remit. Requirements	MSN Message
STATUTE: Miles beyond closest facility, OR **Pick up point outside of U.S.	A0888 on line item for the non-covered mileage	-QM or -QN, origin/destination modifier, and -GY unless condition code 21 claim used	Beneficiary	Bill mileage line item with A0888 -GY and other modifiers as needed to establish liability, line item will be denied; OR bill service on condition code 21 claim, no -GY required, claim will be denied	Group code PR, reason code 96	16.10 "Medicare does not pay for this item or service"; OR, "Medicare no paga por este artículo o servicio"
Beneficiary dies after ambulance is called	Most appropriate ambulance HCPCS mileage code (i.e., ground, air)	-QL unless condition code -21 claim	Provider	Bill mileage line item with -QL as non-covered, line item will be denied	Group Code CO, reason code 96	16.58 "The provider billed this charge as non-covered. You do not have to pay this amount."; OR, "El proveedor facuró este cargo como no cubierto. Usted no tiene que pagar ests cantidad."
Subsidy or government owned Ambulance, Medicare NEVER billed***	A0888 on line item for the non-covered mileage	-QM or -QN, origin/ destination modifier, and -TQ must be used for policy purposes	Provider	Bill mileage line item with A0888, and modifiers as non-covered, line item will be denied	Group Code CO, reason code 96	16.58 "The provider billed this charge as non-covered. You do not have to pay this amount."; OR, "El proveedor facuró este cargo como no cubierto. Usted no tiene que pagar ests cantidad."

* Current ambulance billing requirements state that either the -QM or -QN modifier must be used on services. The -QM is used when the "ambulance service is provided under arrangement by a provider of services," and the -QN when the "ambulance service is provided directly by a provider of services." Line items using either the -QM or -QN modifiers are not subject to the FISS edit associated with FISS reason code 31322 so that these lines items will process to completion. Origin/destination modifiers, also required by current instruction, combine two alpha characters: one for origin, one for destination, and are not non-covered by definition.

** This is the one scenario where the base rate is not paid in addition to mileage, and there are certain exceptions in Canada and Mexico where mileage is covered as described in existing ambulance instructions.

*** If Medicare would normally have been billed, submit mileage charges as covered charges despite subsidies.

Medicare systems may return claims to the provider if they do not comply with the requirements in the table.

© 2019 Optum360, LLC

100-04, 15, 40

Medical Conditions List and Instructions

(Rev.3240, Issued: 04-24-15, Effective: 07-27-15, Implementation: 07-27-15)

See http://www.cms.gov/Center/Provider-Type/Ambulances-Services-Center.html for a medical conditions list and instructions to assist ambulance providers and suppliers to communicate the

patient's condition to Medicare contractors, as reported by the dispatch center and as observed by the ambulance crew. Use of the medical conditions list does not guarantee payment of the claim or payment for a certain level of service.

In addition to reporting one of the medical conditions on the claim, one of the transportation indicators may be included on the claim to indicate why it was necessary for the patient to be transported in a particular way or circumstance. The provider or supplier will place the transportation indicator in the "narrative" field on the claim. Information on the appropriate use of transportation indicators is also available at http://www.cms.gov/Center/Provider-Type/Ambulances-Services-Center.html.

100-04, 16, 60.1.4

Coding Requirements for Specimen Collection

(Rev.3056, Issued: 08-29-14, Effective: 04-01-14, Implementation: 12-01-14)

The following HCPCS codes and terminology must be used:

- 36415 – Collection of venous blood by venipuncture.
- G0471 – Collection of venous blood by venipuncture or urine sample by catheterization from an individual in a skilled nursing facility (SNF) or by a laboratory on behalf of a home health agency (HHA)
- P96I5 – Catheterization for collection of specimen(s).

The allowed amount for specimen collection in each of the above circumstances is included in the laboratory fee schedule distributed annually by CMS.

100-04, 16, 60.2

Travel Allowance

(Rev.4199, Issued: 01-11-19, Effective: 01-01-19, Implementation: 02-12-19)

In addition to a specimen collection fee allowed under §60.1, Medicare, under Part B, covers a specimen collection fee and travel allowance for a laboratory technician to draw a specimen from either a nursing home patient or homebound patient under §1833(h)(3) of the Act and payment is made based on the clinical laboratory fee schedule. The travel allowance is intended to cover the estimated travel costs of collecting a specimen and to reflect the technician's salary and travel costs.

The additional allowance can be made only where a specimen collection fee is also payable, i.e., no travel allowance is made where the technician merely performs a messenger service to pick up a specimen drawn by a physician or nursing home personnel. The travel allowance may not be paid to a physician unless the trip to the home, or to the nursing home was solely for the purpose of drawing a specimen. Otherwise travel costs are considered to be associated with the other purposes of the trip.

The travel allowance is not distributed by CMS. Instead, the carrier must calculate the travel allowance for each claim using the following rules for the particular Code. The following HCPCS codes are used for travel allowances:

Per Mile Travel Allowance (P9603)

- The minimum "per mile travel allowance" is $1.03. The per mile travel allowance is to be used in situations where the average trip to patients' homes is longer than 20 miles round trip, and is to be pro-rated in situations where specimens are drawn or picked up from non-Medicare patients in the same trip. - one way, in connection with medically necessary laboratory specimen collection drawn from homebound or nursing home bound patient; prorated miles actually traveled (carrier allowance on per mile basis); or
- The per mile allowance was computed using the Federal mileage rate plus an additional 45 cents a mile to cover the technician's time and travel costs. Contractors have the option of establishing a higher per mile rate in excess of the minimum ($1.03 a mile in CY 2019) if local conditions warrant it. The minimum mileage rate will be reviewed and updated in conjunction with the clinical lab fee schedule as needed. At no time will the laboratory be allowed to bill for more miles than are reasonable or for miles not actually traveled by the laboratory technician.

Example 1: In CY 2019, a laboratory technician travels 60 miles round trip from a lab in a city to a remote rural location, and back to the lab to draw a single Medicare patient's blood. The total reimbursement would be $61.80 (60 miles x $1.03 a mile), plus the specimen collection fee.

Example 2: In CY 2019, a laboratory technician travels 40 miles from the lab to a Medicare patient's home to draw blood, and then travels an additional 10 miles to a non-Medicare patient's home and then travels 30 miles to return to the lab. The total miles traveled would be 80 miles. The claim submitted would be for one half of the miles traveled or $41.20 (40 x $1.03), plus the specimen collection fee.

Flat Rate (P9604)

The CMS will pay a minimum of $10.30 (based on CY 2019) one way flat rate travel allowance. The flat rate travel allowance is to be used in areas where average trips are less than 20 miles round trip. The flat rate travel fee is to be pro-rated for more than one blood drawn at the same address, and for stops at the homes of Medicare and non-Medicare patients. The laboratory does the pro-ration when the claim is submitted based on the number of patients seen on that trip. The specimen collection fee will be paid for each patient encounter.

This rate is based on an assumption that a trip is an average of 15 minutes and up to 10 miles one way. It uses the Federal mileage rate and a laboratory technician's time of $17.66 an hour, including overhead. Contractors have the option of establishing a flat rate in excess of the minimum of $10.00, if local conditions warrant it. The minimum national flat rate will be reviewed and updated in conjunction with the clinical laboratory fee schedule, as necessitated by adjustments in the Federal travel allowance and salaries.

The claimant identifies round trip travel by use of the LR modifier

Example 3: A laboratory technician travels from the laboratory to a single Medicare patient's home and returns to the laboratory without making any other stops. The flat rate would be calculated as follows: 2 x $10.30 for a total trip reimbursement of $20.60, plus the specimen collection fee.

Example 4: A laboratory technician travels from the laboratory to the homes of five patients to draw blood, four of the patients are Medicare patients and one is not. An additional flat rate would be charged to cover the 5 stops and the return trip to the lab (6 x $10.30 = $61.80). Each of the claims submitted would be for $12.36 ($61.80/5 = $12.36). Since one of the patients is non-Medicare, four claims would be submitted for $12.36 each, plus the specimen collection fee for each.

Example 5: A laboratory technician travels from a laboratory to a nursing home and draws blood from 5 patients and returns to the laboratory. Four of the patients are on Medicare and one is not. The $10.30 flat rate is multiplied by two to cover the return trip to the laboratory (2 x $10.30 = $20.60) and then divided by five (1/5 of $20.60 = $4.12). Since one of the patients is non-Medicare, four claims would be submitted for $4.12 each, plus the specimen collection fee.

If a carrier determines that it results in equitable payment, the carrier may extend the former payment allowances for additional travel (such as to a distant rural nursing home) to all circumstances where travel is required. This might be appropriate, for example, if the carrier's former payment allowance was on a per mile basis. Otherwise, it should establish an appropriate allowance and inform the suppliers in its service area. If a carrier decides to establish a new allowance, one method is to consider developing a travel allowance consisting of:

- The current Federal mileage allowance for operating personal automobiles, plus a personnel allowance per mile to cover personnel costs based upon an estimate of average hourly wages and average driving speed.

Carriers must prorate travel allowance amounts claimed by suppliers by the number of patients (including Medicare and non-Medicare patients) from whom specimens were drawn on a given trip.

The carrier may determine that payment in addition to the routine travel allowance determined under this section is appropriate if:

- The patient from whom the specimen must be collected is in a nursing home or is homebound; and
- The clinical laboratory tests are needed on an emergency basis outside the general business hours of the laboratory making the collection.
- Subsequent updated travel allowance amounts will be issued by CMS via Recurring Update Notification (RUN) on an annual basis.

100-04, 16, 70.8

Certificate of Waiver

(Rev.1652, Issued: 12-19-08, Effective: 01-01-09, Implementation: 01-05-09)

Effective September 1, 1992, all laboratory testing sites (except as provided in 42 CFR 493.3(b)) must have either a CLIA certificate of waiver, certificate for provider-performed microscopy procedures, certificate of registration, certificate of compliance, or certificate of accreditation to legally perform clinical laboratory testing on specimens from individuals in the United States.

The Food and Drug Administration approves CLIA waived tests on a flow basis. The CMS identifies CLIA waived tests by providing an updated list of waived tests to the

Medicare contractors on a quarterly basis via a Recurring Update Notification. To be recognized as a waived test, some CLIA waived tests have unique HCPCS procedure codes and some must have a QW modifier included with the HCPCS code.

For a list of specific HCPCS codes subject to CLIA see http://www.cms.hhs.gov/CLIA/downloads/waivetbl.pdf

100-04, 17, 80.1.1

HCPCS Service Coding for Oral Cancer Drugs

(Rev.1, 10-01-03)

The following codes may be used for drugs other than Prodrugs, when covered:

Generic/Chemical Name	How Supplied	HCPCS
Busulfan	2 mg/ORAL	J8510
Capecitabine	150mg/ORAL	J8520
Capecitabine	500mg/ORAL	J8521
Methotrexate	2.5 mg/ORAL	J8610
Cyclophosphamide *	25 mg/ORAL	J8530
Cyclophosphamide *	(Treat 50 mg. as 2 units 50 mg/ORAL	J8530
Etoposide	50 mg/ORAL	J8560
Melphalan	2 mg/ORAL	J8600
Prescription Drug chemotherapeutic NOC	ORAL	J8999

Each tablet or capsule is equal to one unit, except for 50 mg./ORAL of cyclophosphamide (J8530), which is shown as 2 units. The 25m and 50 mg share the same code.

NOTE: HIPAA requires that drug claims submitted to DMERCs be identified by NDC.

100-04, 17, 80.1.2

HCPCS and NDC Reporting for Prodrugs

(Rev.136, 04-09-04)

FI claims

For oral anti-cancer Prodrugs HCPCS code J8999 is reported with revenue code 0636.

DMERC claims

The supplier reports the NDC code on the claim. The DMERC converts the NDC code to a "WW" HCPCS code for CWF. As new "WW" codes are established for oral anti-cancer drugs they will be communicated in a Recurring Update Notification.

100-04, 17, 80.2.1

HCPCS Codes for Oral Anti-Emetic Drugs

(Rev.3085, Issued: 10-03-14, Multiple effective dates)

The physician/supplier bills for these drugs on Form CMS-1500 or its electronic equivalent, the 837P. The facility bills for these drugs on Form CMS-1450 or its electronic equivalent, the 837I. The following HCPCS codes are assigned:

J8501 APREPITANT, oral, 5 mg

(Note: HCPCS code is effective January 1, 2005, but coverage for aprepitant is effective April 4, 2005. Aprepitant is only covered in combination with a 5HT3 antagonist, and dexamethasone for beneficiaries who have received one or more of the specified anti-cancer chemotherapeutic agents.)

Q0161 CHLORPROMAZINE HYDROCHLORIDE 5mg, oral, FDA-approved prescription anti-emetic, for use as a complete therapeutic substitute for an IV anti-emetic at the time of chemotherapy treatment, not to exceed a 48-hour dosage regimen.

Q0162 ONDANSETRON 1mg, oral, FDA-approved prescription anti-emetic, for use as a complete therapeutic substitute for an IV anti-emetic at the time of chemotherapy treatment, not to exceed a 48-hour dosage regimen.

Q0163 DIPHENHYDRAMINE HYDROCHLORIDE, 50mg, oral, FDA-approved prescription anti-emetic, for use as a complete therapeutic substitute for an IV anti-emetic at time of chemotherapy treatment not to exceed a 48-hour dosage regimen.

Q0164 PROCHLORPERAZINE MALEATE, 5mg, oral, FDA-approved prescription anti-emetic, for use as a complete therapeutic substitute for an IV anti-emetic at the time of chemotherapy treatment, not to exceed a 48-hour dosage regimen.

Q0165 PROCHLORPERAZINE MALEATE, 10mg, oral, FDA-approved prescription anti-emetic, for use as a complete therapeutic substitute for an IV anti-emetic at the time of chemotherapy treatment, not to exceed a 48-hour dosage regimen.

Q0166 GRANISETRON HYDROCHLORIDE, 1mg, oral, FDA-approved prescription anti-emetic, for use as a complete therapeutic substitute for an IV anti-emetic at the time of chemotherapy treatment, not to exceed a 24-hour dosage regimen.

Q0167 DRONABINOL 2.5mg, oral, FDA-approved prescription anti-emetic, for use as a complete therapeutic substitute for an IV anti-emetic at the time of chemotherapy treatment, not to exceed a 48-hour dosage regimen.

Q0168 DRONABINOL 5mg, oral, FDA-approved prescription anti-emetic, for use as a complete therapeutic substitute for an IV anti-emetic at the time of chemotherapy treatment, not to exceed a 48-hour dosage regimen.

Q0169 PROMETHAZINE HYDROCHLORIDE, 12.5mg, oral, FDA-approved prescription anti-emetic, for use as a complete therapeutic substitute for an IV anti-emetic at the time of chemotherapy treatment, not to exceed a 48-hour dosage regimen.

Q0170 PROMETHAZINE HYDROCHLORIDE, 25mg, oral, FDA-approved prescription anti-emetic, for use as a complete therapeutic substitute for an IV anti-emetic at the time of chemotherapy treatment, not to exceed a 48-hour dosage regimen.

Q0171 CHLORPROMAZINE HYDROCHLORIDE, 10mg, oral, FDA-approved prescription anti-emetic, for use as a complete therapeutic substitute for an IV anti-emetic at the time of chemotherapy treatment, not to exceed a 48-hour dosage regimen.

Q0172 CHLORPROMAZINE HYDROCHLORIDE, 25mg, oral, FDA-approved prescription anti-emetic, for use as a complete therapeutic substitute for an IV anti-emetic at the time of chemotherapy treatment, not to exceed a 48-hour dosage regimen.

Q0173 TRIMETHOBENZAMIDE HYDROCHLORIDE, 250mg, oral, FDA-approved prescription anti-emetic, for use as a complete therapeutic substitute for an IV anti-emetic at the time of chemotherapy treatment, not to exceed a 48-hour dosage regimen.

Q0174 THIETHYLPERAZINE MALEATE, 10mg, oral, FDA-approved prescription anti-emetic, for use as a complete therapeutic substitute for an IV anti-emetic at the time of chemotherapy treatment, not to exceed a 48-hour dosage regimen.

Q0175 PERPHENAZINE, 4mg, oral, FDA-approved prescription anti-emetic, for use as a complete therapeutic substitute for an IV anti-emetic at the time of chemotherapy treatment, not to exceed a 48-hour dosage regimen.

Q0176 PERPHENAZINE, 8mg, oral, FDA-approved prescription anti-emetic, for use as a complete therapeutic substitute for an IV anti-emetic at the time of chemotherapy treatment, not to exceed a 48-hours dosage regimen.

Q0177 HYDROXYZINE PAMOATE, 25mg, oral, FDA-approved prescription anti-emetic, for use as a complete therapeutic substitute for an IV anti-emetic at the time of chemotherapy treatment, not to exceed a 48-hour dosage regimen.

Q0178 HYDROXYZINE PAMOATE, 50mg, oral, FDA-approved prescription anti-emetic, for use as a complete therapeutic substitute for an IV anti-emetic at the time of chemotherapy treatment, not to exceed a 48-hour dosage regimen.

Q0179 ONDANSETRON mg, oral, FDA-approved prescription anti-emetic, for use as a complete therapeutic substitute for an IV anti-emetic at the time of chemotherapy treatment, not to exceed a 48-hour dosage regimen.

Q0180 DOLASETRON MESYLATE, 100mg, oral, FDA-approved prescription anti-emetic, for use as a complete therapeutic substitute for an IV anti-emetic at the time of chemotherapy treatment, not to exceed a 24-hour dosage regimen.

Q0181 UNSPECIFIED ORAL DOSAGE FORM, FDA-approved prescription anti-emetic, for use as a complete therapeutic substitute for an IV anti-emetic at the time of chemotherapy treatment, not to exceed a 48-hour dosage regimen.

NOTE: The 24-hour maximum drug supply limitation on dispensing, for HCPCS Codes Q0166 and Q0180, has been established to bring the Medicare benefit as it applies to these two therapeutic entities in conformity with the "Indications and Usage" section of currently FDA-approved product labeling for each affected drug product.

© 2019 Optum360, LLC

100-04, 17, 80.2.4

Billing and Payment Instructions for A/B MACs (A)

(Rev.3085, Issued: 10-03-14, Effective: ICD-10: Upon Implementation of ICD-10; ASC X12: January 1, 2012, Implementation: ICD-10: Upon Implementation of ICD-10; ASC X12: November 4, 2014)

Claims for the oral anti-emetic drug aprepitant, either as a 3-day supply dispensed in a Tri-Pak or as the first day supply (not dispensed in a Tri-Pak), must be billed to the A/B MAC (A) on the ASC 837 institutional claim format or on hard copy Form CMS-1450 with the appropriate cancer diagnosis and HCPCS code or Current Procedural Terminology (CPT) code.

Claims for the second and third dose of the oral anti-emetic drug aprepitant not dispensed in a Tri-Pak must be billed to the DME MAC.

The following payment methodologies apply when hospital and SNF outpatient claims are processed by the A/B MAC (A):

- Based on APC for hospitals subject to the outpatient prospective payment system (OPPS);
- Under current payment methodologies for hospitals not subject to OPPS; or
- On a reasonable cost basis for SNFs.

Institutional providers bill for aprepitant under Revenue Code 0636 (Drugs requiring detailed coding).

NOTE: Inpatient claims submitted for oral anti-emetic drugs are processed under the current payment methodologies.

Medicare contractors shall pay claims submitted for services provided by a CAH as follows: Method I technical services are paid at 101% of reasonable cost; Method II technical services are paid at 101% of reasonable cost, and, Professional services are paid at 115% of the Medicare Physician Fee Schedule Data Base.

100-04, 17, 80.3

Billing for Immunosuppressive Drugs

(Rev.3856, Issued: 09-01-17, Effective: 10-02-17, Implementation: 10-02-17)

Medicare covers a beneficiary's immunosuppressive drugs following a transplant, in accordance with 1861(s)(2)(J) of the Social Security Act, which states that Medicare covers "prescription drugs used in immunosuppressive therapy furnished to an individual who receives an organ transplant for which payment is made under this title."

Medicare pays for FDA approved immunosuppressive drugs and for drugs used in immunosuppressive therapy with specific restrictions. (See 42 CFR 430.10 and the Medicare Benefit Policy Manual, Chapter 15 for detailed coverage requirements.) Generally, contractors pay for self-administered immunosuppressive drugs that are specifically labeled and approved for marketing as such by the FDA, or identified in FDA-approved labeling for use in conjunction with immunosuppressive drug therapy. This benefit is subject to the Part B deductible and coinsurance provision.

Contractors are expected to keep informed of FDA additions to the list of the immunosuppressive drugs and notify providers. Prescriptions for immunosuppressive drugs generally should be non-refillable and limited to a 30-day supply. The 30-day guideline is necessary because dosage frequently diminishes over a period of time, and further, it is not uncommon for the physician to change the prescription from one drug to another. Also, these drugs are expensive and the coinsurance liability on unused drugs could be a financial burden to the beneficiary. Unless there are special circumstances, contractors will not consider a supply of drugs in excess of 30 days to be reasonable and necessary and should deny payment accordingly.

Entities that normally bill the A/B MAC (B) bill the DME MAC. Entities that normally bill the A/B MAC (A) continue to bill the A/B MAC (A), except for hospitals subject to OPPS, which must bill the DME MAC.

Prior to December 21, 2000 coverage was limited to immunosuppressive drugs received within 36 months of a transplant. In practice, ESRD beneficiaries continue to be limited to 36 months of coverage after a Medicare covered kidney transplant because their Medicare entitlement would end 36 months after a successful organ transplant. See 42 CFR 406.13(f)(2). Effective with immunosuppressive drugs furnished on or after December 21, 2000, there is no time limit, but an organ transplant must have occurred for which immunosuppressive therapy is appropriate. That is, the time limit for immunosuppressive drugs was eliminated for transplant beneficiaries that will continue Medicare coverage after 36 months based on disability or age. The date of transplant is reported to the A/B MAC (A) with occurrence code 36.

CWF will edit claim records to determine if a history of a transplant is on record. If not an error will be returned. See Chapter 27 for edit codes and resolution.

As explained below, there are circumstances in which Medicare cannot locate the Medicare claim for the transplant in the claims databases which would have confirmed that Medicare paid for the transplant. In such cases, where the supplier appropriately submits the KX modifier, Medicare makes the assumption that Medicare paid for the transplant, in accordance with the statute, that the supplier has on file documentation that indicates the date of the transplant, and that the services furnished are medically necessary.

The use of the KX modifier is not required. In the case of immunosuppressive drugs, submission of the KX modifier is intended for adjudicating claims when the supplier attests that it maintains documentation that the beneficiary was eligible for Medicare Part A on the date of his/her transplant, but where Medicare cannot identify a claims record indicating the transplant was paid for by fee-for-service Medicare. The additional information provided by the use of the KX modifier permits Medicare to reasonably assume that a Medicare payment for an organ transplant was made.

For claims received on and after July 1, 2008, DME MACs will accept claims for immunosuppressive drugs without a KX modifier but will deny such claims if CMS cannot identify a record of a claim indicating that the transplant was paid for by fee-for-service Medicare.

For claims filed with the KX modifier on and after July 1, 2008, suppliers that furnish an immunosuppressive drug to a Medicare beneficiary, when such drug has been prescribed due to the beneficiary having undergone an organ transplant, must: 1) secure from the prescriber the date of such organ transplant and retain documentation of such transplant date in its files, 2) attest that it has on file documentation that the beneficiary was eligible to receive Medicare Part A benefits at the particular date of the transplant and retain the documentation in its files, and 3) retain such documentation of the beneficiary's transplant date, Medicare Part A eligibility, and that such transplant date precedes the Date of Service (DOS) for furnishing the drug.

Use of the KX modifier permits Medicare to make a reasonable assumption that Medicare paid for the transplant even when the transplant claim does not appear in the claims database. A claim may not appear in the claims database for reasons such as:

1. At the time of the transplant, the beneficiary was enrolled in a Medicare Advantage plan that paid for the transplant. Medicare Advantage data is not included in the Medicare FFS claims database. Although some encounter data may be available, it may be incomplete or may not contain coding information sufficient to identify a transplant claim.
2. There may be instances where claims related to a transplant are old and may not be identifiable in the claims database despite Medicare's payment for the claim.

100-04, 17, 80.4

Billing for Hemophilia Clotting Factors

(Rev.1564, Issued: 07-25-08, Effective: 04-01-08, Implementation: 01-05-09)

Blood clotting factors not paid on a cost or prospective payment system basis are priced as a drug/biological under the drug pricing fee schedule effective for the specific date of service. As of January 1, 2005, the average sales price (ASP) plus 6 percent shall be used.

If a beneficiary is in a covered part A stay in a PPS hospital, the clotting factors are paid in addition to the DRG/HIPPS payment. For FY 2005, this payment is based on 95 percent of AWP. For FY 2006, the add-on payment for blood clotting factor administered to hemophilia inpatients is based on average sales price (ASP) + 6 percent and a furnishing fee. The furnishing fee is updated each calendar year. For a SNF subject to SNF/PPS, the payment is bundled into the SNF/PPS rate.

For hospitals subject to OPPS, the clotting factors, when paid under Part B, are paid the APC. For SNFs the clotting factors, when paid under Part B, are paid based on cost.

Local carriers and Part B MACs shall process non-institutional blood clotting factor claims.

The FIs and Part A MACs shall process institutional blood clotting factor claims (Part A and Part B institutional).

100-04, 17, 80.4.1

Clotting Factor Furnishing Fee

(Rev.3862, Issued: 09-15-17, Effective: 01-01-18, Implementation: 01-02-18)

The Medicare Modernization Act section 303(e)(1) added section 1842(o)(5)(C) of the Social Security Act which requires that, beginning January 1, 2005, a furnishing fee will be paid for items and services associated with clotting factor.

Beginning January 1, 2005, a clotting factor furnishing fee is separately payable to entities that furnish clotting factor unless the costs associated with furnishing the clotting factor is paid through another payment system.

© 2019 Optum360, LLC

The clotting factor furnishing fee is updated each calendar year based on the percentage increase in the consumer price index (CPI) for medical care for the 12-month period ending with June of the previous year. The clotting factor furnishing fees applicable for dates of service in each calendar year (CY) are listed below:

CY 2005 - $0.140 per unit

CY 2006 - $0.146 per unit

CY 2007 - $0.152 per unit

CY 2008 - $0.158 per unit

CY 2009 - $0.164 per unit

CY 2010 - $0.170 per unit

CY 2011 - $0.176 per unit

CY 2012 - $0.181 per unit

CY 2013 - $0.188 per unit

CY 2014 - $0.192 per unit

CY 2015 - $0.197 per unit

CY 2016 - $0.202 per unit

CY 2017 - $0.209 per unit

CY 2018 - $0.215 per unit

Annual updates to the clotting factor furnishing fee are subsequently communicated by a Recurring Update Notification.

CMS includes this clotting factor furnishing fee in the nationally published payment limit for clotting factor billing codes. When the clotting factor is not included on the Average Sales Price (ASP) Medicare Part B Drug Pricing File or Not Otherwise Classified (NOC) Pricing File, the contractor must make payment for the clotting factor as well as make payment for the furnishing fee.

100-04, 17, 80.6

Intravenous Immune Globulin

(Rev.3085, Issued: 10-03-14, Effective: ICD-10: Upon Implementation of ICD-10; ASC X12: January 1, 2012, Implementation: ICD-10: Upon Implementation of ICD-10; ASC X12: November 4, 2014)

Beginning for dates of service on or after January 1, 2004, Medicare pays for intravenous immune globulin administered in the home. (See the Medicare Benefit Policy Manual, Chapter 15 for coverage requirements.) Contractors pay for the drug, but not the items or services related to the administration of the drug when administered in the home, if deemed medically appropriate.

Contractors may pay any entity licensed in the State to furnish intravenous immune globulin. Payment will be furnished to the entity with the authority to furnish the drug. Beneficiaries are ineligible to receive payment for the drug.

Pharmacies and hospitals dispensing intravenous immune globulin for home use would bill the DME MAC. If the beneficiary is receiving treatment in an outpatient hospital, the bill must be sent to the A/B MAC (A). If the beneficiary is receiving treatment in a physician's office, the bill must be sent to the A/B MAC (B). Home Health Agencies dispensing intravenous immune globulin would bill the A/B MAC (HHH). Physicians furnishing intravenous immune globulin for the refilling of an external pump for home infusion would bill the DME MAC.

Effective January 1, 2006, Medicare makes an additional payment once per day per beneficiary for preadministration-related services whenever a beneficiary receives intravenous immune globulin.

100-04, 17, 80.12

Claims Processing Rules for ESAs Administered to Cancer

Patients for Anti-Anemia Therapy

(Rev.3721, Issued: 02-24-17, Effective: 05-25-17, Implementation: 05-25-17)

The national coverage determination (NCD) titled, "The Use of ESAs in Cancer and Other Neoplastic Conditions" lists coverage criteria for the use of ESAs in patients who have cancer and experience anemia as a result of chemotherapy or as a result of the cancer itself. The full NCD can be viewed in Publication 100-03 of the NCD Manual, section 110.21.

Effective for claims with dates of service on and after January 1, 2008, non-ESRD ESA services for HCPCS J0881 or J0885 billed with modifier EC (ESA, anemia, non-chemo/radio) shall be denied when any one of the following diagnosis codes is present on the claim:

ICD-9-CM Applicable

- any anemia in cancer or cancer treatment patients due to folate deficiency (281.2),
- B-12 deficiency (281.1, 281.3),
- iron deficiency (280.0-280.9),
- hemolysis (282.0, 282.2, 282.9, 283.0, 283.2, 283.9-283.10, 283.19), or
- bleeding (280.0, 285.1),
- anemia associated with the treatment of acute and chronic myelogenous leukemias (CML, AML) (205.00-205.21, 205.80-205.91); or
- erythroid cancers (207.00-207.81).

ICD-10-CM Applicable

- any anemia in cancer or cancer treatment patients due to folate deficiency - (D52.0, D52.1, D52.8, or D52.9),
- B-12 deficiency - (D51.1, D51.2, D51.3, D51.8, D51.9, or D53.1),
- iron deficiency - (D50.0, D50.1, D50.8, and D50.9),
- hemolysis - (D55.0, D55.1, D58.0, D58.9, D59.0, D59.1, D59.2, D59 4, D59.5, D59.6, D59.8, or D59.9),
- bleeding - (D50.0, D62),
- anemia associated with the treatment of acute and chronic myelogenous leukemias (CML, AML) - (C92.00, C92.01, C92.02, C92.10, C92.11, C92.12, C92.20, C92.21, C92.40, C92.41, C92.42, C92.50, C92.51, C92.52, C92.60, C92.61, C92.62, C92.90, C92.91, C92.A0, C92.A1, C92.A2, C92Z0, C92Z1, or C92Z2), or
- erythroid cancers - (C94.00, C94.01, C94.02, C94.20, C94.21, C94.22, C94.30, C94.31, C94.80, C94.81, D45).

Effective for claims with dates of service on and after January 1, 2008, contractors shall deny non-ESRD ESA services for HCPCS J0881 or J0885 billed with modifier EC (ESA, anemia, non-chemo/radio) for:

- any anemia in cancer or cancer treatment patients due to bone marrow fibrosis,
- anemia of cancer not related to cancer treatment,
- prophylactic use to prevent chemotherapy-induced anemia,
- prophylactic use to reduce tumor hypoxia,
- patients with erythropoietin-type resistance due to neutralizing antibodies; and
- anemia due to cancer treatment if patients have uncontrolled hypertension.

Effective for claims with dates of service on and after January 1, 2008, non-ESRD ESA services for HCPCS J0881 or J0885 billed with modifier EB (ESA, anemia, radio-induced), shall be denied.

Effective for claims with dates of service on and after January 1, 2008, contractors shall deny non-ESRD ESA services for HCPCS J0881 or J0885 billed with modifier EA (ESA, anemia, chemo-induced) for anemia secondary to myelosuppressive anticancer chemotherapy in solid tumors, multiple myeloma, lymphoma, and lymphocytic leukemia when a hemoglobin 10.0g/dL or greater or hematocrit 30.0% or greater is reported.

NOTE: ESA treatment duration for each course of chemotherapy includes the 8 weeks following the final dose of myelosuppressive chemotherapy in a chemotherapy regime.

Effective for claims with dates of service on and after January 1, 2008, Medicare contractors shall have discretion to establish local coverage policies for those indications not included in NCD 110.21.

Denials of claims for ESAs are based on reasonable and necessary determinations established by NCD 110.21. A provider may have the beneficiary sign an Advanced Beneficiary Notice, making the beneficiary liable for services not deemed reasonable and necessary and thus not covered by Medicare.

The contractor shall use the following remittance advice messages and associated codes when rejecting/denying claims under this policy. This CARC/RARC combination is compliant with CAQH CORE Business Scenario Three.

Group Code: PR or CO
CARC: 50
RARC: N/A
MSN: 15.20

Medicare contractors have the discretion to conduct medical review of claims and reverse the automated adjudication if the medical review results in a determination of clinical necessity.

 © 2019 Optum360, LLC

100-04, 17, 90.3

Hospital Outpatient Payment Under OPPS for New, Unclassified Drugs and Biologicals After FDA Approval But Before Assignment of a Product-Specific Drug or Biological HCPCS Code

(Rev.3085, Issued: 10-03-14, Multiple effective dates)

Section 621(a) of the MMA amends Section 1833(t) of the Social Security Act by adding paragraph (15), Payment for New Drugs and Biologicals Until HCPCS Code Assigned. Under this provision, payment for an outpatient drug or biological that is furnished as part of covered outpatient department services for which a product-specific HCPCS code has not been assigned shall be paid an amount equal to 95 percent of average wholesale price (AWP). This provision applies only to payments under the hospital outpatient prospective payment system (OPPS).

Beginning January 1, 2004, hospital outpatient departments may bill for new drugs and biologicals that are approved by the FDA on or after January 1, 2004, for which a product-specific HCPCS code has not been assigned. Beginning on or after the date of FDA approval, hospitals may bill for the drug or biological using HCPCS code C9399, Unclassified drug or biological.

Hospitals report in the ASC X12 837 institutional claim format in specific locations, or in the "Remarks" section of Form CMS-1450:

1. the National Drug Code (NDC),

2. the quantity of the drug that was administered, expressed in the unit of measure applicable to the drug or biological, and

3. the date the drug was furnished to the beneficiary. Contractors shall manually price the drug or biological at 95 percent of AWP. They shall pay hospitals 80 percent of the calculated price and shall bill beneficiaries 20 percent of the calculated price, after the deductible is met. Drugs and biologicals that are manually priced at 95 percent of AWP are not eligible for outlier payment.

HCPCS code C9399 is only to be reported for new drugs and biologicals that are approved by FDA on or after January 1, 2004, for which there is no HCPCS code that describes the drug.

100-04, 18, 1.2

Table of Preventive and Screening Services

(Rev.4127, Issued: 09-05-18, Effective: 01-01-19, Implementation: 01-07-19)

Service	CPT/ HCPCS	Long Descriptor	USPSTF Rating	Coins./ Deductible
Initial Preventive Physical Examination, IPPE	G0402	Initial preventive physical examination; face to face visits, services limited to new beneficiary during the first 12 months of Medicare enrollment	*Not Rated	WAIVED
	G0403	Electrocardiogram, routine ECG with 12 leads; performed as a screening for the initial preventive physical examination with interpretation and report		Not Waived
	G0404	Electrocardiogram, routine ECG with 12 leads; tracing only, without interpretation and report, performed as a screening for the initial preventive physical examination		Not Waived
	G0405	Electrocardiogram, routine ECG with 12 leads; interpretation and report only, performed as a screening for the initial preventive physical examination		Not Waived
Ultrasound Screening for Abdominal Aortic Aneurysm (AAA) furnished prior to January 1, 2017	G0389	Ultrasound, B-scan and /or real time with image documentation; for abdominal aortic aneurysm (AAA) ultrasound screening	B	WAIVED
	76706	Ultrasound, abdominal aorta, real time with image documentation, screening study for abdominal aortic aneurysm (AAA)		WAIVED
Cardio-vascular Disease Screening	80061	Lipid panel	A	WAIVED
	82465	Cholesterol, serum or whole blood, total		WAIVED
	83718	Lipoprotein, direct measurement; high density cholesterol (hdl cholesterol)		WAIVED
	84478	Triglycerides		WAIVED
Diabetes Screening Tests	82947	Glucose; quantitative, blood (except reagent strip)	B	WAIVED
	82950	Glucose; post glucose dose (includes glucose)		WAIVED
	82951	Glucose; tolerance test (gtt), three specimens (includes glucose)	*Not Rated	WAIVED
Diabetes Self-Management Training Services (DSMT)	G0108	Diabetes outpatient self-management training services, individual, per 30 minutes	*Not Rated	Not Waived
	G0109	Diabetes outpatient self-management training services, group session (2 or more), per 30 minutes		Not Waived
Medical Nutrition Therapy (MNT) Services	97802	Medical nutrition therapy; initial assessment and intervention, individual, face-to-face with the patient, each 15 minutes	B	WAIVED
	97803	Medical nutrition therapy; re-assessment and intervention, individual, face-to-face with the patient, each 15 minutes		WAIVED
	97804	Medical nutrition therapy; group (2 or more individual(s)), each 30 minutes		WAIVED
	G0270	Medical nutrition therapy; reassessment and subsequent intervention(s) following second referral in same year for change in diagnosis, medical condition or treatment regimen (including additional hours needed for renal disease), individual, face to face with the patient, each 15 minutes	B	WAIVED
	G0271	Medical nutrition therapy, reassessment and subsequent intervention(s) following second referral in same year for change in diagnosis, medical condition, or treatment regimen (including additional hours needed for renal disease), group (2 or more individuals), each 30 minutes		WAIVED
Screening Pap Test	G0123	Screening cytopathology, cervical or vaginal (any reporting system), collected in preservative fluid, automated thin layer preparation, screening by cytotechnologist under physician supervision	A	WAIVED
	G0124	Screening cytopathology, cervical or vaginal (any reporting system), collected in preservative fluid, automated thin layer preparation, requiring interpretation by physician		WAIVED

© 2019 Optum360, LLC

Service	CPT/ HCPCS	Long Descriptor	USPSTF Rating	Coins./ Deductible
Screening Pap Test (continued)	G0141	Screening cytopathology smears, cervical or vaginal, performed by automated system, with manual rescreening, requiring interpretation by physician	A	WAIVED
	G0143	Screening cytopathology, cervical or vaginal (any reporting system), collected in preservative fluid, automated thin layer preparation, with manual screening and rescreening by cytotechnologist under physician supervision	A	WAIVED
	G0144	Screening cytopathology, cervical or vaginal (any reporting system), collected in preservative fluid, automated thin layer preparation, with screening by automated system, under physician supervision	A	WAIVED
	G0145	Screening cytopathology, cervical or vaginal (any reporting system), collected in preservative fluid, automated thin layer preparation, with screening by automated system and manual rescreening under physician supervision	A	WAIVED
	G0147	Screening cytopathology smears, cervical or vaginal, performed by automated system under physician supervision	A	WAIVED
	G0148	Screening cytopathology smears, cervical or vaginal, performed by automated system with manual rescreening	A	WAIVED
	P3000	Screening papanicolaou smear, cervical or vaginal, up to three smears, by technician under physician supervision		WAIVED
	P3001	Screening papanicolaou smear, cervical or vaginal, up to three smears, requiring interpretation by physician		WAIVED
	Q0091	Screening papanicolaou smear; obtaining, preparing and conveyance of cervical or vaginal smear to laboratory		WAIVED
Screening Pelvic Exam	G0101	Cervical or vaginal cancer screening; pelvic and clinical breast examination	A	WAIVED
Screening Mammo-graphy	77052	Computer-aided detection (computer algorithm analysis of digital image data for lesion detection) with further physician review for interpretation, with or without digitization of film radiographic images; screening mammography (list separately in addition to code for primary procedure)	B	WAIVED
	77057	Screening mammography, bilateral (2-view film study of each breast)	B	WAIVED
	77063	Screening digital breast tomosynthesis, bilateral		WAIVED

Service	CPT/ HCPCS	Long Descriptor	USPSTF Rating	Coins./ Deductible
Bone Mass Measure-ment	G0130	Single energy x-ray absorptiometry (sexa) bone density study, one or more sites; appendicular skeleton (peripheral) (e.g., radius, wrist, heel)		WAIVED
	77078	Computed tomography, bone mineral density study, 1 or more sites; axial skeleton (e.g., hips, pelvis, spine)	B	WAIVED
	77079	Computed tomography, bone mineral density study, 1 or more sites; appendicular skeleton (peripheral) (e.g., radius, wrist, heel)		WAIVED
	77080	Dual-energy x-ray absorptiometry (dxa), bone density study, 1 or more sites; axial skeleton (e.g., hips, pelvis, spine)		WAIVED
	77081	Dual-energy x-ray absorptiometry (dxa), bone density study, 1 or more sites; appendicular skeleton (peripheral) (e.g., radius, wrist, heel)		WAIVED
	77083	Radiographic absorptiometry (e.g., photo densitometry, radiogrammetry), 1 or more sites		WAIVED
	77085	Dual-energy X-ray absorptiometry (DXA), bone density study, 1 or more sites, axial skeleton, (e.g., hips, pelvis, spine), including vertebral fracture assessment.		WAIVED
	76977	Ultrasound bone density measurement and interpretation, peripheral site(s), any method		WAIVED

NOTE: Anesthesia services furnished in conjunction with and in support of a screening colonoscopy are reported with CPT code 00812 and coinsurance and deductible are waived. When a screening colonoscopy becomes a diagnostic colonoscopy, anesthesia services are reported with CPT code 00811 and with the PT modifier; only the deductible is waived.

Coinsurance and deductible are waived for moderate sedation services (reported with G0500 or 99153) when furnished in conjunction with and in support of a screening colonoscopy service and when reported with modifier 33. When a screening colonoscopy becomes a diagnostic colonoscopy, moderate sedation services (G0500 or 99153) are reported with only the PT modifier; only the deductible is waived.

Colorectal Cancer Screening	G0104	Colorectal cancer screening; flexible sigmoidoscopy	A	WAIVED
	G0105	Colorectal cancer screening; colonoscopy on individual at high risk		WAIVED
	G0106	Colorectal cancer screening; alternative to G0104, screening sigmoidoscopy, barium enema	*Not Rated	Coins. Applies & Ded. is waived
	G0120	Colorectal cancer screening; alternative to G0105, screening colonoscopy, barium enema.		Coins. Applies & Ded. is waived

© 2019 Optum360, LLC

Service	CPT/ HCPCS	Long Descriptor	USPSTF Rating	Coins./ Deductible
Colorectal Cancer Screening (continued)	G0121	Colorectal cancer screening; colonoscopy on individual not meeting criteria for high risk	A	WAIVED
	82270	Blood, occult, by peroxidase activity (e.g., guaiac), qualitative; feces, consecutive		WAIVED
	G0328	Colorectal cancer screening; fecal occult blood test, immunoassay, 1-3 simultaneous		WAIVED
Prostate Cancer Screening	G0102	Prostate cancer screening; digital rectal examination	D	Not Waived
	G0103	Prostate cancer screening; prostate specific antigen test (PSA)		WAIVED
Glaucoma Screening	G0117	Glaucoma screening for high risk patients furnished by an optometrist or ophthalmologist	I	Not Waived
	G0118	Glaucoma screening for high risk patient furnished under the direct supervision of an optometrist or ophthalmologist		Not Waived
Influenza Virus Vaccine	90630	Influenza virus vaccine, quadrivalent (IIV4), split virus, preservative free, for intradermal use	B	WAIVED
	90653	Influenza virus vaccine, inactivated, subunit, adjuvanted, for intramuscular use		WAIVED
	90654	Influenza virus vaccine, split virus, preservative free, for intradermal use, for adults ages 18-64		WAIVED
	90655	Influenza virus vaccine, split virus, preservative free, when administered to children 6-35 months of age, for intramuscular use		WAIVED
	90656	Influenza virus vaccine, split virus, preservative free, when administered to individuals 3 years and older, for intramuscular use		WAIVED
	90657	Influenza virus vaccine, split virus, when administered to children 6-35 months of age, for intramuscular use		WAIVED
	90858	Influenza virus vaccine, trivalent (IIV3), split virus, 0.5 mL dosage, for intramuscular use		WAIVED
	90660	Influenza virus vaccine, live, for intranasal use		WAIVED
	90661	Influenza virus vaccine, derived from cell cultures, subunit, preservative and antibiotic free, for intramuscular use		WAIVED
	90662	Influenza virus vaccine, split virus, preservative free, enhanced immunogenicity via increased antigen content, for intramuscular use		WAIVED
	90672	Influenza virus vaccine, live, quadrivalent, for intranasal use		WAIVED
	90673	Influenza virus vaccine, trivalent, derived from recombinant DNA (RIV3), hemagglutinin (HA) protein only, preservative and antibiotic free, for intramuscular use		WAIVED

Service	CPT/ HCPCS	Long Descriptor	USPSTF Rating	Coins./ Deductible
Influenza Virus Vaccine (continued)	90674	Influenza virus vaccine, quadrivalent (ccIIV4), derived from cell cultures, subunit, preservative and antibiotic free, 0.5 mL dosage, for intramuscular use	B	WAIVED
	90685	Influenza virus vaccine, quadrivalent, split virus, preservative free, when administered to children 6- 35 months of age, for intramuscular use		WAIVED
	90686	Influenza virus vaccine, quadrivalent, split virus, preservative free, when administered to individuals 3 years of age and older, for intramuscular use		WAIVED
	90687	Influenza virus vaccine, quadrivalent, split virus, when administered to children 6-35 months of age, for intramuscular use		WAIVED
	90688	Influenza virus vaccine, quadrivalent, split virus, when administered to individuals 3 years of age and older, for intramuscular use		WAIVED
	90689	Influenza virus vaccine, quadrivalent (IIV4), inactivated, adjuvanted, preservative free, 0.25mL dosage, for Intramuscular use		WAIVED
	90756	Influenza virus vaccine, quadrivalent (ccIIV4), derived from cell cultures, subunit, antibiotic free, 0.5mL dosage, for intramuscular use		WAIVED
	G0008	Administration of influenza virus vaccine		WAIVED
Pneumo-coccal Vaccine	90669	Pneumococcal conjugate vaccine, polyvalent, when administered to children younger than 5 years, for intramuscular use	B	WAIVED
	90670	Pneumococcal conjugate vaccine, 13 valent, for intramuscular use		WAIVED
	90732	Pneumococcal polysaccharide vaccine, 23-valent, adult or immunosuppressed patient dosage, when administered to individuals 2 years or older, for subcutaneous or intramuscular use		WAIVED
	G0009	Administration of pneumococcal vaccine		WAIVED
Hepatitis B Vaccine	90739	Hepatitis B vaccine, adult dosage (2 dose schedule), for intramuscular use	A	WAIVED
	90740	Hepatitis B vaccine, dialysis or immunosuppressed patient dosage (3 dose schedule), for intramuscular use		WAIVED
	90743	Hepatitis B vaccine, adolescent (2 dose schedule), for intramuscular use		WAIVED

© 2019 Optum360, LLC

Service	CPT/ HCPCS	Long Descriptor	USPSTF Rating	Coins./ Deductible
Hepatitis B Vaccine (continued)	90744	Hepatitis B vaccine, pediatric/adolescent dosage (3 dose schedule), for intramuscular use	A	WAIVED
	90746	Hepatitis B vaccine, adult dosage, for intramuscular use		WAIVED
	90747	Hepatitis B vaccine, dialysis or immunosuppressed patient dosage (4 dose schedule), for intramuscular use		WAIVED
	G0010	Administration of Hepatitis B vaccine		WAIVED
Hepatitis C Virus Screening	G0472	Screening for Hepatitis C antibody	B	WAIVED
HIV Screening	G0432	Infectious agent antigen detection by enzyme immunoassay (EIA) technique, qualitative or semi-qualitative, multiple- step method, HIV-1 or HIV-2, screening	A	WAIVED
	G0433	Infectious agent antigen detection by enzyme- linked immunosorbent assay (ELISA) technique, antibody, HIV-1 or HIV-2, screening		WAIVED
	G0435	Infectious agent antigen detection by rapid antibody test of oral mucosa transudate, HIV-1 or HIV- 2 , screening		WAIVED
Smoking Cessation for services furnished prior to October 1, 2016	G0436	Smoking and tobacco cessation counseling visit for the asymptomatic patient; intermediate, greater than 3 minutes, up to 10 minutes	A	WAIVED
	G0437	Smoking and tobacco cessation counseling visit for the asymptomatic patient intensive, greater than 10 minutes		WAIVED
Smoking Cessation for services furnished on or after October 1, 2016	99406	Smoking and tobacco cessation counseling visit for the asymptomatic patient; intermediate, greater than 3 minutes, up to 10 minutes	A	WAIVED
	99407	Smoking and tobacco cessation counseling visit for the asymptomatic patient intensive, greater than 10 minutes		
Annual Wellness Visit	G0438	Annual wellness visit, including PPPS, first visit	*Not Rated	WAIVED
	G0439	Annual wellness visit, including PPPS, subsequent visit		WAIVED
Intensive Behavioral Therapy for Obesity	G0447	Face-to-Face Behavioral Counseling for Obesity, 15 minutes	B	WAIVED
	G0473	Face-to-face behavioral counseling for obesity, group (2-10), 30 minute(s)		
Lung Cancer Screening	G0296	Counseling visit to discuss need for lung cancer screening (LDCT) using low dose CT scan (service is for eligibility determination and shared decision making)	B	WAIVED
	G0297	Low dose CT scan (LDCT) for lung cancer screening		

100-04, 18, 10.1.2

Influenza Virus Vaccine

(Rev.2253, Issued: 07-08-11, Effective: 08-08-11, Implementation: 08-08-11)

Effective for services furnished on or after May 1, 1993, the influenza virus vaccine and its administration is covered when furnished in compliance with any applicable State law. Typically, this vaccine is administered once a flu season. Medicare does not require for coverage purposes that a doctor of medicine or osteopathy order the vaccine. Therefore, the beneficiary may receive the vaccine upon request without a physician's order and without physician supervision. Since there is no yearly limit, A/B MACs (A) and (B) determine whether such services are reasonable and allow payment if appropriate.

See Pub. 100-02, Medicare Benefit Policy Manual, Chapter 15, Section 50.4.4.2 for additional coverage requirements for influenza virus vaccine.

100-04, 18, 10.2.1

Healthcare Common Procedure Coding System (HCPCS) and Diagnosis Codes

(Rev.4100, Issued: 08-03-18; Effective: 01-01-19; Implementation: 01-07-19)

Vaccines and their administration are reported using separate codes. The following codes are for reporting the vaccines only.

HCPCS	Definition
90630	Influenza virus vaccine, quadrivalent (IIV4), split virus, preservative free, for intradermal use
90653	Influenza virus vaccine, inactivated, subunit, adjuvanted, for intramuscular use
90654	Influenza virus vaccine, split virus, preservative-free, for intradermal use, for adults ages 18 – 64;
90655	Influenza virus vaccine, split virus, preservative free, for children 6- 35 months of age, for intramuscular use;
90656	Influenza virus vaccine, split virus, preservative free, for use in individuals 3 years and above, for intramuscular use;
90657	Influenza virus vaccine, split virus, for children 6-35 months of age, for intramuscular use;
90658	Influenza virus vaccine, trivalent (IIV3), split virus, 0.5 mL dosage, for intramuscular use
90660	Influenza virus vaccine, live, for intranasal use;
90661	Influenza virus vaccine, derived from cell cultures, subunit, preservative and antibiotic free, for intramuscular use
90662	Influenza virus vaccine, split virus, preservative free, enhanced immunogenicity via increased antigen content, for intramuscular use
90669	Pneumococcal conjugate vaccine, polyvalent, for children under 5 years, for intramuscular use
90670	Pneumococcal conjugate vaccine, 13 valent, for intramuscular use
90672	Influenza virus vaccine, live, quadrivalent, for intranasal use
90673	Influenza virus vaccine, trivalent, derived from recombinant DNA (RIV3), hemagglutinin (HA) protein only, preservative and antibiotic free, for intramuscular use
90674	Influenza virus vaccine, quadrivalent (ccIIV4), derived from cell cultures, subunit, preservative and antibiotic free, 0.5 mL dosage, for intramuscular use
90682	Influenza virus vaccine, quadrivalent (RIV4), derived from recombinant DNA, hemagglutinin (HA) protein only, preservative and antibiotic free, for intramuscular use
90685	Influenza virus vaccine, quadrivalent, split virus, preservative free, when administered to children 6-35 months of age, for intramuscular use
90686	Influenza virus vaccine, quadrivalent, split virus, preservative free, when administered to individuals 3 years of age and older, for intramuscular use
90687	Influenza virus vaccine, quadrivalent, split virus, when administered to children 6-35 months of age, for intramuscular use
90688	Influenza virus vaccine, quadrivalent, split virus, when administered to individuals 3 years of age and older, for intramuscular use
90689	Influenza virus vaccine, quadrivalent (IIV4), inactivated, adjuvanted, preservative free, 0.25mL dosage, for intramuscular use
90732	Pneumococcal polysaccharide vaccine, 23-valent, adult or immunosuppressed patient dosage, for use in individuals 2 years or older, for subcutaneous or intramuscular use;
90739	Hepatitis B vaccine, adult dosage (2 dose schedule), for intramuscular use
90740	Hepatitis B vaccine, dialysis or immunosuppressed patient dosage (3 dose schedule), for intramuscular use;
90743	Hepatitis B vaccine, adolescent (2 dose schedule), for intramuscular use;

© 2019 Optum360, LLC

HCPCS	Definition
90744	Hepatitis B vaccine, pediatric/adolescent dosage (3 dose schedule), for intramuscular use;
90746	Hepatitis B vaccine, adult dosage, for intramuscular use; and
90747	Hepatitis B vaccine, dialysis or immunosuppressed patient dosage (4 dose schedule), for intramuscular use.
90756	Influenza virus vaccine, quadrivalent (ccIIV4), derived from cell cultures, subunit, antibiotic free, 0.5mL dosage, for intramuscular use

The following codes are for reporting administration of the vaccines only. The administration of the vaccines is billed using:

HCPCS	Definition
G0008	Administration of influenza virus vaccine;
G0009	Administration of pneumococcal vaccine; and
*G0010	Administration of hepatitis B vaccine.
*90471	Immunization administration. (For OPPS hospitals billing for the hepatitis B vaccine administration)
*90472	Each additional vaccine. (For OPPS hospitals billing for the hepatitis B vaccine administration)

*** NOTE:** For claims with dates of service prior to January 1, 2006, OPPS and non-OPPS hospitals report G0010 for hepatitis B vaccine administration. For claims with dates of service January 1, 2006 until December 31, 2010, OPPS hospitals report 90471 or 90472 for hepatitis B vaccine administration as appropriate in place of G0010. Beginning January 1, 2011, providers should report G0010 for billing under the OPPS rather than 90471 or 90472 to ensure correct waiver of coinsurance and deductible for the administration of hepatitis B vaccine.

One of the following diagnosis codes must be reported as appropriate. If the sole purpose for the visit is to receive a vaccine or if a vaccine is the only service billed on a claim, the applicable following diagnosis code may be used.

ICD-9-CM Diagnosis Code	Description
V03.82	Pneumococcus
V04.81**	Influenza
V06.6***	Pneumococcus and Influenza
V05.3	Hepatitis B

**Effective for influenza virus claims with dates of service October 1, 2003 and later.

***Effective October 1, 2006, providers may report ICD-9-CM diagnosis code V06.6 on claims for pneumococcus and/or influenza virus vaccines when the purpose of the visit was to receive both vaccines.

NOTE: ICD-10-CM diagnosis code Z23 may be used for an encounter for immunizations effective October 1, 2015, when ICD-10 was implemented.

If a diagnosis code for pneumococcus, hepatitis B, or influenza virus vaccination is not reported on a claim, contractors may not enter the diagnosis on the claim. Contractors must follow current resolution processes for claims with missing diagnosis codes.

If the diagnosis code and the narrative description are correct, but the HCPCS code is incorrect, the A/B MAC (A or B) may correct the HCPCS code and pay the claim. For example, if the reported diagnosis code is V04.81 and the narrative description (if annotated on the claim) says "flu shot" but the HCPCS code is incorrect, contractors may change the HCPCS code and pay for the flu vaccine. Effective October 1, 2006, A/B MACs (B) should follow the instructions in Pub. 100-04, Chapter 1, Section 80.3.2.1.1 (A/B MAC (B) Data Element Requirements) for claims submitted without a HCPCScode.

Claims for hepatitis B vaccinations must report the I.D. Number of the referring physician. In addition, if a doctor of medicine or osteopathy does not order the influenza virus vaccine, the A/B MACs (A) claims require:

- UPIN code SLF000 to be reported on claims submitted prior to May 23, 2008, when Medicare began accepting NPIs, only
- The provider's own NPI to be reported in the NPI field for the attending physician on claims submitted on or after May 23, 2008, when NPI requirements were implemented.

100-04, 18, 10.2.2.1

Payment for Pneumococcal Pneumonia Virus, Influenza Virus, and Hepatitis B Virus Vaccines and Their Administration on Institutional Claims

(Rev.3754, Issued: 04-21-17, Effective: 07-01-17, Implementation: 07-03-17)

Payment for Vaccines

Payment for these vaccines is as follows:

Facility	Type of Bill	Payment
Hospitals, other than Indian Health Service (IHS) Hospitals and Critical Access Hospitals (CAHs)	12x, 13x	Reasonable cost
IHS Hospitals	12x, 13x, 83x	95% of AWP
IHS CAHs	85x	95% of AWP
CAHs Method I and Method II	85x	Reasonable cost
Skilled Nursing Facilities	22x, 23x	Reasonable cost
Home Health Agencies	34x	Reasonable cost
Hospices	081x, 082x	95% of the AWP
Comprehensive Outpatient Rehabilitation Facilities	75x	95% of the AWP
Independent Renal Dialysis Facilities	72x	95% of the AWP
Hospital-based Renal Dialysis Facilities	72x	Reasonable cost

Payment for Vaccine Administration

Payment for the administration of Influenza Virus and PPV vaccines is as follows:

Facility	Type of Bill	Payment
Hospitals, other than IHS Hospitals and CAHs	12x, 13x	Outpatient Prospective Payment System (OPPS) for hospitals subject to OPPS Reasonable cost for hospitals not subject to OPPS
IHS Hospitals	12x, 13x, 83x	MPFS as indicated in guidelines below.
IHS CAHs	85x	MPFS as indicated in guidelines below.
CAHs Method I and II	85x	Reasonable cost
Skilled Nursing Facilities	22x, 23x	MPFS
Home Health Agencies	34x	OPPS
Hospices	081x, 082x	MPFS
Comprehensive Outpatient Rehabilitation Facilities	75x	MPFS
Independent RDFs	72x	MPFS
Hospital-based RDFs	72x	Reasonable cost

Payment for the administration of Hepatitis B vaccine is as follows:

Facility	Type of Bill	Payment
Hospitals other than IHS hospitals and CAHs	12x, 13x	Outpatient Prospective Payment System (OPPS) for hospitals subject to OPPS Reasonable cost for hospitals not subject to OPPS
IHS Hospitals	12x, 13x, 83x	MPFS
CAHs	85x	Reasonable cost
Method I and II		
IHS CAHs	85x	MPFS
Skilled Nursing Facilities	22x, 23x	MPFS
Home Health Agencies	34x	OPPS
Hospices	081x, 082x	MPFS
Comprehensive Outpatient Rehabilitation Facilities	75x	MPFS
Independent RDFs	72x	MPFS
Hospital-based RDFs	72x	Reasonable cost

© 2019 Optum360, LLC

100-04, 18, 10.2.5.2

Carrier/AB MAC Payment Requirements

(Rev.1278; Issued: 06-29-07; Effective Date: 07-01-07; Implementation Date: 07-30-07)

Payment for pneumococcal, influenza virus, and hepatitis B vaccines follows the same standard rules that are applicable to any injectable drug or biological. (See chapter 17 for procedures for determining the payment rates for pneumococcal and influenza virus vaccines.) Effective for claims with dates of service on or after February 1, 2001, Sec.114, of the Benefits Improvement and Protection Act of 2000 mandated that all drugs and biologicals be paid based on mandatory assignment. Therefore, all providers of influenza virus and pneumococcal vaccines must accept assignment for the vaccine.

Prior to March 1, 2003, the administration of pneumococcal, influenza virus, and hepatitis B vaccines, (HCPCS codes G0008, G0009, and G0010), though not reimbursed directly through the MPFS, were reimbursed at the same rate as HCPCS code 90782 on the MPFS for the year that corresponded to the date of service of the claim.

Prior to March 1, 2003, HCPCS codes G0008, G0009, and G0010 are reimbursed at the same rate as HCPCS code 90471. Assignment for the administration is not mandatory, but is applicable should the provider be enrolled as a provider type "Mass Immunization Roster Biller," submits roster bills, or participates in the centralized billing program.

Carriers/AB MACs may not apply the limiting charge provision for pneumococcal, influenza virus vaccine, or hepatitis B vaccine and their administration in accordance with Secs.1833(a)(1) and 1833(a)(10)(A) of the Social Security Act (the Act.) The administration of the influenza virus vaccine is covered in the influenza virus vaccine benefit under Sec.1861(s)(10)(A) of the Act, rather than under the physicians' services benefit. Therefore, it is not eligible for the 10 percent Health Professional Shortage Area (HPSA) incentive payment or the 5 percent Physician Scarcity Area (PSA) incentive payment.

No Legal Obligation to Pay Nongovernmental entities that provide immunizations free of charge to all patients, regardless of their ability to pay, must provide the immunizations free of charge to Medicare beneficiaries and may not bill Medicare. (See Pub. 100-02, Medicare Benefit Policy Manual, chapter 16.) Thus, for example, Medicare may not pay for influenza virus vaccinations administered to Medicare beneficiaries if a physician provides free vaccinations to all non-Medicare patients or where an employer offers free vaccinations to its employees. Physicians also may not charge Medicare beneficiaries more for a vaccine than they would charge non-Medicare patients. (See Sec.1128(b)(6)(A) of the Act.)

When an employer offers free vaccinations to its employees, it must also offer the free vaccination to an employee who is also a Medicare beneficiary. It does not have to offer free vaccinations to its non-Medicare employees.

Nongovernmental entities that do not charge patients who are unable to pay or reduce their charges for patients of limited means, yet expect to be paid if the patient has health insurance coverage for the services provided, may bill Medicare and expect payment.

Governmental entities (such as PHCs) may bill Medicare for pneumococcal, hepatitis B, and influenza virus vaccines administered to Medicare beneficiaries when services are rendered free of charge to non-Medicare beneficiaries.

100-04, 18, 10.3.1.1

Centralized Billing for Influenza Virus and Pneumococcal Vaccines to Medicare Carriers/AB MACs

(Rev.3329, Issued: 08-14-15, Effective: 01-01-12, Implementation: 09-14-15)

The CMS currently authorizes a limited number of providers to centrally bill for influenza virus and pneumococcal immunization claims. Centralized billing is an optional program available to providers who qualify to enroll with Medicare as the provider type "Mass Immunization Roster Biller," as well as to other individuals and entities that qualify to enroll as regular Medicare providers. Centralized billers must roster bill, must accept assignment, and must bill electronically.

To qualify for centralized billing, a mass immunizer must be operating in at least three payment localities for which there are three different contractors processing claims. Individuals and entities providing the vaccine and administration must be properly licensed in the State in which the immunizations are given and the contractor must verify this through the enrollment process.

Centralized billers must send all claims for influenza virus and pneumococcal immunizations to a single contractor for payment, regardless of the jurisdiction in which the vaccination was administered. (This does not include claims for the Railroad Retirement Board, United Mine Workers or Indian Health Services. These claims must continue to go to the appropriate processing entity.) Payment is made based on the payment locality where the service was provided. This process is only available for claims for the influenza virus and pneumococcal vaccines and their administration. The general coverage and coding rules still apply to these claims.

This section applies only to those individuals and entities that provide mass immunization services for influenza virus and pneumococcal vaccinations and that have been authorized by CMS to centrally bill. All other providers, including those individuals and entities that provide mass immunization services that are not authorized to centrally bill, must continue to bill for these claims to their regular carrier/AB MAC per the instructions in Sec.10.3.1 of this chapter.

The claims processing instructions in this section apply only to the designated processing contractor. However, all carriers/AB MACs must follow the instructions in Sec.10.3.1.1.J, below, "Provider Education Instructions for All Carriers/AB MACs." A. Processing Contractor Trailblazers Health Enterprises is designated as the sole contractor for the payment of influenza virus and pneumococcal claims for centralized billers from October 1, 2000, through the length of the contract. The CMS central office will notify centralized billers of the appropriate contractor to bill when they receive their notification of acceptance into the centralized billing program.

B. Request for Approval

Approval to participate in the CMS centralized billing program is a two part approval process. Individuals and corporations who wish to enroll as a CMS mass immunizer centralized biller must send their request in writing. CMS will complete Part 1 of the approval process by reviewing preliminary demographic information included in the request for participation letter. Completion of Part 1 is not approval to set up vaccination clinics, vaccinate beneficiaries, and bill Medicare for reimbursement. All new participants must complete Part 2 of the approval process (Form CMS-855 Application) before they may set up vaccination clinics, vaccinate Medicare beneficiaries, and bill Medicare for reimbursement. If an individual or entity's request is approved for centralized billing, the approval is limited to 12 months from September to August 31 of the next year. It is the responsibility of the centralized biller to reapply for approval each year. The designated contractor shall provide in writing to CMS and approved centralized billers notification of completion and approval of Part 2 of the approval process. The designated contractor may not process claims for any centralized biller who has not completed Parts 1 and 2 of the approval process. If claims are submitted by a provider who has not received approval of Parts 1 and 2 of the approval process to participate as a centralized biller, the contractor must return the claims to the provider to submit to the local carrier/AB MAC for payment.

C. Notification of Provider Participation to the Processing Contractor

Before September 1 of every year, CMS will provide the designated contractor with the names of the entities that are authorized to participate in centralized billing for the 12 month period beginning September 1 and ending August 31 of the next year.

D. Enrollment

Though centralized billers may already have a Medicare provider number, for purposes of centralized billing, they must also obtain a provider number from the processing contractor for centralized billing through completion of the Form CMS-855 (Provider Enrollment Application). Providers/suppliers are encouraged to apply to enroll as a centralized biller early as possible. Applicants who have not completed the entire enrollment process and received approval from CMS and the designated contractor to participate as a Medicare mass immunizer centralized biller will not be allowed to submit claims to Medicare for reimbursement.

Whether an entity enrolls as a provider type "Mass Immunization Roster Biller" or some other type of provider, all normal enrollment processes and procedures must be followed. Authorization from CMS to participate in centralized billing is dependent upon the entity's ability to qualify as some type of Medicare provider. In addition, as under normal enrollment procedures, the contractor must verify that the entity is fully qualified and certified per State requirements in each State in which they plan to operate.

The contractor will activate the provider number for the 12-month period from September 1 through August 31 of the following year. If the provider is authorized to participate in the centralized billing program the next year, the contractor will extend the activation of the provider number for another year. The entity need not re-enroll with the contractor every year. However, should there be changes in the States in which the entity plans to operate, the contractor will need to verify that the entity meets all State certification and licensure requirements in those new States.

E. Electronic Submission of Claims on Roster Bills

Centralized billers must agree to submit their claims on roster bills in an Electronic Media Claims standard format using the appropriate version of American National Standards Institute (ANSI) format. Contractors should refer to the appropriate ANSI Implementation Guide to determine the correct location for this information on electronic claims. The processing contractor must provide instructions on acceptable

 © 2019 Optum360, LLC

roster billing formats to the approved centralized billers. Paper claims will not be accepted.

F. Required Information on Roster Bills for Centralized Billing

In addition to the roster billing instructions found in Sec.10.3.1 of this chapter, centralized billers must complete on the electronic format the area that corresponds to Item 32 and 33 on Form CMS 1500 (08-05). The contractor must use the ZIP Code in Item 32 to determine the payment locality for the claim. Item 33 must be completed to report the provider of service/supplier's billing name, address, ZIP Code, and telephone number. In addition, the NPI of the billing provider or group must be appropriately reported.

For electronic claims, the name, address, and ZIP Code of the facility are reported in:

- The HIPAA compliant ANSI X12N 837: Claim level loop 2310D NM101=FA. When implemented, the facility (e.g., hospitals) NPI will be captured in the loop 2310D NM109 (NM108=XX) if one is available. Prior to NPI, enter the tax information in loop 2310D NM109 (NM108=24 or 34) and enter the Medicare legacy facility identifier in loop 2310D REF02 (REF01=1C). Report the address, city, state, and ZIP Code in loop 2310D N301 and N401, N402, and N403. Facility data is not required to be reported at the line level for centralized billing.

G. Payment Rates and Mandatory Assignment

The payment rates for the administration of the vaccinations are based on the Medicare Physician Fee Schedule (MPFS) for the appropriate year. Payment made through the MPFS is based on geographic locality. Therefore, payments vary based on the geographic locality where the service was performed.

The HCPCS codes G0008 and G0009 for the administration of the vaccines are not paid on the MPFS. However, prior to March 1, 2003, they must be paid at the same rate as HCPCS code 90782, which is on the MPFS. The designated contractor must pay per the correct MPFS file for each calendar year based on the date of service of the claim. Beginning March 1, 2003, HCPCS codes G0008, G0009, and G0010 are to be reimbursed at the same rate as HCPCS code 90471.

In order to pay claims correctly for centralized billers, the designated contractor must have the correct name and address, including ZIP Code, of the entity where the service was provided.

The following remittance advice and Medicare Summary Notice (MSN) messages apply:

- Claim adjustment reason code 16, "Claim/service lacks information which is needed for adjudication. At least one Remark Code must be provided (may be comprised of either the Remittance Advice Remark Code or NCPDP Reject Reason Code.)" and Remittance advice remark code MA114, "Missing/incomplete/invalid information on where the services were furnished." and MSN 9.4 - "This item or service was denied because information required to make payment was incorrect." The payment rates for the vaccines must be determined by the standard method used by Medicare for reimbursement of drugs and biologicals. (See chapter 17 for procedures for determining the payment rates for vaccines.) Effective for claims with dates of service on or after February 1, 2001, Sec.114, of the Benefits Improvement and Protection Act of 2000 mandated that all drugs and biologicals be paid based on mandatory assignment. Therefore, all providers of influenza virus and pneumococcal vaccines must accept assignment for the vaccine. In addition, as a requirement for both centralized billing and roster billing, providers must agree to accept assignment for the administration of the vaccines as well. This means that they must agree to accept the amount that Medicare pays for the vaccine and the administration. Also, since there is no coinsurance or deductible for the influenza virus and pneumococcal benefit, accepting assignment means that Medicare beneficiaries cannot be charged for the vaccination.

H. Common Working File Information

To identify these claims and to enable central office data collection on the project, special processing number 39 has been assigned. The number should be entered on the HUBC claim record to CWF in the field titled Demonstration Number.

I. Provider Education Instructions for the Processing Contractor

The processing contractor must fully educate the centralized billers on the processes for centralized billing as well as for roster billing. General information on influenza virus and pneumococcal coverage and billing instructions is available on the CMS Web site for providers.

J. Provider Education Instructions for All Carriers/AB MACs

By April 1 of every year, all carriers/AB MACs must publish in their bulletins and put on their Web sites the following notification to providers. Questions from interested providers should be forwarded to the central office address below. Carriers/AB MACs must enter the name of the assigned processing contractor where noted before sending.

NOTIFICATION TO PROVIDERS

Centralized billing is a process in which a provider, who provides mass immunization services for influenza virus and pneumococcal pneumonia virus (PPV) immunizations, can send all claims to a single contractor for payment regardless of the geographic locality in which the vaccination was administered. (This does not include claims for the Railroad Retirement Board, United Mine Workers or Indian Health Services. These claims must continue to go to the appropriate processing entity.) This process is only available for claims for the influenza virus and pneumococcal vaccines and their administration. The administration of the vaccinations is reimbursed at the assigned rate based on the Medicare physician fee schedule for the appropriate locality. The vaccines are reimbursed at the assigned rate using the Medicare standard method for reimbursement of drugs and biologicals.

Individuals and entities interested in centralized billing must contact CMS central office, in writing, at the following address by June 1 of the year they wish to begin centrally billing.

Center for Medicare & Medicaid Services Division of Practitioner Claims Processing Provider Billing and Education Group 7500 Security Boulevard Mail Stop C4-10-07 Baltimore, Maryland 21244 By agreeing to participate in the centralized billing program, providers agree to abide by the following criteria.

CRITERIA FOR CENTRALIZED BILLING

To qualify for centralized billing, an individual or entity providing mass immunization services for influenza virus and pneumococcal vaccinations must provide these services in at least three payment localities for which there are at least three different contractors processing claims.

Individuals and entities providing the vaccine and administration must be properly licensed in the State in which the immunizations are given.

Centralized billers must agree to accept assignment (i.e., they must agree to accept the amount that Medicare pays for the vaccine and the administration).

NOTE: The practice of requiring a beneficiary to pay for the vaccination upfront and to file their own claim for reimbursement is inappropriate. All Medicare providers are required to file claims on behalf of the beneficiary per Sec.1848(g)(4)(A) of the Social Security Act and centralized billers may not collect any payment.

The contractor assigned to process the claims for centralized billing is chosen at the discretion of CMS based on such considerations as workload, user-friendly software developed by the contractor for billing claims, and overall performance. The assigned contractor for this year is [Fill in name of contractor.]

The payment rates for the administration of the vaccinations are based on the Medicare physician fee schedule (MPFS) for the appropriate year. Payment made through the MPFS is based on geographic locality. Therefore, payments received may vary based on the geographic locality where the service was performed. Payment is made at the assigned rate.

The payment rates for the vaccines are determined by the standard method used by Medicare for reimbursement of drugs and biologicals. Payment is made at the assigned rate.

Centralized billers must submit their claims on roster bills in an approved Electronic Media Claims standard format. Paper claims will not be accepted.

Centralized billers must obtain certain information for each beneficiary including name, health insurance number, date of birth, sex, and signature. [Fill in name of contractor] must be contacted prior to the season for exact requirements. The responsibility lies with the centralized biller to submit correct beneficiary Medicare information (including the beneficiary's Medicare Health Insurance Claim Number) as the contractor will not be able to process incomplete or incorrect claims.

Centralized billers must obtain an address for each beneficiary so that a Medicare Summary Notice (MSN) can be sent to the beneficiary by the contractor. Beneficiaries are sometimes confused when they receive an MSN from a contractor other than the contractor that normally processes their claims which results in unnecessary beneficiary inquiries to the Medicare contractor. Therefore, centralized billers must provide every beneficiary receiving an influenza virus or pneumococcal vaccination with the name of the processing contractor. This notification must be in writing, in the form of a brochure or handout, and must be provided to each beneficiary at the time he or she receives the vaccination.

Centralized billers must retain roster bills with beneficiary signatures at their permanent location for a time period consistent with Medicare regulations. [Fill in name of contractor] can provide this information.

Though centralized billers may already have a Medicare provider number, for purposes of centralized billing, they must also obtain a provider number from [Fill in name of contractor]. This can be done by completing the Form CMS-855 (Provider Enrollment Application), which can be obtained from [Fill in name of contractor].

© 2019 Optum360, LLC

If an individual or entity's request for centralized billing is approved, the approval is limited to the 12 month period from September 1 through August 31 of the following year. It is the responsibility of the centralized biller to reapply to CMS CO for approval each year by June 1. Claims will not be processed for any centralized biller without permission from CMS.

Each year the centralized biller must contact [Fill in name of contractor] to verify understanding of the coverage policy for the administration of the pneumococcal vaccine, and for a copy of the warning language that is required on the roster bill.

The centralized biller is responsible for providing the beneficiary with a record of the pneumococcal vaccination.

The information in items 1 through 8 below must be included with the individual or entity's annual request to participate in centralized billing:

1. Estimates for the number of beneficiaries who will receive influenza virus vaccinations;
2. Estimates for the number of beneficiaries who will receive pneumococcal vaccinations;
3. The approximate dates for when the vaccinations will be given;
4. A list of the States in which influenza virus and pneumococcal clinics will be held;
5. The type of services generally provided by the corporation (e.g., ambulance, home health, or visiting nurse);
6. Whether the nurses who will administer the influenza virus and pneumococcal vaccinations are employees of the corporation or will be hired by the corporation specifically for the purpose of administering influenza virus and pneumococcal vaccinations;
7. Names and addresses of all entities operating under the corporation's application;
8. Contact information for designated contact person for centralized billing program.

100-04, 18, 10.4

CWF Edits

(Rev.1617, Issued: 10-24-08, Effective: 04-06-09, Implementation: 04-06-09)

In order to prevent duplicate payments for influenza virus and pneumococcal vaccination claims by the local contractor/AB MAC and the centralized billing contractor, effective for claims received on or after July 1, 2002, CWF has implemented a number of edits.

NOTE: 90659 was discontinued December 31, 2003.

CWF returns information in Trailer 13 information from the history claim. The following fields are returned to the contractor:

- Trailer Code;
- Contractor Number;
- Document Control Number;
- First Service Date;
- Last Service Date;
- Provider, Physician, Supplier Number;
- Claim Type; Procedure code;
- Alert Code (where applicable); and,
- More history (where applicable.)

100-04, 18, 10.4.1

CWF Edits on A/B MAC (A) Claims

(Rev.4100, Issued: 08-03-18; Effective: 01-01-19; Implementation: 01-07-19)

In order to prevent duplicate payment by the same A/B MAC (A), CWF edits by line item on the A/B MAC (A) number, the beneficiary Health Insurance Claim (HIC) number, and the date of service, the influenza virus procedure codes 90630, 90653, 90654, 90655, 90656, 90657, 90658, 90660, 90661, 90662, 90672, 90673, 90674, 90682, 90685, 90686, 90687, 90688, 90689, or 90756 and the pneumococcal procedure codes 90669, 90670, or 90732, and the administration codes G0008 or G0009.

If CWF receives a claim with either HCPCS codes 90630, 90653, 90654, 90655, 90656, 90657, 90658, 90658, 90660, 90661, 90662, 90672, 90673, 90674, 90682, 90685, 90686, 90687, 90688, 90689, or 90756 and it already has on record a claim with the same HIC number, same A/B MAC (A) number, same date of service, and any one of those HCPCS codes, the second claim submitted to CWF rejects.

If CWF receives a claim with HCPCS codes 90669, 90670, or 90732 and it already has on record a claim with the same HIC number, same A/B MAC (A) number, same date of service, and the same HCPCS code, the second claim submitted to CWF rejects when all four items match.

If CWF receives a claim with HCPCS administration codes G0008 or G0009 and it already has on record a claim with the same HIC number, same A/B MAC (A) number, same date of service, and same procedure code, CWF rejects the second claim submitted when all four items match.

CWF returns to the A/B MAC (A) a reject code "7262" for this edit. A/B MACs (A) must deny the second claim and use the same messages they currently use for the denial of duplicate claims.

100-04, 18, 10.4.2

CWF Edits on A/B MAC (B) Claims

(Rev.4100, Issued: 08-03-18; Effective: 01-01-19; Implementation: 01-07-19)

In order to prevent duplicate payment by the same A/B MAC (B), CWF will edit by line item on the A/B MAC (B) number, the HIC number, the date of service, the influenza virus procedure codes 90630, 90653, 90654, 90655, 90656, 90657, 90658, 90660, 90661, 90662, 90672, 90673, 90674, 90682, 90685, 90686, 90687, 90688, 90689, or 90756; the pneumococcal procedure codes 90669, 90670, or 90732; and the administration code G0008 or G0009.

If CWF receives a claim with either HCPCS codes 90630, 90653, 90654, 90655, 90656, 90657, 90658, 90660, 90661, 90662, 90672, 90673, 90674, 90682, 90685, 90686, 90687, 90688, 90689, or 90756 and it already has on record a claim with the same HIC number, same A/B MAC (B) number, same date of service, and any one of those HCPCS codes, the second claim submitted to CWF will reject.

If CWF receives a claim with HCPCS codes 90669, 90670, or 90732 and it already has on record a claim with the same HIC number, same A/B MAC (B) number, same date of service, and the same HCPCS code, the second claim submitted to CWF will reject when all four items match.

If CWF receives a claim with HCPCS administration codes G0008 or G0009 and it already has on record a claim with the same HIC number, same A/B MAC (B) number, same date of service, and same procedure code, CWF will reject the second claim submitted.

CWF will return to the A/B MAC (B) a specific reject code for this edit. A/B MACs (B) must deny the second claim and use the same messages they currently use for the denial of duplicate claims.

In order to prevent duplicate payment by the centralized billing contractor and local A/B MAC (B), CWF will edit by line item for A/B MAC (B) number, same HIC number, same date of service, the influenza virus procedure codes 90630, 90653, 90654, 90655, 90656, 90657, 90658, 90660, 90661, 90662, 90672, 90673, 90674, 90682, 90685, 90686, 90687, 90688, 90689, or 90756; the pneumococcal procedure codes 90669, 90670, or 90732; and the administration code G0008 or G0009.

If CWF receives a claim with either HCPCS codes 90630, 90653, 90654, 90655, 90656, 90657, 90658, 90660, 90661, 90662, 90672, 90673, 90674, 90682, 90685, 90686, 90687, 90688, 90689, or 90756 and it already has on record a claim with a different A/B MAC (B) number, but same HIC number, same date of service, and any one of those same HCPCS codes, the second claim submitted to CWF will reject.

If CWF receives a claim with HCPCS codes 90669, 90670, or 90732 and it already has on record a claim with the same HIC number, different A/B MAC (B) number, same date of service, and the same HCPCS code, the second claim submitted to CWF will reject.

If CWF receives a claim with HCPCS administration codes G0008 or G0009 and it already has on record a claim with a different A/B MAC (B) number, but the same HIC number, same date of service, and same procedure code, CWF will reject the second claim submitted.

CWF will return a specific reject code for this edit. A/B MACs (B) must deny the second claim. For the second edit, the reject code should automatically trigger the following Medicare Summary Notice (MSN) and Remittance Advice (RA) messages.

MSN: 7.2 – "This is a duplicate of a claim processed by another contractor. You should receive a Medicare Summary Notice from them."

Claim Adjustment Reason Code 18 – Exact duplicate claim/service

100-04, 18, 10.4.3

CWF Crossover Edits A/B MAC (B) Claims

(Rev.4100, Issued: 08-03-18; Effective: 01-01-19; Implementation: 01-07-19)

When CWF receives a claim from the A/B MAC (B), it will review Part B outpatient claims history to verify that a duplicate claim has not already been posted.

CWF will edit on the beneficiary HIC number; the date of service; the influenza virus procedure codes 90630, 90653, 90654, 90655, 90656, 90657, 90658, 90660, 90661,

© 2019 Optum360, LLC

90662, 90672, 90673, 90674, 90682, 90685, 90686, 90687, 90688, 90689, or 90756; the pneumococcal procedure codes 90669, 90670, or 90732; and the administration code G0008 or G0009.

CWF will return a specific reject code for this edit. A/B MACs (B) must deny the second claim and use the same messages they currently use for the denial of duplicate claims.

100-04, 18, 20

Mammography Services (Screening and Diagnostic)

(Rev.1387, Issued: 12-07-07, Effective: 04-01-08, Implementation: 04-07-08)

A. Screening Mammography Beginning

January 1, 1991, Medicare provides Part B coverage of screening mammographies for women. Screening mammographies are radiologic procedures for early detection of breast cancer and include a physician's interpretation of the results. A doctor's prescription or referral is not necessary for the procedure to be covered.

Whether payment can be made is determined by a woman's age and statutory frequency parameter. See Pub. 100-02, Medicare Benefit Policy Manual, chapter 15, section 280.3 for additional coverage information for a screening mammography.

Section 4101 of the Balanced Budget Act (BBA) of 1997 provides for annual screening mammographies for women over age 39 and waives the Part B deductible. Coverage applies as follows:

Age Groups	Screening Period
Under age 35	No payment allowed for screening mammography.
35-39	Baseline (pay for only one screening mammography performed on a woman between her 35th and 40th birthday)
Over age 39	Annual 11 full months have elapsed following the month of last screening

NOTE: Count months between screening mammographies beginning the month after the date of the examination. For example, if Mrs. Smith received a screening mammography examination in January 2005, begin counting the next month (February 2005) until 11 months have elapsed. Payment can be made for another screening mammography in January 2006.

B. Diagnostic Mammography

A diagnostic mammography is a radiological mammogram and is a covered diagnostic test under the following conditions: A patient has distinct signs and symptoms for which a mammogram is indicated; A patient has a history of breast cancer; or A patient is asymptomatic, but based on the patient's history and other factors the physician considers significant, the physician's judgment is that a mammogram is appropriate.~Beginning January 1, 2005, Medicare Prescription Drug, Improvement, and Modernization Act (MMA) of 2003, Sec. 644, Public Law 108-173 has changed the way Medicare pays for diagnostic mammography. Medicare will pay based on the MPFS in lieu of OPPS or the lower of the actual change.

100-04, 18, 20.2

HCPCS and Diagnosis Codes for Mammography Services

(Rev.3844, Issued: 08-18-17, Effective: 01-01-18, Implementation: 01-02-18)

The following HCPCS codes are used to bill for mammography services.

HCPCS	Definition
77065* (G0206*)	Diagnostic mammography, including computer-aided detection (CAD) when performed; unilateral
77066* (G0204*)	Diagnostic mammography, including computer-aided detection (CAD) when performed; bilateral
77067* (G0202*)	Screening mammography, bilateral (2-view study of each breast), including computer-aided detection (CAD) when performed
77063**	Screening Breast Tomosynthesis; bilateral (list separately in addition to code for primary procedure).
G0279**	Diagnostic digital breast tomosynthesis, unilateral or bilateral (List separately in addition to code for primary procedure)

***NOTE:** For claims with dates of service January 1, 2017 through December 31, 2017 providers report HCPCS codes G0202, G0204, and G0206. For claims with dates of service on or after January 1, 2018 providers report CPT codes 77067, 77066, and 77065 respectively.

****NOTE:** HCPCS codes 77063 and G0279 are effective for claims with dates of service on or after January 1, 2015.

New Modifier "-GG": Performance and payment of a screening mammography and diagnostic mammography on same patient same day - This is billed with the Diagnostic Mammography code to show the test changed from a screening test to a diagnostic test. A/B MACs (A) and (B) will pay both the screening and diagnostic mammography tests. This modifier is for tracking purposes only. This applies to claims with dates of service on or after January 1, 2002.

A. Diagnosis for Services On or After January 1, 1998

The BBA of 1997 eliminated payment based on high-risk indicators. However, to ensure proper coding, one of the following diagnosis codes should be reported on screening mammography claims as appropriate:

ICD-9-CM

V76.11 - "Special screening for malignant neoplasm, screening mammogram for high-risk patients" or;

V76.12 - "Special screening for malignant neoplasm, other screening mammography."

ICD-10-CM

Z12.31 - Encounter for screening mammogram for malignant neoplasm of breast.

Beginning October 1, 2003, A/B MACs (B) are not permitted to plug the code for a screening mammography when the screening mammography claim has no diagnosis code. Screening mammography claims with no diagnosis code must be returned as unprocessable for assigned claims. For unassigned claims, deny the claim.

In general, providers report diagnosis codes in accordance with the instructions in the appropriate ASC X12 837 claim technical report 3 (institutional or professional) and the paper claim form instructions found in chapters 25 (institutional) and 26 (professional).

In addition, for institutional claims, providers report diagnosis code V76.11 or V76.12 (ICD-9-CM) or Z12.31 (if ICD-10-CM is applicable) in "Principal Diagnosis Code" if the screening mammography is the only service reported on the claim. If the claim contains other services in addition to the screening mammography, these diagnostic codes V76.11 or V76.12 (ICD-9-CM) or Z12.31 (ICD-10-CM) are reported, as appropriate, in "Other Diagnostic Codes." NOTE: Information regarding the form locator number that corresponds to the principal and other diagnosis codes is found in chapter 25.

A/B MACs (B) receive this diagnosis in field 21 and field 24E with the appropriate pointer code of Form CMS-1500 or in Loop 2300 of ASC- X12 837 professional claim format.

Diagnosis codes for a diagnostic mammography will vary according to diagnosis.

100-04, 18, 20.2.2

Screening Digital Breast Tomosynthesis

(Rev.3844, Issued: 08-18-17, Effective: 01-01-18, Implementation: 01-02-18)

When denying claim lines for HCPCS code 77063 that are not submitted with the diagnosis code V76.11 or V76.12, the contractor shall use the following remittance advice messages and associated codes when rejecting/denying claims under this policy. This CARC/RARC combination is compliant with CAQH CORE Business Scenario Three.

CARC: 167

RARC: N386

MSN: 14.9

Group Code PR (Patient Responsibility) assigning financial responsibility to the beneficiary (if a claim is received with a GA modifier indicating a signed ABN is on file).

Group Code CO (Contractual Obligation) assigning financial liability to the provider (if a claim is received with a GZ modifier indicating no signed ABN is on file).

When denying claim lines for HCPCS code G0279 that are not submitted with HCPCS 77066 or 77065

100-04, 18, 20.4

Billing Requirements - FI/A/B MAC Claims

(Rev.3844, Issued: 08-18-17, Effective: 01-01-18, Implementation: 01-02-18)

A/B MACs use the weekly-updated MQSA file to verify that the billing facility is certified by the FDA to perform mammography services, and has the appropriate certification to perform the type of mammogram billed (film and/or digital). (See §20.1.) A/B MACs (A) use the provider number submitted on the claim to identify the facility and use the MQSA data file to verify the facility's certification(s). A/B MAC (A) complete the following activities in processing mammography claims:

- If the provider number on the claim does not correspond with a certified mammography facility on the MQSA file, then A/B MACs (A) deny the claim.
- When a film mammography HCPCS code is on a claim, the claim is checked for a "1" film indicator.

© 2019 Optum360, LLC

- If a film mammography HCPCS code comes in on a claim and the facility is certified for film mammography, the claim is paid if all other relevant Medicare criteria are met.
- If a film mammography HCPCS code is on a claim and the facility is certified for digital mammography only, the claim is denied.
- When a digital mammography HCPCS code is on a claim, the claim is checked for "2" digital indicator.
- If a digital mammography HCPCS code is on a claim and the facility is certified for digital mammography, the claim is paid if all other relevant Medicare criteria are met.
- If a digital mammography HCPCS code is on a claim and the facility is certified for film mammography only, the claim is denied.

NOTE: The Common Working File (CWF) no longer receives the mammography file for editing purposes.

Except as provided in the following sections for RHCs and FQHCs, the following procedures apply to billing for screening mammographies:

The technical component portion of the screening mammography is billed on Form CMS-1450 under bill type 12X, 13X, 14X**, 22X, 23X or 85X using revenue code 0403 and HCPCS code 77067* (G0202*).

The technical component portion of the diagnostic mammography is billed on Form CMS-1450 under bill type 12X, 13X, 14X**, 22X, 23X or 85X using revenue code 0401 and HCPCS code 77065* (G0206*),* 77066*(G0204).

Separate bills are required for claims for screening mammographies with dates of service prior to January 1, 2002. Providers include on the bill only charges for the screening mammography. Separate bills are not required for claims for screening mammographies with dates of service on or after January 1, 2002.

See separate instructions below for rural health clinics (RHCs) and federally qualified health centers (FQHCs).

* For claims with dates of service January 1, 2017 through December 31, 2017, providers report CPT codes G0202, G0204, and G0206. For claims with dates of service January 1, 2018 and later, providers report CPT codes 77067, 77066, and 77065 respectively.

** For claims with dates of service April 1, 2005 and later, hospitals bill for all mammography services under the 13X type of bill or for dates of service April 1, 2007 and later, 12X or 13X as appropriate. The 14X type of bill is no longer applicable. Appropriate bill types for providers other than hospitals are 22X, 23X, and 85X.

In cases where screening mammography services are self-referred and as a result an attending physician NPI is not available, the provider shall duplicate their facility NPI in the attending physician identifier field on the claim.

100-04, 18, 20.5

Billing Requirements - A/B MAC (B) Claims

(Rev.3329, Issued: 08-14-15, Effective: 01-01-12, Implementation: 09-14-15)

Contractors use the weekly-updated file to verify that the billing facility is certified by the FDA to perform mammography services, and has the appropriate certification to perform the type of mammogram billed (film and/or digital). A/B MACs (B) match the FDA

assigned, 6-digit mammography certification number on the claim to the FDA mammography certification number appearing on the file for the billing facility. A/B MACs (B) complete the following activities in processing mammography claims:

- If the claim does not contain the facility's 6-digit certification number, then A/B MACs (B) return the claim as unprocessable.
- If the claim contains a 6-digit certification number that is reported in the proper field or segment (as specified in the previous bullet) but such number does not correspond to the number specified in the MQSA file for the facility, then A/B MACs (B) deny the claim.
- When a film mammography HCPCS code is on a claim, the claim is checked for a "1" film indicator.
- If a film mammography HCPCS code comes in on a claim and the facility is certified for film mammography, the claim is paid if all other relevant Medicare criteria are met.
- If a film mammography HCPCS code is on a claim and the facility is certified for digital mammography only, the claim is denied.
- When a digital mammography HCPCS code is on a claim, the claim is checked for "2" digital indicator.
- If a digital mammography HCPCS code is on a claim and the facility is certified for digital mammography, the claim is paid if all other relevant Medicare criteria are met.
- Process the claim to the point of payment based on the information provided on the claim and in A/B MAC (B) claims history.
- Identify the claim as a screening mammography claim by the CPT-4 code and diagnosis code(s) listed on the claim.
- Assign physician specialty code 45 to facilities that are certified to perform only screening mammography.
- Ensure that entities that bill globally for screening mammography contain a blank in modifier position #1.
- Ensure that entities that bill for the technical component use only HCPCS modifier "-TC."
- Ensure that physicians who bill the professional component separately use HCPCS modifier "-26."
- Ensure all those who are qualified include the 6-digit FDA-assigned certification number of the screening center on the claim. Providers report this number in item 32 on the paper 1500 claim form. A/B MACs (B) retain this number in their provider files.
- When a mammography claim contains services subject to the anti-markup payment limitation and the service was acquired from another billing jurisdiction, the provider must submit their own NPI with the name, address, and ZIP code of the performing physician/supplier.
- Refer to Pub. 100-04, chapter 1, section 10.1.1.1., for claims processing instructions for payment jurisdiction.
- Beginning October 1, 2003, A/B MACs (B) are no longer permitted to add the diagnosis code for a screening mammography when the screening mammography claim has no diagnosis code. Screening mammography claims with no diagnosis code must be returned as unprocessable for assigned claims. For unassigned claims, deny the claim.

A/B MAC (B) Provider Education

- Educate providers that when a screening mammography turns to a diagnostic mammography on the same day for the same beneficiary, add the "-GG" modifier to the diagnostic code and bill both codes on the same claim. Both services are reimbursable by Medicare.
- Educate providers that they cannot bill an add-on code without also billing for the appropriate mammography code. If just the add-on code is billed, the service will be denied. Both the add-on code and the appropriate mammography code should be on the same claim.
- Educate providers to submit their own NPI in place of an attending/referring physician NPI in cases where screening mammography services are self-referred.

100-04, 18, 60

Colorectal Cancer Screening

(Rev.3848, Issued: 08- 25-17, Effective: 09-26-17, Implementation: 09- 26-17)

See the Medicare Benefit Policy Manual, Chapter 15, and the Medicare National Coverage Determinations (NCD) Manual, Chapter 1, Section 210.3 for Medicare Part B coverage requirements and effective dates of colorectal cancer screening services.

Effective for services furnished on or after January 1, 1998, payment may be made for colorectal cancer screening for the early detection of cancer. For screening colonoscopy services (one of the types of services included in this benefit) prior to July 2001, coverage was limited to high-risk individuals. For services July 1, 2001, and later screening colonoscopies are covered for individuals not at high risk.

The following services are considered colorectal cancer screening services:

- Fecal-occult blood test (FOBT),1-3 simultaneous determinations (guaiac-based);
- Flexible sigmoidoscopy;
- Colonoscopy; and,
- Barium enema

Effective for services on or after January 1, 2004, payment may be made for the following colorectal cancer screening service as an alternative for the guaiac-based FOBT, 1-3 simultaneous determinations:

- Fecal-occult blood test, immunoassay, 1-3 simultaneous determinations

Effective for claims with dates of service on or after October 9, 2014, payment may be made for colorectal cancer screening using the Cologuard™ multitarget stool DNA (sDNA) test:

G0464 (Colorectal cancer screening; stool-based DNA and fecal occult hemoglobin (e.g., KRAS, NDRG4 and BMP3).

Note: HCPCS code G0464 expired on December 31, 2015 and has been replaced in the 2016 Clinical Laboratory Fee Schedule with CPT code 81528, Oncology

© 2019 Optum360, LLC

(colorectal) screening, quantitative real-time target and signal amplification of 10 DNA markers (KRAS mutations, promoter methylation of NDRG4 and BMP3) and fecal hemoglobin, utilizing stool, algorithm reported as a positive or negative result.

100-04, 18, 60.1

(Rev.3848, Issued: 08- 25-17, Effective: 09-26-17, Implementation: 09-26-17)

Payment

Payment is under the Medicare Physician Fee Schedule (MPFS) except as follows:

- FOBTs [CPT 82270* (HCPCS G0107*) and HCPCS G0328] are paid under the clinical laboratory fee schedule (CLFS) except reasonable cost is paid to all non-outpatient prospective payment system (OPPS) hospitals, including Critical Access Hospitals (CAHs), but not Indian Health Service (IHS) hospitals billing on type of bill (TOB) 83X. IHS hospitals billing on TOB 83X are paid the Ambulatory Surgery Center (ASC) payment amount. Other IHS hospitals (billing on TOB 13X) are paid the Office of Management and Budget (OMB)-approved all-inclusive rate (AIR), or the facility specific per visit amount as applicable. Deductible and coinsurance do not apply for these tests. See section A below for payment to Maryland waiver hospitals on TOB 13X. Payment to all hospitals for non-patient laboratory specimens on TOB 14X will be based on the CLFS, including CAHs and Maryland waiver hospitals.
- For claims with dates of service on or after January 1, 2015 through December 31, 2015, the Cologuard™ multitarget sDNA test (HCPCS G0464) is paid under the CLFS.

Note: For claims with dates of service October 9, 2014 thru December 31, 2014, HCPCS code G0464 is paid under local contractor pricing.

- For claims with dates of service on or after January 1, 2016, CPT code 81528 replaces G0464 on the CLFS.
- Flexible sigmoidoscopy (code G0104) is paid under OPPS for hospital outpatient departments and on a reasonable cost basis for CAHs; or current payment methodologies for hospitals not subject to OPPS.
- Colonoscopies (G0105 and G0121) and barium enemas (G0106 and G0120) are paid under OPPS for hospital outpatient departments and on a reasonable costs basis for CAHs or current payment methodologies for hospitals not subject to OPPS. Also colonoscopies may be done in an Ambulatory Surgical Center (ASC) and when done in an ASC the ASC rate applies. The ASC rate is the same for diagnostic and screening colonoscopies. The ASC rate is paid to IHS hospitals when the service is billed on TOB 83x.

Prior to January 1, 2007, deductible and coinsurance apply to HCPCS codes G0104, G0105, G0106, G0120, and G0121. Beginning with services provided on or after January 1, 2007, Section 5113 of the Deficit Reduction Act of 2005 waives the requirement of the annual Part B deductible for these screening services. Coinsurance still applies. Coinsurance and deductible applies to the diagnostic colorectal service codes listed below.

The following screening codes must be paid at rates consistent with the diagnostic codes indicated.

Screening Code	Diagnostic Code
G0104	45330
G0105 and G0121	45378
G0106 and G0120	74280

A. Special Payment Instructions for TOB 13X Maryland Waiver Hospitals

For hospitals in Maryland under the jurisdiction of the Health Services Cost Review Commission, screening colorectal services HCPCS G0104, G0105, G0106, 82270* (G0107*), G0120, G0121, G0328, G0464 and 81528 are paid according to the terms of the waiver, that is 94% of submitted charges minus any unmet existing deductible, co-insurance and non-covered charges. Maryland Hospitals bill TOB 13X for outpatient colorectal cancer screenings.

B. Special Payment Instructions for Non-Patient Laboratory Specimen (TOB 14X) for all hospitals

Payment for colorectal cancer screenings (CPT 82270* (HCPCS G0107*), HCPCS G0328, and G0464 (Effective January 1, 2016, HCPCS G0464 is discontinued and replaced with CPT 81528) to a hospital for a non-patient laboratory specimen (TOB 14X), is the lesser of the actual charge, the fee schedule amount, or the National Limitation Amount (NLA), (including CAHs and Maryland Waiver hospitals). Part B deductible and coinsurance do not apply.

***NOTE:** For claims with dates of service prior to January 1, 2007, physicians, suppliers, and providers report HCPCS code G0107. Effective January 1, 2007, code G0107 is discontinued and replaced with CPT code 82270.

100-04, 18, 60.1.1

Deductible and Coinsurance

(Rev.3848, Issued: 08- 25-17, Effective: 09-26-17, Implementation: 09-26-17)

There is no deductible and no coinsurance or copayment for the FOBTs (HCPCS G0107, G0328), flexible sigmoidoscopies (G0104), colonoscopies on individuals at high risk (HCPCS G0105), or colonoscopies on individuals not meeting criteria of high risk (HCPCS G0121). When a screening colonoscopy becomes a diagnostic colonoscopy anesthesia code 00810 should be submitted with only the -PT modifier and only the deductible will be waived.

Prior to January 1, 2007 deductible and coinsurance apply to other colorectal procedures (HCPCS G0106 and G0120). After January 1, 2007, the deductible is waived for those tests. Coinsurance applies.

Effective January 1, 2015, coinsurance and deductible are waived for anesthesia services CPT 00810, Anesthesia for lower intestinal endoscopic procedures, endoscope introduced distal to duodenum, when performed for screening colonoscopy services and when billed with Modifier 33.

Effective for claims with dates of service on and after October 9, 2014, deductible and coinsurance do not apply to the Cologuard™ multitarget sDNA screening test (HCPCS G0464 (Effective January 1, 2016, HCPCS G0464 is discontinued and replaced with CPT 81528)).

NOTE: A 25% coinsurance applies for all colorectal cancer screening colonoscopies (HCPCS G0105 and G0121) performed in ASCs and non-OPPS hospitals effective for services performed on or after January 1, 2007. The 25% coinsurance was implemented in the OPPS PRICER for OPPS hospitals effective for services performed on or after January 1, 1999.

A 25% coinsurance also applies for colorectal cancer screening sigmoidoscopies (HCPCS G0104) performed in non-OPPS hospitals effective for services performed on or after January 1, 2007. Beginning January 1, 2008, colorectal cancer screening sigmoidoscopies (HCPCS G0104) are payable in ASCs, and a 25% coinsurance applies. The 25% coinsurance for colorectal cancer screening sigmoidoscopies was implemented in the OPPS PRICER for OPPS hospitals effective for services performed on or after January 1, 1999.

100-04, 18, 60.2

HCPCS Codes, Frequency Requirements, and Age Requirements (If Applicable)

(Rev.3848, Issued: 08- 25-17, Effective: 09-26-17, Implementation: 09- 26-17)

Effective for services furnished on or after January 1, 1998, the following codes are used for colorectal cancer screening services:

- CPT 82270* (HCPCS G0107*) - Colorectal cancer screening; fecal-occult blood tests, 1-3 simultaneous determinations;
- HCPCS G0104 - Colorectal cancer screening; flexible sigmoidoscopy;
- HCPCS G0105 - Colorectal cancer screening; colonoscopy on individual at high risk;
- HCPCS G0106 - Colorectal cancer screening; barium enema; as an alternative to HCPCS G0104, screening sigmoidoscopy;
- HCPCS G0120 - Colorectal cancer screening; barium enema; as an alternative to HCPCS G0105, screening colonoscopy.

Effective for services furnished on or after July 1, 2001, the following codes are added for colorectal cancer screening services:

- HCPCS G0121 - Colorectal cancer screening; colonoscopy on individual not meeting criteria for high risk.
- HCPCS G0122 - Colorectal cancer screening; barium enema (noncovered).

Effective for services furnished on or after January 1, 2004, the following code is added for colorectal cancer screening services as an alternative to CPT 82270* (HCPCS G0107*):

- HCPCS G0328 - Colorectal cancer screening; immunoassay, fecal-occult blood test, 1-3 simultaneous determinations.

Effective for services furnished on or after October 9, 2014, the following code is added for colorectal cancer screening services:• HCPCS G0464 – Colorectal cancer screening; stool-based DNA and fecal occult hemoglobin (e.g., KRAS, NDRG4 and BMP3) Effective January 1, 2016, HCPCS G0464 is discontinued and replaced with CPT 81528.

*NOTE: For claims with dates of service prior to January 1, 2007, physicians, suppliers, and providers report HCPCS G0107. Effective January 1, 2007, HCPCS G0107 is discontinued and replaced with CPT 82270.

© 2019 Optum360, LLC

G0104 - Colorectal Cancer Screening; Flexible Sigmoidoscopy

Screening flexible sigmoidoscopies (HCPCS G0104) may be paid for beneficiaries who have attained age 50, when performed by a doctor of medicine or osteopathy at the frequencies noted below.

For claims with dates of service on or after January 1, 2002, contractors pay for screening flexible sigmoidoscopies (HCPCS G0104) for beneficiaries who have attained age 50 when these services were performed by a doctor of medicine or osteopathy, or by a physician assistant, nurse practitioner, or clinical nurse specialist (as defined in §1861(aa)(5) of the Social Security Act (the Act) and in the Code of Federal Regulations (CFR) at 42 CFR 410.74, 410.75, and 410.76) at the frequencies noted above. For claims with dates of service prior to January 1, 2002, Medicare Administrative Contractors (MACs) pay for these services under the conditions noted only when a doctor of medicine or osteopathy performs them.

For services furnished from January 1, 1998, through June 30, 2001, inclusive:

- Once every 48 months (i.e., at least 47 months have passed following the month in which the last covered screening flexible sigmoidoscopy was performed).

For services furnished on or after July 1, 2001:

- Once every 48 months as calculated above unless the beneficiary does not meet the criteria for high risk of developing colorectal cancer (refer to §60.3 of this chapter) and he/she has had a screening colonoscopy (HCPCS G0121) within the preceding 10 years. If such a beneficiary has had a screening colonoscopy within the preceding 10 years, then he or she can have covered a screening flexible sigmoidoscopy only after at least 119 months have passed following the month that he/she received the screening colonoscopy (HCPCS G0121).

NOTE: If during the course of a screening flexible sigmoidoscopy a lesion or growth is detected which results in a biopsy or removal of the growth; the appropriate diagnostic procedure classified as a flexible sigmoidoscopy with biopsy or removal along with modifier –PT should be billed and paid rather than HCPCS G0104.

HCPCS G0105 - Colorectal Cancer Screening; Colonoscopy on Individual at High Risk

Screening colonoscopies (HCPCS G0105) may be paid when performed by a doctor of medicine or osteopathy at a frequency of once every 24 months for beneficiaries at high risk for developing colorectal cancer (i.e., at least 23 months have passed following the month in which the last covered HCPCS G0105 screening colonoscopy was performed). Refer to §60.3 of this chapter for the criteria to use in determining whether or not an individual is at high risk for developing colorectal cancer.

NOTE: If during the course of the screening colonoscopy, a lesion or growth is detected which results in a biopsy or removal of the growth, the appropriate diagnostic procedure classified as a colonoscopy with biopsy or removal along with modifier –PT should be billed and paid rather than HCPCS G0105.

A. Colonoscopy Cannot be Completed Because of Extenuating Circumstances

1. A/B MACs (A)

When a covered colonoscopy is attempted but cannot be completed because of extenuating circumstances, Medicare will pay for the interrupted colonoscopy as long as the coverage conditions are met for the incomplete procedure. However, the frequency standards associated with screening colonoscopies will not be applied by the common working file (CWF). When a covered colonoscopy is next attempted and completed, Medicare will pay for that colonoscopy according to its payment methodology for this procedure as long as coverage conditions are met, and the frequency standards will be applied by CWF. This policy is applied to both screening and diagnostic colonoscopies. When submitting a facility claim for the interrupted colonoscopy, providers are to suffix the colonoscopy

Use of HCPCS codes with a modifier of –73 or –74 is appropriate to indicate that the procedure was interrupted. Payment for covered incomplete screening colonoscopies shall be consistent with payment methodologies currently in place for complete screening colonoscopies, including those contained in 42 CFR 419.44(b). In situations where a CAH has elected payment Method II for CAH patients, payment shall be consistent with payment methodologies currently in place as outlined in chapter 3 of this manual. As such, instruct CAHs that elect Method II payment to use modifier –53 to identify an incomplete screening colonoscopy (physician professional service(s) billed in revenue code 096X, 097X, and/or 098X). Such CAHs will also bill the technical or facility component of the interrupted colonoscopy in revenue code 075X (or other appropriate revenue code) using the -73 or -74 modifier as appropriate.

Note that Medicare would expect the provider to maintain adequate information in the patient's medical record in case it is needed by the contractor to document the incomplete procedure.

2. A/B MACs (B)

When a covered colonoscopy is attempted but cannot be completed because of extenuating circumstances (see chapter 12), Medicare will pay for the interrupted colonoscopy at a rate consistent with that of a flexible sigmoidoscopy as long as coverage conditions are met for the incomplete procedure. When a covered colonoscopy is next attempted and completed, Medicare will pay for that colonoscopy according to its payment methodology for this procedure as long as coverage conditions are met. This policy is applied to both screening and diagnostic colonoscopies. When submitting a claim for the interrupted colonoscopy, professional providers are to suffix the colonoscopy code with modifier of –53 to indicate that the procedure was interrupted. When submitting a claim for the facility fee associated with this procedure, ASCs are to suffix the colonoscopy code with modifier –73 or –74 as appropriate. Payment for covered screening colonoscopies, including that for the associated ASC facility fee when applicable, shall be consistent with payment for diagnostic colonoscopies, whether the procedure is complete or incomplete.

Note that Medicare would expect the provider to maintain adequate information in the patient's medical record in case it is needed by the contractor to document the incomplete procedure.

HCPCS G0106 - Colorectal Cancer Screening; Barium Enema; as an Alternative to HCPCS G0104, Screening Sigmoidoscopy

Screening barium enema examinations may be paid as an alternative to a screening sigmoidoscopy (HCPCS G0104). The same frequency parameters for screening sigmoidoscopies (see those codes above) apply.

In the case of an individual aged 50 or over, payment may be made for a screening barium enema examination (HCPCS G0106) performed after at least 47 months have passed following the month in which the last screening barium enema or screening flexible sigmoidoscopy was performed. For example, the beneficiary received a screening barium enema examination as an alternative to a screening flexible sigmoidoscopy in January 1999. Start count beginning February 1999. The beneficiary is eligible for another screening barium enema in January 2003.

The screening barium enema must be ordered in writing after a determination that the test is the appropriate screening test. Generally, it is expected that this will be a screening double contrast enema unless the

individual is unable to withstand such an exam. This means that in the case of a particular individual, the attending physician must determine that the estimated screening potential for the barium enema is equal to or greater than the screening potential that has been estimated for a screening flexible sigmoidoscopy for the same individual. The screening single contrast barium enema also requires a written order from the beneficiary's attending physician in the same manner as described above for the screening double contrast barium enema examination.

CPT 82270* **(HCPCS G0107*) - Colorectal Cancer Screening; Fecal-Occult Blood Test, 1-3 Simultaneous Determinations**

Effective for services furnished on or after January 1, 1998, screening FOBT (CPT 82270* (HCPCS G0107*) may be paid for beneficiaries who have attained age 50, and at a frequency of once every 12 months (i.e., at least 11 months have passed following the month in which the last covered screening FOBT was performed). This screening FOBT means a guaiac-based test for peroxidase activity, in which the beneficiary completes it by taking samples from two different sites of three consecutive stools. This screening requires a written order from the beneficiary's attending physician, or additionally, effective for dates of service on or after January 27, 2014, the beneficiary's attending physician assistant, nurse practitioner, or clinical nurse specialist. (The term "attending physician" is defined to mean a doctor of medicine or osteopathy (as defined in §1861(r)(1) of the Act) who is fully knowledgeable about the beneficiary's medical condition, and who would be responsible for using the results of any examination performed in the overall management of the beneficiary's specific medical problem.)

Effective for services furnished on or after January 1, 2004, payment may be made for an immunoassay-based FOBT (HCPCS G0328, described below) as an alternative to the guaiac-based FOBT, CPT 82270* (HCPCS G0107*). Medicare will pay for only one covered FOBT per year, either CPT 82270* (HCPCS G0107*) or HCPCS G0328, but not both.

*NOTE: For claims with dates of service prior to January 1, 2007, physicians, suppliers, and providers report HCPCS G0107. Effective January 1, 2007, HCPCS G0107 is discontinued and replaced with CPT 82270.

HCPCS G0328 - Colorectal Cancer Screening; Immunoassay, Fecal-Occult Blood Test, 1-3 Simultaneous Determinations

Effective for services furnished on or after January 1, 2004, screening FOBT, (HCPCS G0328) may be paid as an alternative to CPT 82270* (HCPCS G0107*) for beneficiaries who have attained age 50. Medicare will pay for a covered FOBT (either CPT 82270*

 © 2019 Optum360, LLC

(HCPCS G0107*) or HCPCS G0328, but not both) at a frequency of once every 12 months (i.e., at least 11 months have passed following the month in which the last covered screening FOBT was performed).

Screening FOBT, immunoassay, includes the use of a spatula to collect the appropriate number of samples or the use of a special brush for the collection of samples, as determined by the individual manufacturer's instructions. This screening requires a written order from the beneficiary's attending physician, or, additionally, effective for claims with dates of service on or after January 27, 2014, the beneficiary's attending physician assistant, nurse practitioner, or clinical nurse specialist. (The term "attending physician" is defined to mean a doctor of medicine or osteopathy (as defined in §1861(r)(1) of the Act) who is fully knowledgeable about the beneficiary's medical condition, and who would be responsible for using the results of any examination performed in the overall management of the beneficiary's specific medical problem.)

HCPCS G0120 - Colorectal Cancer Screening; Barium Enema; as an Alternative to HCPCS G0105, Screening Colonoscopy

Screening barium enema examinations may be paid as an alternative to a screening colonoscopy (HCPCS G0105) examination. The same frequency parameters for screening colonoscopies (see those codes above) apply.

In the case of an individual who is at high risk for colorectal cancer, payment may be made for a screening barium enema examination (HCPCS G0120) performed after at least 23 months have passed following the month in which the last screening barium enema or the last screening colonoscopy was performed. For example, a beneficiary at high risk for developing colorectal cancer received a screening barium enema examination (HCPCS G0120) as an alternative to a screening colonoscopy (HCPCS G0105) in January 2000. Start counts beginning February 2000. The beneficiary is eligible for another screening barium enema examination (HCPCS G0120) in January 2002.

The screening barium enema must be ordered in writing after a determination that the test is the appropriate screening test. Generally, it is expected that this will be a screening double contrast enema unless the individual is unable to withstand such an exam. This means that in the case of a particular individual, the attending physician must determine that the estimated screening potential for the barium enema is equal to or greater than the screening potential that has been estimated for a screening colonoscopy, for the same individual. The screening single contrast barium enema also requires a written order from the beneficiary's attending physician in the same manner as described above for the screening double contrast barium enema examination.

HCPCS G0121 - Colorectal Screening; Colonoscopy on Individual Not Meeting Criteria for High Risk - Applicable On and After July 1, 2001

Effective for services furnished on or after July 1, 2001, screening colonoscopies (HCPCS G0121) performed on individuals not meeting the criteria for being at high risk for developing colorectal cancer (refer to §60.3 of this chapter) may be paid under the following conditions:

- At a frequency of once every 10 years (i.e., at least 119 months have passed following the month in which the last covered HCPCS G0121 screening colonoscopy was performed.)
- If the individual would otherwise qualify to have covered a HCPCS G0121 screening colonoscopy based on the above but has had a covered screening flexible sigmoidoscopy (HCPCS G0104), then he or she may have covered a HCPCS G0121 screening colonoscopy only after at least 47 months have passed following the month in which the last covered HCPCS G0104 flexible sigmoidoscopy was performed.

NOTE: If during the course of the screening colonoscopy, a lesion or growth is detected which results in a biopsy or removal of the growth, the appropriate diagnostic procedure classified as a colonoscopy with biopsy or removal along with modifier –PT should be billed and paid rather than HCPCS G0121.

HCPCS G0464 - Multitarget Stool DNA (sDNA) Colorectal Cancer Screening Test - CologuardTM

Effective for dates of service on or after October 9, 2014, colorectal cancer screening using the CologuardTM multitarget sDNA test (G0464) is covered once every 3 years for Medicare beneficiaries that meet all of the following criteria:

- Ages 50 to 85 years,
- Asymptomatic (no signs or symptoms of colorectal disease including but not limited to lower gastrointestinal pain, blood in stool, positive guaiac fecal occult blood test or fecal immunochemical test), and,
- At average risk of developing colorectal cancer (no personal history of adenomatous polyps, colorectal cancer, or inflammatory bowel disease, including Crohn's Disease and ulcerative colitis; ?no family history of colorectal cancers or adenomatous polyps, familial adenomatous polyposis, or hereditary nonpolyposis colorectal cancer). See Pub. 100-03, Medicare National Coverage Determinations Manual, Chapter 1, Section 210.3, for complete coverage requirements.

Effective for claims with dates of service on or after October 9, 2014, providers shall report the following diagnosis codes when submitting claims for the Cologuard™ multitarget sDNA test:

ICD-9: V76.41 and V76.51, or,

ICD-10: Z12.11 and Z12.12

NOTE: Effective January 1, 2016, HCPCS G0464 is discontinued and replaced with CPT 81528.

HCPCS G0122 - Colorectal Cancer Screening; Barium Enema

The code is not covered by Medicare.

100-04, 18, 60.6

Billing Requirements for Claims Submitted to A/B MACs (A)

(Rev.3848, Issued: 08- 25-17, Effective: 09-26-17, Implementation: 09- 26-17)

Follow the general bill review instructions in Chapter 25. Hospitals use the ANSI X12N 837I to bill the FI or on the hardcopy Form CMS-1450. Hospitals bill revenue codes and HCPCS codes as follows:

Screening Test/Procedure	Revenue Code	HCPCS Code	TOB
FOBT	030X	82270*** (G0107***), G0328	12X, 13X, 14X**, 22X, 23X, 83X, 85X
Barium enema	032X	G0106, G0120, G0122	12X, 13X, 22X, 23X, 85X****
Flexible Sigmoidoscopy	*	G0104	12X, 13X, 22X, 23X, 83X, 85X****
Colonoscopy-high risk	*	G0105, G0121	12X, 13X, 22X, 23X, 83X, 85X****
Multitarget sDNA - CologuardTM	030X	(G0464*****), 81528*****	13X, 14X**, 85X

* The appropriate revenue code when reporting any other surgical procedure.

** 14X is only applicable for non-patient laboratory specimens.

*** For claims with dates of service prior to January 1, 2007, physicians, suppliers, and providers report HCPCS code G0107. Effective January 1, 2007, code G0107, is discontinued and replaced with CPT code 82270.

**** CAHs that elect Method II bill revenue code 096X, 097X, and/or 098X for professional services and 075X (or other appropriate revenue code) for the technical or facility component.

***** Effective January 1, 2016, HCPCS G0464 is discontinued and replaced with CPT 81528

Special Billing Instructions for Hospital Inpatients

When these tests/procedures are provided to inpatients of a hospital or when Part A benefits have been exhausted, they are covered under this benefit. However, the provider bills on bill type 12X using the discharge date of the hospital stay to avoid editing in the Common Working File (CWF) as a result of the hospital bundling rules.

100-04, 18, 60.7

Medicare Summary Notice (MSN) Messages

(Rev.3848, Issued: 08- 25-17, Effective: 09-26-17, Implementation: 09- 26-17)

The following Medicare Summary Notice (MSN) messages are used (See Chapter 21 for the Spanish versions of these messages):

A. If a claim for a screening FOBT, a screening flexible sigmoidoscopy, or a barium enema is being denied because of the age of the beneficiary, use:

   18.13 - This service is not covered for patients under 50 years of age.

B. If the claim for a screening FOBT, a screening colonoscopy, a screening flexible sigmoidoscopy, or a barium enema is being denied because the time period between the same test or procedure has not passed, use:

   18.14 - Service is being denied because it has not been (12, 24, 48, 120) months since your last (test/procedure) of this kind.

C. If the claim is being denied for a screening colonoscopy or a barium enema because the beneficiary is not at a high risk, use:

   18.15 - Medicare covers this procedure only for patients considered to be at a high risk for colorectal cancer.

D. If the claim is being denied because payment has already been made for a screening FOBT (CPT 82270* (HCPCS G0107*) or HCPCS G0328), flexible sigmoidoscopy (HCPCS G0104), screening colonoscopy (HCPCS G0105), or a screening barium enema (HCPCS G0106 or G0120), use:

© 2019 Optum360, LLC

18.16 - This service is denied because payment has already been made for a similar procedure within a set timeframe.

NOTE: MSN message 18.16 should only be used when a certain screening procedure is performed as an alternative to another screening procedure. For example: If the claims history indicates a payment has been made for HCPCS G0120 and an incoming claim is submitted for HCPCS G0105 within 24 months, the incoming claim should be denied.

E. If the claim is being denied for a non-covered screening procedure code such as HCPCS G0122, use:

16.10 - Medicare does not pay for this item or service.

If an invalid procedure code is reported, the contractor will return the claim as unprocessable to the provider under current procedures.

*NOTE: For claims with dates of service prior to January 1, 2007, physicians, suppliers, and providers report HCPCS G0107. Effective January 1, 2007, HCPCS G0107 is discontinued and replaced with CPT 82270.

F. If denying claims for Cologuard™ multitarget sDNA screening test (HCPCS G0464 Effective January 1, 2016, HCPCS G0464 has been discontinued and replaced with CPT 81528) when furnished more than once in a 3-year period [at least 2 years and 11 full months (35 months total) must elapse from the date of the last screening], use:

15.19 - Local Coverage Determinations (LCDs) help Medicare decide what is covered. An LCD was used for your claim. You can compare your case to the LCD, and send information from your doctor if you think it could change our decision. Call 1-800-MEDICARE (1-800-633-4227) for a copy of the LCD.

Spanish Version - Las Determinaciones Locales de Cobertura (LCDs en inglés) le ayudan a decidir a Medicare lo que está cubierto. Un LCD se usó para su reclamación. Usted puede comparar su caso con la determinación y enviar información de su médico si piensa que puede cambiar nuestra decisión. Para obtener una copia del LCD, llame al 1-800-MEDICARE (1-800-633-4227).

15.20 - The following policies NCD 210.3 were used when we made this decision

Spanish Version – "Las siguientes políticas NCD210.3 fueron utilizadas cuando se tomó esta decisión"

NOTE: Due to system requirement, FISS has combined messages 15.19 and 15.20 so that, when used for the same line item, both messages will appear on the same MSN.

G. If denying claims for Cologuard™ multitarget sDNA screening test (HCPCS G0464 Effective January 1, 2016, HCPCS G0464 has been discontinued and replaced with CPT 81528) because the beneficiary is not between the ages of 50 and 85, use:

15.19 - Local Coverage Determinations (LCDs) help Medicare decide what is covered. An LCD was used for your claim. You can compare your case to the LCD, and send information from your doctor if you think it could change our decision. Call 1-800-MEDICARE (1-800-633-4227) for a copy of the LCD.

Spanish Version - Las Determinaciones Locales de Cobertura (LCDs en inglés) le ayudan a decidir a Medicare lo que está cubierto. Un LCD se usó para su reclamación. Usted puede comparar su caso con la determinación y enviar información de su médico si piensa que puede cambiar nuestra decisión. Para obtener una copia del LCD, llame al 1-800-MEDICARE (1-800-633-4227).

15.20 - The following policies NCD 210.3 were used when we made this decision.

Spanish Version – "Las siguientes políticas NCD 210.3 fueron utilizadas cuando se tomó esta decision."

NOTE: Due to system requirement, FISS has combined messages 15.19 and 15.20 so that, when used for the same line item, both messages will appear on the same MSN.

H. If denying claims for Cologuard™ multitarget sDNA screening test (HCPCS G0464 Effective January 1, 2016, HCPCS G0464 has been discontinued and replaced with CPT 81528) because the claim does not contain all of the ICD-9 or ICD-10 diagnosis codes required, use:

15.19 - Local Coverage Determinations (LCDs) help Medicare decide what is covered. An LCD was used for your claim. You can compare your case to the LCD, and send information from your doctor if you think it could change our decision. Call 1-800-MEDICARE (1-800-633-4227) for a copy of the LCD.

Spanish Version - Las Determinaciones Locales de Cobertura (LCDs en inglés) le ayudan a decidir a Medicare lo que está cubierto. Un LCD se usó para su reclamación. Usted puede comparar su caso con la determinación y enviar información de su médico si piensa que puede cambiar nuestra decisión. Para obtener una copia del LCD, llame al 1-800-MEDICARE (1-800-633-4227).

15.20 - The following policies 210.3 were used when we made this decision

Spanish Version – "Las siguientes políticas NCD210.3 fueron utilizadas cuando se tomó esta decisión"

NOTE: Due to system requirement, FISS has combined messages 15.19 and 15.20 so that, when used for the same line item, both messages will appear on the same MSN.

I. If denying claims for Cologuard™ multitarget sDNA screening test (HCPCS G0464 Effective January 1, 2016, HCPCS G0464 has been discontinued and replaced with CPT 81528) on institutional claims when submitted on a TOB other than 13X, 14X, and 85X, use:

21.25 - This service was denied because Medicare only covers this service in certain settings.

Spanish Version: "El servicio fue denegado porque Medicare solamente lo cubre en ciertas situaciones."

100-04, 18, 70.1.1

HCPCS and Diagnosis Coding

(Rev.3329, Issued: 08-14-15, Effective: 01-01-12, Implementation: 09-14-15)

The following HCPCS codes should be reported when billing for screening glaucoma services:

G0117 - Glaucoma screening for high-risk patients furnished by an optometrist (physician for A/B MAC (B)) or ophthalmologist.

G0118 - Glaucoma screening for high-risk patients furnished under the direct supervision of an optometrist (physician for A/B MAC (B) or ophthalmologist.

The A/B MAC (B) claims type of service for the above G codes is: TOS Q.

Glaucoma screening claims should be billed using screening ("V") code V80.1 (Special Screening for Neurological, Eye, and Ear Diseases, Glaucoma), or if ICD-10-CM is applicable, diagnosis code Z13.5 (encounter for screening for eye and ear disorders). Claims submitted without a screening diagnosis code may be returned to the provider as unprocessable (refer to chapter 1 of this manual for more information about incomplete or invalid claims).

100-04, 18, 80

Initial Preventive Physical Examination (IPPE)

(Rev.3096, Issued: 10-17-14, Effective: 01-27-14, Implementation: 11-18-14)

(NOTE: For billing and payment requirements for the Annual Wellness Visit, see chapter 18, section 140, of this chapter.)

Background: Sections 1861(s)(2)(w) and 1861(ww) of the Social Security Act (and implementing regulations at 42 CFR 410.16, 411.15(a)(1), and 411.15(k)(11)) authorize coverage under Part B for a one-time initial preventive physical examination (IPPE) for new Medicare beneficiaries that meet certain eligibility requirements.

Coverage: As described in implementing regulations at 42 CFR 410.16, 411.15(a)(1), and 411.15(k)(11), the IPPE may be performed by a doctor of medicine or osteopathy as defined in section 1861 (r)(1) of the Social Security Act (the Act) or by a qualified nonphysician practitioner (NPP) (physician assistant, nurse practitioner, or clinical nurse specialist), not later than 12 months after the date the individual's first coverage begins under Medicare Part B. (See section 80.3 for a list of bill types of facilities that can bill A/B MACs for this service.)

The IPPE includes:

(1) review of the individual's medical and social history with attention to modifiable risk factors for disease detection,

(2) review of the individual's potential (risk factors) for depression or other mood disorders,

(3) review of the individual's functional ability and level of safety;

(4) an examination to include measurement of the individual's height, weight, body mass index, blood pressure, a visual acuity screen, and other factors as deemed appropriate, based on the beneficiary's medical and social history;

(5) end-of-life planning, upon agreement of the individual.

(6) education, counseling, and referral, as deemed appropriate, based on the results of the review and evaluation services described in the previous 5 elements, and

(7) education, counseling, and referral including a brief written plan (e.g., a checklist or alternative) provided to the individual for obtaining appropriate screening and other preventive services, which are separately covered under Medicare Part B.

Medicare will pay for only one IPPE per beneficiary per lifetime. The Common Working File (CWF) will edit for this benefit.

The IPPE does not include other preventive services that are currently separately covered and paid under Medicare Part B. (That is: pneumococcal, influenza and

 © 2019 Optum360, LLC

hepatitis B vaccines and their administration, screening mammography, screening pap smear and screening pelvic examinations, prostate cancer screening tests, colorectal cancer screening tests, diabetes outpatient self-management training services, bone mass measurements, glaucoma screening, medical nutrition therapy for individuals with diabetes or renal disease, cardiovascular screening blood tests, diabetes screening tests, screening ultrasound for abdominal aortic aneurysms, an electrocardiogram, and additional preventive services covered under Medicare Part B through the Medicare national coverage determination process.)

For the physician/practitioner billing correct coding and payment policy, refer to chapter 12, section 30.6.1.1, of this manual.

100-04, 18, 80.1

Healthcare Common Procedure Coding System (HCPCS) Coding for the IPPE

(Rev.2159, Issued: 02-15-11, Effective: 01-01-11, Implementation: 04-04-11)

The HCPCS codes listed below were developed for the IPPE benefit effective January 1, 2005, for individuals whose initial enrollment is on or after January 1, 2005.

G0344: Initial preventive physical examination; face-to-face visit, services limited to new beneficiary during the first 6 months of Medicare enrollment

Short Descriptor: Initial Preventive Exam

G0366: Electrocardiogram, routine ECG with 12 leads; performed as a component of the initial preventive examination with interpretation and report

Short Descriptor: EKG for initial prevent exam

G0367: tracing only, without interpretation and report, performed as a component of the initial preventive examination

Short Descriptor: EKG tracing for initial prev

G0368: interpretation and report only, performed as a component of the initial preventive examination

Short Descriptor: EKG interpret & report preve

The following new HCPCS codes were developed for the IPPE benefit effective January 1, 2009, and replaced codes G0344, G0366, G0367, and G0368 shown above beginning with dates of service on or after January 1, 2009:

G0402: Initial preventive physical examination; face-to-face visit, services limited to new beneficiary during the first 12 months of Medicare enrollment

Short Descriptor: Initial Preventive exam

G0403: Electrocardiogram, routine ECG with 12 leads; performed as a screening for the initial preventive physical examination with interpretation and report

Short Descriptor: EKG for initial prevent exam

G0404: Electrocardiogram, routine ECG with 12 leads; tracing only, without interpretation and report, performed as a screening for the initial preventive physical examination

Short Descriptor: EKG tracing for initial prev

G0405: Electrocardiogram, routine ECG with 12 leads; interpretation and report only, performed as a screening for the initial preventive physical examination

Short Descriptor: EKG interpret & report preve

100-04, 18, 80.2

A/B Medicare Administrative Contractor (MAC) and Contractor Billing Requirements

(Rev.3329, Issued: 08-14-15, Effective: 01-01-12, Implementation: 09-14-15)

Effective for dates of service on and after January 1, 2005, through December 31, 2008, contractors shall recognize the HCPCS codes G0344, G0366, G0367, and G0368 shown above in §80.1 for an IPPE. The type of service (TOS) for each of these codes is as follows:

G0344: TOS = 1

G0366: TOS = 5

G0367: TOS = 5

G0368: TOS = 5

Contractors shall pay physicians or qualified nonphysician practitioners for only one IPPE performed not later than 6 months after the date the individual's first coverage begins under Medicare Part B, but only if that coverage period begins on or after January 1, 2005.

Effective for dates of service on and after January 1, 2009, contractors shall recognize the HCPCS codes G0402, G0403, G0404, and G0405 shown above in §80.1 for an IPPE. The TOS for each of these codes is as follows:

G0402: TOS = 1

G0403: TOS = 5

G0404: TOS = 5

G0405: TOS = 5

Under the MIPPA of 2008, contractors shall pay physicians or qualified nonphysician practitioners for only one IPPE performed not later than 12 months after the date the individual's first coverage begins under Medicare Part B only if that coverage period begins on or after January 1, 2009.

Contractors shall allow payment for a medically necessary Evaluation and Management (E/M) service at the same visit as the IPPE when it is clinically appropriate. Physicians and qualified nonphysician practitioners shall use CPT codes 99201-99215 to report an E/M with CPT modifier 25 to indicate that the E/M is a significant, separately identifiable service from the IPPE code reported (G0344 or G0402, whichever applies based on the date the IPPE is performed). Refer to chapter 12, § 30.6.1.1, of this manual for the physician/practitioner billing correct coding and payment policy regarding E/M services.

If the EKG performed as a component of the IPPE is not performed by the primary physician or qualified NPP during the IPPE visit, another physician or entity may perform and/or interpret the EKG. The referring physician or qualified NPP needs to make sure that the performing physician or entity bills the appropriate G code for the screening EKG, and not a CPT code in the 93000 series. Both the IPPE and the EKG should be billed in order for the beneficiary to receive the complete IPPE service. Effective for dates of service on and after January 1, 2009, the screening EKG is optional and is no longer a mandated service of an IPPE if performed as a result of a referral from an IPPE.

Should the same physician or NPP need to perform an additional medically necessary EKG in the 93000 series on the same day as the IPPE, report the appropriate EKG CPT code(s) with modifier 59, indicating that the EKG is a distinct procedural service.

Physicians or qualified nonphysician practitioners shall bill the contractor the appropriate HCPCS codes for IPPE on the Form CMS-1500 claim or an approved electronic format. The HCPCS codes for an IPPE and screening EKG are paid under the Medicare Physician Fee Schedule (MPFS). The appropriate deductible and coinsurance applies to codes G0344, G0366, G0367, G0368, G0403, G0404, and G0405. The deductible is waived for code G0402 but the coinsurance still applies.

100-04, 18, 80.3.3

Outpatient Prospective Payment System (OPPS) Hospital Billing

(Rev.2159, Issued: 02-15-11, Effective: 01-01-11, Implementation: 04-04-11)

Hospitals subject to OPPS (TOBs 12X and 13X) must use modifier -25 when billing the IPPE G0344 along with the technical component of the EKG, G0367, on the same claim. The same is true when billing IPPE code G0402 along with the technical component of the screening EKG, code G0404. This is due to an OPPS Outpatient Code Editor (OCE) which contains an edit that requires a modifier -25 on any evaluation and management (E/M) HCPCS code if there is also a status "S" or "T" HCPCS procedure code on the claim.

100-04, 18, 80.4

Coinsurance and Deductible

(Rev.2159, Issued: 02-15-11, Effective: 01-01-11, Implementation: 04-04-11)

The Medicare deductible and coinsurance apply for the IPPE provided before January 1, 2009.

The Medicare deductible is waived effective for the IPPE provided on or after January 1, 2009. Coinsurance continues to apply for the IPPE provided on or after January 1, 2009.

As a result of the Affordable Care Act, effective for the IPPE provided on or after January 1, 2011, the Medicare deductible and coinsurance (for HCPCS code G0402 only) are waived.

100-04, 18, 120.1

Coding and Payment of DSMT Services

(Rev.1255, Issued: 05-25-07; Effective: 07-01-07; Implementation: 07-02-07)

The following HCPCS codes are used to report DSMT:

- G0108 - Diabetes outpatient self-management training services, individual, per 30 minutes.
- G0109 - Diabetes outpatient self-management training services, group session (2 or more), per 30 minutes.

The type of service for these codes is 1.

© 2019 Optum360, LLC

Payment to physicians and providers for outpatient DSMT is made as follows:

Type of Facility	Payment Method	Type of Bill
Physician (billed to the carrier)	MPFS	NA
Hospitals subject to OPPS	MPFS	12X, 13X
Method I and Method II Critical Access Hospitals (CAHs) (technical services)	101% of reasonable cost	12X and 85X
Indian Health Service (IHS) providers billing hospital outpatient Part B	OMB-approved outpatient per visit all inclusive rate (AIR)	13X
IHS providers billing inpatient Part B	All-inclusive inpatient ancillary per diem rate	12X
IHS CAHs billing outpatient Part B	101% of the all-inclusive facility specific per visit rate	85X
IHS CAHs billing inpatient Part B	101% of the all-inclusive facility specific per diem rate	12X
FQHCs*	All-inclusive encounter rate with other qualified services. Separate visit payment available with HCPCS.	73X
Skilled Nursing Facilities **	MPFS non-facility rate	22X, 23X
Maryland Hospitals under jurisdiction of the Health Services Cost Review Commission (HSCRC)	94% of provider submitted charges in accordance with the terms of the Maryland Waiver	12X, 13X
Home Health Agencies (can be billed only if the service is provided outside of the treatment plan)	MPFS non-facility rate	34X

* Effective January 1, 2006, payment for DSMT provided in an FQHC that meets all of the requirements as above, may be made in addition to one other visit the beneficiary had during the same day, if this qualifying visit is billed on TOB 73X, with HCPCS G0108 or G0109, and revenue codes 0520, 0521, 0522, 0524, 0525, 0527, 0528, or 0900.

** The SNF consolidated billing provision allows separate part B payment for training services for beneficiaries that are in skilled Part A SNF stays, however, the SNF must submit these services on a 22 bill type. Training services provided by other provider types must be reimbursed by X the SNF.

NOTE: An ESRD facility is a reasonable site for this service, however, because it is required to provide dietician and nutritional services as part of the care covered in the composite rate, ESRD facilities are not allowed to bill for it separately and do not receive separate reimbursement. Likewise, an RHC is a reasonable site for this service, however it must be provided in an RHC with other qualifying services and paid at the all-inclusive encounter rate.

Deductible and co-insurance apply.

100-04, 18, 130.1

Healthcare Common Procedure Coding System (HCPCS) for HIV Screening Tests

(Rev.3835, Issued: 08-16-17, Effective: 04-13-15, Implementation: 10-02-17)

Effective for claims with dates of service on and after December 8, 2009, implemented with the April 5, 2010, IOCE, the following HCPCS codes are to be billed for human immunodeficiency virus (HIV) screening:

- G0432- Infectious agent antibody detection by enzyme immunoassay (EIA) technique, HIV-1 and/or HIV-2, screening,
- G0433 - Infectious agent antibody detection by enzyme-linked immunosorbent assay (ELISA) technique, HIV-1 and/or HIV-2, screening, and,
- G0435 - Infectious agent antibody detection by rapid antibody test, HIV-1 and/or HIV-2, screening.

In addition to the above codes, effective for claims with dates of service on or after April 13, 2015, the following HCPCS code may be billed for HIV screening:

- G0475 - HIV antigen/antibody, combination assay, screening

100-04, 18, 130.2

Billing Requirements

(Rev.3835, Issued: 08-16-17, Effective: 04-13-15, Implementation: 10-02-17)

Medicare Administrative Contractors (MACs) shall recognize the above HCPCS codes for HIV screening in accordance with Publication 100-03, Medicare National Coverage Determinations Manual, section 210.7.

Effective for claims with dates of service on and after December 8, 2009, MACs shall pay for voluntary HIV screening as follows:

- A maximum of once annually for beneficiaries at increased risk for HIV infection (11 full months must elapse following the month the previous test was performed in order for the subsequent test to be covered), and,
- A maximum of three times per term of pregnancy for pregnant Medicare beneficiaries beginning with the date of the first test when ordered by the woman's clinician.

Claims that are submitted for HIV screening shall be submitted in the following manner:

For beneficiaries reporting increased risk factors, claims shall contain HCPCS code G0432, G0433, or G0435 with diagnosis code V73.89 (Special screening for other specified viral disease) as primary, and V69.8 (Other problems related to lifestyle), as secondary.

For beneficiaries not reporting increased risk factors, claims shall contain HCPCS code G0432, G0433, or G0435 with diagnosis code V73.89 only.

For pregnant Medicare beneficiaries, claims shall contain HCPCS code G0432, G0433, or G0435 with diagnosis code V73.89 as primary, and one of the following ICD-9 diagnosis codes: V22.0 (Supervision of normal first pregnancy), V22.1 (Supervision of other normal pregnancy), or V23.9 (Supervision of unspecified high-risk pregnancy), as secondary.

Effective for claims with dates of service on or after April 13, 2015, MACs shall also pay for voluntary, HIV screening as follows (replacing ICD-9 with ICD-10 beginning October 1, 2015):

For pregnant Medicare beneficiaries, claims shall contain HCPCS codes G0432, G0433, G0435, or G0475 or CPT-80081 with primary ICD-9/ICD-10 diagnosis code V73.89/Z11.4, along with one of the following ICD-9/ICD-10 diagnosis codes as secondary listed below, and allow no more than 3 HIV screening tests during each term of pregnancy beginning with the date of the 1st test:

ICD-9: V22.0 Supervision of normal first pregnancy

ICD-10: Z34.00 Encounter for supervision of normal first pregnancy, unspecified trimester

Z34.01 Encounter for supervision of normal first pregnancy, first trimester

Z34.02 Encounter for supervision of normal first pregnancy, second trimester

Z34.03 Encounter for supervision of normal first pregnancy, third trimester

ICD-9: V22.1 Supervision of other normal pregnancy

ICD-10: Z34.80 Encounter for supervision of other normal pregnancy, unspecified trimester

Z34.81 Encounter for supervision of other normal pregnancy, first trimester

Z34.82 Encounter for supervision of other normal pregnancy, second trimester

Z34.83 Encounter for supervision of other normal pregnancy, third trimester

Z34.90 Encounter for supervision of normal pregnancy, unspecified, unspecified trimester

Z34.91 Encounter for supervision of normal pregnancy, unspecified, first trimester

Z34.92 Encounter for supervision of normal pregnancy, unspecified, second trimester

Z34.93 Encounter for supervision of normal pregnancy, unspecified, third trimester

ICD-9: V23.9 Supervision of unspecified high-risk pregnancy

ICD-10: O09.90 Supervision of high risk pregnancy, unspecified, unspecified trimester

O09.91 Supervision of high risk pregnancy, unspecified, first trimester

O09.92 Supervision of high risk pregnancy, unspecified, second trimester

O09.93 Supervision of high risk pregnancy, unspecified, third trimester

© 2019 Optum360, LLC

For non-pregnant Medicare beneficiaries, claims shall contain HCPCS code G0432, G0433, G0435, or G0475 for beneficiaries between 15 and 65 years of age one time per annum with ICD-9/ICD-10 diagnosis code V73.89/Z11.4 as primary regardless of risk factors. If primary ICD-9/ICD-10 diagnosis code V73.89/Z11.4 is not present and the beneficiary is between 15 and 65 years of age, or the service is billed more than one time per annum, the detail line shall be denied.

For non-pregnant Medicare beneficiaries, claims shall contain HCPCS code G0432, G0433, G0435, or G0475 for beneficiaries less than 15 and greater than 65 years of age one time per annum with ICD-9/ICD-10 diagnosis code V73.89/ Z11.4 as primary, and one of the following secondary ICD-9/ICD-10 diagnosis codes:

V69.8 (Other problems related to lifestyle)/Z72.89 (Other problems related to lifestyle)

Z72.51 (High risk heterosexual behavior)

Z72.52 (High risk homosexual behavior)

Z72.53 (High risk bisexual behavior)

If ICD-9/ICD-10 diagnosis code V73.89/Z11.4 is not present as primary and one of the ICD-9/ICD-10 secondary codes listed above is not present and the beneficiary is less than 15 or greater than 65 years of age, or the service is billed more than one time per annum, the detail line shall be denied.

100-04, 18, 130.3

Payment Method

(Rev.3835, Issued: 08-16-17, Effective: 04-13-15, Implementation: 10-02-17)

Payment for HIV screening, HCPCS codes G0432, G0433, G0435, is under the Medicare Clinical Laboratory Fee Schedule (CLFS) for Types of Bill (TOB) 12X, 13X, 14X, 22X, and 23X beginning January 1, 2011. For TOB 85X payment is based on reasonable cost. Deductible and coinsurance do not apply. Between December 8, 2009, and April 4, 2010, these services can be billed with unlisted procedure code 87999. Between April 5, 2010, and January 1, 2011, HCPCS codes G0432, G0433, and G0435 will be contractor priced.

Payment for HIV screening, HCPCS code G0475, for institutional claims will be under the Medicare CLFS for TOB 12X, 13X, 14X, 22X, and 23X for claims on or after January 1, 2017. For TOB 85X payment is based on reasonable cost.

Effective for claims with date of service from April 13, 2015 through December 31, 2016, HCPCS code G0475 will be contractor priced. Beginning with date of service January 1, 2017 and after, HCPCS code G0475 will be priced and paid according to the CLFS.

HCPCS code G0475 will be included in the January 2017 CLFS, January 1, 2016 IOCE, the January 2016 OPPS and January 1, 2016 MPFSD. HCPCS code G0475 will be effective retroactive to April 13, 2015 in the IOCE & OPPS.

A/B MACs (B) shall only accept claims submitted with a G0475, G0432, G0433, or G0435 with a Place of Service (POS) Code equal to 81 Independent Lab, and 11, Office.

Deductible and coinsurance do not apply.

100-04, 18, 130.4

Diagnosis Code Reporting

(Rev.3461; Issued: 02-05-16; Effective: 04-13-15; Implementation: 03-07-16)

A claim that is submitted for HIV screening shall be submitted with one or more of the following diagnosis codes in the header and pointed to the line item:

a. For claims where increased risk factors are reported: V73.89 as primary and V69.8 as secondary.

b. For claims where increased risk factors are NOT reported: V73.89 as primary only.

c. For claims for pregnant Medicare beneficiaries, the following diagnosis codes shall be submitted in addition to V73.89 to allow for more frequent screening than once per 12-month period:

V22.0 – Supervision of normal first pregnancy, or,

V22.1 – Supervision of other normal pregnancy, or,

V23.9 - Supervision of unspecified high-risk pregnancy).

100-04, 18, 130.5

Diagnosis Code Reporting

(Rev.3835, Issued: 08-16-17, Effective: 04-13-15, Implementation: 10-02-17)

A claim that is submitted for HIV screening shall be submitted with one or more of the following diagnosis codes in the header and pointed to the line item:

a. For claims where increased risk factors are reported: ICD-9/ICD-10 diagnosis code V73.89/Z11.4 as primary and ICD-9/ICD-10 diagnosis code V69.8/Z72.89, Z72.51, Z72.52, or Z72.53, as secondary.

b. For claims where increased risk factors are NOT reported: ICD-9/ICD-10 diagnosis code V73.89/Z11.4 as primary only.

c. For claims for pregnant Medicare beneficiaries, the following secondary diagnosis codes shall be submitted in addition to primary ICD-9/ICD-10 diagnosis code V73.89/Z11.4 to allow for more frequent screening than once per 12-month period:

ICD-9: V22.0 Supervision of normal first pregnancy

ICD-10: Z34.00 Encounter for supervision of normal first pregnancy, unspecified trimester

Z34.01 Encounter for supervision of normal first pregnancy, first trimester

Z34.02 Encounter for supervision of normal first pregnancy, second trimester

Z34.03 Encounter for supervision of normal first pregnancy, third trimester

ICD-9: V22.1 Supervision of other normal pregnancy

ICD-10: Z34.80 Encounter for supervision of other normal pregnancy, unspecified trimester

Z34.81 Encounter for supervision of other normal pregnancy, first trimester

Z34.82 Encounter for supervision of other normal pregnancy, second trimester

Z34.83 Encounter for supervision of other normal pregnancy, third trimester

Z34.90 Encounter for supervision of normal pregnancy, unspecified, unspecified trimester

Z34.91 Encounter for supervision of normal pregnancy, unspecified, first trimester

Z34.92 Encounter for supervision of normal pregnancy, unspecified, second trimester

Z34.93 Encounter for supervision of normal pregnancy, unspecified, third trimester

ICD-9: V23.9 Supervision of unspecified high-risk pregnancy

ICD-10: O09.90 Supervision of high risk pregnancy, unspecified, unspecified trimester

O09.91 Supervision of high risk pregnancy, unspecified, first trimester

O09.92 Supervision of high risk pregnancy, unspecified, second trimester

O09.93 Supervision of high risk pregnancy, unspecified, third trimester

100-04, 18, 140

Annual Wellness Visit (AWV)

(Rev.2159, Issued: 02-15-11, Effective: 01-01-11, Implementation: 04-04-11)

Pursuant to section 4103 of the Affordable Care Act of 2010, the Centers for Medicare & Medicaid Services (CMS) amended section 411.15(a)(1) and 411.15(k)(15) of 42 CFR (list of examples of routine physical examinations excluded from coverage) effective for services furnished on or after January 1, 2011. This expanded coverage is subject to certain eligibility and other limitations that allow payment for an annual wellness visit (AWV), including personalized prevention plan services (PPPS), for an individual who is no longer within 12 months after the effective date of his or her first Medicare Part B coverage period, and has not received either an initial preventive physical examination (IPPE) or an AWV within the past 12 months.

The AWV will include the establishment of, or update to, the individual's medical/family history, measurement of his/her height, weight, body-mass index (BMI) or waist circumference, and blood pressure (BP), with the goal of health promotion and disease detection and encouraging patients to obtain the screening and preventive services that may already be covered and paid for under Medicare Part B. CMS amended 42 CFR §§411.15(a)(1) and 411.15(k)(15) to allow payment on or after January 1, 2011, for an AWV (as established at 42 CFR 410.15) when performed by qualified health professionals.

Coverage is available for an AWV that meets the following requirements:

1. It is performed by a health professional;

2. It is furnished to an eligible beneficiary who is no longer within 12 months after the effective date of his/her first Medicare Part B coverage period, and he/she has not received either an IPPE or an AWV providing PPPS within the past 12 months.

See Pub. 100-02,Medicare Benefit Policy Manual, chapter 15, section 280.5, for detailed policy regarding the AWV, including definitions of: (1) detection of cognitive impairment, (2) eligible beneficiary, (3) establishment of, or an update to, an individual's medical/family history, (4&5) first and subsequent AWVs providing PPPS, (6) health professional, and, (7) review of an individual's functional ability/level of safety.

© 2019 Optum360, LLC

100-04, 18, 140.1

Healthcare Common Procedure Coding System (HCPCS) Coding for the AWV

(Rev.2159, Issued: 02-15-11, Effective: 01-01-11, Implementation: 04-04-11)

HCPCS codes listed below were developed for the AWV benefit effective January 1, 2011, for individuals whose initial enrollment is on or after January 1, 2011.

G0438 - Annual wellness visit; includes a personalized prevention plan of service (PPPS); first visit

G0439 – Annual wellness visit; includes a personalized prevention plan of service (PPPS); subsequent visit

100-04, 18, 140.5

Coinsurance and Deductible

(Rev.2159, Issued: 02-15-11, Effective: 01-01-11, Implementation: 04-04-11)

Sections 4103 and 4104 of the Affordable Care Act provide for a waiver of Medicare coinsurance/copayment and Part B deductible requirements for the AWV effective for services furnished on or after January 1, 2011.

100-04, 18, 140.6

Common Working File (CWF) Edits

(Rev.2575, Issued: 10-26-12, Effective: 04-01-13, Implementation: 04-01-13)

Effective for claims with dates of service on and after January 1, 2011, CWF shall reject:

- AWV claims for G0438 when a previous (first) AWV, HCPCS code G0438, is paid in history regardless of when it occurred.
- AWV claims when a previous AWV, G0438 or G0439, is paid in history within the previous 12 months.
- Beginning January 1, 2011, AWV claims when a previous IPPE, HCPCS code G0402, is paid in history within the previous 12 months.
- AWV claims (G0438 and G0439) billed for a date of service within 12 months after the effective date of a beneficiary's first Medicare Part B coverage period.

The following change shall be effective for claims processed on or after April 1, 2013. Typically, when a preventive service is posted to a beneficiary's utilization history, separate entries are posted for a "professional" service (the professional claim for the delivery of the service itself) and a "technical" service (the institutional claims for a facility fee). However, in the case of AWV services, since there is no separate payment for a facility fee, the AWV claim will be posted as the "professional" service only, regardless of whether it is paid on a professional claim or an institutional claim.

100-04, 18, 140.8

Advance Care Planning (ACP) as an Optional Element of an Annual Wellness Visit (AWV)

(Rev.3428 Issued: 12-22-15, Effective: 01-01-16, Implementation: 01-04-16)

For services furnished on or after January 1, 2016, Advance Care Planning (ACP) is treated as a preventive service when furnished with an AWV. The Medicare coinsurance and Part B deductible are waived for ACP when furnished as an optional element of an AWV.

The codes for the optional ACP services furnished as part of an AWV are 99497 (Advance care planning including the explanation and discussion of advance directives such as standard forms (with completion of such forms, when performed), by the physician or other qualified health professional; first 30 minutes, face-to-face with the patient, family member(s) and/or surrogate;) and an add-on code 99498 (each additional 30 minutes (List separately in addition to code for primary procedure)). When ACP services are provided as a part of an AWV, practitioners would report CPT code 99497 (and add-on CPT code 99498 when applicable) for the ACP services in addition to either of the AWV codes (G0438 or G0439).

The deductible and coinsurance for ACP will only be waived when billed with modifier 33 on the same day and on the same claim as an AWV (code G0438 or G0439), and must also be furnished by the same provider. Waiver of the deductible and coinsurance for ACP is limited to once per year. Payment for an AWV is limited to once per year. If the AWV billed with ACP is denied for exceeding the once per year limit, the deductible and coinsurance will be applied to the ACP.

Also see Pub. 100-02, Medicare Benefit Policy Manual, chapter 15, section 280.5.1 for more information.

100-04, 18, 160

Intensive Behavioral Therapy (IBT) for Cardiovascular Disease (CVD)

(Rev.2432, Issued: 03-23-12, Effective: 11-08-11, Implementation: 12-27-11 non-shared system edits, 0)

For services furnished on or after November 8, 2011, the Centers for Medicare & Medicaid Services (CMS) covers intensive behavioral therapy (IBT) for cardiovascular disease (CVD). See National Coverage Determinations (NCD) Manual (Pub. 100-03) §210.11 for complete coverage guidelines.

100-04, 18, 160.1

Coding Requirements for IBT for CVD Furnished on or After November 8, 2011

(Rev.2432, Issued: 03-23-12, Effective: 11-08-11, Implementation: 12-27-11 non-shared system edits, 0)

The following is the applicable Healthcare Procedural Coding System (HCPCS) code for IBT for CVD:

G0446: Annual, face-to-face intensive behavioral therapy for cardiovascular disease, individual, 15 minutes

Contractors shall not apply deductibles or coinsurance to claim lines containing HCPCS code G0446.

100-04, 18, 160.2.1

Correct Place of Service (POS) Codes for IBT for CVD on Professional Claims

(Rev.2432, Issued: 03-23-12, Effective: 11-08-11, Implementation: 12-27-11 non-shared system edits, 0)

Contractors shall pay for IBT CVD, G0446 only when services are provided at the following POS:

- 11- Physician's Office
- 22-Outpatient Hospital
- 49- Independent Clinic
- 72-Rural Health Clinic

Claims not submitted with one of the POS codes above will be denied.

The following messages shall be used when Medicare contractors deny professional claims for incorrect POS:

Claim Adjustment Reason Code (CARC) 58: "Treatment was deemed by the payer to have been rendered in an inappropriate or invalid place of service." NOTE: Refer to the 835 Healthcare Policy Identification Segment (loop 2110 Service Payment Information REF), if present.

Remittance Advice Remark Code (RARC) N428: "Not covered when performed in this place of service."

Medicare Summary Notice (MSN) 21.25: "This service was denied because Medicare only covers this service in certain settings."

Spanish Version: El servicio fue denegado porque Medicare solamente lo cubre en ciertas situaciones."

Group Code PR (Patient Responsibility) assigning financial liability to the beneficiary, if a claim is received with a GA modifier indicating a signed ABN is on file.

Group Code CO (Contractual Obligation) assigning financial liability to the provider, if a claim is received with a GZ modifier indicating no signed ABN is on file.

100-04, 18, 160.2.2

Provider Specialty Edits for IBT for CVD on Professional Claims

(Rev.2432, Issued: 03-23-12, Effective: 11-08-11, Implementation: 12-27-11 non-shared system edits, 0)

Contractors shall pay claims for HCPCS code G0446 only when services are submitted by the following provider specialty types found on the provider? enrollment record:

- 01= General Practice
- 08 = Family Practice
- 11= Internal Medicine
- 16 = Obstetrics/Gynecology
- 37= Pediatric Medicine
- 38 = Geriatric Medicine
- 42= Certified Nurse Midwife
- 50 = Nurse Practitioner
- 89 = Certified Clinical Nurse Specialist
- 97= Physician Assistant

Contractors shall deny claim lines for HCPCS code G0446 performed by any other provider specialty type other than those listed above.

The following messages shall be used when Medicare contractors deny IBT for CVD claims billed with invalid provider specialty types:

CARC 185: "The rendering provider is not eligible to perform the service billed."

© 2019 Optum360, LLC

NOTE: Refer to the 835 Healthcare Policy Identification Segment (loop 2110 Service Payment Information REF), if present.

RARC N95: "This provider type/provider specialty may not bill this service."

MSN 21.18: "This item or service is not covered when performed or ordered by this provider."

Spanish version: "Este servicio no esta cubierto cuando es ordenado o rendido por este proveedor."

Group Code PR (Patient Responsibility) assigning financial liability to the beneficiary, if a claim is received with a GA modifier indicating a signed ABN is on file.

Group Code CO (Contractual Obligation) assigning financial liability to the provider, if a claim is received with a GZ modifier indicating no signed ABN is on file.

100-04, 18, 160.3

Correct Types of Bill (TOB) for IBT for CVD on Institutional Claims

(Rev.2432, Issued: 03-23-12, Effective: 11-08-11, Implementation: 12-27-11 non-shared system edits, 0)

Effective for claims with dates of service on and after November 8, 2011, the following types of bill (TOB) may be used for IBT for CVD: 13X, 71X, 77X, or 85X. All other TOB codes shall be denied.

The following messages shall be used when Medicare contractors deny claims for G0446 when submitted on a TOB other than those listed above:

CARC 170: Payment is denied when performed/billed by this type of provider. Note: Refer to the 835 Healthcare Policy Identification Segment (loop 2110 Service Payment Information REF), if present.

RARC N428: Not covered when performed in this place of service."

MSN 21.25: "This service was denied because Medicare only covers this service in certain settings."

Spanish Version: El servicio fue denegado porque Medicare solamente lo cubre en ciertas situaciones."

Group Code PR (Patient Responsibility) assigning financial liability to the beneficiary, if a claim is received with a GA modifier indicating a signed ABN is on file.

Group Code CO (Contractual Obligation) assigning financial liability to the provider, if a claim is received with a GZ modifier indicating no signed ABN is on file.

100-04, 18, 160.4

Frequency Edits for IBT for CVD Claims

(Rev.2432, Issued: 03-23-12, Effective: 11-08-11, Implementation: 12-27-11 non-shared system edits)

A/B MACs (A) and (B) shall allow claims for G0446 no more than once in a 12-month period.

NOTE: 11 full months must elapse following the month in which the last G0446 IBT for CVD took place.

MACs shall deny claims IBT for CVD claims that exceed one (1) visit every 12 months.

A/B MACs (A) and (B) shall allow one professional service and one facility fee claim for each visit.

The following messages shall be used when A/B MACs (A) and (B) deny IBT for CVD claims that exceed the frequency limit:

CARC 119: "Benefit maximum for this time period or occurrence has been reached."

RARC N362: "The number of days or units of service exceeds our acceptable maximum."

MSN 20.5: "These services cannot be paid because your benefits are exhausted at this time."

Spanish Version: "Estos servicios no pueden ser pagados porque sus beneficios se han agotado."

Group Code PR (Patient Responsibility) assigning financial liability to the beneficiary, if a claim is received with a GA modifier indicating a signed ABN is on file.

Group Code CO (Contractual Obligation) assigning financial liability to the provider, if a claim is received with a GZ modifier indicating no signed ABN is on file.

100-04, 18, 160.5

Common Working File (CWF) Edits for IBT for CVD Claims

(Rev.2432, Issued: 03-23-12, Effective: 11-08-11, Implementation: 12-27-11 non-shared system edits, 0)

When applying frequency limitations to G0446, CWF shall allow both a claim for the professional service and a claim for the facility fee. CWF shall identify the following institutional claims as facility fee claims for screening services: TOB 13X, TOB85X when the revenue code is not 096X, 097X, or 098X. CWF shall identify all other claims as professional service claims for screening services.

NOTE: This does not apply to RHCs and FQHCs.

100-04, 18, 170.1

Healthcare Common Procedure Coding System (HCPCS) Codes for Screening for STIs and HIBC to Prevent STIs

(Rev.2476 Issued: 05-23-12)

Effective for claims with dates of service on and after November 8, 2011, the claims processing instructions for payment of screening tests for STI will apply to the following HCPCS codes:

- Chlamydia: 86631, 86632, 87110, 87270, 87320, 87490, 87491, 87810, 87800 (used for combined chlamydia and gonorrhea testing)
- Gonorrhea: 87590, 87591, 87850, 87800 (used for combined chlamydia and gonorrhea testing)
- Syphilis: 86592, 86593, 86780
- Hepatitis B: (hepatitis B surface antigen): 87340, 87341

Effective for claims with dates of service on and after November 8, 2011, implemented with the January 2, 2012, IOCE, the following HCPCS code is to be billed for HIBC to prevent STIs:

G0445 high-intensity behavioral counseling to prevent sexually transmitted infections, face-to-face, individual, includes: education, skills training, and guidance on how to change sexual behavior, performed semi-annually, 30 minutes.

100-04, 18, 170.2

Diagnosis Code Reporting

(Rev.3329, Issued: 08-14-15, Effective: 01-01-12, Implementation: 09-14-15)

A claim that is submitted for screening chlamydia, gonorrhea, syphilis, and/or hepatitis B shall be submitted with one or more of the following diagnosis codes in the header and pointed to the line item:

a. For claims for screening for chlamydia, gonorrhea, and syphilis in women at increased risk who are not pregnant use the following ICD-9-CM diagnosis codes:
   - V74.5 - Screening, bacterial - sexually transmitted; and
   - V69.8 - Other problems related to lifestyle as secondary. (This diagnosis code is used to indicate high/increased risk for STIs).

Effective with the implementation of ICD-10, use the following ICD-10-CM diagnosis codes:

- Z11.3 - Encounter for screening for infections with a predominantly sexual mode of transmission; and • any of
  - Z72.89 - Other problems related to lifestyle ,
  - Z72.51 - High risk heterosexual behavior,
  - Z72.52 - High risk homosexual behavior, or
  - Z72.53 - High risk bisexual behavior. (These diagnosis codes are used to indicate high/increased risk for STIs).

b. For claims for screening for syphilis in men at increased risk use the following ICD-9-CM diagnosis codes:
   - V74.5 - Screening, bacterial - sexually transmitted; and
   - V69.8 - Other problems related to lifestyle as secondary.

Effective with the implementation of ICD-10, use the following ICD-10-CM diagnosis codes:

- Z11.3 - Encounter for screening for infections with a predominantly sexual mode of transmission; and
- any of
  - Z72.89 - Other problems related to lifestyle ,
  - Z72.51 - High risk heterosexual behavior,
  - Z72.52 - High risk homosexual behavior, or
  - Z72.53 - High risk bisexual behavior.

c. For claims for screening for chlamydia and gonorrhea in pregnant women at increased risk for STIs use the following ICD-9-CM diagnosis codes, if applicable:
   - V74.5 - Screening, bacterial - sexually transmitted; and
   - V69.8 - Other problems related to lifestyle, and
   - one of,
     - V22.0 - Supervision of normal first pregnancy, or
     - V22.1 - Supervision of other normal pregnancy, or,

© 2019 Optum360, LLC

- V23.9 - Supervision of unspecified high-risk pregnancy. Effective with the implementation of ICD-10, use ICD-10-CM diagnosis code Z11.3 - Encounter for screening for infections with a predominantly sexual mode of transmission; and one of:

- Z72.89 - Other problems related to lifestyle,
- Z72.51 - High risk heterosexual behavior,
- Z72.52 - High risk homosexual behavior, or
- Z72.53 - High risk bisexual behavior.

and also one of the following.

Code	Description
Z34.00	Encounter for supervision of normal first pregnancy, unspecified trimester
Z34.01	Encounter for supervision of normal first pregnancy, first trimester
Z34.02	Encounter for supervision of normal first pregnancy, second trimester
Z34.03	Encounter for supervision of normal first pregnancy, third trimester
Z34.80	Encounter for supervision of other normal pregnancy, unspecified trimester
Z34.81	Encounter for supervision of other normal pregnancy, first trimester
Z34.82	Encounter for supervision of other normal pregnancy, second trimester
Z34.83	Encounter for supervision of other normal pregnancy, third trimester
Z34.90	Encounter for supervision of normal pregnancy, unspecified, unspecified trimester
Z34.91	Encounter for supervision of normal pregnancy, unspecified, first trimester
Z34.92	Encounter for supervision of normal pregnancy, unspecified, second trimester
Z34.93	Encounter for supervision of normal pregnancy, unspecified, third trimester
O09.90	Supervision of high risk pregnancy, unspecified, unspecified trimester
O09.91	Supervision of high risk pregnancy, unspecified, first trimester
O09.92	Supervision of high risk pregnancy, unspecified, second trimester
O09.93	Supervision of high risk pregnancy, unspecified, third trimester

d. For claims for screening for syphilis in pregnant women use the following ICD-9-CM diagnosis codes:

- V74.5 - Screening, bacterial - sexually transmitted; and
- V22.0 - Supervision of normal first pregnancy, or,
- V22.1 - Supervision of other normal pregnancy, or,
- V23.9 - Supervision of unspecified high-risk pregnancy.

Effective with the implementation of ICD-10, use the following ICD-10-CM diagnosis codes:

- Z11.3 - Encounter for screening for infections with a predominantly sexual mode of transmission;
- and one of

Code	Description
Z34.00	Encounter for supervision of normal first pregnancy, unspecified trimester
Z34.01	Encounter for supervision of normal first pregnancy, first trimester
Z34.02	Encounter for supervision of normal first pregnancy, second trimester
Z34.03	Encounter for supervision of normal first pregnancy, third trimester
Z34.80	Encounter for supervision of other normal pregnancy, unspecified trimester
Z34.81	Encounter for supervision of other normal pregnancy, first trimester
Z34.82	Encounter for supervision of other normal pregnancy, second trimester
Z34.83	Encounter for supervision of other normal pregnancy, third trimester
Z34.90	Encounter for supervision of normal pregnancy, unspecified, unspecified trimester
Z34.91	Encounter for supervision of normal pregnancy, unspecified, first trimester
Z34.92	Encounter for supervision of normal pregnancy, unspecified, second trimester
Z34.93	Encounter for supervision of normal pregnancy, unspecified, third trimester
O09.90	Supervision of high risk pregnancy, unspecified, unspecified trimester
O09.91	Supervision of high risk pregnancy, unspecified, first trimester
O09.92	Supervision of high risk pregnancy, unspecified, second trimester
O09.93	Supervision of high risk pregnancy, unspecified, third trimester

e. For claims for screening for syphilis in pregnant women at increased risk for STIs use the following ICD-9-CM diagnosis codes:

- V74.5 - Screening, bacterial - sexually transmitted; and
- V69.8 - Other problems related to lifestyle, and,
- V22.0 - Supervision of normal first pregnancy, or
- V22.1 - Supervision of other normal pregnancy, or,
- V23.9 - Supervision of unspecified high-risk pregnancy.

Effective with the implementation of ICD-10, use the following ICD-10-CM diagnosis codes: • Z11.3 - Encounter for screening for infections with a predominantly sexual mode of transmission;

- and any of:
  - Z72.89 - Other problems related to lifestyle, or
  - Z72.51 - High risk heterosexual behavior, or
  - Z72.52 - High risk homosexual behavior, or
  - Z72.53 - High risk bisexual behavior

and also one of the following:

Code	Description
Z34.00	Encounter for supervision of normal first pregnancy, unspecified trimester
Z34.01	Encounter for supervision of normal first pregnancy, first trimester
Z34.02	Encounter for supervision of normal first pregnancy, second trimester
Z34.03	Encounter for supervision of normal first pregnancy, third trimester
Z34.80	Encounter for supervision of other normal pregnancy, unspecified trimester
Z34.81	Encounter for supervision of other normal pregnancy, first trimester
Z34.82	Encounter for supervision of other normal pregnancy, second trimester
Z34.83	Encounter for supervision of other normal pregnancy, third trimester
Z34.90	Encounter for supervision of normal pregnancy, unspecified, unspecified trimester
Z34.91	Encounter for supervision of normal pregnancy, unspecified, first trimester
Z34.92	Encounter for supervision of normal pregnancy, unspecified, second trimester
Z34.93	Encounter for supervision of normal pregnancy, unspecified, third trimester
O09.90	Supervision of high risk pregnancy, unspecified, unspecified trimester
O09.91	Supervision of high risk pregnancy, unspecified, first trimester
O09.92	Supervision of high risk pregnancy, unspecified, second trimester
O09.93	Supervision of high risk pregnancy, unspecified, third trimester

f. For claims for screening for hepatitis B in pregnant women use the following ICD-9-CM diagnosis codes:

- V73.89 - Screening, disease or disorder, viral, specified type NEC; and
- V22.0 - Supervision of normal first pregnancy, or,
- V22.1 - Supervision of other normal pregnancy, or,
- V23.9 - Supervision of unspecified high-risk pregnancy.

Effective with the implementation of ICD-10, use the following ICD-10-CM diagnosis codes:

- Z11.59 - Encounter for screening for other viral diseases, and any of
- Z34.00 - Encounter for supervision of normal first pregnancy, unspecified trimester, or

© 2019 Optum360, LLC

- Z34.80 - Encounter for supervision of other normal pregnancy, unspecified trimester, or
- • Z34.90 - Encounter for supervision of normal pregnancy, unspecified, unspecified trimester, or
- O09.90 - Supervision of high risk pregnancy, unspecified, unspecified trimester.

g. For claims for screening for hepatitis B in pregnant women at increased risk for STIs use the following ICD-9-CM diagnosis codes:

- V73.89 - Screening, disease or disorder, viral, specified type NEC; and
- V 69.8 - Other problems related to lifestyle, and,
- V22.0 - Supervision of normal first pregnancy, or,
- V22.1 - Supervision of other normal pregnancy, or,
- V23.9 - Supervision of unspecified high-risk pregnancy.

Effective with the implementation of ICD-10, use the following ICD-10-CM diagnosis codes: • Z11.59 - Encounter for screening for other viral diseases, and • Z72.89 - Other problems related to lifestyle, and

- any of
  - Z72.51 - High risk heterosexual behavior, or
  - Z72.52 - High risk homosexual behavior, or
  - Z72.53 - High risk bisexual behavior; • and also one of the following:

Code	Description
Z34.00	Encounter for supervision of normal first pregnancy, unspecified trimester
Z34.01	Encounter for supervision of normal first pregnancy, first trimester
Z34.02	Encounter for supervision of normal first pregnancy, second trimester
Z34.03	Encounter for supervision of normal first pregnancy, third trimester
Z34.80	Encounter for supervision of other normal pregnancy, unspecified trimester
Z34.81	Encounter for supervision of other normal pregnancy, first trimester
Z34.82	Encounter for supervision of other normal pregnancy, second trimester
Z34.83	Encounter for supervision of other normal pregnancy, third trimester
Z34.90	Encounter for supervision of normal pregnancy, unspecified, unspecified trimester
Z34.91	Encounter for supervision of normal pregnancy, unspecified, first trimester
Z34.92	Encounter for supervision of normal pregnancy, unspecified, second trimester
Z34.93	Encounter for supervision of normal pregnancy, unspecified, third trimester
O09.90	Supervision of high risk pregnancy, unspecified, unspecified trimester
O09.91	Supervision of high risk pregnancy, unspecified, first trimester
O09.92	Supervision of high risk pregnancy, unspecified, second trimester
O09.93	Supervision of high risk pregnancy, unspecified, third trimester

100-04, 18, 170.3

Billing Requirements

(Rev.3329, Issued: 08-14-15, Effective: 01-01-12, Implementation: 09-14-15)

Effective for dates of service November 8, 2011, and later, contractors shall recognize HCPCS code G0445 for HIBC. Medicare shall cover up to two occurrences of G0445 when billed for HIBC to prevent STIs. A claim that is submitted with HCPCS code G0445 for HIBC shall be submitted with ICD-9 diagnosis code V69.8.

Medicare contractors shall pay for screening for chlamydia, gonorrhea, and syphilis (As indicated by the presence of ICD-9 diagnosis code V74.5); and/or hepatitis B (as indicated by the presence of ICD-9 diagnosis code V73.89) as follows:

- One annual occurrence of screening for chlamydia, gonorrhea, and syphilis (i.e., 1 per 12-month period) in women at increased risk who are not pregnant,
- One annual occurrence of screening for syphilis (i.e., 1 per 12-month period) in men at increased risk,
- Up to two occurrences per pregnancy of screening for chlamydia and gonorrhea in pregnant women who are at increased risk for STIs and continued increased risk for the second screening,
- One occurrence per pregnancy of screening for syphilis in pregnant women,
- Up to an additional two occurrences per pregnancy of screening for syphilis in pregnant women if the beneficiary is at continued increased risk for STIs,
- One occurrence per pregnancy of screening for hepatitis B in pregnant women, and,
- One additional occurrence per pregnancy of screening for hepatitis B in pregnant women who are at continued increased risk for STIs.

100-04, 18, 170.4

Types of Bill (TOBs) and Revenue Codes

(Rev.2476 Issued: 05-23-12)

The applicable types of bill (TOBs) for HIBC screening, HCPCS code G0445, are: 13X, 71X, 77X, and 85X.

On institutional claims, TOBs 71X and 77X, use revenue code 052X to ensure coinsurance and deductible are not applied.

Critical access hospitals (CAHs) electing the optional method of payment for outpatient services report this service under revenue codes 096X, 097X, or 098X.

100-04, 18, 170.4.1

Payment Method

(Rev.2476 Issued: 05-23-12)

Payment for HIBC is based on the all-inclusive payment rate for rural health clinics (TOBs 71X) and federally qualified health centers (TOB 77X). Hospital outpatient departments (TOB 13X) are paid based on the outpatient prospective payment system and CAHs (TOB 85X) are paid based on reasonable cost. CAHs electing the optional method of payment for outpatient services are paid based on 115% of the lesser of the Medicare Physician Fee Schedule (MPFS) amount or submitted charge.

Effective for dates of service on and after November 8, 2011, deductible and coinsurance do not apply to claim lines with G0445.

HCPCS code G0445 may be paid on the same date of service as an annual wellness visit, evaluation and management (E&M) code, or during the global billing period for obstetrical care, but only one G0445 may be paid on any one date of service. If billed on the same date of service with an E&M code, the E&M code should have a distinct diagnosis code other than the diagnosis code used to indicate high/increased risk for STIs for the G0445 service. An E&M code should not be billed when the sole reason for the visit is HIBC to prevent STIs.

For Medicare Part B physician and non-practitioner claims, payment for HIBC to prevent STIs is based on the MPFS amount for G0445.

100-04, 18, 170.5

Specialty Codes and Place of Service (POS)

(Rev.2476 Issued: 05-23-12)

Medicare provides coverage for screening for chlamydia, gonorrhea, syphilis, and/or hepatitis B and HIBC to prevent STIs only when ordered by a primary care practitioner (physician or non-physician) with any of the following specialty codes:

- 01-General Practice
- 08-Family Practice
- 11-Internal Medicine
- 16-Obstetrics/Gynecology
- 37-Pediatric Medicine
- 38-Geriatric Medicine
- 42-Certified Nurse Midwife
- 50-Nurse Practitioner
- 89-Certified Clinical Nurse Specialist
- 97-Physician Assistant

Medicare provides coverage for HIBC to prevent STIs only when provided by a primary care practitioner (physician or non-physician) with any of the specialty codes identified above.

Medicare provides coverage for HIBC to prevent STIs only when the POS billed is 11, 22, 49, or 71.

100-04, 18, 180

Alcohol Screening and Behavioral Counseling Interventions in Primary Care to Reduce Alcohol Misuse

(Rev.2433, Issued: 03-26-12, Effective: 10-14-11, Implementation: 12-27-11 non-system changes, 04-02)

The United States Preventive Services Task Force (USPSTF) defines alcohol misuse as risky, hazardous, or harmful drinking which places an individual at risk for future problems with alcohol consumption. In the general adult population, alcohol consumption becomes risky or hazardous when consuming:

© 2019 Optum360, LLC

- Greater than 7 drinks per week or greater than 3drinks per occasion for women and persons greater than 65 years old.
- Greater than 14 drinks per week or greater than 4 drinks per occasion for men 65 years old and younger.

100-04, 18, 180.1

Policy

(Rev.2433, Issued: 03-26-12, Effective: 10-14-11, Implementation: 12-27-11 non-system changes, 04-02)

Claims with dates of service on and after October 14, 2011, the Centers for Medicare & Medicaid Services (CMS) will cover annual alcohol misuse screening (HCPCS code G0442) consisting of 1 screening session, and for those that screen positive, up to 4 brief, face-to-face behavioral counseling sessions (HCPCS code G0443) per 12-month period for Medicare beneficiaries, including pregnant women.

Medicare beneficiaries that may be identified as having a need for behavioral counseling sessions include those:

- Who misuse alcohol, but whose levels or patterns of alcohol consumption do not meet criteria for alcohol dependence (defined as at least three of the following: tolerance, withdrawal symptoms, impaired control, preoccupation with acquisition and/or use, persistent desire or unsuccessful efforts to quit, sustains social, occupational, or recreational disability, use continues despite adverse consequences); and,
- Who are competent and alert at the time that counseling is provided; and,
- Whose counseling is furnished by qualified primary care physicians or other primary care practitioners in a primary care setting.

Once a Medicare beneficiary has agreed to behavioral counseling sessions, the counseling sessions are to be completed based on the 5As approach adopted by the United States Preventive Services Task Force (USPSTF.) The steps to the 5As approach are listed below.

1. Assess: Ask about/assess behavioral health risk(s) and factors affecting choice of behavior change goals/methods.
2. Advise: Give clear, specific, and personalized behavior change advice, including information about personal health harms and benefits.
3. Agree: Collaboratively select appropriate treatment goals and methods based on the patient? interest in and willingness to change the behavior.
4. Assist: Using behavior change techniques (self-help and/or counseling), aid the patient in achieving agreed-upon goals by acquiring the skills, confidence, and social/environmental supports for behavior change, supplemented with adjunctive medical treatments when appropriate.
5. Arrange: Schedule follow-up contacts (in person or by telephone) to provide ongoing assistance/support and to adjust the treatment plan as needed, including referral to more intensive or specialized treatment.

100-04, 18, 180.2

Institutional Billing Requirements

(Rev.2433, Issued:-3-26-12, Effective: 10-14-11, Implementation: 12-27-11 non-system changes, 04-02-)

For claims with dates of service on and after October 14, 2011, Medicare will allow coverage for annual alcohol misuse screening, 15 minutes, G0442, and brief, face-to-face behavioral counseling for alcohol misuse, 15 minutes, G0443 for:

- Rural Health Clinics (RHCs) - type of bill (TOB) 71X only -based on the all-inclusive payment rate
- Federally Qualified Health Centers (FQHCs) - TOB 77X only-based on the all-inclusive payment rate
- Outpatient hospitals ?TOB 13X - based on Outpatient Prospective Payment System (OPPS)-Critical Access Hospitals (CAHs) - TOB 85X-based on reasonable cost
- CAH Method II-TOB 85X - based on 115% of the lesser of the Medicare Physician Fee Schedule (MPFS) amount or actual charge as applicable with revenue codes 096X, 097X, or 098X.

For RHCs and FQHCs the alcohol screening/counseling is not separately payable with another face-to-face encounter on the same day. This does not apply to the Initial Preventive Physical Examination (IPPE), unrelated services denoted with modifier 59, and 77X claims containing Diabetes Self Management Training (DSMT) and Medical Nutrition Therapy (MNT)services. DSMT and MNT apply to FQHCs only. However, the screening/counseling sessions alone when rendered as a face-to-face visit with a core practitioner do constitute an encounter and is paid based on the all-inclusive payment rate.

Note: For outpatient hospital settings, as in any other setting, services covered under this NCD must be provided by a primary care provider.

Claims submitted with alcohol misuse screening and behavioral counseling HCPCS codes G0442 and G0443 on a TOB other than 13X, 71X, 77X, and 85X will be denied.

Effective October 14, 2011, deductible and co-insurance should not be applied for line items on claims billed for alcohol misuse screening G0442 and behavioral counseling for alcohol misuse G0443.

100-04, 18, 180.3

Professional Billing Requirements

(Rev.2433, Issued:-3-26-12, Effective: 10-14-11, Implementation: 12-27-11 non-system changes, 04-02-)

For claims with dates of service on or after October 14, 2011, CMS will allow coverage for annual alcohol misuse screening, 15 minutes, G0442, and behavioral counseling for alcohol misuse, 15 minutes, G0443, only when services are submitted by the following provider specialties found on the provider's enrollment record:

- 01 - General Practice
- 08 - Family Practice
- 11 - Internal Medicine
- 16 - Obstetrics/Gynecology
- 37 - Pediatric Medicine
- 38 - Geriatric Medicine
- 42 - Certified Nurse-Midwife
- 50 - Nurse Practitioner
- 89 - Certified Clinical Nurse Specialist
- 97 - Physician Assistant

Any claims that are not submitted from one of the provider specialty types noted above will be denied.

For claims with dates of service on and after October 14, 2011, CMS will allow coverage for annual alcohol misuse screening, 15 minutes, G0442, and behavioral counseling for alcohol misuse, 15 minutes, G0443, only when submitted with one of the following place of service (POS) codes:

- 11 - Physician's Office
- 22 - Outpatient Hospital
- 49 - Independent Clinic
- 71 - State or local public health clinic or

Any claims that are not submitted with one of the POS codes noted above will be denied.

The alcohol screening/counseling services are payable with another encounter/visit on the same day. This does not apply to RHCs and FQHCs.

100-04, 18, 180.4

Claim Adjustment Reason Codes, Remittance Advice Remark Codes, Group Codes, and Medicare Summary Not

(Rev.2433, Issued: 03-26-12 , Effective: 10-14-11, Implementation: 12-27-11 non-system changes, 04-0)

Contractors shall use the appropriate claim adjustment reason codes (CARCs), remittance advice remark codes (RARCs), group codes, or Medicare summary notice (MSN) messages when denying payment for alcohol misuse screening and alcohol misuse behavioral counseling sessions:

- For RHC and FQHC claims that contain screening for alcohol misuse HCPCS code G0442 and alcohol misuse counseling HCPCS code G0443 with another encounter/visit with the same line item date of service, use group code CO and reason code:
  - Claim Adjustment Reason Code (CARC) 97-The benefit for this service is included in the payment/allowance for another service/procedure that has already been adjudicated. Note: Refer to the 835 Healthcare Policy Identification Segment (loop 2110 Service Payment Information REF) if present
- Denying claims containing HCPCS code G0442 and HCPCS code G0443 submitted on a TOB other than 13X, 71X, 77X, and 85X:
  - Claim Adjustment Reason Code (CARC) 5 - The procedure code/bill type is inconsistent with the place of service. Note: Refer to the 835 Healthcare Policy Identification Segment (loop 2110 Service Payment Information REF) if present
  - Remittance Advice Remark Code (RARC) M77 -Missing/incomplete/invalid place of service

© 2019 Optum360, LLC

- Group Code PR (Patient Responsibility) assigning financial liability to the beneficiary, if a claim is received with a GA modifier indicating a signed ABN is on file.
- Group Code CO (Contractual Obligation) assigning financial liability to the provider, if a claim is received with a GZ modifier indicating no signed ABN is on file. NOTE: For modifier GZ, use CARC 50 and MSN 8.81 per instructions in CR 7228/TR 2148.

- Denying claims that contains more than one alcohol misuse behavioral counseling session G0443 on the same date of service:
  - Medicare Summary Notice (MSN) 15.6-The information provided does not support the need for this many services or items within this period of time.
  - Claim Adjustment Reason Code (CARC) 151-Payment adjusted because the payer deems the information submitted does not support this many/frequency of services.
  - Remittance Advice Remark Code (RARC) M86-Service denied because payment already made for same/similar procedure within set time frame.
  - Group Code PR (Patient Responsibility) assigning financial liability to the beneficiary, if a claim is received with a GA modifier indicating a signed ABN is on file.
  - Group Code CO (Contractual Obligation) assigning financial liability to the provider, if a claim is received with a GZ modifier indicating no signed ABN is on file. NOTE: For modifier GZ, use CARC 50 and MSN 8.81 per instructions in CR 7228/TR 2148.
- Denying claims that are not submitted from the appropriate provider specialties:
  - Medicare Summary Notice (MSN) 21.18-This item or service is not covered when performed or ordered by this provider.
  - Claim Adjustment Reason Code (CARC) 185 - The rendering provider is not eligible to perform the service billed. NOTE: Refer to the 835 Healthcare Policy Identification Segment (loop 2110 Service Payment Information REF), if present.
  - Remittance Advice Remark Code (RARC) N95 - This provider type/provider specialty may not bill this service.
  - Group Code PR (Patient Responsibility) assigning financial liability to the beneficiary, if a claim is received with a GA modifier indicating a signed ABN is on file.
  - Group Code CO (Contractual Obligation) assigning financial liability to the provider, if a claim is received with a GZ modifier indicating no signed ABN is on file. NOTE: For modifier GZ, use CARC 50 and MSN 8.81 per instructions in CR 7228/TR 2148.
- Denying claims without the appropriate POS code:
  - Medicare Summary Notice (MSN) 21.25-This service was denied because Medicare only covers this service in certain settings.
  - Claim Adjustment Reason Code (CARC) 58 -Treatment was deemed by the payer to have been rendered in an inappropriate or invalid place of service. Note: Refer to the 835 Healthcare Policy Identification Segment (loop 2110 Service Payment Information REF) if present.
  - Remittance Advice Remark Code (RARC) N428-Not covered when performed in this place of service.
  - Group Code PR (Patient Responsibility) assigning financial liability to the beneficiary, if a claim is received with a GA modifier indicating a signed ABN is on file.
  - Group Code CO (Contractual Obligation) assigning financial liability to the provider, if a claim is received with a GZ modifier indicating no signed ABN is on file. NOTE: For modifier GZ, use CARC 50 and MSN 8.81 per instructions in CR 7228/TR 2148.
- Denying claims for alcohol misuse screening HCPCS code G0442 more than once in a 12-month period, and denying alcohol misuse counseling sessions HCPCS code G0443 more than four times in the same 12-month period:
  - Medicare Summary Notice (MSN) 20.5-These services cannot be paid because your benefits are exhausted at this time.
  - Claim Adjustment Reason Code (CARC) 119-Benefit maximum for this time period or occurrence has been reached.
  - Remittance Advice Remark Code (RARC) N362-The number of Days or Units of service exceeds our acceptable maximum.
  - Group Code PR (Patient Responsibility) assigning financial liability to the beneficiary, if a claim is received with a GA modifier indicating a signed ABN is on file.
  - Group Code CO (Contractual Obligation) assigning financial liability to the provider, if a claim is received with a GZ modifier indicating no signed ABN is on file. NOTE: For modifier GZ, use CARC 50 and MSN 8.81 per instructions in CR 7228/TR 2148.

100-04, 18, 180.5

CWF Requirements

(Rev.2433, Issued:-3-26-12, Effective: 10-14-11, Implementation: 12-27-11 non-system changes, 04-02-)

When applying frequency, CWF shall count 11 full months following the month of the last alcohol misuse screening visit, G0442, before allowing subsequent payment of another G0442 screening. Additionally, CWF shall create an edit to allow alcohol misuse brief behavioral counseling, HCPCS G0443, no more than 4 times in a 12-month period. CWF shall also count four alcohol misuse counseling sessions HCPCS G0443 in the same 12-month period used for G0442 counting from the date the G0442 screening session was billed.

When applying frequency limitations to G0442 screening on the same date of service as G0443 counseling, CWF shall allow both a claim for the professional service and a claim for a facility fee. CWF shall identify the following institutional claims as facility fee claims for screening services: TOB 13X, TOB 85X when the revenue code is not 096X, 097X, or 098X. CWF shall identify all other claims as professional service claims for screening services (professional claims, and institutional claims with TOB 71X, 77X, and 85X when the revenue code is 096X, 097X, or 098X). NOTE: This does not apply to RHCs and FQHCs.

100-04, 18, 190

Screening for Depression in Adults (Effective October 14, 2011)

(Rev.2359, Issued: 11-23-11, Effective: 10-14-11, Implementation: 12-27-11 non-shared system edits/0)

A. Coverage Requirements

Effective October 14, 2011, the Centers for Medicare & Medicaid Services (CMS) will cover annual screening up to 15 minutes for Medicare beneficiaries in primary care settings that have staff-assisted depression care supports in place to assure accurate diagnosis, effective treatment, and follow-up. Various screening tools are available for screening for depression. CMS does not identify specific depression screening tools. Rather, the decision to use a specific tool is at the discretion of the clinician in the primary care setting. Screening for depression is non-covered when performed more than one time in a 12-month period. The Medicare coinsurance and Part B deductible are waived for this preventive service.

Additional information on this National Coverage Determination (NCD) for Screening for Depression in Adults can be found in Publication 100-03, NCD Manual, Section 210.9.

100-04, 18, 190.1

A/B MAC and Carrier Billing Requirements

(Rev.2431, Issued: 03-23-12, Effective: 10-14-11, Implementation: 12-27-11 non-shared system edits/0)

Effective October 14, 2011, contractors shall recognize new HCPCS G0444, annual depression screening, 15 minutes.

100-04, 18, 190.2

Frequency

(Rev.2431, Issued: 03-23-12, Effective: 10-14-11, Implementation: 12-27-11 non-shared system edits/0)

A/B MACs (B) shall pay for annual depression screening, G0444, no more than once in a 12-month period.

NOTE: 11 full months must elapse following the month in which the last annual depression screening took place.

100-04, 18, 190.3

Place of Service (POS)

(Rev.2431, Issued: 03-23-12, Effective: 10-14-11, Implementation: 12-27-11 non-shared system edits/0)

A/B MACs (B) shall pay for annual depression screening claims, G0444, only when services are provided at the following places of service (POS):

- 11–Office
- 22–Outpatient Hospital
- 49–Independent Clinic

© 2019 Optum360, LLC

- 71–State or Local Public Health Clinic

100-04, 18, 200

Intensive Behavioral Therapy for Obesity (Effective November 29, 2011)

(Rev.2421, Issued: 03-07-12, Effective: 11-29-11, Implementation: 03-06-12, for non-shared system edi)

The United States Preventive Services Task Force (USPSTF) found good evidence that body mass index (BMI) is a reliable and valid indicator for identifying adults at increased risk for mortality and morbidity due to overweight and obesity. It also good evidence that high intensity counseling combined with behavioral interventions in obese adults (as defined by a BMI =30 kg/m2) produces modest, sustained weight loss.

100-04, 18, 200.1

Policy

(Rev.3329, Issued: 08-14-15, Effective: 01-01-12, Implementation: 09-14-15)

For services furnished on or after November 29, 2011, the Centers for Medicare & Medicaid Services (CMS) will cover Intensive Behavioral Therapy for Obesity. Medicare beneficiaries with obesity (BMI =30 kg/m2) who are competent and alert at the time that counseling is provided and whose counseling is furnished by a qualified primary care physician or other primary care practitioner in a primary care setting are eligible for:

- One face-to-face visit every week for the first month;
- One face-to-face visit every other week for months 2-6;
- One face-to-face visit every month for months 7-12, if the beneficiary meets the 3kg (6.6 lbs) weight loss requirement during the first six months as discussed below. The counseling sessions are to be completed based on the 5As approach adopted by the United States Preventive Services Task Force (USPSTF.) The steps to the 5As approach are listed below:

1. Assess: Ask about/assess behavioral health risk(s) and factors affecting choice of behavior change goals/methods.
2. Advise: Give clear, specific, and personalized behavior change advice, including information about personal health harms and benefits.
3. Agree: Collaboratively select appropriate treatment goals and methods based on the patient's interest in and willingness to change the behavior.
4. Assist: Using behavior change techniques (self-help and/or counseling), aid the patient in achieving agreed-upon goals by acquiring the skills, confidence, and social/environmental supports for behavior change, supplemented with adjunctive medical treatments when appropriate.
5. Arrange: Schedule follow-up contacts (in person or by telephone) to provide ongoing assistance/support and to adjust the treatment plan as needed, including referral to more intensive or specialized treatment.

Medicare will cover Face-to-Face Behavioral Counseling for Obesity, 15 minutes, G0447, along with 1 of the ICD-9 codes for BMI 30.0-BMI 70 (V85.30-V85.39 and V85.41-V85.45), up to 22 sessions in a 12-month period for Medicare beneficiaries. The Medicare coinsurance and Part B deductible are waived for this preventive service.

Contractors shall note the appropriate ICD-10 code(s) that are listed below for future implementation. Contractors shall track the ICD-10 codes and ensure that the updated edit is turned on as part of the ICD-10 implementation effective October 1, 2013.

ICD-10	Description
Z68.30	BMI 30.0-30.9, adult
Z68.31	BMI 31.0-31.9, adult
Z68.32	BMI 32.0-32.9, adult
Z68.33	BMI 33.0-33.9, adult
Z68.34	BMI 34.0-34.9, adult
Z68.35	BMI 35.0-35.9, adult
Z68.36	BMI 36.0-36.9, adult
Z68.37	BMI 37.0-37.9, adult
Z68.38	BMI 38.0-38.9, adult
Z68.39	BMI 39.0-39.9, adult
Z68.41	BMI 40.0-44.9, adult
Z68.42	BMI 45.0-49.9, adult
Z68.43	BMI 50.0-59.9, adult
Z68.44	BMI 60.0-69.9, adult
Z68.45	BMI 70 or greater, adult

See National Coverage Determinations (NCD) Manual (Pub. 100-03) §210.12 for complete coverage guidelines.

100-04, 18, 200.2

Institutional Billing Requirements

(Rev.3232, Issued: 04-03-15, Effective: 01-01-15, Implementation: 01-05-15)

Effective for claims with dates of service on and after November 29, 2011, providers may use the following types of bill (TOB) when submitting HCPCS code G0447: 13x, 71X, 77X, or 85X. Service line items on other TOBs shall be denied.

The service shall be paid on the basis shown below:

- Rural Health Clinics (RHCs) - type of bill (TOB) 71X only —based on the all-inclusive payment rate
- Federally Qualified Health Centers (FQHCs) - TOB 77X only —based on the all-inclusive payment rate
- Outpatient hospitals —TOB 13X - based on Outpatient Prospective Payment System (OPPS)
- Critical Access Hospitals (CAHs) - TOB 85X —based on reasonable cost
- CAH Method II —TOB 85X - based on 115% of the lesser of the Medicare Physician Fee Schedule (MPFS) amount or actual charge as applicable with revenue codes 096X, 097X, or 098X.

For RHCs and FQHCs, obesity counseling is not separately payable with another face-to-face encounter on the same day. This does not apply to claims for the Initial Preventive Physical Examination (IPPE), claims with unrelated services denoted with modifier 59, and FQHC claims containing Diabetes Self Management Training (DSMT) and Medical Nutrition Therapy (MNT) services. However, the counseling sessions alone when rendered as a face-to-face visit with a core practitioner do constitute an encounter and are paid based on the all-inclusive payment rate.

Note: For outpatient hospital settings, as in any other setting, services covered under this NCD must be provided by a primary care provider.

100-04, 18, 200.3

Professional Billing Requirements

(Rev.3329, Issued: 08-14-15, Effective: 01-01-12, Implementation: 09-14-15)

For claims with dates of service on or after November 29, 2011, CMS will allow coverage for Face-to-Face Behavioral Counseling for Obesity, 15 minutes, G0447, along with 1 of the ICD-9 codes for BMI 30.0-BMI 70 (V85.30-V85.39 and V85.41-V85.45), only when services are submitted by the following provider specialties found on the provider? enrollment record:

- 01 - General Practice
- 08 - Family Practice
- 11 - Internal Medicine
- 16 - Obstetrics/Gynecology
- 37 - Pediatric Medicine
- 38 - Geriatric Medicine
- 50 - Nurse Practitioner
- 89 - Certified Clinical Nurse Specialist
- 97 - Physician Assistant

Any claims that are not submitted from one of the provider specialty types noted above will be denied.

For claims with dates of service on or after November 29, 2011, CMS will allow coverage for Face-to-Face Behavioral Counseling for Obesity, 15 minutes, G0447, along with 1 of the ICD-9 codes for BMI 30.0-BMI 70 (V85.30-V85.39 and V85.41-V85.45), only when submitted with one of the following place of service (POS) codes:

- 11- Physician's Office
- 22- Outpatient Hospital
- 49- Independent Clinic
- 71- State or Local Public Health Clinic

Any claims that are not submitted with one of the POS codes noted above will be denied.

© 2019 Optum360, LLC

100-04, 18, 200.4

Claim Adjustment Reason Codes (CARCs), Remittance Advice Remark Codes (RARCs), Group Codes, and Medicare Summary Notice (MSN) Messages

(Rev.3329, Issued: 08-14-15, Effective: 01-01-12, Implementation: 09-14-15)

Contractors shall use the appropriate claim adjustment reason codes (CARCs), remittance advice remark codes (RARCs), group codes, or Medicare summary notice (MSN) messages when denying payment for obesity counseling sessions:

- Denying services submitted on a TOB other than 13X, 71X, 77X, and 85X: CARC 5 - The procedure code/bill type is inconsistent with the place of service.
  - Note: Refer to the 835 Healthcare Policy Identification Segment (loop 2110 Service Payment Information REF), if present.
  - RARC M77 - Missing/incomplete/invalid place of service
  - MSN 21.25: "This service was denied because Medicare only covers this service in certain settings."
  - Group Code PR (Patient Responsibility) assigning financial responsibility to the beneficiary (if a claim is received with a GA modifier indicating a signed ABN is on file).
  - Group Code CO (Contractual Obligation) assigning financial liability to the provider (if a claim is received with a GZ modifier indicating no signed ABN is on file).
  - NOTE: For modifier GZ, use CARC 50 and MSN 8.81 per instructions in CR 7228/TR 2148.
- For RHC and FQHC services that contain HCPCS code G0447 with another encounter/visit with the same line item date of service: Claim Adjustment Reason Code (CARC) 97
  - The benefit for this service is included in the payment/allowance for another service/procedure that has already been adjudicated. Note: Refer to the 835 Healthcare Policy Identification Segment (loop 2110 Service Payment Information REF) if present
  - Group Code CO (Contractual Obligation)
- Denying services for obesity counseling sessions HCPCS code G0447 with 1 of the ICD-9 codes (V85.30-V85.39 or V85.41-V85.45) for more than 22 times in the same 12-month period:
  - CARC 119-Benefit maximum for this time period or occurrence has been reached.
  - RARC N362 - The number of days or units of service exceeds our acceptable maximum.
  - MSN 20.5 - These services cannot be paid because your benefits are exhausted at this time.
  - Group Code PR (Patient Responsibility) assigning financial responsibility to the beneficiary (if a claim is received with a GA modifier indicating a signed ABN is on file).
  - Group Code CO (Contractual Obligation) assigning financial liability to the provider (if a claim is received with a GZ modifier indicating no signed ABN is on file).
  - NOTE: For modifier GZ, use CARC 50 and MSN 8.81 per instructions in CR 7228/TR 2148. -
- Denying claim lines for obesity counseling sessions HCPCS code G0447 without 1 of the appropriate ICD-9 codes (V85.30-V85.39 or V85.41-V85.45):
  - CARC 167 - This (these) diagnosis(es) is (are) not covered.
  - Note: Refer to the 835 Healthcare Policy Identification Segment (loop 2110 Service Payment Information REF), if present.
  - RARC N386 -This decision was based on a National Coverage Determination (NCD). An NCD provides a coverage determination as to whether a particular item or service is covered. A copy of this policy is available at www.cms.gov/mcd/search.asp. If you do not have web access, you may contact the contractor to request a copy of the NCD.
  - MSN 14.9 - Medicare cannot pay for this service for the diagnosis shown on the claim.
  - Group Code PR (Patient Responsibility) assigning financial responsibility to the beneficiary (if a claim is received with a GA modifier indicating a signed ABN is on file).
  - Group Code CO (Contractual Obligation) assigning financial liability to the provider (if a claim is received with a GZ modifier indicating no signed ABN is on file).
  - NOTE: For modifier GZ, use CARC 50 and MSN 8.81 per instructions in CR 7228/TR 2148.
- Denying claim lines without the appropriate POS code: CARC 58 —Treatment was deemed by the payer to have been rendered in an inappropriate or invalid place of service. Note: Refer to the 835 Healthcare Policy Identification Segment (loop 2110 Service Payment Information REF), if present.
  - RARC N428 - Not covered when performed in certain settings.
  - MSN 21.25 - This service was denied because Medicare only covers this service in certain settings.
  - Group Code PR (Patient Responsibility) assigning financial responsibility to the beneficiary (if a claim is received with a GA modifier indicating a signed ABN is on file).
  - Group Code CO (Contractual Obligation) assigning financial liability to the provider (if a claim is received with a GZ modifier indicating no signed ABN is on file).
  - NOTE: For modifier GZ, use CARC 50 and MSN 8.81 per instructions in CR 7228/TR 2148.
- Denying claim lines that are not submitted from the appropriate provider specialties: CARC 185 - The rendering provider is not eligible to perform the service billed. NOTE: Refer to the 835 Healthcare Policy Identification Segment (loop 2110 Service Payment Information REF), if present.
  - RARC N95 - This provider type/provider specialty may not bill this service.
  - MSN 21.18 - This item or service is not covered when performed or ordered by this provider.
  - Group Code PR (Patient Responsibility) assigning financial responsibility to the beneficiary (if a claim is received with a GA modifier indicating a signed ABN is on file).
  - Group Code CO (Contractual Obligation) assigning financial liability to the provider (if a claim is received with a GZ modifier indicating no signed ABN is on file).
  - NOTE: For modifier GZ, use CARC 50 and MSN 8.81 per instructions in CR 7228/TR 2148.

100-04, 18, 200.5

Common Working File (CWF) Edits

(Rev.3329, Issued: 08-14-15, Effective: 01-01-12, Implementation: 09-14-15)

When applying frequency, CWF shall count 22 counseling sessions of G0447, along with 1 ICD-9 code from V85.30-V85.39 or V85.41-V85.45 in a 12-month period. When applying frequency limitations to G0447 counseling CWF shall allow both a claim for the professional service and a claim for a facility fee. CWF shall identify the following institutional claims as facility fee claims for this service: TOB 13X, TOB 85X when the revenue code is not 096X, 097X, or 098X. CWF shall identify all other claims as professional service claims. NOTE: This does not apply to RHCs and FQHCs.

100-04, 18, 210

210 – Screening for Hepatitis C Virus (HCV)

(Rev.3215, Issued: 03-11-15, Multiple effective dates)

Effective for services furnished on or after June 2, 2014, an initial screening for hepatitis C virus (HCV) is covered for adults at high risk for HCV infection. "High risk" is defined as persons with a current or past history of illicit injection drug use and persons who have a history of receiving a blood transfusion prior to 1992.

A. Frequency

A single, one-time screening test is covered for adults who do not meet the high risk definition above, but who were born from 1945 through 1965.

Repeat screening for high risk persons is covered annually only for persons who have had continued illicit injection drug use since the prior negative screening test.

NOTE: Annual means a full 11 months must elapse following the month in which the previous negative screening took place.

B. Determination of High Risk for Hepatitis C Disease

The determination of "high risk for HCV" is identified by the primary care physician or practitioner who assesses the patient's history, which is part of any complete medical history, typically part of an annual wellness visit, and considered in the development of a comprehensive prevention plan. The medical record should be a reflection of the service provided.

© 2019 Optum360, LLC

NOTE: See Pub. 100-03, Medicare National Coverage Determinations (NCD) Manual §210.13 for complete coverage guidelines.

NOTE: Beneficiary coinsurance and deductibles do not apply to claim lines containing HCPCS G0472, hepatitis C antibody screening for individual at high risk and other covered indication(s).

Screening for Hepatitis C Virus (HCV)

100-04, 18, 210.2

Professional Billing Requirements

(Rev.3215, Issued: 03-11-15, Multiple effective dates)

For claims with dates of service on or after June 2, 2014, Medicare will allow coverage for HCV screening, HCPCS G0472, only when services are ordered by the following provider specialties found on the provider's enrollment record:

01 - General Practice

08 - Family Practice

11 - Internal Medicine

16 - Obstetrics/Gynecology

37 - Pediatric Medicine

38 - Geriatric Medicine

42 - Certified Nurse Midwife

50 - Nurse Practitioner

89 - Certified Clinical Nurse Specialist

97 - Physician Assistant

HCV screening services ordered by providers other than the specialty types noted above will be denied.

For claims with dates of service on or after June 2, 2014, Medicare will allow coverage for HCV screening, HCPCS G0472, only when submitted with one of the following place of service (POS) codes:

11 - Physician's Office

22 - Outpatient Hospital

49 - Independent Clinic

71 - State or Local Public Health Clinic

81 - Independent Laboratory

HCV screening claims submitted without one of the POS codes noted above will be denied.

100-04, 18, 210.3

Claim Adjustment Reason Codes (CARCs), Remittance Advice Remark Codes (RARCs), Group Codes, and Medicare Summary Notice (MSN) Messages

(Rev.3393, Issued: 11-05-15, Effective: 06- 02-14, Implementation: 04-04-16)

Contractors shall use the appropriate claim adjustment reason codes (CARCs), remittance advice remark codes (RARCs), group codes, or Medicare summary notice (MSN) messages when denying payment for HCV screening, HCPCS G0472:

- Denying services submitted on a TOB other than 13X, 14X or 85X:

  CARC 170 - Payment is denied when performed/billed by this type of provider. Note: Refer to the 835 Healthcare Policy Identification Segment (loop 2110 Service Payment Information REF), if present.

  RARC N95 – This provider type/provider specialty may not bill this service.

  MSN 21.25: This service was denied because Medicare only covers this service in certain settings.

  Spanish Version: "El servicio fue denegado porque Medicare solamente lo cubre en ciertas situaciones."

  Group Code CO (Contractual Obligation) assigning financial liability to the provider (if a claim is received with a GZ modifier indicating no signed ABN is on file).

  NOTE: For modifier GZ, use CARC 50, Group Code CO, and MSN 8.81.

- Denying services where previous HCV screening, HCPCS G0472, is paid in history for claims with dates of service on and after June 2, 2014, and the patient is not deemed high risk by the presence of ICD-9 diagnosis code V69.8, other problems related to lifestyle/ICD-10 diagnosis code Z72.89, other problems related to lifestyle (once ICD-10 is implemented), and ICD-9 diagnosis code 304.91, unspecified drug dependence, continuous/ICD-10 diagnosis code F19.20, other psychoactive substance dependence, uncomplicated (once ICD-10 is implemented):

  CARC 119 – Benefit maximum for this time period or occurrence has been reached.

  RARC N386 - This decision was based on a National Coverage Determination (NCD). An NCD provides a coverage determination as to whether a particular item or service is covered. A copy of this policy is available at www.cms.gov/mcd/search.asp. If you do not have web access, you may contact the contractor to request a copy of the NCD.

  MSN 15.20 – The following policies NCD210.13 were used when we made this decision.

  Spanish Version – Las siguientes politicas NCD210.13 fueron utilizadas cuando se tomo esta decision.

  MSN 15.19 - Local Coverage Determinations (LCDs) help Medicare decide what is covered. An LCD was used for your claim. You can compare your case to the LCD, and send information from your doctor if you think it could change our decision. Call 1-800-MEDICARE (1-800-633-4227) for a copy of the LCD.

  Spanish Version - Las Determinaciones Locales de Cobertura (LCDs en inglés) le ayudan a decidir a Medicare lo que está cubierto. Un LCD se usó para su reclamación. Usted puede comparar su caso con la determinación y enviar información de su médico si piensa que puede cambiar nuestra decisión. Para obtener una copia del LCD, llame al 1-800-MEDICARE (1-800-633-4227).

  NOTE: Due to system requirement, FISS has combined messages 15.19 and 15.20 so that, when used for the same line item, both messages will appear on the same MSN.

  Group Code CO assigning financial liability to the provider (if a claim is received with a GZ modifier indicating no signed ABN is on file).

  NOTE: For modifier GZ, use CARC 50, Group Code CO, and MSN 8.81.

  NOTE: This edit shall be overridable.

- Denying services for HCV screening, HCPCS G0472, for beneficiaries at high risk who have had continued illicit drug use since the prior negative screening test, when claims are not submitted with ICD-9 diagnosis code V69.8/ICD-10 diagnosis code Z72.89 (once ICD-10 is implemented), and ICD-9 diagnosis code 304.91/ICD-10 diagnosis code F19.20 (once ICD-10 is implemented), and/or 11 full months have not passed since the last negative HCV screening test:

  CARC 167 – This (these) diagnosis(es) is (are) not covered. Note: Refer to the 835 Healthcare Policy Identification Segment (loop 2110 Service Payment Information REF), if present.

  RARC N386 - This decision was based on a National Coverage Determination (NCD). An NCD provides a coverage determination as to whether a particular item or service is covered. A copy of this policy is available at www.cms.gov/mcd/search.asp. If you do not have web access, you may contact the contractor to request a copy of the NCD.

  MSN 15.20 – The following policies NCD210.13 were used when we made this decision.

  Spanish Version – Las siguientes politicas NCD210.13 fueron utilizadas cuando se tomo esta decision.

  MSN 15.19 - Local Coverage Determinations (LCDs) help Medicare decide what is covered. An LCD was used for your claim. You can compare your case to the LCD, and send information from your doctor if you think it could change our decision. Call 1-800-MEDICARE (1-800-633-4227) for a copy of the LCD.

  Spanish Version - Las Determinaciones Locales de Cobertura (LCDs en inglés) le ayudan a decidir a Medicare lo que está cubierto. Un LCD se usó para su reclamación. Usted puede comparar su caso con la determinación y enviar información de su médico si piensa que puede cambiar nuestra decisión. Para obtener una copia del LCD, llame al 1-800-MEDICARE (1-800-633-4227).

  NOTE: Due to system requirement, FISS has combined messages 15.19 and 15.20 so that, when used for the same line item, both messages will appear on the same MSN.

  Group Code CO assigning financial liability to the provider (if a claim is received with a GZ modifier indicating no signed ABN is on file).

  NOTE: For modifier GZ, use CARC 50, Group Code CO, and MSN 8.81.

  NOTE: This edit shall be overridable.

- Denying services for HCV screening, HCPCS G0472, for beneficiaries who do not meet the definition of high risk, but who were born from 1945 through 1965, when claims are submitted more than once in a lifetime:

© 2019 Optum360, LLC

CARC 119: "Benefit maximum for this time period or occurrence has been reached."

RARC N386: "This decision was based on a National Coverage Determination (NCD). An NCD provides a coverage determination as to whether a particular item or service is covered. A copy of this policy is available at www.cms.gov/mcd/search.asp. If you do not have web access, you may contact the contractor to request a copy of the NCD."

MSN 15.20 – The following policies NCD210.13 were used when we made this decision.

Spanish Version – Las siguientes politicas NCD210.13 fueron utilizadas cuando se tomo esta decision.

MSN 15.19 - Local Coverage Determinations (LCDs) help Medicare decide what is covered. An LCD was used for your claim. You can compare your case to the LCD, and send information from your doctor if you think it could change our decision. Call 1-800-MEDICARE (1-800-633-4227) for a copy of the LCD.

Spanish Version - Las Determinaciones Locales de Cobertura (LCDs en inglés) le ayudan a decidir a Medicare lo que está cubierto. Un LCD se usó para su reclamación. Usted puede comparar su caso con la determinación y enviar información de su médico si piensa que puede cambiar nuestra decisión. Para obtener una copia del LCD, llame al 1-800-MEDICARE (1-800-633-4227).

NOTE: Due to system requirement, FISS has combined messages 15.19 and 15.20 so that, when used for the same line item, both messages will appear on the same MSN.

Group Code CO assigning financial liability to the provider (if a claim is received with a GZ modifier indicating no signed ABN is on file).

NOTE: For modifier GZ, use CARC 50, Group Code CO, and MSN 8.81.

NOTE: This edit shall be overridable.

- Denying claim lines for HCV screening, HCPCS G0472, without the appropriate POS code:

  CARC 171 – Payment is denied when performed by this type of provider on this type of facility. Note: Refer to the 835 Healthcare Policy Identification Segment (loop 2110 Service Payment Information REF), if present.

  RARC N428 - Not covered when performed in certain settings.

  MSN 21.25 - This service was denied because Medicare only covers this service in certain settings.

  Spanish Version: "El servicio fue denegado porque Medicare solamente lo cubre en ciertas situaciones."

  Group Code CO assigning financial liability to the provider (if a claim is received with a GZ modifier indicating no signed ABN is on file).

  NOTE: For modifier GZ, use CARC 50, Group Code CO, and MSN 8.81.

- Denying claim lines for HCV screening, HCPCS G0472, that are not ordered by an appropriate provider specialty:

  CARC 184 - The prescribing/ordering provider is not eligible to prescribe/order the service billed. NOTE: Refer to the 835 Healthcare Policy Identification Segment (loop 2110 Service Payment Information REF), if present.

  RARC N574 – Our records indicate the ordering/referring provider is of a type/specialty that cannot order or refer. Please verify that the claim ordering/referring provider information is accurate or contact the ordering/referring provider.

  MSN 21.18 - This item or service is not covered when performed or ordered by this provider.

  Group Code CO assigning financial liability to the provider (if a claim is received with a GZ modifier indicating no signed ABN is on file).

  NOTE: For modifier GZ, use CARC 50, Group Code CO, and MSN 8.81.

- Denying claim lines for HCV screening, HCPCS G0472, if beneficiary born prior to 1945 and after 1965 who are not at high risk (absence of V69.8 /ICD-10 diagnosis code Z72.89 (once ICD-10 is implemented) or 304.91/ ICD-10 diagnosis code F19.20 (once ICD-10 is implemented)):

  CARC 96 - Non-covered charge(s). At least one Remark Code must be provided (may be comprised of either the NCPDP Reject Reason [sic] Code, or Remittance Advice Remark Code that is not an ALERT.) Note: Refer to the 835 Healthcare Policy Identification Segment (loop 2110 Service Payment Information REF), if present.

  RARC N386 - This decision was based on a National Coverage Determination (NCD). An NCD provides a coverage determination as to whether a particular item or service is covered. A copy of this policy is available at www.cms.gov/mcd/search.asp. If you do not have web access, you may contact the contractor to request a copy of the NCD.

  MSN 15.19 - Local Coverage Determinations (LCDs) help Medicare decide what is covered. An LCD was used for your claim. You can compare your case to the

  LCD, and send information from your doctor if you think it could change our decision. Call 1-800-MEDICARE (1-800-633-4227) for a copy of the LCD.

  Spanish Version - Las Determinaciones Locales de Cobertura (LCDs en inglés) le ayudan a decidir a Medicare lo que está cubierto. Un LCD se usó para su reclamación. Usted puede comparar su caso con la determinación y enviar información de su médico si piensa que puede cambiar nuestra decisión. Para obtener una copia del LCD, llame al 1-800-MEDICARE (1-800-633-4227).

  MSN 15.20 – The following policies NCD210.13 were used when we made this decision.

  Spanish Version – Las siguientes politicas NCD210.13 fueron utilizadas cuando se tomo esta decision.

  NOTE: Due to system requirement, FISS has combined messages 15.19 and 15.20 so that, when used for the same line item, both messages will appear on the same MSN.

  Group Code CO assigning financial liability to the provider (if a claim is received with a GZ modifier indicating no signed ABN is on file).

100-04, 18, 210.4

Common Working File (CWF) Edits

(Rev.3285, Issued: 06-19-15, Effective: 06-02-14, Implementation: For FISS shared system edits, spli)

The common working file (CWF) shall apply the following frequency limitations to HCV screening, HCPCS G0472:

One initial HCV screening, HCPCS G0472, for beneficiaries at high risk, when claims are submitted with ICD-9 diagnosis code V69.8/ICD-10 diagnosis code Z72.89 (once ICD-10 is implemented),

Annual HCV screening, HCPCS G0472, when claims are submitted with ICD-9 diagnosis code V69.8/ICD-10 diagnosis code Z72.89 (once ICD-10 is implemented), and ICD-9 diagnosis code 304.91/ICD-10 diagnosis code F19.20 (once ICD-10 is implemented),

Once in a lifetime HCV screening, HCPCS G0472, for beneficiaries who are not high risk who were born from 1945 through 1965.

NOTE: These edits shall be overridable.

NOTE: HCV screening, HCPCS G0472 is not a covered service for beneficiaries born prior to 1945 and after 1965 who are not at high risk (absence of V69.8/ICD-10 diagnosis code Z72.89 (once ICD-10 is implemented) and/or 304.91/ ICD-10 diagnosis code F19.20 (once ICD-10 is implemented)).

100-04, 18, 230

Screening for Hepatitis B Virus (HBV)

(Rev.3831, Iss: 8-4-17, Eff: 9-28-16, Imp: 10- 2- 17, 10-2-17- analysis/design; 1/2/18 test/imp)

Effective for services furnished on or after September 28, 2016, an initial screening for hepatitis B virus infection (HBV) is covered for asymptomatic, non-pregnant adolescents and adults at high risk for HBV infection. "High risk" is defined as persons born in countries and regions with high prevalence of HBV infection (i.e., ≥ 2%), US-born persons not vaccinated as infants whose parents were born in regions with a very high prevalence of HBV infection (i.e., ≥ 8%), HIV-positive persons, men who have sex with men, injection drug users, household contacts or sexual partners of persons with HBV infection.

In addition, CMS has determined that repeated screening would be appropriate annually only for beneficiaries with continued high risk (men who have sex with men, injection drug users, household contacts or sexual partners of persons with HBV infection) who do not receive hepatitis B vaccination.

A screening test at the first prenatal visit is covered for pregnant women and then rescreening at time of delivery for those with new or continuing risk factors. In addition, CMS has determined that screening during the first prenatal visit would be appropriate for each pregnancy, regardless of previous hepatitis B vaccination or previous negative hepatitis B surface antigen (HBsAg) test results. See section 170 of this chapter for coverage and billing instructions for pregnant beneficiaries.

Effective for claims with dates of service on or after September 28, 2016, the claims processing instructions for payment of screening for hepatitis B virus will apply to the following HCPCS and CPT codes:

© 2019 Optum360, LLC

- HBV screening for asymptomatic, non-pregnant adolescents and adults at high risk - code G0499
- HBV screening for pregnant women – CPT codes 86704, 86706, 87340 and 87341

A. Frequency

HBV screening for asymptomatic, non-pregnant adolescents and adults at high risk (HCPCS code G0499)

- A single, one-time screening test is covered for asymptomatic, non pregnant adolescents and adults who do meet the high risk definition above.
- Repeat screening for high risk persons is covered annually only for persons who have continued high risk who do not receive hepatitis B vaccination .

Note: Annual means a full 11 months must elapse following the month in which the previous negative screening took place.

Note for ESRD: Effective for claims with dates of service on or after September 28, 2016 submitted with G0499 – "HepB screen high risk indiv, for asymptomatic non-pregnant beneficiaries" and ICD-10 diagnosis code N18.6, End Stage Renal Disease, all of the preceding requirements shall be bypassed and the claim shall be allowed to pay, no matter what other ICD-10 diagnosis codes may appear on the claim.

HBV screening for pregnant women (CPT codes 86704, 86706, 87340 and 87341)

- One occurrence per pregnancy of screening for HBV in pregnant women, and?
- One additional occurrence per pregnancy of screening for HBV in pregnant women who are at continued risk

B. Determination of High Risk for Hepatitis B Disease

The determination of "high risk for HBV" is identified by the primary care physician or practitioner who assesses the patient's history, which is part of any complete medical history, typically part of an annual wellness visit, and considered in the development of a comprehensive prevention plan. The medical record should be a reflection of the service provided.

Note: See Pub. 100-03, Medicare National Coverage Determinations (NCD) Manual §210.6 for complete coverage guidelines.

100-04, 18, 230.1

Institutional Billing Requirements

(Rev.3831, Iss: 8-4-17, Eff: 9-28-16, Imp: 10- 2- 17, 10-2-17- analysis/design; 1/2/18 test/imp)

Effective for claims with dates of service on or after September 28, 2016, providers may use the following types of bill (TOBs) when submitting claims for HBV screening, HCPCS G0499, 86704, 86706, 87340, and 87341: 13X, 14X, 72X, and 85X. Deductible and coinsurance do not apply. Service line-items on other TOBs shall be denied.

The service shall be paid on the basis shown below:

- Outpatient hospitals – TOB 13X - based on Outpatient Prospective Payment System
- Non-patient laboratory specimen – TOB 14X – based on laboratory fee schedule
- End Stage Renal Disease facilities (ESRDs) – TOB 72X – based on ESRD PPS when submitted with code G0499 and diagnosis code N18.6. HBV is not separately payable for (ESRD TOB 72X) unless reported with Modifier AY.
- Critical Access Hospitals (CAHs) - TOB 85X – based on reasonable cost when the revenue code is not 096X, 097X, and 098X

Note: For outpatient hospital settings, as in any other setting, services covered under this NCD must be provided by a primary care provider.

NOTE: Beneficiary coinsurance and deductibles do not apply to claim lines containing HCPCS G0499, and CPT codes 86704, 86706, 87340, and 87341.

NOTE: Medicare Administrative Contractors shall contractor-price HBV screening claims, HCPCS G0499, with dates of service September 28, 2016 through December 31, 2017.

100-04, 18, 230.2

Professional Billing Requirements

(Rev.3831, Iss: 8-4-17, Eff: 9-28-16, Imp: 10- 2- 17, 10-2-17- analysis/design; 1/2/18 test/imp)

For claims with dates of service on or after September 28, 2016, CMS will allow coverage for HBV screening, CPT codes 86704, 86706, 87340, 87341, and HCPCS G0499, only when services are ordered by the following provider specialties found on the provider's enrollment record:

01 - General Practice

08 - Family Practice

11 - Internal Medicine

16 - Obstetrics/Gynecology

37 - Pediatric Medicine

38 - Geriatric Medicine

42 – Certified Nurse Midwife

50 - Nurse Practitioner

89 - Certified Clinical Nurse Specialist

97 - Physician Assistant

Claims ordered by providers other than the specialty types noted above will be denied.

For claims with dates of service on or after September 28, 2016, CMS will allow coverage for HBV screening, 86704, 86706, 87340, 87341, and G0499, only when submitted with one of the following place of service (POS) codes:

11 – Physician's Office

19- Off Campus Outpatient Hospital

22 – On Campus Outpatient Hospital

49 – Independent Clinic

71 – State or Local Public Health Clinic

81-Independent Laboratory

Claims submitted without one of the POS codes noted above will be denied.

NOTE: Beneficiary coinsurance and deductibles do not apply to claim lines containing CPT codes 86704, 86706, 87340, 87341, and HCPCS G0499.

NOTE: Medicare Administrative Contractors shall contractor-price HBV screening claims, HCPCS G0499, with dates of service September 28, 2016 through December 31, 2017.

100-04, 18, 230.3

Diagnosis Code Reporting Requirements

(Rev.3831, Iss: 8-4-17, Eff: 9-28-16, Imp: 10- 2- 17, 10-2-17- analysis/design; 1/2/18 test/imp)

For claims with dates of service on or after September 28, 2016, CMS will allow coverage for HBV screening, HCPCS G0499, only when services are reported with both of the following diagnosis codes denoting high risk:

- Z11.59 Encounter for screening for other viral disease and
- Z72.89 Other Problems related to life style For claims with dates of service on or after September 28, 2016, CMS will allow coverage for HBV screening, HCPCS G0499, for subsequent visits only when services are reported with one of the following diagnosis code:
- Z11.59, and one of the high risk codes below
- F11.10-F11.99
- F13.10-F13.99
- F14.10-F14.99
- F15.10-F15.99
- Z20.2
- Z20.5
- Z72.52
- Z72.53
- For claims with dates of service on or after September 28, 2016, CMS will allow coverage for HBV screening (CPT codes 86704, 86706, 87340 and 87341) in pregnant women only when services are reported with one of the following diagnosis codes:
- Z11.59 - Encounter for screening for other viral diseases, and one of the following
- Z34.00 - Encounter for supervision of normal first pregnancy, unspecified trimester,
- Z34.80 - Encounter for supervision of other normal pregnancy, unspecified trimester,
- Z34.90 - Encounter for supervision of normal pregnancy, unspecified, unspecified trimester,
- O09.90 - Supervision of high risk pregnancy, unspecified, unspecified trimester. For claims with dates of service on or after September 28, 2016, CMS will allow coverage for HBV screening (CPT codes 86704, 86706, 87340 and 87341) in pregnant women at high risk only when services are reported with one of the following diagnosis codes:

© 2019 Optum360, LLC

- Z11.59 - Encounter for screening for other viral diseases, and
- Z72.89 - Other problems related to lifestyle,
- and also one of the following

Code	Description
Z34.00	Encounter for supervision of normal first pregnancy, unspecified trimester
Z34.01	Encounter for supervision of normal first pregnancy, first trimester
Z34.02	Encounter for supervision of normal first pregnancy, second trimester
Z34.03	Encounter for supervision of normal first pregnancy, third trimester
Z34.80	Encounter for supervision of other normal pregnancy, unspecified trimester
Z34.81	Encounter for supervision of other normal pregnancy, first trimester
Z34.82	Encounter for supervision of other normal pregnancy, second trimester
Z34.83	Encounter for supervision of other normal pregnancy, third trimester
Z34.90	Encounter for supervision of normal pregnancy, unspecified, unspecified trimester
Z34.91	Encounter for supervision of normal pregnancy, unspecified, first trimester
Z34.92	Encounter for supervision of normal pregnancy, unspecified, second trimester
Z34.93	Encounter for supervision of normal pregnancy, unspecified, third trimester
O09.90	Supervision of high risk pregnancy, unspecified, unspecified trimester
O09.91	Supervision of high risk pregnancy, unspecified, first trimester
O09.92	Supervision of high risk pregnancy, unspecified, second trimester
O09.93	Supervision of high risk pregnancy, unspecified, third trimester

100-04, 20, 20

Calculation and Update of Payment Rates

(Rev.1, 10-01-03)
B3-5017, PM B-01-54, 2002 PEN Fee Schedule

Section1834 of the Act requires the use of fee schedules under Medicare Part B for reimbursement of durable medical equipment (DME) and for prosthetic and orthotic devices, beginning January 1 1989. Payment is limited to the lower of the actual charge for the equipment or the fee established.

Beginning with fee schedule year 1991, CMS calculates the updates for the fee schedules and national limitation amounts and provides the contractors with the revised payment amounts. The CMS calculates most fee schedule amounts and provides them to the carriers, DMERCs, FIs and RHHIs. However, for some services CMS asks carriers to calculate local fee amounts and to provide them to CMS to include in calculation of national amounts. These vary from update to update, and CMS issues special related instructions to carriers when appropriate.

Parenteral and enteral nutrition services paid on and after January 1, 2002 are paid on a fee schedule. This fee schedule also is furnished by CMS. Prior to 2002, payment amounts for PEN were determined under reasonable charge rules, including the application of the lowest charge level (LCL) restrictions.

The CMS furnishes fee schedule updates (DMEPOS, PEN, etc.) at least 30 days prior to the scheduled implementation. FIs use the fee schedules to pay for covered items, within their claims processing jurisdictions, supplied by hospitals, home health agencies, and other providers. FIs consult with DMERCs and where appropriate with carriers on filling gaps in fee schedules.

The CMS furnishes the fee amounts annually, or as updated if special updates should occur during the year, to carriers and FIs, including DMERCs and RHHIs, and to other interested parties (including the Statistical Analysis DMERC (SADMERC), Railroad Retirement Board (RRB), Indian Health Service, and United Mine Workers).

100-04, 20, 20.4

Contents of Fee Schedule File

(Rev.1, 10-01-03) PM A-02-090

The fee schedule file provided by CMS contains HCPCS codes and related prices subject to the DMEPOS fee schedules, including application of any update factors and any changes to the national limited payment amounts. The file does not contain fees for drugs that are necessary for the effective use of DME. It also does not include fees for items for which fee schedule amounts are not established. See Chapter 23 for a description of pricing for these. The CMS releases via program issuance, the gap-filled amounts and the annual update factors for the various DMEPOS payment classes:

- IN = Inexpensive/routinely purchased...DME;
- FS = Frequency Service...DME;
- CR = Capped Rental...DME;
- OX = Oxygen and Oxygen Equipment...OXY;
- OS = Ostomy, Tracheostomy and Urologicals...P/O;
- S/D = Surgical Dressings...S/D;
- P/O = Prosthetics and Orthotics...P/O;
- SU = Supplies...DME; and
- TE = TENS...DME

The RHHIs need to retrieve data from all of the above categories. Regular FIs need to retrieve data only from categories P/O, S/D and SU. FIs need to retrieve the SU category in order to be able to price supplies on Part B SNF claims.

100-04, 20, 30.1.2

Transcutaneous Electrical Nerve Stimulator (TENS)

(Rev.2605, Issued: 11-30-12, Effective: 06-08-12, Implementation: 01-07-13)

In order to permit an attending physician time to determine whether the purchase of a TENS is medically appropriate for a particular patient, contractors pay 10 percent of the purchase price of the item for each of 2 months. The purchase price and payment for maintenance and servicing are determined under the same rules as any other frequently purchased item, except that there is no reduction in the allowed amount for purchase due to the two months rental.

Effective June 8, 2012, CMS will allow coverage for TENS use in the treatment of chronic low back pain (CLBP) only under specific conditions which are described in the NCD Manual, Pub. 100-03, chapter 1 Section 160.27.

100-04, 20, 30.6

Oxygen and Oxygen Equipment

(Rev.2465, Issued: 05-11-12, Effective: 10-01-12, Implementation: 10-01-12)

For oxygen and oxygen equipment, contractors pay a monthly fee schedule amount per beneficiary. Unless otherwise noted below, the fee covers equipment, contents and supplies. Payment is not made for purchases of this type of equipment.

When an inpatient is not entitled to Part A, payment may not be made under Part B for DME or oxygen provided in a hospital or SNF. (See the Medicare Benefit Policy Manual, Chapter 15) Also, for outpatients using equipment or receiving oxygen in the hospital or SNF and not taking the equipment or oxygen system home, the fee schedule does not apply.

There are a number of billing considerations for oxygen claims. The chart in §130.6 indicates what amounts are payable under which situations.

Effective for claims on or after February 14, 2011, payment for the home use of oxygen and oxygen equipment when related to the treatment of cluster headaches is covered under a National Coverage Determination (NCD). For more information, refer to chapter 1, section 240.2.2, Publication 100-03, of the National Coverage Determinations Manual.

100-04, 20, 30.9

Payment of DMEPOS Items Based on Modifiers

(Rev.3824, Issued: 08-02-17; Effective: 07-01-17, Implementation: 07-03-17)

The following modifiers were added to the HCPCS to identify supplies and equipment that may be covered under more than one DMEPOS benefit category:

- AU Item furnished in conjunction with a urological, ostomy, or tracheostomy supply;
- AV Item furnished in conjunction with a prosthetic device, prosthetic or orthotic; and
- AW Item furnished in conjunction with a surgical dressing.

Codes A4450 and A4452 are the only codes that have been identified at this time that would require use of all three of the above listed modifiers. Providers must report these modifiers on claims for items identified by codes A4450 and A4452 that are furnished on or after January 1, 2005. Modifier AU may also be applicable to code A4217. Providers must report modifier AU on claims for items identified by code A4217 that are furnished in conjunction with a urological, ostomy, or tracheostomy supply on or after January 1, 2005. Items identified by code A4217 that are furnished in conjunction with durable medical equipment are reported without a modifier. In the future, other codes may be identified as codes that must be submitted with these modifiers. Medicare contractors base payment for the codes A4217, A4450, and A4452 on the presence or absence of these modifiers.

Codes L8040 thru L8047 describe facial prostheses. Providers must report the following modifiers on claims for replacement of these items:

- KM Replacement of facial prosthesis including

- g new impression/moulage; and
- KN Replacement of facial prosthesis using previous mastermodel.

Providers must report these modifiers on claims for replacement of items identified by codes L8040 thru L8047 that are furnished on or after January 1, 2005. Medicare contractors base payment for the codes L8040 thru L8047 on the presence of these modifiers. These modifiers are only used when the prostheses is being replaced.

In accordance with section 302(c) of the Medicare Prescription Drug, Improvement, and Modernization Act of 2003 (MMA), the fee schedule update factors for 2004 thru 2008 for durable medical equipment (DME), other than items designated as class III devices by the Food and Drug Administration (FDA), are equal to 0 percent. The HCPCS codes for DME designated as class III devices by the FDA are identified on the DMEPOS fee schedule available on the above mentioned web site by presence of the KF modifier.

Elevating/stair climbing power wheelchairs are class III devices. Suppliers billing the DMERCs must submit claims for the base power wheelchair portion of this device using HCPCS code K0011 (programmable power wheelchair base) with modifier KF for claims submitted on or after April 1, 2004, with dates of service on or after January 1, 2004. For claims with dates of service on or after January 1, 2004, the elevation feature for this device should be billed using HCPCS code E2300 and the stair climbing feature for this device should be billed using HCPCS code A9270.

Regional home health intermediaries (RHHIs) will not be able to implement the KF modifier until January 1, 2005. Therefore, for claims with dates of service prior to January 1, 2005, HHAs must submit claims for the base power wheelchair portion of stair climbing wheelchairs with HCPCS code E1399. For claims with dates of service on or after January 1, 2005, HHAs must submit claims for the base power wheelchair portion of stair climbing wheelchairs with HCPCS code K0011 with modifier KF.

The fee schedule amounts for K0011 with and without the KF modifier appear on the fee schedule file referenced at www.cms.hhs.gov/providers/pufdownload/default.asp#dme. For claims with dates of service prior to January 1, 2005, RHHIs should pay claims for stair climbing wheelchair bases billed with code E1399 using the fee schedule amounts for K0011 with the KF modifier. All other claims for programmable power wheelchair bases should be paid using the fee schedule amounts for K0011 without the KF modifier.

Effective for claims with dates of service on or after January 1, 2005, HHAs must submit modifier KF along with the applicable HCPCS code for all DME items classified by the FDA as class III devices.

The following modifier was added to the HCPCS in 2007 as a placeholder modifier:

- KU DMEPOS Item Subject to DMEPOS Competitive Bidding Program Number 3

The DMEPOS fee schedules are updated on an annual basis in accordance with the statute and regulations. The update process for the DMEPOS fee schedule is located in Pub.100-04, Medicare Claims Processing Manual, chapter 23, section 60. Payment on a fee schedule basis is required for certain durable medical equipment (DME) by §1834(a) of the Social Security Act. Section1834(a)(1)(F)(ii) of the Act mandates adjustments to the fee schedule amounts for certain DME items furnished on or after January 1, 2016, including wheelchair accessories and seat and back cushions, in areas that are not competitive bid areas, based on information from competitive bidding programs (CBPs) for DME.

Section 2 of the Patient Access and Medicare Protection Act (PAMPA) mandates that the adjusted fee schedule amounts for 2016 described above are not be applied to wheelchair accessories and seat and back cushions furnished in connection with Group 3 complex rehabilitative power wheelchairs described by codes K0848 through K0864 of the Healthcare Common Procedure Coding System (HCPCS). Although this change is effective January 1, 2016, it is not being implemented until July 1, 2016. Until these changes are implemented, payment for these items will be based on the adjusted fee schedule amounts.

Providers/suppliers can submit claims for these items with dates of service on or after January 1, 2016, prior to July 1, 2016, but payment will be based on the adjusted fee schedule amounts. On or after July 1, 2016, providers/suppliers can adjust previously paid claims with dates of service on or after January 1, 2016, for the corrected fee payment.

Providers/suppliers must use modifier "KU" for claims submitted on or after July 1, 2016, with dates of service on or after January 1, 2016, and before January 1, 2017, for any HCPCS code describing a wheelchair accessory or seat or back cushion when furnished in connection with a Group 3 complex rehabilitative power wheelchair.

Section 16005 of the 21st Century Cures Act modifies section 2(a) of the PAMPA to require that the adjusted fee schedule amounts for 2017, described in section 1834(a)(1(F)(ii) of the Act, are not to be applied to wheelchair accessories and seat and back cushions furnished in connection with Group 3 complex rehabilitative power wheelchairs (described by HCPCS codes K0848 through K0864) prior to July 1, 2017. Therefore, providers/suppliers should continue the use of the KU modifier on claim line items for these accessories with dates of service after June 30, 2017. Effective July 1, 2017, CMS has taken into consideration the exclusion at section 1847(a)(2)(A) of the Act to revise the policy. As a result, payment for these items furnished in connection with a Group 3 complex rehabilitative power wheelchair and billed with the KU modifier will be based on the unadjusted fee schedule amounts updated in accordance with section 1834(a)(14) of the Act.

100-04, 20, 100

General Documentation Requirements

(Rev.1, 10-01-03)

B3-4107.1, B3-4107.8, HHA-463, Medicare Handbook for New Suppliers: Getting Started, B-02-31

Benefit policies are set forth in the Medicare Benefit Policy Manual, Chapter 15, §§110-130.

Program integrity policies for DMEPOS are set forth in the Medicare Program Integrity Manual, Chapter 5.

See Chapter 21 for applicable MSN messages.

See Chapter 22 for Remittance Advice coding.

100-04, 20, 100.2

Certificates of Medical Necessity (CMN)

(Rev.1, 10-01-03)

B3-3312

For certain items or services billed to the DME Regional Carrier (DMERC), the supplier must receive a signed Certificate of Medical Necessity (CMN) from the treating physician. CMNs are not required for the same items when billed by HHAs to RHHIs. Instead, the items must be included in the physician's signed orders on the home health plan of care. See the Medicare Program Integrity Manual, Chapter 6.

The FI will inform other providers (see §01 for definition pf provider) of documentation requirements.

Contractors may ask for supporting documentation beyond a CMN.

Refer to the local DMERC Web site described in §10 for downloadable copies of CMN forms.

See the Medicare Program Integrity Manual, Chapter 5, for specific Medicare policies and instructions on the following topics:

- Requirements for supplier retention of original CMNs
- CMN formats, paper and electronic
- List of currently approved CMNs and items requiring CMNs
- Supplier requirements for submitting CMNs
- Requirements for CMNs to also serve as a physician's order
- Civil monetary penalties for violation of CMN requirements
- Supplier requirements for completing portions of CMNs
- Physician requirements for completing portions of CMNs

100-04, 20, 130.2

Billing for Inexpensive or Other Routinely Purchased DME

(Rev.4027; Issued: 04-27-18; Effective: 10-01-18; Implementation: 10-01-18)

This is equipment with a purchase price not exceeding $150, or equipment that the Secretary determines is acquired by purchase at least 75 percent of the time, or equipment that is an accessory used in conjunction with a nebulizer, aspirator, or ventilators that are either continuous airway pressure devices or intermittent assist devices with continuous airway pressure devices. Effective October 1, 2015, this category also includes speech generating devices and accessories necessary for the effective use of speech generating devices. Suppliers and providers other than HHAs bill the DME MAC or, in the case of implanted DME only, the A/B MAC (B). HHAs bill the A/B MAC (HHH) or the DME MAC.

Effective for items and services furnished after January 1, 1991, Medicare DME does not include seat lift chairs. Only the seat lift mechanism is defined under Medicare as DME. Therefore, seat lift coverage is limited to the seat lift mechanism. If a seat lift chair is provided to a beneficiary, A/B MACs (A), and (HHH), and DME MACs pay only for the lift mechanism portion of the chair. Some lift mechanisms are equipped with a seat that is considered an integral part of the lift mechanism. A/B MACs (A) and (HHH), and DME MACs do not pay for chairs (HCPCS code E0620) furnished on or after January 1, 1991. The appropriate HCPCS codes for seat lift mechanisms are E0627, E0628, and E0629.

© 2019 Optum360, LLC

For TENS, suppliers and providers other than HHAs bill the DME MAC. HHAs bill the A/B MAC (HHH) using revenue code 0291 for the 2-month rental period (see §30.1.2), billing each month as a separate line item and revenue code 0292 for the actual purchase along with the appropriate HCPCS code.

100-04, 20, 130.3

Billing for Items Requiring Frequent and Substantial Servicing

(Rev.1, 10-01-03)

A3-3629, B3-4107.8

These are items such as intermittent positive pressure breathing (IPPB) machines and ventilators, excluding ventilators that are either continuous airway pressure devices or intermittent assist devices with continuous airway pressure devices.

Suppliers and providers other than HHAs bill the DMERC. HHAs bill the RHHI.

100-04, 20, 130.4

Billing for Certain Customized Items

(Rev.1, 10-01-03)

A3-3629, B3-4107.8

Due to their unique nature (custom fabrication, etc.), certain customized DME cannot be grouped together for profiling purposes. Claims for customized items that do not have specific HCPCS codes are coded as E1399 (miscellaneous DME). This includes circumstances where an item that has a HCPCS code is modified to the extent that neither the original terminology nor the terminology of another HCPCS code accurately describes the modified item.

Suppliers and providers other than HHAs bill the DMERC or local carrier. HHAs bill their RHHI, using revenue code 0292 along with the HCPCS.

100-04, 20, 130.5

Billing for Capped Rental Items (Other Items of DME)

(Rev.1, 10-01-03)

A3-3629, B3-4107.8

These are DME items, other than oxygen and oxygen equipment, not covered by the above categories. Suppliers and providers other than HHAs bill the DMERC. HHAs bill the RHHIs.

100-04, 20, 130.6

Billing for Oxygen and Oxygen Equipment

(Rev.3895, Issued: 10-27-17, Effective: 04-01-18, Implementation: 04- 02-18)

The following instructions apply to all claims from providers and suppliers to whom payment may be made for oxygen. The chart in §130.6.1 indicates what is payable under which situation.

A. Monthly Billing

Fee schedule payments for stationary oxygen system rentals are all inclusive and represent a monthly allowance per beneficiary. Accordingly, a supplier must bill on a monthly basis for stationary oxygen equipment and contents furnished during a rental month.

A portable equipment add-on is also payable when portable oxygen is prescribed and it is determined to be medically necessary in accordance with Medicare coverage requirements. The portable add-on must be claimed in order to be paid. (See §30.6.)

B. HCPCS Codes

The HCPCS codes must be used to report the service. One month of service equals one unit.

C. Use of Payment Modifiers and Revenue Codes for Payment Adjustments

The monthly payment amount for stationary oxygen is subject to adjustment depending on the amount of oxygen prescribed (liters per minute (LPM)), and whether or not portable oxygen is also prescribed. (See §30.6.) HHAs billing the A/B MAC (HHH) for stationary equipment, supplies, or contents, which are not eligible for payment adjustment, bill under revenue code 0601. Claims must indicate the appropriate HCPCS modifier described below, if applicable.

- If the prescribed amount of oxygen is less than 1 LPM, suppliers use the modifier "QE"; HHAs use revenue code 0602. The monthly payment amount for stationary oxygen is reduced by 50 percent.
- If the prescribed amount of oxygen is greater than 4 LPM, suppliers use the modifier "QG"; HHAs use revenue code 0603. The monthly payment amount for stationary oxygen is increased by 50 percent.
- If the prescribed amount of oxygen exceeds 4 LPM and portable oxygen is prescribed, suppliers use the modifier "QF"; HHAs use revenue code 0604. The monthly payment for stationary oxygen is increased by the higher of 50 percent of the monthly stationary oxygen payment amount, or, the fee schedule amount for the portable oxygen add-on. (A separate monthly payment is not allowed for the portable equipment.) Effective April 1, 2017, the modifier "QF" must be used with both the stationary and portable oxygen equipment codes.

Effective April 1, 2017, portable oxygen "QF" modifier fee schedule amounts will be added to the DMEPOS fee schedule file. The portable oxygen "QF" fee schedule amounts will represent the higher of 1) 50 percent of the monthly stationary oxygen payment amount or 2) the fee schedule amount for the portable oxygen add-on.

There are three claims processing scenarios:

Scenario 1 – A claim for stationary oxygen equipment is submitted with the QG modifier. The history is reviewed and it is discovered that portable oxygen equipment was billed AND paid within the last 30 days prior to the stationary oxygen equipment's date of service. Since we have already paid the portable add-on, we can't pay the volume adjustment add-on, therefore billing with QG modifier is inappropriate and the claim should be returned as unprocessable.

Scenario 2 – A claim for stationary oxygen equipment is submitted with the QG modifier and within 30 days, a claim for portable oxygen equipment is received. In this case we have already paid the volume add-on so the portable equipment add – on is returned as unprocessable.

Scenario 3 – A claim for stationary oxygen equipment is submitted with the QG modifier AND the portable oxygen equipment comes in with the same date of service. In this case EVERYTHING is returned as unprocessable due to the incorrect use of the modifier and neither is valid.

NOTE: All these claims are being returned as unprocessable since there is no way for Medicare to know whether the first claim submitted was billed incorrectly or if the subsequent claim was billed incorrectly.

Contractors shall use the following messages for claims that are returned as unprocessable:

Group Code: CO (Contractual Obligation)

CARC 4 - The procedure code is inconsistent with the modifier used or a required modifier is missing. Note: Refer to the 835 Healthcare Policy Identification Segment (loop 2110 Service Payment Information REF), if present.

RARC MA130 - Your claim contains incomplete and/or invalid information, and no appeal rights are afforded because the claim is unprocessable. Please submit a new claim with the complete/correct information.

The following three new pricing modifiers are added to the HCPCS file effective April 1, 2018:

QA PRESCRIBED AMOUNTS OF STATIONARY OXYGEN FOR DAYTIME USE WHILE AT REST AND NIGHTTIME USE DIFFER AND THE AVERAGE OF THE TWO AMOUNTS IS LESS THAN 1 LITER PER MINUTE (LPM)

QB PRESCRIBED AMOUNTS OF STATIONARY OXYGEN FOR DAYTIME USE WHILE AT REST AND NIGHTTIME USE DIFFER AND THE AVERAGE OF THE TWO AMOUNTS EXCEEDS 4 LITERS PER MINUTE

(LPM) AND PORTABLE OXYGEN IS PRESCRIBED

QR PRESCRIBED AMOUNTS OF STATIONARY OXYGEN FOR DAYTIME USE WHILE AT REST AND NIGHTTIME USE DIFFER AND THE AVERAGE OF THE TWO AMOUNTS IS GREATER THAN 4 LITERS PER MINUTE (LPM)

Additionally, the existing QE, QF, and QG modifiers are revised to clarify that the prescribed flow rate at rest is used in accordance with regulations at 42 CFR 414.226(e)(3). This section instructs that if the prescribed flow rate is different for the patient at rest than for the patient at exercise, the flow rate for the patient at rest is used. Effective April 1, 2018, the modifiers are revised to read:

QE PRESCRIBED AMOUNT OF STATIONARY OXYGEN WHILE AT REST IS LESS THAN 1 LITER PER MINUTE (LPM)

QF PRESCRIBED AMOUNT OF STATIONARY OXYGEN WHILE AT REST EXCEEDS 4 LITERS PER MINUTE (LPM) AND PORTABLE OXYGEN IS PRESCRIBED

QG PRESCRIBED AMOUNT OF STATIONARY OXYGEN WHILE AT REST IS GREATER THAN 4 LITERS PER MINUTE (LPM)

Beginning April 1, 2018, claims for monthly oxygen volume adjustments must indicate the appropriate HCPCS modifier described below as applicable. Oxygen fee schedule amounts are adjusted as follows:

If the prescribed amount of oxygen is less than 1 LPM, suppliers use either of the following modifiers with the stationary oxygen HCPCS code:

- The modifier "QE" PRESCRIBED AMOUNT OF STATIONARY OXYGEN WHILE AT REST IS LESS THAN 1 LITER PER MINUTE (LPM); HHAs use revenue code 0602. The monthly payment amount for stationary oxygen is reduced by 50 percent.

- The modifier "QA" PRESCRIBED AMOUNTS OF STATIONARY OXYGEN FOR DAYTIME USE WHILE AT REST AND NIGHTTIME USE DIFFER AND THE AVERAGE OF THE TWO AMOUNTS IS LESS THAN 1 LITER PER MINUTE (LPM); The monthly payment amount for stationary oxygen is reduced by 50 percent. This modifier is used when the prescribed flow rate is different for nighttime use and daytime use and the average of the two flow rates is used in determining the volume adjustment.

If the prescribed amount of oxygen is greater than 4 LPM, suppliers use either of the following modifiers with the stationary oxygen HCPCS code:

- The modifier "QG" PRESCRIBED AMOUNT OF STATIONARY OXYGEN WHILE AT REST IS GREATER THAN 4 LITERS PER MINUTE (LPM); HHAs use revenue code 0603. The monthly payment amount for stationary oxygen is increased by 50 percent.
- The modifier "QR" PRESCRIBED AMOUNTS OF STATIONARY OXYGEN FOR DAYTIME USE WHILE AT REST AND NIGHTTIME USE DIFFER AND THE AVERAGE OF THE TWO AMOUNTS IS GREATER THAN 4 LITERS PER MINUTE (LPM); HHAs use revenue code 0603. The monthly payment amount for stationary oxygen is increased by 50 percent.

If the prescribed amount of oxygen is greater than 4 LPM and portable oxygen is prescribed, suppliers use either of the following modifiers with both the stationary and portable oxygen HCPCS code:

- The modifier "QF" PRESCRIBED AMOUNT OF STATIONAY OXYGEN WHILE AT REST EXCEEDS 4 LITERS PER MINUTE (LPM) AND PORTABLE OXYGEN IS PRESCRIBED; HHAs use revenue code 0604. If the prescribed flow rate differs between stationary and portable oxygen equipment, the flow rate for the stationary equipment is used. The monthly payment for stationary oxygen is increased by the higher of 50 percent of the monthly stationary oxygen payment amount, or the fee schedule amount for the portable oxygen add-on. A separate monthly payment is not allowed for the portable equipment. Effective April 1, 2017, the modifier "QF" must be used with both the stationary and portable oxygen equipment codes.
- The modifier "QB" PRESCRIBED AMOUNTS OF STATIONARY OXYGEN FOR DAYTIME USE WHILE AT REST AND NIGHTTIME USE DIFFER AND THE AVERAGE OF THE TWO AMOUNTS EXCEEDS 4 LITERS PER MINUTE (LPM) AND PORTABLE OXYGEN IS PRESCRIBED; HHAs use revenue code 0604. If the prescribed flow rate differs between stationary and portable oxygen equipment, the flow rate for the stationary equipment is used. The monthly payment for stationary oxygen is increased by the higher of 50 percent of the monthly stationary payment amount, or the fee schedule amount for the portable oxygen add-on. A separate monthly payment is not allowed for the portable equipment. Effective April 1, 2018, the modifier "Q??" must be used with both the stationary and portable oxygen equipment codes. The stationary and portable oxygen equipment QB fee schedule amounts will be added to the

DMEPOS fee schedule file effective 4/1/2018.

The stationary oxygen QF and QB fee schedule amounts on the DMEPOS fee schedule file represent 100 percent of the stationary oxygen allowed fee schedule amount. The portable oxygen equipment add-on QF and QB fee schedule amount on the file by state represent the higher of:

1. 50 percent of the monthly stationary oxygen payment amount (codes E0424, E0439, E1390 or E1391); or
2. The fee schedule amount for the portable oxygen add-on (codes E0431, E0433, E0434, E1392 or K0738).

D. Conserving Device Modifier

The HHA's and suppliers must indicate if an oxygen conserving device is being used with an oxygen delivery system by using HCPCS modifier "QH".

E. DME MACs Only

For all States that have licensure/certification requirements for the provision of oxygen and/or oxygen related products, DME MACs shall process claims for oxygen and oxygen related products only when an oxygen specialty code is assigned to the DMEPOS supplier by the NSC and is forwarded to the DME MACs from the NSC.

This specialty shall be licensed and/or certified by the State when applicable. This specialty shall bill for Medicare-covered services and/or products when State law permits such entity to furnish oxygen and/or oxygen related products.

100-04, 20, 160.2

160.2 - Special Considerations for SNF Billing for TPN and EN Under Part B

(Rev.2993, Effective: ASC X12 – 01-01-12, ICD-10 – Upon Implementation of ICD-10; Implementation: ASC X12 – 08-25-14, ICD-10 – Upon Implementation of ICD-10)

The HCPCS code and any appropriate modifiers are required.

SNFs bill the A/B MAC (B) for TPN and EN under Part B, using the ASC X12 837 professional claim format, or the Form CMS-1500 paper claim if applicable.

The following HCPCS codes apply.

B4034 B4035 B4036 B4081 B4082 B4083 B4084 B4085 B4150 B4151 B4152 B4153 B4154 B4155 B4156 B4164 B4168 B4172 B4176 B4178 B4180 B4184 B4186 B4189 B4193 B4197 B4199 B4216 B4220 B4222 B4224 B5000 B5100 B5200 B9000 B9002 B9004 B9006 E0776XA B9098 B9099

For SNF billing for PEN, a SNF includes the charges for PEN items it supplies beneficiaries under Part A on its Part A bill. The services of SNF personnel who administer the PEN therapy are considered routine and are included in the basic Part A payment for a covered stay. SNF personnel costs to administer PEN therapy are not covered under the Part B prosthetic device benefit.

If TPN supplies, equipment and nutrients qualify as a prosthetic device and the stay is not covered by Part A, they are covered by Part B. Part B coverage applies regardless of whether the TPN items were furnished by the SNF or an outside supplier. The Part B TPN bill must be sent to the DME Medicare Administrative Contractor regardless of whether supplied by the SNF or an outside supplier.

Enteral nutrients provided during a stay that is covered by Part A are classified as food and included in the routine Part A payment sent to the SNF. (See the Medicare Provider Reimbursement Manual, §2203.1E.)

Parenteral nutrient solutions provided during a covered Part A SNF stay are classified as intravenous drugs. The SNF must bill these services as ancillary charges. (See the Medicare Provider Reimbursement Manual, §2203.2.)

100-04, 20, 170

Billing for Splints and Casts

(Rev.2993, Effective: ASC X12 – 01-01-12, ICD-10 – Upon Implementation of ICD- 10; Implementation: ASC X12 – 08-25-14, ICD-10 – Upon Implementation of ICD- 10)

The cost of supplies used in creating casts are not included in the payment amounts for the CPT codes for fracture management and for casts and splints. Thus, for settings in which CPT codes are used to pay for services that include the provision of a cast or splint, supplies maybe billed with separate CPCS codes. The work and practice expenses involved with the creation of the cast or splint are included in the payment for the code for that service.

For claims with dates of service on or after July 1, 2001, jurisdiction for processing claims for splints transferred from the DME MACs to the A/B MAC (B). The A/B MACs (B) have jurisdiction for processing claims for splints and casts, which includes codes for splints that may have previously been billed to the DME MACs.

Jurisdiction for slings is jointly maintained by the A/B MACs (B) (for physician claims) and the DME MACs (for supplier claims). Notwithstanding the above where the beneficiary receives the service from any of the following providers claims jurisdiction is with the A/B MAC (A). An exception to this is hospital outpatient services and hospital inpatient Part B services, which are included in the OPPS payment and are billed to the A/B MAC (A) using the ASC X12 837 institutional claim format or Form CMS- 1450).

Other providers and suppliers that normally bill the A/B MAC (A) for services bill the A/B MAC (B) for splints and casts.

100-04, 20, 180

Billing for Home Infusion Therapy Services

(Rev.4112, Issued: 08-10-18, Effective: 01-01-19, Implementation: 01-07-19)

Effective January 1, 2019 and until the implementation of the full home infusion therapy benefit, Medicare makes separate temporary transitional payments for Home Infusion Therapy (HIT) services to eligible home infusion suppliers (i.e., a licensed pharmacy that provides external infusion pumps and external infusion pump supplies). This payment amount covers the cost of professional services, including nursing services, training and education (not otherwise paid for as durable medical equipment), remote monitoring, and monitoring services for the provision of home infusion therapy furnished by a qualified home infusion with administration of certain transitional home infusion drugs administered through an item of DME.

Temporary transitional payments are made for HIT services based on the home infusion drug provided. Home infusion drugs are assigned to three payment categories, determined by the Healthcare Common Procedure Coding System (HCPCS) J-code. Each DME MAC maintains a list of drugs that are administered through an item of DME and HIT payment is made for days on which home infusion therapy services are furnished by skilled professionals in the individual's home on the day of infusion drug administration.

Temporary Transitional Payment Categories for Home Infusion Therapy Services, by Infusion Drug (J-Code)

© 2019 Optum360, LLC

Category 1

J-Code	Description
J0133	Injection, acyclovir, 5 mg
J0285	Injection, amphotericin b, 50 mg
J0287	Injection, amphotericin b lipid complex, 10 mg
J0288	Injection, amphotericin b cholesteryl sulfate complex, 10 mg
J0289	Injection, amphotericin b liposome, 10 mg
J0895	Injection, deferoxamine mesylate, 500 mg
J1170	Injection, hydromorphone, up to 4 mg
J1250	Injection, dobutamine hydrochloride, per 250 mg
J1265	Injection, dopamine hcl, 40 mg
J1325	Injection, epoprostenol, 0.5 mg
J1455	Injection, foscarnet sodium, per 1000 mg
J1457	Injection, gallium nitrate, 1 mg
J1570	Injection, ganciclovir sodium, 500 mg
J2175	Injection, meperidine hydrochloride, per 100 mg
J2260	Injection, milrinone lactate, 5 mg
J2270	Injection, morphine sulfate, up to 10 mg
J2274	Injection, morphine sulfate, preservative-free for epidural or intrathecal use, 10 mg
J2278	Injection, ziconotide, 1 microgram
J3010	Injection, fentanyl citrate, 0.1 mg
J3285	Injection, treprostinil, 1 mg

Category 2

J-Code	Description
J1555 JB	Injection, immune globulin (cuvitru), 100 mg
J1559 JB	Injection, immune globulin (hizentra), 100 mg
J1561 JB	Injection, immune globulin, (gamunex-c/gammaked), non-lyophilized (e.g., liquid), 500 mg
J1562 JB	Injection, immune globulin (vivaglobin), 100 mg
J1569 JB	Injection, immune globulin, (gammagard liquid), non-lyophilized, (e.g., liquid), 500 mg

100-04, 23, 30.2

MPFSDB Record Layout

(Rev.4298, Issued: 05-03-19, Effective: 01-01-19, Implementation 10-07-19)

The CMS MPFSDB includes the total fee schedule amount, related component parts, and payment policy indicators. The record layout is provided in the Addendum below.

Addendum - MPFSDB File Record Layout and Field Descriptions

(Rev.4298, Issued: 05-03-19, Effective: 01-01-19, Implementation 10-07-19)

The CMS MPFSDB includes the total fee schedule amount, related component parts, and payment policy indicators. The record layout is provided below. *Beginning with the 2019 MPFSDB, and thereafter, the MPFSDB File Record Layout will no longer be revised annually in this section for the sole purpose of changing the calendar year, but will only be revised when there is a change to a field. Previous MPFSDB file layouts (for 2018 and prior) can be found on the CMS web site on the Physician Fee Schedule web page at: https://www.cms.gov/Medicare/Medicare-Fee-for-Service-Payment/PhysicianFeeSched/index.html.*

MPFSDB File Layout

HEADER RECORD

FIELD #	DATA ELEMENT NAME	LOCATION	PIC
1	Header ID	1-4	x(4) Value "Head"
2	Header Number	5	x(1)
3	Data Set Name	6-50	x(45)
4	Record Length	51-53	x(3)
5	Filler	54-54	x(1)
6	Block size	55-58	x(4)
7	Filler	59-59	x(1)
8	Number of Records Number does not include this header record.	60-69	9(10)
9	Date Created	70-77	x(8) YYYYMMDD
10	Blanks	78-345	x(268)

DATA RECORD

FIELD # & ITEM	LENGTH & PIC
1 File Year This field displays the effective year of the file.	4 Pic x(4)
2 A/B MAC (B) Number This field represents the 5-digit number assigned to the A/B MAC (B).	5 Pic x(5)
3 Locality This 2-digit code identifies the pricing locality used.	2 Pic x(2)
4 HCPCS Code This field represents the procedure code. Each A/B MAC (B) Current Procedural Terminology (CPT) code (other than codes for Multianalyte Assays with Algorithmic Analyses (MAAA) and Proprietary Laboratory Analyses (PLA)) and alpha-numeric HCPCS codes other than B, C, E, K and L codes will be included. The standard sort for this field is blanks, alpha, and numeric in ascending order. Note: MAAA and PLA are alpha-numeric CPT codes.	5 Pic x(5)
5 Modifier For diagnostic tests, a blank in this field denotes the global service and the following modifiers identify the components: 26 = Professional component TC = Technical component For services other than those with a professional and/or technical component, a blank will appear in this field with one exception: the presence of CPT modifier -53 which indicates that separate Relative Value Units (RVUs) and a fee schedule amount have been established for procedures which the physician terminated before completion. This modifier is used only with colonoscopy through stoma code 44388, colonoscopy code 45378 and screening colonoscopy codes G0105 and G0121. Any other codes billed with modifier -53 are subject to medical review and priced by individual consideration. Modifier-53 = Discontinued Procedure - Under certain circumstances, the physician may elect to terminate a surgical or diagnostic procedure. Due to extenuating circumstances, or those that threaten the well being of the patient, it may be necessary to indicate that a surgical or diagnostic procedure was started but discontinued.	2 Pic x(2)
6 Descriptor This field will include a brief description of each procedure code.	50 Pic x(50)
7 Code Status This 1 position field provides the status of each code under the full fee schedule. Each status code is explained in §30.2.2.	1 Pic x(1)

© 2019 Optum360, LLC

FIELD # & ITEM	LENGTH & PIC
8 Conversion Factor This field displays the multiplier which transforms relative values into payment amounts. The file will contain the conversion factor for the File Year which will reflect all adjustments.	8 Pic 9(4)v9999
9 Update Factor This update factor has been included in the conversion factor in Field 8.	6 Pic 9(2)v9999
10 Work Relative Value Unit This field displays the unit value for the physician work RVU.	9 Pic 9(7)v99
11 Filler	9 Pic 9(7)v99
12 Malpractice Relative Value Unit This field displays the unit value for the malpractice expense RVU.	9 Pic 9(7)v99
13 Work Geographic Practice Cost Indices (GPCIs) This field displays a work geographic adjustment factor used in computing the fee schedule amount.	5 Pic 99v999
14 Practice Expense GPCI This field displays a practice expense geographic adjustment factor used in computing the fee schedule amount.	5 Pic 99v999
15 Malpractice GPCI This field displays a malpractice expense geographic adjustment factor used in computing the fee schedule amount.	5 Pic 99v999
16 Global Surgery This field provides the postoperative time frames that apply to payment for each surgical procedure or another indicator that describes the applicability of the global concept to the service. 000 = Endoscopic or minor procedure with related preoperative and postoperative relative values on the day of the procedure only included in the fee schedule payment amount; evaluation and management services on the day of the procedure generally not payable. 010 = Minor procedure with preoperative relative values on the day of the procedure and postoperative relative values during a 10-day postoperative period included in the fee schedule amount; evaluation and management services on the day of the procedure and during this 10-day postoperative period generally not payable. 090 = Major surgery with a 1-day preoperative period and 90-day postoperative period included in the fee schedule payment amount. MMM = Maternity codes; usual global period does not apply. XXX = Global concept does not apply. YYY = A/B MAC (B) determines whether global concept applies and establishes postoperative period, if appropriate, at time of pricing. ZZZ = Code related to another service and is always included in the global period of the other service. (Note: Physician work is associated with intra-service time and in some instances the post service time.)	3 Pic x(3)
17 Preoperative Percentage (Modifier 56) This field contains the percentage (shown in decimal format) for the preoperative portion of the global package. For example, 10 percent will be shown as 010000. The total of fields 17, 18, and 19 will usually equal one. Any variance is slight and results from rounding.	6 Pic 9v9(5)
18 Intraoperative Percentage (Modifier 54) This field contains the percentage (shown in decimal format) for the intraoperative portion of the global package including postoperative work in the hospital. For example, 63 percent will be shown as 063000. The total of fields 17, 18, and 19 will usually equal one. Any variance is slight and results from rounding.	6 Pic 9v9(5)

FIELD # & ITEM	LENGTH & PIC
19 Postoperative Percentage (Modifier 55) This field contains the percentage (shown in decimal format) for the postoperative portion of the global package that is provided in the office after discharge from the hospital. For example, 17 percent will be shown as 017000. The total of fields 17, 18, and 19 will usually equal one. Any variance is slight and results from rounding.	6 Pic 9v9(5)

20

Professional Component (PC)/Technical Component (TC) Indicator

0 = Physician service codes: This indicator identifies codes that describe physician services. Examples include visits, consultations, and surgical procedures. The concept of PC/TC does not apply since physician services cannot be split into professional and technical components. Modifiers 26 & TC cannot be used with these codes. The total Relative Value Units (RVUs) include values for physician work, practice expense and malpractice expense. There are some codes with no work RVUs.

1 = Diagnostic tests or radiology services: This indicator identifies codes that describe diagnostic tests, e.g., pulmonary function tests, or therapeutic radiology procedures, e.g., radiation therapy. These codes generally have both a professional and technical component. Modifiers 26 and TC can be used with these codes.

The total RVUs for codes reported with a 26 modifier include values for physician work, practice expense, and malpractice expense.

The total RVUs for codes reported with a TC modifier include values for practice expense and malpractice expense only. The total RVUs for codes reported without a modifier equals the sum of RVUs for both the professional and technical component.

2 = Professional component only codes: This indicator identifies stand alone codes that describe the physician work portion of selected diagnostic tests for which there is an associated code that describes the technical component of the diagnostic test only and another associated code that describes the global test.

An example of a professional component only code is 93010, Electrocardiogram; interpretation and report. Modifiers 26 and TC cannot be used with these codes. The total RVUs for professional component only codes include values for physician work, practice expense, and malpractice expense.

3 = Technical component only codes: This indicator identifies stand alone codes that describe the technical component (i.e., staff and equipment costs) of selected diagnostic tests for which there is an associated code that describes the professional component of the diagnostic tests only.

An example of a technical component code is 93005, Electrocardiogram, tracing only, without interpretation and report. It also identifies codes that are covered only as diagnostic tests and therefore do not have a related professional code. Modifiers 26 and TC cannot be used with these codes.

The total RVUs for technical component only codes include values for practice expense and malpractice expense only.

4 = Global test only codes: This indicator identifies stand alone codes for which there are associated codes that describe: a) the professional component of the test only and b) the technical component of the test only. Modifiers 26 and TC cannot be used with these codes. The total RVUs for global procedure only codes include values for physician work, practice expense, and malpractice expense. The total RVUs for global procedure only codes equals the sum of the total RVUs for the professional and technical components only codes combined.

5 = Incident to codes: This indicator identifies codes that describe services covered incident to a physicians service when they are provided by auxiliary personnel employed by the physician and working under his or her direct supervision.

Payment may not be made by A/B MACs (B) for these services when they are provided to hospital inpatients or patients in a hospital outpatient department. Modifiers 26 and TC cannot be used with these codes.

6 = Laboratory physician interpretation codes: This indicator identifies clinical laboratory codes for which separate payment for interpretations by laboratory physicians may be made. Actual performance of the tests is paid for under the lab fee schedule. Modifier TC cannot be used with these codes. The total RVUs for laboratory physician interpretation codes include values for physician work, practice expense and malpractice expense.

7 = Private practice therapist's service: Payment may not be made if the service is provided to either a hospital outpatient or a hospital inpatient by a physical therapist, occupational therapist, or speech-language pathologist in private practice.

© 2019 Optum360, LLC

FIELD # & ITEM	LENGTH & PIC
20 Professional Component (PC)/Technical Component (TC) Indicator *(continued)* 8 = Physician interpretation codes: This indicator identifies the professional component of clinical laboratory codes for which separate payment may be made only if the physician interprets an abnormal smear for hospital inpatient. This applies only to code 85060. No TC billing is recognized because payment for the underlying clinical laboratory test is made to the hospital, generally through the PPS rate. No payment is recognized for code 85060 furnished to hospital outpatients or non-hospital patients. The physician interpretation is paid through the clinical laboratory fee schedule payment for the clinical laboratory test. 9 = Concept of a professional/technical component does not apply.	
21 Multiple Procedure (Modifier 51) Indicator indicates which payment adjustment rule for multiple procedures applies to the service. 0 = No payment adjustment rules for multiple procedures apply. If procedure is reported on the same day as another procedure, base payment on the lower of: (a) the actual charge or (b) the fee schedule amount for the procedure. 1 = Standard payment adjustment rules in effect before January 1, 1996, for multiple procedures apply. In the 1996 MPFSDB, this indicator only applies to codes with procedure status of "D." If a procedure is reported on the same day as another procedure with an indicator of 1,2, or 3, rank the procedures by fee schedule amount and apply the appropriate reduction to this code (100 percent, 50 percent, 25 percent, 25 percent, 25 percent, and by report). Base payment on the lower of: (a) the actual charge or (b) the fee schedule amount reduced by the appropriate percentage. 2 = Standard payment adjustment rules for multiple procedures apply. If procedure is reported on the same day as another procedure with an indicator of 1, 2, or 3, rank the procedures by fee schedule amount and apply the appropriate reduction to this code (100 percent, 50 percent, 50 percent, 50 percent, 50 percent, and by report). Base payment on the lower of: (a) the actual charge or (b) the fee schedule amount reduced by the appropriate percentage. 3 = Special rules for multiple endoscopic procedures apply if procedure is billed with another endoscopy in the same family (i.e., another endoscopy that has the same base procedure). The base procedure for each code with this indicator is identified in field 31G. Apply the multiple endoscopy rules to a family before ranking the family with other procedures performed on the same day (for example, if multiple endoscopies in the same family are reported on the same day as endoscopies in another family or on the same day as a non-endoscopic procedure). If an endoscopic procedure is reported with only its base procedure, do not pay separately for the base procedure. Payment for the base procedure is included in the payment for the other endoscopy. 4 = Subject to 25% reduction of the TC diagnostic imaging (effective for services January 1, 2006 through June 30, 2010). Subject to 50% reduction of the TC diagnostic imaging (effective for services July 1, 2010 and after). Subject to 25% reduction of the PC of diagnostic imaging (effective for services January 1, 2012 through December 31, 2016). Subject to 5% reduction of the PC of diagnostic imaging (effective for services January 1, 2017 and after). 5 = Subject to 20% reduction of the practice expense component for certain therapy services furnished in office and other non-institutional settings, and 25% reduction of the practice expense component for certain therapy services furnished in institutional settings (effective for services January 1, 2011 and after). Subject to 50% reduction of the practice expense component for certain therapy services furnished in both institutional and non-institutional settings (effective for services April 1, 2013 and after). 6 = Subject to 25% reduction of the TC diagnostic cardiovascular services (effective for services January 1, 2013 and after). 7 = Subject to 20% reduction of the TC diagnostic ophthalmology services (effective for services January 1, 2013 and after). 9 = Concept does not apply.	

FIELD # & ITEM	LENGTH & PIC
22 Bilateral Surgery Indicator (Modifier 50) This field provides an indicator for services subject to a payment adjustment. 0 = 150 percent payment adjustment for bilateral procedures does not apply. If procedure is reported with modifier -50 or with modifiers RT and LT, base payment for the two sides on the lower of: (a) the total actual charge for both sides or (b) 100 percent of the fee schedule amount for a single code. Example: The fee schedule amount for code XXXXX is $125. The physician reports code XXXXX-LT with an actual charge of $100 and XXXXX-RT with an actual charge of $100. Payment would be based on the fee schedule amount ($125) since it is lower than the total actual charges for the left and right sides ($200). The bilateral adjustment is inappropriate for codes in this category because of (a) physiology or anatomy or (b) because the code descriptor specifically states that it is a unilateral procedure and there is an existing code for the bilateral procedure. 1 = 150 percent payment adjustment for bilateral procedures applies. If code is billed with the bilateral modifier or is reported twice on the same day by any other means (e.g., with RT and LT modifiers or with a 2 in the units field), base payment for these codes when reported as bilateral procedures on the lower of: (a) the total actual charge for both sides or (b) 150 percent of the fee schedule amount for a single code. If code is reported as a bilateral procedure and is reported with other procedure codes on the same day, apply the bilateral adjustment before applying any applicable multiple procedure rules. 2 = 150 percent payment adjustment for bilateral procedure does not apply. RVUs are already based on the procedure being performed as a bilateral procedure. If procedure is reported with modifier -50 or is reported twice on the same day by any other means (e.g., with RT and LT modifiers with a 2 in the units field), base payment for both sides on the lower of (a) the total actual charges by the physician for both sides or (b) 100 percent of the fee schedule amount for a single code. Example: The fee schedule amount for code YYYYY is $125. The physician reports code YYYYY-LT with an actual charge of $100 and YYYYY-RT with an actual charge of $100. Payment would be based on the fee schedule amount ($125) since it is lower than the total actual charges for the left and right sides ($200). The RVUs are based on a bilateral procedure because: (a) the code descriptor specifically states that the procedure is bilateral; (b) the code descriptor states that the procedure may be performed either unilaterally or bilaterally; or (c) the procedure is usually performed as a bilateral procedure. 3 = The usual payment adjustment for bilateral procedures does not apply. If procedure is reported with modifier -50 or is reported for both sides on the same day by any other means (e.g., with RT and LT modifiers or with a 2 in the units field), base payment for each side or organ or site of a paired organ on the lower of: (a) the actual charge for each side or (b) 100% of the fee schedule amount for each side. If procedure is reported as a bilateral procedure and with other procedure codes on the same day, determine the fee schedule amount for a bilateral procedure before applying any applicable multiple procedure rules. Services in this category are generally radiology procedures or other diagnostic tests which are not subject to the special payment rules for other bilateral procedures. 9 = Concept does not apply.	1 Pic (x)1

© 2019 Optum360, LLC

FIELD # & ITEM	LENGTH & PIC
23 Assistant at Surgery This field provides an indicator for services where an assistant at surgery is never paid for per IOM. 0 = Payment restriction for assistants at surgery applies to this procedure unless supporting documentation is submitted to establish medical necessity. 1 = Statutory payment restriction for assistants at surgery applies to this procedure. Assistant at surgery may not be paid. 2 = Payment restriction for assistants at surgery does not apply to this procedure. Assistant at surgery may be paid. 9 = Concept does not apply. 24 Co-Surgeons (Modifier 62) This field provides an indicator for services for which two surgeons, each in a different specialty, may be paid. 0 = Co-surgeons not permitted for this procedure. 1 = Co-surgeons could be paid; supporting documentation required to establish medical necessity of two surgeons for the procedure. 2 = Co-surgeons permitted; no documentation required if two specialty requirements are met. 9 = Concept does not apply.	1 Pic (x)1
25 Team Surgeons (Modifier 66) This field provides an indicator for services for which team surgeons may be paid. 0 = Team surgeons not permitted for this procedure. 1 = Team surgeons could be paid; supporting documentation required to establish medical necessity of a team; pay by report. 2 = Team surgeons permitted; pay by report. 9 = Concept does not apply.	1 Pic (x)1 9 Pic 9(7)v99
26 Filler	1 Pic (x)1
27 Site of Service Differential For 1999 and beyond, the site of service differential no longer applies. The following definitions will apply for all years after 1998: 0 = Facility pricing does not apply. 1 = Facility pricing applies. 9 = Concept does not apply. 28 Non-Facility Fee Schedule Amount This field shows the fee schedule amount for the non-facility setting. This amount equals Field 34. **Note**: Field 33 D indicates if an additional adjustment should be applied to this formula. Non-Facility Pricing Amount for *the File Year* [(Work RVU * Work GPCI) + (Non-Facility PE RVU * PE GPCI) + (MP RVU * MP GPCI)] * Conversion Factor	1 Pic (x)1

FIELD # & ITEM	LENGTH & PIC
29 Facility Fee Schedule Amount This field shows the fee schedule amount for the facility setting. This amount equals Field 35. **Note:** Field 33D indicates if an additional adjustment should be applied to this formula. Facility Pricing Amount for *the File Year* [(Work RVU * Work GPCI) + (Facility PE RVU * PE GPCI) + (MP RVU * MP GPCI)] * Conversion Factor Place of service codes to be used to identify facilities. 02 – Telehealth-Medicare pays telehealth services at the facility rate. 19 – Off Campus-Outpatient Hospital 21 - Inpatient Hospital 22 – On Campus-Outpatient Hospital 23 - Emergency Room - Hospital	9 Pic 9(7)v99
24 - Ambulatory Surgical Center – In a Medicare approved ASC, for an approved procedure on the ASC list, Medicare pays the lower facility fee to physicians. Beginning with dates of service January 1, 2008, in a Medicare approved ASC, for procedures NOT on the ASC list of approved procedures, contractors will also pay the lower facility fee to physicians. 26 - Military Treatment Facility 31 - Skilled Nursing Facility 34 - Hospice 41 - Ambulance - Land 42 - Ambulance Air or Water 51 - Inpatient Psychiatric Facility 52 - Psychiatric Facility Partial Hospitalization 53 - Community Mental Health Center 56 - Psychiatric Residential Treatment Facility 61 - Comprehensive Inpatient Rehabilitation Facility	
29A Anti-markup Test Indicator This field providers an indicator for Anti-markup Test HCPCS codes: '1' = Anti-markup Test HCPCS. '9' = Concept does not apply.	1 Pic x
30 Record Effective Date This field identifies the effective date for the MPFSDB record for each HCPCS. The field is in YYYYMMDD format. NOTE: This is not the date the HCPCS code was created. It is the date the code was updated or added to the MPFSDB file for the current file year. This field is set to January 1 for all codes during the annual update process.	8 Pic x(8)
31 Filler	28 Pic x(28)
31EE Reduced therapy fee schedule amount	9Pic(7)v99
31DD Filler	1Pic x(2)
31CC Imaging Cap Indicator A value of "1" means subject to OPPS payment cap determination. A value of "9" means not subject to OPPS payment cap determination.	1Pic x(1)
31BB Non-Facility Imaging Payment Amount	9Pic(7)v99
31AA Facility Imaging Payment Amount	9Pic(7)v99

© 2019 Optum360, LLC

FIELD # & ITEM	LENGTH & PIC
31A Physician Supervision of Diagnostic Procedures This field is for use in post payment review. 01 = Procedure must be performed under the general supervision of a physician. 02 = Procedure must be performed under the direct supervision of a physician. 03 = Procedure must be performed under the personal supervision of a physician. (Diagnostic imaging procedures performed by a Registered Radiologist Assistant (RRA) who is certified and registered by The American Registry of Radiologic Technologists (ARRT) or a Radiology Practitioner Assistant (RPA) who is certified by the Certification Board for Radiology Practitioner Assistants (CBRPA), and is authorized to furnish the procedure under state law, may be performed under direct supervision.) 04 = Physician supervision policy does not apply when procedure is furnished by a qualified, independent psychologist or a clinical psychologist; otherwise must be performed under the general supervision of a physician. 05 = Not subject to supervision when furnished personally by a qualified audiologist, physician or non physician practitioner. Direct supervision by a physician is required for those parts of the test that may be furnished by a qualified technician when appropriate to the circumstances of the test. 06 = Procedure must be personally performed by a physician or a physical therapist (PT) who is certified by the American Board of Physical Therapy Specialties (ABPTS) as a qualified electrophysiological clinical specialist and is permitted to provide the procedure under State law. Procedure may also be performed by a PT with ABPTS certification without physician supervision. 21 = Procedure may be performed by a technician with certification under general supervision of a physician; otherwise must be performed under direct supervision of a physician. Procedure may also be performed by a PT with ABPTS certification without physician supervision. 22 = May be performed by a technician with on-line real-time contact with physician. 66 = May be personally performed by a physician or by a physical therapist with ABPTS certification and certification in this specific procedure. 6A = Supervision standards for level 66 apply; in addition, the PT with ABPTS certification may personally supervise another PT, but only the PT with ABPTS certification may bill. 77 = Procedure must be performed by a PT with ABPTS certification (TC & PC) or by a PT without certification under direct supervision of a physician (TC & PC), or by a technician with certification under general supervision of a physician (TC only; PC always physician). 7A = Supervision standards for level 77 apply; in addition, the PT with ABPTS certification may personally supervise another PT, but only the PT with ABPTS certification may bill. 09 = Concept does not apply.	2 Pic x(2)
31B This field has been deleted to allow for the expansion of field 31A.	
31C Facility Setting Practice Expense Relative Value Units	9 Pic(7)v99
31D Non-Facility Setting Practice Expense Relative Value Units	9 Pic(7)v99
31E Filler	9 Pic(7)v99
31F Filler Reserved for future use.	1 Pic x(1)

FIELD # & ITEM	LENGTH & PIC
31G Endoscopic Base Codes This field identifies an endoscopic base code for each code with a multiple surgery indicator of 3.	5 Pic x(5)
32A 1996 Transition/Fee Schedule Amount This field is no longer applicable since transitioning ended in 1996. This field will contain a zero.	9 Pic 9(7)v99
32B 1996 Transition/Fee Schedule This field is no longer applicable since transitioning ended in 1996. This field will contain spaces.	1 Pic x(1)
32C 1996 Transition/Fee Schedule Amount When Site or Service Differential Applies This field is no longer applicable since transitioning ended in 1996. This field will contain a zero. 33A Units Payment Rule Indicator Reserved for future use. 9 = Concept does not apply.	9 Pic 9(7)v99
33B Mapping Indicator This field is no longer applicable since transitioning ended in 1996.	1 Pic x(1)
3 Pic x (3)	
This field will contain spaces.	
33C Anti-markup Locality—Informational Use—Locality used for reporting utilization of anti-markup services. NOT FOR A/B MAC (B) USE: These Medicare Advantage encounter pricing localities are for Shared System Maintainer purposes only. The locality values were developed to facilitate centralized processing of encounter data by the Medicare Advantage organizations.	2 Pic x(2)
33D Calculation Flag This field is informational only; the SSMs do not need to add this field. The intent is to assist A/B MACs (B) to understand how the fee schedule amount in fields 28 and 29 are calculated. The MMA mandates an additional adjustment to selected HCPCS codes. A value of "1" indicates an additional fee schedule adjustment of 1.32 in 2004 and 1.03 in 2005. A value of "0" indicates no additional adjustment needed. A value of "2" indicates an additional fee schedule adjustment of 1.05 effective 7/1/2008.	1 Pic x(1)
33 E Diagnostic Imaging Family Indicator For services effective January 1, 2011, and after, family indicators 01 - 11 will not be populated. 01 = Family 1 Ultrasound (Chest/Abdomen/Pelvis – Non Obstetrical 02 = Family 2 CT and CTA (Chest/Thorax/Abd/Pelvis) 03 = Family 3 CT and CTA (Head/Brain/Orbit/Maxillofacial/Neck) 04 = Family 4 MRI and MRA (Chest/Abd/Pelvis) 05 = Family 5 MRI and MRA (Head/Brain/Neck) 06 = Family 6 MRI and MRA (spine) 07 = Family 7 CT (spine) 08 = Family 8 MRI and MRA (lower extremities) 09 = Family 9 CT and CTA (lower extremities) 10 = Family 10 Mr and MRI (upper extremities and joints) 11 = Family 11 CT and CTA (upper extremities) 88 = Subject to the reduction of the TC diagnostic imaging (effective for services January 1, 2011, and after). Subject to the reduction of the PC diagnostic imaging (effective for services January 1, 2012 and after). 99 = Concept Does Not Apply	2Pic x(2)

© 2019 Optum360, LLC

FIELD # & ITEM	LENGTH & PIC
33F Performance Payment Indicator (For future use) 33G National Level Future Expansion	1 Pic x (1)
34 Non-Facility Fee Schedule Amount This field replicates field 28.	9 Pic 9(7)v99
35 Facility Fee Schedule Amount This field replicates field 29.	9 Pic 9(7)v99
36 Filler	1 Pic x(1)
37 Future Local Level Expansion** The Updated 1992 Transition Amount was previously stored in this field. A/B MACs (B) can continue to maintain the updated transition amount in this field.	7 Pic x(7)
38A Future Local Level Expansion** The adjusted historical payment basis (AHPB) was previously stored in this field. A/B MACs (B) can continue to maintain the AHPB in this field.	7 Pic x(7)
38 B Filler This field was originally established for 15 spaces. Since AHPB data will only use 7 of the 15 spaces, A/B MACs (B) have 8 remaining spaces for their purposes. ** These fields will be appended by each A/B MAC (B) at the local level.	8 Pix x(8)

100-04, 23, 60.3

(Rev.4130, Issued: 09-14-18, Effective: 06-11-18, Implementation: 10-15-18)

The DME MACs and Part B MACs must gap-fill the DMEPOS fee schedule for items for which charge data were unavailable during the fee schedule data base year using the fee schedule amounts for comparable equipment, using properly calculated fee schedule amounts from a neighboring DME MAC or Part BMAC area, or using supplier price lists

with prices in effect during the fee schedule data base year. Data base "year" refers to the time period mandated by the statute and/or regulations from which Medicare allowed charge data is to be extracted in order to compute the fee schedule amounts for the various DMEPOS payment categories. For example, the fee schedule base year for inexpensive or routinely purchased durable medical equipment is the 12 month period ending June 30, 1987. Supplier price lists include catalogues and other retail price lists (such as internet retail prices) that provide information on commercial pricing for the item. Potential appropriate sources for such commercial pricing information can also include verifiable information from supplier invoices and non-Medicare payer data (e.g., fee schedule amounts comprised of the median of the commercial pricing information adjusted as described below). Mail order catalogs are particularly suitable sources of price information for items such as urological and ostomy supplies which require constant replacement. DME MACs will gap-fill based on current instructions released each year for implementing and updating the new year's payment amounts.

If the only available price information is from a period other than the base period, apply the deflation factors that are included in the current year implementation instructions against current pricing in order to approximate the base year price for gap-filling purposes.

The deflation factors for gap-filling purposes are:

Year*	OX	CR	PO	SD	PE	SC	IL
1987	0.965	0.971	0.974	n/a	n/a	n/a	n/a
1988	0.928	0.934	0.936	n/a	n/a	n/a	n/a
1989	0.882	0.888	0.890	n/a	n/a	n/a	n/a
1990	0.843	0.848	0.851	n/a	n/a	n/a	n/a
1991	0.805	0.810	0.813	n/a	n/a	n/a	n/a
1992	0.781	0.786	0.788	n/a	n/a	n/a	n/a
1993	0.758	0.763	0.765	0.971	n/a	n/a	n/a
1994	0.740	0.745	0.747	0.947	n/a	n/a	n/a
1995	0.718	0.723	0.725	0.919	n/a	n/a	n/a
1996	0.699	0.703	0.705	0.895	0.973	n/a	n/a
1997	0.683	0.687	0.689	0.875	0.951	n/a	n/a
1998	0.672	0.676	0.678	0.860	0.936	n/a	n/a
1999	0.659	0.663	0.665	0.844	0.918	n/a	n/a
2000	0.635	0.639	0.641	0.813	0.885	n/a	n/a
2001	0.615	0.619	0.621	0.788	0.857	n/a	n/a
2002	0.609	0.613	0.614	0.779	0.848	n/a	n/a
2003	0.596	0.600	0.602	0.763	0.830	n/a	n/a
2004	0.577	0.581	0.582	0.739	0.804	n/a	n/a
2005	0.563	0.567	0.568	0.721	0.784	n/a	n/a
2006	0.540	0.543	0.545	0.691	0.752	n/a	n/a
2007	0.525	0.529	0.530	0.673	0.732	n/a	n/a
2008	0.500	0.504	0.505	0.641	0.697	n/a	n/a
2009	0.508	0.511	0.512	0.650	0.707	n/a	n/a
2010	0.502	0.506	0.507	0.643	0.700	n/a	n/a
2011	0.485	0.488	0.490	0.621	0.676	n/a	n/a
2012	0.477	0.480	0.482	0.611	0.665	n/a	n/a
2013	0.469	0.472	0.473	0.600	0.653	n/a	0.983
2014	0.459	0.462	0.464	0.588	0.640	0.980	0.963
2015	0.459	0.462	0.463	0.588	0.639	0.978	0.962
2016	0.454	0.457	0.458	0.582	0.633	0.969	0.952
2017	0.447	0.450	0.451	0.572	0.623	0.953	0.937
2018	0.435	0.437	0.439	0.556	0.605	0.927	0.911

* Year price in effect

Payment Category Key:

OX	Oxygen & oxygen equipment (DME)
CR	Capped rental (DME)
IN	Inexpensive/routinely purchased (DME)
FS	Frequently serviced (DME)
SU	DME supplies
PO	Prosthetics & orthotics
SD	Surgical dressings
OS	Ostomy, tracheostomy, and urological supplies
PE	Parental and enteral nutrition
TS	Therapeutic Shoes
SC	Splints and Casts
IL	Intraocular Lenses inserted in a physician's office IN, FS, OS and SU category deflation factors=PO deflation factors

After deflation, the result must be increased by 1.7 percent and by the cumulative covered item update to complete the gap-filling (e.g., an additional .6 percent for a 2002 DME fee).

Note that when gap-filling for capped rental items, it is necessary to first gap-fill the purchase price then compute the base period fee schedule at 10 percent of the base period purchase price.

For used equipment, establish fee schedule amounts at 75 percent of the fee schedule amount for new equipment.

When gap-filling, for those DME MAC or Part B MAC areas where a sales tax was imposed in the base period, add the applicable sales tax, e.g., five percent, to the gap-filled amount where the gap-filled amount does not take into account the sales tax, e.g., where the gap-filled amount is computed from pre-tax price lists or from another DME MAC or Part B MAC area without a sales tax. Likewise, if the gap-filled amount is calculated from another DME MAC's or Part B MAC's fees where a sales tax

© 2019 Optum360, LLC

is imposed, adjust the gap- filled amount to reflect the applicable local sales tax circumstances.

Contractors send their gap-fill information to CMS. After receiving the gap-filled base fees each year,CMS develops national fee schedule floors and ceilings and new fee schedule amounts for these codes and releases them as part of the July update file each year and during the quarterly updates.

100-04, 32, 11.1

Electrical Stimulation

(Rev.371, Issued 11-19-04, Effective: 04-01-05, Implementation: 04-04-05)

A. Coding Applicable to Carriers & Fiscal Intermediaries (FIs)

Effective April 1, 2003, a National Coverage Decision was made to allow for Medicare coverage of Electrical Stimulation for the treatment of certain types of wounds. The type of wounds covered are chronic Stage III or Stage IV pressure ulcers, arterial ulcers, diabetic ulcers and venous stasis ulcers. All other uses of electrical stimulation for the treatment of wounds are not covered by Medicare. Electrical stimulation will not be covered as an initial treatment modality.

The use of electrical stimulation will only be covered after appropriate standard wound care has been tried for at least 30 days and there are no measurable signs of healing. If electrical stimulation is being used, wounds must be evaluated periodically by the treating physician but no less than every 30 days by a physician. Continued treatment with electrical stimulation is not covered if measurable signs of healing have not been demonstrated within any 30-day period of treatment. Additionally, electrical stimulation must be discontinued when the wound demonstrates a 100% epithelialzed wound bed.

Coverage policy can be found in Pub. 100-03, Medicare National Coverage Determinations Manual, Chapter 1, Section 270.1 (http://www.cms.hhs.gov/manuals/103_cov_determ/ncd103index.asp)

The applicable Healthcare Common Procedure Coding System (HCPCS) code for Electrical Stimulation and the covered effective date is as follows:

HCPCS	Definition	Effective Date
G0281	Electrical Stimulation, (unattended), to one or more areas for chronic Stage III and Stage IV pressure ulcers, arterial ulcers, diabetic ulcers and venous stasis ulcers not demonstrating measurable signs of healing after 30 days of conventional care as part of a therapy plan of care.	04/01/2003

Medicare will not cover the device used for the electrical stimulation for the treatment of wounds. However, Medicare will cover the service. Unsupervised home use of electrical stimulation will not be covered.

B. FI Billing Instructions

The applicable types of bills acceptable when billing for electrical stimulation services are 12X, 13X, 22X, 23X, 71X, 73X, 74X, 75X, and 85X. Chapter 25 of this manual provides general billing instructions that must be followed for bills submitted to FIs. FIs pay for electrical stimulation services under the Medicare Physician Fee Schedule for a hospital, Comprehensive Outpatient Rehabilitation Facility (CORF), Outpatient Rehabilitation Facility (ORF), Outpatient Physical Therapy (OPT) and Skilled Nursing Facility (SNF).

Payment methodology for independent Rural Health Clinic (RHC), provider-based RHCs, free-standing Federally Qualified Health Center (FQHC) and provider based FQHCs is made under the all-inclusive rate for the visit furnished to the RHC/FQHC patient to obtain the therapy service. Only one payment will be made for the visit furnished to the

RHC/FQHC patient to obtain the therapy service. As of April 1, 2005, RHCs/FQHCs are no longer required to report HCPCS codes when billing for these therapy services.

Payment Methodology for a Critical Access Hospital (CAH) is on a reasonable cost basis unless the CAH has elected the Optional Method and then the FI pays115% of the MPFS amount for the professional component of the HCPCS code in addition to the technical component.

In addition, the following revenues code must be used in conjunction with the HCPCS code identified:

Revenue Code	Description
420	Physical Therapy
430	Occupational Therapy
520	Federal Qualified Health Center *
521	Rural Health Center *
977, 978	Critical Access Hospital- method II CAH professional services only

* NOTE: As of April 1, 2005, RHCs/FQHCs are no longer required to report HCPCS codes when billing for these therapy services.

C. Carrier Claims

Carriers pay for Electrical Stimulation services billed with HCPCS codes G0281 based on the MPFS. Claims for Electrical Stimulation services must be billed on Form CMS-1500 or the electronic equivalent following instructions in chapter 12 of this manual (http://www.cms.hhs.gov/manuals/104_claims/clm104c12.pdf).

D. Coinsurance and Deductible

The Medicare contractor shall apply coinsurance and deductible to payments for these therapy services except for services billed to the FI by FQHCs. For FQHCs, only co-insurance applies.

100-04, 32, 11.2

Electromagnetic Therapy

(Rev.2998, Iss.7/25/14 Eff. w/imp. I-10; 01-01-12 - ASC X12, Imp. 8/25/14 ASC X12; w/imp. I-10)

A. HCPCS Coding Applicable to A/B MACs (A and B)

Effective July 1, 2004, a National Coverage Decision was made to allow for Medicare coverage of electromagnetic therapy for the treatment of certain types of wounds. The type of wounds covered are chronic Stage III or Stage IV pressure ulcers, arterial ulcers, diabetic ulcers and venous stasis ulcers. All other uses of electromagnetic therapy for the treatment of wounds are not covered by Medicare. Electromagnetic therapy will not be covered as an initial treatment modality.

The use of electromagnetic therapy will only be covered after appropriate standard wound care has been tried for at least 30 days and there are no measurable signs of healing. If electromagnetic therapy is being used, wounds must be evaluated periodically by the treating physician but no less than every 30 days. Continued treatment with electromagnetic therapy is not covered if measurable signs of healing have not been demonstrated within any 30-day period of treatment. Additionally, electromagnetic therapy must be discontinued when the wound demonstrates a 100% epithelialzed wound bed.

Coverage policy can be found in Pub. 100-03, Medicare National Coverage Determinations Manual, Chapter 1 section 270.1. (http://www.cms.hhs.gov/manuals/103_cov_determ/ncd103index.asp)

The applicable Healthcare Common Procedure Coding System (HCPCS) code for Electrical Stimulation and the covered effective date is as follows:

HCPCS	Definition	Effective Date
G0329	ElectromagneticTherapy, to one or more areas for chronic Stage III and Stage IV pressure ulcers, arterial ulcers, diabetic ulcers and venous stasis ulcers not demonstrating measurable signs of healing after 30 days of conventional care as part of a therapy plan of care.	07/01/2004

Medicare will not cover the device used for the electromagnetic therapy for the treatment of wounds. However, Medicare will cover the service. Unsupervised home use of electromagnetic therapy will not be covered.

B. A/B MAC (A) Billing Instructions

The applicable types of bills acceptable when billing for electromagnetic therapy services are 12X, 13X, 22X, 23X, 71X, 73X, 74X, 75X, and 85X. Chapter 25 of this manual provides general billing instructions that must be followed for bills submitted to A/B MACs (A). A/B MACs (A) pay for electromagnetic therapy services under the Medicare Physician Fee Schedule for a hospital, CORF, ORF, and SNF.

Payment methodology for independent (RHC), provider-based RHCs, free-standing FQHC and provider based FQHCs is made under the all-inclusive rate for the visit furnished to the RHC/FQHC patient to obtain the therapy service. Only one payment will be made for the visit furnished to the RHC/FQHC patient to obtain the therapy service. As of April 1, 2005, RHCs/FQHCs are no longer required to report HCPCS codes when billing for the therapy service.

Payment Methodology for a CAH is payment on a reasonable cost basis unless the CAH has elected the Optional Method and then the A/B MAC (A) pays pay 115% of the MPFS amount for the professional component of the HCPCS code in addition to the technical component.

© 2019 Optum360, LLC

In addition, the following revenues code must be used in conjunction with the HCPCS code identified:

Revenue Code	Description
420	Physical Therapy
430	Occupational Therapy
520	Federal Qualified Health Center *
521	Rural Health Center *
977, 978	Critical Access Hospital- method II CAH professional services only

* NOTE: As of April 1, 2005, RHCs/FQHCs are no longer required to report HCPCS codes when billing for the therapy service.

C. A/B MAC (B) Claims

A/B MACs (B) pay for Electromagnetic Therapy services billed with HCPCS codes G0329 based on the MPFS. Claims for electromagnetic therapy services must be billed using the ASC X12 837 professional claim format or Form CMS-1500 following instructions in chapter 12 of this manual (www.cms.hhs.gov/manuals/104_claims/clm104index.asp).

Payment information for HCPCS code G0329 will be added to the July 2004 update of the Medicare Physician Fee Schedule Database (MPFSD).

D. Coinsurance and Deductible

The Medicare contractor shall apply coinsurance and deductible to payments for electromagnetic therapy services except for services billed to the A/B MAC (A) by FQHCs. For FQHCs only co-insurance applies.

100-04, 32, 11.3.1

Policy

(Rev.2720, Issued: 06-10-2013, Effective: 08-02-12, Implementation: 07-01- 13)

Effective for claims with dates of service on or after August 2, 2012, contractors shall accept and pay for autologous platelet-rich plasma (PRP) only for the treatment of chronic non-healing diabetic, venous and/or pressure wounds only in the context of an approved clinical study in accordance with the coverage criteria outlined in Pub 100-03, chapter 1, section 270.3, of the NCD Manual.

100-04, 32, 11.3.2

Healthcare Common Procedure Coding System (HCPCS) Codes and Diagnosis Coding

(Rev.2998, Iss.7/25/14 Eff. w/imp. I-10; 01-01-12 - ASC X12, Imp. 8/25/14 ASC X12; w/imp. I-10)

HCPCS Code

Effective for claims with dates of service on or after August 2, 2012 Medicare providers shall report HCPCS code G0460 for PRP services.

If ICD-9 Diagnosis coding is applicable

For claims with dates of service on or after August 2, 2012, PRP, for the treatment of chronic non-healing diabetic, venous and/or pressure wounds only in the context of an approved clinical study must be billed using the following ICD codes:

- V70.7
- ICD-9 code from the approved list of diagnosis codes maintained by the Medicare contractor.

If ICD-10 Diagnosis coding is applicable

For claims with dates of service on or after the implementation of ICD-10, ICD-10 CM diagnosis coding is applicable.

- Z00.6
- ICD-10 code from the approved list of diagnosis codes maintained by the Medicare contractor.

Additional billing requirement:

The following modifier and condition code shall be reported when billing for PRP services only in the context of an approved clinical study:

- Q0 modifier
- Condition code 30 (for institutional claims only)
- Value Code D4 with an 8-digit clinical trial number. NOTE: This is optional and only applies to Institutional claims.

100-04, 32, 11.3.3

Types of Bill (TOB)

(Rev.2720, Issued: 06-10-2013, Effective: 08-02-12, Implementation: 07-01-13)

The applicable TOBs for PRP services are: 12X, 13X, 22X, 23X, 71X, 75X, 77X, and 85X.

100-04, 32, 11.3.5

Place of Service (POS) for Professional Claims

(Rev.2720, Issued: 06-10-2013, Effective: 08-02-12, Implementation: 07-01- 13)

Effective for claims with dates of service on or after August 2, 2012, place of service codes 11, 22, and 49 shall be used for PRP services.

100-04, 32, 11.3.6

Medicare Summary Notices (MSNs), Remittance Advice Remark Codes (RARCs), Claim Adjustment Reason Codes (CARCs) and Group Codes

(Rev.2998, Iss.7/25/14 Eff. w/imp. I-10; 01-01-12 - ASC X12, Imp. 8/25/14 ASC X12; w/imp. I-10)

Contractors shall use the following messages when returning to provider/returning as unprocessable claims when required information is not included on claims for autologous platelet-rich plasma (PRP) for the treatment of chronic non-healing diabetic, venous and/or pressure wounds only in the context of an approved clinical study:

CARC 16 - Claim/service lacks information or has submission/billing error(s) which is (are) needed for adjudication. At least one Remark Code must be provided (may be comprised of either the NCPDP Reject Reason Code, or Remittance Advice Remark Code that is not an ALERT.) NOTE: Refer to the 835 Healthcare Policy Identification Segment (loop 2110 Service Payment Information REF), if present.

RARC MA130 – Your claim contains incomplete and/or invalid information, and no appeal rights are afforded because the claim is unprocessable. Please submit a new claim with the complete/correct information.

Contractors shall deny claims for RPR services, HCPCS code G0460, when services are provided on other than TOBs 12X, 13X, 22X, 23X, 71X, 75X, 77X, and 85X using:

MSN 21.25: "This service was denied because Medicare only covers this service in certain settings."

Spanish Version: "El servicio fue denegado porque Medicare solamente lo cubre en ciertas situaciones."

CARC 58: "Treatment was deemed by the payer to have been rendered in an inappropriate or invalid place of service. NOTE: Refer to the 832 Healthcare Policy Identification Segment (loop 2110 Service payment Information REF), if present.

RARC N428: "Service/procedure not covered when performed in this place of service."

Group Code – CO (Contractual Obligation)

Contractors shall deny claims for PRP services for POS other than 11, 22, or 49 using the following:

MSN 21.25: "This service was denied because Medicare only covers this service in certain settings."

Spanish Version: "El servicio fue denegado porque Medicare solamente lo cubre en ciertas situaciones."

CARC 58: "Treatment was deemed by the payer to have been rendered in an inappropriate or invalid place of service. NOTE; Refer to the 835 Healthcare Policy Identification Segment (loop 2110 Service payment Information REF), if present.

RARC N428: "Service/procedure not covered when performed in this place of service."

Group Code – CO (Contractual Obligation)

100-04, 32, 40.1

Coverage Requirements

(Rev.125, 03-26-04)

Effective January 1, 2002, sacral nerve stimulation is covered for the treatment of urinary urge incontinence, urgency-frequency syndrome and urinary retention. Sacral nerve stimulation involves both a temporary test stimulation to determine if an implantable stimulator would be effective and a permanent implantation in appropriate candidates. Both the test and the permanent implantation are covered.

The following limitations for coverage apply to all indications:

- Patient must be refractory to conventional therapy (documented behavioral, pharmacologic and/or surgical corrective therapy) and be an appropriate surgical candidate such that implantation with anesthesia can occur.
- Patients with stress incontinence, urinary obstruction, and specific neurologic diseases (e.g., diabetes with peripheral nerve involvement) that are associated with secondary manifestations of the above three indications are excluded.
- Patient must have had a successful test stimulation in order to support subsequent implantation. Before a patient is eligible for permanent implantation, he/she must demonstrate a 50% or greater improvement through test stimulation. Improvement is measured through voiding diaries.

© 2019 Optum360, LLC

- Patient must be able to demonstrate adequate ability to record voiding diary data such that clinical results of the implant procedure can be properly evaluated.

100-04, 32, 60.4.1

Allowable Covered Diagnosis Codes

(Rev.2998, Issued: 07-25-14, Effective: Upon implementation of ICD-10; 01-01-12)

For services furnished on or after July 1, 2002, the applicable ICD-9-CM diagnosis code for this benefit is V43.3, organ or tissue replaced by other means; heart valve.

For services furnished on or after March 19, 2008, the applicable ICD-9-CM diagnosis codes for this benefit are:

V43.3 (organ or tissue replaced by other means; heart valve),

289.81 (primary hypercoagulable state),

451.0-451.9 (includes 451.11, 451.19, 451.2, 451.80-451.84, 451.89) (phlebitis & thrombophlebitis),

453.0-453.3 (other venous embolism & thrombosis),

453.40-453.49 (includes 453.40-453.42, 453.8-453.9) (venous embolism and thrombosis of the deep vessels of the lower extremity, and other specified veins/unspecified sites)

415.11-415.12, 415.19 (pulmonary embolism & infarction) or,

427.31 (atrial fibrillation (established) (paroxysmal)).

100-04, 32, 70

Billing Requirements for Islet Cell Transplantation for Beneficiaries in a National Institutes of Health (NIH) Clinical Trial

(Rev.986, Issued: 06-16-06, Effective: 05-01-06, Implementation: 07-31-06)

For services performed on or after October 1, 2004, Medicare will cover islet cell transplantation for patients with Type I diabetes who are participating in an NIH sponsored clinical trial. See Pub 100-04 (National Coverage Determinations Manual) section 260.3.1 for complete coverage policy.

The islet cell transplant may be done alone or in combination with a kidney transplant. Islet recipients will also need immunosuppressant therapy to prevent rejection of the transplanted islet cells. Routine follow-up care will be necessary for each trial patient. See Pub 100-04, section 310 for further guidance relative to routine care. All other uses for islet cell services will remain non-covered.

100-04, 32, 80

Billing of the Diagnosis and Treatment of Peripheral Neuropathy with Loss of Protective Sensation in People with Diabetes

(Rev.498, Issued: 03-11-05, Effective/Implementation: N/A)

Coverage Requirements - Peripheral neuropathy is the most common factor leading to amputation in people with diabetes. In diabetes, peripheral neuropathy is an anatomically diffuse process primarily affecting sensory and autonomic fibers; however, distal motor findings may be present in advanced cases. Long nerves are affected first, with symptoms typically beginning insidiously in the toes and then advancing proximally. This leads to loss of protective sensation (LOPS), whereby a person is unable to feel minor trauma from mechanical, thermal, or chemical sources. When foot lesions are present, the reduction in autonomic nerve functions may also inhibit wound healing.

Peripheral neuropathy with LOPS, secondary to diabetes, is a localized illness of the feet and falls within the regulation's exception to the general exclusionary rule (see 42 C.F.R. Sec.411.15(l)(l)(i)). Foot exams for people with diabetic peripheral neuropathy with LOPS are reasonable and necessary to allow for early intervention in serious complications that typically afflict diabetics with the disease.

Effective for services furnished on or after July 1, 2002, Medicare covers, as a physician service, an evaluation (examination and treatment) of the feet no more often than every 6 months for individuals with a documented diagnosis of diabetic sensory neuropathy and LOPS, as long as the beneficiary has not seen a foot care specialist for some other reason in the interim. LOPS shall be diagnosed through sensory testing with the 5.07 monofilament using established guidelines, such as those developed by the National Institute of Diabetes and Digestive and Kidney Diseases guidelines. Five sites should be tested on the plantar surface of each foot, according to the National Institute of Diabetes and Digestive and Kidney Diseases guidelines. The areas must be tested randomly since the loss of protective sensation may be patchy in distribution, and the patient may get clues if the test is done rhythmically. Heavily callused areas should be avoided. As suggested by the American Podiatric Medicine Association, an absence of sensation at two or more sites out of 5 tested on either foot when tested with the 5.07 Semmes-Weinstein monofilament must be present and documented to diagnose peripheral neuropathy with loss of protective sensation.

100-04, 32, 80.2

Applicable HCPCS Codes

(Rev.498, Issued: 03-11-05, Effective/Implementation: N/A)

G0245 - Initial physician evaluation and management of a diabetic patient with diabetic sensory neuropathy resulting in a loss of protective sensation (LOPS) which must include:

1. The diagnosis of LOPS;

2. A patient history;

3. A physical examination that consists of at least the following elements:

(a) visual inspection of the forefoot, hindfoot, and toe web spaces,

(b) evaluation of a protective sensation,

(c) evaluation of foot structure and biomechanics,

(d) evaluation of vascular status and skin integrity,

(e) evaluation and recommendation of footwear, and

4. Patient education.

G0246 - Follow-up physician evaluation and management of a diabetic patient with diabetic sensory neuropathy resulting in a loss of protective sensation (LOPS) to include at least the following:

1. a patient history;

2. a physical examination that includes:

(a) visual inspection of the forefoot, hindfoot, and toe web spaces,

(b) evaluation of protective sensation,

(c) evaluation of foot structure and biomechanics,

(d) evaluation of vascular status and skin integrity,

(e) evaluation and recommendation of footwear, and

3. patient education.

G0247 - Routine foot care by a physician of a diabetic patient with diabetic sensory neuropathy resulting in a LOPS to include if present, at least the following:

(1) local care of superficial (i.e., superficial to muscle and fascia) wounds;

(2) debridement of corns and calluses; and

(3) trimming and debridement of nails.

NOTE: Code G0247 must be billed on the same date of service with either G0245 or G0246 in order to be considered for payment.

The short descriptors for the above HCPCS codes are as follows:

G0245 - INITIAL FOOT EXAM PTLOPS

G0246 - FOLLOWUP EVAL OF FOOT PT LOP

G0247 - ROUTINE FOOTCARE PT W LOPS

100-04, 32, 80.3

80.3 - Diagnosis Codes

(Rev.2998, Issued: 07-25-14, Effective: Upon implementation of ICD-10; 01-01-12 - ASC X12, Implementation: 08-25-2014 - ASC X12; Upon Implementation of ICD-10)

Diagnosis Codes.--Providers should report one of the following diagnosis codes in conjunction with this benefit:

- If ICD-9-CM is applicable - 250.60, 250.61, 250.62, 250.63, and 357.2.
- If ICD-10-CM is applicable - E08.40, E0.842, E09.40, E09.42, E10.40, E10.41, E10.42, E10.43, E10.44, E10.49, E10.610, E11.40, E11.41, E11.42, E11.43, E11.44, E11.49, E11.610, E13.40, E13.41, E13.42, E13.43, E13.44, E13.49, E13.610

Coverage policy can be found in Pub. 100-03, Medicare National Coverage Determinations Manual, Chapter 1, section 70.2.1 Diabetic neuropathy w/ LOPs. (http://www.cms.hhs.gov/manuals/103_cov_determ/ncd103index.asp

100-04, 32, 80.6

80.6 - Editing Instructions for A/B MACs (A)

(Rev.2998, Issued: 07-25-14, Effective: Upon implementation of ICD-10; 01-01-12 - ASC X12, Implementation: 08-25-2014 - ASC X12; Upon Implementation of ICD-10)

Edit 1 - Implement diagnosis to procedure code edits to allow payment only for the LOPS codes, G0245, G0246, and G0247 when submitted with one of the following diagnosis codes

- If ICD-9-CM is applicable: 250.60, 250.61, 250.62, 250.63, or 357.2.
- If ICD-10-CM is applicable: E08.40, E08.42, E09.40, E09.42, E10.40, E10.41, E10.42, E10.43, E10.44, E10.49, E10.610, E11.40, E11.41, E11.42, E11.43, E11.44, E11.49, E11.610, E13.40, E13.41, E13.42, E13.43, E13.44, E13.49, E13.610

© 2019 Optum360, LLC

Deny these services when submitted without one of the appropriate diagnoses.

Use the same messages you currently use for procedure to diagnosis code denials. Edit 2 – Deny G0247 if it is not submitted on the same claim as G0245 or G0246.

Use MSN 21.21 - This service was denied because Medicare only covers this service under certain circumstances.

Use RA claim adjustment reason code 107 - The related or qualifying claim/service was not identified on this claim. NOTE: Refer to the 835 Healthcare Policy Identification Segment (loop 2110 Service Payment Information REF), if present.

100-04, 32, 80.8

CWF Utilization Edits

(Rev.1742, Issued: 05-22-09, Effective: 06-08-09, Implementation: 06-08-09)

Edit 1 - Should CWF receive a claim from an FI for G0245 or G0246 and a second claim from a contractor for either G0245 or G0246 (or vice versa) and they are different dates of service and less than 6 months apart, the second claim will reject. CWF will edit to allow G0245 or G0246 to be paid no more than every 6 months for a particular beneficiary, regardless of who furnished the service. If G0245 has been paid, regardless of whether it was posted as a facility or professional claim, it must be 6 months before G0245 can be paid again or G0246 can be paid. If G0246 has been paid, regardless of whether it was posted as a facility or professional claim, it must be 6 months before G0246 can be paid again or G0245 can be paid. CWF will not impose limits on how many times each code can be paid for a beneficiary as long as there has been 6 months between each service.

The CWF will return a specific reject code for this edit to the contractors and FIs that will be identified in the CWF documentation. Based on the CWF reject code, the contractors and FIs must deny the claims and return the following messages:

> MSN 18.4 -- This service is being denied because it has not been __ months since your last examination of this kind (NOTE: Insert 6 as the appropriate number of months.)
>
> RA claim adjustment reason code 96 - Non-covered charges, along with remark code M86 - Service denied because payment already made for same/similar procedure within set time frame.

Edit 2

The CWF will edit to allow G0247 to pay only if either G0245 or G0246 has been submitted and accepted as payable on the same date of service. CWF will return a specific reject code for this edit to the contractors and FIs that will be identified in the CWF documentation. Based on this reject code, contractors and FIs will deny the claims and return the following messages:

> MSN 21.21 - This service was denied because Medicare only covers this service under certain circumstances.
>
> RA claim adjustment reason code 107 - The related or qualifying claim/service was not identified on this claim.

Edit 3

Once a beneficiary's condition has progressed to the point where routine foot care becomes a covered service, payment will no longer be made for LOPS evaluation and management services. Those services would be considered to be included in the regular exams and treatments afforded to the beneficiary on a routine basis. The physician or provider must then just bill the routine foot care codes, per Pub 100-02, Chapter 15, Sec.290.

The CWF will edit to reject LOPS codes G0245, G0246, and/or G0247 when on the beneficiary's record it shows that one of the following routine foot care codes were billed and paid within the prior 6 months: 11055, 11056, 11057, 11719, 11720, and/or 11721.

The CWF will return a specific reject code for this edit to the contractors and FIs that will be identified in the CWF documentation. Based on the CWF reject code, the contractors and FIs must deny the claims and return the following messages:

> MSN 21.21 - This service was denied because Medicare only covers this service under certain circumstances.
>
> The RA claim adjustment reason code 96 - Non-covered charges, along with remark code M86 - Service denied because payment already made for same/similar procedure within set time frame.

100-04, 32, 110.5

DMERC Billing Instructions

(Rev.816, Issued: 01-20-06, Effective: 04-27-05, Implementation: 04-03-06)

Effective for dates of service on or after April 27, 2005, DMERCs shall allow payment for ultrasonic osteogenic stimulators with the following HCPCS codes:

- E0760 for low intensity ultrasound (include modifier "KF"), or;
- E1399 for other ultrasound stimulation (include modifier "KF")

100-04, 32, 120.1

Payment for Services and Supplies

(Rev.1430; Issued: 02-01-08; Effective: 01-01-08; Implementation: 03-03-08)

For an IOL inserted following removal of a cataract in a hospital, on either an outpatient or inpatient basis, that is paid under the hospital Outpatient Prospective Payment System (OPPS) or the Inpatient Prospective Payment System (IPPS), respectively; or in a Medicare-approved ambulatory surgical center (ASC) that is paid under the ASC fee schedule:

Medicare does not make separate payment to the hospital or ASC for an IOL inserted subsequent to extraction of a cataract. Payment for the IOL is packaged into the payment for the surgical cataract extraction/lens replacement procedure.

Any person or ASC, who presents or causes to be presented a bill or request for payment for an IOL inserted during or subsequent to cataract surgery for which payment is made under the ASC fee schedule, is subject to a civil money penalty.

For a P-C IOL or A-C IOL inserted subsequent to removal of a cataract in a hospital, on either an outpatient or inpatient basis, that is paid under the OPPS or the IPPS, respectively; or in a Medicare-approved ASC that is paid under the ASC fee schedule:

The facility shall bill for the removal of a cataract with insertion of a conventional IOL, regardless of whether a conventional, P-C IOL, or A-C IOL is inserted. When a beneficiary receives a P-C or A-C IOL following removal of a cataract, hospitals and ASCs shall report the same CPT code that is used to report removal of a cataract with insertion of a conventional IOL. Physicians, hospitals and ASCs may also report an additional HCPCS code, V2788, to indicate any additional charges that accrue when a P-C IOL or A-C IOL is inserted in lieu of a conventional IOL until Janaury 1, 2008. Effective for A-C IOL insertion services on or after January 1, 2008, physicians, hospitals and ASCs should use V2787 to report any additional charges that accrue. On or after January 1, 2008, physicians, hospitals, and ASCs should continue to report HCPCS code V2788 to indicate any additional charges that accrue for insertion of a P-C IOL. See Section 120.2 for coding guidelines.

There is no Medicare benefit category that allows payment of facility charges for services and supplies required to insert and adjust a P-C or A-C IOL following removal of a cataract that exceed the facility charges for services and supplies required for the insertion and adjustment of a conventional IOL.

There is no Medicare benefit category that allows payment of facility charges for subsequent treatments, services and supplies required to examine and monitor the beneficiary who receives a P-C or A-C IOL following removal of a cataract that exceeds the facility charges for subsequent treatments, services and supplies required to examine and monitor a beneficiary after cataract surgery followed by insertion of a conventional IOL.

A - For a P-C IOL or A-C IOL inserted in a physician's office

A physician shall bill for a conventional IOL, regardless of a whether a conventional, P-C IOL, or A-C IOL is inserted (see section 120.2, General Billing Requirements)

There is no Medicare benefit category that allows payment of physician charges for services and supplies required to insert and adjust a P-C or A-C IOL following removal of a cataract that exceed the physician charges for services and supplies for the insertion and adjustment of a conventional IOL.

There is no Medicare benefit category that allows payment of physician charges for subsequent treatments, service and supplies required to examine and monitor a beneficiary following removal of a cataract with insertion of a P-C or A-C IOL that exceed physician charges for services and supplies to examine and monitor a beneficiary following removal of a cataract with insertion of a conventional IOL.

B - For a P-C IOL or A-C IOL inserted in a hospital

A physician may not bill Medicare for a P-C or A-C IOL inserted during a cataract procedure performed in a hospital setting because the payment for the lens is included in the payment made to the facility for the surgical procedure.

There is no Medicare benefit category that allows payment of physician charges for services and supplies required to insert and adjust a P-C or A-C IOL following removal of a cataract that exceed the physician charges for services and supplies required for the insertion of a conventional IOL.

C - For a P-C IOL or A-C IOL inserted in an Ambulatory Surgical Center

Refer to Chapter 14, Section 40.3 for complete guidance on payment for P-C IOL or A-C IOL in Ambulatory Surgical Centers.

100-04, 32, 120.2

Coding and General Billing Requirements

(Rev.1430; Issued: 02-01-08; Effective: 01-01-08; Implementation: 03-03-08)

Physicians and hospitals must report one of the following Current Procedural Terminology (CPT) codes on the claim:

© 2019 Optum360, LLC

- 66982 - Extracapsular cataract removal with insertion of intraocular lens prosthesis (one stage procedure), manual or mechanical technique (e.g., irrigation and aspiration or phacoemulsification), complex requiring devices or techniques not generally used in routine cataract surgery (e.g., iris expansion device, suture support for intraocular lens, or primary posterior capsulorrhexis) or performed on patients in the amblyogenic development stage.
- 66983 - Intracapsular cataract with insertion of intraocular lens prosthesis (one stage procedure)
- 66984 - Extracapsular cataract removal with insertion of intraocular lens prosthesis (one stage procedure), manual or mechanical technique (e.g., irrigation and aspiration or phacoemulsification)
- 66985 - Insertion of intraocular lens prosthesis (secondary implant), not associated with concurrent cataract extraction
- 66986 - Exchange of intraocular lens

In addition, physicians inserting a P-C IOL or A-C IOL in an office setting may bill code V2632 (posterior chamber intraocular lens) for the IOL. Medicare will make payment for the lens based on reasonable cost for a conventional IOL. Place of Service (POS) = 11.

Effective for dates of service on and after January 1, 2006, physician, hospitals and ASCs may also bill the non-covered charges related to the P-C function of the IOL using HCPCS code V2788. Effective for dates of service on and after January 22, 2007 through January 1, 2008, non-covered charges related to A-C function of the IOL can be billed using HCPCS code V2788. The type of service indicator for the non-covered billed charges is Q. (The type of service is applied by the Medicare carrier and not the provider). Effective for A-C IOL insertion services on or after January 1, 2008, physicians, hospitals and ASCs should use V2787 rather than V2788 to report any additional charges that accrue.

When denying the non-payable charges submitted with V2787 or V2788, contractors shall use an appropriate Medical Summary Notice (MSN) such as 16.10 (Medicare does not pay for this item or service) and an appropriate claim adjustment reason code such as 96 (non-covered charges) for claims submitted with the non-payable charges.

Hospitals and physicians may use the proper CPT code(s) to bill Medicare for evaluation and management services usually associated with services following cataract extraction surgery, if appropriate.

A - Applicable Bill Types

The hospital applicable bill types are 12X, 13X, 83X and 85X.

B - Other Special Requirements for Hospitals

Hospitals shall continue to pay CAHs method 2 claims under current payment methodologies for conditional IOLs.

100-04, 32, 130

External Counterpulsation (ECP) Therapy

(Rev.898, Issued: 03-31-06; Effective/Implementation Dates: 03-31-06)

Commonly referred to as enhanced external counterpulsation, is a non-invasive outpatient treatment for coronary artery disease refractory medical and/or surgical therapy. Effective for dates of service July 1, 1999, and after, Medicare will cover ECP when its use is in patients with stable angina (Class III or Class IV, Canadian Cardiovascular Society Classification or equivalent classification) who, in the opinion of a cardiologist or cardiothoracic surgeon, are not readily amenable to surgical intervention, such as PTCA or cardiac bypass, because:

- Their condition is inoperable, or at high risk of operative complications or post-operative failure;
- Their coronary anatomy is not readily amenable to such procedures; or
- They have co-morbid states that create excessive risk.

(Refer to Publication 100-03, section 20.20 for further coverage criteria.)

100-04, 32, 130.1

Billing and Payment Requirements

(Rev.898, Issued: 03-31-06; Effective/Implementation Dates: 03-31-06)

Effective for dates of service on or after January 1, 2000, use HCPCS code G0166 (External counterpulsation, per session) to report ECP services. The codes for external cardiac assist (92971), ECG rhythm strip and report (93040 or 93041), pulse oximetry (94760 or 94761) and plethysmography (93922 or 93923) or other monitoring tests for examining the effects of this treatment are not clinically necessary with this service and should not be paid on the same day, unless they occur in a clinical setting not connected with the delivery of the ECP. Daily evaluation and management service, e.g., 99201-99205, 99211-99215, 99217-99220, 99241-99245, cannot be billed with the ECP treatments. Any evaluation and management service must be justified with adequate documentation of the medical necessity of the visit. Deductible and coinsurance apply.

100-04, 32, 140.2.2.1

Correct Place of Service (POS) Code for CR and ICR Services on Professional Claims

(Rev.3058, Issued: 08-29-14, Effective: 02-18-14, Implementation: 08- 18-14))

Effective for claims with dates of service on and after January 1, 2010, place of service (POS) code 11 shall be used for CR and ICR services provided in a physician's office and POS 22 shall be used for services provided in a hospital outpatient setting. All other POS codes shall be denied. Contractors shall adjust their prepayment procedure edits as appropriate.

The following messages shall be used when contractors deny CR and ICR claims for POS:

Claim Adjustment Reason Code (CARC) 171 – Payment is denied when performed/billed by this type of provider in this type of facility.

NOTE: Refer to the 832 Healthcare Policy Identification Segment (loop 2110 Service payment Information REF), if present.

Remittance Advice Remark Code (RARC) N428 - Service/procedure not covered when performed in this place of service.

Medicare Summary Notice (MSN) 21.25 - This service was denied because Medicare only covers this service in certain settings.

Group Code PR (Patient Responsibility) - Where a claim is received with the GA modifier indicating that a signed ABN is on file.

Group Code CO (Contractor Responsibility) – Where a claim is received with the GZ modifier indicating that no signed ABN is on file.

100-04, 32, 140.2.2.2

140.2.2.2 – Requirements for CR and ICR Services on Institutional Claims

(Rev.3084, Issued: 10-03-14, Effective: 05-06-14, Implementation: 11-04-14)

Effective for claims with dates of service on and after January 1, 2010, contractors shall pay for CR and ICR services when submitted on Types of Bill (TOBs) 13X and 85X only. All other TOBs shall be denied.

The following messages shall be used when contractors deny CR and ICR claims for TOBs other than 13X and 85X:

Claim Adjustment Reason Code (CARC) 171 – Payment is denied when performed/billed by this type of provider in this type of facility. NOTE: Refer to the 835 Healthcare Policy Identification Segment (loop 2110 Service Payment Information REF), if present.

Remittance Advice Remark Code (RARC) N428 - Service/procedure not covered when performed in this place of service.

Medicare Summary Notice (MSN) 21.25 - This service was denied because Medicare only covers this service in certain settings.

Group Code PR (Patient Responsibility) – Where a claim is received with the GA modifier indicating that a signed ABN is on file.

Group Code CO (Contractor Responsibility) – Where a claim is received with the GZ modifier indicating that no signed ABN is on file.

100-04, 32, 140.3

Intensive Cardiac Rehabilitation Program Services Furnished On or After January 1, 2010

(Rev.4222, Issued: 02-01-19, Effective: 02-09-18, Implementation: 03-19-19)

As specified at 42 CFR 410.49, Medicare covers intensive cardiac rehabilitation items and

services for patients who have experienced one or more of the following:

- • An acute myocardial infarction within the preceding 12 months;
- • A coronary artery bypass surgery;
- • Current stable angina pectoris;
- • Heart valve repair or replacement;
- • Percutaneous transluminal coronary angioplasty or coronary stenting;
- • A heart or heart-lung transplant.

Effective February 9, 2018, section 51004 of the Bipartisan Budget Act (BBA) of 2018, Pub. L. No. 115-123 (2018), amended section 1861(eee)(4)(B) of the Social Security Act to expand coverage in an intensive cardiac rehabilitation program to additional conditions:

- *table, chronic heart failure defined as patients with left ventricular ejection fraction of 35% or less and New York Heart Association (NYHA) class II to IV symptoms despite being on optimal heart failure therapy for at least 6 weeks; or*

© 2019 Optum360, LLC

- *Any additional condition for which the Secretary has determined that a cardiac rehabilitation program shall be covered, unless the Secretary determines, using the same process used to determine that the condition is covered for a cardiac rehabilitation program, that such coverage is not supported by the clinical evidence.*

***NOTE**: CMS plans to amend our intensive cardiac rehabilitation regulations specified at 42 CFR 410.49 to reflect this expanded coverage. CMS anticipates that the changes will be included in the 2020 Medicare Physician Fee Schedule notice of proposed rulemaking. However, because the expanded coverage under the statutory change was effective on enactment, expanded coverage for these conditions will be made effective for services furnished on or after February 9, 2018.*

Intensive cardiac rehabilitation programs must include the following components:

- Physician-prescribed exercise each day cardiac rehabilitation items and services are furnished;
- Cardiac risk factor modification, including education, counseling, and behavioral intervention at least once during the program, tailored to patients' individual needs;
- Psychosocial assessment;
- • Outcomes assessment; and,
- An individualized treatment plan detailing how components are utilized for each patient.

Intensive cardiac rehabilitation programs must be approved by Medicare. In order to be approved, a program must demonstrate through peer-reviewed published research that it has accomplished one or more of the following for its patients:

- • Positively affected the progression of coronary heart disease;
- • Reduced the need for coronary bypass surgery; and,
- • Reduced the need for percutaneous coronary interventions.

An intensive cardiac rehabilitation program must also demonstrate through peer-reviewed published research that it accomplished a statistically significant reduction in five or more of the following measures for patients from their levels before cardiac rehabilitation services to after cardiac rehabilitation services:

- Low density lipoprotein;
- Triglycerides;
- Body mass index;
- Systolic blood pressure;
- Diastolic blood pressure; and,
- The need for cholesterol, blood pressure, and diabetes medications.

Intensive cardiac rehabilitation items and services must be furnished in a physician's office or a hospital outpatient setting. All settings must have a physician immediately available and accessible for medical consultations and emergencies at all times items and services are being furnished under the program. This provision is satisfied if the physician meets the requirements for direct supervision of physician office services as specified at 42 CFR 410.26 and for hospital outpatient therapeutic services as specified at 42 CFR 410.27. As specified at 42 CFR 410.49(f)(2), ICR program sessions are limited to 72 1-hour sessions, up to 6 sessions per day, over a period of up to 18 weeks.

100-04, 32, 140.3.1

Coding Requirements for Intensive Cardiac Rehabilitation Services Furnished On or After January 1, 2010

(Rev.1882, Issued: 12-21-09; Effective Date: 01-01-10; Implementation Date: 01-04-10)

The following are the applicable HCPCS codes for intensive cardiac rehabilitation services:

G0422 (Intensive cardiac rehabilitation; with or without continuous ECG monitoring, with exercise, per hour, per session)

G0423 (Intensive cardiac rehabilitation; with or without continuous ECG monitoring, without exercise, per hour, per session)

Effective for dates of service on or after January 1, 2010, hospitals and practitioners may report a maximum of 6 1-hour sessions per day. In order to report one session of cardiac rehabilitation services in a day, the duration of treatment must be at least 31 minutes. Additional sessions of intensive cardiac rehabilitation services beyond the first session may only be reported in the same day if the duration of treatment is 31 minutes or greater beyond the hour increment. In other words, in order to report 6 sessions of intensive cardiac rehabilitation services on a given date of service, the first five sessions would account for 60 minutes each and the sixth session would account for at least 31 minutes. If several shorter periods of intensive cardiac rehabilitation services are furnished on a given day, the minutes of service during those periods must be added together for reporting in 1-hour session increments.

Example: If the patient receives 20 minutes of intensive cardiac rehabilitation services in the day, no intensive cardiac rehabilitation session may be reported because less than 31 minutes of services were furnished.

Example: If a patient receives 20 minutes of intensive cardiac rehabilitation services in the morning and 35 minutes of intensive cardiac rehabilitation services in the afternoon of a single day, the hospital or practitioner would report 1 session of intensive cardiac rehabilitation services under 1 unit of the appropriate HCPCS G-code for the total duration of 55 minutes of intensive cardiac rehabilitation services on that day.

Example: If the patient receives 70 minutes of intensive cardiac rehabilitation services in the morning and 25 minutes of intensive cardiac rehabilitation services in the afternoon of a single day, the hospital or practitioner would report two sessions of intensive cardiac rehabilitation services under the appropriate HCPCS G-code(s) because the total duration of intensive cardiac rehabilitation services on that day of 95 minutes exceeds 90 minutes.

Example: If the patient receives 70 minutes of intensive cardiac rehabilitation services in the morning and 85 minutes of intensive cardiac rehabilitation services in the afternoon of a single day, the hospital or practitioner would report three sessions of intensive cardiac rehabilitation services under the appropriate HCPCS G-code(s) because the total duration of intensive cardiac rehabilitation services on that day is 155 minutes, which exceeds 150 minutes and is less than 211 minutes.

100-04, 32, 180.4

Claim Adjustment Reason Codes, Remittance Advice Remark Codes, Group Codes, and Medicare Summary Notice Messages

(Rev 2544, Issued: 09-13-2012, Effective: 10-01-2012, Implementation: 10-01-2012)

Contractors shall use the appropriate claim adjustment reason codes (CARCs), remittance advice remark codes (RARCs), group codes, or Medicare summary notice (MSN) messages when denying payment for alcohol misuse screening and alcohol misuse behavioral counseling sessions:

- For RHC and FQHC claims that contain screening for alcohol misuse HCPCS code G0442 and alcohol misuse counseling HCPCS code G0443 with another encounter/visit with the same line item date of service, use group code CO and reason code:
  - Claim Adjustment Reason Code (CARC) 97 – The benefit for this service is included in the payment/allowance for another service/procedure that has already been adjudicated. Note: Refer to the 835 Healthcare Policy Identification Segment (loop 2110 Service Payment Information REF) if present
- Denying claims containing HCPCS code G0442 and HCPCS code G0443 submitted on a TOB other than 13X, 71X, 77X, and 85X:
  - Claim Adjustment Reason Code (CARC) 5 - The procedure code/bill type is inconsistent with the place of service. Note: Refer to the 835 Healthcare Policy Identification Segment (loop 2110 Service Payment Information REF) if present
  - Remittance Advice Remark Code (RARC) M77 – Missing/incomplete/invalid place of service
  - Group Code PR (Patient Responsibility) assigning financial liability to the beneficiary, if a claim is received with a GA modifier indicating a signed ABN is on file.
  - Group Code CO (Contractual Obligation) assigning financial liability to theprovider, if a claim is received with a GZ modifier indicating no signed ABN is on file.

NOTE: For modifier GZ, use CARC 50 and MSN 8.81 per instructions in CR 7228/TR 2148.

- Denying claims that contains more than one alcohol misuse behavioral counseling session G0443 on the same date of service:
  - Medicare Summary Notice (MSN) 15.6 – The information provided does not support the need for this many services or items within this period of time.
  - Claim Adjustment Reason Code (CARC) 151 – Payment adjusted because the payer deems the information submitted does not support this many/frequency of services.
  - Remittance Advice Remark Code (RARC) M86 – Service denied because payment already made for same/similar procedure within set time frame.

© 2019 Optum360, LLC

- Group Code PR (Patient Responsibility) assigning financial liability to the beneficiary, if a claim is received with a GA modifier indicating a signed ABN is on file.
- Group Code CO (Contractual Obligation) assigning financial liability to the provider, if a claim is received with a GZ modifier indicating no signed ABN is on file.

NOTE: For modifier GZ, use CARC 50 and MSN 8.81 per instructions in CR 7228/TR 2148.

- Denying claims that are not submitted from the appropriate provider specialties:
  - Medicare Summary Notice (MSN) 21.18 – This item or service is not covered when performed or ordered by this provider.
  - Claim Adjustment Reason Code (CARC) 185 - The rendering provider is not eligible to perform the service billed. NOTE: Refer to the 835 Healthcare Policy Identification Segment (loop 2110 Service Payment Information REF), if present.
  - Remittance Advice Remark Code (RARC) N95 - This provider type/provider specialty may not bill this service.
  - Group Code PR (Patient Responsibility) assigning financial liability to the beneficiary, if a claim is received with a GA modifier indicating a signed ABN is on file.
  - Group Code CO (Contractual Obligation) assigning financial liability to the provider, if a claim is received with a GZ modifier indicating no signed ABN is on file.

NOTE: For modifier GZ, use CARC 50 and MSN 8.81 per instructions in CR 7228/TR 2148.

- Denying claims without the appropriate POS code:
  - Medicare Summary Notice (MSN) 21.25 – This service was denied because Medicare only covers this service in certain settings.
  - Claim Adjustment Reason Code (CARC) 58 – Treatment was deemed by the payer to have been rendered in an inappropriate or invalid place of service.

Note: Refer to the 835 Healthcare Policy Identification Segment (loop 2110 Service Payment Information REF) if present.

  - Remittance Advice Remark Code (RARC) N428 – Not covered when performed in this place of service.
  - Group Code PR (Patient Responsibility) assigning financial liability to the beneficiary, if a claim is received with a GA modifier indicating a signed ABN is on file.
  - Group Code CO (Contractual Obligation) assigning financial liability to the provider, if a claim is received with a GZ modifier indicating no signed ABN is on file.

NOTE: For modifier GZ, use CARC 50 and MSN 8.81 per instructions in CR 7228/TR 2148.

- Denying claims for alcohol misuse screening HCPCS code G0442 more than once in a 12-month period, and denying alcohol misuse counseling sessions HCPCS code G0443 more than four times in the same 12-month period:
  - Medicare Summary Notice (MSN) 20.5 – These services cannot be paid because your benefits are exhausted at this time.
  - Claim Adjustment Reason Code (CARC) 119 – Benefit maximum for this time period or occurrence has been reached.
  - Remittance Advice Remark Code (RARC) N362 – The number of Days or Units of service exceeds our acceptable maximum.
  - Group Code PR (Patient Responsibility) assigning financial liability to the beneficiary, if a claim is received with a GA modifier indicating a signed ABN is on file.
  - Group Code CO (Contractual Obligation) assigning financial liability to the provider, if a claim is received with a GZ modifier indicating no signed ABN is on file.

NOTE: For modifier GZ, use CARC 50 and MSN 8.81 per instructions in CR 7228/TR 2148.

- Denying claims for alcohol misuse counseling session HCPCS code G0443 when there is no claim in history for the screening service HCPCS code G0442 in the prior 12 months:
  - Medicare Summary Notice (MSN) 16.26 – Medicare does not pay for services or items related to a procedure that has not been approved or billed.
  - Claim Adjustment Reason Code (CARC) B15 – This service/procedure requires that a qualifying service/procedure be received and covered. The qualifying other service/procedure has not been received/adjudicated. Note: Refer to the 835 Healthcare Policy Identification Segment (loop 2110 Service Payment Information REF), if present.
  - Remittance Advice Remark Code (RARC) M16 – Alert: Please see our web site, mailings, or bulletins for more details concerning this policy/procedure/decision.
  - Group Code PR (Patient Responsibility) assigning financial liability to the beneficiary, if a claim is received with a modifier indicating a signed ABN is on file.
  - Group Code CO (Contractual Obligation) assigning financial liability to the provider, if a claim is received without a modifier indicating no signed ABN is on file.

100-04, 32, 180.5

Additional CWF and Contractor Requirements

(Rev 2544, Issued: 09-13-2012, Effective: 10-01-2012, Implementation: 10-01-2012)

- When applying frequency, CWF shall count 11 full months following the month of the last alcohol misuse screening visit, G0442, before allowing subsequent payment of another G0442 screening.
- CWF shall reject incoming claims when G0443 PROF is billed if four G0443 services have been billed and posted to the BEHV auxiliary file within the 12 month period.
- CWF shall continue to reject incoming claims with consistency error code '32#3' when HCPCS code G0442 PROF and HCPCS code G0443 PROF are billed on same day for TOB 71X, 77X, 85X with 096X, 097X and 098X.
- Contractors and CWF shall use the last date of G0442 PROF for counting the 12-month period for G0443 PROF services.
  - Contractors and CWF shall apply all the same TOBs (13x,71x, 77x and 85x with Rev.Code 96, 97 and 98) POS (11, 22, 49 and 71), no deductible/co-insurance and institutional/professional processing for G0443 that was implemented for G0442 in CR 7633.
- If a claim with G0442 is cancelled, CWF shall do a look back for claims with G0443 and create an IUR (Information Unsolicited Response) along with a Trailer '24' back to the contractor to reject the G0443 claim(s) paid within the 12 month period of the G0442 claims.
- CWF shall display the number of counseling sessions remaining for G0443 PROF on all CWF provider query screens (HUQA, HIQA, HIQH, ELGA, ELGB, ELGH).
- CWF shall display the remaining PROF services counting DOWN from four (4) for the HCPCS code 'G0443' on the MBD/NGD extract file.
  - CWF shall calculate a next eligible date for G0442 PROF and G0443 PROF for a given beneficiary.
  - The calculation shall include all applicable factors including beneficiary Part B entitlement status, beneficiary claims history and utilization rules.
  - When there is no next eligible date, the CWF provider query screens shall display an 8-position alpha code in the date field to indicate why there is not a next eligible date.
  - Any change to beneficiary master data or claims data that would result in a change to any next eligible date shall result in an update to the beneficiary's next eligible date.

NOTE: If G0442 is not paid, the beneficiary is not eligible for G0443.

  - CWF shall create a utility to remove previously posted G0442 TECH for the AUX file.
  - CWF shall remove G0442/G0443 TECH from editing, MBD, NGD, Provider Inquiry screens and all other applicable areas (i.e., HICR) previously done under CR 7633.

Frequency Requirements

When applying frequency, CWF shall count 11 full months following the month of the last alcohol misuse screening visit, G0442, before allowing subsequent payment of another G0442 screening. Additionally, CWF shall create an edit to allow alcohol misuse brief behavioral counseling, HCPCS G0443, no more than 4 times in a 12-month period. CWF shall also count four alcohol misuse counseling sessions HCPCS G0443 in the same 12- month period used for G0442 counting from the date the G0442 screening session was billed.

When applying frequency limitations to G0442 screening on the same date of service as G0443 counseling, CWF shall allow both a claim for the professional service and a

© 2019 Optum360, LLC

claim for a facility fee. CWF shall identify the following institutional claims as facility fee claims for screening services: TOB 13X, TOB 85X when the revenue code is not 096X, 097X, or 098X. CWF shall identify all other claims as professional service claims for screening services (professional claims, and institutional claims with TOB 71X, 77X, and 85X when the revenue code is 096X, 097X, or 098X).

NOTE: This does not apply to RHCs and FQHCs.

100-04, 32, 250.1

Coverage Requirements

(Rev.1889, Issued: 01-08-10; Effective Date: 08-03-09; Implementation Date: 04-05-10)

Effective August 3, 2009, pharmacogenomic testing to predict warfarin responsiveness is covered only when provided to Medicare beneficiaries who are candidates for anticoagulation therapy with warfarin; i.e., have not been previously tested for CYP2C9 or VKORC1 alleles; and have received fewer than five days of warfarin in the anticoagulation regimen for which the testing is ordered; and only then in the context of a prospective, randomized, controlled clinical study when that study meets certain criteria as outlined in Pub 100-03, section 90.1, of the NCD Manual.

NOTE: A new temporary HCPCS Level II code effective August 3, 2009, G9143, warfarin responsiveness testing by genetic technique using any method, any number of specimen(s), was developed to enable implementation of CED for this purpose.

100-04, 32, 250.2

Billing Requirements

(Rev.1889, Issued: 01-08-10; Effective Date: 08-03-09; Implementation Date: 04-05-10)

Institutional clinical trial claims for pharmacogenomic testing for warfarin response are identified through the presence of all of the following elements:

Value Code D4 and 8-digit clinical trial number (when present on the claim) - Refer to Transmittal 310, Change Request 5790, dated January 18, 2008;

ICD-9 diagnosis code V70.7 - Refer to Transmittal 310, Change Request 5790, dated January 18, 2008;

Condition Code 30 - Refer to Transmittal 310, Change Request 5790, dated January 18, 2008;

HCPCS modifier Q0: outpatient claims only - Refer to Transmittal 1418, Change Request 5805, dated January 18, 2008; and,

HCPCS code G9143 (mandatory with the April 2010 Integrated Outpatient Code Editor (IOCE) and the January 2011 Clinical Laboratory Fee Schedule (CLFS) updates. Prior to these times, any trials should bill FIs for this test as they currently do absent these instructions, and the FIs should process and pay those claims accordingly.)

Practitioner clinical trial claims for pharmacogenomic testing for warfarin response are identified through the presence of all of the following elements:

ICD-9 diagnosis code V70.7;

8-digit clinical trial number(when present on the claim);

HCPCS modifier Q0; and HCPCS code G9143 (to be carrier priced for claims with dates of service on and after August 3, 2009, that are processed prior to the January 2011 CLFS update.)

100-04, 32, 260.1

Policy

(Rev.2105, Issued: 11-24-10, Effective: 03-23-10, Implementation: 07-06-10)

The Centers for Medicare & Medicaid Services (CMS) received a request for national coverage of treatments for facial lipodystrophy syndrome (LDS) for human immunodeficiency virus (HIV)-infected Medicare beneficiaries. Facial LDS is often characterized by a loss of fat that results in a facial abnormality such as severely sunken cheeks. This fat loss can arise as a complication of HIV and/or highly active antiretroviral therapy. Due to their appearance and stigma of the condition, patients with facial LDS may become depressed, socially isolated, and in some cases may stop their HIV treatments in an attempt to halt or reverse this complication.

Effective for claims with dates of service on and after March 23, 2010, dermal injections for facial LDS are only reasonable and necessary using dermal fillers approved by the Food and Drug Administration for this purpose, and then only in HIV-infected beneficiaries who manifest depression secondary to the physical stigmata of HIV treatment.

100-04, 32, 260.2.1

Healthcare Common Procedural Coding System (HCPCS), Applicable Diagnosis Codes and Procedure Code

(Rev.3050, Iss. 08/22/14, Eff. 9/23/14, I-10 W/imp. I-1; Imp.9/23/14, I-10 W/imp. I-10)

A - Hospital Outpatient Claims

For hospital outpatient claims, hospitals must bill covered dermal injections for treatment of facial LDS by having all of the required elements on the claim:

- A line with HCPCS codes Q2026 or Q2027 with a Line Item Date of service (LIDOS) on or after March 23, 2010,
- A line with HCPCS code G0429 with a LIDOS on or after March 23, 2010,
- If ICD-9-CM is applicable, ICD-9-CM diagnosis codes 042 (HIV) and 272.6 (Lipodystrophy) or,
- If ICD-10-CM is applicable, ICD-10-CM diagnosis codes B20 Human Immunodeficiency Virus (HIV) disease and E88.1 Lipodystrophy, not elsewhere classified The applicable NCD is 250.5 Facial Lipodystrophy.

B - Outpatient Prospective Payment System (OPPS) Hospitals or Ambulatory Surgical Centers (ASCs):

For line item dates of service on or after March 23, 2010, and until HCPCS codes Q2026 and Q2027 are billable, facial LDS claims shall contain a temporary HCPCS code C9800, instead of HCPCS G0429 and HCPCS Q2026/Q2027, as shown above.

C - Hospital Inpatient Claims

Hospitals must bill covered dermal injections for treatment of facial LDS by having all of the required elements on the claim:

- Discharge date on or after March 23, 2010,
- If ICD-9-CM is applicable,
  - ICD-9-CM procedure code 86.99 (other operations on skin and subcutaneous tissue, i.e., injection of filler material), or
  - ICD-9-CM diagnosis codes 042 (HIV) and 272.6 (Lipodystrophy)
- If ICD-10-PCS is applicable, o ICD-10-PCS procedure code 3E00XGC Introduction of Other Therapeutic Substance into Skin and Mucous Membrances, External Approach, or
  - ICD-10-CM diagnosis codes B20 Human Immundodeficiency Virus [HIV] disease and E88.1 Lipodystrophy not elsewhere classified.

A diagnosis code for a comorbidity of depression may also be required for coverage on an outpatient and/or inpatient basis as determined by the individual Medicare contractor's policy.

100-04, 32, 260.2.2

Practitioner Billing Instructions

(Rev.2998, Iss.7/25/14 Eff. w/imp. I-10; 01-01-12 - ASC X12, Imp. 8/25/14 ASC X12; w/imp. I-10)

Practitioners must bill covered claims for dermal injections for treatment of facial LDS by having all of the required elements on the claim:

Performed in a non-facility setting:

- A line with HCPCS codes Q2026 or Q2027 with a LIDOS on or after March 23, 2010,
- A line with HCPCS code G0429 with a LIDOS on or after March 23, 2010,
- If ICD-9-CM applies, diagnosis codes 042 (HIV) and 272.6 (Lipodystrophy) or,
- If ICD-10-CM applies, diagnosis codes B20 Human Immunodeficiency Virus (HIV) disease and E88.1 (Lipodystrophy not elsewhere classified).

NOTE: A diagnosis code for a comorbidity of depression may also be required for coverage based on the individual Medicare contractor's policy.

Performed in a facility setting:

- A line with HCPCS code G0429 with a LIDOS on or after March 23, 2010,
- If ICD-9 applies, ICD-9-CM diagnosis codes 042 (HIV) and 272.6 (Lipodystrophy) or
- If ICD-10 applies, ICD-10-CM diagnosis codes B20 Human Immundodeficiency Virus (HIV) disease and E88.1 (Lipodystrophy not elsewhere classified).

NOTE: A diagnosis code for a comorbidity of depression may also be required for coverage based on the individual Medicare contractor's policy.

100-04, 32, 280.1

Autologous Cellular Immunotherapy Treatment of Prostate Cancer

(Rev.2380, Issued: 01-06-12, Effective: 06-30-11, Implementation: 08-08-11)

Effective for services furnished on or after June 30, 2011, a National Coverage Determination (NCD) provides coverage of sipuleucel-T (PROVENGE®) for patients

© 2019 Optum360, LLC

with asymptomatic or minimally symptomatic metastatic, castrate-resistant (hormone refractory) prostate cancer. Conditions of Medicare Part A and Medicare Part B coverage for sipuleucel-T are located in the Medicare NCD Manual, Publication 100-03, section 110.22.

100-04, 32, 280.2

Healthcare Common Procedure Coding System (HCPCS) Codes and Diagnosis Coding

(Rev.2380, Issued: 01-06-12, Effective: 06-30-11, Implementation: 08-08-11)

HCPCS Codes

Effective for claims with dates of service on June 30, 2011, Medicare providers shall report one of the following HCPCS codes for PROVENGE®:

- C9273 - Sipuleucel-T, minimum of 50 million autologous CD54+ cells activated with PAP-GM-CSF, including leukapheresis and all other preparatory procedures, per infusion, or
- J3490 - Unclassified Drugs, or
- J3590 - Unclassified Biologics.

NOTE: Contractors shall continue to process claims for HCPCS code C9273, J3490, and J3590, with dates of service June 30, 2011, as they do currently.

Effective for claims with dates of service on and after July 1, 2011, Medicare providers shall report the following HCPCS code:

- Q2043 - Sipuleucel-T, minimum of 50 million autologous CD54+ cells activated with PAP-GM-CSF, including leukapheresis and all other preparatory procedures, per infusion; short descriptor, Sipuleucel-T auto CD54+.

ICD-9 Diagnosis Coding

For claims with dates of service on and after July 1, 2011, for PROVENGE®, the on-label indication of asymptomatic or minimally symptomatic metastatic, castrate-resistant (hormone refractory) prostate cancer, must be billed using ICD-9 code 185 (malignant neoplasm of prostate) and at least one of the following ICD-9 codes:

ICD-9	Description
196.1	Secondary and unspecified malignant neoplasm of intrathoracic lymph nodes
196.2	Secondary and unspecified malignant neoplasm of intra-abdominal lymph nodes
196.5	Secondary and unspecified malignant neoplasm of lymph nodes of inguinal region and lower limb
196.6	Secondary and unspecified malignant neoplasm of intrapelvic lymph nodes
196.8	Secondary and unspecified malignant neoplasm of lymph nodes of multiple sites
196.9	Secondary and unspecified malignant neoplasm of lymph node site unspecified – The spread of cancer to and establishment in the lymph nodes.
197.0	Secondary malignant neoplasm of lung – Cancer that has spread from the original (primary) tumor to the lung. The spread of cancer to the lung. This may be from a primary lung cancer, or from a cancer at a distant site.
197.7	Malignant neoplasm of liver secondary – Cancer that has spread from the original (primary) tumor to the liver. A malignant neoplasm that has spread to the liver from another (primary) anatomic site. Such malignant neoplasms may be carcinomas (e.g., breast, colon), lymphomas, melanomas, or sarcomas.
198.0	Secondary malignant neoplasm of kidney – The spread of the cancer to the kidney. This may be from a primary kidney cancer involving the opposite kidney, or from a cancer at a distant site.
198.1	Secondary malignant neoplasm of other urinary organs
198.5	Secondary malignant neoplasm of bone and bone marrow —Cancer that has spread from the original (primary) tumor to the bone. The spread of a malignant neoplasm from a primary site to the skeletal system. The majority of metastatic neoplasms to the bone are carcinomas.
198.7	Secondary malignant neoplasm of adrenal gland
198.82	Secondary malignant neoplasm of genital organs

Coding for Off-Label PROVENGE® Services

The use of PROVENGE® off-label for the treatment of prostate cancer is left to the discretion of the Medicare Administrative Contractors. Claims with dates of service on and after July 1, 2011, for PROVENGE® paid off-label for the treatment of prostate cancer must be billed using either ICD-9 code 233.4 (carcinoma in situ of prostate), or ICD-9 code 185 (malignant neoplasm of prostate) in addition to HCPCS Q2043.

Effective with the implementation date for ICD-10 codes, off-label PROVENGE® services must be billed with either ICD-10 code D075(carcinoma in situ of prostate), or C61 (malignant neoplasm of prostate) in addition to HCPCS Q2043.

ICD-10 Diagnosis Coding

Contractors shall note the appropriate ICD-10 code(s) that are listed below for future implementation. Contractors shall track the ICD-10 codes and ensure that the updated edit is turned on as part of the ICD-10 implementation effective October 1, 2013.

ICD-10	Description
C61	Malignant neoplasm of prostate (for on-label or off-label indications)
D075	Carcinoma in situ of prostate (for off-label indications only)
C77.1	Secondary and unspecified malignant neoplasm of intrathoracic lymph nodes
C77.2	Secondary and unspecified malignant neoplasm of intra-abdominal lymph nodes
C77.4	Secondary and unspecified malignant neoplasm of inguinal and lower limb lymph nodes
C77.5	Secondary and unspecified malignant neoplasm of intrapelvic lymph nodes
C77.8	Secondary and unspecified malignant neoplasm of lymph nodes of multiple regions
C77.9	Secondary and unspecified malignant neoplasm of lymph node, unspecified
C78.00	Secondary malignant neoplasm of unspecified lung
C78.01	Secondary malignant neoplasm of right lung
C78.02	Secondary malignant neoplasm of left lung
C78.7	Secondary malignant neoplasm of liver
C79.00	Secondary malignant neoplasm of unspecified kidney and renal pelvis
C79.01	Secondary malignant neoplasm of right kidney and renal pelvis
C79.02	Secondary malignant neoplasm of left kidney and renal pelvis
C79.10	Secondary malignant neoplasm of unspecified urinary organs
C79.11	Secondary malignant neoplasm of bladder
C79.19	Secondary malignant neoplasm of other urinary organs
C79.51	Secondary malignant neoplasm of bone
C79.52	Secondary malignant neoplasm of bone marrow
C79.70	Secondary malignant neoplasm of unspecified adrenal gland
C79.71	Secondary malignant neoplasm of right adrenal gland
C79.72	Secondary malignant neoplasm of left adrenal gland
C79.82	Secondary malignant neoplasm of genital organs

100-04, 32, 280.4

Payment Method

(Rev.2380, Issued: 01-06-12, Effective: 06-30-11, Implementation: 08-08-11)

Payment for PROVENGE® is as follows:

- TOBs 12X, 13X, 22X and 23X - based on the Average Sales Price (ASP) + 6%,
- TOB 85X – based on reasonable cost,
- TOBs 71X and 77X – based on all-inclusive rate.

For Medicare Part B practitioner claims, payment for PROVENGE® is based on ASP + 6%.

Contractors shall not pay separately for routine costs associated with PROVENGE®, HCPCS Q2043, except for the cost of administration. (Q2043 is all-inclusive and represents all routine costs except for its cost of administration).

100-04, 32, 280.5

Medicare Summary Notices (MSNs), Remittance Advice Remark Codes (RARCs), Claim Adjustment Reason Codes (CARCs), and Group Codes

(Rev.2394, Issued: 01-25-12, Effective: 06-30-11 for-(claims with dates of service on or after 07-01)

Contractors shall use the following messages when denying claims for the on-label indication for PROVENGE®, HCPCS Q2043, submitted without ICD-9-CM diagnosis code 185 and at least one diagnosis code from the ICD-9 table in Section 280.2 above: MSN 14.9 - Medicare cannot pay for this service for the diagnosis shown on the claim.

Spanish Version - Medicare no puede pagar por este servicio debido al diagnóstico indicado en la reclamación.

© 2019 Optum360, LLC

RARC 167 - This (these) diagnosis (es) are not covered. Note: Refer to the 835 Healthcare Policy Identification segment (loop 2110 Service Payment Information REF), if present.

Group Code – CO (Contractual Obligation)

Contractors shall use the following messages when denying claims for the off-label indication for PROVENGE®, HCPCS Q2043, submitted without ICD-9-CM diagnosis code 233.4:

MSN 14.9 - Medicare cannot pay for this service for the diagnosis shown on the claim.

Spanish Version - Medicare no puede pagar por este servicio debido al diagnóstico indicado en la reclamación.

RARC 167 - This (these) diagnosis (es) are not covered. Note: Refer to the 835 Healthcare Policy Identification segment (loop 2110 Service Payment Information REF), if present.

Group Code – CO (Contractual Obligation)

For claims with dates of service on or after July 1, 2012, processed on or after July 2, 2012, when denying claims for PROVENGE®, HCPCS Q2043® that exceed three (3) services in a patient's lifetime, contractors shall use the following messages:

MSN 20.5 - These services cannot be paid because your benefits are exhausted at this time.

Spanish Version - Estos servicios no pueden ser pagados porque sus beneficios se han agotado.

RARC N362 - The number of Days or Units of Service exceeds our acceptable maximum.

CARC 149 - Lifetime benefit maximum has been reached for this service/benefit category.

Group Code – CO (Contractual Obligation)

100-04, 32, 300

Billing Requirements for Ocular Photodynamic Therapy (OPT) with Verteporfin

(Rev.2728, Issued: 06-14-13-Effective: 04-03-13, Implementation: 07-16-13)

Ocular Photodynamic Therapy (OPT) is used in the treatment of ophthalmologic diseases; specifically, for age-related macular degeneration (AMD), a common eye disease among the elderly. OPT involves the infusion of an intravenous photosensitizing drug called Verteporfin, followed by exposure to a laser. For complete Medical coverage guidelines, see National Coverage Determinations (NCD) Manual (Pub 100-03) ? 80.2 through 80.3.1.

100-04, 32, 300.1

(Rev.2728, Issued: 06-14-13, Effective: 04-03-13, Implementation: 07-16-13)

Coding Requirements for OPT with Verteporfin

The following are applicable Current Procedural Terminology (CPT) codes for OPT with Verteporfin:

67221- Destruction of localized lesion of choroid (e.g. choroidal neovascularization); photodynamic therapy (includes intravenous infusion)

67225- Destruction of localized lesion of choroid (e.g. choroidal neovascularization); photodynamic therapy, second eye, at single session (List separately in addition to code for primary eye treatment)

The following are applicable Healthcare Common Procedure Coding System (HCPCS) code for OPT with Verteporfin:

J3396- Injection, Verteporfin, 0.1 mg

100-04, 32, 300.2

Claims Processing Requirements for OPT with Verteporfin Services on Professional Claims and Outpatient Facility Claims

(Rev.2728, Issued: 06-14-13, Effective: 04-03-13, Implementation: 07-16-13)

OPT with Verteporfin is a covered service when billed with ICD-9-CM code 362.52 (Exudative Senile Macular Degeneration of Retina (Wet)) or ICD-10-CM code H35.32 (Exudative Age-related Macular Degeneration).

Coverage is denied when billed with either ICD-9-CM code 362.50 (Macular Degeneration (Senile), Unspecified) or 362.51 (Non-exudative Senile Macular Degeneration) or their equivalent ICD-10-CM code H35.30 (Unspecified Macular Degeneration) or H35.31 (Non-exudative Age-Related Macular Degeneration).

OPT with Verteporfin for other ocular indications are eligible for local coverage determinations through individual contractor discretion.

Payment for OPT service (CPT code 67221/67225) must be billed on the same claim as the drug (J3396) for the same date of service.

Claims for OPT with Verteporfin for dates of service prior to April 3, 2013 are covered at the initial visit as determined by a fluorescein angiogram (FA) CPT code 92235 . Subsequent follow-up visits also require a FA prior to treatment.

For claims with dates of service on or after April 3, 2013, contractors shall accept and process claims for subsequent follow-up visits with either a FA, CPT code 92235, or optical coherence tomography (OCT), CPT codes 92133 or 92134, prior to treatment.

Regardless of the date of service of the claim, the FA or OCT is not required to be submitted on the claim for OPT and can be maintained in the patient? file for audit purposes.

100-04, 32, 310

Transesophageal Doppler Used for Cardiac Monitoring

(Rev.2743, Issued: 07-25-13, Effective: 07-01-01-13, Implementation, 08-29-13)

Effective May 17, 2007, Transesophageal Doppler used for cardiac monitoring is covered for ventilated patients in the ICU and operative patients with a need for intra-operative fluid optimization was deemed reasonable and necessary. See National Coverage Determinations Manual (Pub. 100-03) ?220.5, for complete coverage guidelines.

A new Healthcare Common Procedure Coding System (HCPCS) code, G9157, Transesophageal Doppler used for cardiac monitoring, will be made effective for use for dates of service on or after January 1, 2013.

100-04, 32, 310.2

Coding Requirements for Transesophageal Doppler Cardiac Monitoring Furnished On or After January 1, 2013

(Rev.2743, Issued: 07-25-13, Effective: 07-01-01-13, Implementation, 08-26-13)

After January 1, 2013, the applicable HCPCS code for Transesophageal Doppler cardiac monitoring is:

HCPCS G9157: Transesophageal Doppler used for cardiac monitoring

Contractors shall allow HCPCS G9157 to be billed when services are provided in POS 21 for ventilated patients in the ICU or for operative patients with a need for intra-operative fluid optimization.

Contractors shall deny HCPCS 76999 when billed for Esophageal Doppler for ventilated patients in the ICU or for operative patients with a need for intra-operative fluid optimization using the following messages:

CARC 189: "'Not otherwise classified' or 'unlisted' procedure code (CPT/HCPCS) was billed when there is a specific procedure code for this procedure/service."

RARC M20: "Missing/incomplete/invalid HCPCS."

MSN 16.13: "The code(s) your provider used is/are not valid for the date of service billed."

(English version) or "El/los código(s) que usó su proveedor no es/son válido(s) en la fecha de servicio facturada." (Spanish version).

Group Code: Contractual Obligation (CO)

100-04, 32, 310.3

Correct Place of Service (POS) Code for Transesophageal Doppler Cardiac Monitoring Services on Professional Claims

(Rev..2743, Issued: 07-25-13, Effective: 07-01-01-13, Implementation, 08-29-13)

Contractors shall pay for Transesophageal Doppler cardiac monitoring, G9157, only when services are provided at POS 21.

Contractors shall deny HCPCS G9157 when billed globally in any POS other than 21 for ventilated patients in the ICU or for operative patients with a need for intra-operative fluid optimization using the following messages:

CARC 58: "Treatment was deemed by the payer to have been rendered in an inappropriate or invalid place of service. Note: Refer to the 835 Healthcare Policy Identification Segment (loop 2110 Service Payment Information REF), if present.

MSN 16.2: This service cannot be paid when provided in this location/facility.

Group Code: CO

100-04, 32, 320.3.5

Replacement Accessories and Supplies for External VADs or Any VAD

(Rev.3054, Issued: 08-29-14, Effective: 10-30- 13, Implementation: 09-30-14)

Effective April 1, 2013, claims for replacement of accessories and supplies for VADs implanted in patients who were not eligible for coverage under Medicare Part A or had other insurance that paid for the device and hospital stay at the time that the device was implanted, but are now eligible for coverage of the replacement supplies and accessories under Part B, should be submitted using HCPCS code Q0509. Those claims will be manually reviewed. In rare instances it may be appropriate to pay for replacement of supplies and accessories for external VADs used by patient who are

 © 2019 Optum360, LLC

discharged from the hospital. In addition, in some rare instances, it may be necessary for a patient to have an emergency back-up controller for an external VAD. Coverage of these items is at the discretion of the contractor. Claims for replacement of supplies and accessories used with an external VAD that are furnished by suppliers should be billed to the B MACs. Claims for replacement of supplies and accessories used with an external VAD that are furnished by hospitals and other providers should be billed to the A MACs. Effective April 1, 2013, these items should be billed using code Q0507 so that the claims can be manually reviewed.

Claims for replacement supplies or accessories used with VADs that do not have specific HCPCS codes and do not meet the criteria of codes Q0507 and Q0509 should be billed using code Q0508.

Claims Coding

HCPCS	Definition	Effective Date
Q0507	Miscellaneous Supply Or Accessory For Use With An External Ventricular Assist Device	April 1, 2013
Q0508	Miscellaneous Supply or Accessory For Use With An Implanted Ventricular Assist Device	April 1, 2013
Q0509	Miscellaneous Supply Or Accessory For Use With Any Implanted Ventricular Assist Device For Which Payment Was Not Made Under Medicare Part A	April 1, 2013

100-04, 32, 330.1

Claims Processing Requirements for Percutaneous Image-guided Lumbar Decompression (PILD) for Lumbar Spinal Stenosis (LSS) on Professional Claims

(Rev.3811, Issued: 07-25-17, Effective: 12-07-16, Implementation: 06-27-17)

For claims with dates of service on or after January 9, 2014, PILD (procedure code 0275T) is a covered service when billed as part of a clinical trial approved by CMS. The description for CPT 0275T is "Percutaneous laminotomy/laminectomy (intralaminar approach) for decompression of neural elements, (with or without ligamentous resection, discectomy, facetectomy and/or foraminotomy", any method, under indirect image guidance (e.g., fluoroscopic, CT), with or without the use of an endoscope, single or multiple levels, unilateral or bilateral; lumbar".

For claims with dates of service on or after January 1, 2015, PILD (procedure code G0276) is a covered service when billed as part of a clinical trial approved by CMS. HCPCS G0276 is "Blinded procedure for lumbar stenosis, percutaneous image-guided lumbar decompression (PILD), or placebo control, performed in an approved coverage with evidence development (CED) clinical trial".

The claim may only contain one of these procedure codes, not both. To use G0276, the procedure must be performed in an approved CED clinical trial that is randomized, blinded, and contains a placebo control arm of the trial. CMS will cover procedure code 0275T for PILD only when the procedure is performed with any other CED approved clinical trial. Regardless of the type of CED approved clinical trial (e.g. G0276 vs 0275T), PILD is only covered when billed for the ICD-9 diagnosis of 724.01-724.03 or the ICD-10 diagnosis of M48.05-M48.07, when billed in places of service 22 (Outpatient) or 24 (Ambulatory Surgical Center), when billed along with V70.7 (ICD-9) or Z00.6 (ICD-10) in either the primary/secondary positions, and when billed with modifier Q0.

Additionally, per Transmittal 2805 (Change Request 8401), issued October 30, 2013, all claims for clinical trials must contain the 8 digit clinical trial identifier number.

The following message(s) shall be used to notify providers of return situations that may occur:

Professional Claims 8-digit Clinical Trial Number

For PILD claims with procedure code 0275T with dates of service on or after January 9, 2014, or for claims with procedure code G0276 with dates of service on or after January 1, 2015, contractors shall pay for PILD only when billed with the numeric, 8-digit clinical trial identifier number preceded by the two alpha characters "CT" when placed in Field 19 of paper Form CMS-1500, or when entered without the "CT" prefix in the electronic 837P in Loop 2300 REF02 (REF01=P4). Claims for PILD which are billed without an 8-digit clinical trial identifier number shall be returned as unprocessable.

The following messages shall be used when Medicare contractors return PILD claims billed without an 8-digit clinical trial identifier number as unprocessable:

Claims Adjustment Reason Code 16: "Claim/service lacks information or has submission/billing error(s) which is needed for adjudication".

Remittance Advice Remark Code N721: "This service is only covered when performed as part of a clinical trial."

Remittance Advice Remark Code MA50: "Missing/incomplete/invalid Investigational Device Exemption number or Clinical Trial number."

Remittance Advice Remark Code N704: "Alert: You may not appeal this decision but can resubmit this claim/service with corrected information if warranted."

Professional Claims Place of Service – 22 or 24

For PILD claims with procedure code 0275T with dates of service on or after January 9, 2014, or for claims with procedure code G0276 with dates of service on or after January 1, 2015, contractors shall pay for PILD for LSS claims only when billed in place of service 22 or 24. Claims for PILD which are billed in any other place of service shall be returned as unprocessable.

The following messages shall be used when Medicare contractors return PILD claims not billed in place of service 22 or 24:

Claims Adjustment Reason Code 58: "Treatment was deemed by the payer to have been rendered in an inappropriate or invalid place of service."

Remittance Advice Remark Code N704: "Alert: You may not appeal this decision but can resubmit this claim/service with corrected information if warranted."

Professional Claims Modifier – Q0

For PILD claims with procedure code 0275T with dates of service on or after January 9, 2014, or for claims with procedure code G0276 with dates of service on or after January 1, 2015, contractors shall pay for PILD for LSS claims only when billed with modifier Q0.

Claims for PILD which are billed without modifier Q0 shall be returned as unprocessable.

The following messages shall be used when Medicare contractors return PILD claims billed without modifier Q0 as unprocessable:

Claims Adjustment Reason Code 4: "The procedure code is inconsistent with the modifier used or a required modifier is missing."

Remittance Advice Remark Code N657: "This should be billed with the appropriate code for these services."

Remittance Advice Remark Code N704: "Alert: You may not appeal this decision but can resubmit this claim/service with corrected information if warranted."

Non-covered Diagnosis

For PILD claims with procedure code 0275T with dates of service on or after January 9, 2014, or for claims with procedure code G0276 with dates of service on or after January 1, 2015, contractors shall pay for PILD for LSS claims only when billed with the ICD-9 diagnosis of 724.01-724.03 or the ICD-10 diagnosis of M48.05-M48.07.

The following messages shall be used when Medicare contractors return PILD claims, billed without the covered diagnosis, as unprocessable:

Claims Adjustment Reason Code B22: "This payment is adjusted based on the diagnosis."

Remittance Advice Remark Code N704: "Alert: You may not appeal this decision but can resubmit this claim/service with corrected information if warranted."

Clinical Trial Diagnosis

For PILD claims with procedure code 0275T with dates of service on or after January 9, 2014, or for claims with procedure code G0276 with dates of service on or after January 1, 2015, contractors shall pay for PILD only when billed with the ICD-9 diagnosis of V70.7 (ICD-9) or Z00.6 (ICD-10) in either the primary or secondary positions. The following messages shall be used when Medicare contractors return PILD claims, billed without the clinical trial diagnosis, as unprocessable:

Claims Adjustment Reason Code B22: "This payment is adjusted based on the diagnosis."

Remittance Advice Remark Code N704: "Alert: You may not appeal this decision but can resubmit this claim/service with corrected information if warranted."

100-04, 32, 330.2

Claims Processing Requirements for PILD for Outpatient Facilities

(Rev.3811, Issued: 07-25-17, Effective: 12- 07-16, Implementation: 06-27-17)

Hospital Outpatient facilities shall bill for percutaneous image-guided lumbar decompression (PILD) procedure code 0275T effective on or after January 9, 2014, or procedure code G0276 effective on or after January 1, 2015, for lumbar spinal stenosis (LSS) on a 13X or 85X TOB. Refer to Section 69 of this chapter for further guidance on billing under CED.

Effective for dates of service on or after December 7, 2016, Medicare will cover PILD under CED for beneficiaries with LSS who are enrolled in a CMS-approved prospective longitudinal study for PILD procedures using a FDA-approved/cleared device that completed a CMS-approved randomized, controlled clinical trial (RCT) that met the

© 2019 Optum360, LLC

criteria listed in the January 2014 NCD (see CR 8757, transmittal # 2959, dated May 16, 2014).

Hospital outpatient procedures for PILD shall be covered when billed with:

- ICD-9 V70.7 (ICD-10 Z00.6) and Condition Code 30.
- Modifier Q0
- An 8-digit clinical trial identifier number listed on the CMS Coverage with Evidence Development website

Hospital outpatient procedures for PILD shall be rejected when billed without:

- ICD-9 V70.7 (ICD-10 Z00.6) and Condition Code 30.
- Modifier Q0
- An 8-digit clinical trial identifier number listed on the CMS Coverage with Evidence Development website

Claims billed by hospitals not participating in the trial /registry, shall be rejected with the following message:

CARC: 50 -These are non-covered services because this is not deemed a "medical necessity" by the payer.

RARC N386 - This decision was based on a National Coverage Determination (NCD). An NCD provides a coverage determination as to whether a particular item or service is covered. A copy of this policy is available at http://www.cms.hhs.gov/mcd/search.asp. If you do not have web access, you may contact the contractor to request a copy of the NCD.

Group Code –Contractual Obligation (CO)
MSN 16.77 – This service/item was not covered because it was not provided as part of a qualifying trial/study. (Este servicio/artículo no fue cubierto porque no estaba incluido como parte de un ensayo clínico/estudio calificado.)

100-04, 36, 50.14

Purchased Accessories & Supplies for Use With Grandfathered Equipment

(Rev.2231, Issued: 05-27-11, Effective: 08-28-11, Implementation: 08-28-11)

Non-contract grandfathered suppliers must use the KY modifier on claims for CBA-residing beneficiaries with dates of service on or after January 1, 2011, for purchased, covered accessories or supplies furnished for use with rented grandfathered equipment. The following HCPCS codes are the codes for which use of the KY modifier is authorized:

Continuous Positive Airway Pressure Devices, Respiratory Assistive Devices, and Related Supplies and Accessories – A4604, A7030, A7031, A7032, A7033, A7034, A7035, A7036, A7037, A7038, A7039, A7044, A7045, A7046, E0561, and E0562

Hospital Beds and Related Accessories – E0271, E0272, E0280, and E0310

Walkers and Related Accessories – E0154, E0156, E0157 and E0158 Grandfathered suppliers that submit claims for the payment of the aforementioned purchased accessories and supplies for use with grandfathered equipment should submit the applicable single payment amount for the accessory or supply as their submitted charge on the claim. Non-contract grandfathered suppliers should be aware that purchase claims submitted for these codes without the KY modifier will be denied. In addition, claims submitted with the KY modifier for HCPCS codes other than those listed above will be denied.

After the rental payment cap for the grandfathered equipment is reached, the beneficiary must obtain replacement supplies and accessories from a contract supplier. The supplier of the grandfathered equipment is no longer permitted to furnish the supplies and accessories once the rental payment cap is reached.

100-04, 36, 50.15

Hospitals Providing Walkers and Related Accessories to Their Patients on the Date of Discharge

(Rev.2231, Issued: 05-27-11, Effective: 08-28-11, Implementation: 08-28-11)

Hospitals may furnish walkers and related accessories to their own patients for use in the home during an admission or on the date of discharge and receive payment at the applicable single payment amount, regardless of whether the hospital is a contract supplier or not. Separate payment is not made for walkers furnished by a hospital for use in the hospital, as payment for these items is included in the Part A payment for inpatient hospital services.

To be paid for walkers as a non-contract supplier, the hospital must use the modifier J4 in combination with the following HCPCS codes: A4636; A4637; E0130; E0135; E0140; E0141; E0143; E0144; E0147; E0148; E0149; E0154; E0155; E0156; E0157; E0158; and E0159. Under this exception, hospitals are advised to submit the claim for the hospital stay before or on the same day that they submit the claim for the walker to ensure timely and accurate claims processing.

Hospitals that are located outside a CBA that furnish walkers and/or related accessories to travelling beneficiaries who live in a CBA must affix the J4 modifier to claims submitted for these items.

The J4 modifier should not be used by contract suppliers.

100-08, 15, 4.2.8

Cardiac Rehabilitation (CR) and Intensive Cardiac Rehabilitation (ICR)

(Rev.530, Issued: 07-18-14, Effective: 02-18-14, Implementation: 08-18-14)

A. General Background Information
Effective January 1, 2010, Medicare Part B covers Cardiac Rehabilitation (CR) and Intensive Cardiac Rehabilitation (ICR) program services for beneficiaries who have experienced one or more of the following:

- An acute myocardial infarction within the preceding 12 months;
- A coronary artery bypass surgery;
- Current stable angina pectoris;
- Heart valve repair or replacement;
- Percutaneous transluminal coronary angioplasty or coronary stenting;
- A heart or heart-lung transplant; or,
- A stable, chronic heart failure defined as patients with left ventricular ejection fraction of 35% or less and New York Heart Association (NYHA) class II to IV symptoms despite being on optimal heart failure therapy for at least 6 weeks (effective February 18, 2014).

ICR programs must be approved by the Centers for Medicare & Medicaid Services (CMS) through the national coverage determination (NCD) process and must meet certain criteria for approval. Individual sites wishing to provide ICR services via an approved ICR program must enroll with their local Medicare Administrative Contractor (MAC) as an ICR program supplier.

B. ICR Enrollment
In order to enroll as an ICR site, a supplier must complete a Form CMS-855B, with the supplier type of "Other" selected. MACs shall verify that the ICR program is approved by CMS through the NCD process. A list of approved ICR programs will be identified through the NCD listings, the CMS Web site and the Federal Register. MACs shall use one of these options to verify that the ICR program has met CMS approval.

ICR suppliers shall be enrolled using specialty code 31. ICR suppliers must separately enroll each of their practice locations. Therefore, each enrolling ICR supplier can only have one practice location on its CMS-855B enrollment application and shall receive its own Provider Transaction Account Number. MACs shall only accept and process reassignments (855R's) to ICR suppliers for physicians defined in 1861(r)(1) of the Social Security Act.

C. Additional Information
For more information on ICR suppliers, refer to:

- 42 CFR §410.49
- Pub. 100-04, Medicare Claims Processing Manual, chapter 32, section 140
- Pub. 100-02, Medicare Benefit Policy Manual, chapter 15, section 232

Pub. 100-03, National Coverage Determinations Manual, chapter 1, part 1, section 20.10

© 2019 Optum360, LLC

Appendix 5 — HCPCS Changes for 2020

NEW CODES

A4226 Supplies for maintenance of insulin infusion pump with dosage rate adjustment using therapeutic continuous glucose sensing, per week

A9590 Iodine I-131, iobenguane, 1 mCi

B4187 Omegaven, 10 g lipids

C1734 Orthopedic/device/drug matrix for opposing bone-to-bone or soft tissue-to bone (implantable)

C1824 Generator, cardiac contractility modulation (implantable)

C1839 Iris prosthesis

C1982 Catheter, pressure generating, one-way valve, intermittently occlusive

C2596 Probe, image guided, robotic, waterjet ablation

C9041 Injection, coagulation factor xa (recombinant), inactivated (andexxa), 10 mg

C9046 Cocaine hydrochloride nasal solution for topical administration, 1 mg

C9047 Injection, caplacizumab-yhdp, 1 mg

C9054 Injection, lefamulin (Xenleta), 1 mg

C9055 Injection, brexanolone, 1 mg

C9756 Intraoperative near-infrared fluorescence lymphatic mapping of lymph node(s) (sentinel or tumor draining) with administration of indocyanine green (ICG) (list separately in addition to code for primary procedure)

C9757 Laminotomy (hemilaminectomy), with decompression of nerve root(s), including partial facetectomy, foraminotomy and excision of herniated intervertebral disc, and repair of annular defect with implantation of bone anchored annular closure device, including annular defect measurement, alignment and sizing assessment, and image guidance; one interspace, lumbar

C9758 Blinded procedure for NYHA Class III/IV heart failure; transcatheter implantation of interatrial shunt or placebo control, including right heart catheterization, transesophageal echocardiography (TEE)/intracardiac echocardiography (ICE), and all imaging with or without guidance (e.g., ultrasound, fluoroscopy), performed in an approved investigational device exemption (IDE) study

E0787 External ambulatory infusion pump, insulin, dosage rate adjustment using therapeutic continuous glucose sensing

E2398 Wheelchair accessory, dynamic positioning hardware for back

G1000 Clinical Decision Support Mechanism Applied Pathways, as defined by the Medicare Appropriate Use Criteria Program

G1001 Clinical Decision Support Mechanism eviCore, as defined by the Medicare Appropriate Use Criteria Program

G1002 Clinical Decision Support Mechanism MedCurrent, as defined by the Medicare Appropriate Use Criteria Program

G1003 Clinical Decision Support Mechanism Medicalis, as defined by the Medicare Appropriate Use Criteria Program

G1004 Clinical Decision Support Mechanism National Decision Support Company, as defined by the Medicare Appropriate Use Criteria Program

G1005 Clinical Decision Support Mechanism National Imaging Associates, as defined by the Medicare Appropriate Use Criteria Program

G1006 Clinical Decision Support Mechanism Test Appropriate, as defined by the Medicare Appropriate Use Criteria Program

G1007 Clinical Decision Support Mechanism AIM Specialty Health, as defined by the Medicare Appropriate Use Criteria Program

G1008 Clinical Decision Support Mechanism Cranberry Peak, as defined by the Medicare Appropriate Use Criteria Program

G1009 Clinical Decision Support Mechanism Sage Health Management Solutions, as defined by the Medicare Appropriate Use Criteria Program

G1010 Clinical Decision Support Mechanism Stanson, as defined by the Medicare Appropriate Use Criteria Program

G1011 Clinical Decision Support Mechanism, qualified tool not otherwise specified, as defined by the Medicare Appropriate Use Criteria Program

G2021 Health care practitioners rendering treatment in place (TIP)

G2022 A model participant (ambulance supplier/provider), the beneficiary refuses services covered under the model (transport to an alternate destination/treatment in place)

G2058 Chronic care management services, each additional 20 minutes of clinical staff time directed by a physician or other qualified health care professional, per calendar month (list separately in addition to code for primary procedure). (Do not report G2058 for care management services of less than 20 minutes additional to the first 20 minutes of chronic care management services during a calendar month.) (Use G2058 in conjunction with 99490.) (Do not report 99490, G2058 in the same calendar month as 99487, 99489, 99491.)

G2061 Qualified nonphysician health care professional online assessment, for an established patient, for up to 7 days, cumulative time during the 7 days; 5-10 minutes

G2062 Qualified nonphysician health care professional online assessment service, for an established patient, for up to 7 days, cumulative time during the 7 days; 11-20 minutes

G2063 Qualified nonphysician qualified health care professional assessment service, for an established patient, for up to 7 days, cumulative time during the 7 days; 21 or more minutes

G2064 Comprehensive care management services for a single high risk disease, e.g., principal care management, at least 30 minutes of physician or other qualified health care professional time per calendar month with the following elements: one complex chronic condition lasting at least 3 months, which is the focus of the care plan, the condition is of sufficient severity to place patient at risk of hospitalization or have been the cause of a recent hospitalization, the condition requires development or revision of disease specific care plan, the condition requires frequent adjustments in the medication regimen, and/or the management of the condition is unusually complex due to comorbidities

G2065 Comprehensive care management for a single high risk disease services, e.g., principal care management, at least 30 minutes of clinical staff time directed by a physician or other qualified health care professional, per calendar month with the following elements: one complex chronic condition lasting at least 3 months, which is the focus of the care plan, the condition is of sufficient severity to place patient at risk of hospitalization or have been cause of a recent hospitalization, the condition requires development or revision of disease-specific care plan, the condition requires frequent adjustments in the medication regimen, and/or the management of the condition is unusually complex due to comorbidities

© 2019 Optum360, LLC

NEW CODES (continued)

G2066 Interrogation device evaluation(s), (remote) up to 30 days; implantable cardiovascular physiologic monitor system, implantable loop recorder system, or subcutaneous cardiac rhythm monitor system, remote data acquisition(s), receipt of transmissions and technician review, technical support and distribution of results

G2067 Medication assisted treatment, methadone; weekly bundle including dispensing and/or administration, substance use counseling, individual and group therapy, and toxicology testing, if performed (provision of the services by a Medicare-enrolled opioid treatment program)

G2068 Medication assisted treatment, buprenorphine (oral); weekly bundle including dispensing and/or administration, substance use counseling, individual and group therapy, and toxicology testing if performed (provision of the services by a Medicare-enrolled opioid treatment program)

G2069 Medication assisted treatment, buprenorphine (injectable); weekly bundle including dispensing and/or administration, substance use counseling, individual and group therapy, and toxicology testing if performed (provision of the services by a Medicare-enrolled opioid treatment program)

G2070 Medication assisted treatment, buprenorphine (implant insertion); weekly bundle including dispensing and/or administration, substance use counseling, individual and group therapy, and toxicology testing if performed (provision of the services by a Medicare-enrolled opioid treatment program)

G2071 Medication assisted treatment, buprenorphine (implant removal); weekly bundle including dispensing and/or administration, substance use counseling, individual and group therapy, and toxicology testing if performed (provision of the services by a Medicare-enrolled opioid treatment program)

G2072 Medication assisted treatment, buprenorphine (implant insertion and removal); weekly bundle including dispensing and/or administration, substance use counseling, individual and group therapy, and toxicology testing if performed (provision of the services by a Medicare-enrolled opioid treatment program)

G2073 Medication assisted treatment, naltrexone; weekly bundle including dispensing and/or administration, substance use counseling, individual and group therapy, and toxicology testing if performed (provision of the services by a Medicare-enrolled opioid treatment program)

G2074 Medication assisted treatment, weekly bundle not including the drug, including substance use counseling, individual and group therapy, and toxicology testing if performed (provision of the services by a Medicare-enrolled opioid treatment program)

G2075 Medication assisted treatment, medication not otherwise specified; weekly bundle including dispensing and/or administration, substance use counseling, individual and group therapy, and toxicology testing, if performed (provision of the services by a Medicare-enrolled opioid treatment program)

G2076 Intake activities, including initial medical examination that is a complete, fully documented physical evaluation and initial assessment by a program physician or a primary care physician, or an authorized health care professional under the supervision of a program physician qualified personnel that includes preparation of a treatment plan that includes the patient's short-term goals and the tasks the patient must perform to complete the short-term goals; the patient's requirements for education, vocational rehabilitation, and employment; and the medical, psycho-social, economic, legal, or other supportive services that a patient needs, conducted by qualified personnel (provision of the services by a Medicare-enrolled opioid treatment program); list separately in addition to code for primary procedure

G2077 Periodic assessment; assessing periodically by qualified personnel to determine the most appropriate combination of services and treatment (provision of the services by a Medicare-enrolled opioid treatment program); list separately in addition to code for primary procedure

G2078 Take home supply of methadone; up to 7 additional day supply (provision of the services by a Medicare-enrolled opioid treatment program); list separately in addition to code for primary procedure

G2079 Take home supply of buprenorphine (oral); up to 7 additional day supply (provision of the services by a Medicare-enrolled opioid treatment program); list separately in addition to code for primary procedure

G2080 Each additional 30 minutes of counseling in a week of medication assisted treatment, (provision of the services by a Medicare-enrolled opioid treatment program); list separately in addition to code for primary procedure

G2081 Patients age 66 and older in institutional special needs plans (SNP) or residing in long-term care with a POS code 32, 33, 34, 54 or 56 for more than 90 days during the measurement period

G2082 Office or other outpatient visit for the evaluation and management of an established patient that requires the supervision of a physician or other qualified health care professional and provision of up to 56 mg of esketamine nasal self administration, includes 2 hours post administration observation

G2083 Office or other outpatient visit for the evaluation and management of an established patient that requires the supervision of a physician or other qualified health care professional and provision of greater than 56 mg esketamine nasal self administration, includes 2 hours post administration observation

G2086 Office-based treatment for opioid use disorder, including development of the treatment plan, care coordination, individual therapy and group therapy and counseling; at least 70 minutes in the first calendar month

G2087 Office-based treatment for opioid use disorder, including care coordination, individual therapy and group therapy and counseling; at least 60 minutes in a subsequent calendar month

G2088 Office-based treatment for opioid use disorder, including care coordination, individual therapy and group therapy and counseling; each additional 30 minutes beyond the first 120 minutes (list separately in addition to code for primary procedure)

G2089 Most recent hemoglobin A1c (HbA1c) level 7.0% to 9.0%

G2090 Patients 66 years of age and older with at least one claim/encounter for frailty during the measurement period and a dispensed medication for dementia during the measurement period or the year prior to the measurement period

G2091 Patients 66 years of age and older with at least one claim/encounter for frailty during the measurement period and either one acute inpatient encounter with a diagnosis of advanced illness or two outpatient, observation, ED or nonacute inpatient encounters on different dates of service with an advanced illness diagnosis during the measurement period or the year prior to the measurement period

G2092 Angiotensin converting enzyme (ACE) inhibitor or angiotensin receptor blocker (ARB) or angiotensin receptor-neprilysin inhibitor (ARNI) therapy prescribed or currently being taken

G2093 Documentation of medical reason(s) for not prescribing ACE inhibitor or ARB or ARNI therapy (e.g., hypotensive patients who are at immediate risk of cardiogenic shock, hospitalized patients who have experienced marked azotemia, allergy, intolerance, other medical reasons)

G2094 Documentation of patient reason(s) for not prescribing ACE inhibitor or ARB or ARNI therapy (e.g., patient declined, other patient reasons)

G2095 Documentation of system reason(s) for not prescribing ACE inhibitor or ARB or ARNI therapy (e.g., other system reasons)

G2096 Angiotensin converting enzyme (ACE) inhibitor or angiotensin receptor blocker (ARB) or angiotensin receptor-neprilysin inhibitor (ARNI) therapy was not prescribed, reason not given

© 2019 Optum360, LLC

NEW CODES (continued)

G2097 Children with a competing diagnosis for upper respiratory infection within 3 days of diagnosis of pharyngitis (e.g., intestinal infection, pertussis, bacterial infection, Lyme disease, otitis media, acute sinusitis, acute pharyngitis, acute tonsillitis, chronic sinusitis, infection of the pharynx/larynx/tonsils/adenoids, prostatitis, cellulitis, mastoiditis, or bone infections, acute lymphadenitis, impetigo, skin staph infections, pneumonia/gonococcal infections, venereal disease (syphilis, chlamydia, inflammatory diseases [female reproductive organs]), infections of the kidney, cystitis or UTI

G2098 Patients 66 years of age and older with at least one claim/encounter for frailty during the measurement period and a dispensed medication for dementia during the measurement period or the year prior to the measurement period

G2099 Patients 66 years of age and older with at least one claim/encounter for frailty during the measurement period and either one acute inpatient encounter with a diagnosis of advanced illness or two outpatient, observation, ED or nonacute inpatient encounters on different dates of service with an advanced illness diagnosis during the measurement period or the year prior to the measurement period

G2100 Patients 66 years of age and older with at least one claim/encounter for frailty during the measurement period and a dispensed medication for dementia during the measurement period or the year prior to the measurement period

G2101 Patients 66 years of age and older with at least one claim/encounter for frailty during the measurement period and either one acute inpatient encounter with a diagnosis of advanced illness or two outpatient, observation, ED or nonacute inpatient encounters on different dates of service with an advanced illness diagnosis during the measurement period or the year prior to the measurement period

G2102 Dilated retinal eye exam with interpretation by an ophthalmologist or optometrist documented and reviewed

G2103 Seven standard field stereoscopic photos with interpretation by an ophthalmologist or optometrist documented and reviewed

G2104 Eye imaging validated to match diagnosis from seven standard field stereoscopic photos results documented and reviewed

G2105 Patients age 66 or older in institutional special needs plans (SNP) or residing in long-term care with POS code 32, 33, 34, 54 or 56 for more than 90 days during the measurement period

G2106 Patients 66 years of age and older with at least one claim/encounter for frailty during the measurement period and a dispensed medication for dementia during the measurement period or the year prior to the measurement period

G2107 Patients 66 years of age and older with at least one claim/encounter for frailty during the measurement period and either one acute inpatient encounter with a diagnosis of advanced illness or two outpatient, observation, ED or nonacute inpatient encounters on different dates of service with an advanced illness diagnosis during the measurement period or the year prior to the measurement period

G2108 Patients age 66 or older in institutional special needs plans (SNP) or residing in long-term care with POS code 32, 33, 34, 54 or 56 for more than 90 days during the measurement period

G2109 Patients 66 years of age and older with at least one claim/encounter for frailty during the measurement period and a dispensed medication for dementia during the measurement period or the year prior to the measurement period

G2110 Patients 66 years of age and older with at least one claim/encounter for frailty during the measurement period and either one acute inpatient encounter with a diagnosis of advanced illness or two outpatient, observation, ED or nonacute inpatient encounters on different dates of service with an advanced illness diagnosis during the measurement period or the year prior to the measurement period

G2112 Patient receiving <=5 mg daily prednisone (or equivalent), or RA activity is worsening, or glucocorticoid use is for less than 6 months

G2113 Patient receiving >5 mg daily prednisone (or equivalent) for longer than 6 months, and improvement or no change in disease activity

G2114 Patients 66-80 years of age with at least one claim/encounter for frailty during the measurement period and a dispensed medication for dementia during the measurement period or the year prior to the measurement period

G2115 Patients 66 years of age and older with at least one claim/encounter for frailty during the measurement period and a dispensed medication for dementia during the measurement period or the year prior to the measurement period

G2116 Patients 66 years of age and older with at least one claim/encounter for frailty during the measurement period and either one acute inpatient encounter with a diagnosis of advanced illness or two outpatient, observation, ED or nonacute inpatient encounters on different dates of service with an advanced illness diagnosis during the measurement period or the year prior to the measurement period

G2117 Patients 66-80 years of age with at least one claim/encounter for frailty during the measurement period and either one acute inpatient encounter with a diagnosis of advanced illness or two outpatient, observation, ED or nonacute inpatient encounters on different dates of service with an advanced illness diagnosis during the measurement period or the year prior to the measurement period

G2118 Patients 81 years of age and older with evidence of frailty during the measurement period

G2119 Within the past 2 years, calcium and/or vitamin D optimization has been ordered or performed

G2120 Within the past 2 years, calcium and/or vitamin D optimization has not been ordered or performed

G2121 Psychosis, depression, anxiety, apathy, and impulse control disorder assessed

G2122 Psychosis, depression, anxiety, apathy, and impulse control disorder not assessed

G2123 Patients 66-80 years of age and had at least one claim/encounter for frailty during the measurement period and either one acute inpatient encounter with a diagnosis of advanced illness or two outpatient, observation, ED or nonacute inpatient encounters on different dates of service with an advanced illness diagnosis during the measurement period or the year prior to the measurement period

G2124 Patients 66-80 years of age and had at least one claim/encounter for frailty during the measurement period and a dispensed dementia medication

G2125 Patients 81 years of age and older with evidence of frailty during the measurement period

G2126 Patients 66 years of age or older and had at least one claim/encounter for frailty during the measurement period and either one acute inpatient encounter with a diagnosis of advanced illness or two outpatient, observation, ED or nonacute inpatient encounters on different dates of service with an advanced illness diagnosis during the measurement period or the year prior to the measurement period

G2127 Patients 66 years of age or older and had at least one claim/encounter for frailty during the measurement period and a dispensed dementia medication

G2128 Documentation of medical reason(s) for not on a daily aspirin or other antiplatelet (e.g., history of gastrointestinal bleed, intracranial bleed, blood disorders, idiopathic thrombocytopenic purpura (ITP), gastric bypass or documentation of active anticoagulant use during the measurement period)

G2129 Procedure related BP's not taken during an outpatient visit. Examples include same day surgery, ambulatory service center, GI, lab, dialysis, infusion center, chemotherapy

G2130 Patients age 66 or older in institutional special needs plans (SNP) or residing in long-term care with POS code 32, 33, 34, 54 or 56 for more than 90 days during the measurement period

© 2019 Optum360, LLC

NEW CODES (continued)

G2131 Patients 81 years and older with a diagnosis of frailty

G2132 Patients 66-80 years of age with at least one claim/encounter for frailty during the measurement period and a dispensed medication for dementia during the measurement period or the year prior to the measurement period

G2133 Patients 66-80 years of age with at least one claim/encounter for frailty during the measurement period and either one acute inpatient encounter with a diagnosis of advanced illness or two outpatient, observation, ED or nonacute inpatient encounters on different dates of service with an advanced illness diagnosis during the measurement period or the year prior to the measurement period

G2134 Patients 66 years of age or older with at least one claim/encounter for frailty during the measurement period and a dispensed medication for dementia during the measurement period or the year prior to the measurement period

G2135 Patients 66 years of age or older with at least one claim/encounter for frailty during the measurement period and either one acute inpatient encounter with a diagnosis of advanced illness or two outpatient, observation, ED or nonacute inpatient encounters on different dates of service with an advanced illness diagnosis during the measurement period or the year prior to the measurement period

G2136 Back pain measured by the visual analog scale (VAS) at 3 months (6 to 20 weeks) postoperatively was less than or equal to 3.0 or back pain measured by the visual analog scale (VAS) within 3 months preoperatively and at 3 months (6 to 20 weeks) postoperatively demonstrated an improvement of 5.0 points or greater

G2137 Back pain measured by the visual analog scale (VAS) at 3 months (6 to 20 weeks) postoperatively was greater than 3.0 and back pain measured by the visual analog scale (VAS) within 3 months preoperatively and at 3 months (6 to 20 weeks) postoperatively demonstrated a change of less than an improvement of 5.0 points

G2138 Back pain as measured by the visual analog scale (VAS) at 1 year (9 to 15 months) postoperatively was less than or equal to 3.0 or back pain measured by the visual analog scale (VAS) within 3 months preoperatively and at 1 year (9 to 15 months) postoperatively demonstrated a change of 5.0 points or greater

G2139 Back pain measured by the visual analog scale (VAS) pain at 1 year (9 to 15 months) postoperatively was greater than 3.0 and back pain measured by the visual analog scale (VAS) within 3 months preoperatively and at 1 year (9 to 15 months) postoperatively demonstrated a change of less than 5.0

G2140 Leg pain measured by the visual analog scale (VAS) at 3 months (6 to 20 weeks) postoperatively was less than or equal to 3.0 or leg pain measured by the visual analog scale (VAS) within 3 months preoperatively and at 3 months (6 to 20 weeks) postoperatively demonstrated an improvement of 5.0 points or greater

G2141 Leg pain measured by the visual analog scale (VAS) at 3 months (6 to 20 weeks) postoperatively was greater than 3.0 and leg pain measured by the visual analog scale (VAS) within 3 months preoperatively and at 3 months (6 to 20 weeks) postoperatively demonstrated less than an improvement of 5.0 points

G2142 Functional status measured by the Oswestry Disability Index (ODI version 2.1a) at 1 year (9 to 15 months) postoperatively was less than or equal to 22 or functional status measured by the ODI version 2.1a within 3 months preoperatively and at 1 year (9 to 15 months) postoperatively demonstrated a change of 30 points or greater

G2143 Functional status measured by the Oswestry Disability Index (ODI version 2.1a) at 1 year (9 to 15 months) postoperatively was greater than 22 and functional status measured by the ODI version 2.1a within 3 months preoperatively and at 1 year (9 to 15 months) postoperatively demonstrated a change of less than 30 points

G2144 Functional status measured by the Oswestry Disability Index (ODI version 2.1a) at 3 months (6 to 20 weeks) postoperatively was less than or equal to 22 or functional status measured by the ODI version 2.1a within 3 months preoperatively and at 3 months (6 to 20 weeks) postoperatively demonstrated a change of 30 points or greater

G2145 Functional status measured by the Oswestry Disability Index (ODI version 2.1a) at 3 months (6 to 20 weeks) postoperatively was greater than 22 and functional status measured by the ODI version 2.1a within 3 months preoperatively and at 3 months (6 to 20 weeks) postoperatively demonstrated a change of less than 30 points

G2146 Leg pain as measured by the visual analog scale (VAS) at 1 year (9 to 15 months) postoperatively was less than or equal to 3.0 or leg pain measured by the visual analog scale (VAS) within 3 months preoperatively and at 1 year (9 to 15 months) postoperatively demonstrated an improvement of 5.0 points or greater

G2147 Leg pain measured by the visual analog scale (VAS) at 1 year (9 to 15 months) postoperatively was greater than 3.0 and leg pain measured by the visual analog scale (VAS) within 3 months preoperatively and at 1 year (9 to 15 months) postoperatively demonstrated less than an improvement of 5.0 points

G2148 Performance met: multimodal pain management was used

G2149 Documentation of medical reason(s) for not using multimodal pain management (e.g., allergy to multiple classes of analgesics, intubated patient, hepatic failure, patient reports no pain during PACU stay, other medical reason(s))

G2150 Performance not met: multimodal pain management was not used

G2151 Patients with diagnosis of a degenerative neurological condition such as ALS, MS, Parkinson's diagnosed at any time before or during the episode of care

G2152 Performance met: the residual change score is equal to or greater than 0

G2153 In hospice or using hospice services during the measurement period

G2154 Patient received at least one Td vaccine or one Tdap vaccine between nine years prior to the start of the measurement period and the end of the measurement period

G2155 Patient had history of at least one of the following contraindications any time during or before the measurement period: anaphylaxis due to Tdap vaccine, anaphylaxis due to Td vaccine or its components; encephalopathy due to Tdap or Td vaccination (post tetanus vaccination encephalitis, post diphtheria vaccination encephalitis or post pertussis vaccination encephalitis)

G2156 Patient did not receive at least one Td vaccine or one Tdap vaccine between nine years prior to the start of the measurement period and the end of the measurement period; or have history of at least one of the following contraindications any time during or before the measurement period: anaphylaxis due to Tdap vaccine, anaphylaxis due to Td vaccine or its components; encephalopathy due to Tdap or Td vaccination (post tetanus vaccination encephalitis, post diphtheria vaccination encephalitis or post pertussis vaccination encephalitis)

G2157 Patients received both the 13-valent pneumococcal conjugate vaccine and the 23-valent pneumococcal polysaccharide vaccine at least 12 months apart, with the first occurrence after the age of 60 before or during the measurement period

G2158 Patient had prior pneumococcal vaccine adverse reaction any time during or before the measurement period

G2159 Patient did not receive both the 13-valent pneumococcal conjugate vaccine and the 23-valent pneumococcal polysaccharide vaccine at least 12 months apart, with the first occurrence after the age of 60 before or during measurement period; or have prior pneumococcal vaccine adverse reaction any time during or before the measurement period

G2160 Patient received at least one dose of the herpes zoster live vaccine or two doses of the herpes zoster recombinant vaccine (at least 28 days apart) anytime on or after the patient's 50th birthday before or during the measurement period

 © 2019 Optum360, LLC

NEW CODES (continued)

G2161 Patient had prior adverse reaction caused by zoster vaccine or its components any time during or before the measurement period

G2162 Patient did not receive at least one dose of the herpes zoster live vaccine or two doses of the herpes zoster recombinant vaccine (at least 28 days apart) anytime on or after the patient's 50th birthday before or during the measurement period; or have prior adverse reaction caused by zoster vaccine or its components any time during or before the measurement period

G2163 Patient received an influenza vaccine on or between July 1 of the year prior to the measurement period and June 30 of the measurement period

G2164 Patient had a prior influenza virus vaccine adverse reaction any time before or during the measurement period

G2165 Patient did not receive an influenza vaccine on or between July 1 of the year prior to the measurement period and June 30 of the measurement period; or did not have a prior influenza virus vaccine adverse reaction any time before or during the measurement period

G2166 Patient refused to participate at admission and/or discharge; patient unable to complete the neck FS PROM at admission or discharge due to cognitive deficit, visual deficit, motor deficit, language barrier, or low reading level, and a suitable proxy/recorder is not available; patient self discharged early; medical reason

G2167 Performance not met: the residual change score is less than 0

J0121 Injection, omadacycline, 1 mg

J0122 Injection, eravacycline, 1 mg

J0179 Injection, brolucizumab-dbll, 1 mg

J0222 Injection, patisiran, 0.1 mg

J0291 Injection, plazomicin, 5 mg

J0593 Injection, lanadelumab-flyo, 1 mg (code may be used for medicare when drug administered under direct supervision of a physician, not for use when drug is self-administered)

J0642 Injection, levoleucovorin (khapzory), 0.5 mg

J1096 Dexamethasone, lacrimal ophthalmic insert, 0.1 mg

J1097 Phenylephrine 10.16 mg/ml and ketorolac 2.88 mg/ml ophthalmic irrigation solution, 1 ml

J1303 Injection, ravulizumab-cwvz, 10 mg

J1444 Injection, ferric pyrophosphate citrate powder, 0.1 mg of iron

J1943 Injection, aripiprazole lauroxil, (aristada initio), 1 mg

J1944 Injection, aripiprazole lauroxil, (aristada), 1 mg

J2798 Injection, risperidone, (perseris), 0.5 mg

J3031 Injection, fremanezumab-vfrm, 1 mg (code may be used for medicare when drug administered under the direct supervision of a physician, not for use when drug is self-administered)

J3111 Injection, romosozumab-aqqg, 1 mg

J7208 Injection, factor viii, (antihemophilic factor, recombinant), pegylated-aucl, (jivi), 1 i.u.

J7314 Injection, fluocinolone acetonide, intravitreal implant (yutiq), 0.01 mg

J7331 Hyaluronan or derivative, synojoynt, for intra-articular injection, 1 mg

J7332 Hyaluronan or derivative, triluron, for intra-articular injection, 1 mg

J7401 Mometasone furoate sinus implant, 10 micrograms

J7677 Revefenacin inhalation solution, fda-approved final product, non-compounded, administered through dme, 1 microgram

J9030 Bcg live intravesical instillation, 1 mg

J9036 Injection, bendamustine hydrochloride, (belrapzo/bendamustine), 1 mg

J9118 Injection, calaspargase pegol-mknl, 10 units

J9119 Injection, cemiplimab-rwlc, 1 mg

J9199 Injection, gemcitabine HCl (Infugem), 200 mg

J9204 Injection, mogamulizumab-kpkc, 1 mg

J9210 Injection, emapalumab-lzsg, 1 mg

J9269 Injection, tagraxofusp-erzs, 10 micrograms

J9309 Injection, polatuzumab vedotin-piiq, 1 mg

J9313 Injection, moxetumomab pasudotox-tdfk, 0.01 mg

J9356 Injection, trastuzumab, 10 mg and hyaluronidase-oysk

K1001 Electronic positional obstructive sleep apnea treatment, with sensor, includes all components and accessories, any type

K1002 Cranial electrotherapy stimulation (CES) system, includes all supplies and accessories, any type

K1003 Whirlpool tub, walk in, portable

K1004 Low frequency ultrasonic diathermy treatment device for home use, includes all components and accessories

K1005 Disposable collection and storage bag for breast milk, any size, any type, each

L2006 Knee-ankle-foot (KAF) device, any material, single or double upright, swing and/or stance phase microprocessor control with adjustability, includes all components (e.g., sensors, batteries, charger), any type activation, with or without ankle joint(s), custom fabricated

L8033 Nipple prosthesis, custom fabricated, reusable, any material, any type, each

M1106 The start of an episode of care documented in the medical record

M1107 Documentation stating patient has a diagnosis of a degenerative neurological condition such as ALS, MS, or Parkinson's diagnosed at any time before or during the episode of care

M1108 Ongoing care not indicated, patient seen only one to two visits (e.g., home program only, referred to another provider or facility, consultation only)

M1109 Ongoing care not indicated, patient discharged after only one to two visits due to specific medical events, documented in the medical record that make the treatment episode impossible such as the patient becomes hospitalized or scheduled for surgery or hospitalized

M1110 Ongoing care not indicated, patient self-discharged early and seen only one to two visits (e.g., financial or insurance reasons, transportation problems, or reason unknown)

M1111 The start of an episode of care documented in the medical record

M1112 Documentation stating patient has a diagnosis of a degenerative neurological condition such as ALS, MS, or Parkinson's diagnosed at any time before or during the episode of care

M1113 Ongoing care not indicated, patient seen only one to two visits (e.g., home program only, referred to another provider or facility, consultation only)

M1114 Ongoing care not indicated, patient discharged after only one to two visits due to specific medical events, documented in the medical record that make the treatment episode impossible such as the patient becomes hospitalized or scheduled for surgery or hospitalized

M1115 Ongoing care not indicated, patient self-discharged early and seen only one to two visits (e.g., financial or insurance reasons, transportation problems, or reason unknown)

M1116 The start of an episode of care documented in the medical record

M1117 Documentation stating patient has a diagnosis of a degenerative neurological condition such as ALS, MS, or Parkinson's diagnosed at any time before or during the episode of care

© 2019 Optum360, LLC

NEW CODES (continued)

M1118 Ongoing care not indicated, patient seen only one to two visits (e.g., home program only, referred to another provider or facility, consultation only)

M1119 Ongoing care not indicated, patient discharged after only one to two visits due to specific medical events, documented in the medical record that make the treatment episode impossible such as the patient becomes hospitalized or scheduled for surgery or hospitalized

M1120 Ongoing care not indicated, patient self-discharged early and seen only one to two visits (e.g., financial or insurance reasons, transportation problems, or reason unknown)

M1121 The start of an episode of care documented in the medical record

M1122 Documentation stating patient has a diagnosis of a degenerative neurological condition such as ALS, MS, or Parkinson's diagnosed at any time before or during the episode of care

M1123 Ongoing care not indicated, patient seen only one to two visits (e.g., home program only, referred to another provider or facility, consultation only)

M1124 Ongoing care not indicated, patient discharged after only one to two visits due to specific medical events, documented in the medical record that make the treatment episode impossible such as the patient becomes hospitalized or scheduled for surgery

M1125 Ongoing care not indicated, patient self-discharged early and seen only one to two visits (e.g., financial or insurance reasons, transportation problems, or reason unknown)

M1126 The start of an episode of care documented in the medical record

M1127 Documentation stating patient has a diagnosis of a degenerative neurological condition such as ALS, MS, or Parkinson's diagnosed at any time before or during the episode of care

M1128 Ongoing care not indicated, patient seen only one to two visits (e.g., home program only, referred to another provider or facility, consultation only)

M1129 Ongoing care not indicated, patient discharged after only one to two visits due to specific medical events, documented in the medical record that make the treatment episode impossible such as the patient becomes hospitalized or scheduled for surgery

M1130 Ongoing care not indicated, patient self-discharged early and seen only one to two visits (e.g., financial or insurance reasons, transportation problems, or reason unknown)

M1131 Documentation stating patient has a diagnosis of a degenerative neurological condition such as ALS, MS, or Parkinson's diagnosed at any time before or during the episode of care

M1132 Ongoing care not indicated, patient seen only one to two visits (e.g., home program only, referred to another provider or facility, consultation only)

M1133 Ongoing care not indicated, patient discharged after only one to two visits due to specific medical events, documented in the medical record that make the treatment episode impossible such as the patient becomes hospitalized or scheduled for surgery

M1134 Ongoing care not indicated, patient self-discharged early and seen only one to two visits (e.g., financial or insurance reasons, transportation problems, or reason unknown

M1135 The start of an episode of care documented in the medical record

M1136 The start of an episode of care documented in the medical record

M1137 Documentation stating patient has a diagnosis of a degenerative neurological condition such as ALS, MS, or Parkinson's diagnosed at any time before or during the episode of care

M1138 Ongoing care not indicated, patient seen only one to two visits (e.g., home program only, referred to another provider or facility, consultation only)

M1139 Ongoing care not indicated, patient self-discharged early and seen only one to two visits (e.g., financial or insurance reasons, transportation problems, or reason unknown)

M1140 Ongoing care not indicated, patient discharged after only one to two visits due to specific medical events, documented in the medical record that make the treatment episode impossible such as the patient becomes hospitalized or scheduled for surgery for surgery or hospitalized

M1141 Functional status was not measured by the Oxford Knee Score (OKS) at 1 year (9 to 15 months) postoperatively

M1142 Emergent cases

M1143 Initiated episode of rehabilitation therapy, medical, or chiropractic care for neck impairment

M1144 Ongoing care not indicated, patient seen only one to two visits (e.g., home program only, referred to another provider or facility, consultation only

P9099 Blood component or product not otherwise classified

Q4205 Membrane graft or membrane wrap, per square centimeter

Q4206 Fluid flow or fluid gf, 1 cc

Q4208 Novafix, per square cenitmeter

Q4209 Surgraft, per square centimeter

Q4210 Axolotl graft or axolotl dualgraft, per square centimeter

Q4211 Amnion bio or axobiomembrane, per square centimeter

Q4212 Allogen, per cc

Q4213 Ascent, 0.5 mg

Q4214 Cellesta cord, per square centimeter

Q4215 Axolotl ambient or axolotl cryo, 0.1 mg

Q4216 Artacent cord, per square centimeter

Q4217 Woundfix, biowound, woundfix plus, biowound plus, woundfix xplus or biowound xplus, per square centimeter

Q4218 Surgicord, per square centimeter

Q4219 Surgigraft-dual, per square centimeter

Q4220 Bellacell hd or surederm, per square centimeter

Q4221 Amniowrap2, per square centimeter

Q4222 Progenamatrix, per square centimeter

Q4226 Myown skin, includes harvesting and preparation procedures, per square centimeter

Q5112 Injection, trastuzumab-dttb, biosimilar, (ontruzant), 10 mg

Q5113 Injection, trastuzumab-pkrb, biosimilar, (herzuma), 10 mg

Q5114 Injection, trastuzumab-dkst, biosimilar, (ogivri), 10 mg

Q5115 Injection, rituximab-abbs, biosimilar, (truxima), 10 mg

Q5116 Injection, trastuzumab-qyyp, biosimilar, (trazimera), 10 mg

Q5117 Injection, trastuzumab-anns, biosimilar, (kanjinti), 10 mg

Q5118 Injection, bevacizumab-bvzr, biosimilar, (zirabev), 10 mg

REVISED CODES

B4185 Parenteral nutrition solution, not otherwise specified, 10 g lipids

G8650 Risk adjusted functional status change residual score for the knee impairment not measured because the patient did not complete the knee FS PROM at initial evaluation and/or near discharge, reason not given

G8662 Risk- adjusted functional status change residual score for the low back impairment not measured because the patient did not complete the low back FS PROM at initial evaluation and/or near discharge, reason not given

G8666 Risk adjusted functional status change residual score for the shoulder impairment not measured because the patient did not complete the shoulder FS PROM at initial evaluation and/or near discharge, reason not given

G8670 Risk adjusted functional status change residual score for the elbow, wrist or hand impairment not measured because the patient did not complete the elbow/wrist/hand FS PROM at initial evaluation and/or near discharge, reason not given

© 2019 Optum360, LLC

REVISED CODES (continued)

G8674 Risk adjusted functional status change residual score for the neck, cranium, mandible, thoracic spine, ribs or other general orthopedic impairment not measured because the patient did not complete the general orthopedic FS PROM at initial evaluation and/or near discharge, reason not given

G9239 Documentation of reasons for patient initiating maintenance hemodialysis with a catheter as the mode of vascular access (e.g., patient has a maturing arteriovenous fistula (AVF)/arteriovenous graft (AVG), time limited trial of hemodialysis, other medical reasons, patient declined AVF/AVG, other patient reasons, patient followed by reporting nephrologist for fewer than 90 days, other system reasons)

G9264 Documentation of patient receiving maintenance hemodialysis for greater than or equal to 90 days with a catheter for documented reasons (e.g., other medical reasons, patient declined arteriovenous fistula (AVF)/arteriovenous graft (AVG), other patient reasons)

G9349 CT scan of the paranasal sinuses ordered at the time of diagnosis or received within 28 days after date of diagnosis

G9355 Early elective delivery or early induction not performed (less than 39 weeks gestation)

G9356 Early elective delivery or early induction performed (less than 39 week gestation)

G9359 Documentation of negative or managed positive TB screen with further evidence that TB is not active prior to the treatment with a biologic immune response modifier

G9405 Patient received follow up within 7 days after discharge

G9414 Patient had one dose of meningococcal vaccine (serogroups A, C, W, Y) on or between the patient's 11th and 13th birthdays

G9469 Patients who have received or are receiving corticosteroids greater than or equal to 10 mg/day of prednisone equivalents for 90 or greater consecutive days or a single prescription equating to 900 mg prednisone or greater for all fills

G9510 Adult patients 18 years of age or older with major depression or dysthymia who did not reach remission at 12 months as demonstrated by a 12 month (+/-60 days) PHQ-9 or PHQ-9M score of less than 5. Either PHQ- 9 or PHQ-9M score was not assessed or is greater than or equal to 5

G9519 Patient achieves final refraction (spherical equivalent) +/- 1.0 diopters of their planned refraction within 90 days of surgery

G9520 Patient does not achieve final refraction (spherical equivalent) +/- 1.0 diopters of their planned refraction within 90 days of surgery

G9531 Patient has documentation of ventricular shunt, brain tumor, multisystem trauma, or is currently taking an antiplatelet medication including: abciximab, anagrelide, cangrelor, cilostazol, clopidogrel, dipyridamole, eptifibatide, prasugrel, ticlopidine, ticagrelor, tirofiban, or vorapaxar

G9547 Cystic renal lesion that is simple appearing (Bosniak I or II), or adrenal lesion less than or equal to 1.0 cm or adrenal lesion greater than 1.0 cm but less than or equal to 4.0 cm classified as likely benign by unenhanced CT or washout protocol CT, or MRI with in- and opposed-phase sequences or other equivalent institutional imaging protocols

G9548 Final reports for imaging studies stating no follow up imaging is recommended

G9549 Documentation of medical reason(s) that follow up imaging is indicated (e.g., patient has lymphadenopathy, signs of metastasis or an active diagnosis or history of cancer, and other medical reason(s))

G9550 Final reports for imaging studies with follow up imaging recommended

G9551 Final reports for imaging studies without an incidentally found lesion noted

G9595 Patient has documentation of ventricular shunt, brain tumor, or coagulopathy

G9663 Any fasting or direct LDL-C laboratory test result <= 190 mg/dl

G9727 Patient unable to complete the knee FS PROM at initial evaluation and/or discharge due to blindness, illiteracy, severe mental incapacity or language incompatibility and an adequate proxy is not available

G9729 Patient unable to complete the hip FS PROM at initial evaluation and discharge due to blindness, illiteracy, severe mental incapacity or language incompatibility and an adequate proxy is not available

G9731 Patient unable to complete the ankle/foot FS PROM at initial evaluation and/or discharge due to blindness, illiteracy, severe mental incapacity or language incompatibility and an adequate proxy is not available

G9733 Patient unable to complete the low back FS PROM at initial evaluation and/or discharge due to blindness, illiteracy, severe mental incapacity or language incompatibility and an adequate proxy is not available

G9735 Patient unable to complete the shoulder FS PROM at initial evaluation and/or discharge due to blindness, illiteracy, severe mental incapacity or language incompatibility and an adequate proxy is not available

G9737 Patient unable to complete the elbow/wrist/hand FS PROM at initial evaluation and/or discharge due to blindness, illiteracy, severe mental incapacity or language incompatibility and an adequate proxy is not available

G9739 Patient unable to complete the general orthopedic FS PROM at initial evaluation and/or discharge due to blindness, illiteracy, severe mental incapacity or language incompatibility and an adequate proxy is not available

G9772 Documentation of medical reason(s) for not achieving at least one body temperature measurement equal to or greater than 35.5 degrees Celsius (or 95.9 degrees Fahrenheit) within the 30 minutes immediately before or the 15 minutes immediately after anesthesia end time (e.g., emergency cases, intentional hypothermia, etc.)

G9781 Documentation of medical reason(s) for not currently being a statin therapy user or receive an order (prescription) for statin therapy (e.g., patient with adverse effect, allergy or intolerance to statin medication therapy, patients who are receiving palliative or hospice care, patients with active liver disease or hepatic disease or insufficiency, and patients with end stage renal disease (ESRD))

G9785 Pathology report diagnosing cutaneous basal cell carcinoma, squamous cell carcinoma, or melanoma (to include in situ disease) sent from the pathologist/dermatopathologist to the biopsying clinician for review within 7 days from the time when the tissue specimen was received by the pathologist

G9786 Pathology report diagnosing cutaneous basal cell carcinoma, squamous cell carcinoma, or melanoma (to include in situ disease) was not sent from the pathologist/dermatopathologist to the biopsying clinician for review within 7 days from the time when the tissue specimen was received by the pathologist

G9798 Discharge(s) for AMI between July 1 of the year prior measurement period to June 30 of the measurement period

G9898 Patient age 65 or older in institutional special needs plans (SNP) or residing in long-term care with POS code 32, 33, 34, 54, or 56 for more than 90 days during the measurement period

G9901 Patient age 65 or older in institutional special needs plans (SNP) or residing in long-term care with POS code 32, 33, 34, 54, or 56 for more than 90 days during the measurement period

G9910 Patients age 66 or older in institutional special needs plans (SNP) or residing in long-term care with POS code 32, 33, 34, 54 or 56 for more than 90 days during the measurement period

G9917 Documentation of advanced stage dementia and caregiver knowledge is limited

G9938 Patients age 66 or older in institutional special needs plans (SNP) or residing in long-term care with POS code 32, 33, 34, 54, or 56 for more than 90 days during the measurement period

© 2019 Optum360, LLC

REVISED CODES (continued)

G9942 Patient had any additional spine procedures performed on the same date as the lumbar discectomy/laminectomy

G9948 Patient had any additional spine procedures performed on the same date as the lumbar discectomy/laminectomy

G9949 Leg pain was not measured by the visual analog scale (VAS) at 3 months (6 to 20 weeks) postoperatively

J0641 Injection, levoleucovorin, not otherwise specified, 0.5 mg

J2794 Injection, risperidone (risperdal consta), 0.5 mg

J7311 Injection, fluocinolone acetonide, intravitreal implant (retisert), 0.01 mg

J7313 Injection, fluocinolone acetonide, intravitreal implant (iluvien), 0.01 mg

J9201 Injection, gemcitabine HCl, not otherwise specified, 200 mg

J9355 Injection, trastuzumab, excludes biosimilar, 10 mg

L8032 Nipple prosthesis, prefabricated, reusable, any type, each

M1009 Discharge/discontinuation of the episode of care documented in the medical record

M1010 Discharge/discontinuation of the episode of care documented in the medical record

M1011 Discharge/discontinuation of the episode of care documented in the medical record

M1012 Discharge/discontinuation of the episode of care documented in the medical record

M1013 Discharge/discontinuation of the episode of care documented in the medical record

M1014 Discharge/discontinuation of the episode of care documented in the medical record

M1015 Discharge/discontinuation of the episode of care documented in the medical record

M1043 Functional status was not measured by the Oswestry Disability Index (ODI version 2.1a) at 1 year (9 to 15 months) postoperatively

M1045 Functional status measured by the Oxford Knee Score (OKS) at 1 year (9 to 15 months) postoperatively was greater than or equal to 37

M1046 Functional status measured by the Oxford Knee Score (OKS) at 1 year (9 to 15 months) postoperatively was less than 37

M1049 Functional status was not measured by the Oswestry Disability Index (ODI version 2.1a) at 3 months (6 to 20 weeks) postoperatively

M1052 Leg pain was not measured by the visual analog scale (VAS) at one year (9 to 15 months) postoperatively

Q4122 Dermacell, dermacell awm or dermacell awm porous, per square centimeter

Q4165 Keramatrix or kerasorb, per square centimeter

Q4184 Cellesta or cellesta duo, per square centimeter

Q5105 Injection, epoetin alfa-epbx, biosimilar, (Retacrit) (for ESRD on dialysis), 100 units

Q5106 Injection, epoetin alfa-epbx, biosimilar, (Retacrit) (for non-ESRD use), 1000 units

DELETED CODES

C9035	C9036	C9037	C9038	C9039	C9040	C9042
C9043	C9044	C9045	C9048	C9049	C9050	C9051
C9052	C9141	C9407	C9408	C9447	C9746	G0365
G0515	G8649	G8653	G8657	G8665	G8669	G8673
G8861	G8978	G8979	G8980	G8981	G8982	G8983
G8984	G8985	G8986	G8987	G8988	G8989	G8990
G8991	G8992	G8993	G8994	G8995	G8996	G8997
G8998	G8999	G9017	G9018	G9019	G9020	G9033
G9034	G9035	G9036	G9158	G9159	G9160	G9161
G9162	G9163	G9164	G9165	G9166	G9167	G9168
G9169	G9170	G9171	G9172	G9173	G9174	G9175
G9176	G9186	G9472	G9742	G9743	G9941	G9944
G9947	J1942	J9031	M1000	M1001	M1002	M1030
M1042	M1044	M1047	M1048	M1050	M1053	S1090

© 2019 Optum360, LLC

Appendix 6 — Place of Service and Type of Service

Place-of-Service Codes for Professional Claims

Listed below are place of service codes and descriptions. These codes should be used on professional claims to specify the entity where service(s) were rendered. Check with individual payers (e.g., Medicare, Medicaid, other private insurance) for reimbursement policies regarding these codes. To comment on a code(s) or description(s), please send your request to posinfo@cms.gov.

01	Pharmacy	A facility or location where drugs and other medically related items and services are sold, dispensed, or otherwise provided directly to patients.
02	Telehealth	The location where health services and health related services are provided or received, through telecommunication technology.
03	School	A facility whose primary purpose is education.
04	Homeless shelter	A facility or location whose primary purpose is to provide temporary housing to homeless individuals (e.g., emergency shelters, individual or family shelters).
05	Indian Health Service freestanding facility	A facility or location, owned and operated by the Indian Health Service, which provides diagnostic, therapeutic (surgical and nonsurgical), and rehabilitation services to American Indians and Alaska natives who do not require hospitalization.
06	Indian Health Service provider-based facility	A facility or location, owned and operated by the Indian Health Service, which provides diagnostic, therapeutic (surgical and nonsurgical), and rehabilitation services rendered by, or under the supervision of, physicians to American Indians and Alaska natives admitted as inpatients or outpatients.
07	Tribal 638 freestanding facility	A facility or location owned and operated by a federally recognized American Indian or Alaska native tribe or tribal organization under a 638 agreement, which provides diagnostic, therapeutic (surgical and nonsurgical), and rehabilitation services to tribal members who do not require hospitalization.
08	Tribal 638 Provider-based Facility	A facility or location owned and operated by a federally recognized American Indian or Alaska native tribe or tribal organization under a 638 agreement, which provides diagnostic, therapeutic (surgical and nonsurgical), and rehabilitation services to tribal members admitted as inpatients or outpatients.
09	Prison/correctional facility	A prison, jail, reformatory, work farm, detention center, or any other similar facility maintained by either federal, state or local authorities for the purpose of confinement or rehabilitation of adult or juvenile criminal offenders.
10	Unassigned	N/A
11	Office	Location, other than a hospital, skilled nursing facility (SNF), military treatment facility, community health center, State or local public health clinic, or intermediate care facility (ICF), where the health professional routinely provides health examinations, diagnosis, and treatment of illness or injury on an ambulatory basis.
12	Home	Location, other than a hospital or other facility, where the patient receives care in a private residence.
13	Assisted living facility	Congregate residential facility with self-contained living units providing assessment of each resident's needs and on-site support 24 hours a day, 7 days a week, with the capacity to deliver or arrange for services including some health care and other services.
14	Group home	A residence, with shared living areas, where clients receive supervision and other services such as social and/or behavioral services, custodial service, and minimal services (e.g., medication administration).
15	Mobile unit	A facility/unit that moves from place-to-place equipped to provide preventive, screening, diagnostic, and/or treatment services.
16	Temporary lodging	A short-term accommodation such as a hotel, campground, hostel, cruise ship or resort where the patient receives care, and which is not identified by any other POS code.
17	Walk-in retail health clinic	A walk-in health clinic, other than an office, urgent care facility, pharmacy, or independent clinic and not described by any other place of service code, that is located within a retail operation and provides preventive and primary care services on an ambulatory basis.
18	Place of employment/ worksite	A location, not described by any other POS code, owned or operated by a public or private entity where the patient is employed, and where a health professional provides on-going or episodic occupational medical, therapeutic or rehabilitative services to the individual.
19	Off campus-outpatient hospital	A portion of an off-campus hospital provider based department which provides diagnostic, therapeutic (both surgical and nonsurgical), and rehabilitation services to sick or injured persons who do not require hospitalization or institutionalization.
20	Urgent care facility	Location, distinct from a hospital emergency room, an office, or a clinic, whose purpose is to diagnose and treat illness or injury for unscheduled, ambulatory patients seeking immediate medical attention.

© 2019 Optum360, LLC

21	Inpatient hospital	A facility, other than psychiatric, which primarily provides diagnostic, therapeutic (both surgical and nonsurgical), and rehabilitation services by, or under, the supervision of physicians to patients admitted for a variety of medical conditions.
22	On campus-outpatient hospital	A portion of a hospital's main campus which provides diagnostic, therapeutic (both surgical and nonsurgical), and rehabilitation services to sick or injured persons who do not require hospitalization or institutionalization.
23	Emergency room—hospital	A portion of a hospital where emergency diagnosis and treatment of illness or injury is provided.
24	Ambulatory surgical center	A freestanding facility, other than a physician's office, where surgical and diagnostic services are provided on an ambulatory basis.
25	Birthing center	A facility, other than a hospital's maternity facilities or a physician's office, which provides a setting for labor, delivery, and immediate post-partum care as well as immediate care of new born infants.
26	Military treatment facility	A medical facility operated by one or more of the uniformed services. Military treatment facility (MTF) also refers to certain former US Public Health Service (USPHS) facilities now designated as uniformed service treatment facilities (USTF).
27-30	Unassigned	N/A
31	Skilled nursing facility	A facility which primarily provides inpatient skilled nursing care and related services to patients who require medical, nursing, or rehabilitative services but does not provide the level of care or treatment available in a hospital.
32	Nursing facility	A facility which primarily provides to residents skilled nursing care and related services for the rehabilitation of injured, disabled, or sick persons, or, on a regular basis, health-related care services above the level of custodial care to individuals other than those with intellectual disabilities.
33	Custodial care facility	A facility which provides room, board, and other personal assistance services, generally on a long-term basis, and which does not include a medical component.
34	Hospice	A facility, other than a patient's home, in which palliative and supportive care for terminally ill patients and their families are provided.
35-40	Unassigned	N/A
41	Ambulance—land	A land vehicle specifically designed, equipped and staffed for lifesaving and transporting the sick or injured.
42	Ambulance—air or water	An air or water vehicle specifically designed, equipped and staffed for lifesaving and transporting the sick or injured.
43-48	Unassigned	N/A
49	Independent clinic	A location, not part of a hospital and not described by any other place-of-service code, that is organized and operated to provide preventive, diagnostic, therapeutic, rehabilitative, or palliative services to outpatients only.
50	Federally qualified health center	A facility located in a medically underserved area that provides Medicare beneficiaries preventive primary medical care under the general direction of a physician.
51	Inpatient psychiatric facility	A facility that provides inpatient psychiatric services for the diagnosis and treatment of mental illness on a 24-hour basis, by or under the supervision of a physician.
52	Psychiatric facility-partial hospitalization	A facility for the diagnosis and treatment of mental illness that provides a planned therapeutic program for patients who do not require full time hospitalization, but who need broader programs than are possible from outpatient visits to a hospital-based or hospital-affiliated facility.
53	Community mental health center	A facility that provides the following services: outpatient services, including specialized outpatient services for children, the elderly, individuals who are chronically ill, and residents of the CMHC's mental health services area who have been discharged from inpatient treatment at a mental health facility; 24 hour a day emergency care services; day treatment, other partial hospitalization services, or psychosocial rehabilitation services; screening for patients being considered for admission to state mental health facilities to determine the appropriateness of such admission; and consultation and education services.
54	Intermediate Care Facility/Individuals with Intellectual Disabilities	A facility which primarily provides health-related care and services above the level of custodial care to individuals with Intellectual Disabilities but does not provide the level of care or treatment available in a hospital or SNF.
55	Residential substance abuse treatment facility	A facility which provides treatment for substance (alcohol and drug) abuse to live-in residents who do not require acute medical care. Services include individual and group therapy and counseling, family counseling, laboratory tests, drugs and supplies, psychological testing, and room and board.
56	Psychiatric residential treatment center	A facility or distinct part of a facility for psychiatric care which provides a total 24-hour therapeutically planned and professionally staffed group living and learning environment.
57	Non-residential substance abuse treatment facility	A location which provides treatment for substance (alcohol and drug) abuse on an ambulatory basis. Services include individual and group therapy and counseling, family counseling, laboratory tests, drugs and supplies, and psychological testing.
58-59	Unassigned	N/A
60	Mass immunization center	A location where providers administer pneumococcal pneumonia and influenza virus vaccinations and submit these services as electronic media claims, paper claims, or using the roster billing method. This generally takes place in a mass immunization setting, such as, a public health center, pharmacy, or mall but may include a physician office setting.

© 2019 Optum360, LLC

61	Comprehensive inpatient rehabilitation facility	A facility that provides comprehensive rehabilitation services under the supervision of a physician to inpatients with physical disabilities. Services include physical therapy, occupational therapy, speech pathology, social or psychological services, and orthotics and prosthetics services.
62	Comprehensive outpatient rehabilitation facility	A facility that provides comprehensive rehabilitation services under the supervision of a physician to outpatients with physical disabilities. Services include physical therapy, occupational therapy, and speech pathology services.
63-64	Unassigned	N/A
65	End-stage renal disease treatment facility	A facility other than a hospital, which provides dialysis treatment, maintenance, and/or training to patients or caregivers on an ambulatory or home-care basis.
66-70	Unassigned	N/A
71	State or local public health clinic	A facility maintained by either state or local health departments that provides ambulatory primary medical care under the general direction of a physician.
72	Rural health clinic	A certified facility which is located in a rural medically underserved area that provides ambulatory primary medical care under the general direction of a physician.
73-80	Unassigned	N/A
81	Independent laboratory	A laboratory certified to perform diagnostic and/or clinical tests independent of an institution or a physician's office.
82-98	Unassigned	N/A
99	Other place of service	Other place of service not identified above.

Type of Service

Common Working File Type of Service (TOS) Indicators

For submitting a claim to the Common Working File (CWF), use the following table to assign the proper TOS. Some procedures may have more than one applicable TOS. CWF will reject codes with incorrect TOS designations. CWF will produce alerts on codes with incorrect TOS designations.

The only exceptions to this annual update are:

- Surgical services billed for dates of service through December 31, 2007, containing the ASC facility service modifier SG must be reported as TOS F. Effective for services on or after January 1, 2008, the SG modifier is no longer applicable for Medicare services. ASC providers should discontinue applying the SG modifier on ASC facility claims. The indicator F does not appear in the TOS table because its use depends upon claims submitted with POS 24 (ASC facility) from an ASC (specialty 49). This became effective for dates of service January 1, 2008, or after.
- Surgical services billed with an assistant-at-surgery modifier (80-82, AS,) must be reported with TOS 8. The 8 indicator does not appear on the TOS table because its use is dependent upon the use of the appropriate modifier. (See Pub. 100-04 *Medicare Claims Processing Manual,* chapter 12, "Physician/Practitioner Billing," for instructions on when assistant-at-surgery is allowable.)
- TOS H appears in the list of descriptors. However, it does not appear in the table. In CWF, "H" is used only as an indicator for hospice. The contractor should not submit TOS H to CWF at this time.
- For outpatient services, when a transfusion medicine code appears on a claim that also contains a blood product, the service is paid under reasonable charge at 80 percent; coinsurance and deductible apply. When transfusion medicine codes are paid under the clinical laboratory fee schedule they are paid at 100 percent; coinsurance and deductible do not apply.

Note: For injection codes with more than one possible TOS designation, use the following guidelines when assigning the TOS:

When the choice is L or 1:

- Use TOS L when the drug is used related to ESRD; or
- Use TOS 1 when the drug is not related to ESRD and is administered in the office.

When the choice is G or 1:

- Use TOS G when the drug is an immunosuppressive drug; or
- Use TOS 1 when the drug is used for other than immunosuppression.

When the choice is P or 1:

- Use TOS P if the drug is administered through durable medical equipment (DME); or
- Use TOS 1 if the drug is administered in the office.

The place of service or diagnosis may be considered when determining the appropriate TOS. The descriptors for each of the TOS codes listed in the annual HCPCS update are:

0	Whole blood
1	Medical care
2	Surgery
3	Consultation
4	Diagnostic radiology
5	Diagnostic laboratory
6	Therapeutic radiology
7	Anesthesia
8	Assistant at surgery
9	Other medical items or services
A	Used DME
B	High risk screening mammography
C	Low risk screening mammography
D	Ambulance
E	Enteral/parenteral nutrients/supplies
F	Ambulatory surgical center (facility usage for surgical services)
G	Immunosuppressive drugs
H	Hospice
J	Diabetic shoes
K	Hearing items and services
L	ESRD supplies
M	Monthly capitation payment for dialysis
N	Kidney donor
P	Lump sum purchase of DME, prosthetics, orthotics
Q	Vision items or services
R	Rental of DME
S	Surgical dressings or other medical supplies
U	Occupational therapy
V	Pneumococcal/flu vaccine
W	Physical therapy

© 2019 Optum360, LLC